Molecular and Genetic Basis of Renal Disease

Molecular and Genetic Basis of Renal Disease

A Companion to Brenner & Rector's The Kidney

David B. Mount, MD
Assistant Professor of Medicine
Harvard Medical School
Renal Division, Brigham and Women's Hospital
Division of General Internal Medicine, VA Boston Healthcare System
Boston, Massachusetts

Martin R. Pollak, MD
Associate Professor of Medicine
Harvard Medical School
Renal Division, Brigham and Women's Hospital
Boston, Massachusetts

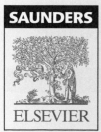

SAUNDERS

ELSEVIER

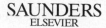

SAUNDERS
ELSEVIER

1600 John F. Kennedy Blvd.
Ste 1800
Philadelphia, PA 19103-2899

Notice

Knowledge and best practice in this field are constantly changing. As new research and experience broaden our knowledge, changes in practice, treatment and drug therapy may become necessary or appropriate. Readers are advised to check the most current, information provided (i) on procedures featured or (ii) by the manufacturer of each product to be administered, to verify the recommended dose or formula, the method and duration of administration, and contraindications. It is the responsibility of the practitioner, relying on his or her own experience and knowledge of the patient, to make diagnoses, to determine dosages and the best treatment for each individual patient, and to take all appropriate safety precautions. To the fullest extent of the law, neither the Publisher nor the Editors assume any liability for any injury and/or damage to persons or property arising out or related to any use of the material contained in this book.

Library of Congress Cataloging-in-Publication Data

Molecular and genetic basis of renal disease / [edited by] David B. Mount, Martin R. Pollak.
    p. ; cm.
  Includes bibliographical references and index.
  ISBN 978-1-4160-0252-9 (alk. paper)
  1. Kidneys—Diseases—Molecular aspects. 2. Kidneys—Diseases—Genetic aspects. I. Mount,
    David B. II. Pollak, Martin R.
  [DNLM: 1. Kidney Diseases—genetics. 2. Kidney Diseases—physiopathology. 3. Genetic
    Predisposition to Disease. 4. Molecular Biology—methods. WJ 300 M718 2008]

RC903.9.M65 2008
616.6'1042—dc22

                                                2006036125

Acquisitions Editor: Susan Pioli
Developmental Editor: Agnes Hunt Byrne
Project Manager: Joan Sinclair
Design Direction: Steven Stave

Printed in China

Last digit is the print number: 9   8   7   6   5   4   3   2   1

Contributors

Seth L. Alper, MD, PhD
Professor of Medicine
Harvard Medical School
Boston, Massachusetts

Thomas Benzing, MD
Renal Division
University Hospital Freiburg
Freiburg, Germany

Joseph V. Bonventre, MD, PhD
Renal Division
Harvard Medical School
Brigham and Women's Hospital;
Division of Health Sciences and Technology
Massachusetts Institute of Technology
Boston, Massachusetts

Matthew Breyer, MD
Professor of Medicine
Vanderbilt University School of Medicine
Nashville, Tennessee;
Senior Medical Fellow II
Biotechnology Discovery Research
Lilly Research Laboratories
Eli Lilly and Company
Indianapolis, Indiana

Josephine P. Briggs, MD
Senior Scientific Officer
Howard Hughes Medical Institute
Chevy Chase, Maryland

Peter M.T. Deen, PhD
Department of Physiology
Nimjegen Center for Molecular Life Sciences
Radboud University
Nimjegen Medical Center
Nimjegen, The Netherlands

Gilbert M. Eisner, MD
Clinical Professor
Department of Medicine
Georgetown University School of Medicine
Washington, DC

David H. Ellison, MD
Professor of Medicine and Physiology and Pharmacology
Head, Division of Nephrology and Hypertension
Oregon Health Sciences University
Portland, Oregon

Ronald J. Falk, MD
Chief and Professor
Department of Medicine
Division of Nephrology and Hypertension
University of North Carolina at Chapel Hill
Chapel Hill, North Carolina

John Feehally, MD, DM, FRCP
Professor of Renal Medicine
University of Leicester Medical School;
Consultant Nephrologist
University Hospitals of Leicester NHS Trust
Leicester, United Kingdom

Robin A. Felder, PhD
Professor of Pathology
School of Medicine
Director, Medical Automation Research Center (MARC)
University of Virginia
Charlottesville, Virginia

Mary H. Foster, MD
Associate Professor
Department of Medicine
Duke University Medical Center;
Chief, Nephrology Section
Durham VAMC
Durham, North Carolina

Alexander Gawlik, MD
Medizinische Klinik II
University Hospital Aachen
Aachen, Germany;
The Samuel Lunenfeld Research Institute
Mount Sinai Hospital
Toronto, Ontario, Canada

Peter C. Harris, PhD
Professor of Biochemistry and Molecular Biology and
    Medicine
Mayo Clinic College of Medicine
Rochester, Minnesota

Raymond Harris, MD
Ann and Roscoe R. Robinson Professor of
    Medicine
Director, Division of Nephrology and
    Hypertension
Department of Medicine
Vanderbilt University School of Medicine
Nashville, Tennessee

Stephen I-Hong Hsu, MD, PhD
Assistant Professor
Harvard Medical School;
Associate Physician
Renal Division
Brigham and Women's Hospital
Boston, Massachusetts

Sabiha M. Hussain, MD
Staff Physician
Department of Nephrology and Hypertension
Allegheny General Hopsital
Pittsburgh, Pennsylvania

J. Ashley Jefferson, MD, MRCP
Assistant Professor
Division of Nephrology
University of Washington
Seattle, Washington

John E. Jones, PhD
Assistant Professor
Molecular Biology and Genetics
Department of Pediatric Nephrology
Georgetown University School of Medicine
Washington, DC

Pedro A. Jose, MD, PhD
Professor of Pediatrics and Physiology and Biophysics
Georgetown University School of Medicine;
Director, Pediatric Nephrology
Georgetown University Medical Center
Washington, DC

Harald W. Jüppner, MD
Associate Professor of Pediatrics
Department of Pediatrics
Harvard Medical School;
Associate Biologist and Chief
Pediatric Nephrology Unit
Massachusetts General Hospital and
   Hospital for Children
Boston, Massachusetts

Raghu Kalluri, PhD
Associate Professor
Harvard Medical School;
Chief, Division of Matrix Biology
Beth Israel Deaconess Medical Center
Boston, Massachusetts

S. Ananth Karumanchi, MD
Associate Professor of Medicine
Harvard Medical School;
Attending Physician, Nephrology
Beth Israel Deaconess Medical Center
Boston, Massachusetts

Sai Ram Keithi-Reddy, MB, BS
Research Fellow in Medicine
Harvard Medical School;

Division of Matrix Biology
Department of Medicine
Beth Israel Deaconess Medical Center
Boston, Massachusetts

Vicki Rubin Kelley, PhD
Associate Professor of Medicine
Department of Pathology
Harvard Medical School
Boston, Massachusetts

Susan M. Kiefer, PhD
Research Assistant Professor of Medicine
Saint Louis University;
Health Science Specialist
Veterans Affairs Medical Center
St. Louis, Missouri

Paul D. Killen, MD
Associate Professor of Pathology
University of Michigan Medical School
Ann Arbor, Michigan

Paul E. Klotman, MD
Professor of Medicine
Mount Sinai School of Medicine
New York, New York

Nine V.A.M. Knoers, MD, PhD
Professor
Department of Human Genetics
Nimjegen Center for Molecular Life Sciences
Radboud University
Nimjegen Medical Center
Nimjegen, The Netherlands

Martin Konrad, MD
Professor of Pediatric Nephrology
Department of Pediatric Nephrology
University Children's Hospital
Münster, Germany

Jordan A. Kreidberg, MD, PhD
Assistant Professor
Department of Pediatrics
Harvard Medical School;
Division of Nephrology
Department of Medicine
Children's Hospital of Boston
Boston, Massachusetts

Christine E. Kurshcat, MD
Research Fellow in Nephrology
Harvard Medical School;
Molecular and Vascular Medicine Unit and Renal
   Division
Beth Israel Deaconess Medical Center
Boston, Massachusetts;
Department of Nephrology
University of Düsseldorf
Düsseldorf, Germany

Charles Y. Kwon, MD
Research Fellow in Pediatrics
Harvard Medical School;
Renal Division
Children's Hospital of Boston;
Renal Division
Brigham and Women's Hospital
Boston, Massachusetts

John N. Lorenz, PhD
Associate Professor
Department of Molecular and Cellular Physiology
College of Medicine
University of Cincinnati
Cincinnati, Ohio

Philip A. Marsden, MD
Professor of Medicine
Oreopoulos-Baxter Division Director of
    Nephrology
University of Toronto;
Kelron Chair in Medical Research
St. Michael's Hospital
Toronto, Ontario, Canada

Charles C. Matouk, MD
Postdoctoral Research Fellow
St. Michael's Hospital
University of Toronto
Toronto, Ontario, Canada

Sharon E. Maynard, MD
Assistant Professor of Medicine
Division of Renal Disease and Hypertension
George Washington University School of
    Medicine;
Consultant Nephrologist
George Washington University Hospital
Washington, DC

Dawn S. Milliner, MD
Professor of Medicine and Pediatrics
Consultant, Division of Nephrology and
    Hypertension and Division of Pediatric
    Nephrology
Mayo Clinic
Rochester, Minnesota

Carla G. Monico, MD
Assistant Professor of Medicine and Pediatrics
Consultant, Division of Nephrology and
    Hypertension and Division of Pediatric
    Nephrology
Mayo Clinic
Rochester, Minnesota

Laurence Morel, PhD
Professor
Department of Pathology, Immunology, and Laboratory
    Medicine
University of Florida
Gainesville, Florida

David B. Mount MD
Assistant Professor of Medicine
Harvard Medical School;
Renal Division, Brigham and Women's Hospital;
Division of General Internal Medicine, VA Boston
    Healthcare System
Boston, Massachusetts

York Pei, MD, FRCP, FACP, FASN
Professor of Medicine
Department of Medicine
University of Toronto
Toronto, Ontario, Canada

Martin R. Pollak MD
Associate Professor of Medicine
Harvard Medical School;
Renal Division, Brigham and Women's Hospital
Boston, Massachusetts

Gloria A. Preston, PhD
Department of Pathology and Laboratory Medicine
Division of Nephrology and Hypertension
UNC Kidney Center
University of North Carolina at Chapel Hill
Chapel Hill, North Carolina

Susan E. Quaggin, MD
Associate Professor
Department of Medicine
The Samuel Lunenfeld Research Institute
Mount Sinai Hospital
University of Toronto;
Division of Nephrology
St. Michael's Hospital
Toronto, Ontario, Canada

Michael Rauchman, MD
Assistant Professor
Department of Internal Medicine and Biochemisty
St. Louis University Health Sciences Center;
Staff Physician
Veterans Affairs Medical Center
St. Louis, Missouri

Joris H. Robben, PhD
Department of Physiology
Nimjegen Center for Molecular Life Sciences
Radboud University
Nimjegen Medical Center
Nimjegen, The Netherlands

Michael J. Ross, MD
Assistant Professor of Medicine
Director, Nephrology Fellowship Program
Mount Sinai School of Medicine
New York, New York

Gillian Rumsby, PhD
Consultant Biochemist
University College London Hospitals
London, England

Paul W. Sanders, MD, FACP
Professor
Division of Nephrology
Department of Medicine
University of Alabama at Birmingham;
Chief, Renal Section
Veterans Affairs Medical Center
Birmingham, Alabama

Jürgen Schnermann, MD
Senior Investigator, Branch Chief
National Institute of Diabetes and Digestive and Kidney
  Diseases
National Institutes of Health
Bethesda, Maryland

Stuart J. Shankland, MD
Professor of Medicine
Belding H. Scribner Endowed Chair in Medicine
Head, Division of Nephrology
University of Washington
Seattle, Washington

James A. Shayman, MD
Professor Internal Medicine and Pharmacology
University of Michigan Medical School;
Associate Vice President for Research, Health Science
University of Michigan
Ann Arbor, Michigan

Rajesh V. Thakker, MD, FRCP, FRCPath
May Professor of Medicine
Nuffield Department of Medicine
University of Oxford;
Consultant Physician and Endocrinologist
Oxford Centre for Diabetes, Endocrinology, and Metabolism
Oxford, United Kingdom

Christie P. Thomas, MB, FRCP, FACP, FASN, FAHA
Professor of Internal Medicine and Molecular Biology
University of Iowa Carver College of Medicine;
Medical Director, Kidney and Pancreas Transplant Program
VA Medical Center and University of Iowa Hospitals and
  Clinics
Iowa City, Iowa

Vicente E. Torres, MD
Professor of Medicine
Mayo Clinic College of Medicine
Rochester, Minnesota

Rodo O. von Vigier, MD
Research Assistant
Department of Pediatrics
University Children's Hospital
Berne, Switzerland

Siegfried Waldegger, MD
Professor of Physiology
Department of Pediatrics
University Children's Hospital
Marburg, Germany

Gerd Walz, MD
Renal Division
University Hospital Freiburg
Freiburg, Germany

Astrid Weins, MD
Postdoctoral Fellow in Medicine
Brigham and Women's Hospital
Boston, Massachusetts

Scott M. Williams, PhD
Associate Professor
Division of Cardiovascular Medicine
Vanderbilt University School of Medicine
Nashville, Tennessee

Ralph Witzgall, MD
Institute for Molecular and Cellular
  Anatomy
University of Regensburg
Regensburg, Germany

Jing Zhou, MD, PhD
Associate Professor of Medicine
Harvard Medical School;
Associate Physician
Brigham and Women's Hospital
Boston, Massachusetts

Contents

Molecular and Genetic Basis of Renal Disease

Color Plates

Plate 1

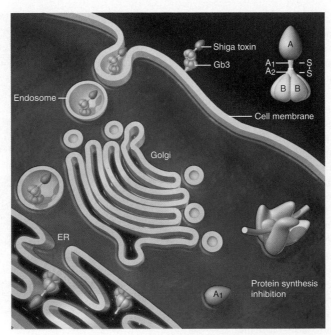

Figure 26-1 Classical paradigm of verotoxin-induced cellular toxicity in diarrhea-associated hemolytic-uremic syndrome. Verotoxins (VTs) are AB_5 exotoxins produced by pathogenic strains of enterohemorrhagic *Escherichia coli*, most prominently *E. coli* O157:H7. They are composed of five identical B subunits noncovalently bonded to a single A subunit in a donut-shaped pentameric ring. The A subunit consists of the enzymatically active A1 fragment and smaller A2 fragment. VT binds to susceptible cell surfaces, particularly endothelial cells, via a Gb_3 glycolipid receptor. This initial binding is followed by receptor-mediated endocytosis, retrograde transport of the toxin through the *trans*-Golgi apparatus and endoplasmic reticulum (ER). During its retrograde transport through the cell's acidic, intracellular compartments, VT is cleaved by furin to release the enzymatically active A1 fragment into the cytosol, where it potently inhibits protein synthesis by a direct and specific activity on ribosomes.

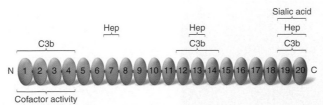

Figure 26-2 Modular organization and critical binding sites of human factor H. Factor H is a plasma-borne regulator of complement activation composed of 20 homologous subunits of approximately 60 amino acids termed short consensus repeats (SCRs) or complement control protein (CCP) modules. C3b, heparin (Hep), and sialic acid binding sites are depicted, as is the functional importance of SCR1-4 in conferring "co-factor activity" to the functional molecule. SCR19-20 represents a mutational "hot spot" in patients with atypical hemolyic-uremic syndrome, comprising over 70% of all disease mutations.

Plate 2

Figure 26-3 Mechanism of action of plasma-borne factor H in protection of endothelial cell surfaces against activation of the alternative pathway of complement in diarrhea-negative hemolytic-uremic syndrome (D-HUS). In the normal individual **(A)**, plasma-borne factor H binds C3b deposited on a damaged (or activated) endothelial cell surface. This interaction is critical in regulating the formation of C3bBb, the alternative pathway C3 convertase, and mitigating complement-mediated host cellular injury. Factor H accomplishes this important task by (1) diminishing factor B binding to C3b, thereby preventing the formation of C3bBb; (2) promoting the dissociation of C3bBb (so-called "decay-accelerating activity"); and (3) acting as a co-factor for factor I in the cleavage of membrane-bound C3b (so-called "co-factor activity"). In a patient with atypical HUS **(B)**, factor H is functionally deficient and cannot efficiently regulate the formation of C3bBb deposited on endothelial surfaces. Membrane-bound C3b is now left unchecked to generate C3bBb in an amplification loop that results in endothelial injury and pathologic thrombosis.

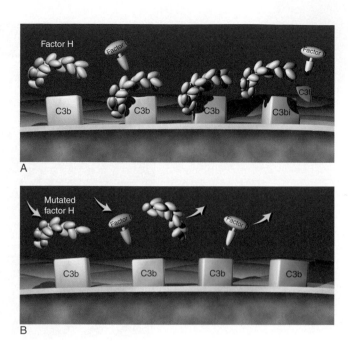

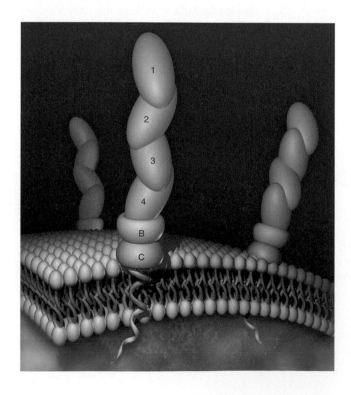

Figure 26-4 Structure of human membrane co-factor protein (MCP, CD46). MCP is a membrane-bound regulator of complement activation that may exist as multiple isoforms in a single cell type. All isoforms share four extracellular, N-terminal SCR domains, akin to those of factor H and other regulators of complement activation. These SCRs are followed by a domain rich in serine, threonine, and proline (STP region), a 12–amino acid juxtamembranous region of unknown sequence homology, transmembrane domain, cytoplasmic anchor, and cytoplasmic tail. The four major isoforms of MCP do not contain the A exon, and all utilize the C exon, while the B exon is alternatively spliced to generate BC- and C-containing STP regions. To date, all disease mutations in atypical hemolytic-uremic syndrome target the shared SCR4 domain.

Plate 3

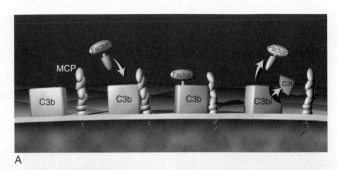

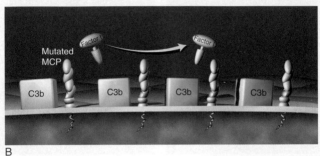

Figure 26-5 Mechanism of action of cell surface human membrane co-factor protein (MCP) in protection of endothelial cells against activation of the alternative pathway of complement in diarrhea-negative hemolytic-uremic syndrome (D-HUS). In the normal individual **(A)**, cell surface MCP binds C3b deposited on a damaged (or activated) endothelial cell surface. This interaction is critical in regulating the formation of C3bBb, the alternative pathway C3 convertase, and mitigating complement-mediated host cellular injury. MCP accomplishes this important task by acting as a co-factor for factor I in the cleavage of membrane-bound C3b, so-called "co-factor activity." In a patient with atypical HUS **(B)**, MCP is functionally deficient and cannot efficiently regulate the formation of C3bBb deposited on endothelial surfaces. All known mutations of the *MCP* gene target the SCR4 domain. As illustrated, the mutant MCP protein is most representative of a T822C transition previously described in two families (see text). Membrane-bound C3b is now left unchecked to generate C3bBb in an amplification loop that results in endothelial injury and pathologic thrombosis.

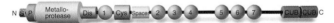

Figure 26-6 Structure of ADAMTS13 (a disintegrin-like and metalloprotease with thrombospondin type I motifs). ADAMTS13 is the plasma-borne von Willebrand factor-protease. It is composed of a series of protein motifs including (from the N-terminus) a signal peptide, propeptide, reprolysin-like metalloprotease domain, disintegrin-like domain, thrombospondin repeat (TSR), cysteine-rich domain, ADAMTS spacer domain, seven additional TSRs, and two CUB (complement components C1r/C1s, urinary epidermal growth factor and bone morphogenic protein-1) domains. Acquired or inherited deficiencies of ADAMTS13 activity are causally linked with thrombotic thrombocytopenic purpura.

Plate 4

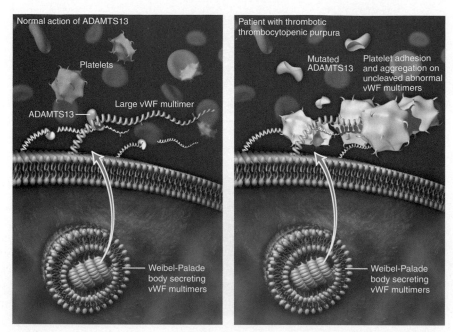

Figure 26-7 Mechanism of action of ADAMTS13 in normal individuals and patients with thrombotic thrombocytopenic purpura (TTP). Secretagogues stimulate endothelial cells to secrete "unusually large" von Willebrand factor (vWF) multimers from their intracellular storage sites, the Weibel-Palade bodies. Attached to the cell surface (and any exposed subendothelial matrix), these vWF multimers uncoil under the influence of high fluid shear stress, exposing sites for attachment of circulating platelets (via an interaction with platelet gp1bα receptors) and cleavage by ADAMTS13. In the normal individual **(A)**, ADAMTS13 successfully competes for target sites on uncoiled, surface-bound vWF multimers and cleaves them to produce characteristic vWF degradation products. In a patient with TTP **(B)**, ADAMTS13 activity is severely deficient and cannot effectively compete with circulating platelets for exposed binding sites. This results in platelet aggregation and pathologic thrombosis.

Plate 5

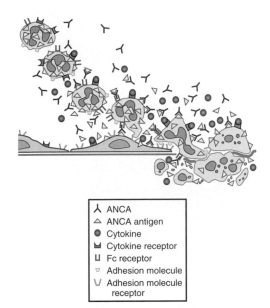

ANCA
ANCA antigen
Cytokine
Cytokine receptor
Fc receptor
Adhesion molecule
Adhesion molecule receptor

Figure 28-1 Schematic of ANCAs and their interaction with neutrophils causing neutrophil degranulation and tissue injury. (From Jennette JC, Falk RJ: Pathogenesis of the vascular and glomerular damage in ANCA-positive vasculitis. Nephrol Dial Transplant 13[Suppl 1]:19, 1998.)

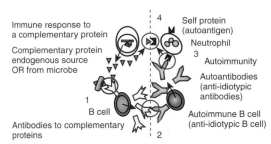

Figure 28-3 Schematic of the theory of autoantigen complementarity. The theory proposes that the immunogen that begins the sequence of events leading to the production of autoantibodies is not the autoantigen or its mimic, but rather its complementary peptide or its mimic. Step 1: The complementary proteins may be introduced by invading microbes or they may be produced by the individual through translation of antisense RNA. An antibody is produced in response to the complementary protein. Step 2: A second antibody is elicited against the first antibody, referred to as an anti-idiotypic response. Step 3: The resultant anti-idiotypic antibodies react with the autoantigen, whose amino acid sequence is complementary to the sequence of the initiating antigen. Step 4: Complementary proteins have a natural affinity because the hydropathy of one is the opposite of the other.

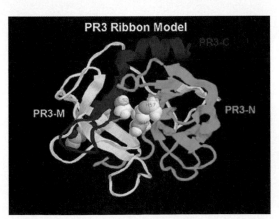

Figure 28-6 Ribbon model of proteinase 3 molecule. The 100–amino acid apoptosis domain appears as the darkest strand.

SECTION 1

The Tools of Molecular Nephrology

Chapter 1

The Impact of Molecular Genetics on Nephrology

Martin R. Pollak and David B. Mount

It is difficult to overstate the impact of the ongoing revolutions in genetics and genomics on biomedical science. In the three decades since the publication of the first edition of Brenner & Rector's *The Kidney,* the scientific and technologic tools available to biologists have transformed renal science. We now know the molecular basis of a large number of inherited kidney diseases and are seeing steady progress in dissecting the genetics of common and complex renal phenotypes. This, in turn, is just now beginning to influence the treatment of patients with kidney disease.

Our rapidly advancing understanding of the pathobiology of polycystic kidney disease (PKD) is among the best examples. When, just over 20 years ago, Reeders et al mapped the *PKD1* locus to chromosome 16, this sort of genome-wide linkage analysis in extended pedigrees was a laborious task based on Southern blot analysis of restriction fragment length polymorphisms.[1] With the subsequent cloning of the autosomal dominant PKD genes *PKD1* and *PKD2*, and the autosomal recessive PKD gene *PKHD1*, investigations into PKD biology have accelerated at a remarkable pace.[2-4] Genetically faithful animal models of human PKD are now being used to examine new approaches to therapy. The role of cilia in mediating cyst formation is becoming increasingly clear. Genetic screens in zebrafish support the notion of ciliary defects as a unifying theme in cystic disease (moving from "Fish to Philosopher" has clearly become an important biologic tool!).[5,6]

Advances in expression cloning methodologies have led to the identification of a many of the transport proteins that are critical components of the renal tubule. Related human genetic studies and genetic manipulations in the mouse have allowed for the integration of these many molecular components into a much deeper understanding of integrated tubule physiology in health and in disease states.

In some cases, molecular advances have led to novel and highly specific treatments. Work on Fabry disease has progressed from an understanding of the genetic basis of this lysosomal storage disease to the development of effective therapy with recombinant α-galactosidase.[7-9] Of course, the best clinical example of how molecular cloning and protein expression has transformed clinical practice in nephrology is recombinant erythropoietin, administered to most end-stage renal disease patients. In this case, molecular cloning has led to a clear improvement in the quality of life for many patients. The ability to clone genes for production of recombinant proteins and expression in cells and animals has also made an enormous indirect impact on biomedical studies. It is rare now to see a research publication that does not in some way utilize reagents developed through molecular genetic technologies.

Understanding even extremely rare forms of inherited diseases can lead to a much deeper understanding of the pathophysiology of common disease. The cloning of the nephrin gene by molecular genetic analysis of families with congenital nephrotic syndrome helped spark an explosion in our understanding of glomerular biology.[10] Our understanding of the acquired forms of thrombotic thrombocytopenic purpura and the hemolytic uremic syndrome has advanced through a better understanding of inherited mutations in *ADAMTS13* and complement factor H.[11,12] Although this has not yet had a significant direct impact on therapy, these molecular advances allow investigations of novel treatment approaches to be much more focused on the underlying pathobiology.

Knowledge of the genetic basis of inherited disease has direct impact on diagnosis. Although genetic testing has yet to become commonplace in the practice of nephrology, molecular genetic analyses can be expected to become increasingly commonplace in guiding the diagnosis of a variety of disorders, from glomerular and cystic disease to electrolyte abnormalities and hypertension. Such testing will lead to more refined diagnoses and, in turn, better therapeutic decisions.

Although we are unable to predict the details, certainly advances in biomedical research will continue to transform the study and understanding of the kidney. We are just now beginning to see the impact of such advances on patient care. The most common forms of kidney disease are clearly multifactorial, involving the interactions of both weak and strong environmental and genetic factors. Integrating laboratory studies of these diseases with epidemiologic observations, population genetics, and the development of therapeutic strategies will be a major challenge for the next several decades.

In this companion volume to *The Kidney*, we have attempted to cover four major topics, reflected in its main sections: I. Tools of Molecular Nephrology, II. Genetic Disorders of Renal Growth and Structure, III. Genetic Disorders of Renal Function, and IV. Acquired and Polygenic Renal Disease. We hope that readers will find this book to be both a useful companion to *The Kidney* as well as an interesting and informative discussion of the major topics in molecular nephrology.

References

1. Reeders ST, et al: A highly polymorphic DNA marker linked to adult polycystic kidney disease on chromosome 16. Nature 317:542–544, 1985.
2. Hughes J, et al: The polycystic kidney disease 1 (*PKD1*) gene encodes a novel protein with multiple cell recognition domains. Nat Genet 10:151–160, 1995.
3. Mochizuki T, et al: *PKD2*, a gene for polycystic kidney disease that encodes an integral membrane protein. Science 272:1339–1342, 1996.
4. Onuchic LF, et al: *PKHD1*, the polycystic kidney and hepatic disease 1 gene, encodes a novel large protein containing multiple immunoglobulin-like plexin-transcription-factor domains and parallel β-helix 1 repeats. Am J Hum Genet 70:1305–1317, 2002.
5. Sun Z, et al: A genetic screen in zebrafish identifies cilia genes as a principal cause of cystic kidney. Development 131:4085–4093, 2004.
6. Smith HW: From Fish to Philosopher. Boston, Little, Brown, 1953.
7. Bernstein HS, et al: Fabry disease: Six gene rearrangements and an exonic point mutation in the α-galactosidase gene. J Clin Invest 83:1390–1399, 1989.
8. Eng CM, et al: Safety and efficacy of recombinant human α-galactosidase A–replacement therapy in Fabry's disease. N Engl J Med 345:9–16, 2001.
9. Schiffmann R, et al: Enzyme replacement therapy in Fabry disease: A randomized controlled trial. JAMA 285:2743–2749, 2001.
10. Kestila M, et al: Positionally cloned gene for a novel glomerular protein—nephrin—is mutated in congenital nephrotic syndrome. Mol Cell 1:575–582, 1998.
11. Warwicker P, et al: Genetic studies into inherited and sporadic hemolytic uremic syndrome. Kidney Int 53:836–844, 1998.
12. Levy GG, et al: Mutations in a member of the *ADAMTS* gene family cause thrombotic thrombocytopenic purpura. Nature 413:488–494, 2001.

Chapter 2

Manipulation of the Mouse Genome: Studying Renal Function and Disease

Alexander Gawlik and Susan E. Quaggin

Complete mapping of the genetic code in several mammalian organisms has led to the need for functional characterization of a vast number of different gene sequences. During the last 10 years new genetic tools have been developed allowing precise genetic targeting in mammals. Investigators can now modify a gene locus by homologous recombination in mouse embryonic stem (ES) cells. Using this technique, studies of loss and gain of function for specific target genes can be performed in vivo. Because of the remarkable similarities between mouse and human gene and cellular functions, the mouse is an excellent model system to study human biology and disease. This has established gene targeting in mice as a widely used and powerful tool for gene function studies.

Although conventional gene targeting within the germline has provided great insight into the biologic functions of many genes, several disadvantages exist. Disruption of gene function in ES cells may result in embryonic or perinatal lethality, preventing the functional characterization of the gene in organs such as the kidney that develop relatively late in fetal life. Additionally, many genes are expressed in multiple cell types, and the resulting knockout phenotypes can be complex and difficult or impossible to dissect. The ability to limit gene targeting to a specific cell type overcomes some of these problems, while the temporal control of gene expression permits more precise dissection of a gene's function. Moreover, if a gene's function depends on tight regulation of its expression, knockout and overexpression studies represent two extremes. In this case, generation of mice with intermediate levels of gene expression is advantageous. Indeed, an ideal tool to manipulate gene function would combine tight control over the spatial and temporal levels of expression with cost effectiveness and efficiency. New developments in genetic engineering should allow realization of many of these criteria.

CONVENTIONAL GENETIC ENGINEERING

In principle, there are three different ways to specifically alter mammalian genomes: Transgene random integration, targeted integration ("knockin"), and targeted deletion ("knockout"). Transgene random integration is used predominantly for overexpression studies. Transgene expression cassettes contain two major components: the transcription unit of a gene of interest and regulatory elements controlling the expression of the transgene. The expression of a gene can be investigated under its own or a heterologous promoter, which can be tissue-specific or broadly expressed. There are no ideal regulatory elements leading to ubiquitous expression, but several fusion proteins direct widespread expression: Examples include the human cytomegalovirus (CMV) enhancer, chicken β-actin promoter and the phosphoglycerate kinase promoter. However, these regulatory sequences lead to broad, but scattered expression, which in addition can be variable in different transgenic lines. The *ROSA26* gene promoter R26 seems to direct generalized and uniform expression.[1]

The dominant technique leading to random integration of a transgene involves microinjection of the construct purified from bacterial DNA sequences into the pronucleus of a developing zygote (Fig. 2-1). Within a 3- to 5-hour period after fertilization before fusion of the male and female pronuclei, DNA can be injected into the larger male pronucleus. Viable eggs are then transferred into the oviducts of pseudopregnant mice. The F0 generation is screened by Southern blot or polymerase chain reaction for the presence of the transgene, and positive animals are called "founders." Usually the F0 generation has multiple integration sites of the transgene. The number of transgenes can be determined by Southern blot analysis of the flanking genomic area. Segregation of independent integration sites starts in the F1 generation, permitting independent transgenic lines for each single integration site to be established. The dramatic differences of transgene expression between the different founder lines are usually due to different integration loci rather than dependence on the number of transgene copies. Transcriptional inactivity in transgenes can be due to insertion into a transcriptionally silent genomic region. Moreover, incorrect spatial expression of the transgene can result from regulatory elements of the flanking sequences. Thus, the investigator must thoroughly evaluate the expression level and locus of the transgene and compare the observed phenotypes of independent transgenic lines.

In contrast to random integration, targeted integration or deletion require the use of ES cells (Fig. 2-2). When a fragment of genomic DNA is introduced into a mammalian cell it can locate and recombine with the endogenous homologous sequence (homologous recombination). Targeting vectors consist of two arms of homology surrounding the mutated area of interest. Possible mutations include the exchange of a coding exon against a positive selection marker or a reporter gene for generation of knockouts, insertion of site-specific recombinases into tissue-specific chromosomal loci, or introduction of point mutations. Electroporation of the linearized construct to ES cells leads to random integration as well as targeted integration by homologous recombination. Positive and negative selection is performed to enrich for ES cells with integration of the transgene at the desired genomic locus. After confirmation of homologous recombination by Southern blot or polymerase chain reaction, targeted ES cells are used to

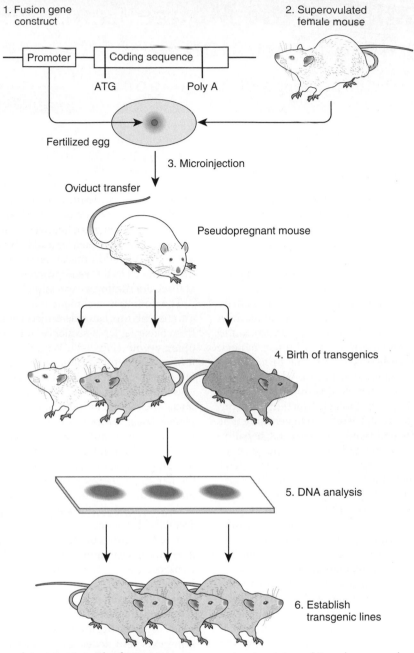

1. Fusion gene construct

Promoter | Coding sequence

ATG   Poly A

Fertilized egg

2. Superovulated female mouse

3. Microinjection

Oviduct transfer

Pseudopregnant mouse

4. Birth of transgenics

5. DNA analysis

6. Establish transgenic lines

Figure 2-1 Basics of pronuclear injection. The fusion gene construct is microinjected into the pronucleus of a fertilized egg. The blastocyst is transferred into the oviduct of a pseudopregnant mouse. After birth the offspring are screened for incorporation of the transgene by Southern blot or polymerase chain reaction. Individual transgenic lines are established from each positive founder.

generate chimeric mice by blastocyst injection or embryo aggregation. Chimeras consist of two different tissues: one derived from the ES cells, the other from the host embryo, as shown by chimeric coat color. Backcrossing the chimera to the host strain eventually leads to mice entirely derived from ES cells in the F1 generation.

In addition to generating knockout animals, gene targeting in ES cells also provides a useful alternative to random integration of transgenes, since expression cassettes can be targeted to a previously characterized genomic locus. Ideally this locus is transcriptionally active and does not influence locus or time of transgene expression. For example, the *Rosa26* locus provides generalized transgene expression and numerous

knockin lines have been generated.[1] The *Hprt* locus has also been used for the integration of transgenes and provides an additional advantage.[2–5] In ES cell lines with a partially deleted *Hprt* locus, expression of hypoxanthine-guanine-phosphoribosyltransferase is no longer possible and cells die after the addition of hypoxanthine-aminopterin-thymidine to the medium. Targeting a transgene into the partially deleted *Hprt* locus restores the expression of *Hprt* by the inclusion of sequences in the targeting vector that complement the deletion. Correctly targeted clones can be enriched by positive selection.

Finally, the addition of docking sites into specific genomic loci of ES cell lines can greatly enhance the targeting frequency (see "Use of Site-Specific Recombinases in the Kidney").

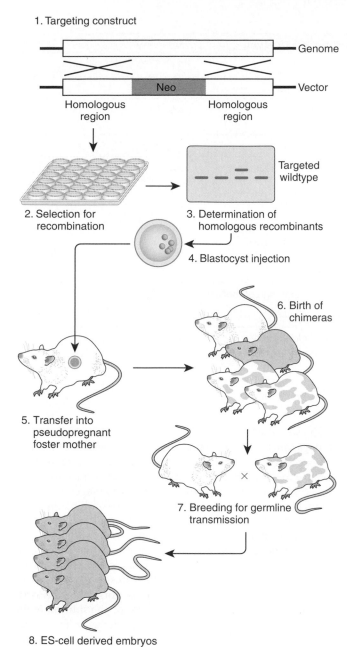

1. Targeting construct

Genome

Neo

Vector

Homologous region

Homologous region

2. Selection for recombination

3. Determination of homologous recombinants

Targeted wildtype

4. Blastocyst injection

5. Transfer into pseudopregnant foster mother

6. Birth of chimeras

7. Breeding for germline transmission

8. ES-cell derived embryos

Figure 2-2 Homologous recombination in ES cells. The targeting construct (vector) consists of the 5′ and 3′ homologous regions surrounding the targeted region of interest. After electroporation into ES cells, colonies surviving positive and negative selection are screened for the desired recombination event by Southern blot. Positive stem cell clones are microinjected into a host blastocyst, which is transferred into a pseudopregnant foster mother. The chimeric offspring are partially derived from ES cells and from the host strain. Breeding of the chimeras to the host strain will result in germline transmission and birth of totally ES cell–derived embryos.

Although this approach is very efficient, ES cells must first be generated to contain docking sites, using homologous recombination.

KIDNEY-SPECIFIC GENE TARGETING

Kidney-Specific Promoters

Several kidney-specific promoters have now been characterized, making it possible to drive gene expression under spatial control (Table 2-1).

Within the tubule, proximal cells can be targeted using a chimeric construct containing a 1,542–base pair (bp) fragment of the 5′ flanking region of the *KAP* gene (kidney androgen-regulated promoter) and the remainder of the human *AGT* structural gene (human angiotensinogen) starting with the last 36 nucleotides of exon II through the poly(A) addition site[6] or 346 bp of the γ-glutamyl transpeptidase type II promoter.[7] Recently a more specific promoter has been described: the mouse *Slc5a2* (Na/glucose cotransporter) 5′ region consisting of the first exon, the first intron, and part of the second exon drives expression specifically in proximal tubule cells.[8]

A 3.0-kilobase (kb) segment of the Tamm-Horsfall protein promoter directs expression to the thick ascending limb of the loop of Henle and early distal convoluted tubules.[9] A 1.34-kb fragment of the Ksp- (kidney-specific) cadherin promoter directs expression to the thick ascending limb of the loop of Henle and collecting ducts of the adult nephron and weakly in other cell types and to the ureteric bud, wolffian duct, müllerian duct, and developing tubules in the mesonephros and metanephros,[10] whereas a 324-bp fragment limits expression to tubular epithelia of the developing kidney and genitourinary tract.[11] The HoxB7 promoter marks the ureteric bud and its derivatives.[12] Principal cells in the renal collecting duct can be targeted using 14 or 9.5 kb of the human aquaporin 2 (*AQP2*) 5′ flanking region.[13,14]

Substantial progress has been made in podocyte-specific gene targeting: 1.25 kb of the human *NPHS1* and 8.3 kb, 5.4 kb, 4.125 kb, and 1.25 kb of the mouse *NPHS1* promoter direct expression to podocytes.[15–17] A podocyte-specific enhancer element from the *NPHS1* gene also directs podocyte-specific gene expression when placed in front of a heterologous promoter.[18] Recently *NPHS2*, another podocyte-specific promoter, has been added to the list.[19]

Despite the growing list of kidney-specific promoters, certain cell types remain untouchable in vivo and include mesangial cells and subpopulations of metanephric mesenchymal cells and their derivatives. Recently, a 2.5-kb promoter fragment from the 5′ flanking region of the megsin gene was described that directs gene expression that is largely restricted to the mesangial cell lineage within the glomerulus in vitro.[20,21] Mesangial cell culture studies have shown that this promoter is functional in vitro.[22] Using the published 5′ flanking fragment that is functional in vitro, we generated a megsin-*lacZ* transgene but were unable to detect any transgene expression within mesangial cells in vivo in 20 individual transgenic founder lines (Gawlik and Quaggin, unpublished data, 2004). Because several genes have been identified that are highly expressed in metanephric mesenchymal cells, it has been possible to generate Cre recombinase lines that express in these cell types, if not through isolated promoters, then through genomic knockin approaches and/or BAC transgenics (see Cre-loxP System).

Table 2-1 Kidney-Specific Promoters

Promoter	Renal Expression	Extrarenal Expression	Reference
Kidney androgen promoter 2	Proximal tubules	Brain	31
γ-Glutamyl transpeptidase	Cortical tubules	None reported	47
Na/glucose cotransporter (Slc5a2)	Proximal tubules	None reported	46
Aquaporin 2	Principal cells of collecting duct	Testis, vas deferens	40,58
Hox-B7	Collecting ducts, ureteric bud, wolffian bud, ureter	Spinal cord, dorsal root ganglia	54
Ksp-cadherin	Renal tubules, collecting ducts, ureteric bud, wolffian duct, mesonephros	Müllerian duct	50
Tamm-Horsfall protein	Thick ascending limbs of loops of Henle	Testis, brain	59
Nephrin	Podocytes	Brain: developing cerebellum	35,57
Podocin	Podocytes	None reported	36
Renin	Juxtaglomerular cells, afferent arterioles	Adrenal gland, testis, sympathetic ganglia, etc.	48

Using these promoters, investigators can determine whether overexpression of their candidate "disease gene" or a dominant-negative version of their protein (one that interferes with the function of the wild-type protein) leads to kidney disease. However, the biologic relevance of these models must be interpreted carefully. In particular, it is difficult to control the level of expression tightly with this approach, and expression of supraphysiologic levels of a gene may not be biologically relevant. Interpretation of experimental results using cell-specific transgene approaches must include these considerations.

ARTIFICIAL CHROMOSOME-BASED STRATEGIES

As discussed above, random integration of plasmid-based constructs frequently leads to different transgene expression levels and incorrect spatial expression. The use of vectors with much larger cloning capacity has allowed researchers to include all transcriptional and post-transcriptional regulatory elements that often are present in intronic sequences or at a considerable distance from the coding region. Besides tightly regulating the transgene expression, the size of artificial chromosome–based vectors minimizes the influence of regulatory sequences in the chromosomal flanking regions. Large-insert clones can be produced using yeast artificial chromosomes (YACs), bacterial artificial chromosomes (BACs), and P1 bacteriophage artificial chromosomes (PACs). In the kidney, PACs containing the entire human renin gene locus have been used to generate transgenic mice. Human renin was only expressed in the kidney and was restricted to juxtaglomerular cells. No positional effects among the lines were reported, and the transgene expression levels correlated strongly with the transgene copy number.[23]

The size of PACs and BACs complicates traditional cloning strategies including restriction digestion and ligation. Plasmid- or phage-based homologous recombination strategies make it possible to modify genes contained in artificial chromosomes. Chi-stimulated recombination, RAC prophage-based ET cloning, and bacteriophage λ-based Red recombination have been used.[24] Using these techniques, artificial chromosomes can be used to target the expression of a gene of interest to a specific tissue: a significant portion of the coding region of a gene encoded on the BAC or PAC is replaced by a complementary DNA of interest, resulting in its expression exclusively in tissues where the BAC or PAC gene is normally expressed. Mullins et al replaced exons III and IV of the murine renin gene encoded on a BAC with the lacZ reporter gene. Transgenic animals expressed β-galactosidase only in renin-expressing cells.[25] Thus artificial chromosomes may help to overcome significant problems of conventional generation of transgenic mice.

USE OF SITE-SPECIFIC RECOMBINASES IN THE KIDNEY

In addition to overexpression studies, investigators often wish to knock down or knock out the function of a specific protein within the kidney. Although expression of a dominant-negative protein may be relevant to human disease or the pathway under study, deletion of a gene within the genome of a specific cell type is also valuable to study gene function. To facilitate the generation of kidney-specific knockouts, site-specific recombinase systems have been used.

Cre-loxP System. Of the recombinase systems available, the Cre-loxP system has been most widely used in mice. Cre

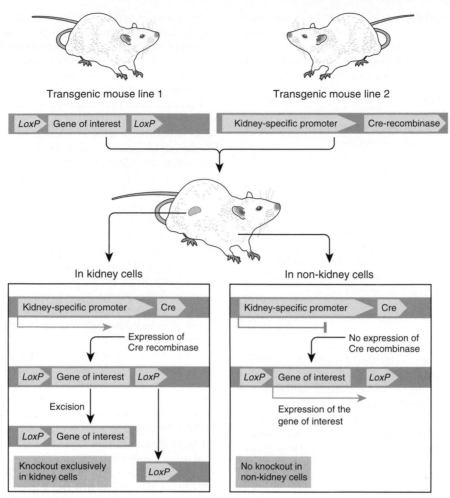

Figure 2-3 Cre-*loxP* system in the kidney. Two transgenic mouse lines are required to achieve a knockout of a gene of interest exclusively in the kidney. One of these lines carries *loxP* sites around a critical portion of, or the entire, gene of interest, the other expresses Cre recombinase under the control of a kidney-specific promoter. After intercrossing, Cre recombinase will excise the floxed gene of interest only in kidney cells. All other cells do not express Cre recombinase.

recombinase (cyclization recombination) is a 38-kDa protein that recognizes a 34-bp DNA target called *loxP* (locus of X-over of P1) and was discovered in the bacteriophage P1.[26,27] This minimal target sequence site is unlikely to occur randomly in the mouse genome and is small enough to be "neutral" when integrated into chromosomal DNA. If two *loxP* sites are located on the same DNA molecule, Cre causes inversion or excision of the intervening DNA segment depending on their respective orientation.

Two transgenic mouse lines are required to facilitate tissue-specific knockouts (Fig. 2-3). The first mouse line expresses Cre recombinase under the control of a tissue-specific promoter. The second carries *loxP* sites around the gene of interest ("floxed gene"). After intercrossing, the gene of interest will be removed selectively from cells expressing Cre recombinase. One or both copies of the gene can be targeted (heterozygosity or homozygosity of the floxed gene, respectively), permitting a crude examination of dosage sensitivity for a specific gene. The Cre-*loxP* system can also be used to activate the expression of genes by excision of a "floxed STOP codon" placed between a highly active promoter and the gene of interest. The advantage of this system over the standard approach using a

cell-specific promoter to directly drive expression of a gene is that it permits robust and reproducible expression of the gene under a well-characterized potent promoter, such as the promoter from the chicken β-actin gene.

Integration of the transgene into an active part of the genome can be rapidly determined using a reporter gene such as *lacZ* or the enhanced green fluorescent protein (EGFP). In a similar manner, activating reporter genes such as *EGFP* makes cell lineage tracing studies possible in vivo. Cells can be tagged at specific time points and their fate followed during development or in disease.[28]

Thus far, kidney-specific Cre mouse lines have been characterized for most of the kidney-specific promoters and exist for γ-glutamyltranspeptidase,[29] *SLC5A3*,[8] Aquaporin 2,[13] HoxB7,[8] Ksp-cadherin,[30] Tamm-Horsfall protein,[31] nephrin,[17] podocin,[32] and renin,[33] and a stromal cell gene BF-2 (Mendelson, unpublished data).

As the number of mouse lines with different floxed genes increases exponentially, it will be possible to determine the role of these genes in podocytes or tubular epithelial cells simply by crossing two mouse strains and analyzing the offspring. In this regard, numerous mouse phenotyping facilities have emerged that permit high-resolution imaging and physiologic analyses. Furthermore, a database has been established by Andras Nagy and colleagues (www.mshri.on.ca/nagy) that describes the characteristics and contacts for many of the transgenic conditional mouse lines currently available.

Flp Recombinase System.
In addition to the Cre-*loxP* system, two other recombinase systems have been used successfully in vivo: the Flp-FRT system from the budding yeast *Saccharomyces cerevisiae*[34] and α-integrase.[35]

Flp recombinase recognizes a 34-bp consensus sequence known as *FRT* and induces recombination between two of these sites. The activities of Cre and Flp have different temperature sensitivities in vitro. Cre was shown to be active over a wider range of temperatures than Flp with a maximal performance at 42°C and therefore offered a theoretical advantage for use in in vivo systems.[36] To improve the activity of Flp, a Flp mutant was developed by introduction of four amino acid changes (Flpe).[37] Flpe has activity in ES cell cultures equivalent to that of Cre and thus should be just as useful for in vivo experiments. Combining both Flp and Cre systems may allow an investigator to target cell lineages that would otherwise be inaccessible.

Integrase System.
Phage integrases also mediate recombination between short sequences of DNA, the phage attachment site (attP), and a short sequence of bacterial DNA, the bacterial attachment site (attB). They are categorized as tyrosine or serine integrases, according to their mode of catalysis. The *Streptomyces* phage-derived φC31, a member of the serine integrase family, has been shown to work efficiently in mammalian cells without any requirement for host cofactors.[35] The ability of phage integrases to unidirectionally and irreversibly integrate an external DNA sequence into the genome makes them useful for genetic engineering in ES cells.[35] Once an "at" site is inserted into a specific chromosomal locus by homologous recombination, any gene of interest may theoretically be integrated into that site at relatively high efficiency. With this strategy, it is possible to insert genes of interest into the same genomic locus so that their effect can be studied and compared in the same context. The biology and applications of phage integrases have recently been reviewed elsewhere.[38]

Caveats.
Despite all of the promising results and insights that recombinase systems have provided, there are several caveats that require consideration. The degree and timing of Cre-mediated excision during embryonic development is critical, because incomplete excision (<100% of targeted cells) might lead to unexpected results, particularly if the gene of interest is a secreted molecule. The presence of residual wild-type cells may produce a different phenotype from that produced by the complete absence of wild-type cells. Although Cre-mediated excision of a floxed reporter allele may be 100%, this can vary from locus to locus.

Efficiency of recombination drops with the distance between *loxP* sites. Although it is not always possible to determine genomic excision for each "floxed" gene in every cell, additional steps such as laser capture microscopy[39] of the cell of interest should be performed to ensure cell-specific and complete excision. The exact stage of Cre-mediated excision during embryonic development of the tissue or cell of interest is also important, and if a gene is expressed before the time of excision, a less severe phenotype may ensue. The stability of the protein and/or gene products may determine this. Though largely theoretical, endogenous pseudo-*loxP* sites that occur naturally in the mammalian genome have been reported; whether any of these sites are associated with genes expressed by renal cells and if recombination of these sites could alter the phenotype of the kidney is not known.

Another theoretical concern in the kidney that has been reported with other tissue-specific promoter-driven Cre systems is that the promoter itself may "mop up" cell-specific transcription factors and alter the phenotype. This is an important consideration that can be overcome by thorough examination of control mice. On occasion, transmission of both the Cre and floxed transgenes through the same germline leads to ubiquitous deletion (i.e., the cell-specific promoter is active within the germ cell leading to widespread excision). This is a major concern if there is a haplo-insufficient phenotype associated with the floxed allele (e.g., vascular endothelial growth factor).[40] Finally, it is mandatory that the investigator periodically check the degree of Cre-mediated excision during a continuing experiment, because activity may decrease in subsequent generations of mice. This can be accomplished by breeding subsequent generations of kidney-specific Cre lines to reporter strains.

From this discussion, it is clear that full characterization of the gene excision in individual Cre lines must be performed. Several excellent reporter mouse strains exist to test cell-specific Cre-mediated excision known as the Z/AP and Z/EG lines.[41,42] In our experience, the Z/EG line that expresses the EGFP subsequent to excision of a floxed STOP allele permits the highest resolution of cell-specific expression when examined using a commercially available antibody to GFP.[17]

Despite the potential pitfalls associated with recombinase systems, as the availability and variety of Cre lines increase, investigators should be able to find lines that suit their experimental needs. In addition, an optimist might consider that mosaic excision or excision after onset of expression of a gene may be desirable—and reveal phenotypes or gene functions that would otherwise be masked by a more complete knockout.

ADDING TEMPORAL CONTROL

The dissection of the role of specific genes in disease requires temporal control of gene expression in addition to tissue specificity. To achieve this goal, tetracycline-sensitive systems have successfully been used in the kidney (Fig. 2-4). Tetracycline binds to the transactivator tTA or "reverse" rtTA. These complexes repress or activate the expression of the gene of interest by binding to the Tet operator (tetO). Shigehara et al[43] recently produced a transgenic line using the human podocin (*NPHS2*) gene promoter to restrict expression of the rtTA cassette to podocytes; they bred these mice with a reporter mouse line that contains the cytomegalovirus minimal promoter and tetO promoter elements together with *lacZ*. Administration of tetracycline in the drinking water or subcutaneously initiated the expression of the *lacZ* reporter gene selectively in podocytes. Replacing *lacZ* by Cre recombinase would allow researchers to benefit from the pool of mouse strains with floxed genes of interest by generating triply transgenic mice that carry the podocyte-specific rtTA, tetracycline-sensitive Cre recombinase transgenes, and the floxed line of interest.

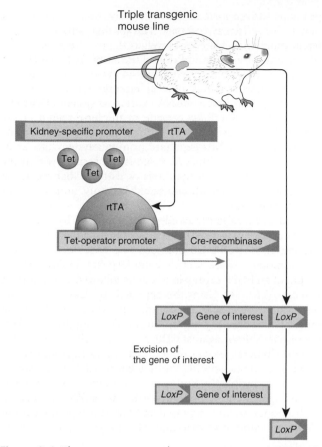

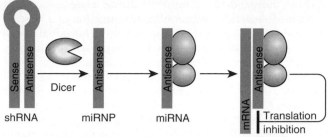

Figure 2-5 Principles of shRNA. Self-complementary short pieces of RNA forming hairpin-like structures (shRNA) activate cytoplasmic Dicer enzymes that cleave the RNA into short pieces (miRNA). miRNAs are incorporated into an miRNA-protein complex (miRNP). The antisense strand guides miRNP to its homologous target mRNA, resulting in inhibition of translation.

Figure 2-4 The reverse tetracycline transactivator (rtTA)–tetO system in the kidney. To achieve inducible knockout of a gene of interest exclusively in the kidney, triple-transgenic mice are generated. The rtTA is expressed under the control of a kidney-specific promoter. Only in the presence of rtTA and tetracycline is the Tet-operator promoter activated, and Cre recombinase is expressed and excises the gene of interest.

RNA INTERFERENCE

Creating knockout animals using homologous recombination in embryonic stem cells is still costly and time consuming. The development of new techniques has made it possible to silence gene expression using short pieces of RNA. RNA interference is a highly conserved mechanism throughout evolution and can be found in plants as well as humans. RNA interference is the process of sequence-specific, post-transcriptional gene silencing initiated by double-stranded RNA (dsRNA) that is homologous in sequence to the silenced gene. The presence of dsRNA in the cytoplasm activates Dicer enzymes that cleave the RNA into short pieces.[48] The mediators of sequence-specific messenger RNA (mRNA) degradation are 21- and 22-nucleotide small interfering RNAs (siRNAs) generated by cleavage from longer dsRNAs.[49]

These siRNAs are incorporated into a multiprotein RNA-inducing silencing complex (RISC). The antisense strand guides RISC to its homologous target mRNA, resulting in cleavage. Unfortunately in mammals the introduction of long dsRNAs leads to a nonspecific inhibitory response mediated through interferon. In 2001, Elbashir et al were able to show that transfection of chemically synthesized siRNAs into mammalian cells effectively silenced the expression of a reporter gene in a sequence-specific manner.[49] These findings have led to widespread application of RNA interference in mammalian species.

Transfection of chemically synthesized siRNA into cells is of a transient nature. To overcome this problem, techniques have been developed using DNA vectors expressing substrates that can be converted into siRNAs in vivo. Expression of these substrates is usually driven by promoters of genes transcribed by RNA polymerase II or III, which produce RNA from a DNA template. To generate dsRNA, transfection with two vectors coding for the sense and antisense strands is necessary. Meanwhile it has been shown that Dicer can process small hairpin RNA (shRNA) structures resulting in the generation of micro-RNAs (miRNAs) (Fig. 2-5). By inhibition of translation, miRNA can effectively silence gene expression, making it possible to target genes using only one vector.[50] These systems can now be used to generate transgenic animals that silence gene expression stably.

Though widely used in vivo, a disadvantage of the tetracycline system is that to knock out a gene of interest in a temporal manner requires generation of triple or quadruple transgenic offspring. Another technique that overcomes this problem and can achieve inducible activity of site-specific recombinases is the development of ligand-regulated forms of Cre and Flpe by fusing a mutant estrogen receptor (ER) ligand binding domain to the C terminus of the enzymes. These fusion proteins are induced by application of the synthetic estrogen antagonist 4-OH tamoxifen but are insensitive to endogenous β-estradiol. Researchers can choose between three different mutant estrogen receptors: Mouse ER[TM],[44] human ER[T],[45] and human ER[T2].[46] CreER[T2] is about 10-fold more sensitive than CreER[T].[47] By placing CreER[T] under the control of a kidney-specific promoter, investigators should be able to generate a simpler system to knock out genes in the kidney in a temporally controlled manner. Although clearly this system would be beneficial, it has not yet been achieved in the kidney. In our own laboratory we generated 12 independent CreER[T2] lines under control of the nephrin promoter (Quaggin, unpublished data, 2004) but were never able to demonstrate excision.

Two independent groups[51,52] demonstrated successful genomic integration and germline transmission of a plasmid expressing siRNA against Ras-gap or Neil-1. Individual ES cell lines were generated that showed varying levels of silencing. Of note, mice derived through germline transmission showed the same level of reduction in the targeted gene as the ES cell line from which they were established. This makes it possible to screen ES cell clones for the desired reduction level (either equal to or less than 100%), permitting the rapid generation of an "allelic series" (i.e., one can look at the phenotype in several lines and determine the effect of more or less expression of a gene on its function). However, the ability to screen expression levels in ES cells before generation of the mouse demands that the gene be expressed in ES cells.

Using pronuclear injection transgenesis, Hasuwa et al[53] accomplished germline transmission of RNA polymerase III (polIII) H1 promoter–driven shRNA expression constructs silencing EGFP expression in *EGFP* transgenic mice to 18%, 4%, and 24% of the control level. Gene silencing by RNA interference exclusively in the kidney might be realized using RNA polymerase II promoters; Ling and Li were able to show that shRNAs transcribed from the CMV promoter could mediate gene silencing.[54] This approach would enable researchers to use any kind of tissue-specific promoter coupled to their shRNA of interest for generation of transgenic mice by simple pronuclear injection.

Additionally, tissue-specific expression can be achieved by the addition of a recombinase system to the siRNA or shRNA plasmid (Fig. 2-6). However, adding *loxP* sites to RNA polIII

promoter–driven systems is challenging, because these promoters are extremely compact. The spacing between the different functional elements as well as the transcriptional start site are critical, and the addition of the 34-bp *loxP* sequence to achieve Cre-inducible shRNA expression would severely impair promoter activity.[55] Kasim et al recently generated a Cre-inducible, polIII-driven shRNA expression system in vitro by placing the *lox*-STOP-*lox* cassette in the loop region of the shRNA.[56] However, because of the palindromic nature of the *loxP* sequence, shRNAs expressed from this system have an 8-bp loop, and the residual *loxP* site is transcribed within the shRNA, resulting in the synthesis of dsRNAs that are 13 bp longer, are less efficient, and could be more prone to nonspecific responses.

Ventura et al elegantly avoided these problems by generating a mutated *loxP* sequence that assumes the function of a specific element of the polIII-U6 promoter, the TATA box, obtaining the promoter activity.[57] The second *loxP* site is placed downstream of an EGFP expression cassette followed by the shRNA sequence (Fig. 2-6). Using this approach in a lentiviral system, the authors were able to conditionally knock down *p53* in mouse embryonic fibroblasts. Moreover, using the same vector with an shRNA against CD8, mouse ES cells were infected and the chimeras were crossed to Cre-expressing mouse lines, resulting in tissue-specific knockdown of CD8. In combination with inducible Cre mouse lines, it should now be possible to have spatial and temporal control over shRNA expression in the kidney, permitting rapid and high-throughput analysis of gene function in a timely and cost-effective manner.

Figure 2-6 Conditional shRNA expression. **A,** A construct driven by the RNA-polymerase III (pol III) U6 promoter is used to express shRNAs only in kidney cells. Two *loxP* sites separated by an 813-bp fragment are placed between sense and antisense regions of shRNA, including six thymines serving as a stop signal for RNA-pol III. In the presence of Cre recombinase the 813-bp fragment is excised and shRNAs with an 8-nucleotide hairpin loop are transcribed. The palindromic region of the *loxP* sequence is transcribed within the dsRNA. **B,** A mutated *loxP* sequence that assumes the function of a specific element of the pol III-U6 promoter was generated. These sites flank the pol III-STOP signal followed by an EGFP expression cassette. Without recombination, EGFP can be expressed. In the presence of Cre, the cell stops making EGFP and in turn starts the production of intact shRNAs with a desired loop sequence.

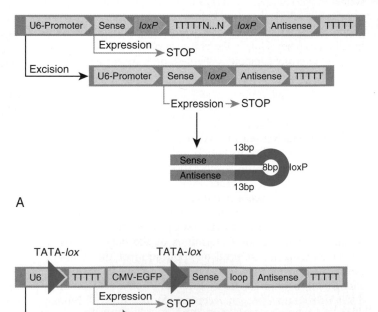

RANDOM MUTAGENESIS

Using the mouse as a model system, standard and conditional gene targeting have provided great insights into our understanding of the function of many genes within the kidney. However, this approach is time consuming, and most knockouts lead to major gene disruptions, which may not be relevant to the subtle gene alterations that underlie human renal disease. Moreover, with many of the complex traits underlying human pathogenesis, predictions about the nature of the genes involved in these diseases are difficult to make.

Whereas in gene targeting experiments the gene is known at the beginning of the experiment (reverse genetics), random mutagenesis represents a complementary phenotype-driven approach (forward genetics). Random mutations are introduced into the genome at high efficiency by chemical mutagenesis. Consecutively, large numbers of animals are screened systematically for specific phenotypes of interest. As soon as a phenotype is identified, test breeding is used to confirm the genetic nature of the trait. The mutated gene is then identified by chromosomal mapping and positional cloning.

The chemical mutagen, N-ethyl-N-nitrosurea (ENU), is one of the most powerful and well-characterized mutagens in the mouse. It acts through random alkylation of nucleic acids, inducing point mutations in spermatogonial stem cells of injected male mice. The mutagenized male will then produce many different mutagenized gametes, with each gamete carrying multiple mutations. Mutations may be complete or partial loss of function, gain of function, or altered function, and can be dominant or recessive. The specific locus mutation frequency of ENU is 1 in 1,000. Assuming a total number of 25,000 to 40,000 genes in the mouse genome, a single treated male mouse should have between 25 and 40 different heterozygous mutagenized genes. In the rare event of a multigenic phenotype, segregation of the mutations in the next generation allows the researcher to focus on monogenic traits. In each generation, 50% of the mutations are lost, and only the mutation underlying the selected phenotype is maintained in the colony.

The screening in ENU mutagenesis experiments can focus on dominant or recessive mutations. Screening for dominant phenotypes is popular, because breeding schemes are simple and a great amount of mutants can be recovered through this approach (Fig. 2-7). About 2% of all F1 mice display a heritable phenotypic abnormality.[58,59]

Because the nature of the mutant phenotypes is random, improved screening techniques to detect subtle phenotypes will result in the recovery of more mutants. Most of the mouse ENU screens thus far are directed toward identification of mouse mutants that serve as models of human disease. Screening focuses on congenital malformations, relevant blood-based biochemical alterations, immunologic defects, and behavior. The Center for Modelling Human Disease in Toronto has recently added a primary renal screen to the ENU mutagenesis project. It includes a laboratory evaluation of plasma creatinine, electrolytes, and urea in blood drawn at 6 weeks of age. Urinalysis is performed by dipstick to detect proteinuria, hematuria, or pyuria. Outliers are retested at 8 weeks of age. The screen already has identified a heritable mouse mutant with glucosuria and isolated glomerulocystic kidney disease ("sweet pee"). None of the known genes for glucosuria or glomerulocystic kidney disease map to the

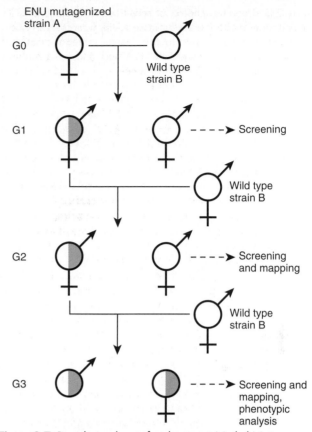

Figure 2-7 Breeding scheme for dominant N-ethyl-N-nitrosourea (ENU) screens. Male strain A mice (G0) are treated with ENU, then bred with wild-type strain B mice to generate G1 mice, which are screened for kidney disease and other phenotypes. Outliers are bred to strain B mice to generate G2 mice, which are phenotypically screened and used for microsatellite mapping. Outliers are again bred for G3 mice, which are used for further microsatellite mapping and in-depth phenotypic analysis.

identified chromosomal region of the new mutation, suggesting the discovery of a new pathophysiologic pathway. These promising results should encourage researchers to use forward genetic approaches to identify new genes responsible for kidney diseases on a broader basis.

Although dominant mutations can unequivocally cause some renal diseases, many others result from interacting mutations in multiple genes that contribute to disease progression. Mutations in "predisposing" genes can be uncovered in "sensitized" mouse strains. G1 ENU-mutagenized males are crossed with females carrying mutations in genes known to predispose to renal disease. G2 animals are phenotypically screened (Fig. 2-8). Using this technique, renal biologists will be able to discover new genes that predispose individuals to their disease of interest.

CONCLUSIONS

New developments in genetic engineering have led to significant improvements in conditional gene targeting in the kidney. Investigators are now able to drive the expression of

Figure 2-8 Breeding scheme for sensitized ENU screens. G1 ENU-mutagenized males are crossed with females carrying mutations in genes known to predispose to renal disease. G2 animals are phenotypically screened and bred further for mapping. G3, mouse with disease.

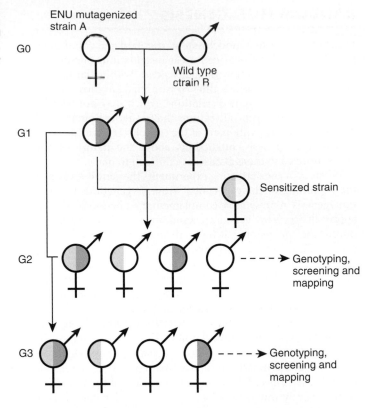

specific genes in specific cell types under temporal control. As the number of cell-specific promoters and Cre lines in the kidneys increases, researchers will be able to target virtually any gene of interest within the kidney. The use of RNA interference will simplify and accelerate this process. Forward genetic approaches like ENU random mutagenesis will supplement conditional gene targeting. In turn, this should lead to great advances in our knowledge about renal physiology, development, and diseases.

References

1. Soriano P: Generalized *lacZ* expression with the *ROSA26* Cre reporter strain. Nat Genet 21:70–71, 1999.
2. Bronson SK, Plaehn EG, Kluckman KD, et al: Single-copy transgenic mice with chosen-site integration. Proc Natl Acad Sci U S A 93:9067–9072, 1996.
3. Cvetkovic B, Yang B, Williamson RA, Sigmund CD: Appropriate tissue- and cell-specific expression of a single-copy human angiotensinogen transgene specifically targeted upstream of the *Hprt* locus by homologous recombination. J Biol Chem 275:1073–1078, 2000.
4. Evans V, Hatzopoulos A, Aird WC, et al: Targeting the *Hprt* locus in mice reveals differential regulation of *Tie2* gene expression in the endothelium. Physiol Genomics 2:67–75, 2000.
5. Guillot PV, Liu L, Kuivenhoven JA, et al: Targeting of human eNOS promoter to the *Hprt* locus of mice leads to tissue-restricted transgene expression. Physiol Genomics 2:77–83, 2000.
6. Lavoie, JL, Lake-Bruse KD, Sigmund CD: Increased blood pressure in transgenic mice expressing both human renin and angiotensinogen in the renal proximal tubule. Am J Physiol Renal Physiol 286:F965–F971, 2004.
7. Sepulveda AR, Huang SL, Lebovitz RM, Lieberman MW: A 346-base pair region of the mouse γ-glutamyl transpeptidase

type II promoter contains sufficient *cis*-acting elements for kidney-restricted expression in transgenic mice. J Biol Chem 272:11959–11967, 1997.
8. Rubera I, Poujeol C, Bertin G, et al: Specific Cre/*lox* recombination in the mouse proximal tubule. J Am Soc Nephrol 15:2050–2056, 2004.
9. Zhu X, Cheng J, Gao J, et al: Isolation of mouse *THP* gene promoter and demonstration of its kidney-specific activity in transgenic mice. Am J Physiol Renal Physiol 282:F608–F617, 2002.
10. Igarashi P, Shashikant CS, Thomson RB, et al: Ksp-cadherin gene promoter. II. Kidney-specific activity in transgenic mice. Am J Physiol 277:F599–F610, 1999.
11. Shao X, Johnson JE, Richardson JA, et al: A minimal Ksp-cadherin promoter linked to a green fluorescent protein reporter gene exhibits tissue-specific expression in the developing kidney and genitourinary tract. J Am Soc Nephrol 13:1824–1836, 2002.
12. Srinivas S, Goldberg MR, Watanabe T, et al: Expression of green fluorescent protein in the ureteric bud of transgenic mice: a new tool for the analysis of ureteric bud morphogenesis. Dev Genet 24:241–251, 1999.
13. Nelson RD, Stricklett P, Gustafson C, et al: Expression of an *AQP2* Cre recombinase transgene in kidney and male reproductive system of transgenic mice. Am J Physiol 275:C216–C226, 1998.
14. Zharkikh L, Zhu X, Stricklett PK, et al: Renal principal cell-specific expression of green fluorescent protein in transgenic mice. Am J Physiol Renal Physiol 283:F1351–F1364, 2002.
15. Wong MA, Cui S, Quaggin SE: Identification and characterization of a glomerular-specific promoter from the human nephrin gene. Am J Physiol Renal Physiol 279:F1027–F1032, 2000.
16. Moeller MJ, Kovari IA, Holzman LB: Evaluation of a new tool for exploring podocyte biology: mouse *Nphs1* 5' flanking region drives *lacZ* expression in podocytes. J Am Soc Nephrol 11:2306–2314, 2000.

17. Eremina V, Wong MA, Cui S, Schwartz L, Quaggin SE: Glomerular-specific gene excision in vivo. J Am Soc Nephrol 13:788–793, 2002.

18. Guo G, Morrison DJ, Licht JD, Quaggin SE: WT1 activates a glomerular-specific enhancer identified from the human nephrin gene. J Am Soc Nephrol 15:2851–2856, 2004.

19. Moeller MJ, Sanden S K, Soofi A, et al: Two gene fragments that direct podocyte-specific expression in transgenic mice. J Am Soc Nephrol 13:1561–1567, 2002.

20. Inagi R, Miyata T, Imasawa T, Nangaku M, Kurokawa K: Mesangial cell-predominant gene, megsin. Nephrol Dial Transplant 17(Suppl 9):32–33, 2002.

21. Inagi R, Miyata T, Suzuki D, et al: Specific tissue distribution of megsin, a novel serpin, in the glomerulus and its up-regulation in IgA nephropathy. Biochem Biophys Res Commun 286:1098–1106, 2001.

22. Inagi R, Miyata T, Nangaku M, et al: Transcriptional regulation of a mesangium-predominant gene, megsin. J Am Soc Nephrol 13:2715–2722, 2002.

23. Sinn PL, Davis DR, Sigmund CD: Highly regulated cell type–restricted expression of human renin in mice containing 140- or 160-kilobase pair P1 phage artificial chromosome transgenes. J Biol Chem 274:35785–35793 1999.

24. Copeland NG, Jenkins NA, Court DL: Recombineering: A powerful new tool for mouse functional genomics. Nat Rev Genet 2:769–779, 2001.

25. Mullins LJ, Payne CM, Kotelevtseva N, et al: Granulation rescue and developmental marking of juxtaglomerular cells using "piggy-BAC" recombination of the mouse ren locus. J Biol Chem 275:40378–40384, 2000.

26. Lakso M, Pichel JG, Gorman JR, et al: Efficient in vivo manipulation of mouse genomic sequences at the zygote stage. Proc Natl Acad Sci U S A 93:5860–5865, 1996.

27. Orban PC, Chui D, Marth JD: Tissue- and site-specific DNA recombination in transgenic mice. Proc Natl Acad Sci U S A 89:6861–6865, 1992.

28. Moeller MJ, Soofi A, Hartmann I, et al: Podocytes populate cellular crescents in a murine model of inflammatory glomerulonephritis. J Am Soc Nephrol 15:61–67, 2004.

29. Iwano M, Plieth D, Danoff TM, et al: Evidence that fibroblasts derive from epithelium during tissue fibrosis. J Clin Invest 110:341–350, 2002.

30. Shao X, Somlo S, Igarashi P: Epithelial-specific Cre/lox recombination in the developing kidney and genitourinary tract. J Am Soc Nephrol 13:1837–1846, 2002.

31. Stricklett PK, Taylor D, Nelson RD, Kohan DE: Thick ascending limb-specific expression of Cre recombinase. Am J Physiol Renal Physiol 285:F33–F39, 2003.

32. Moeller MJ, Sanden SK, Soofi A, et al: Podocyte-specific expression of Cre recombinase in transgenic mice. Genesis 35:39–42, 2003.

33. Sequeira Lopez ML, Pentz ES, Nomasa T, et al: Renin cells are precursors for multiple cell types that switch to the renin phenotype when homeostasis is threatened. Dev Cell 6:719–728, 2004.

34. Dymecki SM: Flp recombinase promotes site-specific DNA recombination in embryonic stem cells and transgenic mice. Proc Natl Acad Sci U S A 93:6191–6196, 1996.

35. Belteki G, Gertsenstein M, Ow DW, Nagy A: Site-specific cassette exchange and germline transmission with mouse ES cells expressing phiC31 integrase. Nat Biotechnol 21:321–324, 2003.

36. Buchholz F, Ringrose L, Angrand PO, et al: Different thermostabilities of Flp and Cre recombinases: implications for applied site-specific recombination. Nucleic Acids Res 24:4256–4262, 1996.

37. Buchholz F, Angrand PO, Stewart AF: Improved properties of Flp recombinase evolved by cycling mutagenesis. Nat Biotechnol 16:657–662, 1998.

38. Groth AC, Calos MP: Phage integrases: Biology and applications. J Mol Biol 335:667–678, 2004.

39. Curran S, McKay JA, McLeod HL, Murray GI: Laser capture microscopy. Mol Pathol 53:64–68, 2000.

40. Carmeliet P, Ferreira V, Breier G, et al: Abnormal blood vessel development and lethality in embryos lacking a single VEGF allele. Nature 380:435–439, 1996.

41. Lobe CG, Koop KE, Kreppner W, et al: Z/AP, a double reporter for Cre-mediated recombination. Dev Biol 208:281–292, 1999.

42. Nolan PM, Peters J, Strivens M, et al: A systematic, genome-wide, phenotype-driven mutagenesis program for gene function studies in the mouse. Nat Genet 25:440–443, 2000.

43. Shigehara T, Zaragoza C, Kitiyakara C, et al: Inducible podocyte-specific gene expression in transgenic mice. J Am Soc Nephrol 14:1998–2003, 2003.

44. Danielian PS, Muccino D, Rowitch DH, et al: Modification of gene activity in mouse embryos in utero by a tamoxifen-inducible form of Cre recombinase. Curr Biol 8:1323–1326, 1998.

45. Logie C, Stewart AF: Ligand-regulated site-specific recombination. Proc Natl Acad Sci U S A 92:5940–5944, 1995.

46. Feil R, Wagner J, Metzger D, Chambon P: Regulation of Cre recombinase activity by mutated estrogen receptor ligand-binding domains. Biochem Biophys Res Commun 237:752–757, 1997.

47. Indra AK, Warot X, Brocard J, et al: Temporally controlled site-specific mutagenesis in the basal layer of the epidermis: comparison of the recombinase activity of the tamoxifen-inducible Cre-ER(T) and Cre-ER(T2) recombinases. Nucleic Acids Res 27:4324–4327, 1999.

48. Bernstein E, Caudy AA, Hammond SM, Hannon GJ: Role for a bidentate ribonuclease in the initiation step of RNA interference. Nature 409:363–366, 2001.

49. Elbashir SM, Harborth J, Lendeckel W, et al: Duplexes of 21-nucleotide RNAs mediate RNA interference in cultured mammalian cells. Nature 411:494–498, 2001.

50. Brummelkamp TR, Bernards R, Agami R: A system for stable expression of short interfering RNAs in mammalian cells. Science 296:550–553, 2002.

51. Carmell MA, Zhang L, Conklin DS, et al: Germline transmission of RNAi in mice. Nat Struct Biol 10:91–92, 2003.

52. Kunath T, Gish G, Lickert H, et al: Transgenic RNA interference in ES cell–derived embryos recapitulates a genetic null phenotype. Nature Biotechnol 21:559–561, 2003.

53. Hasuwa H, Kaseda K, Einarsdottir T, Okabe M: Small interfering RNA and gene silencing in transgenic mice and rats. FEBS Lett 532:227–230, 2002.

54. Ling X, Li F: Silencing of antiapoptotic survivin gene by multiple approaches of RNA interference technology. Biotechniques 36:450–454, 456–460, 2004.

55. Paule MR, White RJ: Survey and summary: transcription by RNA polymerases I and III. Nucleic Acids Res 28:1283–1298, 2000.

56. Kasim V, Miyagishi M, Taira K: Control of siRNA expression utilizing Cre-loxP recombination system. Nucleic Acids Res 3(Suppl):255–256, 2003.

57. Ventura A, Meissner A, Dillon CP, et al: Cre-lox-regulated conditional RNA interference from transgenes. Proc Natl Acad Sci U S A 101:10380–10385, 2004.

58. Hrabe de Angelis MH, Flaswinkel H, Fuchs H, et al: Genome-wide, large-scale production of mutant mice by ENU mutagenesis. Nat Genet 25:444–447, 2000.

59. Nolan PM, Peters J, Strivens M, et al: A systematic, genome-wide, phenotype-driven mutagenesis program for gene function studies in the mouse. Nat Genet 25:440–443, 2000.

Table 3-1 Selection of Targeted Null Mutations as Indicated by Their Protein and Gene Identifications That Are Associated with Cardiorenal Phenotypes in Adult Mice[*]

Protein Product[†]	Gene Symbol	Major Cardiorenal Phenotype	References
Nephrin	Nphs1	Early postnatal death, nephrotic syndrome, edema	Putaala et al: Hum Mol Genet 10:1–8 (2001)
Podocin	Nphs2	Antenatal proteinuria, early renal failure, mesangial expansion	Roselli et al: Mol Cell Biol 24:550–560 (2004)
CD2AP	CD2AP	Renal failure at 6–7 weeks, podocyte abnormalities	Shih et al: Science 286:312–315 (1999)
B7-1	CD80	Protection from LPS-induced nephrotic syndrome	Reiser et al: J Clin Invest 113:1390–1397 (2004)
GLEPP1	Ptpro	Abnormal podocytes, predisposition of hypertension	Wharram et al: J Clin Invest 106:1281–1290 (2000)
Collagen IV	Col4a3	Progressive glomerulonephritis, renal failure	Cosgrove et al: Genes Dev 10:2981–2992 (1996)
Protein kinase C	Prkca	Prevention of diabetic albuminuria	Menne et al: Diabetes 53:2101–2109 (2004)
CFTR	Cftr	Impaired cAMP-mediated Cl⁻ secretion in CCD	Bens et al: Am J Physiol Renal Physiol 281:F434–F442 (2001)
CFEX/PAT1	Slc26a6	Absence of oxalate-stimulated fluid absorption	Wang et al: AJP Cell Physiol (2004)
MinK	KCNE1	Reduced Na⁺ and fluid absorption	Vallon et al: J Am Soc Nephrol 12:2003 (2001)
NKCC1	Slc12a2	Reduced MAP (TCP), reduced venous contractility	Meyer et al: Am J Physiol Heart Circ Physiol 238:H1846–H1855 (2002)
TASK2	Kcnk5	Reduced Na⁺ absorption during HCO₃⁻ administration	Warth et al: Pfluegers Arch 443:171 (2002)
BK$_{Ca}$-β1	Kcnmb1	Increased MAP (AP), smaller rise of GFR, K⁺ excretion after VE	Pluznick et al: Am J Physiol Renal 284:F1274–F1279 (2OC3)
TRPV5	Trpv5	Hypercalciuria, reduced Ca²⁺ absorption in DCT	Hoenderup et al: J Clin Invest 112:1906–1914 (2003)
Sgk1	Sgk	Deficient adaptations of Na⁺ and K⁺ excretion to dietary intake	Huang et al: J Am Soc Nephrol 15:885 (2004)
Pendrin (PDS)	Slc26a4	Absence of CCD HCO₃⁻ secretion	Royeux et al: Proc Natl Acad Sci U S A 98:4221 (2001)
NHERF-1	Slc9a3r	Absence of PKA-mediated inhibition of NHE3	Weinman et al: FEBS Lett 536:141 (2003)
Pept2	Slc15a2	Reduced uptake of filtered dipeptides	Rubio-Aliaga et al: Mol Cell Biol 23:3247 (2003)
Ca²⁺ sensing receptor	Casr	Homozygous mutants not viable, hypercalcemia, hyperparathyroidism	Ho et al: Nat Genet 11:389–394 (1995)

Table 3-1 Selection of Targeted Null Mutations as Indicated by Their Protein and Gene Identifications That Are Associated with Cardiorenal Phenotypes in Adult Mice*—cont'd

Protein Product[†]	Gene Symbol	Major Cardiorenal Phenotype	References
1α-Hydroxylase	Cyp27b1	Hypocalcemia, hyperparathyroidism, rickets	Dardenne et al: Endocrinology 142:3135–3141 (2001)
Vitamin D receptor	Vdr	Failure to thrive after weaning, hypocalcemia	Yoshizawa et al: Nat Genet 6:391–396 (1997)
Oct1/Oct2	Slc22a1/a2	No tubular secretion of organic cations	Jonker et al: Mol Cell Biol 23:7902 (2003)
Adrenomedullin	Adm	Homozygous mutants embryonic lethal, increased MAP (ICP) in heterozygous mutants	Shindo et al: Circulation 104:1964–1971 (2001)
HO-1	Hmox1	Increased severity of renovascular hypertension (TCP)	Wiesel et al: Circ Res 88:1088 (2001)
Caveolin-1	Cav1	Impaired urinary bladder contractions	Lai et al: Neurochem Int 45:1185–1193 (2004)
Gp91 (Phox)	Pirb	Reduced renal vascular resistance	Haque et al: Hypertension 43:335–340 (2004)
Vimentin	Vim	Renal failure and death after partial nephrectomy	Terzi et al: J Clin Invest 100:1520–1528 (1997)
DARPP-32	Ppp1r1b	Increased MAP (TCP), reduced natriuretic response to ANP	Eklof et al: Clin Exp Hypertens 23:449–460 (2001)
5-Lipoxygenase	Alox5	Reduced renal plasma flow, accelerated allograft rejection	Goulet et al: J Immunol 163:359–366 (1999)
Cyp4a14	Cyp4a14	Increased MAP (ICP), increased RVR, reduced autoregulation	Holla et al: Proc Natl Acad Sci U S A 98:5211–5216 (2001)
Epoxide hydrolase	Ephx1	Reduced MAP (TCP) in males	Sinal et al: J Biol Chem 275:40504–40510 (2000)

*Targets that cause mainly developmental changes or that do not show major renal or cardiovascular symptoms are not included. The table does not claim to be complete.
†Protein product names used are those commonly encountered in the physiological literature. Gene names from MGI.
ANP, atrial natriuretic peptide; CD2AP, CD2-associated protein; CFEX/PAT1, chloride/formate exchanger/putative anion transporter; CFTR, cystic fibrosis transmembrane regulator; CCD, cortical collecting duct; Cyp4a14, cytochrome P450 4a14; DARPP, dopamine- and cAMP-regulated phosphoprotein; DCT, distal convoluted tubule; GLEPP1, glomerular epithelial protein 1; GFR, glomerular filtration rate; HO-1, heme oxidase 1; ICP, indwelling catheter pressure; LPS, lipopolysaccharide; MAP, mean arterial pressure; MinK, minimum K channel; NHERF, Na+/H+ exchanger regulating factor; NKCC1, NaK2Cl cotransporter 1; Oct, organic cation transporter; RVR, renal vascular resistance; Sgk, serum- and glucocorticoid-regulated kinase; TASK, twik-related acid-sensitive K+ channel; TCP, tail cuff plethysmography; TRP, transient receptor potential; VE, volume expansion.

fused in situ.[9,10] Hydrogen (H^+) secretion in in vitro–perfused proximal tubules from $NHE3^{-/-}$ mice was reduced by 51% as compared with wild-type tubules.[11] The remaining NHE3-independent $NaHCO_3$ absorption may be driven by H^+-adenosine triphosphatases (ATPases) or by an unidentified amiloride-sensitive pathway that has been observed in tubules from $NHE3^{-/-}$ mice.[11] Formate-, but not oxalate-induced NaCl and fluid absorption was completely abolished in $NHE3^{-/-}$ mice, indicating tight functional coupling between NHE3 and the Cl^-/formate exchanger.[12] In addition to having a reduced basal fluid absorption rate, perfused proximal tubules of $NHE3^{-/-}$ mice have a markedly diminished response of fluid absorption to an increase in tubular flow rate. Thus, the phenomenon of glomerulotubular balance is at least in part the result of flow-dependent stimulation of NHE3.[13] $NHE3^{-/-}$ mice also exhibit a blunted pressure-natriuresis relationship, consistent with a role for this transporter in pressure-dependent changes in proximal reabsorption.[14]

Despite this major transport defect, $NHE3^{-/-}$ mice on a normal NaCl intake can achieve Na^+ balance and are only mildly acidotic, although an increased plasma aldosterone and slightly reduced mean arterial pressure (TCP, AAP, TP) signal the presence of persistent but compensated extracellular volume (ECV) depletion.[9,14] When placed on a low-sodium diet, $NHE3^{-/-}$ mice succumb to progressive volume losses with further decrements in blood pressure, hyperkalemia, acidosis, and salt wasting.[15] However, intolerable salt wasting in these mice is mostly due to lack of intestinal rather than renal NHE3, in that tolerance to a low sodium intake can be restored by transgenic expression of NHE3 in the intestine.[16] $NHE3^{-/-}$ mice have been found to have a 30% to 40% reduction of glomerular filtration rate (GFR), and this reduction of filtered load is largely responsible for the essentially normal flow rates found by micropuncture at the end of the proximal and in the distal tubule.[8,14,16] The reduction in GFR seems to be due to an activation of the TGF mechanism, in that it was only observed when the macula densa (MD) segment was perfused.[8] An increased HCO_3^- reabsorption along cortical and outer medullary collecting ducts was observed in perfused collecting duct segments of $NHE3^{-/-}$ mice, due to an increased H^+-ATPase and hydrogen/potassium (H^+/K^+)-ATPase activity.[17] NHE3-deficient mice exhibit tubular proteinuria, suggesting that NHE3 supports proximal tubular receptor-mediated endocytosis of filtered proteins in vivo.[18] Overall, Na^+ and fluid absorption along the proximal tubule remained unexpectedly high in $NHE3^{-/-}$ mice, inviting a renewed consideration of the quantitative role of individual transporters and transport pathways in proximal Na^+ absorption.

Acid-base or electrolyte balance and plasma aldosterone levels were not measurably changed in $NHE2^{-/-}$ mice, indicating that the NHE2 isoform does not contribute significantly to renal HCO_3^- conservation.[15,19] Nevertheless, NHE2-dependent acidification along the distal tubule seems to limit urinary losses of HCO_3^- in states of elevated distal HCO_3^- delivery, including that caused by the $NHE3$-null mutation.[20]

The overall renal function of $NHE1^{-/-}$ mice has not been studied. However, HCO_3^- absorption in perfused thick ascending limbs of the loop of Henle (TALs) from $NHE1^{-/-}$ mice was reduced by 60%, an effect that was mimicked in wild-type mice by bath addition of amiloride. Thus, basolateral NHE1 seems to regulate the activity of the apical Na^+/H^+ exchanger, probably NHE3.[21]

Sodium/Inorganic Phosphate Cotransporter

Mice with targeted deletion of $Npt2$, the major Na^+/inorganic phosphate (Na^+/P_i) cotransporter in the brush border membrane of proximal tubules, show the expected phosphaturia and hypophosphatemia as well as the resulting changes in vitamin D and calcium metabolism.[22] Heterozygous $Npt2^{+/-}$ mice are only mildly phosphaturic, presumably because Npt2 protein and Na^+/P_i cotransport activity was essentially normal despite a reduction of Npt2 messenger RNA (mRNA).[22] From the magnitude of the functional deficit in $Npt2^{-/-}$ mice one may conclude that Npt2 accounts for about 80% of proximal phosphate transport.[23] Other P_i transporters such as Npt1 are not upregulated in the $Npt2^{-/-}$ mice as compared with controls.[23]

Na+/K+/2Cl– Cotransporter

The dominant role of the $Na^+/K^+/2Cl^-$ cotransporter (NKCC2) in overall NaCl reabsorption along the TAL has been directly demonstrated in mice with targeted deletion of the transporter gene. Mice homozygous for the mutation died within 2 weeks after birth with symptoms of severe volume depletion such as a 200-fold increase in plasma renin concentration (PRC).[24] A small percentage of $NKCC2^{-/-}$ mice could be kept alive by salt supplementation and the administration of indomethacin. The dominant phenotype of adult NKCC2-deficient mice was a marked, vasopressin-resistant polyuria and concentrating defect.[24] Like patients with loss-of-function mutations of NKCC2, $NKCC2^{-/-}$ mice have an increased excretion of prostaglandin E_2 (PGE_2), presumably resulting from activation of COX-2 in TAL cells.[24,25] Mice heterozygous for the $NKCC2$-null mutation ($NKCC2^{+/-}$) have the expected 50% reduction of mRNA expression as compared with wild type, but NKCC2 protein was near normal and no differences in salt balance, PRC, or concentrating capacity were observed between $NKCC2^{+/-}$ and wild-type animals.[26] Similarly, NaCl reabsorption across perfused TAL segments was not measurably altered in $NKCC2^{+/-}$ segments as compared with wild type.[26] It seems to be quite common that heterozygosity, though typically leading to a 50% reduction of mRNA expression, is not associated with corresponding reductions in the expression of the functional protein.

Several isoforms of NKCC2 have been identified that arise from alternative splicing of the mutually exclusive cassette exons A, B, and F.[27] Because the A, B, and F isoforms have been shown to possess different ion affinities, their distinct distribution pattern along the TAL may create an axial pattern of NaCl transport heterogeneities.[28] Mice with a targeted deletion of the B isoform of $NKCC2$ have recently been generated in which the transcription and splicing of the A and F isoforms were maintained.[28b] These mice show a mild concentrating defect and a significant reduction in the dilution of tubular fluid as measured by distal tubule micropuncture.

Renal Outer Medullary K+ Channel

Recycling of K^+ across the apical membrane of TAL cells is required for the maintained activation of NKCC2 and therefore for NaCl transport. In fact, the dominant symptoms associated with loss of function of the renal outer medullary K^+ channel (ROMK), a small-conductance K^+ channel responsible for some part of K^+ recycling, are similar to those caused by NKCC2 deficiency, including a high perinatal mortality due to volume depletion.[29] Those $Romk^{-/-}$ mice that survived to adulthood were hypotensive (TCP) and had a marked reduction in urinary concentrating ability and hydronephrosis. Whole-kidney GFR was drastically reduced but single-nephron GFR was nearly normal, suggesting a decline in the number of functioning nephrons. Cl^- concentration in the distal tubule was somewhat elevated, and net Cl^- reabsorption rate was reduced by about 50%.[29] This relatively well-maintained NaCl absorption is surprising in that patch clamp studies showed not only absence of small-conductance but also of intermediate-conductance K^+ channels in $Romk^{-/-}$ mice.[30,31] Whereas adult $Romk^{-/-}$ mice had a metabolic acidosis, plasma K^+ concentration was not significantly altered, suggesting that K^+ excretion required for K^+ balance was achieved through alternative transport pathways.[29,31]

Chloride Channels

The exceptionally high Cl^- permeability of the thin ascending limbs of Henle's loop is caused by the presence of the CLC-K1 channel. The assumed critical role of Cl^- transport for the operation of the countercurrent mechanism has been established in mice with a deletion of the *CLC-K1* gene.[32] *CLC-K1$^{-/-}$* mice have a vasopressin-resistant polyuria and concentrating defect that did not seem to be due to reduced collecting duct water permeability, because the expression of aquaporin-2 (Aqp2) and the secretion of vasopressin were normal.[33] Accumulation of Na^+, Cl^-, and urea in the renal medulla was markedly reduced under basal conditions and hardly affected by dehydration, suggesting a primary defect in overall countercurrent function.[33] The underlying cause for this defect is presumably the absence of transcellular Cl^- absorption across the thin ascending limbs.[34]

ClC-5 is a Cl^- channel that is abundantly expressed in the kidney, where it is found predominantly in subapical endosomes of proximal tubules and colocalizes with a V-type H^+-ATPase. *ClC-5$^{-/-}$* mice have an impairment of endocytosis that may result from defective acidification of endosomes.[35,36] As a consequence of impaired endocytosis, *ClC-5$^{-/-}$* mice have an increased excretion of endogenous and exogenous low-molecular-weight proteins and of amino acids.[35-37] The phosphaturia of *ClC-5$^{-/-}$* animals has been related to reduced endocytosis of parathyroid hormone (PTH), with the result that concentrations of intraluminal PTH rise to a point where the hormone causes tonic internalization of the Na^+/P_i cotransporter.[36] Intestinal calcium (Ca^{2+}) absorption and plasma Ca^{2+} were found to be unaltered in *ClC-5$^{-/-}$* mice, suggesting that the hypercalciuria resulting from ClC-5 deficiency is of bone or renal rather than intestinal origin.[37,38] Endocytosis of proteins like β-microglobulin, vitamin D–binding protein, retinol-binding protein, and others from the luminal space requires mediation by the megalin/cubilin tandem receptor.[39] Thus, megalin-null mice have major disturbances in both vitamin D and vitamin A metabolism because of deficiencies in endocytotic uptake of vitamin D–binding protein/vitamin D, and retinol-binding protein/retinol complexes.[40,41] Moreover, kidney-specific deletion of megalin has been shown to prevent internalization of the Na^+/P_i cotransporter.[42] A link between the requirements for both megalin and ClC-5 in endocytosis was provided by the finding that *ClC-5$^{-/-}$* mice have reduced levels of megalin and cubilin proteins and a selective deletion of megalin and cubilin from brush border membranes.[36,43] Thus, the impaired endocytosis of *ClC-5$^{-/-}$* mice may result from defective trafficking of megalin and cubilin.

NaCl Cotransporter

Apical thiazide-sensitive NaCl cotransport is the main Na^+ uptake mechanism in the distal convoluted tubule. An early study in mice with targeted deletion of the NaCl cotransporter (NCC) did not show clear symptoms of volume depletion in animals on a standard diet with mean arterial blood pressure (AP) and plasma aldosterone not being different from wild type.[44] More recently, however, a significant increase of plasma aldosterone and a decrease of whole-kidney and single-nephron GFR was reported, suggesting some degree of volume depletion.[45] When $NCC^{-/-}$ mice were fed a low-sodium diet for 2 weeks, their blood pressure (AP) decreased significantly.[44] $NCC^{-/-}$ mice did not show a marked metabolic alkalosis that is typically seen in the human equivalent of Gitelman syndrome, but mice had a reduced plasma magnesium concentration and reduced excretion of calcium.[44] $NCC^{-/-}$ mice were found to have a marked hypertrophy of the connecting tubule and enhanced expression of apical Na^+ channels.[45] Thus, upregulation of connecting tubule NaCl reabsorption seems to be one of the mechanisms compensating for the NCC deficiency, although a marked reduction of GFR also contributes to limiting salt losses.[45]

Epithelial Na+ Channel

The epithelial Na^+ channel (ENaC) is an amiloride-sensitive, multimeric protein consisting of α, β, and γ subunits, which are all required for its full activity. ENaC is expressed in the apical membrane of the collecting duct, and it provides the entry pathway for the movement of Na^+ from lumen to cell. Studies in knockout mice have shown that ENaC, though responsible for only about 2% of total Na^+ absorption, is indispensable for the maintenance of fluid and electrolyte balance. Mice with loss-of-function mutations of the β or γ subunits of *ENaC* die shortly after birth from dehydration and hyperkalemia,[46,47] whereas α-ENaC-deficient mice show a fatal failure to clear the lungs from secreted fluids.[48] Survival and physiological phenotypes of mice heterozygous for ENaC subunits or mineralocorticoid receptor (MR)-null mutations were essentially normal, although in this case the expression of the respective proteins was also reduced.

Partial restoration of *ENaCα* by transgenic expression of the gene in an *ENaCα$^{-/-}$* background reduced perinatal mortality by 50% and generated surviving animals with Na^+ wasting and metabolic acidosis akin to human pseudohypoaldosteronism.[49] Normalization of the electrolyte and acid-base disturbance was observed in adult animals of this strain, indicating that the relative ENaCα deficiency can be compensated with kidney maturation. Transgenic mice with expression of Cre-recombinase under the control of the Hoxb7 promoter were used to generate animals with selective deletion of *ENaC* in collecting ducts.[50] Although amiloride-sensitive currents were completely absent in cortical collecting ducts (CCDs) of these mice, no abnormalities of salt and water homeostasis were observed even under conditions of water deprivation, or the administration of a low-sodium or high-potassium diet.[50]

The somewhat unexpected conclusion would be that the ENaC-expressing nephron segments required for maintaining salt balance must be located upstream from the collecting duct, perhaps in the aldosterone sensitive part of the distal convoluted and connecting tubules. This study provides one of the still few examples of the successful use of the Cre/lox recombination strategy to exert spatial control over the expression of a renal transport protein. A summary of currently available mice in which Cre-recombinase is expressed under the control of a "renal" promoter, and their application for cell-specific recombination, is given in Table 3-2, whereas mice with loxP-flanked sequences are listed in Table 3-3.

A comparably severe phenotype of salt wasting and postnatal mortality has been observed in mice with targeted disruption of the MR gene.[51] Noncompensated volume depletion in $MR^{-/-}$ mice is indicated by the observation that PRC was not different from wild type at birth but had increased 8-fold by day 4, and 440-fold by day 8, the time at which mice began to die.[51] Conversion of corticosterone to the inactive 11-dehydrocorticosterone occurs in aldosterone-sensitive tissue through the action of 11β-hydroxysteroid dehydrogenase type 2 (11β-HSD2). Effective intracellular removal of glucocorticoids is required to maintain the aldosterone sensitivity of MR. Consistent with a role of 11β-HSD2 in preventing a syndrome of apparent mineralocorticoid excess is the observation that $11\beta\text{-}HSD2^{-/-}$ mice are hypokalemic and that they develop marked hypertension (ICP) in the presence of greatly reduced levels of plasma renin and aldosterone.[52]

Table 3-2 Summary of Studies in Which a LoxP-Flanked Target Was Successfully Removed by Cre-Recombinase Expressed by a Promoter That Is Either Kidney-Specific or Highly Active in the Kidney

Promoter	Renal Location	Floxed Target	Reference
SGLT2	Proximal tubule	LacZ	Rubera et al: J Am Soc Nephrol 15:2050–2056 (2004)
γ-Glutamyl transpeptidase	Cortical tubules	GFP	Iwano et al: J Clin Invest 110:341–350 (2002)
AQP2	Collecting duct	ET1	Ahn et al: J Clin Invest 114:504–511 (2004)
Renin	JG cells	LacZ, GFP	Sequeira Lopez et al: Dev Cell 6:719–728 (2004)
Tamm-Horsfall protein	Thick ascending limb	LacZ	Stricklett et al: Am J Physiol 285:F33–F39 (2003)
NPHS2 (podocin)	Podocytes	LacZ	Moeller et al: Genesis 35:39–42 (2003)
Ksp1.3-cadherin	Developing genitourinary tract	Kinesin-II	Lin et al: Proc Natl Acad Sci U S A 100:5286–5291 (2003)
NPHS1 (Nephrin)	Podocytes	VEGF-A	Eremina et al: J Clin Invest 111:707–716 (2003)
Apolipoprotein E	Kidney tubules	Megalin	Leheste et al: Am J Pathol 155:1361–1370 (1999)
HoxB7	Mesonephros, ureteral bud	Sonic hedgehog	Yu et al: Development 129:5301–5312 (2002)
HoxB7	Collecting duct	αENaC	Rubera et al: J Clin Invest 112:554–565 (2003)
Tie1	Endothelial cells	PDGFB	Bjarnegard et al: Development 131:1847–1857 (2003)

Table 3-3 List of Mouse Strains with LoxP-Flanked Genes of Potential Interest for Renal Research

Gene	Reference
Human angiotensinogen	Stec et al: J Biol Chem 274:21285–21290 (1999)
EP4 Receptor	Schneider et al: Genesis 40:7–14 (2004)
Glucocorticoid receptor	Tronche et al: Nat Genet 23:99–103 (1999)
Caveolin 1	Cao et al: Am J Pathol 162:1241–1248 (2003)
GLUT 4	Abel et al: J Clin Invest 104:1703–1714 (1999)
IGF 1	Liu et al: Endocrinology 141:4436–4441 (2000)
Endothelin 1	Ahn et al: J Clin Invest 114:504–511 (2004)
Megalin	Leheste et al: Am J Pathol 155:5301–5312 (2002)
ENaC	Rubera et al: J Clin Invest 112:554–565 (2003)
Calcineurin B1	Neilson et al: Immunity 20:255–266 (2004)
Gsα	Chen et al: Annual meeting Endocrine Society, abstract (2004)

Aquaporins

Mice with an Aqp1 deficiency have a marked, vasopressin-resistant concentrating defect that is due to reduced water permeability of the descending limb of the loops of Henle.[53,54] Osmotic water flux across outer medullary vasa recta was also reduced, which may lead to increased medullary blood flow and contribute to the concentrating defect.[55] Proximal fluid reabsorption of $Aqp1^{-/-}$ mice, assessed either in situ by micropuncture or in the perfused proximal tubule, was reduced by about 50%.[56] Continued salt absorption across a less water-permeable epithelium caused tubular fluid osmolarity to fall below plasma levels.[57] GFR was significantly reduced in $Aqp1^{-/-}$ mice, and the reduced GFR normalized fluid delivery rates to the distal nephron.[56]

Targeted insertion of a point mutation in the $Aqp2$ gene that is associated with nephrogenic diabetes insipidus generated a mouse model with functional Aqp2 deficiency.[58] The appearance of these mice was normal at birth, but the animals failed to thrive and died between days 5 and 6. The major phenotype is a severe concentrating defect with urine osmolarities below isotonicity and absent responses to vasopressin. Plasma osmolarity was significantly elevated, suggesting prerenal failure as the cause of death.[58] A similar phenotype of severe polyuria with early postnatal death was also observed in mice in which a nephrogenic diabetes insipidus resulted from the introduction of a nonsense mutation into the $V2$ vasopressin receptor gene.[59] The severity of the consequences of these forms of nephrogenic diabetes insipidus is somewhat surprising given that newborn mice do not concentrate their urine well and that they do not need to in view of their liquid diet.

Mice with a deficiency of Aqp4, a mercurial-insensitive water channel in the basolateral membrane of collecting duct cells, have a mild impairment in urinary concentrating capacity during water deprivation.[60] The relatively small effect of Aqp4 deficiency on osmotic urine concentration contrasts somewhat with an almost 80% reduction in vasopressin-stimulated water permeability observed in perfused inner medullary collecting ducts.[61] Absence of Aqp3, another basolateral water channel in the collecting duct, is associated with a much more dramatic loss of concentrating ability with urine osmolarity being around or below isotonicity.[62] Aqp3 deficiency, especially on the background of an $Aqp1^{-/-}$ mutation, is associated with hydronephrosis and atrophy of the renal medulla, common consequences of chronic elevations of urine flow in the mouse.[63]

Urea Transporters

Facilitated urea transport by two families of urea transporters is required for the accumulation of urea in the renal inner medulla. Members of the UT-A family are expressed along inner medullary collecting ducts and thin descending limbs of Henle's loop, whereas UT-B type urea transporters in the kidney are found on medullary vasa recta.

Mice with a deletion of the major collecting duct urea transporters UT-A1 and UT-A3 had an increased basal urine flow and a markedly reduced urinary concentrating ability that remained essentially unaltered after 24 hours of water deprivation.[64] Isolated perfused inner medullary collecting ducts of $UT\text{-}A1/3^{-/-}$ mice did not show phloretin-inhibitable and vasopressin-dependent urea transport.[64] Accumulation of urea in the inner medullary tissue was greatly reduced, whereas Na^+, Cl^-, or K^+ contents were unaffected. Although these data confirm that facilitated urea transport through UT-A across inner medullary collecting ducts is critical for medullary urea enrichment, they are difficult to reconcile with the so-called passive concentration of NaCl in the inner medulla.

Mice with loss-of-function mutations of the vascular UT-B urea transporter have a 25% reduction of urinary concentrating ability, and they are able to increase urine osmolarity in response to water deprivation albeit to a lesser extent than wild-type mice.[65] Consistent with this is the finding that papillary urea concentrations were reduced whereas papillary Cl^- concentrations were not significantly different from wild type. In response to an increase in plasma urea concentration by either urea infusion or the administration of a high-protein diet, $UT\text{-}B^{-/-}$ mice were unable to increase overall urinary concentrating ability or to increase urea excretion to the extent seen in wild-type mice.[66] As a result, plasma urea concentrations increased markedly in the knockout animals.[66]

JUXTAGLOMERULAR APPARATUS FUNCTION: TGF, AUTOREGULATION, AND RENIN SECRETION

TGF and Autoregulation

Genetic targeting of proteins believed to be involved in tubuloglomerular feedback (TGF) has helped to elucidate the signaling pathways involved in this homeostatic mechanism. Strong support has been obtained for the hypothesis that adenosine, generated in response to changes in MD transport activity, provides the signal for afferent arteriolar constriction. Two independent laboratories using separately generated mutant mouse lines with targeted deletion of the A1 adenosine receptor (A1AR) have demonstrated a complete absence of TGF responses in micropuncture measurements of stop-flow pressure or single-nephron filtration rate.[67,68] The proximal-distal single-nephron GFR difference, a measure of the basal GFR-suppressing effect of TGF, as well as the TGF-induced oscillations of proximal tubule pressure were abolished in $A1AR^{-/-}$ mice.[69] Finally, the efficiency of both GFR and renal blood flow (RBF) autoregulation was blunted in A1AR-deficient mice.[70] It was concluded that adenosine, as the natural ligand of A1AR, is an obligatory and nonredundant component of the TGF signaling pathway. Absence of TGF regulation makes $A1AR^{-/-}$ mice a unique model to test the physiological role of this regulatory system. This approach was used in studies designed to test the generally accepted notion that the fall of GFR caused by carbonic anhydrase (CA) deficiency results from TGF activation subsequent to increased fluid delivery to the MD. The results of these experiments do not support this concept, however, because the CA inhibitor benzolamide caused identical reductions of GFR and RBF in wild-type and $A1AR^{-/-}$ mice.[71] In a similar approach we have tested our suggestion that the reduction of GFR is the main mechanism that prevents major salt losses in Aqp1-deficient mice.[72] However, when these mice were crossed with $A1AR^{-/-}$ animals that lack TGF regulation of GFR, Aqp1-deficient mice were able to maintain long-term salt balance and blood pressure without a reduction of GFR.[73]

genes have failed to demonstrate a direct correlation between the number of renin genes and PRC or renal renin content.[94,101-103] The implication that the contribution of Ren2 to total plasma renin under basal conditions is relatively small is supported by the finding that PRC is markedly reduced in Ren1d-deficient mice, particularly in female animals,[104,105] and by the early report that removal of the submaxillary glands did not affect plasma renin or plasma Agt, whereas removal of the kidney markedly reduced plasma renin and increased plasma Agt concentrations.[106] In addition, a null mutation of *Ren2* (which depletes submaxillary gland renin) was associated with an increase rather than a fall in PRC, suggesting that the interaction between Ren2 and Ren1 is complex.[107] Arterial blood pressure (ICP, TCP) was only marginally affected in Ren1d-deficient mice, probably reflecting that, in view of the general renin excess, even low levels of renin can generate sufficient amounts of angiotensin II for blood pressure maintenance.[104,105,108]

Although the *Ren1* locus seems to be the primary determinant of basal plasma renin, salivary gland renin and the *Ren2* locus must be considered when designing studies of the RAS in mice, because large amounts of renin can be released from salivary glands and other extrarenal sources during stress.[109,110] This effect is most pronounced in male mice with two renin genes,[111] because *Ren2* gene expression is responsive to androgens.[112]

Genetic RAS Modifications

The use of mice with null mutations of single components of the RAS has provided unique evidence in support of the fundamental importance of this system for the maintenance of body salt balance and arterial blood pressure. Salt depletion (noncompensated in the newborn and compensated in the adult), arterial hypotension, and a concentrating defect form the primary triad characteristic of a genetic loss of RAS function. Whereas the first two symptoms of RAS deficiency are not unexpected, the medullary consequences are surprising and still not completely understood.

Renin

Because of the renin gene duplication in some mouse strains, renin null mutations are most conveniently generated in mice with one renin gene. Homozygous $Ren1c^{-/-}$ mutants usually die shortly after birth.[99] Because they can be rescued by the subcutaneous administration of saline, they apparently succumb to unbalanced NaCl losses, an observation that firmly establishes the necessity of an intact RAS for postnatal salt balance. Surviving reninless mice are severely hypotensive (TCP) and remained polyuric and polydipsic. Renin null mutant mice also show a marked dilatation of the pelvic space and an atrophy of the papilla and medulla.

Angiotensinogen

The consequences of Agt deficiency are similar to those observed in renin null mice. Mice without Agt are born in the expected Mendelian ratio, but postnatal survival is compromised.[98,113] Surviving Agt-deficient mice are polyuric and resistant to vasopressin, and show the typical hydronephrotic syndrome with pelvic space dilatation, papillary effacement,

and cortical thinning.[114,115] In addition, Agt-deficient mice are severely hypotensive (TCP).[98,113,115] From crosses of mice with either disruption or duplication of the *Agt* gene, animals with *Agt* copy numbers ranging from zero to 4 have been generated. Regression analysis showed that blood pressure changed in these animals with a slope of about 8 mmHg per *Agt* copy,[113] although in other studies a reduction in copy number from 1 to zero seems to have a stronger effect, around 20 mmHg.[98,115] With administration of a high-salt diet, arterial blood pressure essentially normalizes, indicating that hypotension is related to salt depletion.[116]

There is less certainty about the role of the RAS in kidney development and maturation. Most evidence suggests that embryonic kidney development is not affected by RAS deficiency, because in general there are no clear morphological abnormalities at birth.[98,115] However, postnatally a slowing of glomerular maturation rate and a medial hyperplasia of interlobular arteries and arterioles have been noted.[113,115] These structural changes resemble those of hypertensive nephrosclerosis, but it is noteworthy that they occur in the absence of angiotensin II and hypertension, both of which are thought to be mediators of vascular remodeling.

Angiotensin-Converting Enzyme

The human *ACE* gene encodes both a somatic enzyme found predominantly in endothelial cells and plasma, and a testis-specific isozyme found exclusively in sperm. Mice with null mutations of the *Ace* gene affecting both isozymes exhibit the expected phenotype of severe arterial hypotension (TCP), postnatal survival problems, and a concentrating defect associated with hydronephrosis and medullary tissue loss.[117,118] Kidney and plasma Ace activities were undetectable in the null mutants,[117,118] but residual levels of angiotensin II were still found.[119,120] A gene titration study has shown that arterial blood pressure (TCP) does not differ significantly between mice with one, two, or three *Ace* gene copies,[121] suggesting that total Ace activity has to be reduced by more than 50% to affect blood pressure. This is probably because Ace activity has to be reduced by more than 50% to reduce plasma angiotensin II.[119] The reduced degradation of bradykinin that one would expect in Ace-deficient mice does not seem to be involved in the hypotension and decreased urinary concentrating ability of these animals, because this phenotype was not altered in bradykinin b_2 receptor/Ace double-knockout mice.[122]

Several mouse strains with genetic *Ace* modifications have been generated to discriminate between effects of membrane-bound, largely endothelial, and serum Ace. One conclusion from these studies is that arterial blood pressure, perhaps not surprisingly, correlates best with plasma angiotensin II (Fig. 3-2), such that a reduction of plasma angiotensin II to less than 30% of control is regularly associated with significant blood pressure reductions.[119,120] Although blood pressure also correlates relatively well with serum Ace activity, levels of kidney Ace seem to be rather unimportant for blood pressure maintenance. For example, kidney Ace including endothelial Ace is virtually absent in two models with ectopic expression of Ace in the liver, but blood pressure (TCP) in these mice was normal.[123,124] A normal blood pressure (TCP) was found in transgenic mice with exclusive expression of Ace in the endothelium, but these mice also had a supranormal plasma Ace activity whereas their kidney Ace was only 20% of

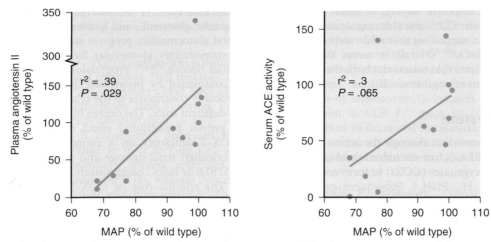

Figure 3-2 Relationship between the percentage change of mean arterial blood pressure (MAP) and the percentage changes of plasma angiotensin II (left) and serum angiotensin-converting enzyme (ACE) activity (right). Changes were normalized for wild-type mice from data obtained in several strains of ACE-transgenic mice[120] and from several strains of recombinant ACE variants.[123,124] Note that the change of blood pressure correlates significantly with plasma angiotensin II but only marginally with serum ACE activity.

normal.[120] Overall, plasma Ace does not seem to correlate well with kidney Ace in these models, and it seems to be plasma Ace, not renal endothelial or proximal tubule Ace, that determines blood pressure.

Male Ace-deficient mice are relatively infertile without showing abnormal counts, morphology, or motility of sperm.[117,118] Studies in mice with selective deletion of somatic Ace or transgenic restitution of germinal Ace have shown that this effect is solely a consequence of the lack of testis Ace and unrelated to somatic Ace.[125,126] Infertility associated with lack of germinal Ace is not a consequence of the lack of angiotensin II, because male Agt-deficient mice are normally fertile although they also lack angiotensin II production. By implication one may conclude that germinal ACE does not seem to affect fertility through hydrolysis of angiotensin I but that it may act on some other substrate or even nonenzymatically.

An ACE homologue, called ACE2, has recently been described that acts as a carboxypeptidase, cleaving a single amino acid from either angiotensin I or angiotensin II generating angiotensins 1-9, or 1-7, respectively.[127,128] Ace2-knockout mice have normal blood pressures (TCP) in the presence of increased levels of angiotensin II. However, cardiac contractility is impaired, as determined echocardiographically as decrements of fractional shortening and shortening velocity, and invasively as decreased dP/dt.[129] The contractility defect was not seen in Ace/Ace2 double-null mutant mice, suggesting that Ace2-dependent cleavage of angiotensin II may normally prevent angiotensin II from reaching pathogenic levels.[129]

Angiotensin II Receptors

Rodents possess three known AT receptors: two isoforms of the AT1 receptor, AT1A and AT1B, which are products of different genes, and the AT2 receptor. The generation of the full RAS knockout triad of salt depletion and poor perinatal survival, arterial hypotension (TCP, ICP), and a concentrating defect with accompanying changes of papillary structure re-

quires deletion of both AT1A and AT1B receptor genes.[130,131] The acute administration of angiotensin II did not affect blood pressure in double AT1 knockouts, arguing against the existence of unrecognized AT receptors.[130,131] An explanation for the characteristic phenotype of the widened renal calyces and papillary atrophy has been provided by studies in AT1 double-knockout mice that show absence of pelvic development, ureteral smooth muscle cell proliferation, and peristaltic ureteral contractions, causing a phenotype that resembles obstructive nephropathy.[132,133] It should be noted that papillary atrophy and calyx dilatation is associated with other states of high urine flow that are not associated with RAS deficiency.

Selective AT1A receptor deficiency is associated with arterial hypotension and markedly reduced pressure (TCP) responses to angiotensin II, but the structure of the kidney including the renal papilla were normal.[134-136] Ambient urine osmolarities of $AT1A^{-/-}$ mice were not different from wild type, although the concentrating ability in response to dehydration was reduced.[137,138] Selective AT1B receptor deficiency, on the other hand, did not cause detectable changes in phenotype as far as tested.[139] It seems that there is a mutual functional compensation among AT1 receptors, but that any compensatory power of the AT1A receptor is considerably stronger. It is likely that this is simply the consequence of the much higher renal expression of the AT1A receptor isoform.[140] Nevertheless, during suppression of endogenous angiotensin II formation, the peptide caused a dose-dependent and losartan-inhibitable increase of blood pressure (TCP) in $AT1A^{-/-}$ mice, demonstrating the pressor potential of AT1B receptors.[141]

Targeted deletion of the AT2 receptor has uncovered a previously unrecognized dilator action of angiotensin II. AT2-knockout mice are slightly hypertensive, by less than 10 mmHg, and respond to angiotensin II with an enhanced pressor response (ICP, TEL).[142-144] Furthermore, chronic infusion of angiotensin II for 7 days at a rate that did not elevate blood pressure in wild-type mice caused a progressive and marked increase of blood pressure in $AT2^{-/-}$ mice that was accompanied by sustained Na^+ retention.[145] The resetting of the

and databases and repositories; will become the site of a knockout mouse model inventory. (www.nih.gov/science/models/mouse/resources/)

NCBI tool called Clonefinder, specific for the mouse genome; useful for identifying clones for any region of the mouse genome; clones can be identified visually using map visualization tools, or specific tools used to search for specific reagents. (www.ncbi.nlm.nih.gov/genome/clone/clonefinder/CloneFinder.html)

National Institute on Ageing clone collection; identification of full-length cDNA clones; clones available without restrictions. (http://lgsun.grc.nia.nih.gov/)

MGC collection of full-length cDNA clones available through the IMAGE consortium; clones available without restrictions. (http://mgc.nci.nih.gov/)

RIKEN collection of full-length cDNA clones; a material transfer agreement with some restrictions is required. (http://genome.gsc.riken.go.jp/FANTOM2CLONES/)

Information about strain characteristics in a searchable form; based on an extensive literature review compiled by Michael Festing, of the Medical Research Council Toxicology Unit[269]; last updated in April 1998; limited information on plasma values and other physiological variables; particularly valuable as a tool to access the older literature for information about strain derivation, behavioral characteristics, immunological properties, and spontaneous tumors and other disorders. (www.informatics.jax.org/external/festing/search_form.cgi)

Jackson Laboratory Phenome project; development of a set of systematic observations on a variety of variables for 40 commonly used mouse strains[270]; community-based project; compiling information provided voluntarily by investigators; database is populated with certain straightforward normative characteristics such as body weight, organ weights including kidney weights, food and water intake, hematological parameters, plasma cholesterol and glucose; some information on tail cuff blood pressures; portal has a variety of easy-to-use analytical tools for comparing parameters in different strains and assessing correlations; descriptions of the methodology used by the project. (www.jax.org/phenome)

The Edinburgh Mouse Atlas project; provides detailed three-dimensional anatomical information about the developing mouse embryo in a database called emap; this data set is linked to the Mouse Gene Expression database maintained by Jackson Laboratories; it is developing detailed information about anatomical patterns of gene expression throughout development; specific patterns of gene expression in the developing kidney and genitourinary tract will soon be added to these electronic resources (URL not yet available). (http://genex.hgu.mrc.ac.uk/)

University of Iowa site with useful information on mouse husbandry and colony maintenance. (http://research.uiowa.edu/animal/)

Eumorphia site, a collection of methods developed for high-throughput screens for European mutagenesis studies. (www.eumorphia.org/EMPReSS/servlet/EMPReSS/Frameset)

Animal Models for Diabetes Complications website; detailed protocols for renal function assessment as well as methods for assessing other complications. (www.amdcc.org/shared/Protocols.aspx)

Maintained by the Academic Medical Center of Amsterdam; collecting information on murine physiology and protocols; still in the construction phase. (www.mousephysio.com)

The landscape of Internet information is continually changing, with new sites and improved access tools becoming available at a rapid pace. Some critical data sets are carefully maintained and continuously updated, whereas other resources are dependent on voluntary efforts, and may languish and become dated or disappear entirely. Thus, although the selected specific sites have been useful to us, the reader will appreciate that this information is, by its nature, selective and vulnerable to rapid obsolescence.

Acknowledgments

Work in the laboratories of the authors was supported by National Institutes of Health/National Institutes of Diabetes and Digestive and Kidney Diseases grant (NIDDK) DK 57552 (J.L.), and by intramural funds from NIDDK (J.S., J.B.).

References

1. Lorenz JN: Considerations for the evaluation of renal function in genetically engineered mice. Curr Opin Nephrol Hypertens 10:65, 2001.
2. Lorenz JN: A practical guide to evaluating cardiovascular, renal, and pulmonary function in mice. Am J Physiol Regul Integr Comp Physiol 282:R1565, 2002.
3. Rao S, Verkman AS: Analysis of organ physiology in transgenic mice. Am J Physiol Cell Physiol 279:C1, 2000.
4. Meneton P, Ichikawa I, Inagami T, Schnermann J: Renal physiology of the mouse. Am J Physiol Renal Physiol 278:F339, 2000.
5. Leiter EH: Mice with targeted gene disruptions or gene insertions for diabetes research: problems, pitfalls, and potential solutions. Diabetologia 45:296, 2002.
6. Thyagarajan T, Totey S, Danton MJ, Kulkarni AB: Genetically altered mouse models: The good, the bad, and the ugly. Crit Rev Oral Biol Med 14:154, 2003.
7. Sigmund CD: Viewpoint: Are studies in genetically altered mice out of control? Arterioscler Thromb Vasc Biol 20:1425, 2000.
8. Lorenz JN, Schultheis PJ, Traynor T, et al: Micropuncture analysis of single-nephron function in NHE3-deficient mice. Am J Physiol Renal Physiol 277:F447, 1999.
9. Schultheis PJ, Clarke LL, Meneton P, et al: Renal and intestinal absorptive defects in mice lacking the NHE3 Na$^+$H$^+$ exchanger. Nat Genet 19:282, 1998.
10. Wang T, Yang, CL, Abbiati, T, et al: Mechanism of proximal tubule bicarbonate absorption in *NHE3* null mice. Am J Physiol 277:F298, 1999.
11. Choi JY, Shah M, Lee MG, et al: Novel amiloride-sensitive sodium-dependent proton secretion in the mouse proximal convoluted tubule. J Clin Invest 105:1141, 2000.
12. Wang T, Yang CL, Abbiati T, et al: Essential role of NHE3 in facilitating formate-dependent NaCl absorption in the proximal tubule. Am J Physiol Renal Physiol 281:F288, 2001.
13. Du Z, Duan Y, Yan Q, et al: Mechanosensory function of microvilli of the kidney proximal tubule. Proc Natl Acad Sci U S A 101:13068, 2004.
14. Noonan WT, Woo AL, Nieman ML, et al: Blood pressure maintenance in NHE3-deficient mice with transgenic expression of NHE3 in small intestine. Am J Physiol Regul Integr Comp Physiol 288:F685, 2005.
15. Ledoussal C, Lorenz JN, Nieman ML, et al: Renal salt wasting in mice lacking NHE3 Na$^+$/H$^+$ exchanger but not in mice lacking NHE2. Am J Physiol Renal Physiol 281:F718, 2001.

16. Woo AL, Noonan WT, Schultheis PJ, et al: Renal function in NHE3-deficient mice with transgenic rescue of small intestinal absorptive defect. Am J Physiol Renal Physiol 284:F1190, 2003.

17. Nakamura S, Amlal H, Schultheis PJ, et al: HCO_3^- reabsorption in renal collecting duct of NHE-3-deficient mouse: A compensatory response. Am J Physiol Renal Physiol 276:F914, 1999.

18. Gekle M, Volker K, Mildenberger S, et al: NHE3 Na^+/H^+ exchanger supports proximal tubular protein reabsorption in vivo. Am J Physiol Renal Physiol 287:F469, 2004.

19. Schultheis PJ, Clarke LL, Meneton P, et al: Targeted disruption of the murine Na^+/H^+ exchanger isoform 2 gene causes reduced viability of gastric parietal cells and loss of net acid secretion. J Clin Invest 101:1243, 1998.

20. Bailey MA, Giebisch G, Abbiati T, et al: NHE2-mediated bicarbonate reabsorption in the distal tubule of *NHE3* null mice. J Physiol 561:765, 2004.

21. Good DW, Watts BA, III, George T, et al: Transepithelial HCO_3^- absorption is defective in renal thick ascending limbs from Na^+/H^+ exchanger *NHE1* null mutant mice. Am J Physiol Renal Physiol 287:F1244, 2004.

22. Beck L, Karaplis AC, Amizuka N, et al: Targeted inactivation of *Npt2* in mice leads to severe renal phosphate wasting, hypercalciuria, and skeletal abnormalities. Proc Natl Acad Sci U S A 95:5372, 1998.

23. Hoag HM, Martel J, Gauthier C, Tenenhouse HS: Effects of *Npt2* gene ablation and low-phosphate diet on renal (Na^+phosphate) cotransport and cotransporter gene expression. J Clin Invest 104:679, 1999.

24. Takahashi N, Chernavvsky DR, Gomez RA, et al: Uncompensated polyuria in a mouse model of Bartter's syndrome. Proc Natl Acad Sci U S A 97:5434, 2000.

25. Wang J-L, Cheng H-F, McKanna JA, Harris RC: Decreased extracellular chloride increases cyclooxygenase-2 (COX-2) expression in cultured cTALH: Possible role of p38 MAP kinase [Abstract]. J Am Soc Nephrol 10:464A, 1999.

26. Takahashi N, Brooks HL, Wade JB, et al: Post-transcriptional compensation for heterozygous disruption of the kidney-specific NaK2Cl cotransporter gene. J Am Soc Nephrol 13:604, 2002.

27. Payne JA, Forbush B: Alternatively spliced isoforms of the putative renal Na-K-Cl cotransporter are differently distributed within the rabbit kidney. Proc Natl Acad Sci U S A 91:4544, 1994.

28. Gimenez I, Isenring P, Forbush B: Spatially distributed alternative splice variants of the renal Na-K-Cl cotransporter exhibit dramatically different affinities for the transported ions. J Biol Chem 277:8767, 2002.

28a. Oppermann M, Mizel D, Huang G, et al: Macula densa control of renin secretion and preglomerular resistance in mice with selective deletion of the B-isoform of the Na,K,2Cl co-transporter. J Am Soc Nephrol 17:2143, 2006.

29. Lorenz JN, Baird NR, Judd LM, et al: Impaired renal NaCl absorption in mice lacking the ROMK potassium channel, a model for type II Bartter's syndrome. J Biol Chem 277:37871, 2002.

30. Lu M, Wang T, Yan Q, et al: ROMK is required for expression of the 70-pS K channel in the thick ascending limb. Am J Physiol Renal Physiol 286:F490, 2004.

31. Lu M, Wang T, Yan Q, et al: Absence of small conductance K^+ channel (SK) activity in apical membranes of thick ascending limb and cortical collecting duct in ROMK (Bartter's) knockout mice. J Biol Chem 277:37881, 2002.

32. Matsumura Y, Uchida S, Kondo Y, et al: Overt nephrogenic diabetes insipidus in mice lacking the CLC-K1 chloride channel. Nat Genet 21:95, 1999.

33. Akizuki N, Uchida S, Sasaki S, Marumo F: Impaired solute accumulation in inner medulla of *Clcnk1⁻/⁻* mice kidney. Am J Physiol Renal Physiol 280:F79, 2001.

34. Liu W, Morimoto T, Kondo Y, et al: Analysis of NaCl transport in thin ascending limb of Henle's loop in CLC-K1 null mice. Am J Physiol Renal Physiol 282:F451, 2002.

35. Gunther W, Piwon N, Jentsch TJ: The ClC-5 chloride channel knock-out mouse—An animal model for Dent's disease. Pflugers Arch 445:456, 2003.

36. Piwon N, Gunther W, Schwake M, et al: ClC-5 Cl^- channel disruption impairs endocytosis in a mouse model for Dent's disease. Nature 408:369, 2000.

37. Wang SS, Devuyst O, Courtoy PJ, et al: Mice lacking renal chloride channel, CLC-5, are a model for Dent's disease, a nephrolithiasis disorder associated with defective receptor-mediated endocytosis. Hum Mol Genet 9:2937, 2000.

38. Silva IV, Cebotaru V, Wang H, et al: The ClC-5 knockout mouse model of Dent's disease has renal hypercalciuria and increased bone turnover. J Bone Miner Res 18:615, 2003.

39. Leheste JR, Rolinski B, Vorum H, et al: Megalin knockout mice as an animal model of low molecular weight proteinuria. Am J Pathol 155:1361, 1999.

40. Nykjaer A, Dragun D, Walther D, et al: An endocytic pathway essential for renal uptake and activation of the steroid 25-(OH) vitamin D_3. Cell 96:507, 1999.

41. Christensen EI, Moskaug JO, Vorum H, et al: Evidence for an essential role of megalin in transepithelial transport of retinol. J Am Soc Nephrol 10:685, 1999.

42. Bachmann S, Schlichting U, Geist B, et al: Kidney-specific inactivation of the megalin gene impairs trafficking of renal inorganic sodium phosphate cotransporter (NaP$_i$-IIa). J Am Soc Nephrol 15:892, 2004.

43. Christensen EI, Devuyst O, Dom G, et al: Loss of chloride channel ClC-5 impairs endocytosis by defective trafficking of megalin and cubilin in kidney proximal tubules. Proc Natl Acad Sci U S A 100:8472, 2003.

44. Schultheis PJ, Lorenz JN, Meneton P, et al: Phenotype resembling Gitelman's syndrome in mice lacking the apical Na^+-Cl^- cotransporter of the distal convoluted tubule. J Biol Chem 273:29150, 1998.

45. Loffing J, Vallon V, Loffing-Cueni D, et al: Altered renal distal tubule structure and renal Na^+ and Ca^{2+} handling in a mouse model for Gitelman's syndrome. J Am Soc Nephrol 15:2276, 2004.

46. McDonald FJ, Yang B, Hrstka RF, et al: Disruption of the β-subunit of the epithelial Na^+ channel in mice: hyperkalemia and neonatal death associated with a pseudo-hypoaldosteronism phenotype. Proc Natl Acad Sci U S A 96:1727, 1999.

47. Barker PM, Nguyen MS, Gatzy JT, et al: Role of γENaC subunit in lung liquid clearance and electrolyte balance in newborn mice. J Clin Invest 102:1634, 1998.

48. Hummler E, Barker P, Gatzy J, et al: Early death due to defective neonatal lung liquid clearance in αENaC-deficient mice. Nat Genet 12:325, 1996.

49. Hummler E, Barker P, Talbot C, et al: A mouse model for the renal salt-wasting syndrome pseudohypoaldosteronism. Proc Natl Acad Sci U S A 94:11710, 1997.

50. Rubera I, Loffing J, Palmer LG, et al: Collecting duct-specific gene inactivation of αENaC in the mouse kidney does not impair sodium and potassium balance. J Clin Invest 112:554, 2003.

51. Berger S, Bleich M, Schmid W, et al: Mineralocorticoid receptor knockout mice: pathophysiology of Na metabolism. Proc Natl Acad Sci U S A 95:9424, 1998.

52. Kotelevtsev Y, Brown RW, Fleming S, et al: Hypertension in mice lacking 11β-hydroxysteroid dehydrogenase type 2. J Clin Invest 103:683, 1999.

53. Ma T, Yang B, Gillespie A, et al: Severely impaired urinary concentrating ability in transgenic mice lacking aquaporin-1 water channels. J Biol Chem 273:4296, 1998.

54. Chou CL, Knepper MA, Hoek AN, et al: Reduced water permeability and altered ultrastructure in thin descending limb of Henle in aquaporin-1 null mice. J Clin Invest 103:491, 1999.

55. Pallone TL, Edwards A, Ma T, et al: Requirement of aquaporin-1 for NaCl-driven water transport across descending vasa recta. J Clin Invest 105:215, 2000.

56. Schnermann J, Chou C-L, Ma T, et al: Defective proximal tubular fluid reabsorption in transgenic aquaporin-1 null mice. Proc Natl Acad Sci U S A 95:9660, 1998.

57. Vallon V, Verkman AS, Schnermann J: Luminal hypotonicity in proximal tubules of aquaporin-1-knockout mice. Am J Physiol Renal Physiol 278:F1030, 2000.

58. Yang B, Gillespie A, Carlson EJ, et al: Neonatal mortality in an aquaporin-2 knock-in mouse model of recessive nephrogenic diabetes insipidus. J Biol Chem 276:2775, 2001.

59. Yun J, Schoneberg T, Liu J, et al: Generation and phenotype of mice harboring a nonsense mutation in the V2 vasopressin receptor gene. J Clin Invest 106:1361, 2000.

60. Ma T, Yang B, Gillespie A, et al: Generation and phenotype of a transgenic knockout mouse lacking the mercurial-insensitive water channel aquaporin-4. J Clin Invest 100:957, 1997.

61. Chou CL, Ma T, Yang B, et al: Fourfold reduction of water permeability in inner medullary collecting duct of aquaporin-4 knockout mice. Am J Physiol 274:C549, 1998.

62. Ma T, Song Y, Yang B, et al: Nephrogenic diabetes insipidus in mice lacking aquaporin-3 water channels. Proc Natl Acad Sci U S A 97:4386, 2000.

63. Yang B, Ma T, Verkman AS: Erythrocyte water permeability and renal function in double knockout mice lacking aquaporin-1 and aquaporin-3. J Biol Chem 276:624, 2001.

64. Fenton RA, Chou CL, Stewart GS, et al: Urinary concentrating defect in mice with selective deletion of phloretin-sensitive urea transporters in the renal collecting duct. Proc Natl Acad Sci U S A 101:7469, 2004.

65. Yang B, Bankir L, Gillespie A, et al: Urea-selective concentrating defect in transgenic mice lacking urea transporter UT-B. J Biol Chem 277:10633, 2002.

66. Bankir L, Chen K, Yang B: Lack of UT-B in vasa recta and red blood cells prevents urea-induced improvement of urinary concentrating ability. Am J Physiol Renal Physiol 286:F144, 2004.

67. Brown R, Ollerstam A, Johansson B, et al: Abolished tubuloglomerular feedback and increased plasma renin in adenosine A1 receptor–deficient mice. Am J Physiol Regul Integr Comp Physiol 281:R1362, 2001.

68. Sun D, Samuelson LC, Yang T, et al: Mediation of tubuloglomerular feedback by adenosine: Evidence from mice lacking adenosine 1 receptors. Proc Natl Acad Sci U S A 98:9983, 2001.

69. Vallon V, Richter K, Huang DY, et al: Functional consequences at the single-nephron level of the lack of adenosine A1 receptors and tubuloglomerular feedback in mice. Pflugers Arch 448:214, 2004.

70. Hashimoto S, Huang YG, Mizel D, et al: Responses of renal blood flow and GFR to blood pressure reduction and volume expansion in adenosine 1 receptor–deficient mice [Abstract]. J Am Soc Nephrol 15:A828, 2004.

71. Hashimoto S, Huang YG, Castrop H, et al: Effect of carbonic anhydrase inhibition on GFR and renal hemodynamics in adenosine-1 receptor–deficient mice. Pflugers Arch 448:621, 2004.

72. Schnermann J: NaCl transport deficiencies—Hemodynamics to the rescue. Pflugers Arch 439:682, 2000.

73. Hashimoto S, Huang Y, Mizel D, et al: Compensation of proximal tubule malabsorption in AQP1-deficient mice without TGF-mediated reduction of GFR. Acta Physiol Scand 181:455, 2004.

74. Schnermann J, Traynor T, Pohl H, et al: Vasoconstrictor responses in thromboxane receptor knockout mice: Tubuloglomerular feedback and ureteral obstruction. Acta Physiol Scand 168:201, 2000.

75. Schnermann JB, Traynor T, Yang T, et al: Absence of tubuloglomerular feedback responses in AT1A receptor–deficient mice. Am J Physiol Renal Physiol 273:F315, 1997.

76. Traynor T, Yang T, Huang YG, et al: Tubuloglomerular feedback in ACE-deficient mice. Am J Physiol Renal Physiol 276:F751, 1999.

77. Traynor T, Yang T, Huang YG, et al: Inhibition of adenosine-1 receptor-mediated preglomerular vasoconstriction in AT1A receptor–deficient mice. Am J Physiol Renal Physiol 275:F922, 1998.

78. Hashimoto S, Adams JW, Bernstein KE, Schnermann J: Micropuncture determination of nephron function in mice without tissue angiotensin converting enzyme. Am J Physiol Renal Physiol 288:F445, 2004.

79. Inscho EW, Cook AK, Imig JD, et al: Physiological role for P2X1 receptors in renal microvascular autoregulatory behavior. J Clin Invest 112:1895, 2003.

80. Castrop H, Huang Y, Hashimoto S, et al: Impairment of tubuloglomerular feedback regulation of GFR in ecto-5′-nucleotidase/CD73-deficient mice. J Clin Invest 114:634, 2004.

81. James PF, Grupp IL, Grupp G, et al: Identification of a specific role for the Na,K-ATPase a2 isoform as a regulator of calcium in the heart. Mol Cell 3:555, 1999.

82. Bell PD, Lapointe JY, Peti-Peterdi J: Macula densa cell signaling. Annu Rev Physiol 65:481, 2003.

83. Wang H, Carretero OA, Garvin JL: Inhibition of apical Na$^+$/H$^+$ exchangers on the macula densa cells augments tubuloglomerular feedback. Hypertension 41:688, 2003.

84. Peti-Peterdi J, Chambrey R, Bebok Z, et al: Macula densa (Na$^+$H$^+$) exchange activities mediated by apical NHE2 and basolateral NHE4 isoforms. Am J Physiol Renal Physiol 278:F452, 2000.

84a. Lorenz JN, Dostanic-Larson I, Shull GE, Lingrel JB: Ouabain inhibits tubuloglomerular feedback in mutant mice with ouabain-sensitive alpha1 Na,K-ATPase. J Am Soc Nephrol 17:2457, 2006.

85. Peti-Peterdi J, Bebok Z, Lapointe JY, Bell PD: Novel regulation of cell Na$^+$ in macula densa cells: Apical Na$^+$ recycling by H-K-ATPase. Am J Physiol Renal Physiol 282:F324, 2002.

86. Meneton P, Schultheis PJ, Greeb J, et al: Increased sensitivity to K$^+$ deprivation in colonic H,K-ATPase-deficient mice. J Clin Invest 101:536, 1998.

87. Vallon V, Traynor T, Barajas L, et al: Feedback control of glomerular vascular tone in neuronal nitric oxide synthase knockout mice. J Am Soc Nephrol 12:1599, 2001.

88. Ren YL, Garvin JL, Ito S, Carretero OA: Role of neuronal nitric oxide synthase in the macula densa. Kidney Int 60:1676, 2001.

89. Ichihara A, Hayashi M, Koura Y, et al: Blunted tubuloglomerular feedback by absence of angiotensin type 1A receptor involves neuronal NOS. Hypertension 40:934, 2002.

90. Schweda F, Wagner C, Kramer BK, et al: Preserved macula densa–dependent renin secretion in A1 adenosine receptor knockout mice. Am J Physiol Renal Physiol 284:F770, 2003.

90a. Kim SM, Mizel D, Huang G, et al: Adenosine as a mediator of macula densa–dependent inhibition of renin secretion. Amer J Physiol Renal Physiol 290:F1016, 2006.

91. Castrop H, Schweda F, Mizel D, et al: Permissive role of nitric oxide in macula densa control of renin secretion. Am J Physiol Renal Physiol 286:F848, 2004.

92. Kurtz A, Wagner C: Role of nitric oxide in the control of renin secretion. Am J Physiol Renal Physiol 275:F849, 1998.

93. Wagner C, Pfeifer A, Ruth P, et al: Role of cGMP-kinase II in the control of renin secretion and renin expression. J Clin Invest 102:1576, 1998.

94. Lantelme P, Rohrwasser A, Gociman B, et al: Effects of dietary sodium and genetic background on angiotensinogen and renin in mouse. Hypertension 39:1007, 2002.

95. Gociman B, Rohrwasser A, Lantelme P, et al: Expression of angiotensinogen in proximal tubule as a function of glomerular filtration rate. Kidney Int 65:2153, 2004.

96. Bouhnik J, Clauser E, Gardes J, et al: Direct radioimmunoassay of rat angiotensinogen and its application to rats in various endocrine states. Clin Sci (Lond) 62:355, 1982.

97. Genain C, Bouhnik J, Tewksbury D, et al: Characterization of plasma and cerebrospinal fluid human angiotensinogen and des-angiotensin I-angiotensinogen by direct radioimmunoassay. J Clin Endocrinol Metab 59:478, 1984.

98. Tanimoto K, Sugiyama F, Goto Y, et al: Angiotensinogen-deficient mice with hypotension. J Biol Chem 269:31334, 1994.

99. Yanai K, Saito T, Kakinuma Y, et al: Renin-dependent cardiovascular functions and renin-independent blood-brain barrier functions revealed by renin-deficient mice. J Biol Chem 275:5, 2000.

100. Poulsen K, Jacobsen J: Inhibition of the enzymatic reaction of renin in aggressive mice. J Hypertens 4:175, 1986.

101. Hansen PB, Yang T, Huang Y, et al: Plasma renin in mice with one or two renin genes. Acta Physiol Scand 181:431, 2004.

102. Ingelfinger JR, Pratt RE, Roth TP, Dzau VJ: Processing of one-chain to two-chain renin in the mouse submandibular gland is influenced by androgen. Pediatr Res 25:332, 1989.

103. Lum C, Shesely EG, Potter DL, Beierwaltes WH: Cardiovascular and renal phenotype in mice with one or two renin genes. Hypertension 43:79, 2004.

104. Clark AF, Sharp MGF, Morley SD, et al: Renin-1 is essential for normal renal juxtaglomerular cell granulation and macula densa morphology. J Biol Chem 272:18185, 1997.

105. Pentz ES, Lopez ML, Kim HS, et al: Ren1d and Ren2 cooperate to preserve homeostasis: Evidence from mice expressing GFP in place of Ren1d. Physiol Genomics 6:45, 2001.

106. Bing J, Poulsen K: The renin system in mice. Effects of removal of kidneys or (and) submaxillary glands in different strains. Acta Pathol Microbiol Scand [A] 79:134, 1971.

107. Sharp MG, Fettes D, Brooker G, et al: Targeted inactivation of the Ren-2 gene in mice. Hypertension 28:1126, 1996.

108. Bertaux F, Colledge WH, Smith SE, et al: Normotensive blood pressure in mice with a disrupted renin Ren-1d gene. Transgenic Res 6:191, 1997.

109. Bing J, Poulsen K: Aggression-provoked renin release from extrarenal and extrasubmaxillary sources in mice. Acta Physiol Scand 107:251, 1979.

110. Poulsen K, Pedersen EB: Increase in plasma renin in aggressive mice originates from kidneys, submaxillary and other salivary glands, and bites. Hypertension 5:180, 1983.

111. Field LJ, McGowan RA, Dickinson DP, Gross KW: Tissue and gene specificity of mouse renin expression. Hypertension 6:597, 1984.

112. Catanzaro DF, Mesterovic N, Morris BJ: Studies of the regulation of mouse renin genes by measurement of renin messenger ribonucleic acid. Endocrinology 117:872, 1985.

113. Kim HS, Krege JH, Kluckman KD, et al: Genetic control of blood pressure and the angiotensinogen locus. Proc Natl Acad Sci U S A 92:2735, 1995.

114. Kihara M, Umemura S, Sumida Y, et al: Genetic deficiency of angiotensinogen produces an impaired urine concentrating ability in mice. Kidney Int 53:548, 1998.

115. Niimura F, Labosky PA, Kakuchi J, et al: Gene targeting in mice reveals a requirement for angiotensin in the development and maintenance of kidney morphology and growth factor regulation. J Clin Invest 96:2947, 1995.

116. Umemura S, Kihara M, Sumida Y, et al: Endocrinological abnormalities in angiotensinogen-gene knockout mice: Studies of hormonal responses to dietary salt loading. J Hypertens 16:285, 1998.

117. Krege JH, John SW, Langenbach LL, et al: Male-female differences in fertility and blood pressure in ACE-deficient mice. Nature 375:146, 1995.

118. Esther CR, Howard TE, Marino EM, et al: Mice lacking angiotensin-converting enzyme have low blood pressure, renal pathology, and reduced male fertility. Lab Invest 74:953, 1996.

119. Cole J, Ertoy D, Lin H, et al: Lack of angiotensin II–facilitated erythropoiesis causes anemia in angiotensin-converting enzyme–deficient mice. J Clin Invest 106:1391, 2000.

120. Kessler SP, des Senanayake P, Scheidemantel TS, et al: Maintenance of normal blood pressure and renal functions are independent effects of angiotensin-converting enzyme. J Biol Chem 278:21105, 2003.

121. Krege JH, Kim H-S, Moyer JS, et al: Angiotensin-converting enzyme gene mutations, blood pressures, and cardiovascular homeostasis. Hypertension 29:150, 1997.

122. Xiao HD, Fuchs S, Cole JM, et al: Role of bradykinin in angiotensin-converting enzyme knockout mice. Am J Physiol Heart Circ Physiol 284:H1969, 2003.

123. Cole J, Quach DL, Sundaram K, et al: Mice lacking endothelial angiotensin-converting enzyme have a normal blood pressure. Circ Res 90:87, 2002.

124. Cole JM, Khokhlova N, Sutliff RL, et al: Mice lacking endothelial ACE: Normal blood pressure with elevated angiotensin II. Hypertension 41:313, 2003.

125. Hagaman JR, Moyer JS, Bachman ES, et al: Angiotensin-converting enzyme and male fertility. Proc Natl Acad Sci U S A 95:2552, 1998.

126. Ramaraj P, Kessler SP, Colmenares C, Sen GC: Selective restoration of male fertility in mice lacking angiotensin-converting enzymes by sperm-specific expression of the testicular isozyme. J Clin Invest 102:371, 1998.

127. Tipnis SR, Hooper NM, Hyde R, et al: A human homolog of angiotensin-converting enzyme. Cloning and functional expression as a captopril-insensitive carboxypeptidase. J Biol Chem 275:33238, 2000.

128. Donoghue M, Hsieh F, Baronas E, et al: A novel angiotensin-converting enzyme–related carboxypeptidase (ACE2) converts angiotensin I to angiotensin 1-9. Circ Res 87:E1, 2000.

129. Crackower MA, Sarao R, Oudit GY, et al: Angiotensin-converting enzyme 2 is an essential regulator of heart function. Nature 417:822, 2002.

130. Oliverio MI, Kim HS, Ito M, et al: Reduced growth, abnormal kidney structure, and type 2 (AT2) angiotensin receptor–mediated blood pressure regulation in mice lacking both AT1A and AT1B receptors for angiotensin II. Proc Natl Acad Sci U S A 95:15496, 1998.

131. Tsuchida S, Matsusaka T, Chen X, et al: Murine double nullizygotes of the angiotensin type 1A and 1B receptor genes duplicate severe abnormal phenotypes of angiotensinogen nullizygotes. J Clin Invest 101:755, 1998.

132. Miyazaki Y, Tsuchida S, Fogo A, Ichikawa I: The renal lesions that develop in neonatal mice during angiotensin inhibition mimic obstructive nephropathy. Kidney Int 55:1683, 1999.

133. Miyazaki Y, Tsuchida S, Nishimura H, et al: Angiotensin induces the urinary peristaltic machinery during the perinatal period. J Clin Invest 102:1489, 1998.

134. Ito M, Oliverio MI, Mannon PJ, et al: Regulation of blood pressure by the type 1A angiotensin II receptor gene. Proc Natl Acad Sci U S A 92:3521, 1995.

135. Oliverio MI, Madsen K, Best CF, et al: Renal growth and development in mice lacking AT1A receptors for angiotensin II. Am J Physiol 274:F43, 1998.

136. Sugaya T, Nishimatsu S, Tanimoto K, et al: Angiotensin II type 1a receptor–deficient mice with hypotension and hyperreninemia. J Biol Chem 270:18719, 1995.

137. Oliverio MI, Delnomdedieu M, Best CF, et al: Abnormal water metabolism in mice lacking the type 1A receptor for ANG II. Am J Physiol Renal Physiol 278:F75, 2000.

138. Mangrum AJ, Gomez RA, Norwood VF: Effects of AT(1A) receptor deletion on blood pressure and sodium excretion during altered dietary salt intake. Am J Physiol Renal Physiol 283:F447, 2002.

139. Chen X, Li W, Yoshida H, et al: Targeting deletion of angiotensin type 1B receptor gene in the mouse. Am J Physiol 272:F299, 1997.

140. Burson JM, Aguilera G, Gross KW, Sigmund CD: Differential expression of angiotensin receptor 1A and 1B in mouse. Am J Physiol 267:E260, 1994.

141. Oliverio MI, Best CF, Kim HS, et al: Angiotensin II responses in AT1A receptor-deficient mice: A role for AT1B receptors in blood pressure regulation. Am J Physiol 272:F515, 1997.

142. Ichiki T, Labosky PA, Shiota C, et al: Effects on blood pressure and exploratory behaviour of mice lacking angiotensin II type-2 receptor. Nature 377:748, 1995.

143. Hein L, Barsh GS, Pratt RE, et al: Behavioural and cardiovascular effects of disrupting the angiotensin II type-2 receptor in mice. Nature 377:744, 1995.

144. Gross V, Milia AF, Plehm R, et al: Long-term blood pressure telemetry in AT2 receptor–disrupted mice. J Hypertens 18:955, 2000.

145. Siragy HM, Inagami T, Ichiki T, Carey RM: Sustained hypersensitivity to angiotensin II and its mechanism in mice lacking the subtype-2 (AT2) angiotensin receptor. Proc Natl Acad Sci U S A 96:6506, 1999.

146. Gross V, Schunck WH, Honeck H, et al: Inhibition of pressure natriuresis in mice lacking the AT2 receptor. Kidney Int 57:191, 2000.

147. Bonventre JV, Huang Z, Taheri MR, et al: Reduced fertility and postischaemic brain injury in mice deficient in cytosolic phospholipase A2. Nature 390:622, 1997.

148. Uozumi N, Kume K, Nagase T, et al: Role of cytosolic phospholipase A_2 in allergic response and parturition. Nature 390:618, 1997.

149. Downey P, Sapirstein A, O'Leary E, et al: Renal concentrating defect in mice lacking group IV cytosolic phospholipase A_2. Am J Physiol Renal Physiol 280:F607, 2001.

150. Dinchuk JE, Car BD, Focht RJ, et al: Renal abnormalities and an altered inflammatory response in mice lacking cyclooxygenase II. Nature 378:406, 1995.

151. Langenbach R, Morham SG, Tiano HF, et al: Prostaglandin synthase 1 gene disruption in mice reduces arachidonic acid–induced inflammation and indomethacin-induced gastric ulceration. Cell 83:483, 1995.

152. Athirakul K, Kim HS, Audoly LP, et al: Deficiency of COX-1 causes natriuresis and enhanced sensitivity to ACE inhibition. Kidney Int 60:2324, 2001.

153. Qi Z, Hao CM, Langenbach RI, et al: Opposite effects of cyclooxygenase-1 and -2 activity on the pressor response to angiotensin II. J Clin Invest 110:61, 2002.

154. Norwood VF, Morham SG, Smithies O: Postnatal development and progression of renal dysplasia in cyclooxygenase-2 null mice. Kidney Int 58:2291, 2000.

155. Morham SG, Langenbach R, Loftin CD, et al: Prostaglandin synthase 2 gene disruption causes severe renal pathology in the mouse. Cell 83:473, 1995.

156. Yang T, Huang YG, Ye W, et al: Influence of genetic background and gender on hypertension and renal failure in COX-2–deficient mice. Am J Physiol Renal Physiol 288:F1125, 2004.

157. Yang T, Endo Y, Huang YG, et al: Renin expression in COX-2 knockout mice on normal or low-salt diets. Am J Physiol Renal Physiol 279:F819, 2000.

158. Cheng HF, Wang JL, Zhang MZ, et al: Genetic deletion of COX-2 prevents increased renin expression in response to ACE inhibition. Am J Physiol Renal Physiol 280:F449, 2001.

159. Cheng HF, Wang SW, Zhang MZ, et al: Prostaglandins that increase renin production in response to ACE inhibition are not derived from cyclooxygenase-1. Am J Physiol Regul Integr Comp Physiol 283:R638, 2002.

160. Lim H, Paria BC, Das SK, et al: Multiple female reproductive failures in cyclooxygenase 2-deficient mice. Cell 91:197, 1997.

161. Loftin CD, Trivedi DB, Tiano HF, et al: Failure of ductus arteriosus closure and remodeling in neonatal mice deficient in cyclooxygenase-1 and cyclooxygenase-2. Proc Natl Acad Sci U S A 98:1059, 2001.

162. Loftin CD, Trivedi DB, Langenbach R: Cyclooxygenase-1-selective inhibition prolongs gestation in mice without adverse effects on the ductus arteriosus. J Clin Invest 110:549, 2002.

163. Fujino T, Nakagawa N, Yuhki K, et al: Decreased susceptibility to renovascular hypertension in mice lacking the prostaglandin I2 receptor IP. J Clin Invest 114:805, 2004.

164. Yokoyama C, Yabuki T, Shimonishi M, et al: Prostacyclin-deficient mice develop ischemic renal disorders, including nephrosclerosis and renal infarction. Circulation 106:2397, 2002.

165. Schweda F, Klar J, Narumiya S, et al: Stimulation of renin release by prostaglandin E_2 is mediated by EP2 and EP4 receptors in mouse kidneys. Am J Physiol Renal Physiol 287:F427, 2004.

166. Audoly LP, Ruan X, Wagner VA, et al: Role of EP(2) and EP(3) PGE(2) receptors in control of murine renal hemodynamics. Am J Physiol Heart Circ Physiol 280:H327, 2001.

167. Imig JD, Breyer MD, Breyer RM: Contribution of prostaglandin EP(2) receptors to renal microvascular reactivity in mice. Am J Physiol Renal Physiol 283:F415, 2002.

168. Fleming EF, Athirakul K, Oliverio MI, et al: Urinary concentrating function in mice lacking EP3 receptors for prostaglandin E2. Am J Physiol 275:F955, 1998.

169. Tilley SL, Audoly LP, Hicks EH, et al: Reproductive failure and reduced blood pressure in mice lacking the EP2 prostaglandin E2 receptor. J Clin Invest 103:1539, 1999.

170. Audoly LP, Tilley SL, Goulet J, et al: Identification of specific EP receptors responsible for the hemodynamic effects of PGE2. Am J Physiol 277:H924, 1999.

171. Kennedy CR, Zhang Y, Brandon S, et al: Salt-sensitive hypertension and reduced fertility in mice lacking the prostaglandin EP2 receptor. Nat Med 5:217, 1999.

172. Segi E, Sugimoto Y, Yamasaki A, et al: Patent ductus arteriosus and neonatal death in prostaglandin receptor EP4-deficient mice. Biochem Biophys Res Commun 246:7, 1998.

173. Thomas DW, Mannon RB, Mannon PJ, et al: Coagulation defects and altered hemodynamic responses in mice lacking receptors for thromboxane A2. J Clin Invest 102:1994, 1998.

174. Francois H, Athirakul K, Mao L, et al: Role for thromboxane receptors in angiotensin-II-induced hypertension. Hypertension 43:364, 2004.

175. Kawada N, Dennehy K, Solis G, et al: TP receptors regulate renal hemodynamics during angiotensin II slow pressor response. Am J Physiol Renal Physiol 287:F753, 2004.

176. Boffa JJ, Just A, Coffman TM, Arendshorst WJ: Thromboxane receptor mediates renal vasoconstriction and contributes to acute renal failure in endotoxemic mice. J Am Soc Nephrol 15:2358, 2004.

177. Sugimoto Y, Segi E, Tsuboi K, et al: Female reproduction in mice lacking the prostaglandin F receptor. Roles of

prostaglandin and oxytocin receptors in parturition. Adv Exp Med Biol 449:317, 1998.

178. Tsuboi K, Sugimoto Y, Iwane A, et al: Uterine expression of prostaglandin H2 synthase in late pregnancy and during parturition in prostaglandin F receptor–deficient mice. Endocrinology 141:315, 2000.

179. Stocco C, Djiane J, Gibori G: Prostaglandin F2α (PGF2α) and prolactin signaling: PGF2α-mediated inhibition of prolactin receptor expression in the corpus luteum. Endocrinology 144:3301, 2003.

180. Huang PL, Huang Z, Mashimo H, et al: Hypertension in mice lacking the gene for endothelial nitric oxide synthase. Nature 377:239, 1995.

181. Shesely EG, Maeda N, Kim H-S, et al: Elevated blood pressure in mice lacking endothelial nitric oxide synthase. Proc Natl Acad Sci U S A 93:13176, 1996.

182. Kurihara N, Alfie ME, Sigmon DH, et al: Role of nNOS in blood pressure regulation in eNOS null mutant mice. Hypertension 32:856, 1998.

183. Godecke A, Decking UK, Ding Z, et al: Coronary hemodynamics in endothelial NO synthase knockout mice. Circ Res 82:186, 1998.

184. Beierwaltes WH, Potter DL, Shesely EG: Renal baroreceptor-stimulated renin in the eNOS knockout mouse. Am J Physiol Renal Physiol 282:F59, 2002.

185. Stauss HM, Godecke A, Mrowka R, et al: Enhanced blood pressure variability in eNOS knockout mice. Hypertension 33:1359, 1999.

186. Kojda G, Laursen JB, Ramasamy S, et al: Protein expression, vascular reactivity and soluble guanylate cyclase activity in mice lacking the endothelial nitric oxide synthase: Contributions of NOS isoforms to blood pressure and heart rate control. Cardiovasc Res 42:206, 1999.

187. Brandes RP, Schmitz-Winnenthal FH, Feletou M, et al: An endothelium-derived hyperpolarizing factor distinct from NO and prostacyclin is a major endothelium-dependent vasodilator in resistance vessels of wild-type and endothelial NO synthase knockout mice. Proc Natl Acad Sci U S A 97:9747, 2000.

188. Sun D, Huang A, Smith CJ, et al: Enhanced release of prostaglandins contributes to flow-induced arteriolar dilation in eNOS knockout mice. Circ Res 85:288, 1999.

188a. Schnermann J, Huang YG, Briggs JP: Angiotensin II blockade causes acute renal failure in eNOS-deficient mice. J Renin-Angiotensin-Aldosterone System 2 (Suppl. 1): S199, 2001.

188b. Wang W, Mitra A, Poole B, et al: Endothelial nitric oxide synthase-deficient mice exhibit increased susceptibility to endotoxin-induced acute renal failure. Am J Physiol Renal Physiol 287:F1044, 2004.

189. Patzak A, Mrowka R, Storch E, et al: Interaction of angiotensin II and nitric oxide in isolated perfused afferent arterioles of mice. J Am Soc Nephrol 12:1122, 2001.

190. Wagner C, Godecke A, Ford M, et al: Regulation of renin gene expression in kidneys of eNOS- and nNOS-deficient mice. Pflugers Arch 439:567, 2000.

191. Chang B, Mathew R, Palmer LS, et al: Nitric oxide in obstructive uropathy: Role of endothelial nitric oxide synthase. J Urol 168:1801, 2002.

192. Yamasowa H, Shimizu S, Inoue T, et al: Endothelial nitric oxide contributes to the renal protective effects of ischemic preconditioning. J Pharmacol Exp Ther 312:153, 2005.

193. Wang W, Mitra A, Poole B, et al: Endothelial nitric oxide synthase–deficient mice exhibit increased susceptibility to endotoxin-induced acute renal failure. Am J Physiol Renal Physiol 287:F1044, 2004.

194. Knowles JW, Reddick RL, Jennette JC, et al: Enhanced atherosclerosis and kidney dysfunction in ($eNOS^{-/-}poe^{-/-}$) mice are ameliorated by enalapril treatment. J Clin Invest 105:451, 2000.

195. Plato CF, Shesely EG, Garvin JL: eNOS mediates L-arginine-induced inhibition of thick ascending limb chloride flux. Hypertension 35:319, 2000.

196. Ortiz PA, Hong NJ, Wang D, Garvin JL: Gene transfer of eNOS to the thick ascending limb of eNOS-KO mice restores the effects of L-arginine on NaCl absorption. Hypertension 42:674, 2003.

197. Barouch LA, Harrison RW, Skaf MW, et al: Nitric oxide regulates the heart by spatial confinement of nitric oxide synthase isoforms. Nature 416:337, 2002.

198. Wang T, Inglis FM, Kalb RG: Defective fluid and HCO_3^- absorption in proximal tubule of neuronal nitric oxide synthase–knockout mice. Am J Physiol Renal Physiol 279:F518, 2000.

199. Jumrussirikul P, Dinerman J, Dawson TM, et al: Interaction between neuronal nitric oxide synthase and inhibitory G protein activity in heart rate regulation in conscious mice. J Clin Invest 102:1279, 1998.

200. Choate JK, Danson EJ, Morris JF, Paterson DJ: Peripheral vagal control of heart rate is impaired in neuronal NOS knockout mice. Am J Physiol Heart Circ Physiol 281:H2310, 2001.

201. Wang T: Role of iNOS and eNOS in modulating proximal tubule transport and acid-base balance. Am J Physiol Renal Physiol 283:F658, 2002.

202. Ullrich R, Bloch KD, Ichinose F, et al: Hypoxic pulmonary blood flow redistribution and arterial oxygenation in endotoxin-challenged NOS2-deficient mice. J Clin Invest 104:1421, 1999.

203. John SW, Krege JH, Oliver PM, et al: Genetic decreases in atrial natriuretic peptide and salt-sensitive hypertension. Science 267:679, 1995.

204. John SW, Veress AT, Honrath U, et al: Blood pressure and fluid-electrolyte balance in mice with reduced or absent ANP. Am J Physiol 271:R109, 1996.

205. Veress AT, Chong CK, Field LJ, Sonnenberg H: Blood pressure and fluid-electrolyte balance in ANF-transgenic mice on high- and low-salt diets. Am J Physiol 269:R186, 1995.

206. Field LJ, Veress AT, Steinhelper ME, et al: Kidney function in ANF-transgenic mice: Effect of blood volume expansion. Am J Physiol 260:R1, 1991.

207. Melo LG, Veress AT, Chong CK, et al: Salt-sensitive hypertension in ANP knockout mice: Potential role of abnormal plasma renin activity. Am J Physiol 274:R255, 1998.

208. Melo LG, Veress AT, Chong CK, et al: Salt-sensitive hypertension in ANP knockout mice is prevented by AT1 receptor antagonist losartan. Am J Physiol 277:R624, 1999.

209. Nakagawa M, Tanaka I, Mukoyama M, et al: Monoclonal antibody against brain natriuretic peptide and characterization of brain natriuretic peptide–transgenic mice. J Hypertens 19:475, 2001.

210. Ogawa Y, Tamura N, Chusho H, Nakao K: Brain natriuretic peptide appears to act locally as an antifibrotic factor in the heart. Can J Physiol Pharmacol 79:723, 2001.

211. Suganami T, Mukoyama M, Sugawara A, et al: Overexpression of brain natriuretic peptide in mice ameliorates immune-mediated renal injury. J Am Soc Nephrol 12:2652, 2001.

212. Lopez MJ, Wong SK, Kishimoto I, et al: Salt-resistant hypertension in mice lacking the guanylyl cyclase-A receptor for atrial natriuretic peptide. Nature 378:65, 1995.

213. Oliver PM, John SW, Purdy KE, et al: Natriuretic peptide receptor 1 expression influences blood pressures of mice in a dose-dependent manner. Proc Natl Acad Sci U S A 95:2547, 1998.

214. Oliver PM, Fox JE, Kim R, et al: Hypertension, cardiac hypertrophy, and sudden death in mice lacking natriuretic peptide receptor A. Proc Natl Acad Sci U S A 94:14730, 1997.

Figure 4-1 Kidney development. The derivatives of the metanephric mesenchyme are in *blue* and *gray* shades; those of the ureteric bud are in *gray*. Not drawn to scale. **A,** Condensed mesenchyme (*light blue*) surrounding the epithelial ureteric bud (*gray*). **B,** Pretubular aggregates (*dark blue*) inferior to the branches of the ureteric bud. On the left, the pretubular aggregate is in its pre-induction mesenchymal state. On the right is shown an epithelial aggregate that has undergone the mesenchymal-to-epithelial transformation. **C,** On the left, a simple comma-shaped tubule is present. On the right, an S-shaped tubule is present, with the portions that will contribute to the glomerulus (G), proximal tubule (P), and distal tubule (D) noted. A capillary (*black*) has begun to invade the glomerular cleft. (The epithelial nature of the ureteric bud is omitted for simplicity.) **D,** A maturing nephron connected to a collecting duct. The glomerulus (actually much smaller in relation to the remainder of the nephron) is shown. The glomerular basement membrane is in *green*. Podocytes are *gray*. **E,** Overall structure of the kidney. The cortex is unshaded, outer medulla *gray* and inner medulla *pink*. The branched network of collecting ducts is in *black*, and nephrons are *blue*. The vascular component is omitted. **F,** A scanning electron micrograph of podocytes extending foot processes around a capillary loop. (Redrawn from Kreidberg JA: Integrins in urogenital development. In Danen EHJ [editor]: Integrins and Development. Austin, Tex, Landes Bioscience, 2006, p 168.)

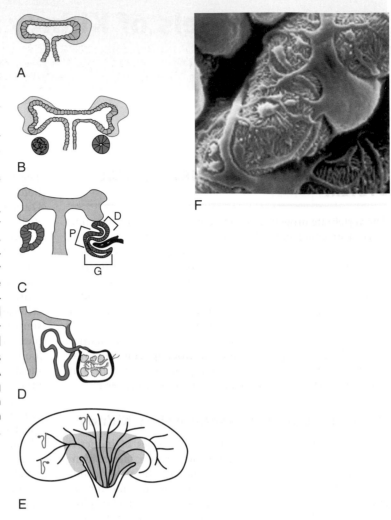

different from those that are active in the tubular portions of the nephron. The collecting ducts are all derived from the original ureteric bud. So, whereas each nephron is an individual unit separately induced and each one originating from a distinct pretubular aggregate, the collecting ducts result from branching morphogenesis beginning with a single epithelial bud. There is, however, considerable remodeling involved in forming collecting ducts from branches of ureteric bud.[6] The branching pattern is highly patterned, with the first several rounds of branching being somewhat symmetrical, followed by additional rounds of asymmetric branching, in which a main trunk of the collecting duct continues to extend toward the periphery of the developing kidney, while smaller buds branch as they induce new nephrons. There is also extensive remodeling to obtain the final structure of the collecting system. Originally, the ureteric bud derivatives are branching within a surrounding mesenchyme. Ultimately, they form a funnel-shaped structure in which a cone-shaped, tightly packed grouping of ducts or papilla, nearly devoid of mesenchymal cells, sits within a funnel or calyx that drains into the ureter. The mouse kidney has a single papilla and calyx, whereas a human kidney has 8 to 10 papillae, each of which drains into a minor calyx, with several minor calyces draining into a smaller number of major calyces.

GENETIC ANALYSIS OF KIDNEY DEVELOPMENT

Much has been learned about the molecular genetic basis of kidney development over the past 15 years. This understanding has primarily been gained through the phenotypic analysis of mice carrying targeted mutations that affect kidney development. Additional information has been gained by identification and study of genes that are expressed in the developing kidney, even though the targeted mutation, or "knockout," either has not yet been done, or the knockout has not affected kidney development or function. The approaches to gene targeting in the kidney have been dealt with extensively in a separate chapter and will not be dealt with further here.

In Vivo Phenotypic Analyses

Renal Agenesis Phenotypes—Absent Ureteric Bud

The first set of phenotypes that were apparent from gene-targeted mice were those that resulted in complete renal agenesis. The knockout of the Wilms' tumor 1 gene, also known as *WT1*, was the first of this group to be reported,[7] followed by many others including *Pax2*,[8] *Eya1*,[9] *Six1*,[10,11] *Sall1*,[12] *Lim1*,[13]

GDNF,[14–16] *GDF11*,[17] *GFRα1*,[18] *Emx2*,[19] gremlin,[20] and *c-Ret*.[21] *GDNF* and *c-Ret* are variable; there is sometimes ureteric bud outgrowth in a minority of embryos. Among this group are putative transcription factors, secreted signaling molecules, a receptor tyrosine kinase, and a co-receptor. In the typical phenotype there is a histologically distinct patch of mesenchyme located in the normal location of the metanephric mesenchyme, but there is no outgrowth of the ureteric bud. Interpretation of these phenotypes involves (1) identification of the expression domains of the mutated gene, (2) analysis of its putative function, and (3) identification of the expression patterns of other genes known to be expressed in the developing kidney. For example, the gene product GDNF (glial cell–derived neurotrophic factor) is a secreted signaling molecule expressed by the metanephric and condensed mesenchyme, which binds the receptor tyrosine kinase c-Ret, and the c-Ret co-receptor, GRFα1, that are expressed at the tip of the ureteric bud.[18,22–24] Thus, it is logical to deduce that GDNF, expressed by the mesenchyme, binds c-Ret and GRFα1, and attracts outgrowth of the ureteric bud from the wolffian duct, and stimulates further growth and branching of the ureteric bud. This conclusion has been supported by additional studies involving the use of beads soaked in GDNF placed adjacent to the ureteric bud, and transgenic mice expressing constitutively active c-Ret.[25–27]

In considering the agenesis phenotypes of transcription factors such as Eya1, Six1, Sall1, Lim1, Wt1, and Pax2, it is more difficult to move from phenotype and genotype to mechanism. Typically, when one of these is "knocked out," the expression patterns of the others are examined. If a particular gene is expressed, it is deduced that this gene is "upstream" of the targeted gene. On the other hand, if a gene is not expressed, it is conversely deduced that this gene is "downstream" of the targeted gene. Although this approach is useful in that it facilitates the proposal of hypotheses that might ultimately be testable in various in vivo and in vitro systems, it must be used cautiously for the following reasons. First, it must be taken into account whether, at a histologic level, the cells that normally express a gene are present and viable. If the cells are absent or undergoing apoptosis, as is common in renal agenesis phenotypes, the absence of gene expression may be a consequence of the complete absence of the cells that normally express that gene. Second, it may be an oversimplification to assume that there are linear upstream and downstream relationships between genes. Gene regulation is likely to be complex, with multiple parallel pathways intersecting at various points. There are multiple levels at which genes can be regulated, including transcription, post-transcription, translation, and post-translation. Moreover, it is emerging that there are multiple mechanisms by which gene expression can be regulated, including transcription factors binding at 5′ ends of genes, chromatin modification through histone acetylation, methylation, and phosphorylation, and localized chromatin winding and unwinding. An additional, as yet unexamined mechanism is whether micro-RNAs, which regulate messenger RNA stability, are involved in kidney development. A third and more obvious issue is whether genes are expressed in the same cell types. For example, if a gene normally expressed in the ureteric bud is knocked out, alterations in gene expression in the mesenchyme are presumably secondary to tissue interactions, rather than being indicative of direct cell-autonomous regulatory effects.

With these caveats in mind, some insights can be discussed with regard to regulatory relationships between different genes that result in renal agenesis phenotypes. *Eya1* and *Six1* mutations are found in humans with branchio-oto-renal syndrome.[28] It is now known, through in vitro experiments, that *Eya1* and Six1 form a regulatory complex that seems to be involved in transcriptional regulation.[29,30] Interestingly, a phosphatase activity is associated with this complex.[30] Moreover, Eya and Six family genes are co-expressed in several tissues in mammals, *Xenopus*, and *Drosophila*, further supporting a functional interaction of these genes.[9,11,31,32] Direct transcriptional targets of this complex seem to include the pro-proliferative factor c-Myc.[30] In the Eya1-deficient urogenital ridge, it has recently been demonstrated that, unlike with some other renal agenesis phenotypes, there is no histologically distinct group of cells in the normal location of the metanephric mesenchyme.[33] Consistent with this finding, Six1 is either not expressed or highly diminished in expression in the location of the metanephric mesenchyme of *Eya1*[−/−] embryos.[30,33] These findings may identify *Eya1* as a gene involved in early commitment of this group of cells to the metanephric lineage. Although *Six1* and *Eya1* may act in a complex together, the Six1 phenotype is somewhat different, in that a histologically distinct mesenchyme is present at E11.5, without an invading ureteric bud, similar to the other renal agenesis phenotypes.[10,11] Eya1 is expressed in the *Six1*[−/−] mesenchyme, suggesting that *Eya1* is upstream of *Six1*. Additionally, Sall and Pax2 are not expressed in the *Six1* mutant mesenchyme, though WT1 is expressed.[10,11,33] Existing discrepancies in the literature about Pax2 expression in *Six1* mutant embryos may reflect the exact position along the anterior-posterior axis of the urogenital ridge of *Six1* mutant embryos from which sections are obtained. In *Pax2*[−/−] embryos, Eya1, Six1, and Sall are expressed.[33] These results are most consistent with the possibility that Eya1, Six1, Sall1, and possibly Pax2 act in a distinct regulatory pathway from Wt1. As emphasized above, although it is fair to conclude that the presence of a gene product in a mutant embryo demonstrates that the mutated gene is not required for expression of the observed gene product, final conclusions about possible interactions between genetic regulatory pathways cannot be based solely on studies of gene expression patterns in mutant embryos and must include additional molecular studies. As an example, through a combination of molecular and in vivo studies, it has been demonstrated that Pax2 appears to act as a transcriptional activator of GDNF.[34]

Early Metanephric Phenotypes—with Ureteric Bud

Additional phenotypes have been obtained that are highly informative about early kidney development. Although these would also be categorized as renal agenesis phenotypes, these are distinguished from the previously discussed phenotypes in that the ureteric bud is present, and may have undergone the first round or two of branching. There are also varying extents of induction of nephrons among these phenotypes. These phenotypes tend more often to be due to the loss of signaling molecules rather than transcription factors.

Mutations of members of the Wnt family are examples of renal agenesis phenotypes where the ureteric bud is present. The Wnt family was originally discovered as the "wingless" mutation in *Drosophila* and in mammals as genes found at retroviral integration sites in mammary tumors in mice. Wnt9b is expressed in the ureteric bud, though not at the very tip.[35] In the absence of Wnt9b, there is outgrowth and the first round of branching of the ureteric bud, and the mesenchyme condenses around the bud, but no pretubular aggregates are formed and no nephrons are induced.[35] These results identified Wnt9b as the prime candidate for the key induction molecule expressed by the ureteric bud and responsible for induction of nephrons. Wnt4 is expressed by cells within the pretubular aggregate that is the precursor of the nephron.[36] In Wnt4 mutant embryos pretubular aggregates are present, but they fail to undergo the mesenchymal-to-epithelial transformation into the tubular precursor of the mature nephron, indicating a role for Wnt4 in the formation of epithelial cells from mesenchyme.[36]

Fibroblast growth factors (FGFs) have been implicated in the very early stages of differentiation of the nephron, even earlier than Wnt4. Conditional mutation of FGF receptors in the mesenchyme results in renal agenesis with a ureteric bud, with expression of early markers such as Eya1 and Six1 in the vicinity of the ureteric bud, but without expression of slightly later markers such as Six2 or Pax2, and no branching of the bud or induction of nephrons.[37] Two groups have published conditional mutations in the *FGF8* gene that eliminate expression of FGF8 in the mesenchyme of the early kidney.[38,39] Failure to properly express FGF8 did not block formation of a Wt1- and Pax2-expressing condensed mesenchyme, but Wnt4-expressing pretubular aggregates were not present, and consequently S-shaped bodies, the precursor of the nephron, never developed.[38,39] Interestingly, these conditionally mutant kidneys were smaller with fewer branches of the collecting ducts, suggesting that nephron differentiation may have a role in driving continued branching morphogenesis of the collecting system.

Bmp7 is a member of another signaling family, the bone morphogenetic proteins. Bmp7 is first expressed in the ureteric bud and then in the condensed mesenchyme.[40,41] In the absence of Bmp7, the first round of nephrons are induced, but there is no further kidney development.[40,41] It has been suggested that this first round of nephrons might result from maternal contribution of Bmp7 across the placenta, and it is not known whether Bmp7 is absolutely required for the induction of nephrons.

A current theme in cell biology is that growth factor signaling often occurs coordinately with signals from the extracellular matrix transduced by adhesion receptors such as members of the integrin family. $\alpha_8\beta_1$ integrin, expressed by cells of the metanephric mesenchyme,[42] binds a novel molecule named nephronectin,[43] expressed on the ureteric bud. In most α_8-integrin mutant embryos, the ureteric bud arrests its outgrowth upon contact with the metanephric mesenchyme.[42] In a small portion of embryos this block is overcome, and a single, usually hypoplastic, kidney develops. Thus, the interaction of $\alpha_8\beta_1$ integrin with nephronectin must have an important role in the continued growth of the ureteric bud into the mesenchyme. This phenotype also implies that there is something about the interaction of ureteric bud cells with the metanephric mesenchyme that distinguishes it from the interaction of the ureteric bud with the undifferentiated mesenchyme of the urogenital ridge, through which it must briefly pass before encountering the metanephric mesenchyme. Whether $\alpha_8\beta_1$ integrin–nephronectin signaling occurs in concert with growth factor signaling is not yet known.

In Vitro Analyses of Early Kidney Development in Organ Culture

Classical Studies

The organ culture system was used extensively in classical studies of embryonic induction. These studies determined such parameters of the induction system as the temporal and physical constraints on exposure of the inductive tissue to the mesenchyme, and the time periods during which various tubular elements of the nephron were first observed in culture.

Mutant Phenotypic Analyses

Organ culture studies have yielded additional information about gene function in early kidney development. As originally shown by Grobstein, Saxen, and colleagues in classical studies of embryonic induction, it is possible to separate the metanephric mesenchyme from the ureteric bud, and use certain other tissues, the best example of which is embryonic neural tube, to induce the mesenchyme to form nephron-like tubules in organotypic culture.[44,45] This experiment is distinguished from placing in culture the whole metanephric rudiment, including the ureteric bud, in that when the whole rudiment is placed in culture, not only do both induction of nephrons and branching of the ureteric bud occur, but the rudiment continues to grow as well. In contrast, when neural tube tissue is used to induce the separated mesenchyme, terminal differentiation of the mesenchyme into tubules occurs, but there is no significant tissue expansion. In renal agenesis situations where there is no outgrowth of the ureteric bud, the mesenchyme can be placed in contact with neural tube to determine whether it has the intrinsic ability to differentiate. In most cases, when the renal agenesis phenotype is due to the absence of a transcription factor, tubular differentiation is not rescued by neural tube, as might be predicted for transcription factors, which would be expected to act in a cell-autonomous fashion.[7] Nevertheless, these experiments have been useful in demonstrating that the gene responsible for the agenesis phenotype is not only involved in stimulating outgrowth the ureteric bud but also has a role in the intrinsic differentiation of the mesenchyme.

In contrast to organ culture results obtained with transcription factor mutants expressed in the metanephric mesenchyme, those using mesenchyme from mutants where the transcription factor is expressed in the ureteric bud, such as Emx2, have yielded the opposite result. Emx2 mesenchyme can be induced to form tubules by embryonic neural tube.[19]

Antisense Oligonucleotides and siRNA in Organ Culture

Several studies have described the use of antisense oligonucleotides and more recently, short interfering RNA (siRNA) molecules, to inhibit gene expression in kidney organ culture. Among the earliest of these was the inhibition of the low-affinity nerve growth factor receptor, p75 or NGFR, by antisense oligonucleotides,[46] a treatment that decreased the growth of the organ culture. A subsequent study could not duplicate this phenotype,[47] although there were possible differences in experimental techniques.[48] An additional study using antisense oligonucleotides to *Pax2* also showed this gene to be crucial in the mesenchymal-to-epithelial transformation.[49] More recently, one report has demonstrated that siRNA to the *Wt1* and *Pax2* genes can inhibit early nephron differentiation.[47,50]

Organ Culture Microinjection.

A novel approach to the organ culture system has also yielded insights about a possible function of the *WT1* gene in early kidney development. A system was established to microinject and electroporate DNA plasmid expression constructs into the condensed mesenchyme of organ cultures.[51] Injection of Pax2 led to increased expression of GDNF, consistent with previously published results from in vitro studies indicating Pax2 was a transcriptional regulator of GDNF.[51] Overexpression of WT1 from an expression construct led to high-level expression of vascular endothelial growth factor A (VEGF-A). The target of VEGF-A appeared to be Flk1 (VEGFR2)–expressing angioblasts at the periphery of the mesenchyme. Blocking signaling through Flk1, if done when the metanephric rudiment was placed in culture, blocked expression of Pax2 and GDNF, and consequently the continued branching of the ureteric bud and induction of nephrons by the bud. Addition of the Flk1 blockade after the organ had been in culture for 48 hours had no effect, indicating that the angioblast-derived signal was required to initiate kidney development but not to maintain continued development. The signal provided by the angioblasts is not yet known, nor is it known whether WT1 is a direct transcriptional activator of VEGF-A. Flk1 signaling is also known to be required to initiate hepatocyte differentiation during liver development.

Genetic Analyses of Nephron Differentiation

Although gene targeting and other analyses have identified many genes involved in the initial induction of the metanephric kidney and the formation of the pretubular aggregate, much less is presently known about how the pretubular aggregate develops into the mature nephron, a process through which a simple tubule elongates, convolutes, and differentiates into multiple distinct segments with different functions. In considering how this segmentation occurs, it has been considered whether there will be similarities to other aspects of development, such as the limb or neural tube, where there is segmentation along various axes.

The Notch group of signaling molecules has been implicated in directing the segmentation of the nephron. Notch family members are transmembrane proteins whose cytoplasmic domains are cleaved by the γ-secretase enzyme, upon the interaction of the extracellular domain with transmembrane ligand proteins of the delta and jagged families, found on adjacent cells.[52] Thus, Notch signaling occurs between adjacent cells, in contrast to signaling by secreted growth factors that may occur at a distance from the growth factor–expressing cells. The cleaved portion of the Notch cytoplasmic domain translocates to the nucleus, where it has a role in directing gene expression. Mice homozygous for a hypomorphic allele of *Notch2* have abnormal glomeruli, with a failure to form a mature capillary tuft.[53,54] Because null mutations of Notch family members usually result in early embryonic lethality, further analysis of Notch family function in kidney development has made use of the organ culture model. When metanephric rudiments are cultured in the presence of a γ-secretase inhibitor,[55,56] there is diminished expression of

podocyte and proximal tubule markers, in comparison with distal tubule markers and branching of the ureteric bud. When the γ-secretase inhibitor is removed, there seems to be a better recovery of expression of proximal tubule markers, in comparison with markers of podocyte differentiation. Similar results were observed in mice carrying targeted mutation of the *PSEN1* and *PSEN2* genes that encode a component of the γ-secretase complex.[57] These results, while requiring confirmation from mice carrying conditional mutations in Notch genes themselves, suggest that Notch signaling is involved in patterning the proximal tubule and glomerulus. Similar results were obtained from mice with mutations in the gene encoding γ-secretase.

There is one example so far of a transcription factor being involved in the differentiation of a specific cell type in the kidney. The phenotype is actually found in the collecting ducts rather than in the nephron itself, but it is discussed in this section because it demonstrates the phenotypic characteristics that investigators expect will be found as additional mutant mice are examined. Two cell types are normally found in the collecting ducts: principal cells that mediate water and salt reabsorption, and intercalated cells that mediate acid-base transport. In the absence of the Foxi1 transcription factor, there is only one cell type present in collecting ducts, and many acid-base-transport proteins normally expressed by intercalated cells are absent.[58]

Several gene-targeted mice have been found to have abnormalities of glomerular development. Those that involve genes that encode podocyte-specific proteins or proteins found in the glomerular basement membrane will be discussed in different chapters. Several transcription factors are known to be expressed in podocytes, whose mutations have resulted in abnormal glomerular development. These include Pod1,[59] Wt1,[60,61] Kreisler,[62] and Lmx1b.[63,64] A podocyte-specific conditional mutation of Wt1 has not yet been reported. However, expression of a presumed dominant-negative form of Wt1 in podocytes led to abnormal glomerular capillary development, suggesting a role for Wt1 and podocytes in regulating formation of the glomerular vasculature.[61] Nephrin and podocalyxin have also been suggested as targets of the *Wt1* gene.[65–67] Poorly formed glomeruli are found in the absence of Pod1.[59] However, this might not reflect a cell-autonomous function of Pod1, and when *Pod1*-homozygous null embryonic stem cells are used to make chimeric mice, *Pod1*-null cells are excluded from the interstitium but not from glomeruli.[68] *Lmx1b* is a Lim-homeodomain transcription factor implicated as the gene responsible for nail-patella syndrome.[69] Podocytes of Lmx1b-deficient mice fail to form foot processes, and Lmx1b binding sites have been found near the genes encoding podocin and Cd2-AP, two proteins associated with the slit-diaphragm.[63,64] Lmx1b also is apparently involved in regulating expression of components of the mature glomerular basement membrane, including the α_3 and α_4 subunits of type IV collagen.[69,70] Kreisler, a basic leucine zipper protein, is also required for later stages of podocyte differentiation, but less is known about potential targets.

The formation of the glomerular vasculature has also received attention through the study of mutant phenotypes. Mutation of either the platelet-derived growth factor B-subunit (PDGF-B) or the platelet-derived growth factor receptor β result in the failure to form proper glomerular capillaries, and instead the glomerulus resembles a single large glomerular

thrive is a common complication of childhood renal failure. Other manifestations include palpable abdominal masses due to obstructed kidneys, concentrating defects resulting in enuresis, electrolyte disorders, dehydration, hypertension, and urinary tract infections. In more than half of babies with kidney abnormalities, extrarenal manifestations are found and often characterize a syndrome.[1] In addition, specific chromosomal abnormalities may be found with multiple congenital anomalies that also involve the kidney and urinary tract (Table 5-1). Although this chapter will not review extrarenal manifestations in detail, in our discussion of specific syndromes and the accompanying table (Table 5-2) we have highlighted organ system anomalies that are frequently associated with kidney and urinary tract malformations. These phenotypic associations are a potential guide to clinical situations that may prompt screening for kidney and urinary tract disorders. In other instances, an index case leads to screening of family members, some of whom may be affected, albeit with lesser severity, as is commonly seen for VUR. Because there can be considerable variability in expressivity of phenotypes in genetic syndromes, including asymptomatic involvement, screening of family members can be an important means of case finding and may help identify individuals at risk for renal failure and hypertension.

In addition to figuring prominently in human congenital birth defects, the kidney has long been regarded as a premiere model system to study organogenesis and inductive signaling between epithelium and mesenchyme. Classic studies by Grobstein and Saxèn established metanephric organ culture as a critical tool to study nephrogenesis.[5a,6] Landmark observations by Edith Potter characterized the embryological findings in normal and abnormal kidney and urinary tracts in human pathological specimens.[7] Collectively, these pioneering studies have provided a framework for understanding the developmental mechanisms that cause congenital anomalies of the kidney and urinary tract. Several excellent reviews are available that summarize recent exciting findings in the field.[8–12] Below we will discuss the key developmental steps that may be disrupted in the syndromes described later in this chapter.

To understand the developmental mechanisms that lead to anomalies of the kidney and urinary tract we first provide a brief overview of nephrogenesis and highlight the developmental defects to be discussed (Fig. 5-1). The urogenital system is derived predominantly from the intermediate mesoderm of the early embryo (reviewed by Saxen[6]). The earliest morphological event in this process is epithelial transformation of the intermediate mesoderm to form the nephric (wolffian) duct, which extends rostrocaudally in the embryo adjacent to a tract of mesoderm, the nephrogenic cord. The nephric duct induces

Table 5-1 Chromosomal Abnormalities Associated with Renal Developmental Disorders

Syndrome	Renal Defects
Cat eye Partial tetrasomy 22	Agenesis/hypoplasia, hydronephrosis, supernumerary kidneys
DiGeorge 22q11.2 deletion	Agenesis, hypodysplasia, VUR*
Trisomy 18	VACTERL phenotype
Turner XO	Agenesis, cystic dysplasia, horseshoe kidney, malrotation, duplication
Williams 7q11.23 deletion	Agenesis, ectopia, VUR, renovascular hypertension

*These renal phenotypes are specifically attributed to a deletion in the GATA3 gene (see "HDR syndrome" section).
VUR, vesicoureteral reflux.

Table 5-2 Syndromes That Combine Extrarenal Defects with Kidney and Urinary Tract Abnormalities

Hearing Loss	Ocular	Skeletal/Limb	Heart	Genital Tract
Branchio-oto-renal	Alagille	Cornelia de Lange	Alagille	ATR-X
CHARGE	Branchio-oto-renal	Ectodermal dyplasia	Cat eye	CHARGE
Cockayne	Cat eye	Fraser	CHARGE	Fanconi anemia (males)
Cornelia de Lange	CHARGE	Hand-foot-genital/uterus	Cornelia de Lange	Fraser
Fraser	Cockayne	Okihiro/Acrorenal	DiGeorge	Hand-foot-genital/uterus
Hypoparathyroidism-deafness-renal	Fraser	Pallister Hall	Okihiro/Holt-Oram	Kallmann
Kallmann	Okihiro	Rubenstein Taybi	Simpson-Golabi-Behmel	Mayer-Rokitansky-Kuster-Hauser
Okihiro		Smith-Lemli-Opitz	Townes Brocks	MURCS
Renal coloboma		Townes Brocks	Turner	Roberts
Townes Brocks		VATER/VACTERL; Fanconi anemia	VATER/VACTERL	Smith-Lemli-Opitz
			Williams	Townes Brocks
				Turner

MURCS, müllerian duct aplasia, unilateral renal agenesis, and cervicothoracic somite anomalies.

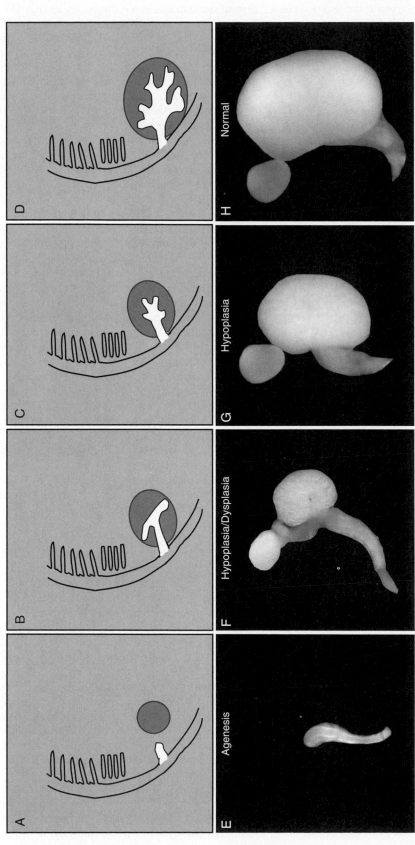

Figure 5-1 Overview of normal kidney development and mechanisms of common nephric defects. **(A–D)** Initial outgrowth of the ureteric bud (white) from the nephric duct is followed by invasion of the metanephric mesenchyme (gray). The initial five or six branches of the ureter form the renal pelvis and calyces. Reiterative branching morphogenesis of the ureter leads to induction of nephrons. **(E–H)** Allelic series of *Sall1* mutants demonstrates the spectrum of renal agenesis and hypoplasia seen in human birth defects. These birth defects occur at an incidence of 1/550 and 1/4,000 live births for unilateral and bilateral renal agenesis, respectively, and 1/750 for hypoplasia/dysplasia. **(E)** In *Sall1-ΔZn²⁻¹⁰* homozygous mutants, the ureter grows out but fails to initiate branching, resulting in renal agenesis. **(F)** Renal hypoplasia in *Sall1-*null homozygous mutants with cystic dysplasia demonstrated by histology[27] where kidneys arrest after initial invasion of the mesenchyme. **(G)** Renal hypoplasia in *Sall1-ΔZn²⁻¹⁰* heterozygotes due to reduced branching morphogenesis (S.K. and M.R., unpublished observations). **(H)** Normal mouse kidney and adrenal at the same developmental stage as the mutants shown (E15).

the adjacent nephrogenic cord mesenchyme to aggregate and transform into epithelial tubules. During its caudal migration the nephric duct induces three embryonic kidneys in the nephrogenic cord: pronephros, mesonephros, and metanephros, in spatial and temporal sequence. Because of the importance of the mesonephros in reproductive tract development, especially in the male, genital duct anomalies may be associated with kidney and urinary tract malformations in some syndromes.

When the nephric duct reaches the level of the developing hind limb, it gives rise to a caudal diverticulum, the ureteric bud, which invades the surrounding metanephric mesenchyme (blastema) at embryonic day 11 (E11) in the mouse and week 4 in humans. Subsequently, the ureter invades the mesenchyme and undergoes branching morphogenesis. Reciprocal inductive interactions between the ureter and blastema lead to formation of all the nephrons that compose the metanephros, the definitive adult kidney. Ultimately, formation of the metanephric kidney therefore depends on initial transformation of intermediate mesoderm to form the nephric duct and its caudal extension to the cloaca where it gives rise to the ureteric bud. *Thus, if there is a defect in formation of the nephric duct, the ureteric bud will not grow out and invade the mesenchyme, resulting in renal agenesis.* For example, in *Pax2* homozygous mutants, the nephric duct does not extend to the cloaca and ultimately causes complete renal agenesis.[13,14] Even if the nephric duct elongates appropriately, an intrinsic defect in this tissue can prevent outgrowth of the ureter as seen in *Ret*[-/-] mice.[15,16]

Abnormalities in the nephric duct or its surrounding undifferentiated mesenchyme may result in ectopic budding of the ureter. This defect could also result in renal hypodysplasia or agenesis, because contact with the mesenchyme is completely or partially impaired. Formation of more than one bud on the nephric duct can lead to *duplications* and *crossed ectopias*, as seen in several mouse mutants.[17–19] Moreover, it has been postulated that ectopic budding of the ureter may in some cases account for a broad range of developmental defects involving the kidney and urinary tract (CAKUT; see "Obstruction, Hydronephrosis, Hydroureter, and Vesicoureteral Reflux").

Defects in the metanephric mesenchyme can also lead to agenesis. The metanephric mesenchyme (blastema) is specified in the posterior intermediate mesoderm before induction by the ureteric bud. By E10.5 to E11.0 in the mouse, it appears as a morphologically discrete group of cells that can be distinguished by expression of unique molecular markers, such as *Pax2*, *Wt1*, and *Eya1*.[6,13,14,20,21] Specification and competency of the mesenchyme is established independent of contact with the ureteric bud.[13] In mice with conditional inactivation of both *Fgfr1* and *Fgfr2* in the mesenchyme, there is no morphologically discrete blastema formed and renal agenesis is observed.[22] Although a distinct metanephric mesenchyme can be observed morphologically in *Wt1*[-/-] mutants, it is not competent to respond to inductive signals, suggesting an intrinsic or autonomous defect.[23] *Thus, if metanephric mesenchyme does not form or is not fully competent to respond to inducer, the ureter cannot induce the blastema, and expected outcomes would be renal agenesis or hypodysplasia.*

Signals from the metanephric mesenchyme are required for outgrowth of the ureteric bud. For example, glial cell line–derived neurotrophic factor (GDNF) is secreted by the metanephric mesenchyme and signals to the ureteric bud via its receptors, RET and GFRα1. Absence of this critical mesenchymal signal results in renal agenesis, because the ureteric bud does not grow out, even though there is no intrinsic defect in the nephric duct.[24,25] *Thus, the absence of mesenchymal signals to the nephric duct that regulate outgrowth of the ureter can lead to renal agenesis.* Recent studies also suggest that distinct molecular events control proper invasion and initial branching of the ureter within the metanephric mesenchyme subsequent to its initial outgrowth from the nephric duct. These events may be cell autonomous in the ureter[26] or depend on signals from the mesenchyme.[27] An example of the latter is the *Sall1* mutant where there is outgrowth of the ureter from the nephric duct, but nephrogenesis arrests early because invasion and initial branching fails (S.K. and M.R., unpublished observations). *Thus, disruption of steps that control invasion of the mesenchyme subsequent to the initial outgrowth of the ureter can also lead to agenesis and hypodysplasia.*

After invasion and initial branching of the ureter within the metanephric blastema, a series of branching events occurs. The developmental and molecular genetic controls of this process are well described in recent reviews.[10,28] Ureteric tips generated by subsequent branching events each induce a cap of mesenchyme to undergo mesenchymal-to-epithelial transformation and differentiation into nephrons. This iterative branching of the ureteric bud occurs for about 15 generations and leads to formation of 300,000 to 1,000,000 nephrons in humans.[29] Thus, there is a direct quantitative relationship between branching of the ureter and nephron number. *Impaired branching morphogenesis is an important mechanism leading to renal hypoplasia, especially in cases of pure hypoplasia (oligomeganephronia or OMN) without dysplasia.* Both defects intrinsic to the ureter and altered signaling from mesenchyme to the branching ureter have been implicated.[15,16,24,25,30,31] Pure renal hypoplasia does occur and, if severe, is termed OMN, a condition that typically leads to secondary focal glomerulosclerosis and renal failure. More commonly, renal hypoplasia is usually associated with some degree of dysplasia both in humans and mouse models, implicating a defect in differentiation of the mesenchyme alone or in combination with a reduction in branching.

Maturation of the ureter is less well understood, although some recent studies have reinvigorated this field.[32,33] Clinically, these disorders are common and are increasingly recognized by finding congenital hydronephrosis during obstetrical ultrasound. In utero obstruction at any level in the urinary tract can significantly impair normal growth and differentiation of the kidney.[34–36] Both anatomical lesions causing mechanical obstruction to urine flow and functional obstruction due to impaired peristalsis can result in severely hypodysplastic kidneys, atrophic kidneys, or enlarged multicystic dysplastic kidneys (MCDK) with minimal or no function. In some cases these kidneys may involute and present as "renal agenesis."[37] *Thus, severe obstruction to urine flow in the fetus is a cause of hypodysplasia and may lead secondarily to atrophy of the kidney.* PUJO and VUR are among the most common defects affecting the urinary tract, and recent studies have advanced our understanding of these disorders (Fig. 5-2). The portion of the elongating ureteric bud that does not invade the metanephric mesenchyme forms the ureter, the muscular conduit that moves urine from the kidney to the bladder. At the distal end, the ureter is initially connected to the urogenital sinus

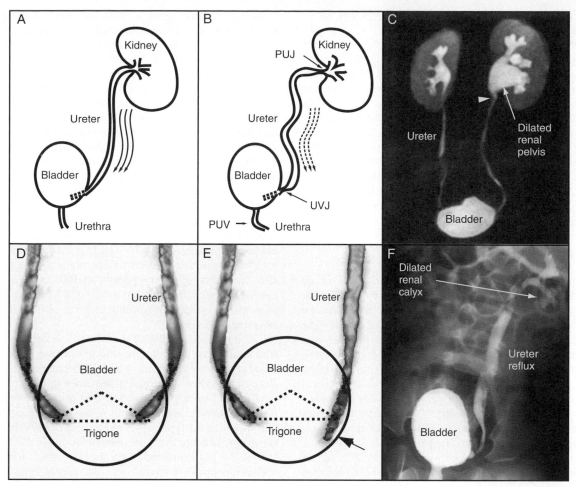

Figure 5-2 Developmental defects of ureter maturation. **A,** Normal urine flow from the kidney requires an intact junction between ureter and pelvis, patent ureter with normal peristalsis, proper insertion of the distal ureters into the bladder, functional bladder, and patent urethra. **B,** Congenital obstruction of the urinary tract occurs most commonly at the pelviureteral junction (PUJ; 1/1500 live births) due to extrinsic compression or abnormal formation of smooth muscle. Ureteral strictures, aperistaltic segments of the ureter near the ureterovesical junction (UVJ), and posterior urethral valves (PUV) in male infants (1/6,500 live births) also cause obstructive uropathy. **C,** Contrast-enhanced computed tomography scan of 5-year-old boy with recurrent abdominal pain showing notching of proximal left ureter (*arrowhead*) and hydronephrosis. **D,** Proper insertion of the ureters into the trigone of the bladder demonstrated by *HoxB7-GFP* transgenic mice. **(E)** Unilateral short intravesical insertion (*arrow*) of the right ureter leading to unilateral vesicoureteral reflux in these mice. **(F)** Voiding cystourethrography demonstrating grade III reflux in an 11-month-old boy (**C,** From McDaniel BB, Jones RA, Scherz H, et al: Dynamic contrast-enhanced MR urography in the evaluation of pediatric hydronephrosis: Part 2, anatomic and functional assessment of uteropelvic junction obstruction. Am J Roentgenol 185:1608, 2005. **D,** Adapted from Murawski IJ, Gupta IR: Vesicoureteric reflux and renal malformations: A developmental problem. Clin Genet 69:105, 2006. **F,** From Lee SK, Chang Y, Park NH, et al: Magnetic resonance voiding cystography in the diagnosis of vesicoureteral reflux: Comparative study with voiding cystourethrography J Magn Reson Imaging 21:406, 2005.)

(future bladder) via the common nephric duct. However, this connection is severed during normal development, and the ureter becomes directly connected to the bladder. *Improper insertion of the distal ureter into the bladder can lead to obstruction at the uterovesical junction and VUR.*

At the proximal end, the pelviureteral junction connects the ureter to the kidney. Corticomedullary patterning occurs relatively late in development and involves remodeling of the initial five or six branches of the ureter to form the renal calyces and pelvis. Conduction of urine down the ureter is initiated by contraction of the renal pelvis. Normal peristalsis of urine depends on proper differentiation of the smooth muscle in the pelvis, where the pacemaker cells are located,

and in the ureter. *Thus, disruption of smooth muscle formation is an important mechanism of functional obstruction of the urinary tract.*

Numerous studies have established a mechanistic framework for understanding developmental defects of the kidney and urinary tract. In the sections that follow, we have not attempted to duplicate an exhaustive overview of the more than 100 syndromes that may involve kidney and urinary tract anomalies.[38] Rather, we discuss specific human syndromes with a goal of highlighting emerging concepts that provide a molecular genetic basis for these congenital disorders and provide new insights into the pathogenesis of their clinical manifestations.

TRANSCRIPTIONAL REGULATORS THAT CAUSE KIDNEY DEFECTS

Proper development of any organ, including the kidney, requires sequentially regulated gene expression. This exquisite regulation is largely carried out by transcription factors that bind unique sequences in promoter regions of target genes and activate or repress transcription through multiprotein co-regulatory complexes (Fig. 5-3). Mutations in a single transcription factor can affect the proper expression of many target genes in different tissues and often lead to multiorgan congenital anomaly syndromes. These are discussed below (Table 5-3). In the next section we expand this list to include those genes that act cooperatively with transcription factors by modifying chromatin structure.

Renal Coloboma Syndrome

Renal coloboma syndrome (RCS; OMIM 120330) is an autosomal dominant syndrome characterized by optic nerve coloboma, renal hypoplasia, and VUR that is caused by mutations in the transcription factor *PAX2*. PAX2 and its eight other family members have been defined by the presence of a highly conserved 128–amino acid paired-box domain in the N-terminal portion of the protein. This domain binds to DNA to allow PAX2 to regulate gene expression of downstream genes during organogenesis. *Pax* genes are highly conserved and are associated with multiple congenital anomalies including Waardenbug syndrome (*PAX3*), aniridia (*PAX6*), and congenital hypothyroidism (*PAX8*).[39]

Deletion of one functional copy of *PAX2* in RCS causes widely varying renal phenotypes ranging from slightly affected to unilateral renal agenesis. RCS patients are identified for *PAX2* mutational analysis by their optic nerve colobomas, proteinuria, and renal insufficiency, and often also have small kidneys (68%), VUR (26%), and high-frequency hearing loss (16%). *PAX2* mutations have also been found in persons with OMN or bilateral renal hypoplasia with no dysplasia (Fig. 5-4), no lower urinary tract anomalies, and no eye malformations.[40] These individuals show a striking reduction in the number of nephrons and compensatory hypertrophy of glomeruli but otherwise have normal kidneys. All affected OMN children develop progressive renal failure leading to end-stage renal disease before mid-adolescence.[41]

Also affecting renal function in individuals with RCS is VUR. PAX2 is expressed throughout the ureter; therefore, a mutation in *PAX2* could also cause malformations at the junction of the bladder and ureter. VUR has been documented in some individuals with RCS[39] and would contribute to renal insufficiency in these patients. Obstruction of the ureter may also occur during embryogenesis in RCS, because a recent patient has been documented with MCDK, which is thought to often arise from congenital ureteral obstruction during early nephrogenesis.[42]

The importance of PAX2 in kidney development has been well established using mouse models. Three mouse models have been described including a large chromosomal deletion of *Pax2* and 7 cM of surrounding sequence in the Krd mouse[43]; *Pax2^{1Neu}*, a 1–base pair insertion that mimics a documented RCS mutation[44]; and *Pax2*-null, a targeted deletion.[14] Deletion of both wild-type copies of *Pax2* results in renal agenesis caused by failure to form the ureteric bud.[14] In the developing kidney, Pax2 is expressed in the wolffian duct, ureteric bud, and metanephric mesenchyme.[45] The loss of Pax2 expression

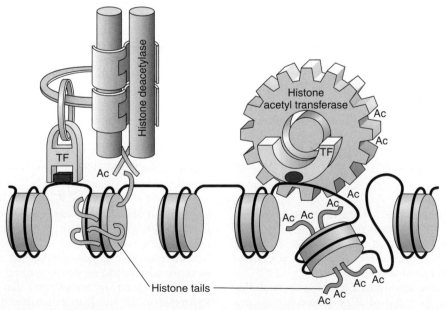

Figure 5-3 Transcriptional regulation and chromatin remodeling. DNA (*black lines*) associates with histones and other proteins to form nucleosomes (*light blue cylinders*). Different modifications of histone tails such as lysine acetylation (*blue*) or deacetylation (*gray*) turns transcription on or off. Mutations in classical sequence-specific transcription factors (TF) are common causes of congenital anomaly syndromes involving the kidney. Regulation of gene expression is mediated by multiprotein coactivator (*gray*) and co-repressor (*blue*) complexes that are recruited by the TF and modify chromatin structure. Recent studies have shown that components of these chromatin-remodeling complexes are also mutated in developmental defects of the kidney and urinary tract.

Table 5-3 Mutations in Transcription Factors Associated with Kidney and Urinary Tract Defects

Syndrome	Inheritance	Gene	Characteristic Features	Renal Phenotypes	Mechanism of Action
Alagille	Autosomal dominant	JAG1	Liver disease, cardiac defects, facial deformity	Agenesis, hypoplasia, cystic dysplasia, PUJO, VUR	Haploinsufficiency
Branchio-oto-renal	Autosomal dominant	EYA-1, SIX-1	Branchial fistula, hearing loss, renal abnormalities	Hypoplasia, VUR	Haploinsufficiency
Hypoparathyroidism-deafness-renal	Autosomal dominant	GATA3	Hypoparathyroidism, hearing loss, renal abnormalities	Agenesis, hypodysplasia, VUR	Haploinsufficiency
Maturity-onset diabetes of the young type V	Autosomal dominant	HNF1β	Early type II diabetes, renal abnormalities	Cystic dysplasia, hypoplasia, glomerulocystic, OMN, agenesis	Haploinsufficiency and gain of function
Okihiro	Autosomal dominant	SALL4	Radial limb defects, Duane eye anomaly	Pelvic or horseshoe kidney, hypoplasia, VUR	Haploinsufficiency
Pallister-Hall	Autosomal dominant	GLI3	Polydactyly, imperforate anus, hypothalamic hamartoma	Agenesis, hydronephrosis, hydroureter, renal ectopia, horseshoe kidney	Dominant truncated protein
Renal coloboma	Autosomal dominant	PAX2	Optic nerve coloboma, renal abnormalities	Hypoplasia, VUR, OMN	Haploinsufficiency
Townes Brocks	Autosomal dominant	SALL1	Hearing loss, triphalangeal thumb, imperforate anus	Agenesis, hypoplasia, posterior urethral valves, VUR, meatal stenosis	Dominant truncated protein and haploinsufficiency

OMN, oligomeganephronia; PUJO, pelviureteral junction obstruction; VUR, vesicoureteral reflux.

causes the wolffian duct to degenerate at E10.5 when the ureteric bud should begin to form.[14] Other tissues derived from the wolffian duct, oviducts, uterus, vagina, epididymis, vas deferens, and seminal vesicles are also not formed, suggesting that *Pax2* is required for proper development of the distal wolffian duct.

The two *Pax* genes, *Pax2* and *Pax8*, have been termed the "master regulators" of nephric development of all three embryonic kidneys—pronephros, mesonephros, and metanephros—which fail to form when both genes are removed.[46] Deletion of *Pax8* alone has no kidney phenotype[47]; therefore, it appears that *Pax2* can completely compensate for the loss of *Pax8* in the kidney. *Pax2* is not required for formation of the proximal nephric duct, but, as discussed above, the definitive metanephric kidney and other distal wolffian duct structures are not formed.[14,44] The uninduced metanephric mesenchyme is present as a discrete cluster of cells in *Pax2*-null embryos, suggesting that *Pax2* plays a role in this tissue after induction by the ureteric bud but is not required for specification of the metanephric mesenchyme.[14] Confirming its role as a master regulator of kidney development, *Pax2* is able to induce nephric (wolffian) duct and mesenchymal condensate structures when ectopically expressed in chick embryo mesoderm.[46] The specification of the nephric lineage by *Pax2*

and *Pax8* underscores the fundamental role of *Pax* genes in determination of a variety of cell lineages including B lymphocytes (*Pax5*), insulin-producing β cells, and somotostatin-expressing δ cells in the pancreas (*Pax4*), and glucagon-synthesizing α cells (*Pax6*) (for review, see Bouchard et al[48]).

Renal hypoplasia found in individuals with RCS and OMN points to a role for *PAX2* in determining nephron number by controlling the extent of arborization of the ureteric bud during development.[49] Most of the documented *PAX2* mutations occur within the paired-box domain, and all are predicted to result in loss of functional PAX2 protein from the mutant allele. One wild-type allele and one mutant allele would therefore produce less than the normal amount of functional PAX2 protein in persons with RCS. This type of dosage sensitivity is termed haploinsufficiency. Haploinsufficiency of *Pax2* causes ureteric bud branches to undergo apoptosis. This results in a 30% to 40% reduction in early nephrogenic epithelial structures in *Pax2*[1Neu] mice.[50] This reduction can be partially rescued by the apoptosis inhibitor V-VAD-fmk, which itself is capable of promoting increased branching in normal kidneys.[51] Reduced nephron number correlates with increased risk of hypertension and susceptibility to renal disease in humans.[5] Severe renal hypoplasia observed in RCS accounts for the high incidence of renal failure in many of these patients.[39]

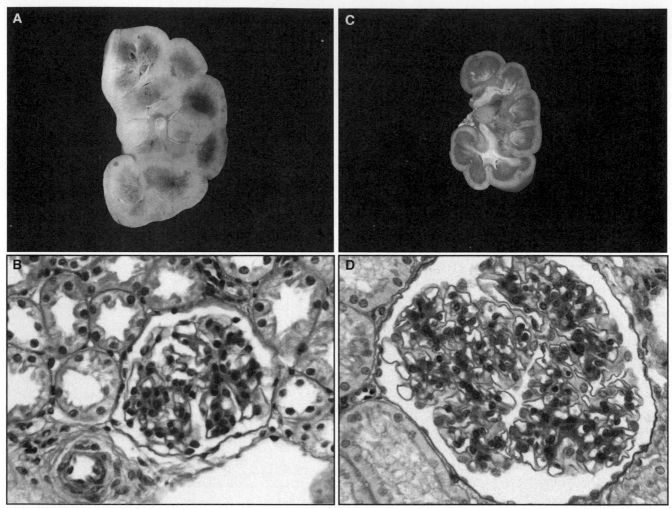

Figure 5-4 Oligomeganephronia. *PAX2* and *HNF1β* mutations can cause a severe reduction in the number of nephrons, but those that form are normal. (**A, B**) Normal gross appearance and renal histology (×25) from an 18-month-old baby. (**C, D**) Gross appearance and renal histopathology from a 2-year-old child with a severely hypoplastic kidney. Histopathology (×25) demonstrated markedly enlarged glomeruli without evidence of dysplasia consistent with oligomeganephronia. (Courtesy of M.C. Gubler, Hospital Necker—Enfants Malades, Universite Rene Descartes, Paris.)

Hypoparathyroidism, Deafness, and Renal Anomaly Syndrome

The syndrome of hypoparathyroidism, deafness, and renal anomaly (HDR; OMIM 146255), also known as Barakat syndrome, was first described in 1977 in two brothers with progressive renal failure, sensorineural deafness, and hypoparathyroidism.[52] These autosomal dominant congenital abnormalities are caused by mutations in the transcription factor GATA3, a potential downstream target of *PAX2-PAX8* in the kidney.[53] These individuals exhibit deafness and hypoparathyroidism, although hypocalcemia is not always symptomatic. Clinical characterization of patients with HDR demonstrates that kidney and urinary tract anomalies also occur in a high (60% to 80%) percentage of cases and that the phenotypic spectrum is quite large. Renal hypodysplasia and agenesis may occur in about one-third of cases,[54] and severe bilateral hypodysplasia with Potter's sequence has been documented in one patient.[55] Deformities of the pelvicalyceal system and VUR also occur. End-stage renal failure has been reported at a frequency of as many as 25% to 30% in two small series, but some of these cases involved patients beyond 60 years of age, raising the possibility that other co-morbid factors independent of HDR may have contributed to renal failure. Nonetheless, clinically significant kidney involvement is clearly a prominent feature of HDR and an important cause of morbidity.

Detailed studies of patients with a syndrome with overlapping phenotype, DiGeorge syndrome, led to the discovery that *GATA3* haploinsufficiency was responsible for HDR.[56] Analysis of DiGeorge patients carrying deletions of two non-overlapping regions on chromosome 10p determined that terminal deletions are associated with HDR, whereas more proximal deletions cause heart malformations and T cell–mediated immune deficiency. Some families with HDR do not have cytogenetic abnormalities involving 10p or detectable *GATA3* mutations, suggesting that this syndrome may be genetically heterogeneous.[54,56] *GATA3* is found on chromosome 10p and belongs to a family of six zinc-finger transcription factors that play critical roles in embryonic development of multiple organs. The family is defined by the presence of two highly conserved C2-C2 zinc-finger domains, with the C-terminal finger mediating DNA binding and the N-terminal finger functioning to stabilize DNA binding and to interact with other proteins such as the "friends of GATA" (FOG) group.[57,58] FOG acts as a co-activator or co-repressor of GATA factors in different developmental contexts.

Deletions of *GATA3* produce typical HDR that is indistinguishable from cases with missense and nonsense mutations. No functional GATA3 transcription factor would be produced by missense mutations that disrupt DNA binding or truncating mutations that are predicted to be degraded by nonsense-mediated decay. Alternatively, truncated proteins could be expressed from some of these mutant alleles, as described for GATA1-associated leukemia in Down syndrome,[59] thereby causing dominant negative or gain-of-function effects. Most truncated proteins would have no ability to bind DNA; however, in a subset of these mutations DNA binding is not affected, but interaction with its co-factor FOG2 (approved gene symbol *ZFPM2*) is impaired.[60] As observed with other syndromes characterized by haploinsufficiency, there is variable expression of the phenotype even within the same family members with identical mutations,[54] and no genotype-phenotype correlation exists.[54,60]

During kidney development, *GATA3* is expressed in the nephric (wolffian) duct and in the ureteric bud at the stage of its initial outgrowth from the nephric duct, but not in the metanephric mesenchyme. This expression pattern in mice and humans is consistent with the range of phenotypes involving the kidney and ureter.[61] The nephric duct does not extend fully to the level of the cloaca in *Gata3⁻/⁻* mice, resulting in no ureteric bud outgrowth,[53] and this mechanism could account for renal agenesis observed in some HDR patients. However, these individuals may also exhibit hypodysplasia, suggesting that GATA3 is also important later in kidney development. Consistent with this idea, *Gata3* expression is detected in the branching ureter that gives rise to the collecting duct and in the extrarenal portion of the ureter.[62,63] Severe renal hypoplasia is observed in *Gata3⁻/⁻* mice that survive past E11.[64] A more complete understanding of the potential role of *Gata3* in branching morphogenesis awaits further studies with conditional gene inactivation.

Branchio-Oto-Renal Syndrome

Branchio-oto-renal syndrome (BOR; OMIM 113650) is an autosomal dominant disorder that results in defective formation of the kidney (agenesis, dysplasia, or hypoplasia) and collecting system abnormalities. These defects are observed with incomplete penetrance and variable expressivity and are associated with other developmental abnormalities such as branchial fistula, hearing loss, and ear deformities. In the *Drosophila* eye, *Pax* is in a genetic pathway with two other transcriptional regulators, eyes absent and sine oculus (for review see Donner and Maas[65]), and orthologues of these genes, *Eya* and *Six*, have been implicated in BOR. Three different loci have been identified, including *EYA1* (BOS1, OMIM 602588), *SIX1* (BOS3, OMIM 608389), and a locus on chromosome 1 that has not yet been identified (BOS2, OMIM 120502). The Eya and Six family members are transcription factors that act in concert to regulate transcription. Eya proteins contain a potent transactivation domain but are not capable of binding to target genes alone. Their binding partners, Six proteins, provide sequence-specific DNA binding by virtue of a Six domain and homeodomain. Eya1 also requires binding to a Six family member to translocate from the cytoplasm to the nucleus where the complex could activate downstream genes.[66]

The mutations that cause BOR in humans are found throughout the 16 exons of the *EYA1* gene and are thought to result in no EYA protein produced from the mutant allele.[67] Like *PAX2* and RCS, haploinsufficiency of *EYA1* causes the developmental defects of the syndrome. Some of the *EYA1* mutations that cause BOR are missense mutations and could produce a mutant protein; however, these mutant EYA proteins have been shown to be compromised in transactivation ability,[68] in binding to Six proteins,[69] or in the catalytic protein phosphatase activity,[68] and could serve as loss-of-function alleles. The only documented *SIX1* mutations causing BOR are missense mutations in the six domain (R110W) or homeodomain (Y129C, delE133). These mutations could also serve as loss-of-function alleles, in that they have been shown to render the protein incapable of properly activating transcription when coexpressed with Eya1.[70] This loss of function could be due to the inability of mutant Six1 to bind Eya1 or to bind Six-specific consensus sites in DNA.

Both *Eya1* and *Six1* are expressed in metanephric mesenchyme and play critical roles in kidney development, because mice that are homozygous null for either *Eya1* or *Six1* do not develop kidneys.[71–73] Loss of either *Eya1* or *Six1* renders the metanephric mesenchyme incapable of signaling properly to the ureteric bud to initiate outgrowth, invasion, and branching. In contrast to *Pax2* mutants, the metanephric mesenchyme does not form in *Eya1* mutants.[21] In *Six1* mutants, the metanephric mesenchyme forms and the ureter grows out, but it fails to branch within the mesenchyme.[73] The lack of inductive signal by the invading ureter causes both mutant mesenchymes to undergo apoptosis by E12.5, when formation of a definitive kidney should be evident. Because kidney development is arrested at a slightly earlier stage in the *Eya1* mutant and these mutants abolish *Six1* expression, but *Six1* mutants retain proper *Eya1* expression, *Eya1* may play a role upstream of *Six1* in the kidney.[73]

The roles of *Eya1* and *Six1* also synergize in the metanephric mesenchyme, because *Eya1⁺/⁻Six1⁺/⁻* double heterozygotes show a significantly higher percentage of agenesis and hypoplasia as compared with either mutation alone.[71,73] The hypoplasia is first detectable at E13.5 when the number of ureteric bud branches is reduced, and is more apparent later in development at E17.5 when a decrease in the number of epithelial tubular structures is apparent in the peripheral nephrogenic zone, where new nephrons form.[73] The observation that these phenotypes are more evident in the double heterozygotes than in animals heterozygous for either Six1 or *Eya1* suggests that these proteins act synergistically to determine nephron number. As has been shown in *Drosophila*, they could achieve this by acting in a complex to modulate Six-responsive genes.[74] Both Eya and Six have been detected by chromatin immunoprecipitation on the promoters of the oncogene *c-Myc* and the growth factor gene *GDNF*.[71] Activation of these genes by this complex could both stimulate proliferation of the metanephric mesenchyme and signal the ureteric bud to branch, two processes that could profoundly affect nephron number. Interestingly, the catalytic phosphatase activity of Eya seems to be critical for its ability to activate transcription and stimulate proliferation, suggesting that phosphorylation controls the activity of this transcriptional complex.[74a]

Townes Brocks Syndrome

Another gene that may control similar steps in mesenchymal growth and signaling is mutated in a syndrome that has considerable phenotypic overlap with BOR, Townes Brocks syndrome (TBS; OMIM 107480). This autosomal dominant congenital disorder results in hearing loss, ear deformities, imperforate anus, triphalangeal thumb, and renal abnormalities. These birth defects are caused by mutations in the SALL1 gene,[75] which may act downstream of Eya1 and Six1 in development of nephrogenic mesenchyme.[73] Carrying one copy of a mutated SALL1 gene leads to renal abnormalities in 60% of individuals with TBS, including renal hypoplasia, unilateral renal agenesis, posterior urethral valves, VUR, and meatal stenosis.[76] Similar to RCS patients, the most common renal abnormality observed in persons with TBS is renal hypoplasia often necessitating renal replacement therapy.[77] The observation that these patients also exhibit lower urinary tract abnormalities suggests that mutant SALL1 expression in the wolffian duct and the urogenital sinus may cause these tissues to develop improperly.

Like Pax, Eya, and Six proteins, Sall proteins are highly conserved from flies to humans and control organogenesis of multiple organs. The SALL1 gene encodes for a transcription factor that contains zinc-finger domains arranged in doublets that are thought to bind DNA via a highly conserved sequence in the second member of each doublet. Binding to the promoter regions of SALL1-responsive genes could repress transcription of these genes via an N-terminal repression domain that recruits a histone-deacetylase repression complex.[78,79] Most of the mutations that cause TBS are clustered around the first double zinc-finger domain. All encode truncating or frameshift mutations that, like RCS and BOR, were thought to produce no functional protein from the mutant allele. However, recent evidence contradicts this hypothesis by showing that a mouse that mimics a mutation found in TBS produces a truncated protein that could act in a dominant negative or gain-of-function fashion.[80] A Sall1-null allele exhibits an exclusively renal phenotype,[27] whereas this mouse model, Sall1-ΔZn, recapitulates all of the characteristic phenotypes of TBS including hearing loss, imperforate anus, limb defects, and kidney abnormalities. Some of these defects, including high-frequency hearing loss and hypoplastic cystic kidneys, are observed in mice carrying one copy of the Sall1-ΔZn allele. This bears a striking similarity to these same abnormalities observed in humans with a single dominant mutant allele of SALL1 and underscores the likelihood that TBS is due to dominant effects of a truncated SALL1 protein. Milder TBS phenotypes have recently been reported in three patients with heterozygous deletions of the SALL1 gene,[81] suggesting that both haploinsufficiency and dominant truncated protein expression are important in the pathogenesis of TBS.

We are just beginning to understand how SALL1 functions normally and how it causes TBS abnormalities. It clearly plays an important role in kidney development, because homozygous Sall1-null and Sall1-ΔZn mice lack kidneys. Like Pax2, it is expressed in both the wolffian duct and the metanephric mesenchyme; however, it is the lack of Sall1 in the mesenchyme that is thought to disrupt kidney development. The ureteric bud grows out from a Sall1-deficient wolffian duct but fails to properly invade the metanephric mesenchyme.[27] Metanephric mesenchyme is formed, but it is smaller and fails to be properly induced by the ureteric bud. As a consequence, kidneys are absent bilaterally (44.4%) or unilaterally (38.9%). The kidneys that do form are extremely small and show disorganized cortical structure, shrunken glomeruli, necrotic proximal tubules, and multiple cysts. This phenotype is more severe in Sall1-ΔZn homozygous mice, where the ureter grows out but does not initiate branching, resulting in complete bilateral renal agenesis.[80] Furthermore, similar to TBS patients, mice carrying one copy of the Sall1-ΔZn allele exhibit renal hypoplasia and cysts. These more severe phenotypes may be due to dominant negative interference of all Sall family members, because truncated Sall1 can bind to the other Sall family members and thereby alter function from these transcription factors and their downstream targets. Further analysis of this model should suggest the precise molecular mechanism by which the truncated protein exerts its deleterious effects on kidney, ear, limb, and anal development.

Okihiro Syndrome

Mutations in a different SALL family member, SALL4, cause a syndrome that is similar to TBS.[82,83] Okihiro or Duane-Radial Ray syndrome (OMIM 607323) is an autosomal dominant disorder characterized by radial limb anomalies and Duane anomaly, an eye movement disorder involving limitation of abduction. Kidney malformations including pelvic kidney, horseshoe kidney, hypoplasia, and VUR are often reported, particularly in a cohort of patients who were previously diagnosed as having "acro-renal-ocular" syndrome.[84,85] Similar to TBS, these individuals also commonly exhibit ear defects including deafness, and heart anomalies, including ventricular septal defect, are more often observed in individuals with Okihiro syndrome.

Identification of SALL4 as the gene mutated in Okihiro syndrome has clarified some clinical overlap in the diagnosis of individuals with Holt-Oram syndrome (OMIM 142900). This syndrome is caused by mutations in the gene for the transcription factor TBX5 and exhibits strikingly similar defects to Okihiro syndrome including limb defects and heart malformations. These patients do not exhibit Duane's anomaly and are therefore diagnosed with Holt-Oram; however, approximately 60% of these individuals do not have TBX5 mutations.[86] A subset of these clinically diagnosed patients has been found to have mutations in SALL4 and have been reclassified by genetic analysis as having Okihiro syndrome. Recently a molecular basis for this clinical overlap has been identified by Koshiba-Takeuchi et al,[87] who found that Sall4 and Tbx5 interact physically and genetically to affect development of the heart and limb. The cooperative association between Sall4 and Tbx5 during limb and heart morphogenesis gives a clear rationale for the phenotypic overlap of these two syndromes and suggests that other Holt-Oram loci may be identified in the TBX-SALL genetic pathway.

The mutations that cause Okihiro syndrome are found throughout the SALL4 gene.[88] Most are nonsense or frameshift mutations that could encode for a mutant protein as is hypothesized for TBS. However, patients with Okihiro syndrome have been described who carry chromosomal deletions of the *SALL4* gene, suggesting that this syndrome is caused by haploinsufficiency. One missense mutation has been described in a family that exhibits atypical symptoms including midline defects such as pituitary hypoplasia and a single central incisor.[89] This mutation is located within a conserved C-terminal zinc finger and would be expected to alter DNA binding. A second family carrying a nonsense mutation that would produce a protein lacking this same zinc-finger motif displays more typical Okihiro phenotypes with milder limb abnormalities, suggesting that there may be both gain-of-function and loss-of-function mutations for this syndrome.[90]

The *Sall4* mouse models support a loss of function mechanism. Mice heterozygous for a *Sall4* truncating allele[87] or a *Sall4-null* allele[90a] recapitulate most features of Okihiro syndrome including digit abnormalities and heart defects, but not renal defects. Renal hypoplasia and agenesis were reported in 40% of *Sall1/Sall4* double heterozygous mice indicating a functional redundancy of these genes in kidney development.[90a] However, a recent report describes similar kidney defects in a different *Sall4+/−* mutant allele demonstrating that kidney development can be perturbed by Sall4 haploinsufficiency.[90b] This discrepancy between the two reported *Sall4-null* alleles is likely attributable to genetic background effects.

Pallister-Hall Syndrome

Mutations in another transcription factor, *GLI3*, which is a key mediator of sonic hedgehog (Shh) signaling, cause the autosomal dominant syndrome Pallister-Hall (PHS; OMIM 146510).[91] This disorder is characterized by postaxial or insertional polydactyly, imperforate anus, hypothalamic hamartoma, and a variety of renal abnormalities.[92] Unilateral or bilateral renal agenesis, dysplasia, hydronephrosis, hydroureter, renal ectopia, and horseshoe kidney have all been described.[93,94] Mutations in *GLI3* are associated with PHS and four other autosomal dominant syndromes, including Greig cephalopolysyndactyly syndrome (OMIM 175700) and three types of isolated polydactyly; however, none of these other syndromes include kidney or urinary tract malformations. This apparent discrepancy was resolved by the realization that mutations in *GLI3* that cause PHS would produce truncated proteins that terminate just after the DNA binding domain that could act as constitutive transcriptional repressors.[92] Therefore, like TBS, PHS is due to dominant effects of a truncated protein. In contrast, loss-of-function mutations and gene deletions support the conclusion that Greig cephalopolysyndactyly syndrome is due to *GLI3* haploinsufficiency.

Both targeted and natural alleles of *Gli3* in mice demonstrate that C-terminally truncated GLI3 mutant proteins, but not null alleles, result in PHS phenotypes including renal malformations.[95] *GLI3* is an orthologue of *Drosophila* cubitus interruptus, a key transducer of the Shh signal within the cell (for review see Villavicencio et al[96]). In the presence of Shh, GLI3 activates downstream target genes, whereas in the absence of Shh, GLI3 is proteolytically cleaved and represses transcription of those same genes. Documented PHS mutations would produce truncated GLI3 protein that would act as a constitutive repressor (GLI3-R) and could downregulate GLI3-responsive genes regardless of the presence of a Shh signal. A PHS mouse model, *Gli3*[Δ699], has been produced that generates a truncated *Gli3* protein and exhibits PHS phenotypes including severe renal hypoplasia and agenesis.[95] In contrast, *Gli3*-null mice have normal kidneys. *Gli2/Gli3* double mutants exhibit horseshoe kidney, suggesting that other *GLI* genes can compensate for the loss of *GLI3* in the kidney in *GLI3* haploinsufficient syndromes.[97] Unfortunately, other than a report showing that *Gli1*, *Gli2*, and *Gli3* are expressed in developing kidney.[98] more detailed studies on the role of *Gli* genes in kidney development are lacking.

Several lines of evidence suggest that disruption of Shh signaling can account at least in part for the PHS phenotypes, including those involving the kidney. *Shh*[−/−] mutants exhibit renal agenesis with approximately 50% penetrance, whereas the remaining mutants showed hypodysplastic kidneys located ectopically in the pelvis.[99] Shh is expressed in the ureteric bud epithelium at E11.5 in the mouse, the time at which the ureteric bud invades and induces the metanephric mesenchyme.[100] This suggests that renal agenesis may result from impaired outgrowth of the ureteric bud or improper invasion of the mesenchyme. However, tissue-specific inactivation of Shh in the ureter does not cause renal agenesis.[100] Thus, the developmental mechanisms that lead to renal agenesis as a consequence of abnormal Shh/Gli signaling have not been fully elucidated.

Renal hypodysplasia in PHS may be the result of reduced branching morphogenesis or, alternatively, a secondary consequence of in utero obstruction. In support of the former hypothesis is the observation that inhibition of Shh signaling acting through its co-receptor smoothened (Smo) results in reduced branching in a GLI3-R–dependent manner.[99] These studies suggest that when *Shh-Smo* is inhibited, GLI3-R is formed and leads to transcriptional repression of downstream targets including *Gli1*, *Gli2*, *Pax2*, *Sall1*, *Myc*, and cyclin D1. As outlined earlier, loss of Pax2 and Sall1 also have profound effects on renal development. Reduced cell proliferation in both the mesenchyme and ureteric bud may account, in part, for hypodysplasia in these mutants. A role for the latter in utero obstruction mechanism is supported by studies in which *Shh* is conditionally inactivated in the ureter.[100] At E14.5 to newborn stage, *Shh* is localized to the distal collecting ducts in the developing inner medulla, renal pelvis and the epithelial layer of the ureter. Inactivation of *Shh* in the ureter resulted in hypoplastic kidneys with loss of the inner medulla, hydronephrosis, and hydroureter.[100] These defects were attributed to reduced proliferation of medullary and periureteral stroma. In addition, defective smooth muscle differentiation in the ureter probably accounts for the hydroureter, as proposed for congenital ureteral strictures in humans.[101,102] These two mechanisms are not mutually exclusive, and thus defective branching morphogenesis and functional ureteral obstruction could both contribute to the observed kidney phenotypes in PHS.

Alagille Syndrome

Alagille syndrome (AGS; OMIM 118450) is an autosomal dominant syndrome that is characterized by liver disease, cardiac defects, and characteristic facies including a prominent forehead and pointed chin. Involvement of one or more additional systems, such as kidney, anterior chamber of the eye, skeleton, vasculature, and pancreas is also common. It represents among the most common forms of genetic liver disease in children and often presents as neonatal jaundice. Cardiac defects are present in 95% or more of patients and typically involve the right side of the heart, ranging in severity from isolated pulmonic stenosis to tetralogy of Fallot. These heart defects and liver failure represent important causes of morbidity and mortality in AGS. In 1987, Alagille reviewed 80 cases of the syndrome that bears his name and noted that 73% of affected individuals had renal anomalies.[103] Subsequent case series involving over 200 patients has confirmed that clinically detectable renal involvement is present at a high (approx. 40% to 50%) frequency in AGS.[104–106] The lower frequency in the more recent series may reflect the inclusion of less severely affected cases that are mutation positive. Lack of detection of subclinical renal involvement is also possible. This has led to the suggestion that individuals with AGS should be screened routinely for renal and urinary tract involvement.[106]

There is an extremely broad spectrum of kidney anomalies associated with AGS, and both infantile and adult-onset renal failure can occur. The spectrum of renal hypoplasia/agenesis with or without cystic dysplasia (multicystic dysplastic kidneys) is well described.[107–109] Though less common, there are also reports of involvement of the ureter and lower urinary tract causing PUJO, VUR, and duplicated collecting system.[110] Renal tubular acidosis may be the most common functional kidney abnormality in these patients.[106] In addition, biopsy-proven glomerular involvement and tubulointerstitial nephritis have been reported.[111] Based on a relatively small number of cases in which biopsies were performed, it seems that mesangial lipidosis is the most common glomerular lesion,[106,112–114] although glomerular sclerosis without lipid deposits is also described. It is not clear if mesangial lipid deposits are secondary to hyperlipidemia in individuals with intrahepatic cholestasis or represent a defect intrinsic to the glomerulus. As discussed below, the gene mutated in AGS, JAG1, clearly has a role in glomerular development. Tubular dilatation was also frequently noted. Thus, the clinical presentation of renal involvement in AGS includes proteinuria, renal insufficiency, and hypertension. The presence of small, cystic, or solitary kidney on routine ultrasonography may also be the first clinical indication of urinary tract involvement. Multicystic dysplastic kidneys have also been detected by prenatal ultrasonography in AGS.[107] Although renal biopsy can be performed safely, AGS is associated with an increased risk of bleeding after invasive procedures, including renal biopsy.[104] There is a single report of successful renal transplantation in a patient with AGS who developed end-stage renal disease.[115] While hypertension can occur as a result of intrinsic renal disease, AGS is associated with vascular anomalies that may involve renal arteries. There are six reported cases of renal artery stenosis in AGS proven by angiography and successful treatment by stenting in one case.[116,117] Thus, evaluation for renovascular disease should be considered in patients with AGS who develop hypertension.

AGS results from mutations in JAG1, which encodes for a ligand of Notch.[118] As is often the case, identification of the genetic cause leads to expansion of the clinical spectrum. For example, there are now reports of isolated cardiac involvement in patients with JAG1 mutations. It has also been known for some time that children severely affected may have a parent with very subtle or even subclinical AGS phenotypes.[119] Individuals with deletions of 20p12 that encompass the entire JAG1 gene express the same phenotype as patients with JAG1 mutations, supporting haploinsufficiency as the mechanism of disease in the majority of patients. Recent studies suggest that mutant JAG1 messenger RNAs (mRNAs) may escape nonsense-mediated decay and potentially produce truncated proteins that would be predicted to have dominant negative effects based on studies in Drosophila and Caenorhabditis elegans.[120] More than 200 unique JAG1 mutations have been described, including small intragenic deletions, insertions, and point mutations, but there is no genotype-phenotype correlation that explains the highly variable expressivity of the phenotype.[121–123] All mutations map to the extracellular or intramembranous domain, and most result in premature stop codons. Thus, if a truncated protein were produced by these mutant alleles, membrane targeting would probably be defective. Similarly, a few missense mutations have been described that result in abnormal glycosylation patterns and defective intracellular trafficking.[124] Mutations in JAG1 account for 70% of AGS cases, suggesting genetic heterogeneity.[105] Other genes in the Notch pathway may be good candidates to account for these cases.

Notch is a highly evolutionarily conserved intercellular signaling pathway that functions in multiple developmental processes in the embryo. A role in regulating kidney or excretory organ formation has been shown in the fly malphigian tubule,[125] Xenopus,[126] and zebrafish pronephros,[127] in addition to mammals. It is thought to play a critical role in organ formation by determining cell fate through lateral inhibition and inductive signaling. Both mechanisms seem to operate in the control of kidney development.[128] Notch ligands are membrane-bound transcription factors that are released by two proteolytic events in response to binding by a ligand such as Jag1. The Notch intracellular domain enters the nucleus where it associates with a co-repressor complex, switching it into an activator of target genes (for review see Mumm and Kopan[129]).

Study of the role of this pathway in kidney development has been somewhat limited by the early embryonic lethality of a number of Notch pathway mouse mutants. Nonetheless, several studies have provided important information on the basis for the kidney phenotypes seen in AGS. Notch2^{del1}, a hypomorphic Notch2 mutant allele in the mouse, exhibits kidney defects involving the glomerulus and renal hypoplasia.[130] Jag1$^{-/-}$ mutants die before metanephric development, so they are not informative. Although AGS is a dominant syndrome attributed to haploinsufficiency, Jag1$^{+/-}$ mutants are normal. However, Jag1/Notch2^{del1} double-heterozygous mice exhibit phenotypes involving the biliary tract, heart, and kidney that resemble those seen in AGS.[131] Other Notch ligands do not genetically interact with Jag1, suggesting that Jag1 signals through Notch2 in the kidney.[131] This also raises the possibility that NOTCH2 is a genetic modifier of the AGS phenotype. Notch2 is expressed in the ureteric bud, whereas Jag1 is expressed in both the ureteric bud and condensing metanephric mesenchyme.[132] Impaired branching morphogenesis could account for the observation that in Notch2$^{del1-/-}$ mice the number of pretubular aggregates is reduced, but those that form appear normal. Consistent with this observation, inhibition of γ-secretase, the protease that performs the intramembranous cleavage to release the intracellular domain of Notch, results in reduced ureteric bud branching.[133]

Altered Ret-GDNF signaling has been noted when the Notch pathway is disrupted in developing kidney,[132] suggesting a plausible molecular mechanism for renal hypoplasia in AGS. However, it is not clear that the degree of impaired branching can account for hypoplasia. The data also suggest that increased apoptosis of nephrogenic progenitors in the periphery of the cortical zone and impaired segmental differentiation of tubular epithelial may contribute to a reduction in nephron number.[130,133,133a]

Notch2 is also expressed in glomerular endothelial cells, whereas Jag1 is detected in podocytes. The glomerular phenotype is thought to result because Jag1 mutant podocytes fail to attract and properly organize glomerular endothelial and mesangial cells, possibly as a result of reduced expression of Vegf and Pdgfrb.[130] There may also be a cell-autonomous requirement for Jag1 in developing podocytes. Pharmacological inhibition or genetic ablation of γ-secretase activity of presenilins also supports a critical role for the Notch pathway in development of glomeruli and proximal tubules.[133,134] Together, these studies in mouse models provide some insight into the molecular pathogenesis of renal hypoplasia, glomerular disease, and renal tubular acidosis in AGS.

Maturity-Onset Diabetes of the Young, Type V

Maturity-onset diabetes of the young (MODY) is a monogenic form of type 2 diabetes mellitus characterized by early age of onset, usually before 25 years of age, and autosomal dominant inheritance. One of the six MODY loci, MODY5 (OMIM 604284), also frequently causes a wide clinical spectrum of renal anomalies, including cystic dysplasia, hypoplasia, glomerulocystic disease, pelvicalyceal abnormalities, OMN, and unilateral agenesis. In the more than 50 reported cases of mutation-positive MODY5, renal involvement has been an almost universal feature, affecting approximately 90% of patients.[135] Thus, structural renal anomalies may be completely or near fully penetrant in this syndrome. Clinical manifestations of MODY5 include chronic renal failure often culminating in end-stage renal disease, proteinuria, renal cysts, small kidneys, transient neonatal renal failure with salt wasting, and pelvicalyceal dilatation without obstruction. Although clinical renal involvement may occur in childhood, it is often not detected before the second decade of life. Because both diabetes mellitus and chronic kidney failure are common in the general population, this syndrome may be overlooked in some individuals.

The diabetic and renal phenotypes characterized by MODY5 are due to mutations in the gene for the transcription factor hepatocyte nuclear factor 1β (HNF1β/TCF2).[136] The kidney abnormalities in MODY5 are considered independent of the effects of diabetes, because they usually predate diagnosis of diabetes and are not associated with the well-known features of diabetic nephropathy such as enlarged kidneys with thickening glomerular basement membranes and arteriolar changes, and high-grade glomerular proteinuria is not typical.[135] In a few cases, MODY5 has also been associated with additional clinical features such as genital müllerian aplasia[137] (vaginal aplasia and rudimentary or bicornate uterus) and liver dysfunction,[138] although these manifestations seem to be less penetrant than the kidney abnormalities. Loss of a closely related family member HNF1α/TCF1 in mice has been shown

to cause a proximal tubule dysfunction resulting in Fanconi syndrome.[139] Mutation of this gene causes autosomal dominant MODY3 in humans. Although these patients do not exhibit renal failure independent of diabetic nephropathy, proximal tubular dysfunction, such as renal glycosuria and Fanconi syndrome, similar to that seen in the mouse mutant, has been described.[140–142] Consistent with this observation, HNF1α expression is restricted to proximal tubules.[139] HNF1β can homodimerize or heterodimerize with HNF1α, the MODY3 gene product; therefore, HNF1β mutant proteins produced in MODY5 could act in a dominant negative fashion to modulate proper HNF function through these physical associations.[143] However, the absence of structural renal defects in MODY3 indicates that these related transcription factors are not functionally redundant in kidney development.

The variable expressivity of renal anomalies may also be compounded by the multiple molecular mechanisms ascribed to MODY5 mutations. Most of the mutations that cause MODY5 are found within the DNA binding domains of the protein and are predicted to cause early truncations, internal deletions, or missense mutations that would abrogate proper DNA binding and activation of downstream target genes.[143] Other mutations remove the nuclear localization signal and cause mislocalization of HNF1β to the cytoplasm.[143] A third type of mutation exhibits a gain-of-function phenotype by causing hyperactivation of downstream genes.[144,145] Germline mosaicism may also contribute to variable expressivity. The transcriptional activity of HNF1β is coordinately regulated by binding to co-repressor and co-activator proteins (see Fig. 5-3). Mutations that increase binding of HNF1β to the co-repressor HDAC1 or decrease binding to the co-activator histone acetyltransferases CBP or PCAF would abrogate transcriptional activation and act as loss-of-function mutations. Conversely, mutations that decrease binding to HDAC or increase binding to histone acetyltransferase (HAT) could act as gain-of-function mutations. Studies from other model organisms are consistent with the possibility that different classes of mutations may account for the variable kidney phenotypes in MODY5. Overexpression of MODY5 mutants and wild-type HNF1β in Xenopus embryos exhibits a dose-responsive block to pronephros development. A gain-of-function mutation effectively blocks formation of nephric precursors; wild-type HNF1β blocks less well, and a loss-of-function mutation blocks to a much lower degree.[144] Furthermore, expression of a human HNF1β mutant with reduced DNA binding leads to reduced nephron number and compensatory hypertrophy in Xenopus, a phenotype strikingly similar to OMN.[144] Thus, results from different mutations of HNF1β may lead to different phenotypic consequences.[146] However, because of the large range of renal anomalies reported for MODY5, a more precise phenotype-genotype correlation awaits detailed phenotypic analysis of additional numbers of patients.

The role of HNF1 in formation of the kidney has yet to be fully elucidated, because mice lacking both copies of the gene die before kidney development.[147] However, renal-specific inactivation of murine HNF1β in developing collecting ducts and thick ascending loops of Henle leads to polycystic kidneys.[148] In a separate in vivo assay, loss of functional HNF1β caused by overexpression of a dominant negative mutant in developing tubules also causes cyst formation.[146] These phenotypes may be explained at least in part by direct transcriptional regulation by HNF1β of Pkd2, Pkhd1, and uromodulin, genes directly implicated in human cystic kidney disease. Loss of *HNF1β* leads to increased proliferation of cystic epithelium[148] and may account for recent observations suggesting that germline mutation of *HNF1β* may predispose to a subtype of renal carcinoma.[149] Cystic disease exhibits varied expressivity in MODY5 by presenting as one or a few isolated cysts detected on renal ultrasonography, MCDK, glomerulocystic disease associated with hypoplastic kidneys, and enlarged polycystic kidneys detected at prenatal ultrasonography.[150] There is also an isolated report of juvenile hyperuricemic nephropathy, a variant of medullary cystic disease, associated with MODY5.[151] These results confirm that *HNF1β* mutations can cause structural developmental defects in the kidney and elucidate the potential molecular mechanisms of cystogenesis associated with MODY5.

Additional roles of *HNF1β* are predicted to account for the other renal phenotypes associated with MODY5. HNF1β is expressed in the wolffian duct, in the ureteric bud, and in differentiated renal tubular epithelium along the entire nephron from proximal tubules to collecting ducts.[152] Therefore, independent roles of HNF1β during different steps of kidney development may account for the wide clinical spectrum of MODY5 anomalies. For example, impaired branching morphogenesis is probably the mechanism of renal hypoplasia and OMN because of a requirement for HNF1β in the ureteric bud. In zebrafish, mutations of *vhnf1*, the *HNF1β* orthologue, disrupt development of the pronephros and lead to development of cysts.[153] In *vhnf1* mutant embryos, *pax2.1* expression is lost in prospective pronephric tubules, sug-gesting that these two genes may function in the same pathway. Human mutations in *PAX2* and *HNF1β* represent the only examples of monogenic OMN, supporting an important role for these genes in determining nephron number.

CHROMATIN REMODELING IN STRUCTURAL RENAL DEFECTS

It has been recognized that the modification of DNA and chromatin is integral to the regulation of gene expression in developing organs. Gene regulation is controlled by multiprotein complexes that include sequence-specific transcription factors in association with co-activators and co-repressors (see Fig. 5-3). Characterization of these complexes has identified a complex set of enzymatic modifications including acetylation, methylation, and ubiquitination that either repress or activate chromatin at selected target genes. As discussed above, several syndromes that prominently affect the kidney and urinary tract, such as TBS[78] and RCS,[154] are due to mutations in sequence-specific DNA binding transcription factors that can associate with co-activator and co-repressor complexes. Recently, mutations in genes encoding chromatin-modifying enzymes or proteins that maintain chromatin structure have been described (for review see Hendrich and Bickmore[155]). Below we discuss the growing number of these chromatin-remodeling syndromes that can result in kidney and urinary tract anomalies (Table 5-4). Because of the often ubiquitous nature of these genes and general involvement in regulation of

Table 5-4 Mutations in Chromatin Remodeling and DNA Repair Factors Associated with Kidney and Urinary Tract Defects

Syndrome	Inheritance	Gene	Characteristic Features	Renal Phenotypes	Mechanism of Action
ATR-X	X-linked	*ATRX*	Mental retardation, α-thalassemia, facial deformities, skeletal defects, genital anomalies	Hypoplasia, agenesis, VUR, hydronephrosis	Not yet determined
CHARGE	Autosomal dominant	*CHD7*	Coloboma, heart defects, choanal atresia, growth retardation, genital anomalies, ear defects/hearing loss	Agenesis, hypodysplasia, hydronephrosis, hydroureter	Haploinsufficiency
Cornelia de Lange	Autosomal dominant	*NIPBL*	Mental retardation, growth retardation, facial deformities, limb defects	Hypoplasia, VUR, pelvic dilatation, ectopia	Haploinsufficiency
Fanconi anemia– VACTERL	Autosomal recessive	Multiple genes (see text)	Bone marrow failure, leukemia, VACTERL phenotype	Agenesis, hypoplasia, pelvic kidney, hydronephrosis	Homozygous loss of function
Rubinstein-Taybi	Autosomal dominant	*CBP* *EP300*	Mental retardation, skeletal anomalies, heart defects	Unilateral agenesis, cystic hypodysplasia, urethral defects	Haploinsufficiency
Roberts	Autosomal recessive	*ESCO2*	Overlaps with Cornelia de Lange	Agenesis, hypodysplasia, hydronephrosis	Homozygous loss of function

VUR, vesicoureteral reflux.

gene expression, these syndromes tend to affect many organs. In some cases (e.g., CHARGE association) the broad range of phenotypes has suggested that perhaps a single gene defect was not responsible.

CHARGE and VATER/VACTERL Associations

CHARGE syndrome (OMIM 214800) defines the nonrandom association of congenital anomalies that include choanal atresia, abnormalities of the external and inner ear, ocular coloboma, and cardiovascular malformations. These individuals can also receive the diagnosis of Hall-Hittner syndrome when they exhibit ocular coloboma, atresia choanae, and hypoplastic semicircular canals.[156] A broad range of renal anomalies occur in CHARGE, including renal agenesis and hypodysplasia, and ureteric defects causing hydronephrosis and hydroureter. Although many occurrences are sporadic, familial occurrence and concordance in monozygotic twins has suggested a genetic basis for this syndrome. Vissers et al[157] demonstrated a 2.3-megabase microdeletion on chromosome 8q12 in affected individuals. Subsequent analysis identified heterozygous missense mutations in *CHD7* in affected patients without the microdeletion. Together, these results indicate that haploinsufficiency for a single gene located on chromosome 8q12, *CHD7*, accounts for the majority of CHARGE cases, including sporadic cases where de novo mutations were demonstrated. However, as previously suggested, other loci are probably causative of the CHARGE phenotype.[158,159] For example, there is one report of a missense mutation in the semaphorin 3E (*SEMA3E*) gene causing CHARGE.[160] Recent analysis of 110 patients with CHARGE syndrome found *CHD7* mutations distributed throughout the gene in 58% of affected individuals. Consistent with these findings, nine different nonsense and splice-site mutations in *Chd7* were associated with CHARGE phenotypes identified in a mouse mutagenesis screen.[161] In contrast to cardiovascular malformations that occur more frequently in *CHD7* mutation–positive cases, kidney and urinary tract anomalies seem to be equally prevalent in mutation positive and negative cases.[162]

CHD7 encodes a member of the chromodomain helicase DNA binding proteins. These proteins regulate chromatin organization and thereby have important effects on gene expression. The chromodomain interacts with methylated histones, DNA, and RNA, and the helicase domain can use adenosine triphosphate to enzymatically unwind nucleosomes. The finding of missense mutations in the helicase domain further supports a critical role for chromatin remodeling in this disorder.[162] *CHD7* is broadly expressed in developing embryos, including all tissues affected in CHARGE syndrome.[157,162] Through their important effects on gene expression, these proteins are thought to control developmental gene expression programs in many different contexts. However, biochemical studies are needed to define the specific roles of CHD7 in remodeling chromatin and regulating gene expression.

VATER/VACTERL (OMIM 192350) association is characterized by a nonrandom pattern of multiple anomalies including vertebral abnormalities, anal atresia, cardiovascular malformations, tracheo-esophageal fistula, and renal and limb defects. Diagnosis requires the presence of at least three of these abnormalities. The majority of occurrences are sporadic, although familial occurrence is documented especially in cases associated with hydrocephalus. In the latter, both autosomal recessive and X-linked inheritance are probable.[163,164] Kidney and urinary tract defects are common and broad spectrum, including renal agenesis/hypoplasia, pelvic kidney, and hydronephrosis that is sometimes the result of urethral atresia. The constellation of findings that define VACTERL can also be seen in other genetically defined multiple anomaly syndromes such as TBS, Holt-Oram, and Smith-Lemli-Opitz, suggesting the possibility that the Shh-Gli[97] and Sall pathways could play a role. Isolated reports have linked other genetic defects to the VACTERL phenotype. These include mutations in mitochondrial DNA,[165] the *PTEN* tumor suppressor gene,[166] and trisomy 18. In addition, infants of diabetic mothers and fetal alcohol syndrome may present with the VATER/VACTERL association, indicating a possible role for teratogens.

Fanconi anemia (OMIM 227650) is an autosomal recessive disorder that has also been linked to VACTERL. This condition is characterized by defects in all bone marrow elements leading to pancytopenia, multiple congenital organ anomalies, pigmentary skin changes, and a later risk of cancer, especially leukemia. Overall, renal anomalies occur in about 22% of patients with Fanconi anemia.[167] Approximately 5% to 10% of individuals with Fanconi anemia display a VACTERL phenotype, and in these cases renal anomalies are present in approximately 65%.[167,168] Radial-ray anomalies are common in Fanconi anemia (~50%), further suggesting a potential link between *SALL4* and VACTERL phenotypes (see Okihiro syndrome, under "Transcriptional Regulators That Cause Kidney Defects"). Although structural anomalies are present at the time of birth, hematological abnormalities may not appear until later in childhood. Thus, this diagnosis should be considered in individuals with multiple anomalies that also involve the kidney and urinary tract. The presence of pigmentary changes, such as café au lait spots, can be an important clue to the diagnosis of Fanconi anemia in VACTERL patients when hematological findings are not yet present.[169] Fanconi anemia is a genetically complex disorder. Eleven complementation groups have been identified for which nine genes have been cloned.[170] A characteristic feature of Fanconi anemia is that cell lines from affected individuals exhibit increased sensitivity to DNA cross-linking agents, chromosomal instability, and prolonged G_2 phase of the cell cycle.[171] Consistent with this observation, many of the protein products of the Fanconi anemia genes exist in a multiprotein complex that plays a key role in DNA repair and maintenance of chromosomal integrity in response to genotoxic stresses (for review see Kennedy and D'Andrea[172]). Therefore, maintenance of genomic integrity seems to be particularly important for ensuring normal renal development.

α-Thalassemia, Mental Retardation, X-linked Syndrome

Individuals with α-thalassemia, mental retardation, X-linked (ATR-X) syndrome (OMIM 301040) typically display moderate to severe mental retardation, α-thalassemia, characteristic facial features, and skeletal and genital anomalies. Renal and urinary tract anomalies occur in about 15% of cases and consist of renal hypoplasia or agenesis, cystic kidneys, VUR, and hydronephrosis.[173] Mutations in *ATRX* cause this dominant syndrome as well as a growing number of syndromes with X-linked mental retardation.[173,174] *ATRX* encodes a large protein of 2,492 amino acids that contains several functional domains predicted by homology. These include an N-terminal plant homeodomain-like (PHD) zinc-finger that is present in many chromatin-remodeling components. At the C-terminal end there is a helicase and a P domain, both of which are conserved motifs found in SWI/SNF2-type adenosine triphosphatase/helicases. As predicted by these functional domains, ATRX has been shown to exhibit chromatin-remodeling activity. Biochemical evidence suggests that this chromatin remodeling is involved in transcriptional repression, because ATRX physically interacts with the homeotic polycomb family repressor enhancer of zeste 2,[175] localizes to transcriptionally quiescent pericentromeric heterochromatin where it associates with heterochromatin protein 1α,[176,177] and is found in punctate nuclear loci containing transcriptional regulatory complexes (PML bodies).[178] However, it is also possible that ATRX can activate expression of some genes. At the cellular level, ATRX has been shown to regulate progenitor cell survival in the central nervous system, where loss of ATRX increased apoptosis of progenitor cells without affecting proliferation.[179] Whether a similar pathogenetic mechanism occurs in other developing tissues is not clear.

More than 50 different mutations have been described in more than 80 families with this syndrome, and overall phenotype-genotype correlation is generally poor.[173] However, missense mutations are clustered in the zinc-finger and helicase domains, suggesting that disruption of regions in the protein known to be involved in chromatin remodeling is sufficient to cause classic ATR-X. Moreover, truncating mutations that result in loss of the C-terminal P domain conserved among SWI/SNF2 proteins may increase the likelihood of severe urogenital anomalies.[173] In the brain, both over-expression and loss of ATRX cause brain abnormalities.[179,180] Because expression of truncated proteins has been demonstrated from ATR-X patients,[177] it remains to be determined whether the absence of ATRX, the presence of a truncated ATRX, or both mechanisms cause the developmental defects seen in patients. There are no studies that examine ATRX function specifically in kidney. Because the abdominal B Hox homeotic gene clusters have been shown to be important for urogenital tract development and are regulated by polycomb in some contexts,[176,177] several of these phenotypes could be caused by improper interactions of mutant ATRX with homeotic polycomb family repressors.

Rubinstein-Taybi Syndrome

Another autosomal dominant syndrome associated with a broad range of congenital anomalies is Rubinstein-Taybi (RSTS; OMIM 180849). Prominent features are mental retardation, skeletal anomalies, and heart defects. Urinary tract anomalies, including unilateral renal agenesis, cystic hypo-dysplasia, and urethral defects, are relatively frequent in this syndrome. Patients with RSTS also exhibit an increased risk of tumor formation. Mutations in the gene encoding the CREB-binding protein (CBP) are responsible for RSTS.[181] CBP is a co-activator molecule for a large number of transcription factors. It possesses intrinsic HAT activity and is thought to positively regulate gene expression through acetylation of

histones thereby opening chromatin structure at selected promoters (see Fig. 5-3). Missense and splice-site mutations in *RSTS* that selectively disrupt the HAT domain and its associated enzymatic activity are sufficient to cause the syndrome.[182,183] Acetylation of transcription factors themselves by CBP can also have important effects on gene expression, with the cell cycle regulator p53 and general transcription factors being important examples of in vivo targets of CBP acetylation.[184,185] Most *RSTS* mutations are thought to occur de novo rather than by germline transmission. Mutations in the closely related *EP300* gene that encodes for the p300 HAT have recently been shown in a subset of patients with RSTS who do not have *CBP* mutations.[186] The presence of micro-deletions that remove the entire *CBP* gene suggests that haploinsufficiency is the cause of the syndrome. However, genetic studies in mice indicate that many of the observed phenotypes are best accounted for by expression of a truncated mutant form of CBP rather than a null allele, raising the possibility that dominant negative effects may occur with some point mutations. Because CBP interacts with many DNA binding proteins, it is unclear at this time what pathways are affected that result in observed urinary tract defects. In *Drosophila*, dCBP is required for induction of the *Bmp* ortho-logue decapentaplegic (*dpp*) expression by sonic hedgehog.[187] Alterations in BMP4 and BMP7 signaling are thus candidates to mediate the renal and skeletal malformations in RSTS.

Cornelia de Lange and Roberts Syndromes

Cornelia de Lange syndrome (CDLS; OMIM 122470) is a multisystem developmental disorder that exhibits characteristic facies, limb defects, mental retardation, and hearing loss. Until recently urinary tract anomalies were not considered a common feature of CDLS. However, this probably reflects case-finding bias. Evaluation of an Italian cohort of 61 unselected CDLS cases[188] identified kidney and urinary tract anomalies in about 40% of cases. Significantly, impaired renal function was detected in about one-third of those cases with renal anomalies. The malformations observed were VUR, pelvic dilatation, small kidneys, and ectopia. Recently, two groups identified mutations in *NIPBL* in patients with classic and mild forms of CDLS.[189,190] Most mutations are predicted to result in premature termination codons. The presence of heterozygous deletions in two individuals with CDLS supports the conclusion that this autosomal dominant syndrome is due to haploinsufficiency for *NIPBL*. This gene encodes for delangin, a homologue of *Drosophila* developmental regulator Nipped-B. Nipped-B is thought to mediate multiple functions in chromatin maintenance, including sister chromatid cohesion, DNA repair, and gene regulation, by facilitating interaction between promoter and long-range enhancers in target genes. Interestingly, in *Drosophila* Nipped-B interacts with genes in the *Notch* pathway and *cut*, both of which have been implicated in mammalian kidney development (for review see Strachan[191] or Dorsett[192]).

Roberts syndrome (OMIM 268300) is an autosomal recessive disorder that displays phenotypic overlap with CDLS. Renal anomalies include renal agenesis, dysplasia, horseshoe kidney, and hydronephrosis. *RBS* chromosomes show a lack of cohesion involving heterochromatic C-banding regions around centromeres and the distal part of the long arm of the

Y chromosome.[193] Vega et al[194] have demonstrated mutations in *ESCO2* in RBS patients. Consistent with these cytogenetic findings, *ESCO2* is similar to a yeast gene with putative acetyltransferase activity and is essential for establishment of sister chromatid cohesion.[195,196] The clinical overlap of these two syndromes suggests that genes involved in sister chromatin cohesion are critical for proper development of multiple organs.

GROWTH FACTORS AND RECEPTORS THAT ALTER KIDNEY MORPHOGENESIS

Numerous growth factors have been implicated in kidney development in mouse models and in vitro studies. However, relatively few mutations in growth factors and their receptors have been found in human syndromes affecting the urinary tract. This may be due to considerable redundancy in these genes as illustrated by the complexity of the more than 20 fibroblast growth factor (FGF) family members and their receptor specificity.[197,198] Alternatively, these genes are critical for many processes in early development that may lead to embryonic lethality. The importance of growth factors for renal development has been more recently highlighted by the identification of human mutations in genes that help regulate the intensity, duration, or range of the growth factor signal. Among these, extracellular matrix (ECM) proteins or their modifying enzymes are increasingly being recognized as playing an important role in this process. Several human syndromes that cause significant renal anomalies are the result of disruption in these genes (Table 5-5). Importantly, those genes involved in Fraser syndrome have established a novel receptor-ligand interaction important for kidney development (Fig. 5-5).

Smith-Lemli-Opitz Syndrome

Smith-Lemli-Optiz syndrome (SLOS; OMIM 270400) is relatively common, with an estimated frequency as high as 1 in 20,000 to 1 in 30,000 in populations of northern and central European background.[199] It is a recessive syndrome that affects multiple organs, exhibits a broad range of clinical severity, and frequently involves the genitourinary tract. Common phenotypic features include behavioral problems, mental retardation, craniofacial anomalies such as cleft palate and midline defects, limb abnormalities, and growth retardation. Many affected individuals exhibit genital tract defects, especially hypospadias and cryptorchidism, findings that may lead to early postnatal diagnosis in boys. Upper urinary tract abnormalities were detected in about 57% of affected children.[200] These include defects that involve the ureter, such as PUJO, hydronephrosis, and VUR. Renal cystic dysplasia, also a common feature of SLOS, could be the result of intrinsic impairment of metanephric development or secondary to severe obstruction occurring in utero. Positional abnormalities of the kidney and renal agenesis also occur in a subset of SLOS patients. Because many of these urinary tract anomalies are associated with significant morbidity and may require specific treatment, children with this diagnosis should be screened with renal ultrasonography.[200] Antenatal detection of renal agenesis with oligohydramnios sequence can also be seen in SLOS.[201]

In the large majority of cases, SLOS results from an inborn error in cholesterol biosynthesis due to a deficiency in 3β-hydroxysterol Δ^7-reductase activity, which results in impaired conversion of 7-dehydrocholesterol to cholesterol.[202–204] Thus far more than 70 mutations have been described in *DHCR7*, the gene encoding for this enzyme. Phenotypic severity correlates best with the degree of reduction in cholesterol

Table 5-5 Mutations in Growth Factor Signaling and Extracellular Matrix Components Associated with Kidney and Urinary Tract Defects

Syndrome	Inheritance	Gene	Characteristic Features	Renal Phenotypes	Mechanism of Action
Fraser	Autosomal recessive	FRAS1 FREM2	Cryptophthalmos, cutaneous syndactyly, urogenital defects	Renal agenesis, cystic dysplasia, hypoplasia, hydronephrosis, bladder agenesis	Loss of function
Kallmann	X-linked or autosomal dominant	KAL1 KAL2	Hypogonadotropic hypogonadism, anosmia	Unilateral renal agenesis, VUR, cystic dysplasia	Loss of function, haploinsufficiency
Mayer-Rokitansky-Kuster-Hauser	ND	ND	Absent vagina, rudimentary uterus	Renal agenesis, ectopy, malrotation	ND
Simpson-Golabi-Behmel	X-linked	GPC-3	Overgrowth/tall stature, supernumerary nipples, heart defects, kidney defects	Medullary cystic dysplasia	Loss of function
Smith-Lemli-Opitz	Autosomal recessive	DHCR7	Mental retardation, craniofacial anomalies, growth retardation, limb defects, genital tract defects	PUJO, hydronephrosis, VUR, cystic dysplasia	Loss of function

ND, not determined; PUJO, pelviureteral junction obstruction; VUR, vesicoureteral reflux.

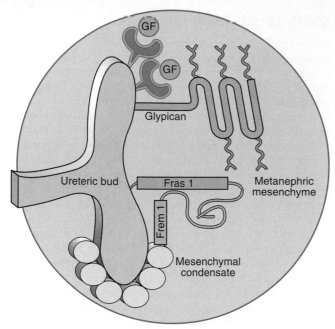

Figure 5-5 Growth factor signaling, co-receptors, and extracellular matrix components. At an early stage of kidney development (mouse E11.5) the ureter (*gray*) has invaded and undergone its initial branching in the metanephric mesenchyme (*blue*). Reciprocal interactions between the mesenchyme and the ureteric bud induce mesenchymal condensates (*light blue cylinders*) to differentiate into nephrons and the ureteric bud to continue branching. Growth factor (GF) signaling systems such as BMP, FGF, and WNT mediate these interactions. In humans, mutations in proteins that modulate this GF signaling such as co-receptors (glypican) and extracellular matrix components (anosmin) cause kidney malformations. Recent genetic studies have also identified novel pathways mediating interactions between the ureteral epithelium and the mesenchyme (Fras/Frem).

levels.[205] Since this discovery, mutations in other genes that affect cholesterol biosynthesis have been shown to similarly affect organ development, further emphasizing the importance of cholesterol in embryonic development. At least two of these syndromes, Antley-Bixler syndrome and the syndrome of congenital hemidysplasia with ichthyosiform erythroderma and limb defects, result in kidney and urinary tract defects including horseshoe kidney and duplications in the former, and renal agenesis and hydronephrosis in the latter.

Several lines of evidence have linked at least some of the abnormalities in SLOS to defective signaling in the SHH growth factor pathway. First, developmental malformations in this syndrome occur in tissues whose normal development depends on proper signaling by the hedgehog family of secreted proteins. Specific anomalies, such as holoprosencephaly and patterning defects of the distal limb, are virtually identical when each of these pathways is disrupted by mutations in mice and humans, as well as by pharmacologic inhibitors of cholesterol biosynthesis. Phenotypes observed in the urogenital tract of SLOS patients are also consistent with an important role for hedgehog family members. Targeted inactivation of *Shh* in the ureteric bud in mouse and mutation of *DHCR7*

in SLOS patients both lead to hydronephrosis. Interestingly, defective development of the proximal ureteric bud into the inner medulla and papilla is a feature that is common to *Shh* inactivation and SLOS.[206]

Biochemical studies also support an important role for sterols in hedgehog signaling. Covalent attachment of cholesterol to Shh is required for the autoprocessing step that results in formation of the mature, cholesterol-modified N-terminal Shh mediated by the C-terminal catalytic domain (for review see Cohen[207]). Shh-N seems to possess all the signaling activity of Shh. Interference with the autoprocessing step was thus hypothesized to provide a biochemical link between SLOS and Shh signaling. However, further studies have indicated that Shh autoprocessing is probably not impaired in the presence of 7-dehydrocholesterol, the precursor that accumulates in SLOS. Rather, it seems that depletion of sterols diminishes the responsiveness of target tissues to the hedgehog signal.[208] When hedgehog binds its receptor, Patched, an associated transmembrane protein, smoothened, is freed to activate hedgehog downstream signaling. Patched contains a sterol-sensing domain that is required for its activity.[209] Sterol depletion, as occurs in SLOS, affects activity of smoothened, thereby reducing hedgehog signaling. Thus, although the mechanism by which sterol depletion affects hedgehog signaling has not been fully elucidated, these important studies establish a novel link between a specific genetically determined metabolic defect, signaling by a developmental morphogen, and multiple congenital malformations, including those affecting the kidney and urinary tract.

Mayer-Rokitansky-Kuster-Hauser Syndrome

Mayer-Rokitansky-Kuster-Hauser syndrome (OMIM 277000) presents as the absence of a vagina and rudimentary uterus in a female with normal karyotype, normal ovaries, and secondary sexual characteristics. Additional abnormalities of the urinary tract are also common, such as renal agenesis, ectopy, or malrotation of one kidney.[210] Recently, this syndrome was postulated to be caused by mutations in the *WNT4* growth factor gene, because a *WNT4* mutation was identified in a sporadic case of a female patient with an absence of vagina and uterus (müllerian duct–derived structures), unilateral renal agenesis, and androgen excess.[211] This was an attractive hypothesis, because *Wnt4* is clearly involved in urogenital development. Targeted disruption of *Wnt4* in mice leads to masculinized müllerian duct–derived structures and early arrest in kidney development due to failure of the mesenchymal-to-epithelial transition.[212,213] The missense mutation identified in the patient was thought to result in misfolding of the protein, leading to defective palmitoylation and impaired secretion. As a result of impaired secretion, the mutant protein would be trapped in the endoplasmic reticulum and may exert dominant negative effects from this mislocalization. The phenotype in this patient is similar to that observed in kidneys and female reproductive tracts in *Wnt4*-null mice.[212,213] Despite the resemblance between this patient's phenotype and that of the Mayer-Rokitansky-Kuster-Hauser syndrome, *WNT4* seems to have been excluded as a major gene in this syndrome.[214] However, it remains to be determined if additional *WNT4* mutations will be identified in humans and if other factors regulating *WNT* signaling are involved in this disorder.

Simpson-Golabi-Behmel Syndrome

In stark contrast to the human syndromes that produce under-developed kidneys, patients with Simpson-Golabi-Behmel syndrome (SGBS; OMIM 312879) develop kidney cystic dysplasia from overgrowth of ureters and collecting ducts. This X-linked syndrome is caused by mutations in the glypican-3 (*GPC3*) gene, which encodes for a haparan sulfate proteoglycan.[215] These mutations are typically microdeletions encompassing one or more of the eight exons and are predicted to produce no functional protein. Loss of expression of *GPC3* causes overgrowth above the 97th percentile, tall stature, "coarse" face, supernumerary nipples, congenital heart defects, generalized muscular hypotonia, and MCDK. There is an increased risk of neoplasia in infancy, particularly Wilms tumor.[216] Cell surface haparan sulfate proteoglycans like GPC3 are well known for their role in controlling growth by acting as co-receptors for growth factor signaling (see Fig. 5-5).[217]

Loss of *Gpc3* in mice recapitulates some of the key features of SGBS, including overgrowth and cystic dysplastic kidneys.[218] Kidney development is accelerated at early stages when *Gpc3*-null mice exhibit larger kidneys with increased numbers of ureteric bud branches. Properly forming mesenchymal structures condense at the sites of ureteric bud tips, and the kidneys appear mature for their gestational age. Overgrowth of the kidney seems to be driven by increased proliferation of the ureteric bud, in that the level of mesenchymal cell proliferation does not differ from wild-type kidneys. Later in development (E16.5), when the kidney should have organized into cortex and medullary compartments, mutant kidneys contain no recognizable medullary collecting system. Instead, numerous cysts occupy the medullary space, which is degenerating rapidly because of an increase in cell death by apoptosis.[219] Ureter overgrowth and formation of medullary cysts seem to be a cell-autonomous effect of loss of *Gpc3* in collecting ducts, although it is also expressed in the metanephric mesenchyme.[218]

SGBS bears strong similarity to another overgrowth syndrome, Beckwith-Wiedemann (OMIM 130650), which is associated with the loss of imprinting of several genes including the insulin-like growth factor IGF2 (reviewed in Li et al[220]). This syndrome also results in enlarged kidneys and Wilms tumor; therefore, the etiology of SGBS was initially hypothesized to be linked to IGF2 signaling. It was proposed that GPC3 serves as a negative regulator of IGF2 signaling by competing for IGF2 binding with its receptor.[215] In the absence of GPC3, IGF2 signaling would be enhanced and overgrowth would occur in a similar paradigm to mice over-expressing IGF2.[221] However, numerous studies have contradicted this hypothesis by demonstrating that GPC3 does not directly affect the IGF signaling pathway.[218,222,223] Instead, it seems to modulate alternative signaling pathways important for kidney development.

Growth factor signaling through haparan sulfate–mediated proteins like Gpc3 is critical for renal development, because a knockout mouse for an enzyme catalyzing the formation of haparan sulfate proteoglycans, haparan sulfate-2-sulfotransferase, exhibits bilateral renal agenesis.[224] The ureter grows out and invades the metanephric mesenchyme but does not branch. This phenotype could be mediated in part by the interaction of Gpc3 and FGF signaling.[223] In support of this, *Fgf10*-null mice exhibit medullary dysplasia.[225] Whereas most

proteins containing haparan sulfate have been shown to activate Fgf signaling, Gpc1 can inhibit Fgf signaling in a haparan sulfate–dependent manner.[226] Therefore, a similar mechanism would suggest that loss of Gpc3 in SGBS would augment FGF signaling and further promote ureter growth and branching. This seems likely, because addition of a similar Fgf, Fgf7, to *Gpc3*-null E12.5 kidney explants stimulates ureter branch point formation fourfold over wild type.[219] Thus, ureter overgrowth and cyst formation in SGBS patients may arise, in part, from increased FGF signaling.

Another growth factor that is probably affected in SGBS patients is the family of bone morphogenetic proteins (BMPs). Loss of one copy of the *Bmp4* gene causes a medullary dysplastic phenotype similar to SGBS,[227] and combining these mice with a *Gpc3*-null allele results in more severe and more penetrant limb defects not seen in either mutant individually.[228] Embryonic kidney explants and collecting duct cell cultures from *Gpc3*-null mice are no longer able to respond properly to Bmps, corroborating the idea that Gpc3 is involved in the Bmp signaling pathway.[219] Loss of one copy of a similar *Bmp* gene, *Bmp2*, combined with the *Gpc3*-null allele results in synergistic increases in ureteric bud proliferation.[229] In these mice, loss of *Gpc3* decreases levels of receptor-phosphorylated Smad1, suggesting that Gpc3 activates the Bmp pathway at the level of the ligand-receptor interaction. These data imply that the hypothesis that glypicans act as co-receptors to promote Bmp signaling in *Drosophila* may be also be true for the vertebrate kidney.[230]

Glypicans have been also been shown to regulate Wnt and hedgehog signaling systems in *Drosophila*.[231,232] The Wnt signaling system is affected in the *Gpc3*-null mouse, and overexpression of Gpc3 in mesothelioma cells has the opposite effect.[233] It is tempting to speculate that Gpc3 modulates Wnt11 activity in the branching ureter tips to control growth and branching as it does when controlling cell polarity in zebrafish.[234] An equally likely mechanism of action is that Gpc3 participates in hedgehog signaling. The growth factor sonic hedgehog is strongly expressed in the medullary collecting ducts, and *Shh* deletion causes a similar disruption of maturation of the renal medulla.[100] The *Drosophila* glypican Dally-like is required for hedgehog signal transduction upstream or at the level of the receptor; therefore, it is possible that deficient hedgehog signaling between the ureter and the medullary mesenchyme triggers apoptosis and cyst formation in the medulla of SGBS patients.[219,235]

Kallmann Syndrome

Kallmann syndrome (KS) is a genetically heterogeneous syndrome caused by mutations in several different loci and is characterized by hypogonadotropic hypogonadism and anosmia. Two loci have been mapped and include an X-linked (*KAL1*; OMIM 308700) and autosomal (*KAL2*; OMIM 147950) form. *KAL1* encodes the anosmin-1 protein, and these mutations account for about 60% of familial KS cases and about 10% to 15% of sporadic cases in males. Mutations in *FGFR1* cause autosomal dominant KAL2 and occur in about 10% of KS cases.[236] Renal agenesis, usually unilateral, may occur in as many as 50% of *KAL1* cases and is predominantly right sided, in contrast to left predominance of sporadic renal agenesis.[237,238] These patients may be at risk for development of hypertension and proteinuria in young adulthood.[239]

Although much less common, VUR and MCDK have also been reported in *KAL1* mutation positive cases. KS patients with no *KAL1* or *KAL2* mutations also exhibit renal agenesis, suggesting there are additional loci that cause KS-associated renal anomalies.[238]

Anosmin-1 is a 680–amino acid protein that contains a whey acidic protein-like domain and four fibronectin-like type III repeats that contain heparan sulfate–binding sequences, suggesting it is an ECM protein. Indeed, immunohistochemical studies confirm that anosmin-1 is present in basement membranes and interstitial matrices in developing organs.[240] *FGFR1* mutations in KS clearly demonstrate a role for this growth factor signaling pathway in this syndrome. Cell culture studies show that wild-type anosmin-1, but not proteins with KS mutations, enhances FGF2/FGFR1 type IIIc pathway activity and mitogenic responses.[241] This effect is dependent on haparan sulfate proteoglycan, a known modulator of FGFR signaling[241–243] via direct interaction of the C-terminal fibronectin repeats in anosmin-1 with haparan sulfate proteoglycan. Together the genetic studies suggest that reductions in FGF signaling cause developmental defects in KS. Thus, other modulators of FGF signaling are good candidates for KS cases in which *KAL1* and *KAL2/FGFR1* mutations are not found.

In the kidney, anosmin-1 is expressed in the mesonephric (wolffian) duct and its adjacent tubules, and in the proximal ureter where it ultimately becomes restricted to medullary collecting ducts.[240] Renal agenesis could be accounted for by a requirement for *KAL1* in the mesonephric duct for outgrowth of the ureteric bud. Renal dysplasia in KS could then reflect a later requirement of *KAL1* in elongation or maintenance of medullary collecting ducts, as has been shown for *GPC3*. Studies in the mouse clearly implicate FGF signaling in kidney development, and thus renal malformations in KAL1 may be due to effects on FGF signaling.[244,245] Consistent with murine data in which *Fgfr1* is dispensable for ureteric bud outgrowth and branching,[245] no kidney and urinary tract malformations have been noted in *KAL2/FGFR1* mutation positive cases.[238] In contrast, conditional ablation of *Fgfr2* in the ureteric bud results in small dysplastic kidneys,[245] and expression of a soluble dominant negative Fgfr2 in transgenic mice results in renal hypodysplasia and complete agenesis.[244] Homozygous deficiency of both *Fgf7* and *Fgf10*, Fgfr2 ligands, also result in hypoplastic kidneys.[197,225,246] Simultaneous deficiency of *Fgfr1* and *Fgfr2* in metanephric mesenchyme results in complete renal agenesis, because the mesenchyme is not properly specified.[22] Therefore, it is likely that anosmin-1 may regulate multiple FGF receptors and thereby affect kidney development.

Fraser Syndrome

Fraser syndrome (OMIM 219000) causes multiple organ defects comprising most commonly cryptophthalmos, cutaneous syndactyly, and urogenital defects. Cryptophthalmos, in which skin covers the globe of the eye, affects the majority (~90%) of patients. Renal agenesis is the most common renal anomaly (45%), and in half of these individuals bilateral agenesis causes perinatal mortality.[247] An additional 12% of affected individuals exhibit hypoplasia of one or both kidneys and less commonly additional urinary tract anomalies such as cystic dysplasia, hypoplasia, or agenesis of the bladder, and hydronephrosis can occur. Thus, overall more than 50% of

Fraser syndrome patients have clinically important renal anomalies that affect kidney function and patient survival.

Several recent studies have significantly advanced our understanding of the pathogenesis of Fraser syndrome. McGregor et al[248] identified homozygous mutations in a gene on chromosome 4 for five pedigrees exhibiting autosomal recessive inheritance of the syndrome. These mutations are located within the *FRAS1* gene and are predicted to produce no functional protein. Similarly, *Fras1*−/−mice recapitulate the human syndrome, suggesting that complete loss of function of *FRAS1* is responsible for Fraser syndrome.[249] This was verified by the discovery that an older model of Fraser syndrome, the blebbed (*bl*) mouse mutant, also carries a *Fras1* mutation.[248,249] *FRAS1* encodes for a predicted protein of 4,007 amino acids that has similarity to a sea urchin ECM component ECM3.

FRAS1 mutations account for about 50% of Fraser syndrome cases; therefore, other genetic loci were also investigated. Other genes that had corresponding mouse models of Fraser syndrome were prime candidates, including the *FRAS*-related gene *FREM1*, and glutamate receptor interacting protein, *GRIP1*, which have been shown to be mutated in the *bat*[250] and the eye blebs (*eb*)[251] mouse models, respectively. Like *Fras1* mutants, these mice exhibit kidney phenotypes including renal agenesis. In developing kidney, they exhibit complementary expression patterns. *Frem1* is expressed at E12.5 in the mesenchyme surrounding the proximal, but not distal branching ureter,[250] and *Fras1* has been localized to the mesonephric duct and basal surface of the ureteric bud.[249] GRIP1 is a PDZ domain protein that co-localizes with FRAS1 to the basal surface of epithelia, including the ureteric bud. GRIP1 can physically interact with FRAS1 via its PDZ domain and is required for proper targeting of FRAS1 to the basal membrane.[251] Despite the strong association between Frem1 and Grip1 mouse models and Fraser syndrome phenotypes, thus far no human mutations have been identified in these genes.

Conversely, two unrelated Fraser syndrome families have been found to have mutations in the *FREM1*-like gene *FREM2*.[252] One of the affected individuals displayed unilateral renal agenesis and severe hypodysplasia on the other side with the ureter directly connected to the vagina. A gene trap mutation in mice that disrupts *Frem2*,[252] and the myelencephalic blebs (*My*) radiation-induced *Frem2* mutant[253] cause phenotypes typical of Fraser syndrome. These mutants, like Fraser patients, exhibit phenotypes in the kidney that range from renal agenesis to cystic kidneys. These families exhibit a missense mutation causing an E1974K amino acid substitution in a calcium-binding cadherin-like domain[252] (CALXβ). This domain may function in cell adhesion and is shared among FRAS1, FREM1, and FREM2.[250] The charge alteration induced by this mutation is predicted to affect Ca^{2+} binding, thereby resulting in a loss of function. These results indicate that the proper function of the CALXβ domain is required for normal kidney development. *FREM2* is strongly expressed in the tips of ureteric buds, similar to *FRAS1*, and in developing epithelial structures in the metanephros as well as in mature collecting ducts, proximal tubules, and renal blood vessels.

These proteins are thought to be involved in ECM interactions between the ureteric bud and the metanephric mesenchyme. This is based on data from *Fras1* and *bl* mutant mice, where ureteric bud outgrowth and invasion of the metanephric mesenchyme seem to occur normally.[249] However, induction of the mesenchyme fails, resulting in apoptosis. Because the basal surface of the ureteric bud contacts the metanephric mesenchyme, these results suggest that Fras1 is involved in signaling from the ureter to the mesenchyme. This phenotype is strikingly similar to *Six1*- or *Sall1*-null mice, suggesting that these transcription factors may control the mesenchymal responses to ureter signaling at a similar time during kidney development. GRIP1 is probably involved in properly localizing both FRAS1 and FREM2 to the basal surface of the ureter and ensuring the correct stoichiometry of ECM components like the chondroitin sulfate proteoglycan NG2 and collagen.[251] According to predicted functional domains in Fras1 and Frem2, their absence from the basal membrane might affect the FGF signaling pathways involved in survival and differentiation of the metanephric mesenchyme, because FGF2 can interact with NG2,[254] and it has been implicated as a ureteric bud–derived survival factor for the mesenchyme.[255] For FRAS1, the furin domain could modulate BMP signaling activity in that a furin cleavage reaction is necessary to release active ligand. Their well described role in kidney development suggests that BMP4 and BMP7 would be good candidates.[256–258] Frem1 lacks the transmembrane domains of Fras1 and Frem2, suggesting it may be a secreted factor. It has been speculated that Frem1 might interact directly with Fras1 and Frem2 in the ECM, thereby mediating epithelial-mesenchymal interactions in the developing kidney. In addition, defective deposition of collagens in basement membranes may contribute to the pathogenesis of Fraser syndrome. Thus, this newly discovered family of ECM proteins seems to have important functions in induction of the metanephric mesenchyme and proper developmental morphogenesis of the branched metanephric kidney.

CONGENITAL DEFECTS AFFECTING THE RENAL VASCULATURE

Several monogenic disorders, especially those affecting the ECM, result in defects of renal vasculature (Table 5-6). The most common abnormality is obstruction of the renal artery manifesting clinically as hypertension of renovascular origin. In addition to causing renal artery stenosis, abnormalities of the vascular wall predispose to aneurysm formation that may be complicated by renal artery rupture and renal infarction.[259–261] These manifestations may present in childhood or be silent until the fourth or fifth decade of life. Typically, these conditions affect normal formation of vessels generally, and manifestations are thus usually not restricted to the vascular bed of the kidney. These include Marfan's syndrome and Ehlers-Danlos syndrome type IV, which are caused by mutations in the genes encoding the ECM proteins fibrillin (*FBS1*) and type III collagen (*COL3AI*) and will not be discussed further. In some cases, the mutated gene regulates multiple aspects of vascular and kidney development. This is the case for Alagille syndrome (see "Transcriptional Regulators That Cause Kidney Defects"), where renal artery stenosis and glomerular sclerosis are accompanied by renal anomalies that span the entire spectrum that characterizes CAKUT. Those monogenic syndromes affecting renal vasculature for which more detailed pathogenic information is available are discussed below.

Table 5-6 Congenital Syndromes Affecting the Renal Vasculature

Syndrome	Gene	OMIM
RTD	REN AGT ANG AGTR1*	267430
Williams	ELN†	194050
Neurofibromatosis type 1	NF1	162200
Marfan's	FBN1	154700
Ehlers-Danlos	COL3A1	130050
Alagille	JAG1	118450
Cutis laxa	ELN1 FBLN5	123700
Fibromuscular dysplasia	ND	135580

*Compound heterozygous or homozygous mutations in any of these genes.
†Contiguous gene deletion. ELN deficiency is thought to cause vascular defects.
ND, not determined.

Williams Syndrome

Williams syndrome (WS; OMIM 194050) is a contiguous gene deletion syndrome of chromosome 7q11.23 that is characterized by typical (elfin) facies, cardiovascular defects, especially supravalvular aortic stenosis, and mental retardation. Renal involvement is common in this syndrome and displays a broad array of defects, of which renal artery stenosis leading to hypertension is probably the most common.[262–264] Hypertension, vascular disease, and possibly reflux nephropathy result in proteinuria and renal insufficiency in some WS patients, especially after the first decade of life.[265] Though less common, structural anomalies of the kidney and urinary tract have been described in WS and include unilateral renal agenesis, crossed fused ectopia, bladder diverticula, and VUR.[262,266] Another feature of WS, hypercalcemia and hypercalciuria, may lead to nephrocalcinosis and contribute to progressive renal failure.[267]

The pathogenesis of this complex disorder is incompletely understood. The gene encoding elastin is deleted in 75% of WS patients and haploinsufficiency at this locus is thought to account for the vascular defects.[268,269] Elastin is an important structural component of the elastic lamina and would be predicted to disrupt the integrity of the blood vessel wall, similar to that observed in Marfan's and Ehlers–Danlos syndromes. In support of this, mutations in elastin (*ELN*) or the elastin-binding protein fibulin 5 (*FBLN5*) cause the heterogeneous disorder cutis laxa (OMIM 123700) and have been associated with fibromuscular dysplasia of renal arteries.[270] Analysis of *Eln*[+/−] mice revealed that structural changes in the wall of large vessels led to alerted vascular compliance. These vascular developmental defects subsequently led to elevated blood pressure in adult mice, suggesting a potentially novel mechanism for initiation of systemic hypertension.[271]

underestimating the frequency of familial PUJO. Analysis of the few reported pedigrees suggests autosomal dominant inheritance with reduced penetrance.[300,301] Linkage to chromosome 6p is implicated in some, but not all reported pedigrees. However, these data also point out that this disorder is genetically heterogeneous, and most cases may be polygenic and involve the interaction of multiple susceptibility loci.[302]

Thus far only one genetic locus, angiotensin type 2 receptor gene (AGTR2) on the X chromosome, has been shown to confer susceptibility for this disorder in humans. A common single-nucleotide polymorphism (SNP) in this gene results in an A→G transition in intron 1. Genotyping of patients with isolated PUJO or MCDK showed that the "G" allele was significantly more prevalent (72% to 74%) in two different cohorts as compared with controls (42%). This SNP occurs at the lariat branch point downstream of the 3′ splice site. Patients with the "G" allele show reduced Agtr2 mRNA expression and inefficient splicing of exon 2,[303] consistent with a functional effect of this SNP. Further support for the role of AGTR2 comes from genetic studies in the mouse. Inactivation of Agtr2 in the mouse results in a low frequency (2% to 20%) of congenital anomalies of the kidney and urinary tract (CAKUT), including PUJO. These phenotypes are dependent on genetic background, suggesting an important role for other genetic modifiers. Thus far only small cohorts of individuals with PUJO have been analyzed. One study confirmed a statistically significant association of PUJO with the "G" allele,[304] whereas a second did not.[305] Together, these results support the conclusion that AGTR2 is probably one of several loci that contributes to the pathogenesis of PUJO, but other genetic and environmental factors remain to be determined.

The developmental mechanisms that lead to PUJO are not well understood, and both structural lesions and functional disturbances have been noted. Extrinsic compression from an angulated lower pole blood vessel that compresses the renal pelvis is thought to constitute a common structural anomaly.[306] It has been observed that the location of ureteral strictures correlates with where fetal blood vessels normally cross the ureter at the pelviureteral junction.[307] This has led to the suggestion that these fetal vessels, which normally undergo involution, may cause extrinsic compression during development thereby resulting in a stricture. However, in many cases no anatomic obstruction is present and functional disturbances that impair peristalsis are thought to cause PUJO. Analysis of surgical specimens obtained at the time of correction of congenital ureteral strictures and PUJO have noted reduction and disorganization of periureteral smooth muscle.[307–310] These anatomic defects could obstruct urine flow because of impaired peristalsis.

Recent studies in the mouse provide support for the hypothesis that impaired peristalsis may be an important developmental mechanism for PUJO. For instance, hydronephrosis in Shh mutant mice results from impaired formation of SMCs that surround the ureter.[100] These SMCs are derived from progenitors in the periureteral mesenchyme and are required for peristalsis and hence propagation of urine down the ureter and into the bladder. Shh is expressed in the urothelium and acts as a paracrine signal to adjacent periureteral mesenchyme where it induces downstream target genes including its receptor patched 1 and the TGFβ family member Bmp4. Shh signaling from epithelium to mesenchyme in the ureter regulates proliferation of smooth muscle (mesenchymal) cell

progenitors and may affect the timing and pattern of SMC differentiation. Interestingly, reports of hydronephrosis and holoprosencephaly in humans have been linked to chromosome 7q abnormalities that are predicted to result in SHH haploinsufficiency, although this region also includes HLXB9, a gene responsible for sacral agenesis that has been associated with bilateral PUJO.[311–313] The association of PUJO with SLOS is also consistent with a role of Shh signaling in this disorder.[200] Heterozygous loss of function of Bmp4 in mice results in a broad range of urinary tract anomalies, including hydroureter.[227,314] Bmp4, a Shh target, is expressed in the periureteral mesenchyme where it regulates SMC differentiation[315] but not SMC progenitor proliferation.[100]

Genes encoding for types 1 and 2 angiotensin receptors, Agtr1 and Agtr2, are also strongly expressed in periureteral mesenchyme, including in the region of the developing renal pelvis. The renal pelvis does not form in mice deficient in Agtr1 and, like the Shh mutant, periureteral smooth muscle is hypoplastic because of reduced proliferation of mesenchymal SMC progenitors.[316] Although a mutation in AGTR2 is linked to susceptibility for PUJO in humans,[303,304] it is not known if a similar defect in SMCs is involved. Nonetheless, these studies suggest that signaling through angiotensin is critical for maturation of the renal pelvis. It is possible that AGTR1 and AGTR2 are functionally redundant in the periureteral mesenchyme, accounting in part for the low frequency of PUJO associated with AGTR2 mutations. At present it is not known if angiotensin signaling acts in a common or parallel pathway with Shh. In a third mouse model of functional obstruction, conditional inactivation of the ubiquitous calcineurin regulatory subunit isoform, Cnb1, in periureteral mesenchyme leads to congenital PUJO.[317] Analysis of this mutant demonstrates that the renal pelvis fails to form as a consequence of reduced proliferation of SMC precursors in the mesenchyme. Thus, in keeping with observations in human pathologic specimens, defects in the ureteric smooth muscle seem to constitute an important influence in functional obstruction of the urinary tract. Future studies will be needed to elucidate the epistatic relationship of these pathways in the ureter, to discover novel genes involved in formation of the renal pelvis and ureter, and to genotype affected individuals to clarify the role of susceptibility loci in human disease.

A few monogenic syndromes have been associated with PUJO (see Table 5-7). Although these cases are rare, they may provide insight into the pathogenesis of the common sporadic form. For example, PUJO has been reported in the hand-foot-uterus syndrome that results from mutations in HOXA13.[318] AbdB Hox genes are expressed in periureteral mesenchyme[319] and have been implicated in kidney development in the mouse,[320,321] suggesting they may play an important role in human CAKUT. In addition, targeted deletion of genes not previously suspected of regulating development of the ureter and causing PUJO or congenital hydronephrosis, such as Scarb2, Foxc1/c2, Gdf11, Id2, and the gene encoding the metalloproteinase Adamts1, represent novel candidates to be investigated.[19,322–325]

Vesicoureteral Reflux

VUR is defined as the retrograde passage of urine from the bladder into the upper urinary tract and represents the most common urologic malformation after hypospadias. This section will focus on the more common primary VUR that is attributed to a congenital anomaly of the ureterovesical junction. Secondary forms that occur as a result of increased intravesical pressure, such as with posterior urethral valves and neurogenic bladder, will not be discussed.

VUR is found in about 1% of all neonates and in 35% to 40% of infants who develop urinary tract infections,[326–331] As with PUJO, detection of prenatal hydronephrosis is often the clue to early diagnosis of VUR in asymptomatic newborns.[332] Confirmation of the diagnosis requires a voiding cystourethrogram to demonstrate reflux of urine from the bladder up into the urinary collecting system (see Fig. 5-2). Postnatal diagnosis is usually made when an infant or child is evaluated for urinary tract infection or as part of a screen of family members of an index case. The severity of reflux is graded I to V on the basis of findings from the voiding cystourethrogram,[333] and the likelihood of spontaneous resolution correlates principally with the severity, especially for mild disease (grades I–II). In more severe reflux (grades III–IV), increased patient age and bilateral reflux significantly reduce the chance of spontaneous resolution.[334] Most cases of bilateral reflux are associated with a more severe grade (III–V). Overall spontaneous resolution occurs in as many as 60% of patients with grade III–V reflux, although grade V reflux rarely resolves without medical intervention. Nevertheless, many patients show some evidence of renal scarring[335] at the time of diagnosis, and these children may be at risk for later development of hypertension and renal failure. The major clinical importance of VUR relates to its association with renal injury culminating in secondary focal glomerulosclerosis, so-called reflux nephropathy, leading to end-stage renal failure. Although the mechanism of renal damage in VUR is controversial, reflux nephropathy remains a major cause of hypertension and renal failure in children. Early detection of VUR followed by antibiotic and even surgical treatment may not prevent progressive renal scarring and dysfunction. Moreover, in some studies reflux grade does not correlate with the degree of renal scarring found on DMSA radionuclide scan.[336] This has led to the plausible hypothesis that patients with VUR who develop kidney failure have associated developmental defects in the kidney.[337–340] In support of this idea is the finding of small kidneys in boys without a history of urinary tract infection who develop reflux nephropathy.[341,342] This view is also consistent with analysis of mouse models of monogenic syndromic VUR, indicating that individual genes regulate multiple independent steps in kidney development leading to small dysplastic kidneys together with lower urinary tract anomalies. Thus, in many cases, reflux of infected urine and damage to the kidney from back pressure may not be the principal cause of progressive renal failure.

Numerous studies support the conclusion that there is a strong genetic predisposition to primary VUR. These include demonstration of a substantially higher risk of VUR in first-degree relatives of an index case and the higher concordance of VUR in monozygotic (~80%) compared with dizygotic (~40%) twins.[343–347] Because invasive screening of asymptomatic family members is impractical and spontaneous resolution occurs at high frequency, accurate case ascertainment limits genetic studies. Nonetheless, it has been possible to analyze kindreds and draw several conclusions. Overall, the data support the conclusion that there is considerable genetic heterogeneity in VUR. Most pedigrees suggest autosomal

dominant inheritance with incomplete penetrance and variable expressivity of the phenotype.[348–350] However, isolated families with recessive and X-linked transmission have also been suggested.[351,352] For some or perhaps many sporadic cases, it also possible that VUR is an oligogenetic or typical polygenic trait, like essential hypertension. Linkage analysis in some human pedigrees mapped VUR loci to chromosomal regions 6p21, 1p13, 10q26, and 19q13.[349,353–356] Lu et al have reported that *Robo2*, a gene that causes ectopic budding and duplication of the ureter in the mouse, is disrupted in primary VUR.[18,357] However, a recent study examined these candidate loci in seven new multigenerational families with multiple affected members and found no evidence of linkage to loci associated with VUR in other studies, including *ROBO2* and genes that cause syndromic VUR.[350] This supports the conclusion that primary VUR exhibits a high degree of genetic heterogeneity, and thus thorough phenotypic evaluation of many pedigrees or single large pedigrees that exhibit high penetrance will be needed to identify responsible genes.

One approach has been to test candidate genes based on the finding of VUR in multiorgan congenital anomaly syndromes due to a single-gene defect. For example, RCS due to *PAX2* mutations causes VUR in humans.[39] However, analysis of kindreds with primary isolated VUR did not identify *PAX2* mutations.[348,358] Similarly, other genetically defined syndromes that result in VUR have not been linked to the more common, sporadic isolated disorder (Table 5-8). Another approach has been to examine human orthologous genes that result in VUR or other defects in formation of the ureter when mutated in the mouse. Although this also represents a reasonable strategy, it too has not resulted in definitive results, with the possible exception of *ROBO2*. For example, *Agtr2* results in CAKUT including VUR in mice, and the human homologue causes increased susceptibility to PUJO in some human cohorts. However, in a study of 88 families with two or more

Table 5-8 Congenital Syndromes Associated with Vesicoureteral Reflux

Syndrome	Gene	OMIM
Branchio-oto-renal	*EYA1* *SIX1*	113650
Cornelia de Lange	*NIPBL*	122470
Hand-foot-genital	*HOXD13*	142989
HDR	*GATA3*	146255
Kallmann	*KAL1*	308700
Renal coloboma	*PAX2*	120330
Townes Brocks	*SALL1*	107480
VACTER, VACTERL	mtDNA, *PTEN*, Fanconi anemia genes	192350
Williams	*ELN**	194050

*Continuous deletion syndrome. It is not clear which gene deletion causes VUR.
mtDNA, mitochondrial DNA genes.
HDR, hypoparathyroidism, deafness, and renal anomaly syndrome.

affected members, *AGTR2* could not be implicated in the pathogenesis of VUR.[359] Some studies have suggested an association between primary VUR and SNPs in the *ACE* and *AGTR2* genes.[360–363] However, in the absence of additional evidence demonstrating plausible biologic effects of these SNPs, these association studies do not establish any causative link between the RAS and VUR. Similarly, although mouse mutagenesis has established a critical role for GDNF-Ret signaling in kidney and lower urinary tract development, no human mutations were found in the single pedigree of primary VUR that has been reported.[364] Targeted inactivation of both uroplakin II and IIIa (*UPIIIa*) in mice results in VUR and one study has reported renal dysplasia in heterozygous *UPIIIa* individuals,[365–367] but analysis of 126 sib pairs with VUR did not find linkage to this locus.[368] Some of the *UPIIIa* affected patients exhibited VUR, but it is not clear if kidney failure in these patients was related to VUR or other associated urinary tract defects.[366]

As with PUJO, studies in engineered mouse mutants have extended important observations from studies of human pathologic specimens and provide novel insights into the pathogenesis of VUR. In general, the data support the long-held view that VUR represents a congenital defect of the UVJ. Normally, a flaplike mechanism compresses the intravesical ureter during bladder contraction, thereby acting as a valve to prevent reflux of urine.[369] Failure of the anti-reflux mechanism in primary VUR is thought to result when the intravesical portion of the ureter is shortened or the ureteral orifices are ectopically placed within the bladder (see Fig. 5-2).[370,371] As already noted, one developmental mechanism proposed to account for abnormalities of the UVJ and associated kidney anomalies is budding of the ureter from the mesonephric duct at a location that is either rostral or caudal to its normal position.[372] This view is supported by some mouse models with VUR, but is not likely to explain most cases of primary VUR. In many of these models, a failure to properly localize GDNF-Ret signaling in the nephric duct leads to ectopic budding of the ureter. However, the GDNF-Ret signaling pathway is also active in the urogenital sinus and regulates maturation of the distal ureter, a developmental process that seems to be temporally and spatially distinct from that controlling the initial site at which the ureter sprouts. Studies of mouse mutants in which retinoic acid signaling is disrupted have provided novel insights into this process. Proper insertion of the distal ureter into the bladder requires a complex series of morphogenetic movements that depend on formation of an epithelial outgrowth at the base of the mesonephric (wolffian) duct termed the trigonal wedge.[32] Failure of this process in retinoic acid receptor *Rara⁻ᐟ⁻ Rarb2⁻ᐟ⁻* double-mutant mice results in hydronephrosis because the ureter does not join the bladder. A similar phenotype is seen in *Ret⁻ᐟ⁻* mice. *Ret* mRNA is expressed at the base of the mesonephric duct, the site where the epithelial wedge forms, and is dependent on vitamin A, suggesting that these genes function in a common pathway to control maturation of the distal ureter. Moreover, more recent studies indicate that contrary to previous views, the trigone of the bladder does not form from the common nephric duct, the posterior part of the mesonephric duct that connects the ureter to the urogenital sinus.[33] Rather apoptosis of the common nephric duct must occur for proper insertion of the ureter into the developing bladder to take place. This process is dependent on retinoic acid signaling from the urogenital sinus. Although human cases of primary VUR or hydronephrosis due to obstruction have not been linked directly to retinoic acid or GDNF-Ret signaling, these studies provide a molecular and developmental framework for understanding these common birth defects. Integration of these studies with data from mouse models that display defects in differentiation of the urogenital sinus, such as Eph/ephrin signaling,[373] suggest other candidate pathways regulate proper insertion of the ureter into the bladder via signaling from the urogenital sinus to the common nephric duct. Future studies are also likely to elucidate the cellular and molecular basis for formation of the trigone, an important structural component of the anti-reflux mechanism.

CONCLUSIONS

In this chapter we have attempted to highlight new insights into our understanding of the molecular pathogenesis of congenital birth defects affecting the kidney and urinary tract. In large part this has been sparked by advances in human and mouse genetics, coupled with classical embryologic approaches and careful phenotypic analysis of patients. The genes responsible for several monogenic syndromes that affect the kidney and urinary tract have now been determined, and progress has been made in dissecting their epistatic relationships. In many cases, this has led to delineation of specific roles of transcription factors and chromatin remodeling complexes in kidney development that were not previously appreciated. Because growth factors can be more readily studied in metanephric organ culture, their role in regulating nephrogenesis has been relatively well studied. However, the recent advances presented in this chapter have identified novel pathways that regulate kidney formation. Identification of genetic defects in these syndromes has also focused attention on the role of low-affinity co-receptors (SGBS), post-translational modifications (SLOS), and ECM components (KS) as key modulators of canonical ligand-receptor signaling pathways (for all three examples, see "Growth Factors and Receptors That Alter Kidney Morphogenesis" above). Where corresponding mouse mutants have been generated, scientists have been able to analyze developmental mechanisms at the molecular level. In some instances, this has even led to important new insights into areas of normal embryology that were previously less amenable to analysis and hence not well understood (see sections on PUJO and VUR in "Obstruction, Hydronephrosis, Hydroureter, and Vesicoureteral Reflux").

The decade ahead also promises to be productive for this line of investigation. With the sequencing of the mouse genome, mutagenesis screens in mouse for kidney defects will become more common and should uncover novel pathways regulating nephrogenesis. Targeted gene knockin in mice is being used to address specific biochemical and cellular functions in vivo.[374,375] Moreover, other model organisms will probably contribute increasingly to our understanding of mammalian organogenesis.[376] However, if these advances are to be translated into preventative and therapeutic interventions, then it will be necessary to make use of emerging cell biologic and proteomics analyses together with traditional biochemical approaches. Importantly, the role of clinicians will also require expansion. More sophisticated phenotypic analyses, including identification of disease biomarkers and noninvasive methods to screen large numbers of patients for kidney and urinary tract defects will help to elucidate such common defects such as VUR, PUJO, and the potential role of reduced nephron number (subclinical renal hypoplasia) in kidney failure.

References

1. California Birth Defects Monitoring Program. Kidney defects. Available at www.cbdmp.org/bd_kidney.htm.
2. March of Dimes. Genital and urinary tract defects. Available at www.marchofdimes.com/printableArticles/681_1215.asp.
3. Lewis MA, Shaw J: Report from the paediatric renal registry. In Ansell D, Burden R, Feest T, et al (editors): The UK Renal Registry: The Fifth Annual Report. Bristol, The Renal Association, 2002, p 253.
4. Rees L: Management of the infant with end-stage renal failure. Nephrol Dial Transplant 17:1564, 2002.
5. Keller G, Zimmer G, Mall G, et al: Nephron number in patients with primary hypertension. N Engl J Med 348:101, 2003.
5a. Grobstein C: Trans-filter induction of tubules in mouse metanephrogenic mesenchyme. Exp Cell Res 10:424, 1956.
6. Saxèn L: Organogenesis of the kidney. Cambridge, Cambridge University Press, 1987.
7. Potter EL: Normal and abnormal development of the kidney. Chicago, Year Book Medical Publishers, 1972.
8. Dressler G: Tubulogenesis in the developing mammalian kidney. Trends Cell Biol 12:390, 2002.
9. Mori K, Yang J, Barasch J: Ureteric bud controls multiple steps in the conversion of mesenchyme to epithelia. Semin Cell Dev Biol 14:209, 2003.
10. Shah MM, Sampogna RV, Sakurai H, et al: Branching morphogenesis and kidney disease. Development 131:1449, 2004.
11. Vainio S, Lin Y: Coordinating early kidney development: lessons from gene targeting. Nat Rev Genet 3:533, 2002.
12. Yu J, McMahon AP, Valerius MT: Recent genetic studies of mouse kidney development. Curr Opin Genet Dev 14:550, 2004.
13. Brophy PD, Ostrom L, Lang KM, Dressler GR: Regulation of ureteric bud outgrowth by Pax2-dependent activation of the glial derived neurotrophic factor gene. Development 128:4747, 2001.
14. Torres M, Gomez-Pardo E, Dressler GR, Gruss P: Pax2 controls multiple steps of urogenital development. Development 121:4057, 1995.
15. Schuchardt A, D'Agati V, Pachnis V, Costantini F: Renal agenesis and hypodysplasia in ret⁻ᵏ⁻ mutant mice result from defects in ureteric bud development. Development 122:1919, 1996.
16. Schuchardt A, D'Agati V, Larsson-Blomberg L, et al: Defects in the kidney and enteric nervous system of mice lacking the tyrosine kinase receptor Ret. Nature 367:380, 1994.
17. Basson MA, Akbulut S, Watson-Johnson J, et al: Sprouty1 is a critical regulator of GDNF/RET-mediated kidney induction. Dev Cell 8:229, 2005.
18. Grieshammer U, Le M, Plump AS, et al: SLIT2-mediated ROBO2 signaling restricts kidney induction to a single site. Dev Cell 6:709, 2004.
19. Kume T, Deng K, Hogan BL: Murine forkhead/winged helix genes Foxc1 (Mf1) and Foxc2 (Mfh1) are required for the early organogenesis of the kidney and urinary tract. Development 127:1387, 2000.
20. Kreidberg JA, Sariola H, Loring JM, et al: WT1 is required for early kidney development. Cell 74:679, 1993.
21. Sajithlal G, Zou D, Silvius D, Xu PX: Eya1 acts as a critical regulator for specifying the metanephric mesenchyme. Dev Biol 284:323, 2005.
22. Poladia DP, Kish K, Kutay B, et al: Role of fibroblast growth factor receptors 1 and 2 in the metanephric mesenchyme. Dev Biol 291:325.
23. Donovan MJ, Natoli TA, Sainio K, et al: Initial differentiation of the metanephric mesenchyme is independent of WT1 and the ureteric bud. Dev Genet 24:252, 1999.
24. Pichel JG, Shen L, Sheng HZ, et al: Defects in enteric innervation and kidney development in mice lacking GDNF. Nature 382:73, 1996.
25. Sanchez MP, Silos-Santiago I, Frisen J, et al: Renal agenesis and the absence of enteric neurons in mice lacking GDNF. Nature 382:70, 1996.
26. Miyamoto N, Yoshida M, Kuratani S, et al: Defects of urogenital development in mice lacking Emx2. Development 124:1653, 1997.
27. Nishinakamura R, Matsumoto Y, Nakao K, et al: Murine homolog of SALL1 is essential for ureteric bud invasion in kidney development. Development 128:3105, 2001.
28. Hu MC, Rosenblum ND: Genetic regulation of branching morphogenesis: Lessons learned from loss-of-function phenotypes. Pediatr Res 54:433, 2003.
29. Nyengaard JR, Bendtsen TF: Glomerular number and size in relation to age, kidney weight, and body surface in normal man. Anat Rec 232:194, 1992.
30. Shakya R, Watanabe T, Costantini F: The role of GDNF/Ret signaling in ureteric bud cell fate and branching morphogenesis. Dev Cell 8:65, 2005.
31. Wong A, Bogni S, Kotka P, et al: Phosphotyrosine 1062 is critical for the in vivo activity of the Ret9 receptor tyrosine kinase isoform. Mol Cell Biol 25:9661, 2005.
32. Batourina E, Choi C, Paragas N, et al: Distal ureter morphogenesis depends on epithelial cell remodeling mediated by vitamin A and Ret. Nat Genet 32:109, 2002.
33. Batourina E, Tsai S, Lambert S, et al: Apoptosis induced by vitamin A signaling is crucial for connecting the ureters to the bladder. Nat Genet 37:1082, 2005.
34. Attar R, Quinn F, Winyard PJ, et al: Short-term urinary flow impairment deregulates PAX2 and PCNA expression and cell survival in fetal sheep kidneys. Am J Pathol 152:1225, 1998.
35. Chevalier RL, Roth K: Obstructive uropathy. In Avner E, Harmon W, Niaudet P (editors): Pediatric Nephrology. Philadelphia, Lippincott Williams & Wilkins, 2004, p 1049.
36. Yang SP, Woolf AS, Quinn F, Winyard PJ: Deregulation of renal transforming growth factor-β1 after experimental short-term ureteric obstruction in fetal sheep. Am J Pathol 159:109, 2001.
37. Mesrobian HG, Rushton HG, Bulas D: Unilateral renal agenesis may result from in utero regression of multicystic renal dysplasia. J Urol 150:793, 1993.
38. Limwongse C, Cassidy SB: Syndromes and malformations of the urinary tract. In Avner E, Harmon W, Niaudet P (editors): Pediatric Nephrology. Philadelphia, Lippincott Williams & Wilkins, 2004, p 93.
39. Eccles MR, Schimmenti LA: Renal-coloboma syndrome: A multi-system developmental disorder caused by PAX2 mutations. Clin Genet 56:1, 1999.
40. Salomon R, Tellier AL, Attie-Bitach T, et al: PAX2 mutations in oligomeganephronia. Kidney Int 59:457, 2001.
41. Drukker A: Oligonephropathy: From a rare childhood disorder to a possible health problem in the adult. Isr Med Assoc J 4:191, 2002.
42. Fletcher J, Hu M, Berman Y, et al: Multicystic dysplastic kidney and variable phenotype in a family with a novel deletion mutation of PAX2. J Am Soc Nephrol 16:2754, 2005.
43. Keller SA, Jones JM, Boyle A, et al: Kidney and retinal defects (Krd), a transgene-induced mutation with a deletion of mouse chromosome 19 that includes the Pax2 locus. Genomics 23:309, 1994.

from ADPKD. Thus, until its diagnostic utility has been formally evaluated as in ultrasonography, it should not be used as the initial imaging modality for diagnosis of ADPKD.

Diagnosis of ADPKD by Genetic Testing

The localization of their gene loci followed by detailed characterization of the genomic structures of *PKD1* and *PKD2* has provided all the essential reagents required for molecular diagnosis of this disease.[7,8,16–19,141,142] Both DNA linkage analysis and gene-based mutation screening can be used for this purpose. As discussed earlier, presymptomatic diagnosis of ADPKD is typically performed by renal ultrasonography. However, there is a role for molecular diagnosis, especially in patients with equivocal imaging results, in those with a negative family history, and in cases when younger at-risk subjects with a negative ultrasound study are being evaluated as potential living-related kidney donors.

DNA Linkage Analysis

This family-based analysis requires both genotype and phenotype data from multiple affected and unaffected members, and the at-risk subject being tested.[138] Typically, polymorphic simple-sequence repeat markers flanking both the *PKD1* and *PKD2* loci are genotyped in the study subjects, and previously affected individuals are used to establish linkage phase in the at-risk subject. Linkage analysis then provides a statistical inference on the likelihood that a specific marker allele co-segregates with the disease. For clinical testing, Bayesian statistical algorithms are used to provide a probability estimate of linkage of the family to a disease locus. When the flanking polymorphic markers are informative, the inheritance of a disease allele can be inferred in an at-risk subject with an error of less than 1%. The major advantage of this method is that when a large family with multiple affected members is available, it is almost always possible to determine whether the test subject is an obligate disease carrier. On the other hand, gene linkage testing requires blood sampling and renal imaging from multiple individuals. It is not expected to be informative in small families or in de novo ADPKD.

Gene-Based Mutation Screening

Despite the challenges imposed by the complexity and size of *PKD1*, mutation screening of the entire coding sequence and splice junctions of both *PKD1* and *PKD2* from DNA templates have now been developed, allowing for comprehensive screening of these genes.[18] To date, approximately 200 different *PKD1* and over 50 *PKD2* mutations have been reported, with most of them predicted to truncate the mutant protein (due to frameshift deletions and insertions, nonsense mutations, or splice defects).[18,80,141–143] Most of these mutations are unique to a single family and scattered throughout these genes with no clear "hot-spots." Thus, exon-by-exon screening of these genes is required to ensure a high sensitivity in detecting disease-causing mutations.

To define the sensitivity of the gene-based diagnosis of ADPKD, mutation screening of both *PKD1* and *PKD2* by denaturing high-performance liquid chromatography (DHPLC) followed by sequencing of PCR fragments with altered DHPLC profiles was performed in a recent study of 45 genetically uncharacterized ADPKD patients.[18] In general, a high rate of missense mutations was detected in *PKD1*, with an average of five per patient. By contrast, only two polymorphisms were detected in the entire patient cohort. Despite a comprehensive screening of the coding sequence and splice junctions of both genes, protein-truncating mutations in *PKD1* and *PKD2* were found in 26 patients and 3 patients, respectively. Thus, the overall sensitivity for detecting a definitive mutation was 64% (29/45). The reasons for the relatively low sensitivity in detecting definitive mutations in this patient cohort are unclear. It is possible that some of the missense mutations identified may in fact be pathogenic. However, in the absence of a valid functional assay, it is difficult to differentiate the disease-causing missense mutations from benign polymorphisms. Additionally, mutations in the gene promoter region, which may affect gene expression, are not screened by the above assays. Currently, gene-based diagnosis of ADPKD is available commercially (Athena Diagnostics, Worcester, MA; http://www.athenadiagnostics.com). The main advantage of this test is that only a blood sample from the test subject is required. On the other hand, it is expensive, and although the sensitivity data for detecting definitive mutations have not been published by the company, a definitive mutation is likely found in no more than approximately two-thirds of the test subjects. Thus, this screen is only useful when the result is positive.

Monitoring Renal Disease Progression

Recent advances in radiologic imaging have made it feasible to examine the renal structural-functional relationship in ADPKD. Using serial ultrasonography, CT scan, or MRI with three-dimensional image reconstruction, these studies provided measures of total kidney size, cystic and noncystic kidney volumes, and noncystic renal parenchymal volume in patients with ADPKD.[83–86] In patients with early or established ADPKD, MRI with three-dimensional image reconstruction appears to provide both a sensitive and accurate measure of renal disease progression. This technique was recently evaluated by the Consortium for Radiological Imaging Studies of Polycystic Kidney Disease (CRISP) in a large multicenter study in which 241 patients 15 to 45 years of age with creatinine clearances greater than 70 mL/min underwent standardized renal MRI, renal iothalamate clearance, and comprehensive clinical evaluation annually for 3 years.[85] In this study, MRI provided reliable and reproducible measurements of total kidney volume, renal cyst and parenchymal volumes, and renal blood flow.[85,86] Inverse correlations were noted in the study cohort between renal structural parameters (total kidney volume and total cyst volume) and function (GFR), although the multivariate coefficient of determination (R^2) of these correlations was only approximately 10%. Older age, hypertension, and higher albumin excretion rate were associated with greater total kidney and renal cyst volumes.[85] Renal blood flow was found to be a significant predictor of GFR, with an R^2 of approximately 25%.[86]

The CRISP study has also documented that changes in total cyst volume and total kidney volume in the study patients were highly correlated ($R^2 = 0.9$) and that both of these measures increased exponentially with time, consistent with an expansion process dependent on growth.[144] Importantly, while the baseline total kidney volume predicted the subsequent rate of

noninvasive methods to screen large numbers of patients for kidney and urinary tract defects will help to elucidate such common defects such as VUR, PUJO, and the potential role of reduced nephron number (subclinical renal hypoplasia) in kidney failure.

References

1. California Birth Defects Monitoring Program. Kidney defects. Available at www.cbdmp.org/bd_kidney.htm.
2. March of Dimes. Genital and urinary tract defects. Available at www.marchofdimes.com/printableArticles/681_1215.asp.
3. Lewis MA, Shaw J: Report from the paediatric renal registry. In Ansell D, Burden R, Feest T, et al (editors): The UK Renal Registry: The Fifth Annual Report. Bristol, The Renal Association, 2002, p 253.
4. Rees L: Management of the infant with end-stage renal failure. Nephrol Dial Transplant 17:1564, 2002.
5. Keller G, Zimmer G, Mall G, et al: Nephron number in patients with primary hypertension. N Engl J Med 348:101, 2003.
5a. Grobstein C: Trans-filter induction of tubules in mouse metanephrogenic mesenchyme. Exp Cell Res 10:424, 1956.
6. Saxèn L: Organogenesis of the kidney. Cambridge, Cambridge University Press, 1987.
7. Potter EL: Normal and abnormal development of the kidney. Chicago, Year Book Medical Publishers, 1972.
8. Dressler G: Tubulogenesis in the developing mammalian kidney. Trends Cell Biol 12:390, 2002.
9. Mori K, Yang J, Barasch J: Ureteric bud controls multiple steps in the conversion of mesenchyme to epithelia. Semin Cell Dev Biol 14:209, 2003.
10. Shah MM, Sampogna RV, Sakurai H, et al: Branching morphogenesis and kidney disease. Development 131:1449, 2004.
11. Vainio S, Lin Y: Coordinating early kidney development: lessons from gene targeting. Nat Rev Genet 3:533, 2002.
12. Yu J, McMahon AP, Valerius MT: Recent genetic studies of mouse kidney development. Curr Opin Genet Dev 14:550, 2004.
13. Brophy PD, Ostrom L, Lang KM, Dressler GR: Regulation of ureteric bud outgrowth by Pax2-dependent activation of the glial derived neurotrophic factor gene. Development 128:4747, 2001.
14. Torres M, Gomez-Pardo E, Dressler GR, Gruss P: Pax2 controls multiple steps of urogenital development. Development 121:4057, 1995.
15. Schuchardt A, D'Agati V, Pachnis V, Costantini F: Renal agenesis and hypodysplasia in ret⁻k⁻ mutant mice result from defects in ureteric bud development. Development 122:1919, 1996.
16. Schuchardt A, D'Agati V, Larsson-Blomberg L, et al: Defects in the kidney and enteric nervous system of mice lacking the tyrosine kinase receptor Ret. Nature 367:380, 1994.
17. Basson MA, Akbulut S, Watson-Johnson J, et al: Sprouty1 is a critical regulator of GDNF/RET-mediated kidney induction. Dev Cell 8:229, 2005.
18. Grieshammer U, Le M, Plump AS, et al: SLIT2-mediated ROBO2 signaling restricts kidney induction to a single site. Dev Cell 6:709, 2004.
19. Kume T, Deng K, Hogan BL: Murine forkhead/winged helix genes Foxc1 (Mf1) and Foxc2 (Mfh1) are required for the early organogenesis of the kidney and urinary tract. Development 127:1387, 2000.
20. Kreidberg JA, Sariola H, Loring JM, et al: WT1 is required for early kidney development. Cell 74:679, 1993.
21. Sajithlal G, Zou D, Silvius D, Xu PX: Eya1 acts as a critical regulator for specifying the metanephric mesenchyme. Dev Biol 284:323, 2005.
22. Poladia DP, Kish K, Kutay B, et al: Role of fibroblast growth factor receptors 1 and 2 in the metanephric mesenchyme. Dev Biol 291:325.
23. Donovan MJ, Natoli TA, Sainio K, et al: Initial differentiation of the metanephric mesenchyme is independent of WT1 and the ureteric bud. Dev Genet 24:252, 1999.
24. Pichel JG, Shen L, Sheng HZ, et al: Defects in enteric innervation and kidney development in mice lacking GDNF. Nature 382:73, 1996.
25. Sanchez MP, Silos-Santiago I, Frisen J, et al: Renal agenesis and the absence of enteric neurons in mice lacking GDNF. Nature 382:70, 1996.
26. Miyamoto N, Yoshida M, Kuratani S, et al: Defects of urogenital development in mice lacking Emx2. Development 124:1653, 1997.
27. Nishinakamura R, Matsumoto Y, Nakao K, et al: Murine homolog of SALL1 is essential for ureteric bud invasion in kidney development. Development 128:3105, 2001.
28. Hu MC, Rosenblum ND: Genetic regulation of branching morphogenesis: Lessons learned from loss-of-function phenotypes. Pediatr Res 54:433, 2003.
29. Nyengaard JR, Bendtsen TF: Glomerular number and size in relation to age, kidney weight, and body surface in normal man. Anat Rec 232:194, 1992.
30. Shakya R, Watanabe T, Costantini F: The role of GDNF/Ret signaling in ureteric bud cell fate and branching morphogenesis. Dev Cell 8:65, 2005.
31. Wong A, Bogni S, Kotka P, et al: Phosphotyrosine 1062 is critical for the in vivo activity of the Ret9 receptor tyrosine kinase isoform. Mol Cell Biol 25:9661, 2005.
32. Batourina E, Choi C, Paragas N, et al: Distal ureter morphogenesis depends on epithelial cell remodeling mediated by vitamin A and Ret. Nat Genet 32:109, 2002.
33. Batourina E, Tsai S, Lambert S, et al: Apoptosis induced by vitamin A signaling is crucial for connecting the ureters to the bladder. Nat Genet 37:1082, 2005.
34. Attar R, Quinn F, Winyard PJ, et al: Short-term urinary flow impairment deregulates PAX2 and PCNA expression and cell survival in fetal sheep kidneys. Am J Pathol 152:1225, 1998.
35. Chevalier RL, Roth K: Obstructive uropathy. In Avner E, Harmon W, Niaudet P (editors): Pediatric Nephrology. Philadelphia, Lippincott Williams & Wilkins, 2004, p 1049.
36. Yang SP, Woolf AS, Quinn F, Winyard PJ: Deregulation of renal transforming growth factor-β1 after experimental short-term ureteric obstruction in fetal sheep. Am J Pathol 159:109, 2001.
37. Mesrobian HG, Rushton HG, Bulas D: Unilateral renal agenesis may result from in utero regression of multicystic renal dysplasia. J Urol 150:793, 1993.
38. Limwongse C, Cassidy SB: Syndromes and malformations of the urinary tract. In Avner E, Harmon W, Niaudet P (editors): Pediatric Nephrology. Philadelphia, Lippincott Williams & Wilkins, 2004, p 93.
39. Eccles MR, Schimmenti LA: Renal-coloboma syndrome: A multi-system developmental disorder caused by PAX2 mutations. Clin Genet 56:1, 1999.
40. Salomon R, Tellier AL, Attie-Bitach T, et al: PAX2 mutations in oligomeganephronia. Kidney Int 59:457, 2001.
41. Drukker A: Oligonephropathy: From a rare childhood disorder to a possible health problem in the adult. Isr Med Assoc J 4:191, 2002.
42. Fletcher J, Hu M, Berman Y, et al: Multicystic dysplastic kidney and variable phenotype in a family with a novel deletion mutation of PAX2. J Am Soc Nephrol 16:2754, 2005.
43. Keller SA, Jones JM, Boyle A, et al: Kidney and retinal defects (Krd), a transgene-induced mutation with a deletion of mouse chromosome 19 that includes the Pax2 locus. Genomics 23:309, 1994.

44. Favor J, Sandulache R, Neuhauser-Klaus A, et al: The mouse *Pax2(1Neu)* mutation is identical to a human *PAX2* mutation in a family with renal-coloboma syndrome and results in developmental defects of the brain, ear, eye, and kidney. Proc Natl Acad Sci U S A 93:13870, 1996.

45. Dressler GR, Deutsch U, Chowdhury K, et al: *Pax2*, a new murine paired-box-containing gene and its expression in the developing excretory system. Development 109:787, 1990.

46. Bouchard M, Souabni A, Mandler M, et al: Nephric lineage specification by *Pax2* and *Pax8*. Genes Dev 16:2958, 2002.

47. Mansouri A, Chowdhury K, Gruss P: Follicular cells of the thyroid gland require *Pax8* gene function. Nat Genet 19:87, 1998.

48. Bouchard M, Schleiffer A, Eisenhaber F, Busslinger M: Evolution and function of *Pax* genes. In Cooper DN (editors): Encyclopedia of the Human Genome. London, Nature Publishing Group, 2003.

49. Porteous S, Torban E, Cho NP, et al: Primary renal hypoplasia in humans and mice with *PAX2* mutations: Evidence of increased apoptosis in fetal kidneys of *Pax2(1Neu)*[+/-] mutant mice. Hum Mol Genet 9:1, 2000.

50. Dziarmaga A, Clark P, Stayner C, et al: Ureteric bud apoptosis and renal hypoplasia in transgenic *PAX2-Bax* fetal mice mimics the renal-coloboma syndrome. J Am Soc Nephrol 14:2767, 2003.

51. Clark P, Dziarmaga A, Eccles M, Goodyer P: Rescue of defective branching nephrogenesis in renal-coloboma syndrome by the caspase inhibitor, Z-VAD-fmk. J Am Soc Nephrol 15:299, 2004.

52. Barakat AY, D'Albora JB, Martin MM, Jose PA: Familial nephrosis, nerve deafness, and hypoparathyroidism. J Pediatr 91:61, 1977.

53. Grote D, Souabni A, Busslinger M, Bouchard M: *Pax 2/8*-regulated Gata3 expression is necessary for morphogenesis and guidance of the nephric duct in the developing kidney. Development 133:53, 2006.

54. Muroya K, Hasegawa T, Ito Y, et al: GATA3 abnormalities and the phenotypic spectrum of HDR syndrome. J Med Genet 38:374, 2001.

55. Bilous RW, Murty G, Parkinson DB, Thakker RV, et al: Brief report: autosomal dominant familial hypoparathyroidism, sensorineural deafness, and renal dysplasia. N Engl J Med 327:1069, 1992.

56. Van Esch H, Groenen P, Nesbit MA, et al: GATA3 haploinsufficiency causes human HDR syndrome. Nature 406:419, 2000.

57. Cantor AB, Orkin SH: Coregulation of GATA factors by the friend of GATA (FOG) family of multitype zinc finger proteins. Semin Cell Dev Biol 16:117, 2005.

58. Tsang AP, Visvader JE, Turner CA, et al: FOG, a multitype zinc finger protein, acts as a cofactor for transcription factor GATA1 in erythroid and megakaryocytic differentiation. Cell 90:109, 1997.

59. Nichols KE, Crispino JD, Poncz M, et al: Familial dyserythropoietic anaemia and thrombocytopenia due to an inherited mutation in *GATA1*. Nat Genet 24:266, 2000.

60. Nesbit MA, Bowl MR, Harding B, et al: Characterization of *GATA3* mutations in the hypoparathyroidism, deafness, and renal dysplasia (HDR) syndrome. J Biol Chem 279:22624, 2004.

61. Debacker C, Catala M, Labastie MC: Embryonic expression of the human *GATA3* gene. Mech Dev 85:183, 1999.

62. Lakshmanan G, Lieuw KH, Lim KC, et al: Localization of distant urogenital system–, central nervous system–, and endocardium-specific transcriptional regulatory elements in the *GATA3* locus. Mol Cell Biol 19:1558, 1999.

63. Labastie MC, Catala M, Gregoire JM, Peault B: The *GATA3* gene is expressed during human kidney embryogenesis. Kidney Int 47:1597, 1995.

64. Lim KC, Lakshmanan G, Crawford SE, et al: *Gata3* loss leads to embryonic lethality due to noradrenaline deficiency of the sympathetic nervous system. Nat Genet 25:209, 2000.

65. Donner AL, Maas RL: Conservation and non-conservation of genetic pathways in eye specification. Int J Dev Biol 48:743, 2004.

66. Ohto H, Kamada S, Tago K, et al: Cooperation of Six and Eya in activation of their target genes through nuclear translocation of Eya. Mol Cell Biol 19:6815, 1999.

67. Chang EH, Menezes M, Meyer NC, et al: Branchio-oto-renal syndrome: The mutation spectrum in *EYA1* and its phenotypic consequences. Hum Mutat 23:582, 2004.

68. Mutsuddi M, Chaffee B, Cassidy J, et al: Using *Drosophila* to decipher how mutations associated with human branchio-oto-renal syndrome and optical defects compromise the protein tyrosine phosphatase and transcriptional functions of eyes absent. Genetics 170:687, 2005.

69. Buller C, Xu X, Marquis V, et al: Molecular effects of *Eya1* domain mutations causing organ defects in BOR syndrome. Hum Mol Genet 10:2775, 2001.

70. Ruf RG, Xu PX, Silvius D, et al: *SIX1* mutations cause branchio-oto-renal syndrome by disruption of EYA1-SIX1-DNA complexes. Proc Natl Acad Sci U S A 101:8090, 2004.

71. Li X, Oghi KA, Zhang J, et al: Eya protein phosphatase activity regulates Six1-Dach-Eya transcriptional effects in mammalian organogenesis. Nature 426:247, 2003.

72. Xu PX, Adams J, Peters H, et al: Eya1-deficient mice lack ears and kidneys and show abnormal apoptosis of organ primordia. Nat Genet 23:113, 1999.

73. Xu PX, Zheng W, Huang L, et al: Six1 is required for the early organogenesis of mammalian kidney. Development 130:3085, 2003.

74. Pignoni F, Hu B, Zavitz KH, et al: The eye-specification proteins So and Eya form a complex and regulate multiple steps in *Drosophila* eye development. Cell 91:881, 1997.

74a. Tootle TL, Silver SJ, Davies EL, et al: The transcription factor Eyes absent is a protein tyrosine phosphatase. Nature 426:299, 2003.

75. Kohlhase J, Wischermann A, Reichenbach H, et al: Mutations in the SALL1 putative transcription factor gene cause Townes-Brocks syndrome. Nat Genet 18:81, 1998.

76. Powell CM, Michaelis RC: Townes-Brocks syndrome. J Med Genet 36:89, 1999.

77. Salerno A, Kohlhase J, Kaplan BS: Townes-Brocks syndrome and renal dysplasia: A novel mutation in the *SALL1* gene. Pediatr Nephrol 14:25, 2000.

78. Kiefer SM, McDill BW, Yang J, Rauchman M: Murine Sall1 represses transcription by recruiting a histone deacetylase complex. J Biol Chem 277:14869, 2002.

79. Netzer C, Rieger L, Brero A, et al: *SALL1*, the gene mutated in Townes-Brocks syndrome, encodes a transcriptional repressor which interacts with TRF1/PIN2 and localizes to pericentromeric heterochromatin. Hum Mol Genet 10:3017, 2001.

80. Kiefer SM, Ohlemiller KK, Yang J, et al: Expression of a truncated Sall1 transcriptional repressor is responsible for Townes-Brocks syndrome birth defects. Hum Mol Genet 12:2221, 2003.

81. Borozdin W, Steinmann K, Albrecht B, et al: Detection of heterozygous *SALL1* deletions by quantitative real time PCR proves the contribution of a SALL1 dosage effect in the pathogenesis of Townes-Brocks syndrome. Hum Mutat 27:211, 2006.

82. Al Baradie R, Yamada K, St Hilaire C, et al: Duane radial ray syndrome (Okihiro syndrome) maps to 20q13 and results from mutations in *SALL4*, a new member of the *SAL* family. Am J Hum Genet 71:1195, 2002.

83. Kohlhase J, Heinrich M, Schubert L, et al: Okihiro syndrome is caused by *SALL4* mutations. Hum Mol Genet 11:2979, 2002.

84. Borozdin W, Wright MJ, Hennekam RC, et al: Novel mutations in the gene *SALL4* provide further evidence for acro-renal-ocular and Okihiro syndromes being allelic entities, and extend the phenotypic spectrum. J Med Genet 41:e102, 2004.

85. Kohlhase J, Schubert L, Liebers M, et al: Mutations at the *SALL4* locus on chromosome 20 result in a range of clinically overlapping phenotypes, including Okihiro syndrome, Holt-Oram syndrome, acro-renal-ocular syndrome, and patients previously reported to represent thalidomide embryopathy. J Med Genet 40:473, 2003.

86. Cross SJ, Ching YH, Li QY, et al: The mutation spectrum in Holt-Oram syndrome. J Med Genet 37:785, 2000.

87. Koshiba-Takeuchi K, Takeuchi JK, Arruda EP, et al: Cooperative and antagonistic interactions between *Sall4* and *Tbx5* pattern the mouse limb and heart. Nat Genet 38:175, 2005.

88. Kohlhase J, Chitayat D, Kotzot D, et al: *SALL4* mutations in Okihiro syndrome (Duane-radial ray syndrome), acro-renal-ocular syndrome, and related disorders. Hum Mutat 26:176, 2005.

89. Miertus J, Borozdin W, Frecer V, et al: A *SALL4* zinc finger missense mutation predicted to result in increased DNA binding affinity is associated with cranial midline defects and mild features of Okihiro syndrome. Hum Genet 119:154, 2006.

90. Terhal P, Rosler B, Kohlhase J: A family with features overlapping Okihiro syndrome, hemifacial microsomia and isolated Duane anomaly caused by a novel *SALL4* mutation. Am J Med Genet A 140:222, 2006.

90a. Sakaki-Yumoto M, Kobayashi C, Sato A, et al: The murine homolog of SALL4, a causative gene in Okihiro syndrome, is essential for embryonic stem cell proliferation, and cooperates will Sall1 in anorectal, heart, brain and kidney development. Development 133:3005, 2006.

90b. Warren M, Wang W, Spiden S, et al: A Sall4 mutant mouse model useful for studying the role of Sall4 in early embryonic development and organogenesis. Genesis 45:51, 2007.

91. Kang S, Graham JM, Jr, Olney AH, Biesecker LG: GLI3 frameshift mutations cause autosomal dominant Pallister-Hall syndrome. Nat Genet 15:266, 1997.

92. Johnston JJ, Olivos-Glander I, Killoran C, et al: Molecular and clinical analyses of Greig cephalopolysyndactyly and Pallister-Hall syndromes: robust phenotype prediction from the type and position of *GLI3* mutations. Am J Hum Genet 76:609, 2005.

93. Hall JG, Pallister PD, Clarren SK, et al: Congenital hypothalamic hamartoblastoma, hypopituitarism, imperforate anus and postaxial polydactyly—A new syndrome? Part I: Clinical, causal, and pathogenetic considerations. Am J Med Genet 7:47, 1980.

94. Pallister PD, Hecht F, Herrman J: Three additional cases of the congenital hypothalamic "hamartoblastoma" (Pallister-Hall) syndrome. Am J Med Genet 33:500, 1989.

95. Bose J, Grotewold L, Ruther U: Pallister-Hall syndrome phenotype in mice mutant for *Gli3*. Hum Mol Genet 11:1129, 2002.

96. Villavicencio EH, Walterhouse DO, Iannaccone PM: The sonic hedgehog-patched-gli pathway in human development and disease. Am J Hum Genet 67:1047, 2000.

97. Kim J, Kim P, Hui CC: The VACTERL association: lessons from the sonic hedgehog pathway. Clin Genet 59:306, 2001.

98. Hui CC, Slusarski D, Platt KA, et al: Expression of three mouse homologs of the *Drosophila* segment polarity gene cubitus interruptus, *Gli*, *Gli2*, and *Gli3*, in ectoderm- and mesoderm-derived tissues suggests multiple roles during postimplantation development. Dev Biol 162:402, 1994.

99. Hu MC, Mo R, Bhella S, et al: GLI3-dependent transcriptional repression of *Gli1*, *Gli2* and kidney patterning genes disrupts renal morphogenesis. Development 133:569, 2006.

100. Yu J, Carroll TJ, McMahon AP: Sonic hedgehog regulates proliferation and differentiation of mesenchymal cells in the mouse metanephric kidney. Development 129:5301, 2002.

101. Culp DA: Congenital anomalies of the ureter. In Bergman H (editors): The Ureter. New York, Springer-Verlag, 1981, p 625.

102. Tanagho EA: Development of the ureter. In Bergman H (editors): The Ureter. New York, Springer-Verlag, 1981, p 1.

103. Alagille D, Estrada A, Hadchouel M, et al: Syndromic paucity of interlobular bile ducts (Alagille syndrome or arteriohepatic dysplasia): Review of 80 cases. J Pediatr 110:195, 1987.

104. Lykavieris P, Hadchouel M, Chardot C, Bernard O: Outcome of liver disease in children with Alagille syndrome: A study of 163 patients. Gut 49:431, 2001.

105. Krantz ID, Colliton RP, Genin A, et al: Spectrum and frequency of jagged1 (*JAG1*) mutations in Alagille syndrome patients and their families. Am J Hum Genet 62:1361, 1998.

106. Emerick KM, Rand EB, Goldmuntz E, et al: Features of Alagille syndrome in 92 patients: frequency and relation to prognosis. Hepatology 29:822, 1999.

107. Martin SR, Garel L, Alvarez F: Alagille's syndrome associated with cystic renal disease. Arch Dis Child 74:232, 1996.

108. Devriendt K, Dooms L, Proesmans W, et al: Paucity of intrahepatic bile ducts, solitary kidney and atrophic pancreas with diabetes mellitus: Atypical Alagille syndrome? Eur J Pediatr 155:87, 1996.

109. LaBrecque DR, Mitros FA, Nathan RJ, et al: Four generations of arteriohepatic dysplasia. Hepatology 2:467, 1982.

110. Dommergues JP, Gubler MC, Habib R, et al: [Renal involvement in the Alagille syndrome]. Arch Pediatr 1:411, 1994.

111. Hyams JS, Berman MM, Davis BH: Tubulointerstitial nephropathy associated with arteriohepatic dysplasia. Gastroenterology 85:430, 1983.

112. Chung-Park M, Petrelli M, Tavill AS, et al: Renal lipidosis associated with arteriohepatic dysplasia (Alagille's syndrome). Clin Nephrol 18:314, 1982.

113. Habib R, Dommergues JP, Gubler MC, et al: Glomerular mesangiolipidosis in Alagille syndrome (arteriohepatic dysplasia). Pediatr Nephrol 1:455, 1987.

114. Russo PA, Ellis D, Hashida Y: Renal histopathology in Alagille's syndrome. Pediatr Pathol 7:557, 1987.

115. Schonck M, Hoorntje S, van Hooff J: Renal transplantation in Alagille syndrome. Nephrol Dial Transplant 13:197, 1998.

116. Berard E, Sarles J, Triolo V, et al: Renovascular hypertension and vascular anomalies in Alagille syndrome. Pediatr Nephrol 12:121, 1998.

117. Hirai H, Santo Y, Kogaki S, et al: Successful stenting for renal artery stenosis in a patient with Alagille syndrome. Pediatr Nephrol 20:831, 2005.

118. Oda T, Elkahloun AG, Pike BL, et al: Mutations in the human *JAGGED1* gene are responsible for Alagille syndrome. Nat Genet 16:235, 1997.

119. Kamath BM, Bason L, Piccoli DA, et al: Consequences of *JAG1* mutations. J Med Genet 40:891, 2003.

120. Boyer J, Crosnier C, Driancourt C, et al: Expression of mutant JAGGED1 alleles in patients with Alagille syndrome. Hum Genet 116:445, 2005.

121. Spinner NB, Colliton RP, Crosnier C, et al: *Jagged1* mutations in Alagille syndrome. Hum Mutat 17:18, 2001.

122. Giannakudis J, Ropke A, Kujat A, et al: Parental mosaicism of *JAG1* mutations in families with Alagille syndrome. Eur J Hum Genet 9:209, 2001.

123. Ropke A, Kujat A, Graber M, et al: Identification of 36 novel Jagged1 (*JAG1*) mutations in patients with Alagille syndrome. Hum Mutat 21:100, 2003.

124. Morrissette JD, Colliton RP, Spinner NB: Defective intracellular transport and processing of *JAG1* missense mutations in Alagille syndrome. Hum Mol Genet 10:405, 2001.

125. Skaer H: Development of malpighian tubules in *Drosophila melanogaster*. In Vize PD, Woolf AS, Bard JBL (editors): The Kidney. London, Academic Press, 2003, p 7.

126. McLaughlin KA, Rones MS, Mercola M: Notch regulates cell fate in the developing pronephros. Dev Biol 227:567, 2000.

127. Zecchin E, Conigliaro A, Tiso N, et al: Expression analysis of jagged genes in zebrafish embryos. Dev Dyn 233:638, 2005.

128. McCright B: Notch signaling in kidney development. Curr Opin Nephrol Hypertens 12:5, 2003.

129. Mumm JS, Kopan R: Notch signaling: From the outside in. Dev Biol 228:151, 2000.

130. McCright B, Gao X, Shen L, et al: Defects in development of the kidney, heart and eye vasculature in mice homozygous for a hypomorphic Notch2 mutation. Development 128:491, 2001.

131. McCright B, Lozier J, Gridley T: A mouse model of Alagille syndrome: Notch2 as a genetic modifier of *Jag1* haploinsufficiency. Development 129:1075, 2002.

132. Kuure S, Sainio K, Vuolteenaho R, et al: Crosstalk between Jagged1 and GDNF/Ret/GFRa1 signalling regulates ureteric budding and branching. Mech Dev 122:765, 2005.

133. Cheng HT, Miner JH, Lin M, et al: γ-Secretase activity is dispensable for mesenchyme-to-epithelium transition but required for podocyte and proximal tubule formation in developing mouse kidney. Development 130:5031, 2003.

133a. Cheng HT, Kim M, Valerius MT, et al: Notch2, but not Notch1, is required for proximal fate acquisition in the mammalian nephron. Development 134:801, 2007.

134. Wang P, Pereira FA, Beasley D, Zheng H: Presenilins are required for the formation of comma- and S-shaped bodies during nephrogenesis. Development 130:5019, 2003.

135. Sagen JV, Bostad L, Njolstad PR, Sovik O: Enlarged nephrons and severe nondiabetic nephropathy in hepatocyte nuclear factor-1β (HNF-1β) mutation carriers. Kidney Int 64:793, 2003.

136. Horikawa Y, Iwasaki N, Hara M, et al: Mutation in hepatocyte nuclear factor-1β gene (*TCF2*) associated with MODY. Nat Genet 17:384, 1997.

137. Lindner TH, Njolstad PR, Horikawa Y, et al: A novel syndrome of diabetes mellitus, renal dysfunction and genital malformation associated with a partial deletion of the pseudo-POU domain of hepatocyte nuclear factor-1β. Hum Mol Genet 8:2001, 1999.

138. Montoli A, Colussi G, Massa O, et al: Renal cysts and diabetes syndrome linked to mutations of the hepatocyte nuclear factor-1β gene: Description of a new family with associated liver involvement. Am J Kidney Dis 40:397, 2002.

139. Pontoglio M, Barra J, Hadchouel M, et al: Hepatocyte nuclear factor 1 inactivation results in hepatic dysfunction, phenylketonuria, and renal Fanconi syndrome. Cell 84:575, 1996.

140. Ellard S: Hepatocyte nuclear factor 1α (HNF-1α) mutations in maturity-onset diabetes of the young. Hum Mutat 16:377, 2000.

141. Menzel R, Kaisaki PJ, Rjasanowski I, et al: A low renal threshold for glucose in diabetic patients with a mutation in the hepatocyte nuclear factor-1α (*HNF-1α*) gene. Diabet Med 15:816, 1998.

142. Stride A, Ellard S, Clark P, et al: β-Cell dysfunction, insulin sensitivity, and glycosuria precede diabetes in hepatocyte nuclear factor-1α mutation carriers. Diabetes Care 28:1751, 2005.

143. Barbacci E, Chalkiadaki A, Masdeu C, et al: *HNF1β/TCF2* mutations impair transactivation potential through altered co-regulator recruitment. Hum Mol Genet 13:3139, 2004.

144. Wild W, Pogge VS, Nastos A, et al: The mutated human gene encoding hepatocyte nuclear factor 1β inhibits kidney formation in developing *Xenopus* embryos. Proc Natl Acad Sci U S A 97:4695, 2000.

145. Yoshiuchi I, Yamagata K, Zhu Q, et al: Identification of a gain-of-function mutation in the *HNF-1β* gene in a Japanese family with MODY. Diabetologia 45:154, 2002.

146. Hiesberger T, Bai Y, Shao X, et al: Mutation of hepatocyte nuclear factor-1β inhibits *Pkhd1* gene expression and produces renal cysts in mice. J Clin Invest 113:814, 2004.

147. Barbacci E, Reber M, Ott MO, et al: Variant hepatocyte nuclear factor 1 is required for visceral endoderm specification. Development 126:4795, 1999.

148. Gresh L, Fischer E, Reimann A, et al: A transcriptional network in polycystic kidney disease. EMBO J 23:1657, 2004.

149. Rebouissou S, Vasiliu V, Thomas C, et al: Germline hepatocyte nuclear factor 1α and 1β mutations in renal cell carcinomas. Hum Mol Genet 14:603, 2005.

150. Bellanné-Chantelot C, Chauveau D, Gautier JF, et al: Clinical spectrum associated with hepatocyte nuclear factor-1β mutations. Ann Intern Med 140:510, 2004.

151. Bingham C, Ellard S, van't Hoff WG, et al: Atypical familial juvenile hyperuricemic nephropathy associated with a hepatocyte nuclear factor-1β gene mutation. Kidney Int 63:1645, 2003.

152. Coffinier C, Barra J, Babinet C, Yaniv M: Expression of the vHNF1/HNF1β homeoprotein gene during mouse organogenesis. Mech Dev 89:211, 1999.

153. Sun Z, Hopkins N: *Vhnf1*, the MODY5 and familial GCKD-associated gene, regulates regional specification of the zebrafish gut, pronephros, and hindbrain. Genes Dev 15:3217, 2001.

154. Eberhard D, Jimenez G, Heavey B, Busslinger M: Transcriptional repression by Pax5 (BSAP) through interaction with corepressors of the Groucho family. EMBO J 19:2292, 2000.

155. Hendrich B, Bickmore W: Human diseases with underlying defects in chromatin structure and modification. Hum Mol Genet 10:2233, 2001.

156. Verloes A: Updated diagnostic criteria for CHARGE syndrome: A proposal. Am J Med Genet A 133:306, 2005.

157. Vissers LE, van Ravenswaaij CM, Admiraal R, et al: Mutations in a new member of the chromodomain gene family cause CHARGE syndrome. Nat Genet 36:955, 2004.

158. Arrington CB, Cowley BC, Nightingale DR, et al: Interstitial deletion 8q11.2–q13 with congenital anomalies of CHARGE association. Am J Med Genet A 133:326, 2005.

159. Lev D, Nakar O, Bar-Am I, et al: CHARGE association in a child with de novo chromosomal aberration 46, X,der(X)t(X;2)(p22.1;q33) detected by spectral karyotyping. J Med Genet 37:E47, 2000.

160. Lalani SR, Safiullah AM, Molinari LM, et al: *SEMA3E* mutation in a patient with CHARGE syndrome. J Med Genet 41:e94, 2004.

161. Bosman EA, Penn AC, Ambrose JC, et al: Multiple mutations in mouse *Chd7* provide models for CHARGE syndrome. Hum Mol Genet 14:3463, 2005.

162. Lalani SR, Safiullah AM, Fernbach SD, et al: Spectrum of *CHD7* mutations in 110 individuals with CHARGE syndrome and genotype-phenotype correlation. Am J Hum Genet 78:303, 2006.

163. Briard ML, Le Merrer M, Plauchu H, et al: [Association of VACTERL and hydrocephalus: A new familial entity]. Ann Genet 27:220, 1984.

164. Evans JA, Stranc LC, Kaplan P, Hunter AG: VACTERL with hydrocephalus: Further delineation of the syndrome(s). Am J Med Genet 34:177, 1989.

165. Damian MS, Seibel P, Schachenmayr W, et al: VACTERL with the mitochondrial np 3243 point mutation. Am J Med Genet 62:398, 1996.

166. Reardon W, Zhou XP, Eng C: A novel germline mutation of the *PTEN* gene in a patient with macrocephaly, ventricular dilatation, and features of VATER association. J Med Genet 38:820, 2001.

167. Giampietro PF, Adler-Brecher B, Verlander PC, et al: The need for more accurate and timely diagnosis in Fanconi anemia: A report from the International Fanconi Anemia Registry. Pediatrics 91:1116, 1993.

168. Faivre L, Guardiola P, Lewis C, et al: Association of complementation group and mutation type with clinical outcome in Fanconi anemia. European Fanconi Anemia Research Group. Blood 96:4064, 2000.

169. Faivre L, Portnoi MF, Pals G, et al: Should chromosome breakage studies be performed in patients with VACTERL association? Am J Med Genet A 137:55, 2005.

170. Levitus M, Rooimans MA, Steltenpool J, et al: Heterogeneity in Fanconi anemia: Evidence for 2 new genetic subtypes. Blood 103:2498, 2004.

171. Soulier J, Leblanc T, Larghero J, et al: Detection of somatic mosaicism and classification of Fanconi anemia patients by analysis of the FA/BRCA pathway. Blood 105:1329, 2005.

172. Kennedy RD, D'Andrea AD: The Fanconi anemia/BRCA pathway: new faces in the crowd. Genes Dev 19:2925, 2005.

173. Gibbons RJ, Higgs DR: Molecular-clinical spectrum of the ATR-X syndrome. Am J Med Genet 97:204, 2000.

174. Gibbons RJ, Picketts DJ, Villard L, Higgs DR: Mutations in a putative global transcriptional regulator cause X-linked mental retardation with α-thalassemia (ATR-X syndrome). Cell 80:837, 1995.

175. Cardoso C, Timsit S, Villard L, et al: Specific interaction between the XNP/ATR-X gene product and the SET domain of the human EZH2 protein. Hum Mol Genet 7:679, 1998.

176. Le Douarin B, Nielsen AL, Garnier JM, et al: A possible involvement of TIF1α and TIF1β in the epigenetic control of transcription by nuclear receptors. EMBO J 15:6701, 1996.

177. McDowell TL, Gibbons RJ, Sutherland H, et al: Localization of a putative transcriptional regulator (*ATRX*) at pericentromeric heterochromatin and the short arms of acrocentric chromosomes. Proc Natl Acad Sci U S A 96:13983, 1999.

178. Tang J, Wu S, Liu H, et al: A novel transcription regulatory complex containing death domain-associated protein and the ATR-X syndrome protein. J Biol Chem 279:20369, 2004.

179. Berube NG, Mangelsdorf M, Jagla M, et al: The chromatin-remodeling protein ATRX is critical for neuronal survival during corticogenesis. J Clin Invest 115:258, 2005.

180. Berube NG, Jagla M, Smeenk C, et al: Neurodevelopmental defects resulting from ATRX overexpression in transgenic mice. Hum Mol Genet 11:253, 2002.

181. Petrij F, Giles RH, Dauwerse HG, et al: Rubinstein-Taybi syndrome caused by mutations in the transcriptional co-activator CBP. Nature 376:348, 1995.

182. Kalkhoven E, Roelfsema JH, Teunissen H, et al: Loss of CBP acetyltransferase activity by PHD finger mutations in Rubinstein-Taybi syndrome. Hum Mol Genet 12:441, 2003.

183. Murata T, Kurokawa R, Krones A, et al: Defect of histone acetyltransferase activity of the nuclear transcriptional coactivator CBP in Rubinstein-Taybi syndrome. Hum Mol Genet 10:1071, 2001.

184. Gu W, Shi XL, Roeder RG: Synergistic activation of transcription by CBP and p53. Nature 387:819, 1997.

185. Imhof A, Yang XJ, Ogryzko VV, et al: Acetylation of general transcription factors by histone acetyltransferases. Curr Biol 7:689, 1997.

186. Roelfsema JH, White SJ, Ariyurek Y, et al: Genetic heterogeneity in Rubinstein-Taybi syndrome: mutations in both the CBP and EP300 genes cause disease. Am J Hum Genet 76:572, 2005.

187. Akimaru H, Chen Y, Dai P, et al: *Drosophila* CBP is a co-activator of cubitus interruptus in hedgehog signalling. Nature 386:735, 1997.

188. Selicorni A, Sforzini C, Milani D, et al: Anomalies of the kidney and urinary tract are common in de Lange syndrome. Am J Med Genet A 132:395, 2005.

189. Krantz ID, McCallum J, Descipio C, et al: Cornelia de Lange syndrome is caused by mutations in *NIPBL*, the human homolog of *Drosophila melanogaster* Nipped-B. Nat Genet 36:631, 2004.

190. Tonkin ET, Wang TJ, Lisgo S, et al: *NIPBL*, encoding a homolog of fungal Scc2-type sister chromatid cohesion proteins and fly Nipped-B, is mutated in Cornelia de Lange syndrome. Nat Genet 36:636, 2004.

191. Strachan T: Cornelia de Lange syndrome and the link between chromosomal function, DNA repair and developmental gene regulation. Curr Opin Genet Dev 15:258, 2005.

192. Dorsett D: Adherin: Key to the cohesin ring and Cornelia de Lange syndrome. Curr Biol 14:R834–R836, 2004.

193. Van Den Berg DJ, Francke U: Roberts syndrome: A review of 100 cases and a new rating system for severity. Am J Med Genet 47:1104, 1993.

194. Vega H, Waisfisz Q, Gordillo M, et al: Roberts syndrome is caused by mutations in *ESCO2*, a human homolog of yeast *ECO1* that is essential for the establishment of sister chromatid cohesion. Nat Genet 37:468, 2005.

195. Skibbens RV, Corson LB, Koshland D, Hieter P: *Ctf7p* is essential for sister chromatid cohesion and links mitotic chromosome structure to the DNA replication machinery. Genes Dev 13:307, 1999.

196. Toth A, Ciosk R, Uhlmann F, et al: Yeast cohesin complex requires a conserved protein, Eco1p(Ctf7), to establish cohesion between sister chromatids during DNA replication. Genes Dev 13:320, 1999.

197. Ornitz DM, Xu J, Colvin JS, et al: Receptor specificity of the fibroblast growth factor family. J Biol Chem 271:15292, 1996.

198. Ornitz DM: FGFs, heparan sulfate and FGFRs: Complex interactions essential for development. Bioessays 22:108, 2000.

199. Ryan AK, Bartlett K, Clayton P, et al: Smith-Lemli-Opitz syndrome: A variable clinical and biochemical phenotype. J Med Genet 35:558, 1998.

200. Joseph DB, Uehling DT, Gilbert E, Laxova R: Genitourinary abnormalities associated with the Smith-Lemli-Opitz syndrome. J Urol 137:719, 1987.

201. Nowaczyk MJ, Eng B, Waye JS, et al: Fetus with renal agenesis and Smith-Lemli-Opitz syndrome. Am J Med Genet A 120:305, 2003.

202. Wassif CA, Maslen C, Kachilele-Linjewile S, et al: Mutations in the human sterol Δ7-reductase gene at 11q12–13 cause Smith-Lemli-Opitz syndrome. Am J Hum Genet 63:55, 1998.

203. Waterham HR, Wijburg FA, Hennekam RC, et al: Smith-Lemli-Opitz syndrome is caused by mutations in the 7-dehydrocholesterol reductase gene. Am J Hum Genet 63:329, 1998.

204. Irons M, Elias ER, Salen G, Tint GS, et al: Defective cholesterol biosynthesis in Smith-Lemli-Opitz syndrome. Lancet 341:1414, 1993.

205. Cunniff C, Kratz LE, Moser A, et al: Clinical and biochemical spectrum of patients with RSH/Smith-Lemli-Opitz syndrome and abnormal cholesterol metabolism. Am J Med Genet 68:263, 1997.

206. Rakheja D, Wilson GN, Rogers BB: Biochemical abnormality associated with Smith-Lemli-Opitz syndrome in an infant

with features of Rutledge multiple congenital anomaly syndrome confirms that the latter is a variant of the former. Pediatr Dev Pathol 6:270, 2003.

207. Cohen MM, Jr.: The hedgehog signaling network. Am J Med Genet A 123:5, 2003.

208. Cooper MK, Wassif CA, Krakowiak PA, et al: A defective response to Hedgehog signaling in disorders of cholesterol biosynthesis. Nat Genet 33:508, 2003.

209. Stone DM, Hynes M, Armanini M, et al: The tumour-suppressor gene patched encodes a candidate receptor for sonic hedgehog. Nature 384:129, 1996.

210. Opitz JM: Vaginal atresia (von Mayer-Rokitansky-Kuster or MRK anomaly) in hereditary renal adysplasia (HRA). Am J Med Genet 26:873, 1987.

211. Biason-Lauber A, Konrad D, Navratil F, Schoenle EJ: A *WNT4* mutation associated with müllerian-duct regression and virilization in a 46,XX woman. N Engl J Med 351:792, 2004.

212. Stark K, Vainio S, Vassileva G, McMahon AP: Epithelial transformation of metanephric mesenchyme in the developing kidney regulated by Wnt-4. Nature 372:679, 1994.

213. Vainio S, Heikkila M, Kispert A, et al: Female development in mammals is regulated by Wnt-4 signalling. Nature 397:405, 1999.

214. Clement-Ziza M, Khen N, Gonzales J, et al: Exclusion of *WNT4* as a major gene in Rokitansky-Kuster-Hauser anomaly. Am J Med Genet A 137:98, 2005.

215. Pilia G, Hughes-Benzie RM, MacKenzie A, et al: Mutations in *GPC3*, a glypican gene, cause the Simpson-Golabi-Behmel overgrowth syndrome. Nat Genet 12:241, 1996.

216. Neri G, Gurrieri F, Zanni G, Lin A: Clinical and molecular aspects of the Simpson-Golabi-Behmel syndrome. Am J Med Genet 79:279, 1998.

217. Selleck SB: Overgrowth syndromes and the regulation of signaling complexes by proteoglycans. Am J Hum Genet 64:372, 1999.

218. Cano-Gauci DF, Song HH, Yang H, et al: Glypican-3-deficient mice exhibit developmental overgrowth and some of the abnormalities typical of Simpson-Golabi-Behmel syndrome. J Cell Biol 146:255, 1999.

219. Grisaru S, Cano-Gauci D, Tee J, et al: Glypican-3 modulates BMP- and FGF-mediated effects during renal branching morphogenesis. Dev Biol 231:31, 2001.

220. Li M, Squire JA, Weksberg R: Molecular genetics of Wiedemann-Beckwith syndrome. Am J Med Genet 79:253, 1998.

221. Eggenschwiler J, Ludwig T, Fisher P, et al: Mouse mutant embryos overexpressing IGF-II exhibit phenotypic features of the Beckwith-Wiedemann and Simpson-Golabi-Behmel syndromes. Genes Dev 11:3128, 1997.

222. Chiao E, Fisher P, Crisponi L, et al: Overgrowth of a mouse model of the Simpson-Golabi-Behmel syndrome is independent of IGF signaling. Dev Biol 243:185, 2002.

223. Song HH, Shi W, Filmus J: OCI-5/rat glypican-3 binds to fibroblast growth factor-2 but not to insulin-like growth factor-2. J Biol Chem 272:7574, 1997.

224. Bullock SL, Fletcher JM, Beddington RS, Wilson VA: Renal agenesis in mice homozygous for a gene trap mutation in the gene encoding heparan sulfate 2-sulfotransferase. Genes Dev 12:1894, 1998.

225. Ohuchi H, Hori Y, Yamasaki M, et al: FGF10 acts as a major ligand for FGF receptor 2 IIIb in mouse multi-organ development. Biochem Biophys Res Commun 277:643, 2000.

226. Bonneh-Barkay D, Shlissel M, Berman B, et al: Identification of glypican as a dual modulator of the biological activity of fibroblast growth factors. J Biol Chem 272:12415, 1997.

227. Miyazaki Y, Oshima K, Fogo A, et al: Bone morphogenetic protein 4 regulates the budding site and elongation of the mouse ureter. J Clin Invest 105:863, 2000.

228. Paine-Saunders S, Viviano BL, Zupicich J, et al: Glypican-3 controls cellular responses to Bmp4 in limb patterning and skeletal development. Dev Biol 225:179, 2000.

229. Hartwig S, Hu MC, Cella C, et al: Glypican-3 modulates inhibitory Bmp2-Smad signaling to control renal development in vivo. Mech Dev 122:928, 2005.

230. Fujise M, Takeo S, Kamimura K, et al: Dally regulates Dpp morphogen gradient formation in the *Drosophila* wing. Development 130:1515, 2003.

231. Baeg GH, Lin X, Khare N, et al: Heparan sulfate proteoglycans are critical for the organization of the extracellular distribution of Wingless. Development 128:87, 2001.

232. Lum L, Yao S, Mozer B, et al: Identification of hedgehog pathway components by RNAi in *Drosophila* cultured cells. Science 299:2039, 2003.

233. Song HH, Shi W, Xiang YY, Filmus J: The loss of glypican-3 induces alterations in Wnt signaling. J Biol Chem 280:2116, 2005.

234. Topczewski J, Sepich DS, Myers DC, et al: The zebrafish glypican knypek controls cell polarity during gastrulation movements of convergent extension. Dev Cell 1:251, 2001.

235. Desbordes SC, Sanson B: The glypican Dally-like is required for Hedgehog signalling in the embryonic epidermis of *Drosophila*. Development 130:6245, 2003.

236. Dode C, Levilliers J, Dupont JM, et al: Loss-of-function mutations in *FGFR1* cause autosomal dominant Kallmann syndrome. Nat Genet 33:463, 2003.

237. Albuisson J, Pecheux C, Carel JC, et al: Kallmann syndrome: 14 novel mutations in *KAL1* and *FGFR1* (*KAL2*). Hum Mutat 25:98, 2005.

238. Sato N, Katsumata N, Kagami M, et al: Clinical assessment and mutation analysis of Kallmann syndrome 1 (KAL1) and fibroblast growth factor receptor 1 (FGFR1, or KAL2) in five families and 18 sporadic patients. J Clin Endocrinol Metab 89:1079, 2004.

239. Duke V, Quinton R, Gordon I, et al: Proteinuria, hypertension and chronic renal failure in X-linked Kallmann's syndrome, a defined genetic cause of solitary functioning kidney. Nephrol Dial Transplant 13:1998, 1998.

240. Hardelin JP, Julliard AK, Moniot B, et al: Anosmin-1 is a regionally restricted component of basement membranes and interstitial matrices during organogenesis: implications for the developmental anomalies of X chromosome-linked Kallmann syndrome. Dev Dyn 215:26, 1999.

241. Gonzalez-Martinez D, Kim SH, et al: Anosmin-1 modulates fibroblast growth factor receptor 1 signaling in human gonadotropin-releasing hormone olfactory neuroblasts through a heparan sulfate-dependent mechanism. J Neurosci 24:10384, 2004.

242. Bulow HE, Hobert O: Differential sulfations and epimerization define heparan sulfate specificity in nervous system development. Neuron 41:723, 2004.

243. Hu Y, Gonzalez-Martinez D, et al: Cross-talk of anosmin-1, the protein implicated in X-linked Kallmann's syndrome, with heparan sulfate and urokinase-type plasminogen activator. Biochem J 384:495, 2004.

244. Celli G, LaRochelle WJ, Mackem S, et al: Soluble dominant-negative receptor uncovers essential roles for fibroblast growth factors in multi-organ induction and patterning. EMBO J 17:1642, 1998.

245. Zhao H, Kegg H, Grady S, et al: Role of fibroblast growth factor receptors 1 and 2 in the ureteric bud. Dev Biol 276:403, 2004.

246. Qiao J, Uzzo R, Obara-Ishihara T, et al: FGF-7 modulates ureteric bud growth and nephron number in the developing kidney. Development 126:547, 1999.

247. Slavotinek AM, Tifft CJ: Fraser syndrome and cryptophthalmos: review of the diagnostic criteria and

evidence for phenotypic modules in complex malformation syndromes. J Med Genet 39:623, 2002.

248. McGregor L, Makela V, Darling SM, et al: Fraser syndrome and mouse blebbed phenotype caused by mutations in *FRAS1/Fras1* encoding a putative extracellular matrix protein. Nat Genet 34:203, 2003.

249. Vrontou S, Petrou P, Meyer BI, et al: Fras1 deficiency results in cryptophthalmos, renal agenesis and blebbed phenotype in mice. Nat Genet 34:209, 2003.

250. Smyth I, Du X, Taylor MS, et al: The extracellular matrix gene *Frem1* is essential for the normal adhesion of the embryonic epidermis. Proc Natl Acad Sci U SA 101:13560, 2004.

251. Takamiya K, Kostourou V, Adams S, et al: A direct functional link between the multi-PDZ domain protein GRIP1 and the Fraser syndrome protein Fras1. Nat Genet 36:172, 2004.

252. Jadeja S, Smyth I, Pitera JE, Taylor MS, et al: Identification of a new gene mutated in Fraser syndrome and mouse myelencephalic blebs. Nat Genet 37:520, 2005.

253. Timmer JR, Mak TW, Manova K, et al: Tissue morphogenesis and vascular stability require the Frem2 protein, product of the mouse myelencephalic blebs gene. Proc Natl Acad Sci U S A 102:11746, 2005.

254. Goretzki L, Burg MA, Grako KA, Stallcup WB: High-affinity binding of basic fibroblast growth factor and platelet-derived growth factor-AA to the core protein of the NG2 proteoglycan. J Biol Chem 274:16831, 1999.

255. Barasch J, Qiao J, McWilliams G, et al: Ureteric bud cells secrete multiple factors, including bFGF, which rescue renal progenitors from apoptosis. Am J Physiol 273:F757–F767, 1997.

256. Dudley AT, Lyons KM, Robertson EJ: A requirement for bone morphogenetic protein-7 during development of the mammalian kidney and eye. Genes Dev 9:2795, 1995.

257. Luo G, Hofmann C, Bronckers AL, et al: BMP-7 is an inducer of nephrogenesis, and is also required for eye development and skeletal patterning. Genes Dev 9:2808, 1995.

258. Oxburgh L, Dudley AT, Godin RE, et al: BMP4 substitutes for loss of BMP7 during kidney development. Dev Biol 286:637, 2005.

259. Baum MA, Harris HW, Jr., Burrows PE, et al: Renovascular hypertension in Marfan syndrome. Pediatr Nephrol 11:499, 1997.

260. Phan TG, Sakulsaengprapha A, Wilson M, Wing R: Ruptured internal mammary artery aneurysm presenting as massive spontaneous haemothorax in a patient with Ehlers-Danlos syndrome. Aust NZ J Med 28:210, 1998.

261. Pope FM, Nicholls AC, Jones PM, et al: EDS IV (acrogeria): New autosomal dominant and recessive types. J R Soc Med 73:180, 1980.

262. Ingelfinger JR, Newburger JW: Spectrum of renal anomalies in patients with Williams syndrome. J Pediatr 119:771, 1991.

263. Morris CA, Demsey SA, Leonard CO, et al: Natural history of Williams syndrome: Physical characteristics. J Pediatr 113:318, 1988.

264. Williams JC, Barratt-Boyes BG, Lowe JB: Supravavular aortic stenosis. Circulation 24:1311, 1961.

265. Biesecker LG, Laxova R, Friedman A: Renal insufficiency in Williams syndrome. Am J Med Genet 28:131, 1987.

266. Babbitt DP, Dobbs J, Boedecker RA: Multiple bladder diverticula in Williams "Elfin-Facies" syndrome. Pediatr Radiol 8:29, 1979.

267. Wiltse HE, Goldbloom RB, Antia AU, et al: Infantile hypercalcemia syndrome in twins. N Engl J Med 275:1157, 1966.

268. Ewart AK, Morris CA, Atkinson D, et al: Hemizygosity at the elastin locus in a developmental disorder, Williams syndrome. Nat Genet 5:11, 1993.

269. Morris CA, Thomas IT, Greenberg F: Williams syndrome: Autosomal dominant inheritance. Am J Med Genet 47:478, 1993.

270. Maxwell E, Esterly NB: Cutis laxa. Am J Dis Child 117:479, 1969.

271. Faury G, Pezet M, Knutsen RH, et al: Developmental adaptation of the mouse cardiovascular system to elastin haploinsufficiency. J Clin Invest 112:1419, 2003.

272. Del Campo M, Antonell A, Magano LF, et al: Hemizygosity at the *NCF1* gene in patients with Williams-Beuren syndrome decreases their risk of hypertension. Am J Hum Genet 78:533, 2006.

273. Culler FL, Jones KL, Deftos LJ: Impaired calcitonin secretion in patients with Williams syndrome. J Pediatr 107:720, 1985.

274. Kitagawa H, Fujiki R, Yoshimura K, et al: The chromatin-remodeling complex WINAC targets a nuclear receptor to promoters and is impaired in Williams syndrome. Cell 113:905, 2003.

275. Elias DL, Ricketts RR, Smith RB, III: Renovascular hypertension complicating neurofibromatosis. Am Surg 51:97, 1985.

276. Criado E, Izquierdo L, Lujan S, et al: Abdominal aortic coarctation, renovascular, hypertension, and neurofibromatosis. Ann Vasc Surg 16:363, 2002.

277. Guthrie GP, Jr, Tibbs PA, McAllister RG, Jr, et al: Hypertension and neurofibromatosis. Case report. Hypertension 4:894, 1982.

278. Han M, Criado E: Renal artery stenosis and aneurysms associated with neurofibromatosis. J Vasc Surg 41:539, 2005.

279. Greene JF, Jr, Fitzwater JE, Burgess J: Arterial lesions associated with neurofibromatosis. Am J Clin Pathol 62:481, 1974.

280. The I, Hannigan GE, Cowley GS, et al: Rescue of a *Drosophila* NF1 mutant phenotype by protein kinase A. Science 276:791, 1997.

281. Hamilton SJ, Friedman JM: Insights into the pathogenesis of neurofibromatosis 1 vasculopathy. Clin Genet 58:341, 2000.

282. Riccardi VM: The vasculopathy of *NF1* and histogenesis control genes. Clin Genet 58:345, 2000.

283. Spencer JA, Hacker SL, Davis EC, et al: Altered vascular remodeling in fibulin-5-deficient mice reveals a role of fibulin-5 in smooth muscle cell proliferation and migration. Proc Natl Acad Sci U S A 102:2946, 2005.

284. Li DY, Brooke B, Davis EC, et al: Elastin is an essential determinant of arterial morphogenesis. Nature 393:276, 1998.

285. Liu X, Wu H, Byrne M, et al: Type III collagen is crucial for collagen I fibrillogenesis and for normal cardiovascular development. Proc Natl Acad Sci U S A 94:1852, 1997.

286. Halpern MM, Sanford HS, Viamonte M, Jr: Renal-artery abnormalities in three hypertensive sisters. Probable familial fibromuscular hyperplasia. JAMA 194:512, 1965.

287. Major P, Genest J, Cartier P, Kuchel O: Hereditary fibromuscular dysplasia with renovascular hypertension. Ann Intern Med 86:583, 1977.

288. Rushton AR: The genetics of fibromuscular dysplasia. Arch Intern Med 140:233, 1980.

289. Gribouval O, Gonzales M, Neuhaus T, et al: Mutations in genes in the renin-angiotensin system are associated with autosomal recessive renal tubular dysgenesis. Nat Genet 37:964, 2005.

290. Marcussen N: Atubular glomeruli in renal artery stenosis. Lab Invest 65:558, 1991.

291. Sequeira Lopez ML, Pentz ES, et al: Embryonic origin and lineage of juxtaglomerular cells. Am J Physiol Renal Physiol 281:F345–F356, 2001.

292. Sequeira Lopez ML, Pentz ES, et al: Renin cells are precursors for multiple cell types that switch to the renin phenotype when homeostasis is threatened. Dev Cell 6:719, 2004.

293. Tufro-McReddie A, Johns DW, Geary KM, et al: Angiotensin II type 1 receptor: Role in renal growth and gene expression during normal development. Am J Physiol 266:F911–F918, 1994.

294. Gao X, Chen X, Taglienti M, et al: Angioblast-mesenchyme induction of early kidney development is mediated by Wt1 and Vegfa. Development 132:5437, 2005.
295. Ichikawa I, Kuwayama F, Pope JC, et al: Paradigm shift from classic anatomic theories to contemporary cell biological views of CAKUT. Kidney Int 61:889, 2002.
296. Johnston JH, Evans JP, Glassberg KI, Shapiro SR: Pelvic hydronephrosis in children: A review of 219 personal cases. J Urol 117:97, 1977.
297. Kelalis PP, Culp OS, Stickler GB, Burke EC: Ureteropelvic obstruction in children: experiences with 109 cases. J Urol 106:418, 1971.
298. Lebowitz RL, Griscom NT: Neonatal hydronephrosis: 146 cases. Radiol Clin North Am 15:49, 1977.
299. Robson WJ, Rudy SM, Johnston JH: Pelviureteric obstruction in infancy. J Pediatr Surg 11:57, 1976.
300. Buscemi M, Shanske A, Mallet E, et al: Dominantly inherited ureteropelvic junction obstruction. Urology 26:568, 1985.
301. Santava A, Utikalova A, Bartova A, et al: Familial hydronephrosis unlinked to the HLA complex. Am J Med Genet 70:118, 1997.
302. Pope JC, Brock JW, III, Adams MC, et al: Congenital anomalies of the kidney and urinary tract—Role of the loss of function mutation in the pluripotent angiotensin type 2 receptor gene. J Urol 165:196, 2001.
303. Nishimura H, Yerkes E, Hohenfellner K, et al: Role of the angiotensin type 2 receptor gene in congenital anomalies of the kidney and urinary tract, CAKUT, of mice and men. Mol Cell 3:1, 1999.
304. Hahn H, Ku SE, Kim KS, et al: Implication of genetic variations in congenital obstructive nephropathy. Pediatr Nephrol 20:1541, 2005.
305. Hiraoka M, Taniguchi T, Nakai H, et al: No evidence for AT2R gene derangement in human urinary tract anomalies. Kidney Int 59:1244, 2001.
306. McDaniel BB, Jones RA, Scherz H, et al: Dynamic contrast-enhanced MR urography in the evaluation of pediatric hydronephrosis: Part 2, anatomic and functional assessment of uteropelvic junction obstruction. Am J Roentgenol 185:1608, 2005.
307. Allen TD: Congenital ureteral strictures. J Urol 104:196, 1970.
308. Foote JW, Blennerhassett JB, Wiglesworth FW, Mackinnon KJ: Observations on the ureteropelvic junction. J Urol 104:252, 1970.
309. Hanna MK: Some observations on congenital ureteropelvic junction obstruction. Urology 12:151, 1978.
310. Zhang PL, Peters CA, Rosen S: Ureteropelvic junction obstruction: morphological and clinical studies. Pediatr Nephrol 14:820, 2000.
311. Lurie IW, Ilyina HG, Podleschuk LV, et al: Chromosome 7 abnormalities in parents of children with holoprosencephaly and hydronephrosis. Am J Med Genet 35:286, 1990.
312. Nowaczyk MJ, Huggins MJ, Tomkins DJ, et al: Holoprosencephaly, sacral anomalies, and situs ambiguus in an infant with partial monosomy 7q/trisomy 2p and SHH and HLXB9 haploinsufficiency. Clin Genet 57:388, 2000.
313. Ross AJ, Ruiz-Perez V, Wang Y, et al: A homeobox gene, HLXB9, is the major locus for dominantly inherited sacral agenesis. Nat Genet 20:358, 1998.
314. Dunn NR, Winnier GE, Hargett LK, et al: Haploinsufficient phenotypes in Bmp4 heterozygous null mice and modification by mutations in Gli3 and Alx4. Dev Biol 188:235, 1997.
315. Raatikainen-Ahokas A, Hytonen M, Tenhunen A, et al: BMP-4 affects the differentiation of metanephric mesenchyme and reveals an early anterior-posterior axis of the embryonic kidney. Dev Dyn 217:146, 2000.
316. Miyazaki Y, Tsuchida S, Nishimura H, et al: Angiotensin induces the urinary peristaltic machinery during the perinatal period. J Clin Invest 102:1489, 1998.
317. Chang CP, McDill BW, Neilson JR, et al: Calcineurin is required in urinary tract mesenchyme for the development of the pyeloureteral peristaltic machinery. J Clin Invest 113:1051, 2004.
318. Donnenfeld AE, Schrager DS, Corson SL: Update on a family with hand-foot-genital syndrome: Hypospadias and urinary tract abnormalities in two boys from the fourth generation. Am J Med Genet 44:482, 1992.
319. Benson GV, Nguyen TH, Maas RL: The expression pattern of the murine Hoxa10 gene and the sequence recognition of its homeodomain reveal specific properties of Abdominal B-like genes. Mol Cell Biol 15:1591, 1995.
320. Patterson LT, Pembaur M, Potter SS: Hoxa11 and Hoxd11 regulate branching morphogenesis of the ureteric bud in the developing kidney. Development 128:2153, 2001.
321. Wellik DM, Hawkes PJ, Capecchi MR: Hox11 paralogous genes are essential for metanephric kidney induction. Genes Dev 16:1423, 2002.
322. Esquela AF, Lee SJ: Regulation of metanephric kidney development by growth/differentiation factor 11. Dev Biol 257:356, 2003.
323. Gamp AC, Tanaka Y, Lullmann-Rauch R, et al: LIMP-2/LGP85 deficiency causes ureteric pelvic junction obstruction, deafness and peripheral neuropathy in mice. Hum Mol Genet 12:631, 2003.
324. Yokoyama H, Wada T, Kobayashi K, et al: A disintegrin and metalloproteinase with thrombospondin motifs (ADAMTS)-1 null mutant mice develop renal lesions mimicking obstructive nephropathy. Nephrol Dial Transplant 17 (Suppl 9):39, 2002.
325. Aoki Y, Mori S, Kitajima K, et al: Id2 haploinsufficiency in mice leads to congenital hydronephrosis resembling that in humans. Genes Cells 9:1287, 2004.
326. Arant BS, Jr: Vesicoureteric reflux and renal injury. Am J Kidney Dis 17:491, 1991.
327. Bailey RR: The relationship of vesico-ureteric reflux to urinary tract infection and chronic pyelonephritis-reflux nephropathy. Clin Nephrol 1:132, 1973.
328. Chapman CJ, Bailey RR, Janus ED, et al: Vesicoureteric reflux: segregation analysis. Am J Med Genet 20:577, 1985.
329. Dillon MJ, Goonasekera CD: Reflux nephropathy. J Am Soc Nephrol 9:2377, 1998.
330. Hiraoka M, Hori C, Tsukahara H, et al: Vesicoureteral reflux in male and female neonates as detected by voiding ultrasonography. Kidney Int 55:1486, 1999.
331. Hoberman A, Charron M, Hickey RW, et al: Imaging studies after a first febrile urinary tract infection in young children. N Engl J Med 348:195, 2003.
332. Brophy MM, Austin PF, Yan Y, Coplen DE: Vesicoureteral reflux and clinical outcomes in infants with prenatally detected hydronephrosis. J Urol 168:1716, 2002.
333. International Reflux Study Committee: Medical versus surgical treatment of primary vesicoureteral reflux. Pediatrics 67:392, 1981.
334. Elder JS, Peters CA, Arant BS, Jr, International Reflux Study Committee: Pediatric Vesicoureteral Reflux Guidelines Panel summary report on the management of primary vesicoureteral reflux in children. J Urol 157:1846, 1997.
335. Upadhyay J, McLorie GA, Bolduc S, et al: Natural history of neonatal reflux associated with prenatal hydronephrosis: Long-term results of a prospective study. J Urol 169:1837, 2003.
336. Wan J, Greenfield SP, Ng M, et al: Sibling reflux: A dual center retrospective study. J Urol 156:677, 1996.
337. Craig JC, Irwig LM, Knight JF, Roy LP: Does treatment of vesicoureteric reflux in childhood prevent end-stage renal

disease attributable to reflux nephropathy? Pediatrics 105:1236, 2000.

338. Marra G, Oppezzo C, Ardissino G, et al: Severe vesicoureteral reflux and chronic renal failure: A condition peculiar to male gender? Data from the ItalKid Project. J Pediatr 144:677, 2004.

339. Moorthy I, Easty M, McHugh K, et al: The presence of vesicoureteric reflux does not identify a population at risk for renal scarring following a first urinary tract infection. Arch Dis Child 90:733, 2005.

340. Wheeler D, Vimalachandra D, Hodson EM, et al: Antibiotics and surgery for vesicoureteric reflux: A meta-analysis of randomised controlled trials. Arch Dis Child 88:688, 2003.

341. Patterson LT, Strife CF: Acquired versus congenital renal scarring after childhood urinary tract infection. J Pediatr 136:2, 2000.

342. Wennerstrom M, Hansson S, Jodal U, Stokland E: Primary and acquired renal scarring in boys and girls with urinary tract infection. J Pediatr 136:30, 2000.

343. Chertin B, Puri P: Familial vesicoureteral reflux. J Urol 169:1804, 2003.

344. Devriendt K, Groenen P, Van Esch H, et al: Vesico-ureteral reflux: a genetic condition? Eur J Pediatr 157:265, 1998.

345. Kaefer M, Curran M, Treves ST, et al: Sibling vesicoureteral reflux in multiple gestation births. Pediatrics 105:800, 2000.

346. Noe HN, Wyatt RJ, Peeden JN, Jr, Rivas ML: The transmission of vesicoureteral reflux from parent to child. J Urol 148:1869, 1992.

347. Uehling DT, Vlach RE, Pauli RM, Friedman AL: Vesicoureteric reflux in sibships. Br J Urol 69:534, 1992.

348. Eccles MR, Bailey RR, Abbott GD, Sullivan MJ: Unravelling the genetics of vesicoureteric reflux: A common familial disorder. Hum Mol Genet 5:1425, 1996.

349. Feather SA, Malcolm S, Woolf AS, et al: Primary, nonsyndromic vesicoureteric reflux and its nephropathy is genetically heterogeneous, with a locus on chromosome 1. Am J Hum Genet 66:1420, 2000.

350. Sanna-Cherchi S, Reese A, Hensle T, et al: Familial vesicoureteral reflux: testing replication of linkage in seven new multigenerational kindreds. J Am Soc Nephrol 16:1781, 2005.

351. Middleton GW, Howards SS, Gillenwater JY: Sex-linked familial reflux. J Urol 114:36, 1975.

352. Pasch A, Hoefele J, Grimminger H, et al: Multiple urinary tract malformations with likely recessive inheritance in a large Somalian kindred. Nephrol Dial Transplant 19:3172, 2004.

353. Groenen PM, Garcia E, Debeer P, et al: Structure, sequence, and chromosome 19 localization of human USF2 and its rearrangement in a patient with multicystic renal dysplasia. Genomics 38:141, 1996.

354. Groenen PM, Vanderlinden G, Devriendt K, et al: Rearrangement of the human CDC5L gene by a t(6;19)(p21;q13.1) in a patient with multicystic renal dysplasia. Genomics 49:218, 1998.

355. Mackintosh P, Almarhoos G, Heath DA: HLA linkage with familial vesicoureteral reflux and familial pelvi-ureteric junction obstruction. Tissue Antigens 34:185, 1989.

356. Ogata T, Muroya K, Sasagawa I, et al: Genetic evidence for a novel gene(s) involved in urogenital development on 10q26. Kidney Int 58:2281, 2000.

357. Lu W, Peters R, Ferguson H, et al: Disruption of ROBO2 is associated with vesicoureteral reflux (Abstract). J Am Soc Nephrol 15:32A, 2004.

358. Choi KL, McNoe LA, French MC, et al: Absence of PAX2 gene mutations in patients with primary familial vesicoureteric reflux. J Med Genet 35:338, 1998.

359. Yoneda A, Cascio S, Oue T, et al: Risk factors for the development of renal parenchymal damage in familial vesicoureteral reflux. J Urol 168:1704, 2002.

360. Liu KP, Lin CY, Chen HJ, et al: Renin-angiotensin system polymorphisms in Taiwanese primary vesicoureteral reflux. Pediatr Nephrol 19:594, 2004.

361. Rigoli L, Chimenz R, di Bella C, et al: Angiotensin-converting enzyme and angiotensin type 2 receptor gene genotype distributions in Italian children with congenital uropathies. Pediatr Res 56:988, 2004.

362. Ohtomo Y, Nagaoka R, Kaneko K, et al: Angiotensin converting enzyme gene polymorphism in primary vesicoureteral reflux. Pediatr Nephrol 16:648, 2001.

363. Yim HE, Jung MJ, Choi BM, et al: Genetic polymorphism of the renin-angiotensin system on the development of primary vesicoureteral reflux. Am J Nephrol 24:178, 2004.

364. Shefelbine SE, Khorana S, Schultz PN, et al: Mutational analysis of the GDNF/RET-GDNFRα signaling complex in a kindred with vesicoureteral reflux. Hum Genet 102:474, 1998.

365. Hu P, Deng FM, Liang FX, et al: Ablation of uroplakin III gene results in small urothelial plaques, urothelial leakage, and vesicoureteral reflux. J Cell Biol 151:961, 2000.

366. Jenkins D, Bitner-Glindzicz M, Malcolm S, et al: De novo Uroplakin IIIa heterozygous mutations cause human renal adysplasia leading to severe kidney failure. J Am Soc Nephrol 16:2141, 2005.

367. Kong XT, Deng FM, Hu P, et al: Roles of uroplakins in plaque formation, umbrella cell enlargement, and urinary tract diseases. J Cell Biol 167:1195, 2004.

368. Kelly H, Ennis S, Yoneda A, et al: Uroplakin III is not a major candidate gene for primary vesicoureteral reflux. Eur J Hum Genet 13:500, 2005.

369. Tanagho EA, Pugh RC: The anatomy and function of the ureterovesical junction. Br J Urol 35:151, 1963.

370. Tanagho EA, Guthrie TH, Lyon RP: The intravesical ureter in primary reflux. J Urol 101:824, 1969.

371. Vermillion CD, Heale WF: Position and configuration of the ureteral orifice and its relationship to renal scarring in adults. J Urol 109:579, 1973.

372. Mackie GG, Stephens FD: Duplex kidneys: a correlation of renal dysplasia with position of the ureteral orifice. J Urol 114:274, 1975.

373. Dravis C, Yokoyama N, Chumley MJ, et al: Bidirectional signaling mediated by ephrin-β2 and Ephβ2 controls urorectal development. Dev Biol 271:272, 2004.

374. Hoch RV, Soriano P: Context-specific requirements for Fgfr1 signaling through Frs2 and Frs3 during mouse development. Development 133:663, 2006.

375. Jain S, Encinas M, Johnson EM, Jr, Milbrandt J: Critical and distinct roles for key RET tyrosine docking sites in renal development. Genes Dev 20:321, 2006.

376. Cagan R: The signals that drive kidney development: A view from the fly eye. Curr Opin Nephrol Hypertens 12:11, 2003.

377. Gicquel C, Rossignol S, Cabrol S, et al: Epimutation of the telomeric imprinting center region on chromosome 11p15 in Silver-Russell syndrome. Nat Genet 37:1003, 2005.

Chapter 6

Autosomal Dominant Polycystic Kidney Disease

Jing Zhou and York Pei

INTRODUCTION

Autosomal dominant polycystic kidney disease (ADPKD) [MIM 173900] is the most common monogenic disorder of the kidney,[1,2] affecting all ethnic groups worldwide with a frequency of 1:400 to 1:1,000.[3–5] In the United States alone, approximately 600,000 people are affected with ADPKD, and each year more than 2,100 of them require renal replacement treatment. These latter patients account for approximately 5% of the burden of end-stage renal disease (ESRD) and incur an annual cost for renal replacement therapy of $1 billion.[6] ADPKD is characterized by progressive formation and enlargement of renal cysts, typically resulting in chronic renal failure by late middle life. It is a multisystemic disorder with potentially serious extrarenal complications such as cardiac valve defects, colonic diverticulosis, abdominal wall hernias, and intracranial arterial aneurysms.[1,2] ADPKD is caused by a mutation in either of two genes, *PKD1* and *PKD2*, which encode polycystins-1 and -2 (PC1 and PC2), respectively. The cystogenic process is highly complex, accompanied by increased proliferation and apoptosis, altered membrane protein sorting, altered secretory function, and disorganization of extracellular matrix in tubular epithelial cells.[1,2] Recent advances from studies of PKD genes and proteins have dramatically increased our understanding of the pathobiology and signaling pathways involved in this disease. In this chapter, we will provide a comprehensive review of the current knowledge of the clinical features, genetics, and molecular and cell biology of ADPKD. Additionally, we will highlight how some of these recent advances are being translated at the bedside toward the development of novel therapies.

GENETIC EPIDEMIOLOGY

ADPKD is inherited as an autosomal dominant trait with complete penetrance, but variable expressivity.[7–9] Although all ethnic groups worldwide are affected, reliable risk estimates for this disease are presently available only in the white population. Two large population-based studies from Copenhagen, Denmark, and Olmsted County, Minnesota, United States, have estimated the prevalence of ADPKD to be 1:1,000 and 1:400, respectively.[3–5,10] The earlier Danish study published in 1957 was based on data derived from clinical cases, autopsy records, and death certificates, and was likely confounded by ascertainment bias for symptomatic cases. Thus, the prevalence of 1:1,000 in this study represents an estimate of the minimum risk.[3] By contrast, a more recent North American study was based on data derived from clinical cases, autopsy

records, and cases detected by family screening, and was modeled for potential cases that would have been missed if all the deaths from the region had been subjected to autopsy. It suggested that only half of the patients with ADPKD were clinically diagnosed during their lifetime and provided a prevalence estimate of 1:400.[4]

ADPKD is genetically heterogeneous. Since the localization of the first disease gene (*PKD1*) locus to the region of the α-globin gene on chromosome 16p13,[7] a second disease gene (*PKD2*) locus was mapped to chromosome 4q21–q23.[8] In the white population, linkage studies suggest that the disease is due to mutations of *PKD1* and *PKD2* in 85% and 15% of ADPKD families, respectively.[11,12] However, there may be an ascertainment bias in favor of identifying families with *PKD1* mutations since patients with *PKD2* mutations have milder clinical disease and tend to be underdiagnosed.[13] Thus, the relative proportion of families with ADPKD due to *PKD2* mutations may be higher than 15%. Virtually all the clinical cases of ADPKD are expected to be due to heterozygous mutations in one of these two known genes. Although subjects affected with homozygous *PKD1* or *PKD2* mutations are predicted to occur in approximately 1 in 250,000 and 1 in 1,000,000 marriages in the general population, respectively, there is no definitive documentation of such individuals.[14,15] Based on the results of *Pkd1*- and *Pkd2*-knockout mice (see later section on Animal Models), mutant homozygotes may be lethal in humans and therefore may not be clinically recognized.[15]

Both *PKD1* and *PKD2* have been identified and characterized. *PKD1* is a large complex gene composed of 46 exons spanning over 52 kb of genomic DNA.[16,17] It encodes an approximately 14-kb transcript that is predicted to translate into a protein of approximately 4,300 amino acids. Interestingly, the entire 5' region of *PKD1* up to exon 33 has been duplicated at six other sites on chromosome 16p.[16,17] The presence of these homologous pseudogenes, with many of them also encoding messenger RNA (mRNA) transcripts, provides a major challenge for genetic analysis of the duplicated region. However, recent development of locus-specific, long-range polymerase chain reaction (PCR) has allowed the complete screening of this gene for mutations.[18] Unlike *PKD1*, *PKD2* is a single-copy gene encoding a 5.3-kb mRNA transcript with 15 exons and is predicted to translate into a protein of 968 amino acids.[19]

In addition to the two known genes, the existence of one or more rare disease genes for ADPKD has been suggested by the observation of several families unlinked to either the *PKD1* or *PKD2* loci.[20–23] However, the absence of linkage in these families does not necessarily imply the presence of another disease gene since a number of potential confounders (genotyping errors, nonpaternity, misdiagnosis, and bilineal disease) could lead to false exclusion of linkage.[24,25] Indeed, recent confirmation of these findings has been lacking, and one such unlinked family was actually found to have bilineal ADPKD from heterozygous *PKD1* and *PKD2* mutations.[26]

CLINICAL FEATURES

Renal Manifestations

Formation of renal cysts is an age-dependent, fully penetrant trait in ADPKD.[27] Typically, a few focal renal cysts are detected in most affected subjects before 30 years of age. However, by the fifth decade of life, hundreds to thousands of cysts will be present in the kidneys of most patients (Fig. 6-1). In patients with established disease, their enlarged kidneys can each measure up to 40 cm in length (compared with 10–12 cm in normal individuals) and weigh up to 8 kg (compared with 400–500 g in normal individuals).[28] The severity of the renal structural abnormality, in turn, correlates with complications such as pain, hematuria, hypertension, and renal insufficiency (Table 6-1).[10]

Renal Pain

Back or flank pain is a common symptom that can affect up to 60% of patients with ADPKD.[27,28] Acute back or flank pain in ADPKD can be due to renal cyst infection, hemorrhage, or nephrolithiasis, and should be differentiated from nonrenal

Table 6-1 Renal Manifestations of ADPKD

Renal functional abnormalities
Urine concentrating defect
Reduced urine ammonium relative to pH
Reduced renal blood flow
Renal pain, caused by
Cyst hemorrhage
Renal calculi
Renal infection
Hematuria, due to
Cyst hemorrhage
Renal calculi
Renal cell carcinoma
Proteinuria
Low-grade (less than 1 g/day)
Hypertension, associated with
Activation of renin-angiotensin system
Impaired endothelial-dependent vascular relaxation
Increased sympathetic nerve activity
Renal disease progression, possibly due to
Compression atrophy
Tubular obstruction
Renal ischemia
Interstitial inflammation
Apoptosis of tubular epithelial cells

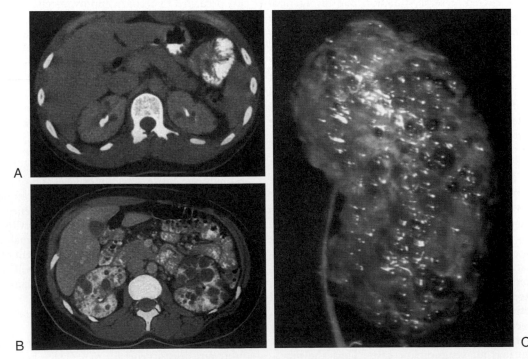

Figure 6-1 Cyst formation in autosomal dominant polycystic kidney disease is a sporadic and age-dependent process. Serial computed tomography scans from a *PKD1* patient showing several renal cysts at age 28 years (*A*) and numerous renal cysts of different sizes and one large liver cyst at age 42 years (*B*). Gross appearance of a severely enlarged polycystic kidney (*C*).

sources such as pain originating from musculoskeletal structures.[29] A small subset of patients with renal enlargement and structural distortion will develop chronic flank, back, or abdominal pain without a specifically identifiable etiology and they are at risk for analgesic dependency. Avoidance of aggravating activities complemented by a supportive attitude on the part of the physician and a multidisciplinary team approach for pain management that utilizes both pharmacologic (nonnarcotic and narcotic analgesics) and nonpharmacological (transcutaneous electrical nerve stimulation, acupuncture, and biofeedback) measures may be helpful.[29] However, surgical decompression may be appropriate in selected patients whose kidneys are grossly distorted by large cysts. This can be done by percutaneous puncture and drainage with alcohol sclerosis. However, the limitation of this approach is that only a few cysts can be drained, and pain recurrence is common. Alternatively, laparoscopic surgical deroofing can be associated with significant pain relief in up to 80% of patients.[30–32] In general, cyst decompression in these patients with moderate renal insufficiency (glomerular filtration rate [GFR] of ~50% or less) does not seem either to improve or impair renal function, but its long-term effects are not known.[30] Nephrectomy is sometimes indicated for patients with advanced renal insufficiency and intractable pain that is unresponsive to the above measures. In this setting, laparoscopic nephrectomy performed by a surgeon who is experienced in this technique may reduce the risk for operative complications.[32–34]

Hematuria

Gross hematuria in ADPKD is usually due to rupture of a cyst into the renal pelvis. It occurs in up to 40% of patients sometime during the course of their disease, and many of them will have recurrent episodes.[10] The differential diagnosis in this setting will include stone, infection, and tumor. If the cyst does not communicate with the collecting system, the patient may present with flank pain without hematuria. Additionally, fever can also occur with cyst hemorrhage, but cyst infection needs to be seriously considered. Occasionally, a ruptured hemorrhagic cyst can result in a severe retroperitoneal bleed, requiring blood transfusion. In this setting, treatment with desmopressin acetate (DDAVP) and aprotinin may be useful,[35] and transcatheter arterial embolization has been used in patients with recurrent and severe hemorrhage.[36] In most patients, however, cyst hemorrhage is self-limiting and generally resolves with supportive measures within 2 to 7 days. When gross hematuria is persistent for longer than 1 week, detailed radiologic investigations should be undertaken to exclude a renal tumor.

Proteinuria

Proteinuria is usually a minor feature of ADPKD since it is a tubular disorder. In one study of 270 patients with ADPKD, for example, only 18% of them excreted more than 300 mg of urinary protein per day. Even in patients with more advanced disease, the mean urinary protein excretion rate was only about 900 mg/day.[37] This observation suggests that secondary focal segmental glomerulosclerosis plays a relatively minor role in the progression of this disease to renal failure.[38] Nephrotic range proteinuria has been rarely reported with ADPKD and usually indicates a superimposed glomerular disease.[39]

Renal Infection

Infection is the second most common cause of death for patients with ADPKD.[28,40] Up to 50% of patients with ADPKD will have one or more episodes of renal infection during their lifetime.[41,42] As in the general population, renal infection will be more likely to occur in women than in men with ADPKD and is caused by gram-negative enteric organisms that ascend from the lower urinary tract. An infected cyst and acute pyelonephritis are the most common renal infections, which are associated with fever and flank pain, with or without bacteremia.[41] The differentiation between these two diagnoses is often difficult. The presence of white cell casts is suggestive of acute pyelonephritis, while identification of a new area of discrete flank tenderness supports the diagnosis of an infected cyst or cyst hemorrhage. Pyuria alone is not a useful laboratory finding since it can be seen in up to 45% of uninfected patients with ADPKD.[41] Radiologic investigations are generally not very helpful in this setting.

Treatment of an infected cyst is complicated by the fact that most renal cysts are not connected to a filtering glomerulus.[43] Thus, antimicrobials must enter the cyst via a mechanism other than glomerular filtration, and lipid-soluble antibiotics are preferable in achieving reliably high therapeutic concentrations within the cyst than water-soluble antibiotics. The major drugs that achieve therapeutic concentrations within the cysts and are active against common gram-negative enteric organisms include trimethoprim-sulfamethoxazole, quinolones, and chloramphenicol.[42] Both trimethoprim-sulfamethoxazole and quinolones are particularly useful since they can achieve high therapeutic concentrations with oral dosing. The optimal duration of treatment for an infected cyst is unclear, but 4 to 6 weeks of antimicrobial treatment may be reasonable. In a patient with recurrent renal infections who is being considered for a kidney transplant, surgical nephrectomy should be considered to minimize the risk of posttransplantation infection under immunosuppressive treatment.

Renal Calculi

Kidney stones occur in approximately 20% of patients with ADPKD.[44] In contrast to the predominance of calcium oxalate stones in the general population, more than 50% of the stones in patients with ADPKD are composed of uric acid, with the remainder due to calcium oxalate.[45] Distal acidification defects, abnormal ammonium transport, low urine pH, and hypocitraturia may be important in the pathogenesis of renal stones in ADPKD.[44,45] The possible presence of a kidney stone should be suspected in any ADPKD patient with acute flank pain. However, establishing the diagnosis by ultrasonography is more difficult because of the presence of large cysts and calcifications in the cyst walls. Most stones can be detected by intravenous pyelography, but CT scan is more sensitive in detecting small or radiolucent stones.[44]

The treatment of obstructing stones in ADPKD includes standard measures such as analgesics for pain relief and hydration to ensure adequate urine flow. However, it may be complicated by the presence of large renal cysts, which make percutaneous nephrostomy or extracorporeal shock-wave lithotripsy (ESWL) harder to perform. Despite this concern, ESWL has been used successfully in patients with small stones

(<2 cm in diameter) in the renal pelvis or calyces. For long-term prevention of recurrent kidney stones, thiazide diuretics may be used in the patients with hypercalciuria, and potassium citrate for patients with uric acid stones and stones associated with hypocitraturia or a distal acidification defect.[44,45]

Renal Cancer

Renal cell carcinoma is an infrequent complication of ADPKD and does not appear to occur with increased frequency compared with the general population.[28,46] However, in ADPKD these tumors are more often bilateral at presentation, multi-centric, and sarcomatoid in type. The diagnosis of renal cell carcinoma is often difficult to establish in ADPKD.[46] Findings such as hematuria and complex renal cysts from hemorrhage are common findings on radiologic imaging in the absence of malignancy. Systemic symptoms (fever, anorexia, fatigue, and weight loss) that are out of proportion with the severity of renal disease, in the absence of sepsis, or with rapid growth of a complex cyst should raise the suspicion for an underlying malignancy. Computed tomography (CT) scan and magnetic resonance imaging (MRI), with and without contrast enhancement, are often useful in distinguishing a malignancy from a complex cyst.[46] Percutaneous aspiration and cytologic examination can be performed on suspicious cysts. Nephrectomy of the involved kidney is indicated when the diagnosis of a non-metastatic renal cell carcinoma is confirmed.

Hypertension

Cardiovascular disease is the most common cause of death in patients with ADPKD.[40] Hypertension is a major modifiable risk factor for both cardiovascular and renal disease progression in ADPKD.[47] It affects 50% to 70% of patients with ADPKD and typically occurs before any significant reduction in GFR.[48–53] In a prospective study of 164 nonazotemic patients with ADPKD and 250 unaffected family members, 62% of patients were found to be hypertensive compared with 22% of their unaffected family members.[50] Similarly, in a longitudinal study of 154 children born with 50% risk for ADPKD, 22% of the clinically affected children were found to be hypertensive at the time of their diagnosis compared with 5% of their clinically unaffected siblings.[51] Additionally, an increased incidence of left ventricular mass was found in children and young adults with ADPKD and normal renal function, but not in their unaffected siblings.[52,53] This surrogate cardiovascular end point, however, could not be reliably predicted by blood pressure readings in the clinic.[52–55] Notably, approximately 20% of the normotensive (as defined by clinic blood pressure readings) patients with ADPKD were found to have left ventricular hypertrophy by echocardiography.[54] In a recent study of 26 young normotensive patients with ADPKD and 26 age- and gender-matched control subjects, 24-hour systolic blood pressure was found to be the only predictor of increased left ventricular mass by multivariate analysis. By contrast, although the absence of normal nocturnal fall of blood pressure was noted in many of the patients ("non-dippers"), it was not predictive of increased left ventricular mass.[55] Although the findings of this study are interesting, the clinical utility of ambulatory blood pressure monitoring in ADPKD remains uncertain at the present time. Further studies with larger patient sample size are required to evaluate the role of this novel technology in identifying high-risk patients for aggressive blood pressure control.

The pathogenesis of hypertension in ADPKD is not well defined. However, activation of the renin-angiotensin-aldosterone system resulting from cyst compression of blood vessels leading to renal ischemia has been proposed as a pathogenic mechanism for this complication.[49] This hypothesis is supported by the documentation of cyst compression of the renal blood vessels from angiographic studies[56] and activation of the renin-angiotensin system in volume-expanded patients at an early stage of ADPKD.[57–60] Additionally, advanced sclerosis of preglomerular arterioles, tubular atrophy, and interstitial fibrosis were pathologic features of ADPKD kidneys from patients with normal renal function or mild renal insufficiency. In these kidneys, global glomerulosclerosis, which is a pathologic feature of renal ischemia, was commonly observed, whereas focal segmental glomerulosclerosis, which is the typical lesion associated with hyperfiltration injury, was absent.[38] Moreover, the presence of renin-containing cells in the attenuated arteries of the cyst walls and surrounding stromal tissue of ADPKD kidneys had been documented by immunohistochemical studies, and active renin was present within the cyst fluid as well.[61] More recently, activation of an intrarenal renin-angiotensin system within the cysts and dilated tubules was documented by a comprehensive study of kidneys from patients with ADPKD.[62] Other mechanisms may contribute to the genesis of hypertension in ADPKD, and they include an increased sympathetic nerve activity and impaired endothelial-dependent relaxation of small resistant blood vessels.[63,64]

Although blood pressure control is of critical importance in reducing renal disease progression and cardiovascular complications in ADPKD, only 30% of patients with well-preserved renal function were found to achieve a target blood pressure below 150/90 mmHg.[65] This degree of blood pressure control is similar to that found in patients with essential hypertension in the National Health and Nutrition Examination Surveys (NHANES) III in the United States.[66] However, with an extensive education program targeting both patients with ADPKD and their primary care physicians, it is possible to improve the rate of blood pressure control to approximately 60%.[65] Nonetheless, evidence-based recommendations for blood pressure treatment in ADPKD are lacking.[49] In particular, it is currently unclear what target range of blood pressure control is most optimal in reducing end-organ damage for this disease. In the Modification of Diet in Renal Disease (MDRD) study, which included 200 patients with ADPKD, aggressive blood pressure control did not affect the rate of loss of GFR compared with standard blood pressure control. However, the average difference of mean arterial blood pressure between aggressive and standard treatment groups was only 4.7 mmHg, instead of the planned target difference of 15 mmHg. Additionally, the study was performed in ADPKD patients with moderately advanced renal disease (GFR <55 mL/min) and with a short duration of follow-up of 2.2 years.[67] In a recent study, 72 ADPKD patients with preserved renal function (creatinine clearance >80 mL/min) were randomized to receive rigorous (<120/80 mmHg) or standard (135–140/85–90 mmHg) blood pressure control, and a mean arterial blood pressure difference of 10 mmHg was achieved between the two study groups over a 7-year period. In spite of this difference, rigorous blood pressure control was associated with a reduction of left ventricular mass ($P < 0.01$), but not with a slower rate of loss of renal function.[68] None of the few available randomized controlled trials conducted in ADPKD to date, however, were designed with adequate power to test the effects of blood pressure control on renal disease progression. It is important to note that more vigorous blood pressure control may not necessarily mean greater clinical benefits. Indeed, a recent meta-analysis of 11 randomized controlled blood pressure trials in nonproteinuric renal diseases suggests that while a systolic blood pressure goal of 110 to 129 mmHg may be beneficial for patients with proteinuria of greater than 1 g/day, lowering of systolic blood pressure to less than 110 mmHg may increase the risk for kidney disease progression.[69] This is particularly relevant for patients with moderate to advanced ADPKD, who are treated with an angiotensin-converting enzyme (ACE) inhibitor or angiotensin receptor blocker (ARB). Acute reversible renal failure has been reported in this setting and may result from the disruption of renal autoregulation via a mechanism similar to that seen in bilateral renal artery stenosis.[70] Recent randomized controlled trials have also shown that pharmacologic interruption of the renin-angiotensin axis confers a class-specific advantage in retarding the progression of both diabetic and nondiabetic proteinuric kidney diseases, and this benefit is most evident in patients with significant proteinuria (2 or more g/day).[69,71,72] However, whether the renoprotective effects of ACE inhibitors or ARBs can be extended to patients with nondiabetic kidney disease with low-grade proteinuria (<1 g/day) is currently unclear.[69] This is relevant for patients with ADPKD, since most of them will not have proteinuria of greater than 0.5 g/day. In a recent meta-analysis of 142 ADPKD patients from randomized controlled trials of nondiabetic kidney disease, treatment with an ACE inhibitor was associated with a small but significant reduction of proteinuria. However, the effect of this therapy on renal disease progression in ADPKD was inconclusive.[73] Until more definitive data are available, it is reasonable to use the guidelines from the seventh report of the Joint National Committee on Prevention, Detection, Evaluation, and Treatment of High Blood Pressure (JNC VII report) for blood pressure management of patients with ADPKD.[74]

Renal Disease Progression

Although ADPKD can present as early as in utero, its progression to ESRD typically occurs in late middle age. In general, considerable inter- and intrafamilial renal disease variability has been well documented.[13,75–80] The probability of ESRD in patients with ADPKD has been estimated to be less than 5% in those younger than 40 years, 25% to 40% by 50 years, 50% to 65% by 60 years, and 60% to 80% by 70 years.[13,47,75,76] Clinically, the most important risk factors for renal disease progression in ADPKD are the PKD1 genotype (see later section on Gene Locus Effect) and age.[13,75,76] Additional risk factors include early diagnosis of ADPKD, hypertension, gross hematuria, multiple pregnancies, and large kidney size.[47,81–86] A gender effect with milder renal disease favoring the female patients is also evident for type 2, but not type 1, ADPKD.[13,75,79,80] By contrast, uninephrectomy in patients with moderately advanced disease (GFR ~50% of normal) did not appear to accelerate the progression of ADPKD.[87]

Extrarenal Manifestations

Polycystic Liver Disease

Polycystic liver disease is the most common extrarenal complication of ADPKD and is associated with both PKD1 and PKD2 genotypes. Hepatic cysts are derived from the biliary epithelia and are commonly found in patients with advanced renal disease. The incidence of hepatic cysts in ADPKD increases from approximately 10% in patients younger than 30 years to greater than 40% in patients older than 60 years.[88,89] Polycystic liver disease associated with ADPKD should be differentiated from autosomal dominant polycystic liver disease (ADPLD), another monogenic disorder due to mutations of at least three distinct genes[90,91] (see Chapter 7). In contrast to ADPKD, patients with ADPLD have few or no renal cysts and are not at risk for progressive renal failure.[90]

Although the incidence of polycystic liver disease in patients with ADPKD is similar between men and women, massive polycystic liver disease occurs almost exclusively in women, particularly those with multiple pregnancies.[88] An increased sensitivity to the growth effects of estrogen has been proposed as a mechanism for massive polycystic liver disease, although other unidentified factors are likely involved in patients with this extreme phenotype.[92,93] Most ADPKD patients with polycystic liver disease will remain asymptomatic with preserved hepatic function. Occasionally, they may experience focal complications such as cyst infection and hemorrhage. Rarely, some patients with severe polycystic liver disease will experience symptoms of a "mass effect" (such as abdominal pain, dyspnea, orthopnea, early satiety, and gastroesophageal reflux), hepatic venous outflow obstruction, and inferior vena caval compression. The treatment of these symptomatic patients includes cyst aspiration with alcohol sclerosis, cyst fenestration, partial liver resection, and liver transplantation.[89,93]

Intracranial Arterial Aneurysms

Ruptured intracranial aneurysm is a rare but devastating complication of ADPKD.[28] Based on three prospective studies, the prevalence of asymptomatic intracranial aneurysm (ICA) in ADPKD has been estimated to be 8%, which is four to five times higher than that seen in the general population.[94–97] Familial clustering of ICA is documented in ADPKD, and the risk for asymptomatic ICA is approximately 20% in patients with a positive family history, compared with approximately 5% in those with a negative family history.[98,99] This complication has been noted in both PKD1 and PKD2.[100,101] Although the cause of ICA in ADPKD is unknown, both PC1 and PC2 (gene products of PKD1 and PKD2, respectively) are highly expressed within arterial smooth muscle cells and myofibroblasts.[102,103] Thus, reduced expression of normal PC in these cells in ADPKD may play a pathogenic role. Indeed, reduced PC2 expression to about half of its normal level in the vascular smooth muscle cells of heterozygous Pkd2 knockout mice (compared with their wild-type littermates) was associated with altered intracellular calcium signaling in vitro.[104] Nonetheless, the relevance of this observation to the pathogenesis of ICA is unclear, and additional factors may be required to explain the focal nature of this complication.

The natural history of ICA in ADPKD remains unclear. The incidence of ruptured ICA in patients with ADPKD is estimated to be approximately 1 in 2,000 person-years, a rate five times higher than that in the general population.[105,106] Given that the prevalence of asymptomatic ICA in ADPKD is also about five times higher than that in the general population,[94–97] the risk for ruptured ICA in ADPKD is comparable with that in the general population. The mean age of rupture of ICA in ADPKD patients is approximately 40 years, which is similar to that observed in other familial forms of ICA, but occurs approximately 10 years earlier than in the general population.[98,105–107] At the time of rupture, half of patients with ICA have normal renal function and 25% of them have normal blood pressure. The middle cerebral artery is usually involved, and one in three patients will have multiple aneurysms. Although it is unclear if hypertension and cigarette smoking are independent risk factors, a family history of ICA is a risk factor of aneurysm rupture in ADPKD.[108]

Clinically, ruptured ICA results in subarachnoid hemorrhage (SAH) and is associated with a sudden and severe headache, often described as "a blow or explosion inside the head" or the "worst headache ever." The headache is often diffuse and may radiate to the occipital or cervical region. However, minor SAH can cause less severe and diffuse headache. In 20% to 50% of patients, a series of "warning headaches" may precede the index episode of bleeding.[109,110] Other symptoms or signs of SAH include nausea and vomiting, photophobia, neck stiffness, lethargy, seizures, and focal neurologic deficits. Noncontrast CT scan is generally used as the first diagnostic test. If SAH is strongly suspected but not confirmed by CT scan, a lumbar puncture should also be performed. The presence of bloody cerebrospinal fluid unrelated to a traumatic tap is indicative of SAH. In such case, emergency neurosurgical consultation is indicated, and four-vessel angiography or CT angiography is indicated to localize the site of rupture.[108] The classical intervention is surgical clipping of the aneurysm, although endovascular embolization has emerged as a promising alternative, especially for older patients.[111,112] Despite these interventions, the morbidity and mortality rates are 35% and 55%, respectively, once an ICA is ruptured.[98,107] Additionally, survivors of a ruptured ICA are at risk for recurrent ICA at the original site or a new site. In a small prospective study of 11 ADPKD patients with ruptured ICA, repeat screening showed that 36% of them either had an increased size of the original ICA or developed a new ICA after a mean follow-up of 15 years. However, all the recurrent ICAs were small (<6 mm in diameter) and none ruptured.[113] In general, any additional intact ICA detected at the time of rupture should be treated whenever feasible, and serial screening of ICA in these patients with MRI or spiral CT scan at intervals of 2 to 3 years is recommended.[108]

The role of radiologic screening for ICA in asymptomatic patients with ADPKD remains unclear and depends on a comparison between the risk (morbidity and mortality) for untreated ICAs and that associated with the screening procedures and subsequent therapeutic interventions, if indicated. Currently, MR angiography (MRA) is the screening test of choice since it is safe and highly sensitive in detecting ICAs greater than 3 mm in diameter. By comparison, conventional intra-arterial angiography, which is still necessary before a therapeutic intervention, carries a 5% risk for complications (including a 0.5% risk for permanent neurologic deficit).[108] The difficulty in recommending screening is that most ICAs detected in this setting are small (<6 mm in diameter) and are presumed to be at low risk for rupture.[114] Moreover, there is an appreciable risk for severe neurologic complications following elective aneurysm surgery.[108] In the International Study of Unruptured Intracranial Aneurysms (ISUIA), a large cohort of patients with at least one unruptured ICA were prospectively followed, with 1,692 patients treated conservatively, 1,917 patients treated with surgical clipping, and 451 patients treated with endovascular embolization.[115] The 5-year cumulative rupture rates depend on the size and location of the ICA (Table 6-2). In patients with asymptomatic ICAs of less than 7 mm and no previous history of SAH, the rupture rate is very low (~0.1% per year), and accordingly, it would be difficult to improve the natural history of these lesions. Importantly, a family history of rupture did not increase the risk in this group. By contrast, in patients with ICAs of the anterior circulation greater than 7 mm and in patients with ICAs of the posterior circulation, the 5-year cumulative rupture rates were higher, but were often equaled or exceeded by the risks associated with surgical or endovascular repair. In patients without previous SAH, the total morbidity and mortality rates at 1 year were approximately 10% with surgical clipping and approximately 9% with endovascular repair. Age was an important predictor of adverse surgical outcome, with a substantial increase in risk for those older than 50 years. Whether the very low risk for rupture in small ICAs found in this study can be extrapolated to patients with ADPKD is unclear. In a recent prospective study of ADPKD patients with an initial negative screen for ICAs, only approximately 3% (2/76) of them developed an ICA on repeat screening after a mean follow-up of 9.8 years, and none of these patients had a rupture. One of these patients without a family history of ICA developed a 2-mm ICA 11 years after his initial screen. A second patient with a positive family history of ICA developed a 10-mm vertebral artery aneurysm, a 10-mm internal carotid artery aneurysm, and a 4-mm middle cerebral artery aneurysm 9.6 years after her initial screen.[115] Notably, a family history of ruptured ICA in two or more affected family members was present in 20% (15/72) of these patients. Similarly, in another prospective study, 21 ADPKD patients with a previously documented asymptomatic ICA underwent repeat MRA screening over a mean follow-up period of approximately 7 years. Only approximately 10% of them developed an increased size of the original ICA or a new ICA, and none of these small ICAs detected on repeat screening (<6 mm in diameter) ruptured.[114] Based on these data, it appears that most ICAs detected by presymptomatic screening in ADPKD patients are small and their risk for rupture is similar to those ICAs seen in the general population. Currently, several experts have recommended that presymptomatic screening of ICAs should be restricted to ADPKD patients with a positive family history of ICAs. In these individuals, serial screening with MRA at 5-year intervals may be adequate.[108,114,115]

Other Vascular Abnormalities

In addition to ICAs, patients with ADPKD may have diffuse arterial dolichoectasias of the anterior and posterior cerebral circulation, which can predispose to arterial dissection and stroke. Aggressive management of hypertension in these patients should be instituted to reduce the risk for dissection.[116,117] There are rare reports of PKD1-linked families in which ADPKD co-segregated with a Marfan-like syndrome and some of the affected members suffered dissection of the aorta

Table 6-2 Five-Year Cumulative Rupture Rates for Asymptomatic Patients with Intracranial Aneurysms

Size of Aneurysm	Site of Aneurysm*	
	Anterior Circulation	Posterior Circulation
< 7 mm	0%	2.5%
7–12 mm	2.6%	14.5%
13–24 mm	14.5%	18.4%
> 25 mm	40%	50%

*The sites of ICAs in the anterior circulation include those in the internal carotid artery, anterior communicating artery, anterior cerebral artery, and middle cerebral artery. The sites of intracranial aneurysms in the posterior circulation include the posterior communicating artery and the arteries in the posterior circulation.
Data derived from the International Study of Unruptured Intracranial Aneurysms (Lancet 362:103–110, 2003).

and other large vessels.[118,119] A recent prospective study, however, found that there was no increase in frequency of abdominal aortic aneurysms in ADPKD patients compared with their unaffected relatives.[120]

Valvular Heart Disease

Mitral valve prolapse is the most common abnormality detected by cardiac echocardiography in up to 30% of patients with ADPKD. Other valvular abnormalities, including mitral sufficiency, aortic insufficiency, tricuspid insufficiency, and tricuspid valve prolapse, also occurred more frequently in patients with ADPKD than their unaffected relatives. Pathologically, valvular tissue in these patients is affected by myxoid degeneration. These findings are consistent with the notion that ADPKD is a systemic connective tissue disorder.[121,122] Most patients are asymptomatic, but an occasional patient may have severe disease requiring valve replacement. Antibiotic prophylaxis is recommended for patients with audible murmurs.

Other Connective Tissue Abnormalities

Colonic diverticulae were found in approximately 80% (10/12) of patients with ADPKD on renal replacement therapy in a retrospective study.[123] By contrast, a more recent study of 55 non-ESRD patients did not show an increased prevalence of diverticular disease in these patients compared to a control group of 71 unaffected family members and randomly selected patients undergoing barium enemas.[124] Based on a recent retrospective review, the prevalence of abdominal wall herniae was increased in 45% (38/85) of patients with ADPKD compared with 8% (7/85) of age- and gender-matched patients with other renal disease.[125] Patients with ADPKD treated with continuous ambulatory peritoneal dialysis are at increased risk for developing an indirect inguinal hernia.[126]

DIAGNOSIS AND MONITORING OF RENAL DISEASE

The diagnosis of overt ADPKD is generally straightforward. Affected patients typically present with enlarged kidneys with multiple cysts bilaterally and a positive family history consistent with autosomal dominant inheritance. Additional

clinical features include the absence of symptoms and signs suggestive of other syndromic forms of renal cystic disease (see Table 6-2), the presence of liver and other extrarenal cysts, and cardiac valve abnormality such as mitral valve prolapse. However, ADPKD will occasionally present very early within the first years of life and may be confused with autosomal recessive polycystic kidney disease (ARPKD) and renal cystic dysplasia. In this setting, the presence of a positive family history and larger renal cyst size will help to differentiate ADPKD from ARPKD, and the presence of malformations and ureteral obstruction will help to differentiate renal cystic dysplasia from ADPKD.[127,128] Additionally, a family history may be absent in 10% to 30% of new patients in whom the diagnosis of ADPKD is first suspected from imaging studies performed to evaluate otherwise unexplained hematuria, abdominal mass, flank pain, or renal insufficiency.[28] In these cases, the finding of ADPKD can be due to a de novo mutation[129] or, more likely, ascertainment of a small PKD2 family with mild renal disease, which is often underdiagnosed.[13] In the latter case, ultrasound examination of both parents may demonstrate multiple renal cysts in one parent. In the case when one or both parents are deceased, review of autopsy reports (if available) may be helpful.

Differential Diagnosis of Renal Cystic Disorders

Renal cysts can be a manifestation of both syndromic and nonsyndromic renal cystic disorders other than ADPKD (Table 6-3).[130] A careful review of the history, clinical examination, and radiologic examination may reveal clinical features of these disorders that are atypical of ADPKD. For example, tuberous sclerosis (TSC) is an autosomal dominant disorder that is frequently associated with seizures, mental retardation, and several characteristic skin lesions (facial angiofibromas, periungual fibroma, hypomelanotic macules, and Shagreen patch). Additionally, the co-existence of renal cysts with angiomyolipomas is pathognomonic of this disorder.[131] However, these clinical features may not be present at the time of diagnosis of the renal cystic disease. Moreover, a rare contiguous gene syndrome has been reported due to gross deletion of both PKD1 and TSC2, which lie in close proximity on chromosome 16p13.3.[132,133] Patients with this syndrome typically present with bilaterally enlarged polycystic kidneys during infancy and progress to ESRD within the first

Table 6-3 Differential Diagnosis of Autosomal Dominant Polycystic Kidney Disease (ADPKD)

Renal Cystic Disorder	Prevalence	Clinical Findings Not Found in ADPKD
Syndromic		
Tuberous sclerosis	~1:10,000	Skin lesions (facial angiofibromas, periungual fibroma, hypomelanotic macules, Shagreen patch); retinal hamartomas; seizures; mental retardation; cortical tuber; subependymal giant cell astrocytoma; cardiac rhabdomyoma; lymphangioleiomyomatosis; renal angiomyolipoma. Contiguous deletion of *PKD1* and *TSC2* results in severe polycystic kidney disease in infancy or early childhood with ESRD typically occurring in the first two decades of life.
Von Hippel-Lindau syndrome	~1:50,000	Central nervous system and retinal hemangioblastoma; pancreatic cysts; pheochromocytoma; renal cell carcinoma occurs in 25%–45% of patients; papillary cystadenoma of epididymis.
Medullary sponge kidney	~1:5,000	Medullary nephrocalcinosis; "paintbrush" appearance of renal papillae on intravenous pyelogram.
Oro-facio-digital syndrome	Very rare	Lethal in affected males; oral anomalies (hyperplastic frenula, cleft tongue, cleft palate or lip, and malposed teeth); facial anomalies (broad nasal root with hypoplasia of nasal alae and malar bones), and digital anomalies.
Nonsyndromic		
Simple renal cysts	Common	Rare under 30 years, but increase in number with age.
Acquired renal cystic disease	Common	Chronic renal insufficiency or ESRD with multiple renal cysts associated with normal-sized or small kidneys.

ESRD, end-stage renal disease.

two decades of life. Clinical features suggestive of tuberous sclerosis were absent in 30% (5/17) of patients, some of whom were mistakenly diagnosed to have ADPKD.[133]

Von Hippel-Lindau syndrome is an autosomal dominant disorder that is associated with retinal and central nervous system hemangioblastomas, renal cell carcinoma, pheochromocytoma, and papillary cystadenomas of the epididymis. The presence of any of these tumors with renal cysts should therefore raise the suspicion of this disorder. Additionally, the presence of multiple pancreatic cysts is rarely found in ADPKD, but is highly characteristic of this disorder. In the absence of solid tumors and pancreatic cysts, however, the renal findings in Von Hippel-Lindau syndrome may mimic that of ADPKD.[134] Medullary sponge kidney is a common developmental disorder characterized by dilated medullary and papillary collecting ducts that give the renal medulla a "spongy" appearance. It is also frequently associated with other congenital defects (e.g., congenital hemi-hypertrophy, Beckwith-Wiedemann syndrome, Ehler-Danlos syndrome, and Marfan syndrome). The main clinical manifestations of this disorder include multiple renal cysts, hematuria, and calcium oxalate renal stones. Medullary nephrocalcinosis is a frequent radiologic feature of this disorder, and on intravenous pyelography, a characteristic "paintbrush" appearance of the renal papillae is seen. Another syndromic renal cystic disorder that can be confused with ADPKD is oro-facio-digital syndrome type 1, a rare X-linked dominant disorder, which is lethal in males. Affected females may have polycystic kidneys that are indistinguishable from ADPKD, as well as liver cysts. However, the presence of oral, facial, and digital anomalies will help to pinpoint the correct diagnosis of this disorder.[128]

Simple renal cysts and acquired renal cystic disease are two common nonsyndromic cystic disorders that may be confused with ADPKD.[135–137] Simple renal cysts are the most common cystic disorder and increase with age in the general population. The prevalence of individuals with one or more simple renal cysts has been estimated to be 0 to 0.22% in those younger than 30 years, approximately 2% in those 30 to 49 years, 11.5% in those 50 to 70 years, and 22% in those older than 70 years.[135,136] Although the presence of simple renal cysts in a subject at 50% risk for ADPKD can lead to a false-positive diagnosis, ultrasonographic diagnostic criteria with increasing stringency in the older subjects have been developed, which performed well in predicting type 1 ADPKD (see below).[138] Acquired renal cystic disease is a common disorder observed in 7% of patients with chronic kidney disease and approximately 20% of patients with ESRD. Despite the presence of multiple renal cysts bilaterally with varying degree of renal insufficiency, the size of the kidneys in this disorder is either normal or small.[137] By contrast, the presence of chronic kidney insufficiency in ADPKD generally denotes advanced disease and is typically associated with large polycystic kidneys several times the normal size. An algorithm for the diagnostic evaluation of ADPKD is shown in Figure 6-2.

Diagnosis of ADPKD by Renal Imaging

Renal ultrasonography is currently widely used for presymptomatic screening of at-risk subjects and for evaluation of potential living-related kidney donors from ADPKD families. Using DNA linkage results as the "gold standard" for disease assignment, age-dependent ultrasonographic diagnostic criteria with high sensitivity and specificity have been derived for individuals born with 50% risk from PKD1 families (Table 6-4).[138] Among at-risk subjects 15 to 29 years of age, the presence of *at least two renal cysts (unilateral or bilateral)* is

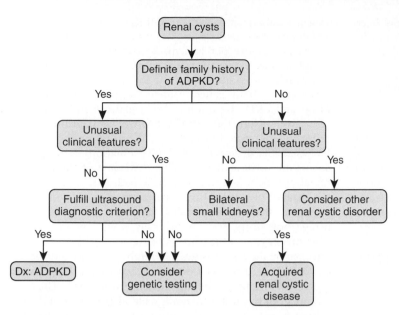

Figure 6-2 Diagnostic algorithm for autosomal dominant polycystic kidney disease. (Adapted from Pei Y: Diagnostic approach in autosomal dominant polycystic kidney disease. Clin J Am Soc Nephrol 1:1108–1114, 2006.)

Table 6-4 Performance Characteristics of Ultrasound Diagnostic Criteria for PKD1 Subjects Born with 50% Risk for Autosomal Dominant Polycystic Kidney Disease

Age Group (years)	Diagnostic Criterion	SEN (%)	SPEC (%)	NPV (%)	PPV (%)
15–29	At least 2 renal cysts (unilateral or bilateral)	~96	100	~97	100
30–59	At least 2 cysts in each kidney	100	100	100	100
60 or older	Four or more cysts in each kidney	100	100	100	100

Data derived from Ravine D, et al: Evaluation of ultrasonographic diagnostic criteria for autosomal dominant polycystic kidney disease 1. Lancet 343:824–827, 1994.
SEN, sensitivity; SPEC, specificity; NPV and PPV, negative and positive predictive value, respectively.

sufficient for diagnosis. This is because simple renal cysts are rare in this age group, making the finding of any renal cyst highly specific for ADPKD. By contrast, more stringent criteria are required for the older age groups because of increasing prevalence of simple renal cysts. Thus, among at-risk subjects 30 to 59 years of age and 60 years or older, the presence of *at least two cysts in each kidney* and *at least four cysts in each kidney*, respectively, are required for the diagnosis. Conversely, in subjects 30 to 59 years of age, the absence of *at least two cysts in each kidney*, which is associated with a false-negative rate of 0%, can be used for disease exclusion.

While the above PKD1 diagnostic criteria are widely used for genetic counseling and for the evaluation of at-risk subjects as living-related kidney donors to their affected relatives, the underlying genotype of most test subjects is seldom known in the clinic setting. Given that PKD2 is a much milder disease,[13,75] the validity of these diagnostic criteria for at-risk subjects of unknown genotype has not been well defined. To address this issue, a multicenter study has recently compared the performance of various ultrasonographic diagnostic criteria in a large cohort of at-risk subjects with PKD1 and PKD2 using their genotype as the "gold-standard" for disease assignment.[139] This study showed that the current diagnostic criteria used for PKD1 maintained high specificity, but suffered from reduced sensitivity (increased false-negative rate) in PKD2. Thus, the commonly used PKD1 criteria are expected

to perform well for diagnosing PKD2. However, further refinement of the current criterion is required for exclusion of PKD2. By simulations, this study also evaluated a number of diagnostic criteria using replicates of PKD1 and PKD2 patients to mimic the case mix seen in clinical practice. From this study, it is expected that a set of refined diagnostic criteria with high sensitivity and specificity will be available in the near future for the evaluation of at-risk subjects from families of undefined ADPKD gene type.

Both CT scan and MRI, with and without contrast enhancement, have been used for diagnosis of ADPKD, generally in the setting when ultrasonography is equivocal.[10,140] These imaging modalities, with improved resolution, can detect cysts of smaller size than ultrasonography. The major disadvantages of CT scan include the risk for exposure to radiation and radiocontrast, which can be associated with a small chance of serious allergic reactions and nephrotoxicity in patients with renal insufficiency. By comparison, MRI, with gadolinium as a contrast agent, has minimal renal toxicity. This agent provides the same information as iodinated compounds do with respect to tubular function and parenchymal volume. Heavy-weighted T2 images also permit the detection of cysts only 2 to 3 mm in diameter with great certainty.[10] Its safety and enhanced sensitivity thus make it a promising imaging modality for ADPKD.[140] However, MRI will likely detect both small simple cysts as well as small cysts arising from ADPKD. Thus, until its diagnostic utility has been formally evaluated as in ultrasonography, it should not be used as the initial imaging modality for diagnosis of ADPKD.

Diagnosis of ADPKD by Genetic Testing

The localization of their gene loci followed by detailed characterization of the genomic structures of *PKD1* and *PKD2* has provided all the essential reagents required for molecular diagnosis of this disease.[7,8,16–19,141,142] Both DNA linkage analysis and gene-based mutation screening can be used for this purpose. As discussed earlier, presymptomatic diagnosis of ADPKD is typically performed by renal ultrasonography. However, there is a role for molecular diagnosis, especially in patients with equivocal imaging results, in those with a negative family history, and in cases when younger at-risk subjects with a negative ultrasound study are being evaluated as potential living-related kidney donors.

DNA Linkage Analysis

This family-based analysis requires both genotype and phenotype data from multiple affected and unaffected members, and the at-risk subject being tested.[138] Typically, polymorphic simple-sequence repeat markers flanking both the *PKD1* and *PKD2* loci are genotyped in the study subjects, and previously affected individuals are used to establish linkage phase in the at-risk subject. Linkage analysis then provides a statistical inference on the likelihood that a specific marker allele co-segregates with the disease. For clinical testing, Bayesian statistical algorithms are used to provide a probability estimate of linkage of the family to a disease locus. When the flanking polymorphic markers are informative, the inheritance of a disease allele can be inferred in an at-risk subject with an error of less than 1%. The major advantage of this method is that when a large family with multiple affected members is available, it is almost always possible to determine whether the test subject is an obligate disease carrier. On the other hand, gene linkage testing requires blood sampling and renal imaging from multiple individuals. It is not expected to be informative in small families or in de novo ADPKD.

Gene-Based Mutation Screening

Despite the challenges imposed by the complexity and size of *PKD1*, mutation screening of the entire coding sequence and splice junctions of both *PKD1* and *PKD2* from DNA templates have now been developed, allowing for comprehensive screening of these genes.[18] To date, approximately 200 different *PKD1* and over 50 *PKD2* mutations have been reported, with most of them predicted to truncate the mutant protein (due to frameshift deletions and insertions, nonsense mutations, or splice defects).[18,80,141–143] Most of these mutations are unique to a single family and scattered throughout these genes with no clear "hot-spots." Thus, exon-by-exon screening of these genes is required to ensure a high sensitivity in detecting disease-causing mutations.

To define the sensitivity of the gene-based diagnosis of ADPKD, mutation screening of both *PKD1* and *PKD2* by denaturing high-performance liquid chromatography (DHPLC) followed by sequencing of PCR fragments with altered DHPLC profiles was performed in a recent study of 45 genetically uncharacterized ADPKD patients.[18] In general, a high rate of missense mutations was detected in *PKD1*, with an average of five per patient. By contrast, only two polymorphisms were detected in the entire patient cohort. Despite a comprehensive screening of the coding sequence and splice junctions of both genes, protein-truncating mutations in *PKD1* and *PKD2* were found in 26 patients and 3 patients, respectively. Thus, the overall sensitivity for detecting a definitive mutation was 64% (29/45). The reasons for the relatively low sensitivity in detecting definitive mutations in this patient cohort are unclear. It is possible that some of the missense mutations identified may in fact be pathogenic. However, in the absence of a valid functional assay, it is difficult to differentiate the disease-causing missense mutations from benign polymorphisms. Additionally, mutations in the gene promoter region, which may affect gene expression, are not screened by the above assays. Currently, gene-based diagnosis of ADPKD is available commercially (Athena Diagnostics, Worcester, MA; http://www.athenadiagnostics.com). The main advantage of this test is that only a blood sample from the test subject is required. On the other hand, it is expensive, and although the sensitivity data for detecting definitive mutations have not been published by the company, a definitive mutation is likely found in no more than approximately two-thirds of the test subjects. Thus, this screen is only useful when the result is positive.

Monitoring Renal Disease Progression

Recent advances in radiologic imaging have made it feasible to examine the renal structural-functional relationship in ADPKD. Using serial ultrasonography, CT scan, or MRI with three-dimensional image reconstruction, these studies provided measures of total kidney size, cystic and noncystic kidney volumes, and noncystic renal parenchymal volume in patients with ADPKD.[83–86] In patients with early or established ADPKD, MRI with three-dimensional image reconstruction appears to provide both a sensitive and accurate measure of renal disease progression. This technique was recently evaluated by the Consortium for Radiological Imaging Studies of Polycystic Kidney Disease (CRISP) in a large multicenter study in which 241 patients 15 to 45 years of age with creatinine clearances greater than 70 mL/min underwent standardized renal MRI, renal iothalamate clearance, and comprehensive clinical evaluation annually for 3 years.[85] In this study, MRI provided reliable and reproducible measurements of total kidney volume, renal cyst and parenchymal volumes, and renal blood flow.[85,86] Inverse correlations were noted in the study cohort between renal structural parameters (total kidney volume and total cyst volume) and function (GFR), although the multivariate coefficient of determination (R^2) of these correlations was only approximately 10%. Older age, hypertension, and higher albumin excretion rate were associated with greater total kidney and renal cyst volumes.[85] Renal blood flow was found to be a significant predictor of GFR, with an R^2 of approximately 25%.[86]

The CRISP study has also documented that changes in total cyst volume and total kidney volume in the study patients were highly correlated ($R^2 = 0.9$) and that both of these measures increased exponentially with time, consistent with an expansion process dependent on growth.[144] Importantly, while the baseline total kidney volume predicted the subsequent rate of increase in kidney volume, decline in GFR was only observed in patients with larger kidneys. Specifically, patients with baseline total kidney volumes of less than 750 mL (or approximately three times the normal size) had a stable GFR over the 3 years of observation. By contrast, patients with baseline total kidney volumes of 750 to 1,500 mL and greater than 1,500 mL had a mean rate of GFR decline of 0.7 and 4.3 mL/min/year, respectively. These findings are consistent with the clinical observation that ADPKD patients with profound distortion of renal structures and significant enlargement of the polycystic kidneys can still have relatively normal GFR. Presumably, renal compensatory mechanisms (resulting in increased single-nephron GFR) exist in these individuals that mitigate the loss of total GFR and mask the progressive destruction of renal structures by the cystic disease in early stages of ADPKD. Reduction in GFR, therefore, is not a sensitive measure of renal disease progression in this disease and reflects relative late events when the renal compensatory mechanisms have been exhausted.[10] Based on these findings, kidney volume progression has now been adapted as a primary end point for three recently launched clinical trials in ADPKD (see discussions below of the HALT, Tolvaptan, and Rapamycin trials).

MOLECULAR AND CELL BIOLOGY OF ADPKD

PC1 and PC2 belong to the polycystin family of integral membrane proteins, which has nine known members and can be divided into two subfamilies based on protein structure and putative function: PC1-like receptor-like molecules that includes PC1, polycystin REJ, polycystin-1L1, polycystin-1L2 and polycystin-1L3; and PC2-like ion channels that includes PC2, polycystin-L, and polycystin-2L2 (Table 6-5).

PC1 is an approximately 4,300-residue receptor-like molecule (Fig. 6-3) with a large extracellular N-terminal domain that contains a number of adhesive domains, 11 transmembrane domains,[145] and a C-terminal cytoplasmic domain of approximately 200 amino acids.[16,17] The leucine-rich repeats and a C-type lectin domain within the N terminus can bind to extracellular components such as collagen I and laminin fragments in vitro.[146,147] There are 14 copies of a novel PKD domain that has homology to immunoglobin-like domains. These domains are likely involved in Ca^{2+}-dependent homophilic interactions.[148] Following these PKD domains is a large approximately 600–amino acid domain, the so-called REJ domain, which shares homology with the receptor of egg jelly in sea urchins.[149] Some evidence suggests that PC1 is cleaved near the GPS domain,[150] a cleavage site found in G protein–coupled receptors (GPCRs). The C-terminal tail of PC1 contains a coiled coil domain that binds to PC2,[151,152] a G protein activation sequence that binds to G proteins.[153–155] It also associates with the regulators of G-protein signaling (RGS proteins).[156] PC1 has a number of phosphorylation sites.[157,158] It is phosphorylated by cyclic adenosine monophosphate (cAMP)–dependent protein kinase A, but not protein kinase C in vitro.[159] Phosphorylation of PC1 is increased in ADPKD cells with putative defective PC1 function.[160] In cultured cells, PC1 appears to associate with the focal adhesion proteins talin, vinculin, p130Cas, FAK, α-actinin, paxillin, and pp60c-src,[158] and with intermediate filaments.[161]

PC2 is a 968-residue protein with six transmembrane domains and a pore region[19,162] (see Fig. 6-3). It was initially identified by its homology with PC1.[162] It shares sequence homology with the transient receptor potential (TRP) family and with Na^+ and K^+ channels, and has been considered as a member of the TRP channel superfamily, named TRPP2.[163] It has a long extracellular loop between the first two transmembrane domains that contains a polycystin motif, conserved in all polycystins.[164] Both N- and C-terminal domains of PC2 are located intracellularly. The C-terminal domain of PC2 contains a Ca^{2+}-binding EF-hand that is important in channel

Table 6-5 Polycystin Protein Family

Protein	Gene	Chromosome Locus	Expression	G-Protein Binding/ Activation	Pore-forming	Reference
PC1-like						
Polycystin-1	PKD1	16p13.3	Widespread	+	−	17,16,154,155
Polycystin-REJ	PKDREJ	22q13	Testis	n.d.	n.d.	309
Polycystin-1L1	PKD1L1	16p12-13	Relatively widespread with higher levels in heart, testis	+	n.d.	310
Polycystin-1L2	PKD1L2	16q23	Relatively widespread with higher levels in heart, testis	+	n.d.	311,312
Polycystin-1L3	PKD1L3	16q22	Relatively widespread, but not in skeletal muscle	n.d.	n.d.	312
PC2-like						
Polycystin-2	PKD2	4q21-23	Widespread	n.d.	+	19,162
Polycystin-L	PKDL	10q24-25	Relatively widespread	n.d.	+	164,231
Polycystin-2L2	PKD2L2	5q31	Heart, testis	n.d.	n.d.	313,314

n.d., not described.

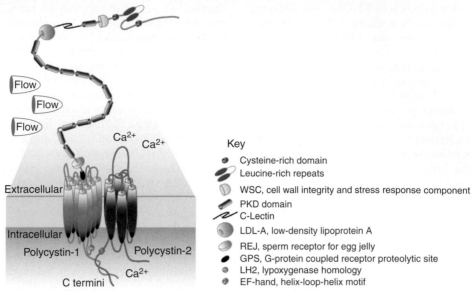

Figure 6-3 A schematic representation of the domain architecture of polycystin-1 (PC1) and -2 (PC2). Respective domains are indicated. Arrow indicates the pore region in PC2 through which the Ca^{2+} ions enter the cell. (Adapted from Nauli SM, Zhou J: Polycystins and mechanosensation in renal and nodal cilia. Bioessays 26:844–856, 2004.)

activation in L-type Ca^{2+} channels, although no evidence supports its importance in modulating channel activity in PC2. PC2 associates with PC1 with its C-terminal tail.[151,152] PC2 is linked to the cytoskeleton, probably through hax-1,[165] tropomyosin-1, and troponin-1.[166,167] There is evidence that PC2 associates with TRPC1, another TRP channel,[168] although the functional significance of these associations is unknown. Recently, PC2 has been found to interact with mDia during cell division[169] and with Id2 to control the cell cycle.[170] Additionally, PC2 interacts with fibrocystin, the protein encoded by PKHD1 that is mutated in the autosomal recessive form of PKD and kinesin-2,[171,172] suggesting that ADPKD and ARPKD share a common signaling pathway.

Molecular Functions of Polycystins

Polycystin-1 as a G Protein–Coupled Receptor

PC1 shares sequence and domain topology with PC2, but it has a large N-terminal domain predicted to be extracellular and a total of 11 transmembrane domains (five more than PC2) (see Fig. 6-3). PC1 homomers do not form ion channels.[154,173] The complex domain structure of PC1 suggests a diverse role as a cell surface receptor involved in cell-cell and cell-matrix interactions. Indeed, PC1 acts as a typical GPCR using Ca^{2+} channels and GIRK K^+ channels as a readout in sympathetic neurons.[154] When expressed alone, PC1 can activate a G-protein signaling pathway by direct binding and activation of heterotrimeric $G\alpha i/o$ proteins[153,154] and consequently modulates voltage-gated Ca^{2+} channels and GIRK K^+ channels via the release of $G\beta\gamma$ subunits.[154] Since PC1, unlike the typical GPCRs that have seven transmembrane domains, has 11 transmembrane domains, it is considered as an untraditional or atypical GPCR. PC2 is known to bind to PC1 in vitro via its C-terminal cytoplasmic tail.[151,152] Co-expression of PC2 with PC1 strongly represses G protein activation by PC1.[154] This

finding has the following implications: (1) since the PC1-PC2 protein complex is normally silent, mutations leading to the distortion of its stoichiometry (e.g., resulting in relative overexpression of PC1 or PC2) may trigger abnormal G-protein signaling and lead to cyst formation in ADPKD[154]; (2) the polycystin protein complex may be activated upon specific physiologic stimulations, which may result in a conformational change of the protein complex, releasing the inhibition of PC2 on PC1, and thus initiating G protein signaling. One way to test this hypothesis is to use an antibody raised to the extracellular domain of PC1 as an artificial stimulation and measure the G protein activation function of PC1 when PC1 and PC2 are co-expressed. This approach has led to the finding that PC1 stimulation simultaneously activates G proteins and the PC2 channel in rat sympathetic neurons, a model cell line that allows robust expression of PC1.[174] Abnormal G protein–mediated signaling may contribute to cyst formation by modulating cellular proliferation, transepithelial fluid secretion, and differentiation mediated by adenylate cyclase and mitogen-activated protein kinase pathways. However, whether PC1 can activate G proteins in a physiologically relevant cell type is currently unknown. Additionally, the physiologic activator of PC1-mediated G-protein signaling is also unknown.

RGS proteins are negative regulators of G-protein signaling by accelerating the intrinsic guanosine triphosphatase (GTPase) activity of specific $G\alpha$ subunits. Although RGS7, a member of the regulators of G-protein signaling (RGS) family, has recently been reported to bind to the C terminus of PC1,[156] the functional activation of Gi/o proteins by full-length PC1 is independent of the RGS protein.[154]

Polycystin-2 Functions as a Ca^{2+}-Permeable Nonselective Cation Channel

The elucidation of the Ca^{2+}-modulated, Ca^{2+}-permeable, cation-selective channel property of polycystin-L (PCL)[175] facilitated the discovery of the function of PC2.[176–178] Like PCL, PC2 is permeable to Ca^{2+}, Na^+, and K^+, and its channel activity is modulated by intracellular Ca^{2+} concentration. The PC2 channel is found within the cell and intracellular membranes. It is insensitive to ryanodine and inositol-triphosphate (IP_3).[176] With its reported endoplasmic reticulum (ER) location, it has been proposed that PC2 is a member of a third class of Ca^{2+} release channels in addition to ryanodine receptors and IP_3 receptors.[176] This hypothesis later gained support from another study using lipid bilayers.[178] PC2 may also contribute to the K^+ influx pathways in the ER that are coupled to Ca^{2+} release as part of a highly cooperative ion-exchange mechanism due to its large K^+ conductance.[176] Mutant PC2 channels appear to have partial function.[179] The Ca^{2+} dependence of the PC2 channel appears to be mediated by serine phosphorylation at position 812[180] (see reviews of polycystin channels[181,182]).

Cellular and Subcellular Localization of Polycystins

Polycystin-1 Expression is Developmentally Regulated

PC1 and PC2 are widely distributed. The subcellular localization of PC1 and PC2 has been controversial. Based on immunolocalization studies in tissues and in cultured cells, PC1 is now generally accepted as a plasma membrane protein. PC1 is found at apical membranes and the adherent and desmosomal junctions.[183–186] More recently it has been found in cilia of inner medullary collecting ducts (IMCD)[187,188] and epithelial cells derived from mouse embryonic kidney (MEK).[189] PC1 is also detected in the cilia of renal tubules in vivo.[189] PC1 is highly expressed in developing tissues and maintained in low-expression levels in adult tissues.[183] In the mouse kidney, PC1 expression is found in nearly all the tubular segments of the nephron. Its expression peaks at embryonic day 15, and 2 weeks after birth it falls to a low level that is maintained in adult life.[184] PC1 is expressed in a number of other tissues, including kidney, liver, pancreatic ducts, and vasculature.[102,183,184,190]

Polycystin-2 Channel Functions at Multiple Subcellular Locations

Unlike PC1, PC2 expression levels do not change strikingly during development. Data on in vivo subcellular location have been controversial since cytoplasmic,[191] apical, and basolateral membrane localization for PC2 have all been reported.[192–194] PC2 was found in the cilia[195] of kidney tubules. In cultured cells, it has been found in the ER, cilia, and plasma membrane.[188,192] A major obstacle in demonstrating PC2 channel function was the absence or the low levels of cell surface expression in common expression systems (e.g., Xenopus oocytes), but Gonzalez-Perrett and colleagues found moderate levels of PC2 channel activity in reconstituted apical membrane vesicles of human placenta syncytiotrophoblasts (hST) and membranes of PC2-expressing, baculovirus-infected Sf9 insect cells.[177]

Recent studies have supported the hypothesis[181] that the subcellular localization of PC2 is cell type specific and dynamic. The PC2 protein and channel properties can be detected on the cell plasma membrane [188] and in the ER[178] of renal tubular epithelia. A number of factors can modulate the PC2 localization. The PC2 channel can be translocated to the cell membrane in the presence of chemical chaperones and proteasome inhibitors and in the presence of PC1 in cultured cells.[176] Its localization to the plasma membrane is in part modulated by phosphorylation at Ser76, a site that is likely phosphorylated by glycogen synthase kinase 3.[196] An acidic cluster in the C terminus of PC2 was recently found to be responsible for its ER, Golgi, and plasma membrane trafficking. Two adaptor proteins called PACS-1 and PACS-2 bind to the acidic cluster in PC2 in a phosphorylation-dependent manner.[197] Another coiled coil domain containing protein, called PIGEA, regulates the ER-Golgi trafficking of PC2 by linking PC2 to GM130, a Golgi matrix protein.[198] More recently, the short sequence RVxP in the N-terminal domain of PC2 has been shown to be required for ciliary targeting of PC2.[199]

Localization of Polycystin-1 and -2— Interdependent or Independent?

PC1 and PC2 physically interact with each other through their C-terminal cytoplasmic domains and regulate each other's subcellular localization. The first evidence came from a co-expression study of PC1 and PC2 in Chinese hamster ovary cells. The researchers suggested that PC1 assists targeting of PC2 to cell plasma membranes.[173] This conclusion was drawn from the observation that single transfection of PC2 results in its accumulation in the ER, whereas co-transfection of PC2 with PC1 results in cell surface expression of both proteins. This result was supported by another study using sympathetic neurons as an expression system.[154] PC2 localization on the plasma membrane and cilia was also abnormal in kidney epithelial cells derived from embryonic day 15.5 homozygous Pkd1 targeted animals.[189] In cyst-lining epithelial cells from human ADPKD, PC2 was absent from cilia in most cells, but remained in some cells.[200] A recent study by Grimm and colleagues proposes that PC2 regulates the subcellular distribution of PC1. In the absence of PC2, PC1 is located on plasma membrane, whereas co-transfection of both results in ER localization of PC1.[201] Geng and colleagues, however, have shown that PC2 remains in the nodal cilia of PC1 knockout mice, suggesting that PC2 targeting is independent of PC1.[199] These researchers also found PC2 in cilia of renal tubular epithelial cells lacking PC1 and proposed that selective PC2 agonists may be effective therapeutic agents for treatment of ADPKD. The localization and functional relationships between PC1 and PC2 deserve further study.

Primary Cilium in ADPKD

The latest research focus of polycystic kidney disease has been on the primary cilium, a thin hairlike structure that typically appears as a single projection from the apical surface of a cell. Primary cilia have a "9 + 0" microtubule arrangement, lack the central pair of microtubules, and thus structurally differentiate themselves from motile cilia. The existence of primary cilia has been documented for decades, yet their functions in the kidney were not known until recently.

Clues for a Role of Primary Cilia in PKD

The assembly and maintenance of eukaryotic flagella or cilia require the movement of proteins along flagellar microtubules, a process named interflagellar transport (IFT). A role for the primary cilia in PKD was initially suggested by observations made during the studies on polycystins and IFT in model organisms: (1) a PC1 homolog, *lov-1*, is localized to cilia of the only ciliated cell type (sensory neurons) in *Caenorhabditis elegans*,[202] and (2) IFT88, a gene responsible for the aflagellar phenotype in a *Chlamedomona* mutant, is homologous to *Tg737* (encoding polaris), whose hypomorphic mutation causes shortened cilia and PKD in mice.[203] Although genetic rescue experiments in the *Tg737* mutant mice restored the length of the primary cilia, they failed to prevent the renal cystic phenotype, thus arguing against defective ciliogenesis as a cause of PKD.[204]

Ciliary Polycystin-1 as a Mechanoreceptor of Urine Flow

What is the function of the primary cilium? Is ciliary dysfunction a general feature of polycystic kidney disease? Do mutations in PC1 and PC2 disrupt this function? Praetorius and Spring suggested that the primary cilium of renal epithelium is mechanically sensitive and serves as a flow sensor. Bending of cilia either by suction with a micropipette or increasing the flow rate of perfusate causes a substantial increase in intracellular calcium.[205] PC1 and PC2 expression in cilia has lended further circumstantial evidence for the role of renal epithelial cilia in human cystic kidney disease.[187,189,195]

To test whether polycystins are involved in the sensing of flow by renal cilia, Nauli and colleagues tested whether cells from PKD kidneys are able to respond to fluid flow. Mouse embryonic kidney (MEK) cells were isolated from mice with targeted *Pkd1* mutations and their normal littermates.[189] Since a defect must be present at or prior to the earliest stage of cyst formation if it is causative for cyst formation, cells from embryonic day 15.5 (E15.5) in *Pkd1* targeted mice, just as cysts begin to appear, were isolated and examined. It was found that while the wild-type MEK cells respond to fluid flow at a rate that is similar to the physiologic urine flow rate of 0.75 dyne/cm^2, *Pkd1* knockout epithelial cells failed to respond to a wide range of fluid flow rates tested. Furthermore, the removal of extracellular Ca^{2+} abolished flow-induced cytosolic Ca^{2+} increase, suggesting that Ca^{2+} influx is required to transduce the mechanical signal into the cell.[189] These data suggest that PC1 mediates a flow-induced Ca^{2+} response.

A Model of Shear Stress Activation of Polycystin-1 and -2 Complex

PC1 is known to interact with PC2, but the impact of this interaction on PC2 channel activity was unknown at the time. The possibility that PC2 functions as a channel within the PC1-PC2 complex through which the Ca^{2+} enters the cell during flow stimulation was tested by the use of blocking antibodies. Wild-type cells pre-incubated with an antibody raised against an extracellular loop of PC2 lost their Ca^{2+} response to flow. By contrast, application of antibodies directed at the intracellular domain of PC2 had no effect on flow-stimulated response. Based on these data, the authors proposed that PC1 and PC2 form a complex in the primary cilia of kidney epithelia where they sense fluid flow and transduce this mechanical signal into a Ca^{2+} signal. In this model, the large extracellular domain of PC1 serves as an extracellular "antenna" for mechanical stress such as urine flow, and subsequent conformational changes of PC1 activate the PC2 channel, resulting in the initial Ca^{2+} entry. Through the use of various inhibitors, it was found that the initial Ca^{2+} entry signals are further amplified through ryanodine receptor–mediated, Ca^{2+}-induced Ca^{2+} release mechanisms[189] (Fig. 6-4). Both the local Ca^{2+} entry and global Ca^{2+} release signals may modulate cellular activities.

A role of polycystins in primary cilia and in mechanosensation is now generally accepted. A number of studies have also shown that both structural and functional abnormalities in primary cilia lead to polycystic kidney disease. For example, conditional inactivation of KIF3A, which encodes a subunit of the kinesin II motor protein that mediates antegrade ciliary IFT, resulted in absence of cilium formation and PKD.[206] Together with the observation that multiple cystogenic proteins are localized to the primary cilia or basal body,[207] the above studies raise the intriguing possibility that ciliary dysfunction may serve as a convergent mechanism for multiple forms of PKD.[208]

Flow-Independent Activation of the Polycystin-2 Channel

A common theme that links the TRP channels is their activation or modulation by phosphatidylinositol signal transduction pathways.[163] Phosphatidylinositol is an important lipid, both as a key membrane constituent and as a participant in essential metabolic processes in all plants and animals. Phosphatidylinositol is generated by the activation of phospholipase C (PLC). Since PC2 is a member of the TRP channel superfamily, Ma and colleagues recently tested the activation of PC2 by PLC and phosphatidylinositol.[209] They searched for components of the PLC activation pathway that have been reported to cause renal cystic disease. Because epidermal growth factor receptor (EGFR)–mutant mice develop dilated collecting tubules,[210] they tested a functional interaction between the EGFR and PC2. Activated EGFR binds PLC and generates IP$_3$ and diacylglycerol (DAG) from phosphatidylinositol-4,5-bisphosphate (PIP$_2$). Activated EGFR also activates phosphoinositide 3-kinase (PI3K) to phosphorylate PIP$_2$ to phosphatidylinositol-3,4,5-triphosphate (PIP$_3$). Using PC2 antibodies as a blocking agent, they found that PC2 mediated EGF-induced currents in LLC-PK$_1$ cells. Moreover, recombinant PC2 co-immunoprecipitated PLC-γ2 and EGFR.[209] It is not known whether endogenous PC2 also co-immunoprecipitates PLC-γ2. Interestingly, PIP$_2$ colocalizes with PC2 in primary cilia of LLC-PK$_1$ cells, suggesting that the EGF-PC2 channel activation pathway is active on primary cilium.

Polycystin Signaling Pathways
Does Fluid Flow Inhibit the Cleavage of the PC1 C-Terminal Cytoplasmic Tail?

An interesting question arising from the ciliary polycystin mechanosensation hypothesis is how the initial calcium signal

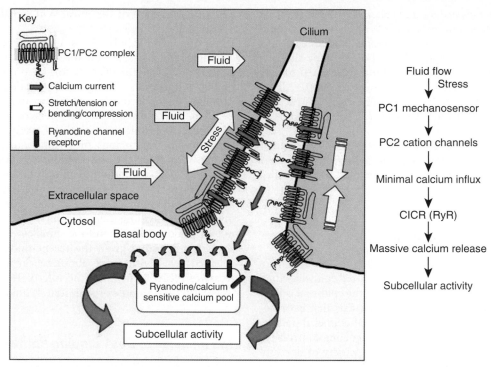

Figure 6-4 Schematic diagram of mechanisms of fluid shear stress–induced calcium signaling in kidney epithelial cells. Cilia act as antennae to sense fluid movement. Polycystin-1 (PC1), with its large extracellular domains, acts as a sensory molecule to fluid shear stress and transduces the signal from the extracellular fluid environment to polycystin-2 (PC2), which allows sufficient calcium influx, in turn, to activate ryanodine receptors through calcium-induced calcium release. The resulting local increase in the cytosolic calcium concentration then regulates numerous cellular/subcellular activities. (Adapted from Nauli SM, et al: Polycystins 1 and 2 mediate mechanosensation in the primary cilium of kidney cells. Nat Genet 33:129–137, 2003.)

triggered by fluid flow shear stress is inferred within a cell. Two recent studies have reported that the C-terminal cytoplasmic tail of PC1 is cleaved under static conditions and proposed that fluid flow inhibits the cleavage of the PC1 C-tail.[211,212] Both groups showed that the cleaved C-tail is translocated to the nucleus, where it initiates nuclear signaling. Chauvet and colleagues observed the cleaved C-tail in kidneys of wild-type animals after unilateral ureteral ligation, and in mice manifesting a conditional inactivation of the KIF3A subunit, which is essential for cilia formation, suggesting that fluid flow normally inhibits the cleavage and that the cleavage occurs under pathologic conditions.[211] Low and colleagues showed that the cleavage of the PC1 tail occurs under static cell culture conditions.[212] It is noteworthy that the cleavage fragments identified by these two groups were of different sizes (34 and 14 kD, respectively), suggesting the presence of two distinct cleavage sites in the C-tail. It appears that the 34-kD nuclear PC1 C-tail can activate the AP1 pathway,[211] while the 14-kD fragment binds to STAT6 (signal transducer amd activator of transcription protein 6) and its co-activator P100 and activates STAT6-dependent gene transcription.[212] It is important to note that ureteral ligation, the method used to study fluid flow by Chauvet and colleagues, may affect a number of factors other than flow and pressure and may initiate nonspecific injury-related events. On the other hand, Low and colleagues induced flow through orbital shaking, a condition with unknown activation status of Ca^{2+} signaling. One of the major current efforts in the field is to identify the downstream signaling cas-

cades that eventually lead to the abnormal cellular behaviors seen in PKD.

PC1 and Wnt Signaling

The Wnt signaling pathway describes a complex network of proteins that can regulate the production of Wnt signaling molecules, their interactions with receptors on target cells, and the physiologic responses of target cells that result from the exposure of cells to the extracellular Wnt ligands. Wnt signaling is best known for its role during development, but may also play a role in normal physiologic processes in adult life. In canonical Wnt signaling, Wnt proteins bind to cell surface receptors of the Frizzled family, causing the receptors to activate dishevelled family of proteins. This activation inhibits the degradation of β-catenin by the GSK3-axin-APC complex and increases the amount of β-catenin that reaches the nucleus where β-catenin interacts with T-cell factor (TCF) family members and activates Wnt target genes.

Early in 1999, Kim and colleagues[213] reported that the membrane-anchored C-tail of PC1 activates Wnt signaling. Their conclusion was based on three major observations: first, the membrane-anchored PC1 C-tail stabilizes β-catenin, an indicator of Wnt signaling; second, the C-tail activates the Siamois promoter reporter construct that contains a β-catenin TCF binding motif, another readout of Wnt signaling, in HEK293 cells; and third, microinjection of the polycystin C-terminal cytoplasmic domain induces dorsalization in zebrafish. In 2004, however, Le and colleagues[214] reported that the PC1 C-tail does not modulate Wnt signaling using a TOP/FOP assay in HEK293 cells and human kidney epithelial cells. These data were supported by another study showing that neither the membrane-anchored nor the cleaved soluble PC1 tail was able to activate Wnt pathway using TOP-, TOP-FLASH as well as Siamois promoter reporter constructs.[212] Therefore, whether PC1 modulates Wnt signaling remains an open question.

Noncanonical Wnt signaling does not involve β-catenin/TCF-mediated transcription. The best characterized noncanonical pathway is involved in a cellular process called planar cell polarity (PCP).

Planar Cell Polarity and PKD

Polarization along the apical/basal axis is a universal feature of epithelial cells and is important for specialized epithelial functions. In addition to apical-basal polarity, the epithelial cells of many tissues are also polarized along an axis that is orthogonal to the apical/basal axis. This form of epithelial polarity is known as PCP or tissue polarity. PCP signaling controls cell division orientation and is involved in a variety of developmental processes that determine cell differentiation fate and contribute to tissue and organ morphogenesis.

Several signaling pathways have been implicated in planar cell polarity. Disruption of noncanonical Wnt signaling results in abnormalities in oriented cell division during zebrafish gastrulation, and indicate that oriented cell division is a driving force for axis elongation.[215] Recent work by Fischer and colleagues shows that lengthening of renal tubules is associated with mitotic orientation of cells along the tubule axis, an intrinsic planar cell polarization process. They described a defect in the mitotic orientation in PCK rats and HNF1β-knockout mice (models of autosomal recessive polycystic kidney disease) before overt tubule dilation and cyst formation,[216] suggesting that defects in PCP are responsible for cyst development. The researchers proposed that orientated cell division dictates the control of tubular lumen size during tubule elongation. The molecular events underlying orientated cell division and tubular lumen size are currently unknown, and no other PCP defects are known to be present in ADPKD.

A study on inversin, a protein involved in left-right asymmetry and kidney cyst formation, has provided some clues about how fluid-flow shear stress may regulate the Wnt signaling pathway.[217] Fluid flow over a kidney cell line increases inversin levels and slightly reduces β-catenin levels (~19%). Inversin facilitates the degradation of cytosolic disheveled 1 that is involved in canonical Wnt signaling, but not plasma membrane-bound disheveled that mediates noncanonical Wnt signaling. Furthermore, they showed that inversin is required for convergent extension movements in gastrulating *Xenopus laevis* embryos, a process mediated by the β-catenin-independent, noncanonical Wnt pathway. Based on these findings, the researchers proposed that inversin serves as a molecular switch between Wnt signaling pathways and that fluid flow terminates canonical Wnt signaling. It remains to be determined whether this cell culture model system adequately reflects the in vivo situation. The BATgal mouse, which allows visualization of β-catenin-dependent Wnt signaling, may provide more insight into the spatial and temporal activation of canonical Wnt signaling during renal development.

An attractive hypothesis is that cilia of renal tubular epithelial cells may sense the direction of primary urine flow and provide a cue for PCP and oriented cell division during tubule enlongation through the function of polycystins. Although the molecular events that mediate polycystins with PCP are currently unknown, interaction of the PC2 C-terminal cytoplasmic tail with the N terminal of mDia1/Drf1 (mammalian Diaphanous or Diaphanous-related formin 1 protein)[169] may serve as one of the links. mDia1 is a member of the RhoA GTPase-binding formin homology protein family that participates in cytoskeletal organization, cytokinesis, and signal transduction. The mDia-PC2 interaction is more prevalent in dividing cells in which endogenous PC2 and mDia1 colocalize to the mitotic spindles. This finding is particularly interesting given the recent finding that PCP and oriented cell division are abnormal in animal models of recessive PKD.[216] However, the role of PC2 in cell division orientation and spindle organization is unknown.

The Inhibitor of DNA Binding Pathway

The Inhibitor of DNA Binding (Id) protein family comprises relatively new transcriptional regulators that belong to the superfamily of helix-loop-helix proteins. There are four members in this family that inhibit differentiation of certain lineages and have the potential to stimulate proliferation. A recent study has shown that PC2 directly associates with Id2 and controls cell cycle progression.[170] Membrane-anchored PC2 sequesters Id2 in the cytosol through direct binding and prevents Id2 nuclear translocation. It is important to note that Id2 binds to phosphorylated PC2 and that the phosphorylation of PC2 is modulated by PC1. Whereas overexpression of PC1 causes an increase in PC2 phosphorylation and PC2-Id2 interaction, mutations in PC1 disrupt this interaction and lead to increased Id2 nuclear accumulation in *Pkd1*-targeted mice and in human ADPKD patients with either *PKD1* or *PKD2* mutations.[170] Nuclear Id2 is known to antagonize the function of E2A/E47-dependent growth suppressive gene transcription and induces cell proliferation. Interestingly, inhibition of Id2 mRNA by RNA interference reversed the proliferative cell cycle profile of *Pkd1* knockout cells to normal,[170] suggesting that methods for modulating Id2 expression levels or subcellular localization may provide a new direction for treatment of ADPKD.

The PC2-Id2 pathway is linked to several other important signaling proteins, some of which have been suspected to play a role in the pathogenesis of PKD. These proteins, which include β-catenin,[218] E-cadherin,[219] c-myc, and Rb,[220] may also contribute to the hyperproliferative phenotype in cyst lining epithelia. β-catenin, which has been found to associate with PC1, can activate transcription of Id2, probably through C-myc, which is overexpressed in cystic kidneys. In addition, a role of Id2 in cell proliferation and differentiation has recently been linked to Smad4-dependent transforming growth factor-β (TGF-β)[219] and bone morphogenesis protein (BMP)–mediated pathways.[221] The effective arrest of cystic disease by a cyclin-dependent kinase inhibitor (roscovitine) in two animal models of PKD (*cpk* and *jck*)[222] supports the notion that dysregulated cell cycle is a proximal cause of cystogenesis.

The JAK-STAT Pathway

STAT proteins are tyrosine phosphorylated by members of the Janus kinase (JAK) family, tyrosine kinase growth factor receptors, nonreceptor tyrosine kinases, and seven transmembrane pass receptors.[223] The JAK-STAT signaling pathway has been described to mediate polycystin signaling.[212,224] At least two STATs are involved, STAT1 and STAT6. A study using full-length PC1 stable cell lines shows that PC1 induces STAT1 activation by direct association and activation of JAK2, and in turn results in an induction of p21 and modulation of cell cycle. The notion that activation of JAK2 by PC1 requires PC2 was based on the observation that the R4227X truncation mutant of PC1 was able to bind but not to activate JAK2 and that full-length PC1 was unable to activate JAK2 in cells lacking PC2.[224] A more recent study shows that the expression of the cleaved C-terminal cytoplasmic tail of PC1 activates STAT6 by directly binding to P100.[208] Because PC1 binds to JAK2 but not JAK1 and its interaction with JAK3 was not tested, Low and colleagues propose that JAK3 may be involved in PC1-dependent activation of STAT6, although phosphorylation of STAT6 by JAK2 when PC1 is activated is not excluded. In this study, a pathologic role of STAT6 was suggested. The researchers examined the localization of STAT6 in human ADPKD kidneys and found an increased expression of STAT6 in the nucleus of cyst lining epithelial cells in ADPKD kidneys. It was proposed that in normal renal tubular lumens with fluid flow and normal PC1, STAT6 is sequestered in the cilia by PC1. Under the absence of urine flow or PC1, or overexpression of mutant PC1, STAT6 translocates from the cilia to the nucleus to initiate STAT6-dependent transcription. Although several factors such as fluid flow, calcium influx, and cytokine stimulation have been speculated to facilitate the activation of the JAK-STAT pathway, the mechanism of STAT6 upregulation and activation in ADPKD remains unclear and requires further study.

The mTOR Pathway

Another recently identified pathway that deserves attention is the mammalian target of rapamycin (mTOR) pathway. Following the effective treatment of the Han:SPRD rat model of PKD with rapamycin, an antiproliferative drug that blocks the mTOR pathway,[225] Shillingford and colleagues[226] explored the possible mechanism underlying this observation. mTOR has essential roles in protein translation, cell growth, and proliferation and is upregulated in a number of tumors. mTOR is regulated by the *TSC2* gene product, tuberin, through the small GTPase Rheb. *TSC2* mutation causes tuberous sclerosis, a genetic disease with renal cysts and tumors in a number of tissues. *TSC2* is localized tail to tail with *PKD1* on chromosome 16p13.3 with about 60 bp apart.[227] Using a tuberin-deficient renal cell line, Kleymenova and colleagues[228] has shown that tuberin expression is required for the plasma membrane targeting of PC1. Shillingford and colleagues recently provided biochemical evidence that the transfected N- but not the C-terminal segment of the PC1 cytoplasmic tail co-immunoprecipitated with endogenous tuberin in MDCK cells. Co-transfection of tuberin with the N-terminal fragment of PC1 shifted tuberin from its punctate cytoplasmic pattern to the Golgi apparatus, where the PC1 fragment is localized. Given the lack of co-immunoprecipitation

data on endogenous proteins, these data suggest that PC1 and tuberin transiently interact and modulate each other's localization. Another interesting finding of this study is the upregulation of the phosphorylated, active form of mTOR and its downstream effector S6K kinase in cyst lining epithelial cells from human ADPKD kidneys. This upregulation was also seen in cysts but not normal tubules in *Pkd1* mutant mice and two other mouse PKD models (*MAL* and *orpk* due to myelin and lymphocyte protein overexpression and mutation in a ciliary protein, Tg737, respectively). The inhibition of mTOR by rapamycin significantly alleviated the cystic phenotype in these animal models. Additionally, in a small retrospective study, reduction of renal cyst volume was noted in renal transplant patients with ADPKD who were treated with rapamycin compared to those without.

Animal Models of ADPKD

Pkd1 and Pkd2 Targeted Mutants

Although there are a number of "spontaneous" animal models of PKD, none are due to mutations in the mouse orthologs of *PKD1* or *PKD2*. Therefore, a number of targeted mutants were made. The first *Pkd1*-targeted mouse mutant, *Pkd1*^{del34}, was created in 1997.[229] Homozygous *Pkd1*^{del34} and *Pkd1*^{null} mice develop polyhydramnios and hydrops fetalis and die perinatally.[229] Kidney development of all homozygotes proceeds normally until embryonic day 15.5, when dilatation of Bowman's space and the proximal tubule is evident. Cyst development soon progresses to the collecting system, and by birth, the entire kidney is cystic (Fig. 6-5). A survivor of *Pkd1*$^{del34/del34}$ lived to 8 days after birth, but developed massive cystic kidneys.[229]

The *del34* mutant was created by a deletion of exon 34 in mouse *Pkd1*. This mutation mimics many mutations found in human patients and is predicted to produce a PC1 protein lacking the C-terminal half of its transmembrane domains and the complete C-terminal cytoplasmic domain.[229] A *null* mutation was later generated by the insertion of a *neomycin* cassette into exon 4 of the mouse *Pkd1* gene, which results in an immediate frame shift and truncates approximately 98% of the PC1 protein. This mutation was generated as a "loss-of-function" animal model of PC1.[230] In homozygosity, both *del34* and *null* germline mutations resulted in severe polycystic kidney and pancreatic disease in utero, providing unequivocal evidence that PC1 plays a key role in kidney and pancreatic development. Unfortunately, these mice, as well as all other *Pkd1* mutants generated later, die between the 13th day of embryonic life and shortly after birth, which greatly limits the use of these animal models for studies of the molecular mechanisms of cystogenesis that occurs mostly in postnatal life in ADPKD. Heterozygotes for either of these mutations gradually develop scattered cysts in the kidney and liver. The kidney cysts range from 2 to greater than 50 per animal in 14- to 20-month-old *del34* mutants. Mice with *Pkd2* mutations develop polycystic kidneys like the *Pkd1* mutants.[231]

In an attempt to develop a better model for ADPKD, the *Cre*-loxP site-specific recombination system has been used to produce mice with tissue- and time-specific deletions. By crossing the "floxed" mice with transgenic mice expressing the *Cre* recombinase in the desired time-specific and/or tissue-specific manner, one can achieve conditional gene

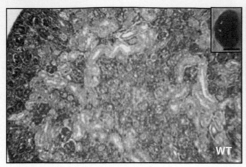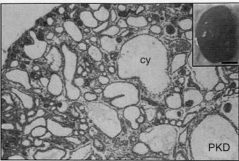

Figure 6-5 Polycystic kidney (PKD) in a *Pkd1^{-/-}*-targeted mouse. Hematoxylin and eosin staining of a kidney section from a wild-type mouse at newborn (*left*) and a cystic kidney from a *Pkd1^{-/-}*-targeted mutant of the same stage (*right*). Insets show that the polycystic kidney is significantly larger than the age-matched wild-type kidney. Cy, cyst. Bar, 5 mm.

inactivation. This approach was recently used to develop a conditional model in which somatic *Pkd1* inactivation was under control of the γGT:Cre[232] and MMTV-*Cre*.[233] Although the MMTV-*Cre* mice were created successfully, only scattered cysts were observed in mice at 20 weeks of age. The lack of a consistent cystic kidney phenotype and the long time needed to develop the phenotype limits the usefulness of this model for phenotypic and experimental studies of ADPKD. γGT:Cre gives a more striking cystic phenotype and appears to be a better model for ADPKD.[232] Animal models with various *Pkd1* or *Pkd2* mutations are summarized in Table 6-6.

The extrarenal phenotypes are also seen in animal models of ADPKD. Liver cyst is the most common extrarenal phenotype in heterozygotes: all *Pkd1*^{del34} heterozygotes eventually develop macroscopic liver cysts.[234] *Pkd2*-mutant mice also develop polycystic liver disease like the *Pkd1* mutants.[231] A fraction of *Pkd1* and *Pkd2* mutants also develop pancreatic cystic disease. In fact, cystic degeneration in homozygous *Pkd1* and *Pkd2* mutants were first seen in the pancreas at E13.5, two stages earlier than in the kidney, consistent with a role of polycystins in mechanosensation in tubular and ductal epithelial cells.

In addition to the cystic phenotype, a small portion of the *Pkd1* and *Pkd2* knockout mice also develop hemorrhage, suggesting a role for polycystins in the maintenance of blood vessel integrity.[104,235] Some studies have also shown cardiac defects in *Pkd1* and *Pkd2* mutants.[236,237] Characterization of *Pkd1* and *Pkd2* knockout mice has also uncovered roles of PCs in skeletal development (personal communication, P. Pennekamp).[230,236]

The vertebrate body plan has conserved handed left-right asymmetry that is apparent in the heart, lungs, and gut. Situs inversus is a condition in which the organs of the chest and abdomen are arranged in a perfect mirror image reversal of the normal positioning. Although there is no report of its association with PKD, recent studies in animal models have suggested a role of PC2 but not PC1 in the determination of left-right body axis.[238] *Pkd2* mutant mice exhibit randomized embryonic turning.[238] This phenotype is not seen in any of the *Pkd1* mutants, providing an example of tissue-specific uncoupling of PC1-PC2 function. The ciliary connection of polycystins has provided some insights into this phenotype. It is believed that ciliary PC2 serves as a mechanosensor sensing nodal flow in the embryonic node.[239,240]

Animal models with various *Pkd1* or *Pkd2* mutations are summarized in Table 6-2.

MECHANISMS OF RENAL DISEASE PROGRESSION

Pathogenic Mechanisms of Renal Disease Progression

The pathophysiology of renal disease progression in ADPKD is not well understood. However, it is ultimately related to the total renal cystic burden, which is determined by both the number and size of individual cysts.[83,84,144] Detailed reconstruction and dissection studies have shown that renal cysts developed initially as saccular outpouchings arising from any nephron segment. Most of these dilated tubules eventually become cysts as a result of cellular proliferation and fluid secretion, and detached from their tubule of origin when enlarged beyond a few millimeters in diameter.[10,43] Cyst formation, however, may only involve 1% to 2% of the nephrons, even with advanced disease.[43,241] Thus, progressive renal failure in ADPKD is not simply due to loss of function of the cystic nephrons.

Histologic studies have shown that tubulo-interstitial inflammation and fibrosis are the best predictors for renal disease progression in ADPKD.[38,242] Additionally, widespread apoptosis involving both cystic and noncystic tubular epithelial cells was commonly observed and may mediate the loss of renal tissue.[243] In the early stages of Han:SPRD rat polycystic kidney disease, detailed micropuncture and microdissection studies have revealed that approximately 40% of renal tubules were obstructed by intraluminal adenomatous polyps or by extrinsic compression from adjacent cysts.[244] Since mechanical stretching of epithelial cells from tubular obstruction and compression is known to activate signaling cascades for inflammation and apoptosis,[245–248] cyst expansion and encroachment upon adjacent parenchyma within the confined renal capsule may cause indirect tissue damage. In this way, individual cyst expansion may amplify their effect to compromise the function of adjacent noncystic renal tubules and glomeruli by distorting the delicate tubulo-interstitial network of capillaries, arterioles, and venules, leading to functional disturbances of the surrounding parenchyma.[10] Consistent with this concept, "atubular glomeruli" (in which the connections between the renal corpuscles and proximal tubules are severed) have been commonly observed in the Han:SPRD rat model.[249] Hypertrophy of nephrons and glomeruli may compensate for the loss of parenchymal mass

Table 6-6 Phenotypes of *Pkd1* and *Pkd2* Knockout Mice

Strain (reference)	Mutation	Allele	EL	K&P Cysts	Edema	Cardiovascular Defects	Skeletal Defects	L-R Defects	Het
*Pkd1*del34 (229,234)	Exon 34 deletion	*Pkd1*tm1Jzh	+	+	+	–	+	–	K.L.P. cysts
*Pkd1*null (230)	Exon 4 insertion	*Pkd1*tm1Jzh	+	+	+	Subcutaneous bleeding seen in <1% of animals	+	–	K.L.P. cysts
*Pkd1*del43 (235)	Exon 43–45 deletion	*Pkd1*tm1Maa	+	+	+	Vascular leak	n.d.	n.d.	n.d.
*Pkd1*del17 (236)	Exon 17–21 deletion	*Pkd1*tm1Rsa	+	+	+	+	+	–	K.L. cysts
Pkd1- (315)	Exon 2–6 deletion	*Pkd1*tm1Shh	+	+	+	Double outlet right ventricle	n.d.	n.d.	n.d.
Pkd1-(316)	Single amino acid substitution	*Pkd1*tm1Bei	+	+	+	n.d.	n.d.	n.d.	K.L.P. cysts
*Pkd1*nl/nl (273)	Insertion of neo cassette in intron 1, cause 80% splicing defects	*Pkd1*nl/nl	–	+	–	Aorta aneurysms	n.d.	n.d.	No cysts
*Pkd1*flox	Exon 2–6 deletion, γGT.Cre	*Pkd1*flox	–	+	–	–	–	–	n.d.
*Pkd1*cond (233)	Exon 2–4, MMTV.Cre	*Pkd1*cond	–	± in K	–	–	–	–	n.d.
*Pkd2*null (237,267)	Exon 1 disruption	*Pkd2*tm1Som	+	+	+	+	n.d.	+	n.d.
*Pkd2*ws25 (237)	Exon 1 duplication causing unstable allele	*Pkd2*tm2Som	+	+	n.d.	n.d.	n.d.	+	K. cysts
*Pkd2*lacZ (238)	Exon 1 deletion with LacZ promoter trap	*Pkd2*tm1Blum	+	+	n.d.	+	+	Randomization, right pulmonary isomerism	n.d.

EL, embryonic lethality with death occurring between embryonic day 13.5 and birth. All mutations are targeted mutations with the exception of one, N-ethyl-nitrosourea induced point mutation (*Pkd1*Bei). K, kidney; L, liver; P, pancreas; L-R defects, left-right asymmetry defects; n.d., not described.

for many years, but ultimately the amount of noncystic parenchyma decreases so that, at the end stage, only the survivor cysts remain. If tubular obstruction and compression are major mechanisms of tissue injury effecting the loss of renal structure and function, therapeutic interventions targeting cyst expansion are expected to delay renal disease progression in ADPKD. Indeed, the recent findings of vasopressin V2 receptor antagonism in a Pkd2 mouse model are consistent with such an effect (see later section on Promising Disease-Modifying Therapies).

Molecular Genetic Basis of Cyst Formation

Focal and sporadic cyst formation is an intriguing feature of ADPKD that occurs in an age-dependent manner.[250] Typically, only a few renal cysts are detected in affected individuals during the first three decades of life. By the fifth decade, however, hundreds to thousands of renal cysts of different sizes can be easily found in most patients (see Fig. 6-1). Additionally, significant within-family renal disease variability is well documented.[78,80] For example, as an extreme example, one dizygotic twin was reported to have bilaterally enlarged polycystic kidneys in utero while the kidneys of his co-twin remained normal up to 5 years of age, yet both twins were affected with the same germline *PKD1* mutation.[251] These findings suggest that additional factor(s) other than the germline mutation of a polycystic kidney disease gene might be required for cystogenesis.

A "Two-Hit" Model for Cystogenesis

To explain the above observations, a "two-hit" model of cystogenesis analogous to Knudson's classic model for carcinogenesis was proposed for ADPKD.[252] According to this model, individual cyst formation is triggered by bi-allelic inactivation of a polycystic kidney disease gene through germline and somatic mutations within an epithelial cell. While the germline PKD mutation is necessary, somatic mutation of a previously normal PKD gene within a single epithelial cell constitutes the second and rate-limiting step in cystogenesis, similar to that seen with numerous tumor suppressor genes in cancer[253,254] (Fig. 6-6). Indeed, recent studies provide strong support that this likely is a major mechanism of cystogenesis in human ADPKD.

Using novel techniques that purified cyst-lining epithelial cells from stromal cells (such as fibroblasts, endothelial cells, and blood leukocytes, which could mask the detection of genetic events in the former cells), two laboratories independently reported that individual PKD1 cystic epithelia derived from a monoclonal origin.[255,256] These studies also showed that gross somatic *PKD1* deletions (i.e., loss of heterozygosity) occurred in approximately 20% of the cysts examined. Additionally, small intragenic somatic *PKD1* mutations were detected in up to 30% of PKD1 liver cysts.[257] Similarly, loss of heterozygosity and small intragenic somatic mutations of *PKD2* were reported in up to 10% and 40% of human PKD2 renal and liver cysts, respectively.[258–260] In general, most somatic mutations detected from different cysts were unique within the same patient. Of interest, almost all germline and somatic mutations reported in the human cyst studies were predicted to truncate the C-terminal portion of the mutant polycystins. In some cysts with loss of heterozygosity at either

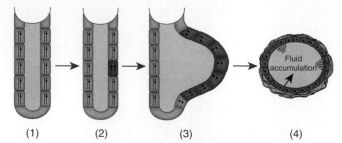

Figure 6-6 A "two-hit" mechanism of cyst formation in autosomal dominant polycystic kidney disease. (1) All epithelial cells in a renal tubule contain an identical germline polycystic kidney disease gene mutation (denoted by the black dot); (2) somatic mutation of the wild-type polycystic kidney disease allele occurs in a single epithelial cell; (3 and 4) monoclonal proliferation of this epithelial cell results in tubular dilatation and cyst formation.

PKD1 or *PKD2* locus, the availability of informative polymorphic markers made it possible to determine the parental origin of these somatic deletions. In other cysts with intragenic mutations, close proximity between the sites of germline and somatic mutations also allowed the same analysis to be performed. In 35 of 35 instances when the parental origin of the somatic polycystin mutations could be determined in individual PKD1 and PKD2 cysts, they were always found to affect the wild-type allele. These data indicate that these somatic "second-hit" events were not random[255–260] (see example in Fig. 6-7). Taken together, these genetic data showed that cyst formation occurs by a molecular recessive mechanism. Moreover, inactivating somatic *PKD1* mutations have been reported in approximately 8% of PKD2 cysts, and conversely, inactivating somatic *PKD2* mutations in approximately 13% of PKD1 cysts.[261,262] Given that PC1 and PC2 have been shown to interact in vitro, a trans-heterozygous two-hit model may provide an additional, albeit minor, mechanism for cystogenesis.

Two concerns have been voiced against the two-hit model.[263] First, it was argued that if the somatic PKD mutation constitutes the rate-limiting step for cystogenesis, then a higher rate of somatic PKD mutations should be reported. However, none of the earlier human cyst studies screened the entire *PKD1* or *PKD2* for somatic mutations. Additionally, *PKD1* mutation screening is technically challenging because of its large size (an open reading frame of ~13 kb) and complexity (with ~75% of the gene duplicated in at least three homologs). To address this issue, a more recent study screened the entire *PKD2* coding sequence and splice junctions in 28 PKD2 renal cysts for somatic mutations. Using single-stranded conformational analysis with a known sensitivity for mutation detection of approximately 75%, inactivating somatic *PKD2* mutations were found in 71% of cysts screened.[261] Thus, when sensitive and comprehensive mutation screening is employed, somatic *PKD2* mutations can be detected in PKD2 cysts at a very high rate. The second concern relates to the detection of PC1 or PC2 immunoreactivity by C-terminal antibodies in a significant number of cystic epithelia, which is unexpected in light of the two-hit model.[191,264]

Although this issue remains unresolved at present, there are several potential explanations. First, in the cases of in-frame

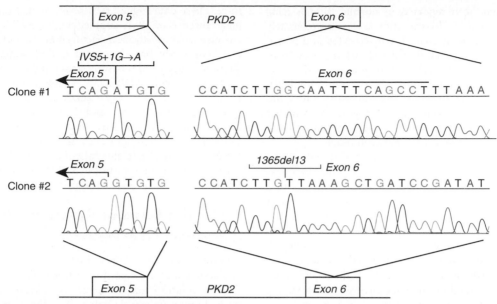

Figure 6-7 Bi-allelic *PKD2* inactivation within a monoclonal population of epithelial cells lining a single renal cyst. Both germline and somatic *PKD2* mutations were identified from the genomic DNA of these purified epithelial cells. Sequence tracings of two genomic clones amplified by long-range polymerase chain reaction contain the sites of germline and somatic *PKD2* mutations. Clone #1 shows the presence of the splice site germline mutation in exon 5 (IVS+1G→A) and normal sequence in exon 6. Clone #2 shows a normal sequence in exon 5 and a somatic mutation in exon 6 (1365del13).

deletions or missense mutations that maintain the mRNA open reading frame of the mutant transcript, the presence of immunoreactivity in a cyst might merely reflect the detection of a nonfunctional protein. Second, in the cases of truncating mutations, alternative readings of the mutant *Pkd1* transcript may allow the near full-length translation of a nonfunctional mutant protein, as shown in the del34 *Pkd1*-knockout mouse model (see Animal models of ADPKD, previous).[230] Third, detection of polycystin immunoreactivity is expected in trans-heterozygous inactivation in approximately 10% of ADPKD cysts.

In light of the above concerns, two recent studies have provided further support of the two-hit model for ADPKD. The first study indicates that the two-hit model is mechanistically linked to primary ciliary dysfunction, which has been recently shown to provide a convergent pathway for multiple renal cystic disorders (see earlier section on Primary Cilium in ADPKD).[200] It showed that both immortalized and primary cultured renal epithelial cells originated from normal or nondilated PKD1 kidney tubules displayed normal ciliary expression of polycystins and response to fluid-flow shear stress. By contrast, cyst-derived immortalized and primary cultured renal epithelial cells, which had undergone bi-allelic *PKD1* inactivation, did not respond to fluid-flow shear stress. The second study examined the gene locus effect on kidney size in the CRISP cohort using MRI for the volumetric measurements and cyst counts.[265] It showed that cyst formation increases with age in both gene types. However, PKD1 kidneys were significantly larger than PKD2 kidneys in age-matched patients, but the rate of cyst growth did not differ between the two gene types. Thus, PKD1 is associated with more severe renal disease because more cysts develop earlier, not because they grow faster (see later section on Gene Locus Effect). In turn, these data fit well with the two-hit model

since *PKD1* is approximately four times larger and is intrinsically more prone to mutation than *PKD2*.[141]

Knockout mouse studies also support the classical two-hit model in ADPKD (see earlier section on Animal Models of ADPKD).[266] *Pkd1* or *Pkd2* heterozygous inactivation in these models leads to focal renal and extrarenal cyst formation during adult life, similar to patients. By contrast, homozygous *Pkd1* or *Pkd2* inactivation is associated with embryonic/perinatal lethality and massive polycystic kidney disease. Of interest is the del34 *Pkd1* model, which was created by deletion of exon 34 and predicted to generate a truncated mutant protein lacking the C-terminal tail.[230] Using an N-terminal antibody, a truncated protein of the predicted size and, unexpectedly, a nearly full-length protein were detected in the mutant homozygotes. These data suggest that alternative readings of the mutant transcript may allow the translation of a nearly full-length mutant protein, and provide a possible explanation for increased PC1 immunoreactivity in the cystic epithelia. Further support of the two-hit hypothesis is provided by *Pkd2* mouse models that carry an unstable allele, ws25, which can undergo somatic rearrangement to generate a normal or null allele.[267] The frequency of renal cysts in these models increases according to the allelic series, with the most severe disease occurring in *Pkd2*[ws25/−], followed by *Pkd2*[ws25/−], *Pkd2*[+/−], and *Pkd2*[+/ws25] mice. Moreover, PC2 immunoreactivity was present in normal tubules, but uniformly negative in cystic epithelia, suggesting that complete loss of this protein was required for cyst development.

Since thousands of cysts can be found in a polycystic kidney with advanced disease, the two-hit model implies a very high rate of somatic mutations in renal epithelial tissue. Indeed, using a functional assay for inactivating mutations in the X-linked hypoxanthine phosphoribosyl transferase (*HPRT*) gene, a high somatic mutation frequency (i.e., ~5–25 mutations/

locus/10^5 cells) has been reported in normal human renal epithelial tissue in vivo.[268] This mutation rate is approximately 20 times higher than in human T lymphocytes and is unexpected, given that renal epithelial cells have a slow proliferation rate. These data therefore suggest an intrinsically higher somatic mutation frequency in the renal epithelia. Because of the high metabolism associated with secretory and resorptive functions, these cells may be exposed to a higher burden of oxidative stress and DNA damage. Alternatively, the efficiency of DNA repair may differ between tissues.

The two-hit model predicts that the somatic mutation of a PKD gene is the rate-limiting step for individual cyst formation. Thus, the cumulative frequency of such events within the kidney is expected to determine the total cyst number over the lifetime of a patient. Accordingly, common environmental factors such as cigarette smoking, food-borne mutagens (heterocyclic amines and polycyclic aromatic hydrocarbons), and folic acid deficiency may modify renal disease severity by modulating the renal somatic burden.[269] Additionally, functional gene variants encoding enzymes involved in detoxifying exogenous and endogenous mutagens (e.g., cytochrome P450 enzyme CYP2D6, and N-acetyltransferase 1 and 2) and in DNA repair may act as genetic modifiers of renal disease in ADPKD[270] (see later section on Modifier Genes).

Other Potential Mechanisms of Cystogenesis

While the classical two-hit model predicts that a complete loss of polycystin function is required for cytogenesis, alterations of polycystin gene dosage have been shown to cause renal cysts in experimental models. For example, transgenic mice overexpressing *Pkd1* caused renal cystic disease, suggesting that a normal level of polycystin is critical to maintain a differentiated tubular epithelial phenotype.[271] However, the relevance of this model to ADPKD is unclear since most cysts developed in these transgenic mice were derived from glomerular origin, and *Tsc2*, another cystogene associated with tuberous sclerosis, was concurrently overexpressed. Moreover, polycystin gene amplification has not been documented in human ADPKD. Two other studies, however, suggest that loss of function beyond a critical threshold, but not complete absence of polycystin, may initiate cystogenesis. The first study compared the renal phenotype between the *Pkd1*+/−, *Pkd2*+/−, and *Pkd1*+/−:*Pkd2*+/− knockout mice.[272] In keeping with the two-hit mechanism of cystogenesis, approximately 70% of kidney cysts in the *Pkd2*+/− mice exhibited uniform loss of PC2. However, the severity of cystic disease in the *Pkd1*+/−:*Pkd2*+/− mice was increased in excess of that predicted by a simple additive effect based on cyst formation in the singly heterozygous mutants. Coupled with the observation that only approximately 5% of the *Pkd1*+/−:*Pkd2*+/− cysts exhibited a complete loss of PC2 expression, this study proposes that the extra-additive effect observed in the transheterozygous mutants might be due to a two-hit mechanism involving a null and a hypomorphic *Pkd* allele. The second study examined the effects of a novel knockout mouse model with a hypomorphic allele, *Pkd1*nl, that is prone to aberrant splicing.[273] Interestingly, most homozygous *Pkd1*nl/*Pkd1*nl mutants retained 10% to 20% of the normally spliced *Pkd1* transcript and were viable despite developing massive polycystic kidneys at birth. Of note, variable PC1 immunostaining was seen in only a small number of cysts in *Pkd1*nl/*Pkd1*nl

mice. These data suggest that severe reduction, but not complete absence of PC1, coupled with possibly other genetic, environmental, or stochastic factors may also induce cystogenesis. A recent study has documented that somatic cytogenetic alterations occurred relatively frequently in the cystic epithelia of patients with ADPKD.[274] Using comparative genomic hybridization (CGH), both genomic deletions (on chromosomes 1p, 9q, 16p, 19, and 22q) and amplifications (on chromosomes 3q and 4q) were detected in multiple cyst samples. While their clinical significance remains uncertain at the present time, these data raise the possibility that additional somatic genetic alterations beyond the second PKD hits may be involved in the initiation or growth of individual cysts.

Molecular Basis of Cyst Growth

A Balancing Act of Proliferation and Apoptosis

A number of cellular defects, including increased proliferation and apoptosis, fluid secretion, extracellular matrix alterations, dedifferentiation, and abnormal polarity, have been observed in the human polycystic kidney.[10] In the context of renal cyst growth, cellular proliferation and apoptosis are clearly of premier importance. These two tightly regulated processes are required for normal development and tissue morphogenesis, and both are perturbed in ADPKD. In the normal adult kidney, tubular epithelial cells are well differentiated and quiescent. By contrast, cyst-lining epithelia in ADPKD are positive for the proliferating cell nuclear antigen (PCNA), indicating that they are actively proliferating. Additionally, increased apoptosis also occurs in both cystic epithelia and noncystic renal tubules.[243] While the molecular mechanisms of renal cyst growth in ADPKD remain incompletely understood, experimental studies have provided some important insights. Specifically, the notion that increased cellular proliferation is a critical first step for cyst growth is exemplified by the development of polycystic kidney disease in transgenic mice overexpressing proto-oncogenes such as *c-myc* or *H-ras*.[275,276] The importance of apoptosis is also highlighted by targeted inactivation of inhibitors of apoptosis (*bcl2* or activating protein 2β) in knockout mice that develop polycystic kidney disease.[277,278] Interestingly, increased cellular proliferation and apoptosis appear coupled in all these models and multiple human renal cystic diseases, suggesting that they may be general mechanisms for cytogenesis. Thus, increased apoptosis may provide a mechanism for the removal of normal parenchymal tissue, thereby allowing the cystic epithelia to proliferate. On the other hand, increased apoptosis in the polycystic kidneys may exert a counterproliferative effect. This is exemplified by reduction of *Pax2* gene dosage in the cpk mouse model, which results in increased apoptosis and amelioration of the renal cystic disease.[279] Although therapeutic strategies are now available to modulate the rate of apoptosis in tubular epithelial cells, further understanding of the complex interaction between proliferation and apoptosis is necessary before these interventions can be exploited for their clinical benefits.[280]

Dysregulation of $[Ca^{2+}]_i$ and $[cAMP]_i$

In vitro studies of cyst-lining epithelial cells from patients with ADPKD have provided strong evidence that dysregulation of $[Ca^{2+}]_i$ and $[cAMP]_i$ modulates cyst growth and transepithelial fluid secretion.[281-283] In these studies, cAMP increased cystic epithelial cell proliferation through activation of the B-Raf/MEK/extracellular signal–regulated kinase (B-Raf/MEK/ ERK) pathway and a number of adenylyl cyclase agonists, including arginine vasopressin (AVP), desmopressin (dDAVP), and a cyst-derived neutral lipid factor, can potentiate this response. By contrast, cAMP had an inhibitory effect on the proliferation of normal kidney tubular epithelial cells. This aberrant mitogenic response to cAMP appears to be related to reduced basal $[Ca^{2+}]_i$, which was approximately 20 nM lower in cystic epithelia than in epithelial cells derived from normal human kidneys or noncystic tubules of ADPKD kidneys. This proliferative phenotype can be induced in normal tubular epithelia by $[Ca^{2+}]_i$ restriction and reversed in cystic epithelia by $[Ca^{2+}]_i$ normalization through pharmacologic manipulations. Thus, the proliferative phenotype of cystic epithelia appears to be triggered by a calcium switch, which may be potentially linked to the loss of polycystin channel function.

Cyst expansion requires cellular proliferation, as well as fluid secretion to fill the enlarging cyst cavity. In vitro studies have shown that cAMP also stimulates apical transepithelial chloride transport through the cystic fibrosis transmembrane conductance regulator (CFTR), and pharmacologic blockade of CFTR appears to inhibit cyst growth in ADPKD.[284] Whether cystic fibrosis confers a renal protective effect in ADPKD is presently unclear, limited by conflicting results from two clinical studies with small sample sizes.[285] A more recent study of metanephric organ culture showed that the cAMP-mediated cystogenic effect can be reduced by pharmacologic CFTR inhibition and abolished in $Cftr^{-/-}$ mice. Interestingly, the $Cftr^{-/-}$ genotype completely suppressed cyst formation in $Pkd1^{-/-}$ embryonic kidneys in response to cAMP, but did not rescue the $Pkd1^{-/-}$ embryos from lethality.[286] Further studies are needed to evaluate the role of CFTR inhibitors as potential therapeutic agents for retarding cyst growth in ADPKD.

More recently, the effect of cAMP on cyst proliferation was confirmed in vivo by three different models of murine polycystic kidney disease. Treatment with a vasopressin V2 receptor (VPV2R) antagonist, OPC31260, was shown to significantly reduce renal cAMP and dramatically inhibit the cystic disease in the PCK rats (model of ARPKD) and pcy mice (model of nephronophthisis).[287] Similarly, this treatment also markedly inhibited the enlargement of renal cysts in $Pkd2^{ws25/-}$ mice, an orthologous model of human ADPKD.[288] Of note, the effects of VPV2R antagonism are restricted to the principal cells of the renal collecting duct, and most of the renal cysts in $Pkd2^{ws25/-}$ mice are derived from the distal nephron. These exciting data provide the basis for a major upcoming randomized clinical trial in ADPKD.

Activation of mTOR Signaling Pathway

The evidence for a novel proliferative pathway involving mTOR activation in ADPKD has been reviewed elsewhere (see earlier section on Polycystin Signaling Pathways).[226] While mTOR inhibition with rapamycin significantly ameliorated the renal cystic disease in both orpk and MAL mice, this antiproliferative effect needs to be confirmed in an orthologous model of ADPKD. Additionally, in a small retrospective study, reduction of total cystic kidney volume was noted in renal transplant patients with ADPKD who were treated with rapamycin compared to those without. Collectively, these promising data provide a strong rationale for two upcoming clinical trials of mTOR inhibitors in ADPKD.

Activation of Epidermal Growth Factor Signaling Pathway

EGF and TGF-α are secreted growth factors that signal through EGFR and the EGFR-related tyrosine kinase receptor, Erb-B2. Both EGF and TGF-α have been shown to modulate cyst growth in vitro through a cAMP-independent mechanism.[282,289] Renal cyst fluid from ADPKD, ARPKD, and multiple PKD animal models contains EGF and EGF-like activities, and EGFR is overexpressed and mislocalized to the apical surface of cystic epithelial cells in both ADPKD and ARPKD. Experimental manipulations of the EGF signaling cascade in three different recessive PKD models suggest that EGF and TGF-α modulate renal cyst growth in vivo.[280,290] Taken together, these data suggest that pharmacologic blockade of EGF signaling may be beneficial in modulating renal cyst growth. However, a recent study shows EGFR tyrosine kinase inhibition was deleterious in PCK rats (orthologous model of ARPKD).[291]

Angiogenesis

Renal cyst growth requires not only increased cellular proliferation, but also an adequate blood supply to provide oxygenation and nutrients to the expanding cell mass. Not surprisingly, recent studies have documented a rich network of blood vessels in the renal cyst walls of ADPKD kidneys.[292,293] Furthermore, a local autocrine/paracrine vascular endothelial growth factor (VEGF) signaling pathway appears to be in place between the cyst-lining epithelial cells and endothelial cells from blood vessels of the supporting stroma. While the primary stimuli for neovascularization have not been defined, local hypoxia and mTOR activation may potentially result in VEGF activation. Further studies are needed to define the role of angiogenesis in cyst expansion and anti-angiogenic treatments as potential therapy for ADPKD.

GENETIC BASIS OF PHENOTYPIC VARIABILITY IN ADPKD

Renal Disease Progression as a Complex Genetic Trait

Renal disease progression in ADPKD is highly variable, with the age of onset of ESRD ranging from childhood to old age.[294] Recent studies have provided important insights into the basis of this phenotypic variability and support the notion that renal disease progression in ADPKD is a complex trait influenced by genetic, environmental, and possibly stochastic factors. Additionally, a poorly understood gender effect favoring female patients is evident for PKD2, but not PKD1.

Gene Locus Effect

The gene locus confers a major effect on interfamilial renal disease variability in ADPKD.[13,75] Specifically, PKD1 patients present with ESRD (median age 53 [95% confidence interval

(CI) 51.2–54.8] vs. 69 [95% CI 66.9–71.3] years) approximately 15 years earlier than PKD2 patients. Based on the disease prevalence of these two gene types, it has been suggested that *PKD1* is inherently more mutagenic with a de novo germline mutation rate four to five times higher than *PKD2*.[141] Several unique features of the *PKD1* locus have been proposed to explain its increased mutagenicity: First, with an open reading frame four times larger than that of *PKD2* (~12 vs. ~3 kb, respectively), it is a larger target for mutations. Second, a long poly-pyrimidine tract on intron 21 may predispose to triplex DNA formation and recombination. Third, the presence of several homologous genes with high sequence similarity may predispose it to mutations from gene conversion. Thus, the locus effect coupled with the two-hit mechanism of cystogenesis would predict a higher cyst number in PKD1 than PKD2. Indeed, this notion is supported by recent data on kidney size variability by disease gene type in the CRISP cohort (see Monitoring Renal Disease Progression, previous).[265]

Allelic Effect

Most *PKD1* and *PKD2* mutations reported to date are protein truncating and predicted to result in a "loss-of-function" effect.[18,80,141–143] Two recent studies have examined whether there is an allelic effect in ADPKD that might influence renal disease severity. The first study examined the genotype-renal functional correlation in approximately 320 patients from 80 families with known *PKD1* mutations.[79] In this study, a positional effect was detected in that patients with germline mutations in the 3′ half of *PKD1* were found to have milder renal disease than patients with mutations in the 5′ half of the gene. However, this effect is rather modest and is translated into an average delay for initiation of ESRD therapy of 3 years. The types (nonsense, frameshift, and missense) of *PKD1* mutations in this study did not influence renal disease severity. By contrast, a second recent study that examined the genotype-renal functional correlation in approximately 410 patients from 71 families with known *PKD2* mutations did not detect a positional effect.[80] Instead, this latter study suggested that most *PKD2* germline mutations were associated with a complete loss-of-function effect. Of note, significant intrafamilial renal disease variability was present in both studies and could confound the assessment of allelic effects. Thus, an allelic effect on renal disease variability in ADPKD, if present, is weak.

Rare Mendelian Syndromes

Two rare mendelian syndromes have been shown to confer large effects on renal disease severity in ADPKD. The first syndrome involved patients with large genomic deletions of both *PKD1* and *TSC2*.[133] *PKD1* and *TSC2* are located in close proximity to each other on chromosome 16p13.3 in a tail-to-tail orientation, and germline mutations of either gene can give rise to a dominantly inherited renal cystic phenotype in ADPKD and tuberous sclerosis, respectively. Patients with contiguous deletions of both genes have a severe renal cystic phenotype: they developed infantile polycystic kidney disease and usually reached ESRD before the second decade of life. This finding suggests an interaction of these two cystogenes and convergence of signaling pathways downstream from their gene products, polycystin and tuberin. Of note, the

extrarenal manifestations of tuberous sclerosis in these patients may not be clinically evident and can be easily missed. Additionally, a family history was not apparent in a high percentage of probands since their affected parents were somatic mosaics with subtle disease. The second syndrome of interest involved bilineal inheritance of two independently segregating *PKD1* and *PKD2* germline mutations in a large family with ADPKD.[26] In this unusual family with at least 28 affected members, two affected individuals were shown to have trans-heterozygous germline *PKD1* and *PKD2* mutations and they both developed ESRD approximately 20 years earlier than other affected family members with either *PKD1* or *PKD2* mutation alone. These rare syndromes provide unique evidence for the role of interaction between cystogenes (*PKD1* with *TSC2*, and *PKD1* with *PKD2*) in modifying renal cystic disease severity.

Modifier Genes

Phenotypic variability of mendelian disorders such as cystic fibrosis and Hirschsprung's disease are in fact complex because of the existence and interaction of genetic and environmental modifiers.[295] Similarly, renal disease progression in ADPKD can be regarded as a complex trait influenced by both environmental and genetic factors. Recent studies have documented significant intrafamilial renal disease variability in ADPKD.[78,80] By controlling for the locus and allelic effects, these studies suggest that renal disease progression in ADPKD may be modified by genetic, environmental, and stochastic factors. The existence of a modifier gene effect on renal disease severity is further supported by increased intraclass correlation in affected twin pairs compared with affected sibling pairs.[296] Additionally, quantitative genetic analysis in two large family-based studies of PKD1 patients has estimated that the modifier gene effect may account for 30% to 40% and 50% to 80% of the variance for creatinine clearance and age at ESRD, respectively.[297,298] Furthermore, genetic background modulates the severity of experimental murine polycystic kidney disease, and a number of modifier gene loci have been mapped in multiple models.[266]

Taken together, the above data strongly implicate the existence of genetic and environmental modifiers of renal disease severity in human ADPKD.[294] Data from the CRISP study further suggests that polycystic kidney expansion is a two-phase process involving cyst initiation and growth.[265] Thus, different modifiers may be involved in each phase of cystogenesis. For example, functional gene variants encoding enzymes involved in detoxifying exogenous and endogenous mutagens, DNA repair, and oxidative metabolism, and environmental procarcinogens (e.g., cigarette smoking, food-borne mutagens, and folic acid deficiency) are strong biologic candidate modifiers for renal cyst number. By contrast, functional gene variants and environmental factors that regulate epithelial cell proliferation and apoptosis may modulate cyst expansion. However, because of the existence of multiple modifiers, each with modest effect, their identification will be challenging. Indeed, several population association studies have recently implicated specific variants of the angiotensin-converting enzyme and endothelial nitric oxide synthase genes as modifiers of renal disease progression in ADPKD. However, these studies are limited by their research design and small patient sample size and have produced conflicting results.[79,299-302] International collaborative research efforts are currently in progress to assemble a large cohort of genetically well-characterized patients to identify major genetic and environmental modifiers of renal disease variability in PKD1. A thorough knowledge of these determinants will allow better patient risk assessment and development of mechanism-based therapeutics for this important disease.

Extrarenal Variability

The molecular basis for extrarenal phenotypic variability in ADPKD is poorly understood. However, a recent retrospective study suggests that patients with mutations located on the 5′ half of *PKD1* may have an increased risk for intracranial arterial aneurysms.[101] By contrast, the type of mutations did not seem to influence the risk for this vascular phenotype. However, the patient sample size is relatively small in this study, and the observed effect is modest so that these findings should be regarded as preliminary.

CLINICAL MANAGEMENT OF ADPKD

Nonspecific Management

A number of nonspecific measures have been recommended for ADPKD.[10,28,280] In general, patients are encouraged to pursue an active lifestyle and participate in regular exercise to maintain optimal general health. However, those with significant renal disease should avoid contact sports to minimize the risk for traumatic cyst rupture. Based on the negative results of the MDRD study, dietary protein restriction as a therapeutic intervention to delay renal disease progression is not recommended.[66] On the other hand, excess protein intake should also be avoided. Although several metabolic and dietary interventions, such as sodium bicarbonate, potassium citrate flax oil, and soy protein, have been shown to be beneficial in experimental PKD, their role for the human disease is less clear since these studies were performed in nonorthologous models of ADPKD.[280] Given the potential role of somatic mutations in cystogenesis, it is prudent for patients with ADPKD to avoid exposure to cigarette smoking, and daily intake of antioxidants such as vitamin C and folic acid may also be considered. Excessive use of caffeine should be avoided since it increases $[cAMP]_i$ by inhibiting phosphodiesterase in vitro.[303] The management of specific complications in ADPKD has been reviewed under their subheadings (see earlier sections on Renal and Extrarenal Manifestations).

As the renal disease progresses, more than half of the patients with ADPKD will eventually require ESRD therapy.[10,28] In general, the treatment of these patients will be the same as those with other kidney diseases. However, peritoneal dialysis may not be ideal for some patients with severely enlarged polycystic kidneys because of incompatibility between the intra-abdominal space requirement and effective peritoneal exchange of fluid and solutes, increased risk for abdominal hernia, and back pain. For patients being considered for renal transplantation, a pretransplantation nephrectomy may be indicated for those with massive polycystic kidneys to better accommodate the allograft, as well as for those with a history of recurrent renal cyst infection. Renal transplant recipients with ADPKD have a twofold increased risk for colonic per-foration compared to those without, reflecting an increased prevalence of diverticulosis.[304] Overall, patients with ADPKD have an excellent survival rate after ESRD and reduced risk for death compared with nondiabetic dialysis patients.[305]

Promising Disease-Modifying Therapies

Advances in our understanding of the molecular pathobiology of ADPKD, coupled by the availability of orthologous animal models for the human disease, have facilitated the testing and identification of several classes of promising candidate drugs in preclinical studies. In turn, we are now witnessing a period of intense translational research when a number of highly promising disease-modifying drugs will be tested in major clinical trials. Based on their results from preclinical studies, most of these candidate drugs are expected to retard renal disease progression by targeting renal cyst growth. Moreover, the fact that several of them (e.g., tolvaptan, octreotide, and rapamycin) have already been approved for other clinical indications would likely facilitate their fast-track approval for clinical trials in ADPKD.[226,306,307]

In the planning of clinical trials for ADPKD, the use of renal function as a primary outcome measure poses a serious methodologic challenge, since decades of normal or near-normal renal function, despite progressive enlargement and distortion of the cystic kidneys, characterize the natural history of this disease.[10] Thus, early intervention trials would require an unrealistic duration of follow-up in order to detect changes in renal function. By contrast, late interventional trials targeting patients with impaired renal function risk passing the "point of no return" for potential therapeutic benefits because of advanced structural disease. Fortunately, MRI-based kidney volume progression, as validated by recent results from CRISP, provides both a sensitive and accurate measure of renal disease progression in ADPKD.[144] Thus, the availability of this surrogate marker of renal disease progression makes it possible to evaluate the efficacy of a promising treatment within a realistic time frame and has now replaced renal function as the gold standard for clinical trials in ADPKD. Ultimately, the clinical efficacy and side effect profile of these novel drugs will determine whether they will be used in the clinical setting. Effective drugs that are safe can be used for long-term and even early "preventive" treatment. By contrast, effective drugs with potentially serious side effects will likely be used as "rescue therapy" for a defined duration in patients with moderate to severe disease.

Clinical Trial of Vasopressin V2 Receptor Antagonism

Based on the promising results of OPC-31260 in *Pkd2*[ws25/−] mice, a phase 3, multicenter, double-blinded, placebo-controlled, parallel-arm trial will begin in 2007 to determine the long-term safety and efficacy of tolvaptan on renal disease progression in ADPKD. In this study, plans are to recruit and randomize at least 1,200 patients to receive either tolvaptan or placebo for three years. The primary clinical outcome of this trial will be the rate of change in kidney volume between tolvaptan and placebo-treated patients over the treatment period. Adult patients with an estimated GFR of 60 mL/min and total kidney volume of over 750 mL will be eligible, and a dose escalation schedule will be used to maximize the pharmacologic effects. Because of the selective expression of vasopressin V2 receptor, tolvaptan is not be expected to have any therapeutic effects in noncollecting duct cysts and extrarenal cysts. The major side effects of this drug include polyuria and dry mouth, but it is otherwise safe and well tolerated in short-term clinical studies.[306]

Clinical Trials of mTOR Inhibition

The discovery that PC1 normally interacts with tuberin, that the disruption of this interaction is associated with mTOR activation in ADPKD, and that mTOR inhibition significantly ameliorates the cystic phenotype in two recessive PKD models has provided a novel therapeutic paradigm for the use of mTOR inhibitors. Interestingly, preliminary data also showed a reduction of cystic kidney volume in renal transplant patients with ADPKD who were treated with rapamycin compared to those without.[226] While these promising findings need to be confirmed in orthologous models of ADPKD, at least three clinical trials of mTOR inhibitors (rapamycin or everolimus) are being organized in Germany, Switzerland, and the United States using similar eligibility criteria as in the tolvaptan study. Compared to vasopressin V2 receptor antagonism, mTOR inhibition is expected to have a more generalized antiproliferative effect targeting renal cysts from all segments of the nephron, as well as extrarenal cysts.[308] On the other hand, long-term treatment with rapamycin may be associated with an increased risk for side effects such as dyslipidemia, thrombocytopenia, impaired wound healing, and immunosuppression, as well as poorly understood idiosyncratic reactions such as proteinuria and interstitial pulmonary fibrosis (Product Monograph, Wyeth Canada).

Clinical Trial of Antagonism of Renin-Angiotensin Axis

The HALT PKD Study is a multicenter, randomized, controlled trial designed to evaluate the efficacy of pharmacologic blockade of the renin-angiotensin system on the progression of cystic disease and the decline in renal function in ADPKD. Study A will test the efficacy of combination therapy with an angiotensin-converting enzyme inhibitor (ACEI) and an angiotensin receptor blocker (ARB) versus monotherapy with an ACEI in approximately 550 patients over 4 years. Patients will also be randomized to two levels of blood pressure control: low blood pressure control defined as 95 to 110/60 to 75 mmHg and standard blood pressure control defined as 120 to 130/70 to 80 mmHg. Additional blood pressure medications will be added per protocol as needed. Patients with early kidney disease (GFR >60 mL/min) will be eligible for this study, and MRI-based kidney volume progression will be used to evaluate the treatment effect. Study B will test the efficacy of combination therapy with an ACEI and an ARB versus monotherapy with an ACEI in approximately 700 patients with more advanced kidney disease as defined by a GFR of 30 to 60 mL/min. All patients will be treated to a standard level of blood pressure control (120–130/70–80 mmHg). Additional blood pressure medications will be added per protocol as needed. The primary end point of this study is the time to doubling of serum creatinine, ESRD, or death. The novel aspect of this trial is that study A will test whether the combination of an ACEI and an ARB has an additive effect compared with ACEI alone in inhibiting renal cyst growth. However, the lack of a control group of patients not treated with ACEI and ARB will make it difficult to conclude any class-specific effect.

Other Promising Candidate Drugs

Several other promising drugs are currently being evaluated in preclinical and phase I/II clinical studies. Somatostatin is a promising candidate with a more generalized inhibitory effect on $[cAMP]_i$ accumulation in both the kidneys and liver. Octreotide, a stable synthetic analog of somatostatin, has been shown to reduce renal and hepatic cyst expansion in PCK rats (personal communication, V. Torres, 2007). These observations are consistent with the inhibition of renal growth in a pilot study of long-acting octreotide (Sandostatin LAR) in ADPKD.[307] Additionally, the potential role of Erb-B1 (EGFR) tyrosine kinase inhibitors and cyclin-dependent kinase inhibitors as novel treatment of ADPKD needs to be further evaluated.

Acknowledgments

This work is supported by grants from the Kidney Foundation of Canada and Canadian Institutes of Health Research (MOP 53324) to Y. Pei, and grants from the National Institutes of Health (NIDDK) 53357, 51050, 074030, and 40703 to J. Zhou.

References

1. Igarashi P, Somlo S: Genetics and pathogenesis of polycystic kidney disease. J Am Soc Nephrol 13:2384–2398, 2002.
2. Ong AC, Harris PC: Molecular pathogenesis of ADPKD: The polycystin complex gets complex. Kidney Int 67:1234–1247, 2005.
3. Dalgaard OZ: Bilateral polycystic disease of the kidneys; a follow-up of two hundred and eighty-four patients and their families. Acta Med Scand Suppl 328:1–255, 1957.
4. Iglesias CG, et al: Epidemiology of adult polycystic kidney disease, Olmsted County, Minnesota: 1935–1980. Am J Kidney Dis 2:630–639, 1983.
5. Levy M, Feingold J: Estimating prevalence in single-gene kidney diseases progressing to renal failure. Kidney Int 58:925–943, 2000.
6. Collins AJ, et al: Excerpts from the United States Renal Data System 2004 annual data report: Atlas of end-stage renal disease in the United States. Am J Kidney Dis 45:A5–A7, 2005.
7. Reeders ST, et al: A highly polymorphic DNA marker linked to adult polycystic kidney disease on chromosome 16. Nature 317:542–544, 1985.
8. Peters DJ, et al: Chromosome 4 localization of a second gene for autosomal dominant polycystic kidney disease. Nat Genet 5:359–362, 1993.
9. Dobin A, et al: Segregation analysis of autosomal dominant polycystic kidney disease. Genet Epidemiol 10:189–200, 1993.
10. Grantham J, Winklhofer F: In Brenner BM (ed): Brenner and Rector's The Kidney. Philadelphia, WB Saunders, 2003, pp 1743–1773.
11. Peters DJ, Sandkuijl LA: Genetic heterogeneity of polycystic kidney disease in Europe. Contrib Nephrol 97:128–139, 1992.
12. Peral B, et al: Estimating locus heterogeneity in autosomal dominant polycystic kidney disease (ADPKD) in the Spanish population. J Med Genet 30:910–913, 1993.
13. Hateboer N, et al: Comparison of phenotypes of polycystic kidney disease types 1 and 2. European PKD1-PKD2 Study Group. Lancet 353:103–107, 1999.

14. Wilkie AO: The molecular basis of genetic dominance. J Med Genet 31:89–98, 1994.
15. Paterson AD, Wang KR, Lupea D, et al: Recurrent fetal loss associated with bilineal inheritance of type 1 autosomal dominant polycystic kidney disease. Am J Kidney Dis 40:16–20, 2002.
16. Hughes J, et al: The polycystic kidney disease 1 (*PKD1*) gene encodes a novel protein with multiple cell recognition domains. Nat Genet 10:151–160, 1995.
17. International Polycystic Kidney Disease Consortium: Polycystic kidney disease: The complete structure of the *PKD1* gene and its protein. Cell 81:289–298, 1995.
18. Rossetti S, et al: A complete mutation screen of the ADPKD genes by DHPLC. Kidney Int 61:1588–1599, 2002.
19. Mochizuki T, et al: *PKD2*, a gene for polycystic kidney disease that encodes an integral membrane protein. Science 272:1339–1342, 1996.
20. Daoust MC, Reynolds DM, Bichet DG, Somlo S: Evidence for a third genetic locus for autosomal dominant polycystic kidney disease. Genomics 25:733–736, 1995.
21. de Almeida S, et al: Autosomal dominant polycystic kidney disease: Evidence for the existence of a third locus in a Portuguese family. Hum Genet 96:83–88, 1995.
22. Turco AE, Clementi M, Rossetti S, et al: An Italian family with autosomal dominant polycystic kidney disease unlinked to either the *PKD1* or *PKD2* gene. Am J Kidney Dis 28:759–761, 1996.
23. Ariza M, et al: A family with a milder form of adult dominant polycystic kidney disease not linked to the *PKD1* (16p) or *PKD2* (4q) genes. J Med Genet 34:587–589, 1997.
24. Paterson AD, Pei Y: Is there a third gene for autosomal dominant polycystic kidney disease? Kidney Int 54:1759–1761, 1998.
25. Paterson AD, Pei Y: PKD3—To be or not to be? Nephrol Dial Transplant 14:2965–2966, 1999.
26. Pei Y, et al: Bilineal disease and trans-heterozygotes in autosomal dominant polycystic kidney disease. Am J Hum Genet 68:355–363, 2001.
27. Milutinovic J, et al: Clinical manifestations of autosomal dominant polycystic kidney disease in patients older than 50 years. Am J Kidney Dis 15:237–243, 1990.
28. Gabow PA: Autosomal dominant polycystic kidney disease. N Engl J Med 329:332–342, 1993.
29. Bajwa ZH, Gupta S, Warfield CA, Steinman TI: Pain management in polycystic kidney disease. Kidney Int 60:1631–1644, 2001.
30. Elzinga LW, et al: Cyst decompression surgery for autosomal dominant polycystic kidney disease. J Am Soc Nephrol 2:1219–1226, 1992.
31. Segura J, King B, Fowsey S, et al: In Watson ML, Torres V (ed): Polycystic Kidney Disease. Oxford, UK, Oxford University Press, 1996, pp 462–480.
32. Badani KK, Hemal AK, Menon M: Autosomal dominant polycystic kidney disease and pain—A review of the disease from aetiology, evaluation, past surgical treatment options to current practice. J Postgrad Med 50:222–226, 2004.
33. Dunn MD, et al: Laparoscopic nephrectomy in patients with end-stage renal disease and autosomal dominant polycystic kidney disease. Am J Kidney Dis 35:720–725, 2000.
34. Lee DI, Clayman RV: Hand-assisted laparoscopic nephrectomy in autosomal dominant polycystic kidney disease. J Endourol 18:379–382, 2004.
35. Zwettler U, Zeier M, Andrassy K, et al: Treatment of gross hematuria in autosomal dominant polycystic kidney disease with aprotinin and desmopressin acetate. Nephron 60:374, 1992.
36. Harley JD, Shen FH, Carter SJ: Transcatheter infarction of a polycystic kidney for control of recurrent hemorrhage. AJR 134:818–820, 1980.
37. Chapman AB, Johnson AM, Gabow PA, Schrier RW: Overt proteinuria and microalbuminuria in autosomal dominant polycystic kidney disease. J Am Soc Nephrol 5:1349–1354, 1994.
38. Zeier M, et al: Renal histology in polycystic kidney disease with incipient and advanced renal failure. Kidney Int 42:1259–1265, 1992.
39. Contreras G, Mercado A, Pardo V, Vaamonde CA: Nephrotic syndrome in autosomal dominant polycystic kidney disease. J Am Soc Nephrol 6:1354–1359, 1995.
40. Fick GM, Johnson AM, Hammond WS, Gabow PA: Causes of death in autosomal dominant polycystic kidney disease. J Am Soc Nephrol 5:2048–2056, 1995.
41. Schwab SJ, Bander SJ, Klahr S: Renal infection in autosomal dominant polycystic kidney disease. Am J Med 82:714–718, 1987.
42. Gibson P, Watson ML: Cyst infection in polycystic kidney disease: A clinical challenge. Nephrol Dial Transplant 13:2455–2457, 1998.
43. Grantham JJ, Geiser JL, Evan AP: Cyst formation and growth in autosomal dominant polycystic kidney disease. Kidney Int 31:1145–1152, 1987.
44. Torres VE, Wilson DM, Hattery RR, Segura JW: Renal stone disease in autosomal dominant polycystic kidney disease. Am J Kidney Dis 22:513–519, 1993.
45. Grampsas SA, et al: Anatomic and metabolic risk factors for nephrolithiasis in patients with autosomal dominant polycystic kidney disease. Am J Kidney Dis 36:53–57, 2000.
46. Keith DS, Torres VE, King BF, et al: Renal cell carcinoma in autosomal dominant polycystic kidney disease. J Am Soc Nephrol 4:1661–1669, 1994.
47. Gabow PA, et al: Factors affecting the progression of renal disease in autosomal-dominant polycystic kidney disease. Kidney Int 41:1311–1319, 1992.
48. Bell PE, et al: Hypertension in autosomal dominant polycystic kidney disease. Kidney Int 34:683–690, 1988.
49. Ecder T, Schrier RW: Hypertension in autosomal-dominant polycystic kidney disease: Early occurrence and unique aspects. J Am Soc Nephrol 12:194–200, 2001.
50. Gabow PA, Ikle DW, Holmes JH: Polycystic kidney disease: Prospective analysis of nonazotemic patients and family members. Ann Intern Med 101:238–247, 1984.
51. Sedman A, et al: Autosomal dominant polycystic kidney disease in childhood: A longitudinal study. Kidney Int 31:1000–1005, 1987.
52. Ivy DD, et al: Cardiovascular abnormalities in children with autosomal dominant polycystic kidney disease. J Am Soc Nephrol 5:2032–2036, 1995.
53. Zeier M, Geberth S, Schmidt KG, et al: Elevated blood pressure profile and left ventricular mass in children and young adults with autosomal dominant polycystic kidney disease. J Am Soc Nephrol 3:1451–1457, 1993.
54. Chapman AB, et al: Left ventricular hypertrophy in autosomal dominant polycystic kidney disease. J Am Soc Nephrol 8:1292–1297, 1997.
55. Valero FA, et al: Ambulatory blood pressure and left ventricular mass in normotensive patients with autosomal dominant polycystic kidney disease. J Am Soc Nephrol 10:1020–1026, 1999.
56. Ettinger A, Kahn PC, Wise HM, Jr: The importance of selective renal angiography in the diagnosis of polycystic disease. J Urol 102:156–161, 1969.
57. Chapman AB, Johnson A, Gabow PA, Schrier RW: The renin-angiotensin-aldosterone system and autosomal dominant polycystic kidney disease. N Engl J Med 323:1091–1096, 1990.
58. Harrap SB, et al: Renal, cardiovascular and hormonal characteristics of young adults with autosomal dominant polycystic kidney disease. Kidney Int 40:501–508, 1991.

59. Barrett BJ, Foley R, Morgan J, et al: Differences in hormonal and renal vascular responses between normotensive patients with autosomal dominant polycystic kidney disease and unaffected family members. Kidney Int 46:1118–1123, 1994.

60. Torres VE, Wilson DM, Burnett JC Jr, et al: Effect of inhibition of converting enzyme on renal hemodynamics and sodium management in polycystic kidney disease. Mayo Clin Proc 66:1010–1017, 1991.

61. Torres VE, et al: Synthesis of renin by tubulocystic epithelium in autosomal-dominant polycystic kidney disease. Kidney Int 42:364–373, 1992.

62. Loghman-Adham M, Soto CE, Inagami T, Cassis L: The intrarenal renin-angiotensin system in autosomal dominant polycystic kidney disease. Am J Physiol Renal Physiol 287:F775–F788, 2004.

63. Klein IH, Ligtenberg G, Oey PL, et al: Sympathetic activity is increased in polycystic kidney disease and is associated with hypertension. J Am Soc Nephrol 12:2427–2433, 2001.

64. Wang D, Iversen J, Wilcox CS, Strandgaard S: Endothelial dysfunction and reduced nitric oxide in resistance arteries in autosomal-dominant polycystic kidney disease. Kidney Int 64:1381–1388, 2003.

65. Ecder T, et al: Progress in blood pressure control in autosomal dominant polycystic kidney disease. Am J Kidney Dis 36:266–271, 2000.

66. Klahr S, et al: Dietary protein restriction, blood pressure control, and the progression of polycystic kidney disease. Modification of Diet in Renal Disease Study Group. J Am Soc Nephrol 5:2037–2047, 1995.

67. Coresh J, et al: Prevalence of high blood pressure and elevated serum creatinine level in the United States: Findings from the third National Health and Nutrition Examination Survey (1988–1994). Arch Intern Med 161:1207–1216, 2001.

68. Schrier R, et al: Cardiac and renal effects of standard versus rigorous blood pressure control in autosomal-dominant polycystic kidney disease: Results of a seven-year prospective randomized study. J Am Soc Nephrol 13:1733–1739, 2002.

69. Jafar TH, et al: Progression of chronic kidney disease: The role of blood pressure control, proteinuria, and angiotensin-converting enzyme inhibition: A patient-level meta-analysis. Ann Intern Med 139:244–252, 2003.

70. Chapman AB, Gabow PA, Schrier RW: Reversible renal failure associated with angiotensin-converting enzyme inhibitors in polycystic kidney disease. Ann Intern Med 115:769–773, 1991.

71. Group AIIDNT: Should all patients with type 1 diabetes mellitus and microalbuminuria receive angiotensin-converting enzyme inhibitors? A meta-analysis of individual patient data. Ann Intern Med 134:370–379, 2001.

72. Maschio G, Marcantoni C, Bernich P: Lessons from large interventional trials on antihypertensive therapy in chronic renal disease. Nephrol Dial Transplant 17(Suppl 11):47–49, 2002.

73. Jafar TH, et al: The effect of angiotensin-converting-enzyme inhibitors on progression of advanced polycystic kidney disease. Kidney Int 67:265–271, 2005.

74. Chobanian AV, et al: The Seventh Report of the Joint National Committee on Prevention, Detection, Evaluation, and Treatment of High Blood Pressure: The JNC 7 report. JAMA 289:2560–2572, 2003.

75. Parfrey PS, et al: The diagnosis and prognosis of autosomal dominant polycystic kidney disease. N Engl J Med 323:1085–1090, 1990.

76. Ravine D, et al: Phenotype and genotype heterogeneity in autosomal dominant polycystic kidney disease. Lancet 340:1330–1333, 1992.

77. Fick GM, Johnson AM, Gabow PA: Is there evidence for anticipation in autosomal-dominant polycystic kidney disease? Kidney Int 45:1153–1162, 1994.

78. Hateboer N, Lazarou LP, Williams AJ, et al: Familial phenotype differences in PKD11. Kidney Int 56:34–40, 1999.

79. Rossetti, S, et al: The position of the polycystic kidney disease 1 (PKD1) gene mutation correlates with the severity of renal disease. J Am Soc Nephrol 13:1230–1237, 2002.

80. Magistroni R, et al: Genotype-renal function correlation in type 2 autosomal dominant polycystic kidney disease. J Am Soc Nephrol 14:1164–1174, 2003.

81. Johnson AM, Gabow PA: Identification of patients with autosomal dominant polycystic kidney disease at highest risk for end-stage renal disease. J Am Soc Nephrol 8:1560–1567, 1997.

82. Fick-Brosnahan GM, Tran ZV, Johnson AM, et al: Progression of autosomal-dominant polycystic kidney disease in children. Kidney Int 59:1654–1662, 2001.

83. Fick-Brosnahan GM, Belz MM, McFann KK, et al: Relationship between renal volume growth and renal function in autosomal dominant polycystic kidney disease: A longitudinal study. Am J Kidney Dis 39:1127–1134, 2002.

84. King BF, Reed JE, Bergstralh EJ, et al: Quantification and longitudinal trends of kidney, renal cyst, and renal parenchyma volumes in autosomal dominant polycystic kidney disease. J Am Soc Nephrol 11:1505–1511, 2000.

85. Chapman AB, et al: Renal structure in early autosomal-dominant polycystic kidney disease (ADPKD): The Consortium for Radiologic Imaging Studies of Polycystic Kidney Disease (CRISP) cohort. Kidney Int 64:1035–1045, 2003.

86. King BF, et al: Magnetic resonance measurements of renal blood flow as a marker of disease severity in autosomal-dominant polycystic kidney disease. Kidney Int 64:2214–2221, 2003.

87. Zeier M, et al: The effect of uninephrectomy on progression of renal failure in autosomal dominant polycystic kidney disease. J Am Soc Nephrol 3:1119–1123, 1992.

88. Gabow PA, et al: Risk factors for the development of hepatic cysts in autosomal dominant polycystic kidney disease. Hepatology 11:1033–1037, 1990.

89. Chauveau D, Fakhouri F, Grunfeld JP: Liver involvement in autosomal-dominant polycystic kidney disease: Therapeutic dilemma. J Am Soc Nephrol 11:1767–1775, 2000.

90. Qian Q, et al: Clinical profile of autosomal dominant polycystic liver disease. Hepatology 37:164–171, 2003.

91. Drenth JP, Martina JA, van de Kerkhof R, et al: Polycystic liver disease is a disorder of cotranslational protein processing. Trends Mol Med 11:37–42, 2005.

92. Sherstha R, et al: Postmenopausal estrogen therapy selectively stimulates hepatic enlargement in women with autosomal dominant polycystic kidney disease. Hepatology 26:1282–1286, 1997.

93. Everson GT, Taylor MR, Doctor RB: Polycystic disease of the liver. Hepatology 40:774–782, 2004.

94. Chapman AB, et al: Intracranial aneurysms in autosomal dominant polycystic kidney disease. N Engl J Med 327:916–920, 1992.

95. Huston J, 3rd, Torres VE, Sulivan PP, et al: Value of magnetic resonance angiography for the detection of intracranial aneurysms in autosomal dominant polycystic kidney disease. J Am Soc Nephrol 3:1871–1877, 1993.

96. Ruggieri PM, et al: Occult intracranial aneurysms in polycystic kidney disease: Screening with MR angiography. Radiology 191:33–39, 1994.

97. Rinkel GJ, Djibuti M, Algra A, van Gijn J: Prevalence and risk of rupture of intracranial aneurysms: A systematic review. Stroke 29:251–256, 1998.

98. Chauveau D, et al: Intracranial aneurysms in autosomal dominant polycystic kidney disease. Kidney Int 45:1140–1146, 1994.

99. Belz MM, et al: Familial clustering of ruptured intracranial aneurysms in autosomal dominant polycystic kidney disease. Am J Kidney Dis 38:770–776, 2001.

100. Watnick T, et al: Mutation detection of PKD1 identifies a novel mutation common to three families with aneurysms and/or very-early-onset disease. Am J Hum Genet 65:1561–1571, 1999.

101. Rossetti S, et al: Association of mutation position in polycystic kidney disease 1 (PKD1) gene and development of a vascular phenotype. Lancet 361:2196–2201, 2003.

102. Griffin MD, Torres VE, Grande JP, Kumar R: Vascular expression of polycystin. J Am Soc Nephrol 8:616–626, 1997.

103. Torres VE, et al: Vascular expression of polycystin-2. J Am Soc Nephrol 12:1–9, 2001.

104. Qian Q, et al: Pkd2 haploinsufficiency alters intracellular calcium regulation in vascular smooth muscle cells. Hum Mol Genet 12:1875–1880, 2003.

105. Schievink WI, Torres VE, Piepgras DG, Wiebers DO: Saccular intracranial aneurysms in autosomal dominant polycystic kidney disease. J Am Soc Nephrol 3:88–95, 1992.

106. Lozano AM, Leblanc R: Familial intracranial aneurysms. J Neurosurg 66:522–528, 1987.

107. Schievink WI: Intracranial aneurysms. N Engl J Med 336:28–40, 1997.

108. Pirson Y, Chauveau D Torres V: Management of cerebral aneurysms in autosomal dominant polycystic kidney disease. J Am Soc Nephrol 13:269–276, 2002.

109. Linn FH, et al: Prospective study of sentinel headache in aneurysmal subarachnoid haemorrhage. Lancet 344:590–593, 1994.

110. Edlow JA, Caplan LR: Avoiding pitfalls in the diagnosis of subarachnoid hemorrhage. N Engl J Med 342:29–36, 2000.

111. Johnston SC, et al: Recommendations for the endovascular treatment of intracranial aneurysms: A statement for healthcare professionals from the Committee on Cerebrovascular Imaging of the American Heart Association Council on Cardiovascular Radiology. Stroke 33:2536–2544, 2002.

112. Molyneux A, et al: International Subarachnoid Aneurysm Trial (ISAT) of neurosurgical clipping versus endovascular coiling in 2,143 patients with ruptured intracranial aneurysms: A randomised trial. Lancet 360:1267–1274, 2002.

113. Belz MM, et al: Recurrence of intracranial aneurysms in autosomal-dominant polycystic kidney disease. Kidney Int 63:1824–1830, 2003.

114. Gibbs GF, et al: Follow-up of intracranial aneurysms in autosomal-dominant polycystic kidney disease. Kidney Int 65:1621–1627, 2004.

115. Wiebers DO, et al: Unruptured intracranial aneurysms: Natural history, clinical outcome, and risks of surgical and endovascular treatment. Lancet 362:103–110, 2003.

116. Schievink WI, Torres VE, Wiebers DO, Huston J, 3rd: Intracranial arterial dolichoectasia in autosomal dominant polycystic kidney disease. J Am Soc Nephrol 8:1298–1303, 1997.

117. Graf S, et al: Intracranial aneurysms and dolichoectasia in autosomal dominant polycystic kidney disease. Nephrol Dial Transplant 17:819–823, 2002.

118. Somlo S, et al: A kindred exhibiting cosegregation of an overlap connective tissue disorder and the chromosome 16 linked form of autosomal dominant polycystic kidney disease. J Am Soc Nephrol 4:1371–1378, 1993.

119. Hateboer N, Buchalter M, Davies SJ, et al: Co-occurrence of autosomal dominant polycystic kidney disease and Marfan syndrome in a kindred. Am J Kidney Dis 35:753–760, 2000.

120. Torra R, et al: Abdominal aortic aneurysms and autosomal dominant polycystic kidney disease. J Am Soc Nephrol 7:2483–2486, 1996.

121. Timio M, et al: The spectrum of cardiovascular abnormalities in autosomal dominant polycystic kidney disease: A 10-year follow-up in a five-generation kindred. Clin Nephrol 37:245–251, 1992.

122. Hossack KF, Leddy CL, Johnson AM, et al: Echocardiographic findings in autosomal dominant polycystic kidney disease. N Engl J Med 319:907–912, 1988.

123. Scheff RT, Zuckerman G, Harter H, et al: Diverticular disease in patients with chronic renal failure due to polycystic kidney disease. Ann Intern Med 92:202–204, 1980.

124. Sharp CK, Zeligman BE, Johnson AM, et al: Evaluation of colonic diverticular disease in autosomal dominant polycystic kidney disease without end-stage renal disease. Am J Kidney Dis 34:863–868, 1999.

125. Morris-Stiff G, Coles G, Moore R, et al: Abdominal wall hernia in autosomal dominant polycystic kidney disease. Br J Surg 84:615–617, 1997.

126. Modi KB, Grant AC, Garret A, Rodger RS: Indirect inguinal hernia in CAPD patients with polycystic kidney disease. Adv Perit Dial 5:84–86, 1989.

127. Fick GM, et al: Characteristics of very early onset autosomal dominant polycystic kidney disease. J Am Soc Nephrol 3:1863–1870, 1993.

128. Fick GM, Gabow PA: Hereditary and acquired cystic disease of the kidney. Kidney Int 46:951–964, 1994.

129. Davies F, et al: Polycystic kidney disease re-evaluated: A population-based study. Q J Med 79:477–485, 1991.

130. Pei Y: Diagnostic approach in autosomal dominant polycystic kidney disease. Clin J Am Soc Nephrol 1:1108–1114, 2006.

131. Sparagana SP, Roach ES: Tuberous sclerosis complex. Curr Opin Neurol 13:115–119, 2000.

132. Brook-Carter PT, et al: Deletion of the TSC2 and PKD1 genes associated with severe infantile polycystic kidney disease—A contiguous gene syndrome. Nat Genet 8:328–332, 1994.

133. Sampson JR, et al: Renal cystic disease in tuberous sclerosis: Role of the polycystic kidney disease 1 gene. Am J Hum Genet 61:843–851, 1997.

134. Michels V: In Watson ML, Torres VE (ed): Polycystic Kidney Disease. Oxford, UK, Oxford University Press, 1996, pp 309–330.

135. McHugh K, Stringer DA, Hebert D, Babiak CA: Simple renal cysts in children: Diagnosis and follow-up with US. Radiology 178:383–385, 1991.

136. Ravine D, Gibson RN, Donlan J, Sheffield LJ: An ultrasound renal cyst prevalence survey: Specificity data for inherited renal cystic diseases. Am J Kidney Dis 22:803–807, 1993.

137. Tantravahi J, Steinman TI: Acquired cystic kidney disease. Semin Dial 13:330–334, 2000.

138. Ravine D, et al: Evaluation of ultrasonographic diagnostic criteria for autosomal dominant polycystic kidney disease 1. Lancet 343:824–827, 1994.

139. Pei Y, Magistroni R, Parfrey P, et al: Unified ultrasonographic diagnostic criteria for autosomal dominant polycystic kidney disease. J Am Soc Nephrol 15:657A, 2004.

140. Nascimento AB, et al: Rapid MR imaging detection of renal cysts: Age-based standards. Radiology 221:628–632, 2001.

141. Rossetti S, et al: Mutation analysis of the entire PKD1 gene: Genetic and diagnostic implications. Am J Hum Genet 68:46–63, 2001.

142. Pei Y, et al: A spectrum of mutations in the polycystic kidney disease-2 (PKD2) gene from eight Canadian kindreds. J Am Soc Nephrol 9:1853–1860, 1998.

143. Deltas CC: Mutations of the human polycystic kidney disease 2 (PKD2) gene. Hum Mutat 18:13–24, 2001.

144. Grantham JJ, et al: Volume progression in polycystic kidney disease. N Engl J Med 354:2122–2130, 2006.

145. Nims N, Vassmer D, Maser RL: Transmembrane domain analysis of polycystin-1, the product of the polycystic kidney

disease-1 (*PKD1*) gene: Evidence for 11 membrane-spanning domains. Biochemistry 42:13035–13048, 2003.

146. Malhas AN, Abuknesha RA, Price RG: Interaction of the leucine-rich repeats of polycystin-1 with extracellular matrix proteins: Possible role in cell proliferation. J Am Soc Nephrol 13:19–26, 2002.

147. Slade MJ, Kirby RB, Pocsi I, et al: Presence of laminin fragments in cyst fluid from patients with autosomal dominant polycystic kidney disease (ADPKD): Role in proliferation of tubular epithelial cells. Biochim Biophys Acta 1401:203–210, 1998.

148. Ibraghimov-Beskrovnaya O, et al: Strong homophilic interactions of the Ig-like domains of polycystin-1, the protein product of an autosomal dominant polycystic kidney disease gene, *PKD1*. Hum Mol Genet 9:1641–1649, 2000.

149. Moy GW, et al: The sea urchin sperm receptor for egg jelly is a modular protein with extensive homology to the human polycystic kidney disease protein, PKD1. J Cell Biol 133:809–817, 1996.

150. Qian F, et al: Cleavage of polycystin-1 requires the receptor for egg jelly domain and is disrupted by human autosomal-dominant polycystic kidney disease 1–associated mutations. Proc Natl Acad Sci U S A 99:16981–16986, 2002.

151. Qian F, et al: PKD1 interacts with PKD2 through a probable coiled-coil domain. Nat Genet 16:179–183, 1997.

152. Tsiokas L, Kim E, Arnould T, et al: Homo- and heterodimeric interactions between the gene products of *PKD1* and *PKD2*. Proc Natl Acad Sci U S A 94:6965–6970, 1997.

153. Parnell SC, et al: The polycystic kidney disease-1 protein, polycystin-1, binds and activates heterotrimeric G-proteins in vitro. Biochem Biophys Res Commun 251:625–631, 1998.

154. Delmas P, et al: Constitutive activation of G-proteins by polycystin-1 is antagonized by polycystin-2. J Biol Chem 277:11276–11283, 2002.

155. Parnell SC, et al: Polycystin-1 activation of c-Jun N-terminal kinase and AP-1 is mediated by heterotrimeric G proteins. J Biol Chem 277:19566–19572, 2002.

156. Kim E, et al: Interaction between RGS7 and polycystin. Proc Natl Acad Sci U S A 96:6371–6376, 1999.

157. Parnell SC, Magenheimer BS, Maser RL, Calvet JP: Identification of the major site of in vitro PKA phosphorylation in the polycystin-1 C-terminal cytosolic domain. Biochem Biophys Res Commun 259:539–543, 1999.

158. Geng L, Burrow CR, Li HP, Wilson PD: Modification of the composition of polycystin-1 multiprotein complexes by calcium and tyrosine phosphorylation. Biochim Biophys Acta 1535:21–35, 2000.

159. Li HP, Geng L, Burrow CR, Wilson PD: Identification of phosphorylation sites in the PKD1-encoded protein C- terminal domain. Biochem Biophys Res Commun 259:356–363, 1999.

160. Roitbak T, et al: A polycystin-1 multiprotein complex is disrupted in polycystic kidney disease cells. Mol Biol Cell 15:1334–1346, 2004.

161. Xu GM, et al: Polycystin-1 interacts with intermediate filaments. J Biol Chem 276:46544–46552, 2001.

162. Schneider MC, et al: A gene similar to *PKD1* maps to chromosome 4q22: A candidate gene for PKD2. Genomics 38:1–4, 1996.

163. Clapham DE, Runnels LW, Strubing C: The TRP ion channel family. Nat Rev Neurosci 2:387–396, 2001.

164. Nomura H, et al: Identification of PKDL, a novel polycystic kidney disease 2–like gene whose murine homologue is deleted in mice with kidney and retinal defects. J Biol Chem 273:25967–25973, 1998.

165. Gallagher AR, Cedzich A, Gretz N, et al: The polycystic kidney disease protein PKD2 interacts with Hax-1, a protein associated with the actin cytoskeleton. Proc Natl Acad Sci U S A 97:4017–4022, 2000.

166. Li Q, Shen PY, Wu G, Chen XZ: Polycystin-2 interacts with troponin I, an angiogenesis inhibitor. Biochemistry 42:450–457, 2003.

167. Li Q, et al: Polycystin-2 associates with tropomyosin-1, an actin microfilament component. J Mol Biol 325:949–962, 2003.

168. Tsiokas L, et al: Specific association of the gene product of *PKD2* with the TRPC1 channel. Proc Natl Acad Sci U S A 96:3934–3939, 1999.

169. Rundle DR, Gorbsky G, Tsiokas L: PKD2 interacts and co-localizes with mDia1 to mitotic spindles of dividing cells: Role of mDia1 in PKD2 localization to mitotic spindles. J Biol Chem 279:29728–29739, 2004.

170. Li X, et al: Polycystin-1 and polycystin-2 regulate the cell cycle through the helix-loop-helix inhibitor Id2. Nat Cell Biol 7:1102–1112, 2005.

171. Wang SZJ, Nauli SM, Li X, et al: Fibrocystin/polyductin, found in the same protein complex with polycystin-2, regulates calcium responses in kidney epithelia. Mol Cell Biol 27:3241–3252, 2007.

172. Wu, Y, et al: Kinesin-2 mediates physical and functional interactions between polycystin-2 and fibrocystin. Hum Mol Genet 15:3280–3292, 2006.

173. Hanaoka K, et al: Co-assembly of polycystin-1 and -2 produces unique cation-permeable currents. Nature 408:990–994, 2000.

174. Delmas P, et al: Gating of the polycystin ion channel signaling complex in neurons and kidney cells. FASEB J 18:740–742, 2004.

175. Chen XZ, et al: Polycystin-L is a calcium-regulated cation channel permeable to calcium ions. Nature 401:383–386, 1999.

176. Vassilev PM, et al: Polycystin-2 is a novel cation channel implicated in defective intracellular Ca^{2+} homeostasis in polycystic kidney disease. Biochem Biophys Res Commun 282:341–350, 2001.

177. Gonzalez-Perret S, et al: Polycystin-2, the protein mutated in autosomal dominant polycystic kidney disease (ADPKD), is a Ca^{2+}-permeable nonselective cation channel. Proc Natl Acad Sci U S A 98:1182–1187, 2001.

178. Koulen P, et al: Polycystin-2 is an intracellular calcium release channel. Nat Cell Biol 4:191–197, 2002.

179. Chen XZ, et al: Transport function of the naturally occurring pathogenic polycystin-2 mutant, R742X. Biochem Biophys Res Commun 282:1251–1256, 2001.

180. Cai Y, et al: Calcium dependence of polycystin-2 channel activity is modulated by phosphorylation at Ser812. J Biol Chem 279:19987–19995, 2004.

181. Stayner C, Zhou J: Polycystin channels and kidney disease. Trends Pharmacol Sci 22:543–546, 2001.

182. Tsiokas L, Kim S, Ong EC: Cell biology of polycystin-2. Cell Signal 19:444–453, 2007.

183. Geng L, et al: Identification and localization of polycystin, the *PKD1* gene product. J Clin Invest 98:2674–2682, 1996.

184. Geng L, et al: Distribution and developmentally regulated expression of murine polycystin. Am J Physiol 272:F451–F459, 1997.

185. Huan Y, van Adelsberg J: Polycystin-1, the *PKD1* gene product, is in a complex containing E-cadherin and the catenins. J Clin Invest 104:1459–1468, 1999.

186. Scheffers MS, et al: Polycystin-1, the product of the polycystic kidney disease 1 gene, co-localizes with desmosomes in MDCK cells. Hum Mol Genet 9:2743–2750, 2000.

187. Yoder BK, Hou X, Guay-Woodford LM: The polycystic kidney disease proteins, polycystin-1, polycystin-2, polaris, and cystin, are co-localized in renal cilia. J Am Soc Nephrol 13:2508–2516, 2002.

188. Luo Y, Vassilev PM, Li X, et al: Native polycystin 2 functions as a plasma membrane Ca^{2+}-permeable cation channel in renal epithelia. Mol Cell Biol 23:2600–2607, 2003.

189. Nauli SM, et al: Polycystins 1 and 2 mediate mechanosensation in the primary cilium of kidney cells. Nat Genet 33:129–137, 2003.

190. Ward CJ, et al: Polycystin, the polycystic kidney disease 1 protein, is expressed by epithelial cells in fetal, adult, and polycystic kidney. Proc Natl Acad Sci U S A 93:1524–1528, 1996.

191. Ong AC, et al: Coordinate expression of the autosomal dominant polycystic kidney disease proteins, polycystin-2 and polycystin-1, in normal and cystic tissue [In Process Citation]. Am J Pathol 154:1721–1729, 1999.

192. Cai Y, et al: Identification and characterization of polycystin-2, the PKD2 gene product. J Biol Chem 274:28557–28565, 1999.

193. Foggensteiner L, et al: Cellular and subcellular distribution of polycystin-2, the protein product of the PKD2 gene. J Am Soc Nephrol 11:814–827, 2000.

194. Obermuller N, et al: The rat pkd2 protein assumes distinct subcellular distributions in different organs. Am J Physiol 277:F914–F925, 1999.

195. Pazour GJ, San Agustin JT, Follit JA, et al: Polycystin-2 localizes to kidney cilia and the ciliary level is elevated in orpk mice with polycystic kidney disease. Curr Biol 12:R378–R380, 2002.

196. Streets AJ, Moon DJ, Kane ME, et al: Identification of an N-terminal glycogen synthase kinase 3 phosphorylation site which regulates the functional localization of polycystin-2 in vivo and in vitro. Hum Mol Genet 15:1465–1473, 2006.

197. Kottgen M, et al: Trafficking of TRPP2 by PACS proteins represents a novel mechanism of ion channel regulation. EMBO J 24:705–716, 2005.

198. Hidaka S, Konecke V, Osten L, Witzgall R: PIGEA-14, a novel coiled-coil protein affecting the intracellular distribution of polycystin-2. J Biol Chem 279:35009–35016, 2004.

199. Geng L, et al: Polycystin-2 traffics to cilia independently of polycystin-1 by using an N-terminal RVxP motif. J Cell Sci 119:1383–1395, 2006.

200. Nauli SM, et al: Loss of polycystin-1 in human cyst-lining epithelia leads to ciliary dysfunction. J Am Soc Nephrol 17:1015–1025, 2006.

201. Grimm DH, et al: Polycystin-1 distribution is modulated by polycystin-2 expression in mammalian cells. J Biol Chem 278:36786–36793, 2003.

202. Barr MM, Sternberg PW: A polycystic kidney-disease gene homologue required for male mating behaviour in C. elegans. Nature 401:386–389, 1999.

203. Pazour GJ, et al: Chlamydomonas IFT88 and its mouse homologue, polycystic kidney disease gene tg737, are required for assembly of cilia and flagella. J Cell Biol 151:709–718, 2000.

204. Brown NE, Murcia NS: Delayed cystogenesis and increased ciliogenesis associated with the re-expression of polaris in Tg737 mutant mice. Kidney Int 63:1220–1229, 2003.

205. Praetorius HA, Spring KR: Bending the MDCK cell primary cilium increases intracellular calcium. J Membr Biol 184:71–79, 2001.

206. Lin F, et al: Kidney-specific inactivation of the KIF3A subunit of kinesin-II inhibits renal ciliogenesis and produces polycystic kidney disease. Proc Natl Acad Sci U S A 100:5286–5291, 2003.

207. Hildebrandt F, Otto E: Cilia and centrosomes: A unifying pathogenic concept for cystic kidney disease? Nat Rev Genet 6:928–940, 2005.

208. Bisgrove BW, Yost HJ: The roles of cilia in developmental disorders and disease. Development 133:4131–4143, 2006.

209. Ma R, et al: PKD2 functions as an epidermal growth factor–activated plasma membrane channel. Mol Cell Biol 25:8285–8298, 2005.

210. Threadgill DW, et al: Targeted disruption of mouse EGF receptor: Effect of genetic background on mutant phenotype. Science 269:230–234, 1995.

211. Chauvet V, et al: Mechanical stimuli induce cleavage and nuclear translocation of the polycystin-1 C terminus. J Clin Invest 114:1433–1443, 2004.

212. Low SH, et al: Polycystin-1, STAT6, and P100 function in a pathway that transduces ciliary mechanosensation and is activated in polycystic kidney disease. Dev Cell 10:57–69, 2006.

213. Kim E, et al: The polycystic kidney disease 1 gene product modulates Wnt signaling. J Biol Chem 274:4947–4953, 1999.

214. Le NH, et al: Aberrant polycystin-1 expression results in modification of activator protein-1 activity, whereas Wnt signaling remains unaffected. J Biol Chem 279:27472–27481, 2004.

215. Gong Y, Mo C, Fraser SE: Planar cell polarity signalling controls cell division orientation during zebrafish gastrulation. Nature 430:689–693, 2004.

216. Fischer E, et al: Defective planar cell polarity in polycystic kidney disease. Nat Genet 38:21–23, 2006.

217. Simons M, et al: Inversin, the gene product mutated in nephronophthisis type II, functions as a molecular switch between Wnt signaling pathways. Nat Genet 37:537–543, 2005.

218. Rockman SP, et al: Id2 is a target of the beta-catenin/T cell factor pathway in colon carcinoma. J Biol Chem 276:45113–45119, 2001.

219. Kondo M, et al: A role for Id in the regulation of TGF-beta-induced epithelial-mesenchymal transdifferentiation. Cell Death Differ 11:1092–1101, 2004.

220. Lasorella A, Noseda M, Beyna M, et al: Id2 is a retinoblastoma protein target and mediates signalling by Myc oncoproteins. Nature 407:592–598, 2000.

221. Kowanetz M, Valcourt U, Bergstrom R, et al: Id2 and Id3 define the potency of cell proliferation and differentiation responses to transforming growth factor beta and bone morphogenetic protein. Mol Cell Biol 24:4241–4254, 2004.

222. Bukanov NO, Smith LA, Klinger KW, et al: Long-lasting arrest of murine polycystic kidney disease with CDK inhibitor roscovitine. Nature 444:949–952, 2006.

223. Calo V, et al: STAT proteins: From normal control of cellular events to tumorigenesis. J Cell Physiol 197:157–168, 2003.

224. Bhunia AK, et al: PKD1 induces p21(waf1) and regulation of the cell cycle via direct activation of the JAK-STAT signaling pathway in a process requiring PKD2. Cell 109:157–168, 2002.

225. Tao Y, Kim J, Schrier RW, Edelstein CL: Rapamycin markedly slows disease progression in a rat model of polycystic kidney disease. J Am Soc Nephrol 16:46–51, 2005.

226. Shillingford JM, et al: The mTOR pathway is regulated by polycystin-1, and its inhibition reverses renal cystogenesis in polycystic kidney disease. Proc Natl Acad Sci U S A 103:5466–5471, 2006.

227. Harris PC, Ward CJ, Peral B, Hughes J: Autosomal dominant polycystic kidney disease: Molecular analysis. Hum Mol Genet 4(Special No):1745–1749, 1995.

228. Kleymenova E, et al: Tuberin-dependent membrane localization of polycystin-1: A functional link between polycystic kidney disease and the TSC2 tumor suppressor gene. Mol Cell 7:823–832, 2001.

229. Lu W, et al: Perinatal lethality with kidney and pancreas defects in mice with a targetted Pkd1 mutation. Nat Genet 17:179–181, 1997.

230. Lu W, et al: Comparison of Pkd1-targeted mutants reveals that loss of polycystin-1 causes cystogenesis and bone defects. Hum Mol Genet 10: 2385–2396, 2001.

231. Wu G, et al: Identification of PKD2L, a human PKD2-related gene: Tissue-specific expression and mapping to chromosome 10q25 [In Process Citation]. Genomics 54:564–568, 1998.

232. Li X, et al: Establishing a polycystin-1 conditional knockout mouse model [Abstract]. J Am Soc Nephrol 2003.

233. Piontek KB, et al: A functional floxed allele of *Pkd1* that can be conditionally inactivated in vivo. J Am Soc Nephrol 15:3035–3043, 2004.

234. Lu W, et al: Late onset of renal and hepatic cysts in *Pkd1*-targeted heterozygotes [Letter]. Nat Genet 21:160–161, 1999.

235. Kim K, Drummond I, Ibraghimov-Beskrovnaya O, et al: Polycystin 1 is required for the structural integrity of blood vessels. Proc Natl Acad Sci U S A 97:1731–1736, 2000.

236. Boulter C, et al: Cardiovascular, skeletal, and renal defects in mice with a targeted disruption of the *Pkd1* gene. Proc Natl Acad Sci U S A 98:12174–12179, 2001.

237. Wu G, et al: Cardiac defects and renal failure in mice with targeted mutations in *Pkd2*. Nat Genet 24:75–78, 2000.

238. Pennekamp P, et al: The ion channel polycystin-2 is required for left-right axis determination in mice. Curr Biol 12:938–943, 2002.

239. McGrath J, Somlo S, Makova S, et al: Two populations of node monocilia initiate left-right asymmetry in the mouse. Cell 114:61–73, 2003.

240. Nauli SM, Zhou J: Polycystins and mechanosensation in renal and nodal cilia. Bioessays 26:844–856, 2004.

241. Birenboim N, Donoso VS, Huseman RA, Grantham JJ: Renal excretion and cyst accumulation of beta2 microglobulin in polycystic kidney disease. Kidney Int 31:85–92, 1987.

242. Welling L, Grantham J: In Tisher CG, Brenner BM (eds): Renal Pathology. Philadelphia, JB Lippincott, 1994, pp 1312–1354.

243. Woo D: Apoptosis and loss of renal tissue in polycystic kidney diseases [see comments]. N Engl J Med 333:18–25, 1995.

244. Tanner GA, Gretz N, Connors BA, et al: Role of obstruction in autosomal dominant polycystic kidney disease in rats. Kidney Int 50:873–886, 1996.

245. Diamond JR, Kees-Folts D, Ding G, et al: Macrophages, monocyte chemoattractant peptide-1, and TGF-beta 1 in experimental hydronephrosis. Am J Physiol 266:F926–F933, 1994.

246. Lee RT, et al: Mechanical deformation promotes secretion of IL-1 alpha and IL-1 receptor antagonist. J Immunol 159:5084–5088, 1997.

247. Klahr S: Obstructive nephropathy. Kidney Int 54:286–300, 1998.

248. Eddy AA: Experimental insights into the tubulointerstitial disease accompanying primary glomerular lesions. J Am Soc Nephrol 5:1273–1287, 1994.

249. Tanner GA, et al: Atubular glomeruli in a rat model of polycystic kidney disease. Kidney Int 62:1947–1957, 2002.

250. Baert L: Hereditary polycystic kidney disease (adult form): A microdissection study of two cases at an early stage of the disease. Kidney Int 13:519–525, 1978.

251. Peral B, et al: A stable, nonsense mutation associated with a case of infantile onset polycystic kidney disease 1 (PKD1). Hum Mol Genet 5:539–542, 1996.

252. Reeders ST: Multilocus polycystic disease [News]. Nat Genet 1:235–237, 1992.

253. Qian F, Germino GG: "Mistakes happen": Somatic mutation and disease. Am J Hum Genet 61:1000–1005, 1997.

254. Pei Y: A "two-hit" model of cystogenesis in autosomal dominant polycystic kidney disease? Trends Mol Med 7:151–156, 2001.

255. Qian F, Watnick TJ, Onuchic LF, Germino GG: The molecular basis of focal cyst formation in human autosomal dominant polycystic kidney disease type I. Cell 87:979–987, 1996.

256. Brasier JL, Henske EP: Loss of the polycystic kidney disease (PKD1) region of chromosome 16p13 in renal cyst cells supports a loss-of-function model for cyst pathogenesis. J Clin Invest 99:194–199, 1997.

257. Watnick TJ, et al: Somatic mutation in individual liver cysts supports a two-hit model of cystogenesis in autosomal dominant polycystic kidney disease. Mol Cell 2:247–251, 1998.

258. Pei Y, et al: Somatic *PKD2* mutations in individual kidney and liver cysts support a "two-hit" model of cystogenesis in type 2 autosomal dominant polycystic kidney disease. J Am Soc Nephrol 10:1524–1529, 1999.

259. Torra R, et al: A loss-of-function model for cystogenesis in human autosomal dominant polycystic kidney disease type 2. Am J Hum Genet 65:345–352, 1999.

260. Koptides M, Hadjimichael C, Koupepidou P, et al: Germinal and somatic mutations in the *PKD2* gene of renal cysts in autosomal dominant polycystic kidney disease. Hum Mol Genet 8:509–513, 1999.

261. Watnick T, et al: Mutations of PKD1 in ADPKD2 cysts suggest a pathogenic effect of trans-heterozygous mutations. Nat Genet 25:143–144, 2000.

262. Koptides M, Mean R, Demetriou K, et al: Genetic evidence for a trans-heterozygous model for cystogenesis in autosomal dominant polycystic kidney disease. Hum Mol Genet 9:447–452, 2000.

263. Ong AC, Harris PC: Molecular basis of renal cyst formation—One hit or two? Lancet 349:1039–1040, 1997.

264. Ong AC, et al: Polycystin-1 expression in PKD1, early-onset PKD1, and TSC2/PKD1 cystic tissue. Kidney Int 56:1324–1333, 1999.

265. Harris PC, et al: Cyst number but not the rate of cystic growth is associated with the mutated gene in autosomal dominant polycystic kidney disease. J Am Soc Nephrol 17:3013–3019, 2006.

266. Guay-Woodford LM: Murine models of polycystic kidney disease: Molecular and therapeutic insights. Am J Physiol Renal Physiol 285:F1034–F1049, 2003.

267. Wu G, et al: Somatic inactivation of Pkd2 results in polycystic kidney disease. Cell 93:177–188, 1998.

268. Martin GM, et al: Somatic mutations are frequent and increase with age in human kidney epithelial cells. Hum Mol Genet 5:215–221, 1996.

269. Perera FP: Environment and cancer: Who are susceptible? Science 278:1068–1073, 1997.

270. Nebert DW: Polymorphisms in drug-metabolizing enzymes: What is their clinical relevance and why do they exist? Am J Hum Genet 60:265–271, 1997.

271. Pritchard L, et al: A human *PKD1* transgene generates functional polycystin-1 in mice and is associated with a cystic phenotype. Hum Mol Genet 9:2617–2627, 2000.

272. Wu G, et al: Trans-heterozygous *Pkd1* and *Pkd2* mutations modify expression of polycystic kidney disease. Hum Mol Genet 11:1845–1854, 2002.

273. Lantinga-van Leeuwen IS, et al: Lowering of Pkd1 expression is sufficient to cause polycystic kidney disease. Hum Mol Genet 13:3069–3077, 2004.

274. Gogusev J, et al: Molecular cytogenetic aberrations in autosomal dominant polycystic kidney disease tissue. J Am Soc Nephrol 14:359–366, 2003.

275. Trudel M, Barisoni L, Lanoix J, D'Agati V: Polycystic kidney disease in SBM transgenic mice: Role of *c-myc* in disease induction and progression. Am J Pathol 152:219–229, 1998.

276. Gilbert E, et al: In vivo effects of activated *H-ras* oncogene expressed in the liver and in urogenital tissues. Int J Cancer 73:749–756, 1997.

277. Veis DJ, Sorenson CM, Shutter JR, Korsmeyer SJ: Bcl-2-deficient mice demonstrate fulminant lymphoid apoptosis, polycystic kidneys, and hypopigmented hair. Cell 75:229–240, 1993.

278. Moser M, et al: Enhanced apoptotic cell death of renal epithelial cells in mice lacking transcription factor AP-2beta. Genes Dev 11:1938–1948, 1997.

279. Ostrom L, Tang MJ, Gruss P, Dressler GR: Reduced *Pax2* gene dosage increases apoptosis and slows the progression of renal cystic disease. Dev Biol 219:250–258, 2000.

280. Qian Q, Harris PC, Torres VE: Treatment prospects for autosomal-dominant polycystic kidney disease. Kidney Int 59:2005–2022, 2001.

281. Belibi FA, et al: Cyclic AMP promotes growth and secretion in human polycystic kidney epithelial cells. Kidney Int 66:964–973, 2004.

282. Yamaguchi T, et al: Cyclic AMP activates B-Raf and ERK in cyst epithelial cells from autosomal-dominant polycystic kidneys. Kidney Int 63:1983–1994, 2003.

283. Yamaguchi T, Hempson SJ, Reif GA, et al: Calcium restores a normal proliferation phenotype in human polycystic kidney disease epithelial cells. J Am Soc Nephrol 17:178–187, 2006.

284. Li H, Findlay IA, Sheppard DN: The relationship between cell proliferation, Cl- secretion, and renal cyst growth: A study using CFTR inhibitors. Kidney Int 66:1926–1938, 2004.

285. Persu A, et al: CF gene and cystic fibrosis transmembrane conductance regulator expression in autosomal dominant polycystic kidney disease. J Am Soc Nephrol 11:2285–2296, 2000.

286. Magenheimer BS, et al: Early embryonic renal tubules of wild-type and polycystic kidney disease kidneys respond to cAMP stimulation with cystic fibrosis transmembrane conductance regulator/Na(+),K(+),2Cl(-) co-transporter-dependent cystic dilation. J Am Soc Nephrol 17:3424–3437, 2006.

287. Gattone VH, 2nd, Wang X, Harris PC, Torres VE: Inhibition of renal cystic disease development and progression by a vasopressin V2 receptor antagonist. Nat Med 9:1323–1326, 2003.

288. Torres VE, et al: Effective treatment of an orthologous model of autosomal dominant polycystic kidney disease. Nat Med 10:363–364, 2004.

289. Sweeney WE, Futey L, Frost P, Avner ED: In vitro modulation of cyst formation by a novel tyrosine kinase inhibitor. Kidney Int 56:406–413, 1999.

290. Richards WG, et al: Epidermal growth factor receptor activity mediates renal cyst formation in polycystic kidney disease. J Clin Invest 101:935–939, 1998.

291. Torres VE, et al: Epidermal growth factor receptor tyrosine kinase inhibition is not protective in PCK rats. Kidney Int 66:1766–1773, 2004.

292. Bello-Reuss E, Holubec K, Rajaraman S: Angiogenesis in autosomal-dominant polycystic kidney disease. Kidney Int 60:37–45, 2001.

293. Wei W, Popov V, Walocha JA, et al: Evidence of angiogenesis and microvascular regression in autosomal-dominant polycystic kidney disease kidneys: A corrosion cast study. Kidney Int 70:1261–1268, 2006.

294. Pei Y: Nature and nurture on phenotypic variability of autosomal dominant polycystic kidney disease. Kidney Int 67:1630–1631, 2005.

295. Dipple KM, McCabe ER: Modifier genes convert "simple" mendelian disorders to complex traits. Mol Genet Metab 71:43–50, 2000.

296. Persu A, et al: Comparison between siblings and twins supports a role for modifier genes in ADPKD. Kidney Int 66:2132–2136, 2004.

297. Fain PR, et al: Modifier genes play a significant role in the phenotypic expression of PKD1. Kidney Int 67:1256–1267, 2005.

298. Paterson AD, et al: Progressive loss of renal function is an age-dependent heritable trait in type 1 autosomal dominant polycystic kidney disease. J Am Soc Nephrol 16:755–762, 2005.

299. Baboolal K, et al: Association of the angiotensin I converting enzyme gene deletion polymorphism with early onset of ESRF in PKD1 adult polycystic kidney disease. Kidney Int 52:607–613, 1997.

300. van Dijk MA, Breuning MH, Peters DJ, Chang PC: The ACE insertion/deletion polymorphism has no influence on progression of renal function loss in autosomal dominant polycystic kidney disease. Nephrol Dial Transplant 15:836–839, 2000.

301. Persu A, et al: Modifier effect of ENOS in autosomal dominant polycystic kidney disease. Hum Mol Genet 11:229–241, 2002.

302. Walker D, et al: The ENOS polymorphism is not associated with severity of renal disease in polycystic kidney disease 1. Am J Kidney Dis 41:90–94, 2003.

303. Belibi FA, et al: The effect of caffeine on renal epithelial cells from patients with autosomal dominant polycystic kidney disease. J Am Soc Nephrol 13:2723–2729, 2002.

304. Andreoni KA, et al: Increased incidence of gastrointestinal surgical complications in renal transplant recipients with polycystic kidney disease. Transplantation 67:262–266, 1999.

305. Perrone RD, Ruthazer R, Terrin NC: Survival after end-stage renal disease in autosomal dominant polycystic kidney disease: Contribution of extrarenal complications to mortality. Am J Kidney Dis 38:777–784, 2001.

306. Schrier RW, et al: Tolvaptan, a selective oral vasopressin V2-receptor antagonist, for hyponatremia. N Engl J Med 355:2099–2112, 2006.

307. Ruggenenti P, et al: Safety and efficacy of long-acting somatostatin treatment in autosomal-dominant polycystic kidney disease. Kidney Int 68:206–216, 2005.

308. Walz G: Therapeutic approaches in autosomal dominant polycystic kidney disease (ADPKD): Is there light at the end of the tunnel? Nephrol Dial Transplant 21:1752–1757, 2006.

309. Hughes J, Ward CJ, Aspinwall R, et al: Identification of a human homologue of the sea urchin receptor for egg jelly: A polycystic kidney disease-like protein. Hum Mol Genet 8:543–549, 1999.

310. Yuasa T, et al: The sequence, expression, and chromosomal localization of a novel polycystic kidney disease 1-like gene, PKD1L1, in human. Genomics 79:376–386, 2002.

311. Yuasa T, Takakura A, Denker BM, et al: Polycystin-1L2 is a novel G-protein-binding protein. Genomics 84:126–138, 2004.

312. Li A, Tian X, Sung SW, Somlo S: Identification of two novel polycystic kidney disease-1–like genes in human and mouse genomes. Genomics 81:596–608, 2003.

313. Guo L, Chen M, Basora N, Zhou J: The human polycystic kidney disease 2–like (PKDL) gene: Exon/intron structure and evidence for a novel splicing mechanism. Mammal Genome 11:46–50, 2000.

314. Veldhuisen B, Spruit L, Dauwerse HG, et al: Genes homologous to the autosomal dominant polycystic kidney disease genes (PKD1 and PKD2). Eur J Hum Genet 7:860–872, 1999.

315. Muto S, et al: Pioglitazone improves the phenotype and molecular defects of a targeted Pkd1 mutant. Hum Mol Genet 11:1731–1742, 2002.

316. Herron BJ, et al: Efficient generation and mapping of recessive developmental mutations using ENU mutagenesis. Nat Genet 30:185–189, 2002.

Chapter 7

Autosomal Recessive Polycystic Kidney Disease

Peter C. Harris and Vicente E. Torres

Autosomal recessive polycystic kidney disease (ARPKD) is predominantly an infantile disorder that results in significant neonatal mortality and childhood renal impairment.[1-4] However, the recent literature indicates that many patients now survive into adulthood, and a proportion are diagnosed only later in life.[5,6] The kidney disease is classically characterized by neonatal bilateral renal enlargement due to fusiform dilatation of the collecting ducts. The other pathognomonic feature of the disease is biliary dysgenesis, resulting in congenital hepatic fibrosis.

Previous names for this disorder, such as infantile polycystic kidney disease or infantile polycystic disease of the kidney and liver, reflected the characteristic neonatal disease, but because there are other causes of early-onset PKD and because this disease can present later in life, ARPKD is now the favored designation. The other commonly used term for this disorder in the older literature is Potter syndrome type 1, reflecting the classification by Osathanondh and Potter[7] of cystic kidneys into four distinct pathoanatomic categories.[8] The disease in type 1 kidneys was described as hyperplasia of the interstitial portion of the collecting ducts and distinct from the focal cyst development found in the more common, predominantly adult disease, that is now termed autosomal dominant polycystic kidney disease (ADPKD; Potter syndrome type 3) and dysplastic kidneys.

ARPKD was probably first recognized as a distinct disease entity at the end of the 19th century[9-11] but the familial nature of the disease, suggesting autosomal recessive inheritance, was not documented until the 1960s.[7,12-15] In 1971 Blyth and Ockenden[16] suggested classification of the disease into four separate clinicopathologic entities, dependent on the age at presentation and severity of renal and liver disease: perinatal, neonatal, infantile, and juvenile. The renal disease was most prominent in the younger age groups with limited liver disease, whereas older patients presented typically with complications of the liver disease and had less marked kidney involvement.[17] Subsequently, it became clear from examples of intrafamilial phenotypic variability that such a strict subdivision was not wholly consistent with the data.[18-21] In recent years, initially from linkage studies and since the identification of the gene (PKHD1) in 2002 by direct mutation analysis, the molecular basis of the disease has now been defined.[22-25] These studies indicate genetic homogeneity, at least for the vast majority of typical ARPKD patients, but marked allelic heterogeneity.[2,4,26] They also confirm that congenital hepatic fibrosis with minimal renal disease can be part of the ARPKD phenotype.[6,23]

PREVALENCE OF ARPKD

In common with many rarer recessive disorders, the incidence of ARPKD has been difficult to estimate, and figures have varied widely from study to study. At the lower end of the scale, extrapolated from European autopsy studies, is a figure of 1/40,000,[8] while at the other extreme, numbers of approximately 1/10,000 have been indicated in more isolated populations where consanguinity may be a factor.[27,28] Recently, considering all the available data, an incidence of 1:20,000 was estimated and a carrier frequency of 1:70 suggested to be considered for genetic counseling purposes.[29] There are little data about the prevalence in non-white populations, but recent molecular data showing marked allelic heterogeneity at PKHD1 and no very common mutation (suggesting a significant level of new mutation) indicate that ARPKD is likely to be found in all racial groups.[2,4]

CLINICAL DESCRIPTION

In the older literature, ARPKD was considered a disease that invariably resulted in neonatal death.[7,30] With an increased appreciation of the phenotypic variability associated with ARPKD and improved clinical practice, the prognosis for this disorder is now not universally so poor.[19,31,32] Nevertheless, the typical disease presentation is of enlarged and cystic kidneys detected in utero or in the perinatal-neonatal period. The most extreme cases have the "Potter's phenotype," consisting of pulmonary hypoplasia (secondary to oligohydramnios), characteristic facies, and spine and limb abnormalities.[33] Present estimates are that approximately 30% of patients die by the neonatal period (although no exact figures are available), primarily of respiratory insufficiency; these figures may be decreasing with improved respiratory care.

Recent comprehensive studies of ARPKD in two North American populations have more clearly defined the childhood disease of perinatal survivors,[31,32] whereas a number of longer term follow-up studies have characterized the disease in adolescents and adults.[5,19,34,35] Overall, these studies indicate that hypertension, renal insufficiency, and portal hypertension are the major disease complications in surviving infants, with liver disease becoming more important in older patients. Between 55% and 86% of patients developed hypertension with elevated levels often seen at birth or at diagnosis. In one study, the average age at onset of hypertension was

16 days in patients diagnosed by the neonatal period,[31] whereas Fonck et al[5] found that no patients developed hypertension after 18 years of age. End-stage renal disease (ESRD) is rare in the neonate and, indeed, during the first year or two of life renal function can improve and renal size relative to body mass often decreases.[36–38] Nevertheless, between 40% and 87% of patients developed chronic renal insufficiency with 15% to 33% progressing to ESRD during follow-up.[5,19,31,32,35] Other renal complications include hyponatremia due to a concentrating defect, as seen in a minority of younger patients, and urinary tract infections, which are common.[19]

As patients age the hepatic disease becomes more evident, with complications of portal hypertension the major complaint in older children and adults; this is seen in 20% to 47% of patients.[5,19,31,32,34,39] The presenting features of liver disease include splenomegaly and/or hepatomegaly, along with complications of bleeding esophageal or gastric varices. Hypersplenism can also develop, resulting in thrombocytopenia, anemia, and leukopenia.[34,40] Recurrent ascending cholangitis is a common and serious complication, especially in patients with dilatation of intrahepatic bile ducts, Caroli disease, that can lead to liver failure.[40–42] A proportion of patients present in later childhood, adolescence, or even adulthood with the complication of liver disease but only minimal renal involvement.[6,23,43] Discussions over many years have questioned whether this isolated congenital hepatic fibrosis and/or Caroli disease is a separate disease entity or part of the spectrum of ARPKD.[44–46] Now, identification of PKHD1 mutations in a

proportion of these patients indicates that this can be part of the ARPKD disease spectrum.[6,23]

Two reports have described ARPKD cases with multiple intracranial aneurysms (ICAs).[47,48] ICAs are known to be associated with ADPKD at a level about 8 times higher than the normal population.[49] However, from the available data, it is not clear if the frequency of ICAs is also elevated in ARPKD, or if these cases are coincidental findings.

DISEASE PATHOLOGY

The disease phenotype is highly variable in ARPKD, with the pathogenic features of the kidney and biliary disease related to the age when the disease manifests.[16]

Kidney

In the most severely affected cases, gross bilateral enlargement of the kidneys, as much as 10 times the normal size, is found (Fig. 7-1A).[7,37,50] The kidneys maintain their reniform shape and are smooth in gross appearance, although a dimpled surface reflecting underlying microcysts may cover the kidney.[7,12] The number and branching of the collecting tubules appear unaltered, suggesting normal early renal development.[7] The renal enlargement is due to fusiform dilatation of collecting ducts to 1 to 2 mm in the cortex and medulla, giving the appearance of a sponge (hence the sometimes used name,

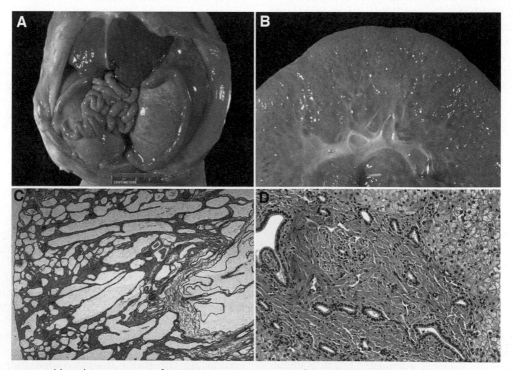

Figure 7-1 Anatomic and histologic images of ARPKD. **A,** Gross image of the perinatal form of ARPKD showing the greatly enlarged kidneys. **B,** Cross-section of neonatal ARPKD kidney showing the spongelike appearance due to dilation of multiple collecting ducts. **C,** Microscopic examination of a longitudinal section of neonatal kidney showing dilated radially distributed cortical collecting ducts and dilated medullary collecting ducts. **D,** Ductal plate malformation in the liver showing proliferation and enlargement of bile ducts and congenital hepatic fibrosis. (Courtesy of Dr. Donna Lager, Department of Laboratory Medicine and Pathology, Mayo Clinic, Rochester, Minnesota.)

sponge kidney[51]) in cross-section (Fig. 7-1B and C). Almost 100% of collecting ducts are affected in the most severely affected cases. Dilatation of the collecting ducts occurs in the fetal period, and the glomeruli and more proximal tubular elements of the nephron appear normal, although they may become crowded. However, there is evidence in early human fetuses (14–24 weeks) that proximal tubule cysts occur (as in some rodent models of recessive PKD[52–54]), but these are no longer evident after 34 weeks' gestation.[55] The dilated collecting ducts are lined by typical cuboidal cells.[12,37] The relative reduction in kidney size seen in many neonate cases as they age occurs as the cystic dilatation becomes limited to medullary ectasia.[37] As a result of these changes the cyst size becomes more variable, with focal cysts as large as 5 cm becoming evident.[56] These changes give the kidneys an appearance similar to that seen in ADPKD.[20,38] In older presenting cases the proportion of dilated collecting ducts may be less than 10%, with renal enlargement less marked or even completely absent. The renal disease may be limited to one or a small number of focal cysts or to renal medullary tubular ectasia that appear as medullary sponge kidney on imaging analysis.[57,58]

Liver

In the liver, the abnormality is of ductal plate malformation and seems to result from an early defect in bile duct development, ductal plate malformation.[46,59,60] The defect is characterized by excessive ductal proliferation, resulting in the production of multiple dilated periportal biliary ductals (Fig. 7-1D). The abnormalities of ductal proliferation are accompanied by anomalous branching of the portal vein and result in congenital hepatic fibrosis.[15,46,61] The portal tracts are often linked by fibrous septa, and the liver takes on a gritty texture. In some cases, Caroli's disease occurs.[58,62] The increasing portal fibrosis with hypoplasia of the small portal vein branches often leads to portal hypertension as the disease develops.

Pancreas

In rare cases, periductal and lobular fibrosis of the pancreas has been associated with ARPKD.[12,63]

Cellular Changes in ARPKD

The liver disease seems to result from an arrest of normal developmental epithelial-mesenchymal interactions that give rise to aberrant bile duct development: the ductal plate malformation.[59] In the kidney the defect seems to occur after the formation of tubules and results in a failure in the terminal differentiation of collecting ducts.[50] Several cellular processes seem to be abnormal in ARPKD, including altered proliferative properties, differentiation arrest, changed polarity and secretory characteristics of the epithelia, and abnormal interactions between the cellular and basement membranes.[64,65]

Animal Models of Recessive PKD

A large number of mouse models of recessively inherited PKD with kidney and liver phenotypes similar to human ARPKD have been described.[66] These models have helped characterize the cellular and biochemical changes associated with PKD and been used to map genetic modifying loci that may have sig-

nificance to human ARPKD.[66–69] However, the mapping and identification of the primary genetic defects in these models showed that none was orthologous to ARPKD, although two have recently been shown to be models of other childhood cystic diseases: *pcy* mouse, adolescent nephronophthisis (type 3) (NPHP3)[70], and the *inv* mouse, infantile nephronophthisis (type 2) (NPHP2).[71]

In 2000, a new model of recessive PKD was identified, the polycystic kidney (PCK) rat.[72–74] Mapping the disease gene showed that it was an orthologous model of ARPKD and led to the identification of human *PKHD1* (see later discussion).[23] This model has progressive renal and biliary cystic disease. Focal renal cysts become evident in collecting ducts, loops of Henle, and distal tubules from 1 week and grow to form large and cystic kidneys within 6 months.[73] Diluted bile ducts are evident in newborn animals and progressive cyst development and expansion occurs in the liver.[73] During this process the biliary tree undergoes extensive remodeling with dilatation, similar to Caroli disease, and later focal budding of cysts from the biliary tree.[75] The biliary disease development is associated with portal fibrosis, but the animals do not develop the fibrous septa and portal hypertension typical of the human disease.[73,74] Overall, the animal model resembles milder cases of ARPKD and is proving to be a very useful model for testing potential therapeutic agent for the disease (see later discussion).

GENETICS

Inheritance

ARPKD is a recessively inherited disorder. Parents of an affected case will usually be unaffected but are obligate carriers of one mutant allele. Siblings of ARPKD patients are at 25% risk of having the disease, with affected individuals usually limited to a single generation. Although there are many examples of families with two or more affected siblings that revealed the genetic nature of the disease,[22] the majority of cases present as isolated individuals with no family history of kidney disease.

Gene Localization

The disease gene, polycystic kidney and hepatic disease 1 (*PKHD1*), was localized to chromosome region 6p21-cen in 1994 using a gene linkage approach.[22] A lod score of 7.42 was obtained by analysis of 12 multiplex and 4 simplex ARPKD families, mainly with milder ARPKD. This location was refined to an interval of 3.8 cM by analysis of additional families, including those with the most severe perinatal form of the disease.[25] These and subsequent linkage studies[26] suggested genetic homogeneity for ARPKD. Additional linkage studies refined the position of the disease gene to within approximately 1 cM, and the physical interval of approximately 1 Mb between the flanking markers, D6S1714 and D6S1024, was cloned and mapped.[76–78] A number of candidate genes within the interval were identified but excluded as *PKHD1*, either by linkage analysis or mutation studies in ARPKD patients.[77,79–81]

Gene Identification

Two different groups, both using positional cloning approaches, identified the gene in 2002.[23,24] One studied the PCK rat.[73,74]

Using a whole-genome mapping approach, the *Pck* gene was localized to a 2.5-cM region of rat chromosome 9, an area syntenic to the ARPKD candidate region on human chromosome 6, indicating that *Pck* and *PKHD1* were probably orthologs.[23] The rat gene was precisely localized (0.35 cM) using markers syntenic to those in the ARPKD candidate region, and a single gene, encoding an approximately 13-kb kidney-expressed transcript, was found to span the candidate region. The human transcript was cloned by a reverse transcription–polymerase chain reaction (RT-PCR) strategy linking predicted exons, and screening for mutations in a group of ARPKD patients revealed a number of pathogenic changes. The mutation in the rat *Pkhd1* ortholog (a splicing change; IVS35-2A→T) was also identified, confirming that the disease gene had been found.[23]

The second group independently identified the gene using a gene linkage and mutation screening approach in humans.[24] A transcriptional map was generated for the candidate region using bioinformatics and RT-PCR. Mutation screening of two separate clones identified ARPKD-associated mutations, and ultimately those clones were found to be part of the same large transcript of *PKHD1*.

Structure of *PKHD1*

PKHD1 is a very large gene with a genomic area of approximately 472 kb and 67 exons.[23,24] The largest open reading frame (ORF) is 12,222 bp, extending from exon 2 to exon 67. The mouse gene has a similar structure, with the longest ORF of 12,177, and covering a genomic region of approximately 500 kb.[82] A common feature of both the human and murine genes is the possibility of extensive alternative splicing.[23,24,82,83] A variety of alternative products have been identified by RT-PCR, and Onuchic et al[24] estimated that a minimum of 86 exons may be involved in various splice forms. However, the physiologic importance of any of these splice forms has yet to be demonstrated, and most studies of the gene and protein have so far concentrated on the sequence associated with the identified ORF.

Mutation Analysis in ARPKD

Several comprehensive mutation screens of the 66 coding exons of *PKHD1* have now been described[2,4,23,24,84,85] (see also references 2 and 4). These have applied strategies for rapid searching all exons for base-pair mismatches by denaturing high-performance liquid chromatography[6,84,85] or SSCP[86] and characterized exons with possible mutations. Mutation detection rates per allele have ranged from 47% to 85%, with two mutations detected in 44.7% of cases, one in 26.5%, and no mutations in 28.8%. The highest detection levels were found in patients with the most severe disease (resulting in perinatal death),[6,86] indicating that some cases with milder ARPKD may not be due to *PKHD1* mutation. It is also likely that mutations were missed in this large and complex gene (possibly in unscreened, alternatively spliced exons). Nevertheless, the present data raise the possibility of genetic heterogeneity in ARPKD, especially in less severely affected cases.[2,87]

One clear message from the mutation screening is that many different mutations cause ARPKD (marked allelic heterogeneity). A total of approximately 300 different muta-

tions have been identified on more than 600 nonconsanguineous alleles, complicating molecular diagnostics for this disorder.[6,84–86] (Also ARPKD Mutation Database [http://www.humgen.rwth-aachen.de].) The mutations are spread widely throughout the coding region of *PKHD1* and are of all possible types (Fig. 7-2). Mutations predicted to truncate the protein by deletion or insertion, nonsense mutation, or splicing changes represent approximately 40% of the different mutations, but the majority are missense changes. A significant number of reported neutral polymorphisms has also complicated the certainty by which a pathogenic missense change can be defined.[2,4] Most mutations have been described in just a single family, but there are several mutations that are more frequent in particular populations (e.g., R496X in Finland and 9689delA in Spain).[6,86] One missense substitution, T36M, has been found on approximately 16% of mutant alleles and seems to be an ancestral mutation that arose in Europe more than 1,000 years ago.[87]

A few, mainly consanguineous, patients are homozygotes, but the vast majority of cases are compound heterozygotes reflecting the wide range of different mutations that cause this disorder.[2,4] Genotype-phenotype studies are complicated by the large number of compound heterozygotes, but it has become clear that patients with two truncating mutations have the most severe form of the disease, resulting in perinatal death.[6,86] Patients with at least one missense change are, on average, less severely affected,[84] indicating that some missense mutations may be hypomorphic alleles that generate some functional protein or some functional protein isoforms.[2,4] Disease variability seen between siblings indicates that genetic modifying and environmental influences also affect the disease phenotype.

THE ARPKD PROTEIN FIBROCYSTIN AND EXPRESSION STUDIES

Fibrocystin Structure

The *PKHD1* gene product fibrocystin (also called polyductin) is predicted to be a large protein (4,074 amino acids [aa]; 447 kDa) with a single transmembrane domain, large extracellular region, and short cytoplasmic tail (Fig. 7-3).[23,24] A large section of the extracellular region consists of multiple copies of a TIG/IPT (immunoglobulin-like fold shared by plexins and transcription factors) domain. This domain consists of 80 to 100 aa, has an immunoglobulin-like fold, and is found in receptor proteins such as Met, various plexins, and Ron, although the precise role of the motif is unknown.[88] There is another significant region of homology, found twice in fibrocystin, termed the TMEM regions A and B, with a protein of unknown function TMEM2 and a protein from the filamentous bacteria *Chloroflexus aurantiacus* (see Fig. 7-3).[23,89] Several parallel β-helix repeats have also been identified in fibrocystin, many overlapping with the TMEM regions.[24,82] Recently, a newly defined domain, PA14, with a β-barrel architecture that may be involved in carbohydrate binding has been identified in fibrocystin (see Fig. 7-3).[90] The overall structure of fibrocystin suggests that it may be a receptor protein taking cues from the extracellular environment and signaling via possible phosphorylation sites in the short cytoplasmic tail.[23]

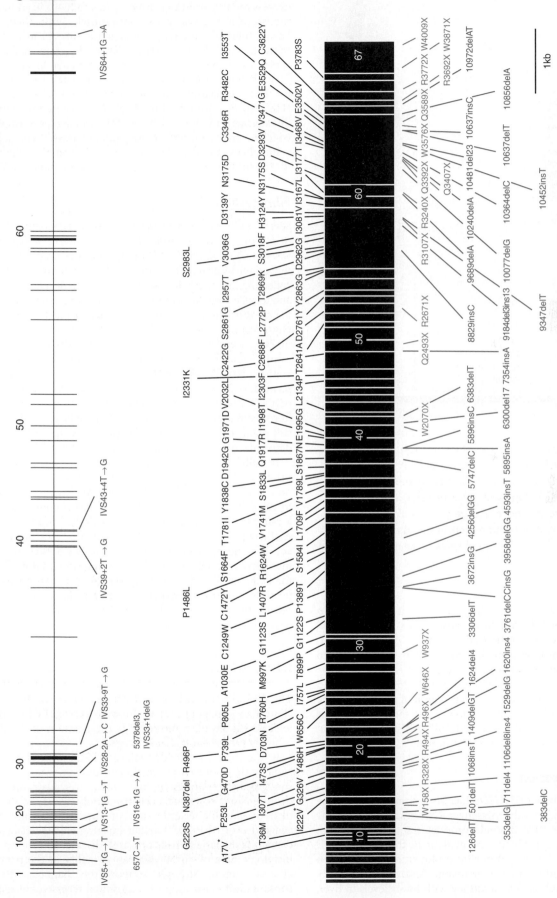

Figure 7-2 The *PKHD1* gene (top) and open reading frame of the transcript (bottom) showing the intron-exon structure. Some of the published mutations found in ARPKD patients are illustrated,6,23,24,84–87 showing that they are found throughout the gene. Unique changes are shown in plain text, and changes found in more than one family are in bold type. Splicing changes (gray) are shown against the gene structure (top), and missense and single amino acid deletions (black), nonsense mutations (light blue), and frameshifting deletions/insertions (blue) against the transcript.

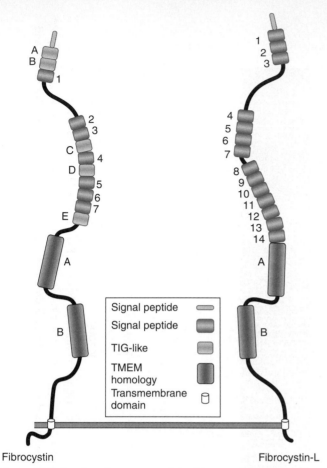

Fibrocystin   Fibrocystin-L

Figure 7-3 Predicted structures of the fibrocystin proteins. The structure of the ARPKD protein, fibrocystin (left), and fibrocystin-like (L) protein (right) illustrating known domains and regions of homology with other proteins (see key for details). Both proteins have a large extracellular region, single transmembrane domain, and short cystoplasmic tail. The function of fibrocystin-L is not known, but it does not seem to be associated with ARPKD.

Fibrocystin was the founding member of a new protein family when first identified because of its unique overall structure. However, a second member of this family, fibrocystin-L, has now been identified.[89] This protein, encoded by *PKHDL1* from chromosome region 8q23, is predicted to be a large protein (4,243 aa; 466 kDa) with 25% identity and 41.5% similarity to the extracellular region of fibrocystin. The function of this protein is unknown, but mutation analysis indicates that it is not associated with ARPKD. Expression studies suggest a role in cellular immunity.[89]

PKHD1 *Expression*

Expression analysis of *PKHD1* has been complicated by the apparent instability of the messenger RNA, resulting in a smear of signal rather than a single product resolved on human northern blots; a problem less evident in the mouse.[23,24,83] Nevertheless, RT-PCR and northern blot studies have shown that *PKHD1*, and the mouse ortholog, *Pkhd1*, are moderately expressed in adult and fetal kidney with lower levels in liver,

pancreas, and probably lung and testis.[23,24] Other sites of expression have been suggested by in situ hybridization in the mouse, including vascular smooth muscle, sympathetic ganglia and trachea,[82] and embryonic neural tube, bronchial buds, midgut, and adrenal cortex.[91] There is some evidence of expression of specific splice forms at particular locations.[82]

Analysis of the *PKHD1* promoter has revealed a binding site for the transcription factor, hepatocyte nuclear factor-1β (HNF-1β).[92,93] Mutation to *HNF-1β* can cause the dominant disease, maturity-onset diabetes of the young type 5 (MODY5), which involves congenital cystic kidney disease.[94] This suggests a link between ARPKD and MODY5, and that the cystic disease in MODY5 may be due to downregulation of *PKHD1*.

Fibrocystin Expression

Several antibodies have been generated to fibrocystin, and these detect one or more large protein products (>400 kDa) by western blot analysis.[91,95–98] Immunohistochemical analysis of the kidney localized fibrocystin to the branching ureteric bud, collecting ducts, and loops of Henle in the developing kidney and to collecting ducts in the adult.[95] The biliary tree was found to be positive in the liver along with pancreatic ducts and islets. Other staining was detected in epithelial structures in the seminiferous tubules and epididymal duct.[95] Fetal expression in murine embryonic neural tube, bronchial buds, and midgut epithelia has been described.[91] Many of the epithelial structures seemed to show apical staining of the protein.[91,95] Analysis of ARPKD tissue suggested a loss or reduction in the level of fibrocystin in the disease tissue.[91,95] In the PCK rat, fibrocystin still seems to be present (or at least some splice forms were detected) but may be expressed at a lower level.[91,95,96]

In cultured renal cells, fibrocystin has been localized to the primary cilium and basal body.[91,95–98] A wealth of evidence now links defects in known ciliary proteins to the development of PKD, and many PKD-associated proteins have been localized to primary cilia or the basal body.[99] Studies with the ADPKD protein, polycystin-1, indicate that this protein may act as a flow sensor on the primary cilia that results in increased intracellular Ca^{2+} levels in response to flow.[100,101] In the PCK rat, the biliary cilia appear shorter than normal and possibly abnormal in structure, with no ciliary localization of fibrocystin.[96] However, the role of fibrocystin in the ciliary-basal axis has yet to be determined.

DIAGNOSIS

The diagnosis of ARPKD is dependent on a combination of clinical and imaging data and may be assisted by histopathologic and molecular studies.[3] The presentation of the disease is highly variable and related to age.

In the infant, bilaterally enlarged kidneys (that are echogenic with a poor corticomedullary differentiation on ultrasonography), pulmonary hypoplasia, oligohydramios, and hypertension, as well as a negative family history of PKD (on ultrasonographic examination of the parents) are highly suggestive of ARPKD.[3] Further imaging evidence suggesting congenital hepatic fibrosis or Caroli disease, and/or especially histologic data of ductal plate abnormality in the patient or affected sibling, strongly support the diagnosis. Parental consanguinity also supports autosomal recessive inheritance, although consanguineous families only account for rare ARPKD cases in western populations.[2,4] Molecular evidence of two pathogenic *PKHD1* mutations is proof of ARPKD.

In utero, an ARPKD diagnosis is suggested by ultrasonographic data indicating enlarged, echogenic kidneys, oligohydramnios, and absence of urine in the bladder in conjunction with a proven negative family history of PKD. However, renal enlargement and increased echogenicity plus the oligohydramnios may not become evident until later in the pregnancy,[102] so molecular genetic testing may be appropriate in a family known to be at risk for ARPKD.

The patient presenting later in childhood or as an adult is more likely to have complications of liver disease than clinical kidney disease. The kidneys may not be so greatly enlarged with evidence of focal macrocysts (≤5 cm). The number of cysts may be small, or even completely absent, and the appearance may be of medullary sponge kidney. The presenting features are often those associated with portal hypertension, including hepatosplenomegaly, hypersplenism, variceal bleeding, and/or cholangitis. Mutation screening may be helpful to obtain a definite diagnosis in these patients.

Imaging

Ultrasonograms of ARPKD infant kidneys show large, echogenic, bilateral organs with poor corticomedullary differentiation (Fig. 7-4A).[103] High-resolution analysis can reveal the characteristic radial array of dilated collecting ducts.[104] In the older patient the kidney is usually less extremely enlarged, and the appearance of focal cysts may more closely resemble those seen in ADPKD.[38] Magnetic resonance (MR) can reveal a hyperintense T2-weighted signal and a radial pattern in the cortex and medulla on rapid aquisition with relaxation enhancement (RARE-MR; Fig. 7-4B and C).[105]

Hepatic disease may be evident on ultrasonography as hepatomegaly, dilated intrahepatic bile ducts (Caroli disease), and increased echogenicity. Caroli disease may be more readily detected by computed tomography (CT) or MR analysis[106] (Fig. 7-4D).

Histology

Histopathologic analysis of liver from biopsy or at autopsy shows a characteristic ductal plate abnormality with bile duct proliferation and ectasia with evidence of hepatic fibrosis.[37] Histologic evidence of congenital hepatic fibrosis is strong evidence of ARPKD, although it is not clear that all isolated congenital hepatic fibrosis without evidence of renal disease is due to *PKHD1* mutation.

Molecular Genetic Testing

Because of the severity of disease in ARPKD, there is significant demand for antenatal diagnostics. This interest is largely among couples with a previously affected pregnancy, either detected in utero (possibly having resulted in termination) or the birth of an affected child (who may have died in the neonatal period).[26] However, there is also demand for molecular diagnostics in older patients with less severe disease to differentiate ARPKD from other causes of childhood PKD. Molecular diagnostics have been offered since *PKHD1* was localized using a linkage-based approach with flanking markers.[26] This method has

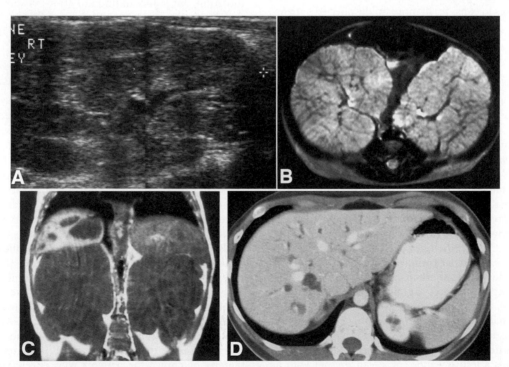

Figure 7-4 **A,** Longitudinal sonographic image of the right kidney illustrating marked enhancement, increased echogenicity, and loss of corticomedullary differentiation in a 40-day-old infant with ARPKD. **B** and **C,** Axial T2- and coronal T1-weighted MR images demonstrating marked bilateral renal enlargement in the same patient. **D,** Axial CT image illustrating intrahepatic dilatation of bile ducts in a 53-year-old woman with Caroli disease.

been highly successful, but material from an affected individual is required and the diagnosis can be complicated by crossovers between the flanking markers. This methodology is not appropriate if there is any doubt about the diagnosis of ARPKD. With the gene discovery, mutation-based diagnostics is now possible, and recently prenatal diagnosis by this approach has been described.[107] This method has the advantage that DNA from a previously affected family member is not required and that patients with an uncertain diagnosis can be tested. However, gene-based diagnostics is complicated by the marked allelic heterogeneity and prevalence of novel missense mutations of uncertain pathogenicity.[2,4] If two clearly pathogenic mutations are identified, the molecular diagnostics is highly reliable, and even if one known mutation is identified, diagnostics will often be possible in combination with a focused linkage approach.[87] The usefulness of this testing may be more limited in cases where one (or even two) novel missense changes of uncertain pathogenicity are detected. Accumulating data on ARPKD-associated missense mutations and neutral polymorphisms should help to differentiate pathogenic changes and aid gene-based diagnostics in the future.[2,4] Because not all *PKHD1* mutations are detected by the existing methodologies, a negative result does not exclude ARPKD.

DIFFERENTIAL DIAGNOSIS

The phenotype of greatly enlarged and echogenic kidneys in the neonate should not be considered pathognomonic for ARPKD, and it is important to consider other possible cystic disorders when making a diagnosis. Furthermore, the phenotype in the ARPKD patient is highly variable, with other possible diagnoses to consider in more mildly affected patients.

ADPKD

ADPKD is a relatively common genetic disorder (incidence 1:500–1:1,000), and rarely (<1%) cases present in utero or in the neonatal period with clinical symptoms very similar to ARPKD.[108,109] Although ADPKD patients will normally have a family history of PKD, an affected parent is only recognized after the diagnosis of a severely affected child in approximately 50% of cases.[110] A false negative renal ultrasonogram result may also be obtained in ADPKD patients younger than 30 years of age[111]; MR may be a more sensitive screening method. In addition, approximately 10% of ADPKD families can be traced to a new mutation, so rare de novo, early-onset ADPKD cases may occur.[112] Rare families with mutation or linkage suggested ARPKD, but renal and/or hepatic cystic disease in a parent, possibly due to co-inheritance with ADPKD,[86,87] shows the potential complications of diagnostics in this disorder and the usefulness of molecular testing. Congenital hepatic fibrosis is not normally part of the ADPKD phenotype, but rare reports of an association have been described.[113,114] Patients with contiguous deletions of the ADPKD gene, *PKD1*, and the adjacent tuberous sclerosis gene, *TSC2*, can present with an ARPKD-like renal phenotype, and the majority are due to de novo mutation and so have a negative family history.[115,116] However, these patients usually have additional lesions typically of TSC.

Other Cystic Diseases

Glomerulocystic kidney disease (GCKD) is a rare disorder that can present in the neonatal period with an ARPKD-like phenotype.[117–119] Microscopically, the disease involves dilatation of the Bowman's capsule but on ultrasonography can resemble the large echogenic kidneys characteristic of ARPKD. About 10% of GCKD patients have evidence of biliary dysgenesis.[120] Nephronophthisis may also be confused with ARPKD.[121] Although in nephronophthisis the kidneys are not usually enlarged, the cystic pattern can be similar to milder ARPKD, and in a minority of cases the disease is associated with congenital hepatic fibrosis.[122]

Syndromic Cystic Dysplasias

Several syndromic congenital hepatorenal disorders can be associated with renal abnormalities and congenital hepatic fibrosis.[123–127] These include Meckel-Gruber syndrome, Bardet-Biedl syndrome, and asphyxiating thoracic dystrophy.[124–127] In most cases these diseases are also associated with many other congenital abnormalities that are not found in ARPKD. Rare families of with ARPKD-like disease and skeletal and facial anomalies[128,129] or recessively inherited renal and hepatic cystic disease with hypoglycemia[87,130] that are unlinked to *PKHD1*, have been described.

In later childhood or adulthood, ARPKD should be considered in patients with medullary sponge kidney, rare renal cysts, or even in the absence of renal disease found in combination with congenital hepatic fibrosis and/or Caroli disease. It is clear from molecular studies that isolated congenital hepatic fibrosis or Caroli disease can be due to *PKHD1* mutation, but failure to find mutations in some cases suggests that it may also have other etiologies.[6,23]

CLINICAL MANAGEMENT

In the severely affected neonate, the primary concern is to stabilize respiratory function by mechanical ventilation. Significant advances in respiratory care in the previous decade have improved survival for these patients. Unilateral or bilateral nephrectomy in cases with greatly enlarged kidneys may be beneficial.[131–133] However, it is likely that there remains a group in which lung development is so compromised as to be incompatible with survival. Mutation studies indicate that patients with two truncating mutations do not survive the neonatal period.[86]

Hypertension is the other disease complication that may require attention early in life. Several different agents, including angiotensin-converting enzyme inhibitors, calcium channel blockers, and β blockers, have been used. Often a combination of drugs is required for effective therapy.[36] As a result of the urine concentrating defect in ARPKD, patients may be prone to dehydration during illnesses associated with fever, nausea, or diarrhea. Transplant is the renal replacement therapy of choice for patients who develop ESRD. Because ARPKD is a recessive disorder, the parents may be suitable living donors. Growth retardation may be significant even in the absence of renal failure[31] and may be alleviated by growth hormone therapy.[134]

Complications of portal hypertension are common, especially in older patients. The progression of this complication may be monitored with serial ultrasonograms and Doppler flow studies. Treatment of varices may require a portocaval shunt or transjugular intrahepatic portosystemic shunt. As the success of living partial liver transplants improves, this may become the treatment of choice in severe cases.

EXPERIMENTAL THERAPIES FOR ARPKD

Because correction of the primary defect in ARPKD, loss of fibrocystin through *PHKD1* mutation, will be difficult to accomplish in the foreseeable future, therapeutic options are focusing on correcting the downstream effects of the disease mutation.[135] In the last few years an increased understanding of the biochemical changes associated with cystogenesis, and the likelihood of a common ciliary-basal body defect in these disorders, has raised the prospects of common treatments for human cystic diseases. Previously, many possible treatments have looked promising in certain animal models, but then proved ineffective in orthologous models to human disease, such as the PCK rat for ARPKD. The epidermal growth factor receptor has been targeted for inhibition because it is mislocalized and upregulated in ARPKD, and positive results were found in the *bpk* and Han:SPRD models of PKD.[136–138] However, this treatment was found to have a deleterious effect in the PCK rat.[139]

Studies of several PKD systems, including ARPKD cells, have suggested that changes in the epithelial cell phenotype, resulting in proliferation and altered fluid secretion, may be associated with reduced intracellular Ca^{2+}.[135,140] This in turn may impede normal regulation of cyclic adenosine monophosphate (cAMP), leading to an increased level and activation of Ras/Raf/MEK/ERK signaling. Strategies have therefore been designed to attempt to correct these defects. The major cAMP agonist in the collecting duct (ARPKD is mainly a disease of the collecting duct in the kidney) is vasopressin, working via the vasopressin V2 receptor. Recent data has shown that a VPV2 antagonist, OPC31260, can lower the concentration of cAMP and markedly inhibit cystogenesis in the PCK rat and other models of PKD.[141,142] A related drug is already in clinical trials for water retention disorders and has shown few side effects. Trials are already underway to determine the effectiveness of this therapy in ADPKD, and this reagent may prove helpful in ARPKD. However, this treatment is only effective in the kidney (where the VPV2R is expressed) and further agents will be needed to target the biliary disease. Furthermore, it will be necessary to develop surrogate markers to monitor disease progression in ARPKD.

References

1. Guay-Woodford L: Autosomal recessive polycystic kidney disease. In Flinter EM, Saggar-Malik A (editors): The Genetics of Renal Disease. Oxford, Oxford University Press, 2003, pp 239–251.
2. Harris PC, Rossetti S: Molecular genetics of autosomal recessive polycystic kidney disease. Mol Genet Metab 81:75–85, 2004.
3. MacRae Dell KM, Avner ED: Autosomal recessive polycystic kidney disease: GeneReviews; Genetic Disease Online Reviews at GeneTests-GeneClinics. University of Washington, Seattle, 2006. Available at http://genetest.org.
4. Bergmann C, Senderek J, Küpper F, et al: *PKHD1* mutations in autosomal recessive polycystic kidney disease (ARPKD). Hum Mutation 23:453–463, 2004.
5. Fonck C, Chauveau D, Gagnadoux MF, et al: Autosomal recessive polycystic kidney disease in adulthood. Nephrol Dial Transplant 16:1648–1652, 2001.
6. Rossetti S, Torra R, Coto E, et al: A complete mutation screen of *PKHD1* in autosomal recessive polycystic kidney pedigrees. Kidney Int 64:391–403, 2003.
7. Osathanondh V, Potter EL: Pathogenesis of polycystic kidneys. Type 1 due to hyperplasia of interstitial portions of the collecting tubules. Arch Pathol 77:466–473, 1964.
8. Zerres K, Volpel M-C, Wei BH: Cystic kidneys. Hum Genet 68:1044–135, 1984.
9. Steiner: Über grosscystische Degeneration der Nieren und der Leber. Dtsch Med Wochenschr 25:677–678, 1899.
10. Couvelaire A: Sur la dégenérescence kystique congénitale des organes glandulaires et an particulier des reins et du foie. Ann Gynécol Obstét 52:453–482, 1899.
11. Torres VE, Watson ML: Polycystic kidney disease: Antiquity to the 20th century. Nephrol Dial Transplant 13:2690–2696, 1998.
12. Lundin PM, Olow I: Polycystic kidneys in newborns, infants and children. A clinical and pathological study. Acta Paediatr 50:185–200, 1961.
13. Heggo O, Natvig JB: Cystic disease of the kidneys. Autopsy report and family study. Acta Pathol Microbiol Scand 64:459–469, 1965.
14. Kerr DN, Harrison CV, Sherlock S, Walker RM: Congenital hepatic fibrosis. Q J Med 30:91–117, 1961.
15. Kerr DN, Warrick CK, Hart-Mercer J: A lesion resembling medullary sponge kidney in patients with congenital hepatic fibrosis. Clin Radiol 13:85–91, 1962.
16. Blyth H, Ockenden BG: Polycystic disease of kidneys and liver presenting in childhood. J Med Genet 8:257–284, 1971.
17. Summerfield JA, Nagafuchi Y, Sherlock S, et al: Hepatobiliary fibropolycystic diseases. A clinical and histological review of 51 patients. J Hepatol 2:141–156, 1986.
18. Deget F, Rudnik-Schoneborn S, Zerres K: Course of autosomal recessive polycystic kidney disease (ARPKD) in siblings: A clinical comparison of 20 sibships. Clin Genet 47:248–253, 1995.
19. Kaplan BS, Fay J, Shah V, et al: Autosomal recessive polycystic kidney disease. Pediatr Nephrol 3:43–49, 1989.
20. Gang DL, Herrin JT: Infantile polycystic disease of the liver and kidneys. Clin Nephrol 25:28–36, 1986.
21. Kaplan BS, Kaplan P, de Chadarevian JP, et al: Variable expression of autosomal recessive polycystic kidney disease and congenital hepatic fibrosis within a family. Am J Med Genet 29:639–647, 1988.
22. Zerres K, Mücher G, Bachner L, et al: Mapping of the gene for autosomal recessive polycystic kidney disease (ARPKD) to chromosome 6p21-cen. Nat Genet 7:429–432, 1994.
23. Ward CJ, Hogan MC, Rossetti S, et al: The gene mutated in autosomal recessive polycystic kidney disease encodes a large, receptor-like protein. Nat Genet 30:1–11, 2002.
24. Onuchic LF, Furu L, Nagasawa Y, et al: *PKHD1*, the polycystic kidney and hepatic disease 1 gene, encodes a novel large protein containing multiple immunoglobulin-like plexin-transcription-factor domains and parallel β-helix 1 repeats. Am J Hum Genet 70:1305–1317, 2002.
25. Guay-Woodford LM, Muecher G, Hopkins SD, et al: The severe perinatal form of autosomal recessive polycystic kidney disease maps to chromosome 6p21.1–p12: Implications for genetic counseling. Am J Hum Genet 56:1101–1107, 1995.
26. Zerres K, Mücher G, Becker J, et al: Prenatal diagnosis of autosomal recessive polycystic kidney disease (ARPKD): Molecular genetics, clinical experience, and fetal morphology. Am J Med Genet 76:137–144, 1998.

27. Lombard EH, Kromberg JG, Thomson PD, et al: Autosomal recessive polycystic kidney disease. Evidence for high frequency of the gene in the Afrikaans-speaking population. S Afr Med J 76:321–323, 1989.

28. Kaariainen H: Polycystic kidney disease in children: A genetic and epidemiological study of 82 Finnish patients. J Med Genet 24:474–481, 1987.

29. Zerres K, Rudnik-Schöneborn S, Steinkamm C, et al: Autosomal recessive polycystic kidney disease. J Mol Med 76:303–309, 1998.

30. Bernstein J: Heritable cystic disorders of the kidney. The mythology of polycystic disease. Pediatr Clin North Am 18:435–444, 1971.

31. Guay-Woodford LM, Desmond RA: Autosomal recessive polycystic kidney disease: The clinical experience in North America. Pediatrics 111:1072–1080, 2003.

32. Capisonda R, Phan V, Traubuci J, et al: Autosomal recessive polycystic kidney disease: Outcomes from a single-center experience. Pediatr Nephrol 18:119–126, 2003.

33. Potter EL: Facial characteristics of infants with bilateral renal agenesis. Am J Obstet Gynecol 51:885–888, 1964.

34. Roy S, Dillon MJ, Trompeter RS, Barratt TM: Autosomal recessive polycystic kidney disease: Long-term outcome of neonatal survivors. Pediatr Nephrol 11:302–306, 1997.

35. Gagnadoux MF, Habib R, Levy M, et al: Cystic renal diseases in children. Adv Nephrol Necker Hosp 18:33–57, 1989.

36. Cole BR, Conley SB, Stapleton FB: Polycystic kidney disease in the first year of life. J Pediatr 111:693–699, 1987.

37. Lieberman E, Salinas-Madrigal L, Gwinn JL, et al: Infantile polycystic disease of the kidneys and liver: Clinical, pathological and radiological correlations and comparison with congenital hepatic fibrosis. Medicine 50:277–318, 1971.

38. Blickman JG, Bramson RT, Herrin JT: Autosomal recessive polycystic kidney disease: Long-term sonographic findings in patients surviving the neonatal period. Am J Roentgenol 164:1247–1250, 1995.

39. Khan K, Schwarzenberg SJ, Sharp HL, et al: Morbidity from congenital hepatic fibrosis after renal transplantation for autosomal recessive polycystic kidney disease. Am J Transplant 2:360–365, 2002.

40. Birnbaum A, Suchy FJ: The intrahepatic cholangiopathies. Semin Liver Dis 18:263–269, 1998.

41. Murray-Lyon IM, Shilkin KB, Laws JW, et al: Non-obstructive dilatation of the intrahepatic biliary tree with cholangitis. Q J Med 41:477–489, 1972.

42. Kashtan CE, Primack WA, Kainer G, et al: Recurrent bacteremia with enteric pathogens in recessive polycystic kidney disease. Pediatr Nephrol 13:678–682, 1999.

43. Adeva M, El-Youssef M, Rossetti S, et al: Clinical spectrum of autosomal recessive polycystic kidney and liver disease, a single center experience. Medicine 85:1–21, 2006.

44. Jorgensen M: A stereological study of intrahepatic bile ducts. 4. Congenital hepatic fibrosis. Acta Pathol Microbiol Scand [A] 82:21–29, 1974.

45. Cole BR: Autosomal recessive polycystic kidney disease. In Gardner KD, Jr., Bernstein J (editors): The Cystic Kidney. Dordrecht, The Netherlands, Kluwer Academic Publishers, 1990, pp 117–146.

46. Desmet VJ: Congenital diseases of intrahepatic bile ducts: Variations on the theme "ductal plate malformation." Hepatology 16:1069–1083, 1992.

47. Lilova MI, Petkov DL: Intracranial aneurysms in a child with autosomal recessive polycystic kidney disease. Pediatr Nephrol 16:1030–1032, 2001.

48. Neumann HP, Krumme B, van Velthoven V, et al: Multiple intracranial aneurysms in a patient with autosomal recessive polycystic kidney disease. Nephrol Dial Transpl 14:936–939, 1999.

49. Pirson Y, Chauveau D, Torres V: Management of cerebral aneurysms in autosomal dominant polycystic kidney disease. J Am Soc Nephrol 13:269–276, 2002.

50. Bernstein J, Slovis TL: Polycystic diseases of the kidney. In Edelmann CM (editor): Pediatric Kidney Disease, Vol. 2, 2nd ed. Boston, Little, Brown, 1992, pp 1139–1157.

51. Sanchez-Lucas JG: [Morphogenesis of the polycystic kidney.] Semin Hop 27:2793–2800, 1951.

52. Nauta J, Ozawa Y, Sweeney WE, Jr., et al: Renal and biliary abnormalities in a new murine model of autosomal recessive polycystic kidney disease. Pediatr Nephrol 7:163–172, 1993.

53. Moyer JH, Lee-Tischler MJ, Kwon H-Y, et al: Candidate gene associated with a mutation causing recessive polycystic kidney disease in mice. Science 263:1329–1333, 1994.

54. Avner ED, Studnicki FE, Young MC, et al: Congenital murine polycystic kidney disease. I. The ontogeny of tubular cyst formation. Pediatr Nephrol 1:587–596, 1987.

55. Nakanishi K, Sweeney WE, Jr., Zerres K, et al: Proximal tubular cysts in fetal human autosomal recessive polycystic kidney disease. J Am Soc Nephrol 11:760–763, 2000.

56. Premkumar A, Berdon WE, Levy J, et al: The emergence of hepatic fibrosis and portal hypertension in infants and children with autosomal recessive polycystic kidney disease. Initial and follow-up sonographic and radiographic findings. Pediatr Radiol 18:123–129, 1988.

57. Welling LW, Grantham JJ: Cystic diseases of the kidney. In Tisher CC, Brenner BM (editors): Renal Pathology with Clinical and Functional Correlations. Philadelphia, Lippincott, 1989, pp 1233–1275.

58. Bernstein J, Viranuvatti V, Boyer JL: What is Caroli's disease? [Letter] Gastroenterology 68:417–419, 1975.

59. Jorgensen MJ: The ductal plate malformation. Acta Pathol Microbiol Scand Suppl 257:1–87, 1977.

60. Bernstein J: Hepatic involvement in hereditary renal syndromes. Birth Defects 23:115–130, 1987.

61. Parker RG: Fibrosis of the liver as a congenital anomaly. J Pathol Bacteriol 71:359–368, 1956.

62. Caroli J: Diseases of intrahepatic bile ducts. Isr J Med Sci 4:21–35, 1968.

63. Uhari M, Herva R: Polycystic kidney disease of perinatal type. Acta Paediatr Scand 68:443–444, 1979.

64. Calvet JP. Polycystic kidney disease: Primary extracellular matrix abnormality or defective cellular differentiation? Kidney Int 43:101–108, 1993.

65. Carone FA, Bacallao R, Kanwar YS: Biology of polycystic kidney disease. Lab Invest 70:437–448, 1994.

66. Guay-Woodford LM: Murine models of polycystic kidney disease: Molecular and therapeutic insights. Am J Physiol Renal Physiol 285:F1034–F1049, 2003.

67. Woo DDL, Nguyen DKP, Khatibi N, Olsen P: Genetic identification of two major modifier loci of polycystic kidney disease progression in PCY mice. J Clin Invest 100:1934–1940, 1997.

68. Iakoubova OA, Dushkin H, Beier DR: Localization of a murine recessive polycystic kidney disease mutation and modifying loci that affect disease severity. Genomics 26:107–114, 1995.

69. Guay-Woodford LM, Wright CJ, Walz G, Churchill GA: Quantitative trait loci modulate renal cystic disease severity in the mouse bpk model. J Am Soc Nephrol 11:1253–1260, 2000.

70. Olbrich H, Fliegauf M, Hoefele J, et al: Mutations in a novel gene, NPHP3, cause adolescent nephronophthisis, tapeto-retinal degeneration and hepatic fibrosis. Nat Genet 34:455–459, 2003.

71. Otto EA, Schermer B, Obara T, et al: Mutations in INVS encoding inversin cause nephronophthisis type 2, linking renal cystic disease to the function of primary cilia and left-right axis determination. Nat Genet 34:413–420, 2003.

72. Katsuyama M, Masuyama T, Komura I, et al: Characterization of a novel polycystic kidney rat model with accompanying polycystic liver. Exp Anim 49:51–55, 2000.

73. Lager DJ, Qian Q, Bengal RJ, et al: The pck rat: A new model that resembles human autosomal dominant polycystic kidney and liver disease. Kidney Int 59:126–136, 2001.

74. Sanzen T, Harada K, Yasoshima M, et al: Polycystic kidney rat is a novel animal model of Caroli's disease associated with congenital hepatic fibrosis. Am J Pathol 158:1605–1612, 2001.

75. Masyuk TV, Huang BQ, Masyuk AI, et al: Biliary dysgenesis in the PCK rat, an orthologous model of autosomal recessive polycystic kidney disease. Am J Pathol 165:1719–1730, 2004.

76. Lens XM, Onuchic LF, Wu G, et al: An integrated genetic and physical map of the autosomal recessive polycystic kidney disease region. Genomics 41:463–466, 1997.

77. Mücher G, Becker J, Knapp M, et al: Fine mapping of the autosomal recessive polycystic kidney disease locus (PKHD1) and the genes MUT, RDS, CSNK2b, and GSTA1 at 6p21.2–p12. Genomics 48:40–45, 1998.

78. Park JH, Dixit MP, Onuchic LF, et al: A 1-Mb BAC/PAC-based physical map of the autosomal recessive polycystic kidney disease gene (PKHD1) region on chromosome 6. Genomics 57:249–255, 1999.

79. Onuchic LF, Mrug M, Lakings AL, et al: Genomic organization of the KIAA0057 gene that encodes a TRAM-like protein and its exclusion as a polycystic kidney and hepatic disease 1 (PKHD1) candidate gene. Mamm Genome 10:1175–1178, 1999.

80. Hofmann Y, Becker J, Wright F, et al: Genomic structure of the gene for the human P1 protein (MCM3) and its exclusion as a candidate for autosomal recessive polycystic kidney disease. Eur J Hum Genet 8:163–166, 2000.

81. Onuchic LF, Mrug M, Hou X, et al: Refinement of the autosomal recessive polycystic kidney disease (PKHD1) interval and exclusion of an EF hand-containing gene as a PKHD1 candidate gene. Am J Med Genet 110:346–352, 2002.

82. Nagasawa Y, Matthiesen S, Onuchic LF, et al: Identification and characterization of Pkhd1, the mouse orthologue of the human ARPKD gene. J Am Soc Nephrol 13:2246–2258, 2002.

83. Xiong H, Chen Y, Yi Y, et al: A novel gene encoding a TIG multiple domain protein is a positional candidate for autosomal recessive polycystic kidney disease. Genomics 80:96–104, 2002.

84. Furu L, Onuchic LF, Gharavi AG, et al: Milder presentation of recessive polycystic kidney disease requires presence of amino acid substitution mutations. J Am Soc Nephrol 14:2004–2014, 2003.

85. Bergmann C, Senderek J, Schneider F, et al: PKHD1 mutations in families requesting prenatal diagnosis for autosomal recessive polycystic kidney disease (ARPKD). Hum Mut 23:487–495, 2004.

86. Bergmann C, Senderek J, Sedlacek B, et al: Spectrum of mutations in the gene for autosomal recessive polycystic kidney disease (ARPKD/PKHD1). J Am Soc Nephrol 14:76–89, 2003.

87. Consugar MB, Anderson SA, Rossetti S, et al: Haplotype analysis improves molecular diagnostics of autosomal recessive polycystic kidney disease. Am J Kidney Dis 45:77–897, 2005.

88. Bork P, Doerks T, Springer TA, Snel B: Domains in plexins: Links to integrins and transcription factors. Trends Biochem Sci 24:261–263, 1999.

89. Hogan MC, Griffin MD, Rossetti S, et al: PKHDL1, a homolog of the autosomal recessive polycystic kidney disease gene, encodes a receptor with inducible T lymphocyte expression. Hum Mol Genet 12:685–689, 2003.

90. Rigden DJ, Mello LV, Galperin MY: The PA14 domain, a conserved all b-domain in bacterial toxins, enzymes, adhesins and signaling molecules. Trends Biochem Sci 29:335–339, 2004.

91. Zhang MZ, Mai W, Li C, et al: PKHD1 protein encoded by the gene for autosomal recessive polycystic kidney disease associates with basal bodies and primary cilia in renal epithelial cells. Proc Natl Acad Sci U S A 101:2311–2316, 2004.

92. Hiesberger T, Bai Y, Shao X, et al: Mutation of hepatocyte nuclear factor-1b inhibits Pkhd1 gene expression and produces renal cysts in mice. J Clin Invest 113:814–825, 2004.

93. Gresh L, Fischer E, Reimann A, et al: A transcriptional network in polycystic kidney disease. EMBO J 23:1657–1668, 2004.

94. Horikawa Y, Iwasaki N, Hara M, et al: Mutation in hepatocyte nuclear factor-1 b gene (TCF2) associated with MODY. Nat Genet 17:384–385, 1997.

95. Ward CJ, Yuan D, Masyuk TV, et al: Cellular and subcellular localization of the ARPKD protein; fibrocystin is expressed on primary cilia. Hum Mol Genet 12:2703–2710, 2003.

96. Masyuk TV, Huang BQ, Ward CJ, et al: Defects in cholangiocyte fibrocystin expression and ciliary structure in the PCK rat. Gastroenterology 125:1303–1310, 2003.

97. Wang S, Luo Y, Wilson PD, et al: The autosomal recessive polycystic kidney disease protein is localized to primary cilia, with concentration in the basal body area. J Am Soc Nephrol 15:592–602, 2004.

98. Menezes LFC, Cai Y, Nagasawa Y, et al: Polyductin, the PKHD1 gene product, comprises isoforms expressed in plasma membrane, primary cilium and cytoplasm. Kidney Int 66:1345–1355, 2004.

99. Calvet JP: New insights into ciliary function: Kidney cysts and photoreceptors. Proc Natl Acad Sci U S A 100:5583–5585, 2003.

100. Nauli SM, Alenghat FJ, Luo Y, et al: Polycystins 1 and 2 mediate mechanosensation in the primary cilium of kidney cells. Nat Genet 33:129–137, 2003.

101. Praetorius HA, Spring KR: Bending the MDCK cell primary cilium increases intracellular calcium. J Membr Biol 184:71–79, 2001.

102. Luthy DA, Hirsch JH: Infantile polycystic kidney disease: Observations from attempts at prenatal diagnosis. Am J Med Genet 20:505–517, 1985.

103. Lonergan GJ, Rice RR, Suarez ES: Autosomal recessive polycystic kidney disease: Radiologic-pathologic correlation. Radiographics 20:837–855, 2000.

104. Jain M, LeQuesne GW, Bourne AJ, Henning P: High-resolution ultrasonography in the differential diagnosis of cystic diseases of the kidney in infancy and childhood: Preliminary experience. J Ultrasound Med 16:235–240, 1997.

105. Kern S, Zimmerhackl LB, Hildebrandt F, et al: Appearance of autosomal recessive polycystic kidney disease in magnetic resonance imaging and RARE-MR-urography. Pediatr Radiol 30:156–160, 2000.

106. Jung G, Benz-Bohm G, Kugel H, et al: MR cholangiography in children with autosomal recessive polycystic kidney disease. Pediatr Radiol 29:463–466, 1999.

107. Zerres K, Senderek J, Rudnik-Schoneborn S, et al: New options for prenatal diagnosis in autosomal recessive polycystic kidney disease by mutation analysis of the PKHD1 gene. Clin Genet 66:53–57, 2004.

108. Zerres K, Rudnik-Schöneborn S, Deget F: German Working Group on Paediatric Nephrology: Childhood onset autosomal dominant polycystic kidney disease in sibs: Clinical picture and recurrence risk. J Med Genet 30:583–588, 1993.

109. Fick GM, Johnson AM, Strain JD, et al: Characteristics of very early onset autosomal dominant polycystic kidney disease. J Am Soc Nephrol 3:1863–1870, 1993.

110. Chapman A: Particular problems in childhood and adolescence in autosomal dominant polycystic kidney disease. In Watson M, Torres V (editors): Polycystic Kidney Disease. Oxford, Oxford University Press, 1996, pp 548–567.

111. Ravine D, Gibson RN, Walker RG, et al: Evaluation of ultrasonographic diagnostic criteria for autosomal dominant polycystic kidney disease 1. Lancet 343:824–827, 1994.

112. Rossetti S, Strmecki L, Gamble V, et al: Mutation analysis of the entire *PKD1* gene: Genetic and diagnostic implications. Am J Hum Genet 68:46–63, 2001.

113. Lipschitz B, Berdon WE, Defelice AR, Levy J: Association of congenital hepatic fibrosis with autosomal dominant polycystic kidney disease. Report of a family with review of literature. Pediatr Radiol 23:131–133, 1993.

114. Cobben JM, Breuning MH, Schoots C, et al: Congenital hepatic fibrosis in autosomal-dominant polycystic kidney disease. Kidney Int 38:880–885, 1990.

115. Sampson JR, Maheshwar MM, Aspinwall R, et al: Renal cystic disease in tuberous sclerosis: The role of the polycystic kidney disease 1 gene. Am J Hum Genet 61:843–851, 1997.

116. Brook-Carter PT, Peral B, Ward CJ, et al: Deletion of the *TSC2* and *PKD1* genes associated with severe infantile polycystic kidney disease—A contiguous gene syndrome. Nat Genet 8:328–332, 1994.

117. Rizzoni G, Loirat C, Levy M, et al: Familial hypoplastic glomerulocystic kidney. A new entity? Clin Nephrol 18:263–268, 1982.

118. Kaplan BS, Gordon I, Pincott J, Barratt TM: Familial hypoplastic glomerulocystic kidney disease: A definite entity with dominant inheritance. Am J Med Genet 34:569–573, 1989.

119. Sharp CK, Bergman SM, Stockwin JM, et al: Dominantly transmitted glomerulocystic kidney disease: a distinct genetic entity. J Am Soc Nephrol 8:77–84, 1997.

120. Bernstein J: Glomerulocystic kidney disease—Nosological considerations. Pediatr Nephrol 7:464–470, 1993.

121. Hildebrandt F, Omram H: New insights: Nephronophthisis-medullary cystic kidney disease. Pediatr Nephrol 16:168–176, 2001.

122. Boichis H, Passwell J, David R, Miller H: Congenital hepatic fibrosis and nephronophthisis. A family study. Q J Med 42:221–233, 1973.

123. Johnson CA, Gissen P, Sergi C: Molecular pathology and genetics of congenital hepatorenal fibrocystic syndromes. J Med Genet 40:311–319, 2003.

124. Blankenberg TA, Ruebner BH, Ellis WG, et al: Pathology of renal and hepatic anomalies in Meckel syndrome. Am J Med Genet Suppl 3:395–410, 1987.

125. Salonen R, Paavola P: Meckel syndrome. J Med Genet 35:497–501, 1998.

126. Katsanis N: The oligogenic properties of Bardet-Biedl syndrome. Hum Mol Genet 13 (Suppl 1):R65–R71, 2004.

127. Yerian LM, Brady L, Hart J: Hepatic manifestations of Jeune syndrome (asphyxiating thoracic dystrophy). Semin Liver Dis 23:195–200, 2003.

128. Hallermann C, Mucher G, Kohlschmidt N, et al: Syndrome of autosomal recessive polycystic kidneys with skeletal and facial anomalies is not linked to the ARPKD gene locus on chromosome 6p. Am J Med Genet 90:115–119, 2000.

129. Gillessen-Kaesbach G, Meinecke P, Garrett C, et al: New autosomal recessive lethal disorder with polycystic kidneys type Potter I, characteristic face, microcephaly, brachymelia, and congenital heart defects. Am J Med Genet 45:511–518, 1993.

130. Müller D, Zimmering M, Roehr CC: Should nifedipine be used to counter low blood sugar levels in children with persistent hyperinsulinaemic hypoglycaemia? Arch Dis Child 89:83–85, 2004.

131. Bean SA, Bednarek FJ, Primack WA: Aggressive respiratory support and unilateral nephrectomy for infants with severe perinatal autosomal recessive polycystic kidney disease. J Pediatr 127:311–313, 1995.

132. Munding M, Al-Uzri A, Gralnek D, Riden D: Prenatally diagnosed autosomal recessive polycystic kidney disease: Initial postnatal management. Urology 54:1097, 1999.

133. Spechtenhauser B, Hochleitner BW, Ellemunter H, et al: Bilateral nephrectomy, peritoneal dialysis and subsequent cadaveric renal transplantation for treatment of renal failure due to polycystic kidney disease requiring continuous ventilation. Pediatr Transplant 3:246–248, 1999.

134. Lilova M, Kaplan BS, Meyers KE: Recombinant human growth hormone therapy in autosomal recessive polycystic kidney disease. Pediatr Nephrol 18:57–61, 2003.

135. Torres VE: Therapies to slow polycystic kidney disease. Nephron Exp Nephrol 98:e1–e7, 2004.

136. Dell KM, Nemo R, Sweeney WE, Jr., et al: A novel inhibitor of tumor necrosis factor-α converting enzyme ameliorates polycystic kidney disease. Kidney Int 60:1240–1248, 2001.

137. Sweeney WE, Jr., Chen Y, Nakanish K, et al: Treatment of polycystic kidney disease with a novel tyrosine kinase inhibitor. Kidney Int 57:33–40, 2000.

138. Sweeney WE, Jr., Hamahira K, Sweeney J, et al: Combination treatment of PKD utilizing dual inhibition of EGF-receptor activity and ligand bioavailability. Kidney Int 64:1310–1319, 2003.

139. Torres VE, Sweeney WE, Jr., Wang X, et al: Epidermal growth factor receptor tyrosine kinase inhibition is not protective in PCK rats. Kidney Int 66:1766–1773, 2004.

140. Belibi FA, Reif G, Wallace DP, et al: Cyclic AMP promotes growth and secretion in human polycystic kidney epithelial cells. Kidney Int 66:964–973, 2004.

141. Gattone VH, 2nd, Wang X, Harris PC, Torres VE: Inhibition of renal cystic disease development and progression by a vasopressin V2 receptor antagonist. Nat Med 9:1323–1326, 2003.

142. Torres VE, Wang X, Qian Q, et al: Effective treatment of an orthologous model of autosomal dominant polycystic kidney disease. Nat Med 10:363–364, 2004.

Chapter 8

Pathogenesis of Nephronophthisis and Medullary Cystic Kidney Disease

Thomas Benzing and Gerd Walz

Nephronophthisis (NPH) and medullary cystic kidney disease (MCKD) constitute a group of renal cystic diseases that share the macroscopic feature of cyst development at the corticomedullary border and in the outer medulla of the kidneys and a common renal histology: tubular basement membrane disintegration, tubular atrophy with cyst formation, interstitial cell infiltration, and fibrosis.[1,2] The initial clinical description —as a renal disease characterized by its occurrence in siblings and its progression to renal failure, with prominent polyuria in the absence of hematuria, heavy proteinuria, and hypertension and small kidneys at autopsy with mainly tubulointerstitial lesions—nicely illustrates the common characteristics of this group of diseases.[3–6] Despite the similarities that led to the description as "NPH/MCKD complex,"[2,7] it is now apparent, that the NPH/MCKD complex is characterized by both clinical as well as genetic heterogeneity.[8,9] Initially much confusion has been caused by the use of two different terms for these diseases, MCKD and NPH.[10] It is now accepted to summarize the autosomal recessive forms as NPH and the less common dominant forms as MCKD (Table 8-1).[8,11]

NPH is the most common genetic cause of end-stage renal disease (ESRD) in children and adolescents, and it was estimated that NPH accounts for about 10% of cases of ESRD in children.[12] According to their clinical presentation (mode of inheritance and age of onset of ESRD), patients have been grouped into three different clinical forms of the NPH disease (infantile, juvenile, and adolescent NPH) and two different forms of MCKD (early adult form and late adult form).[8,13] Because of the extensive genetic heterogeneity, with certainly more than five different loci for NPH (*NPHP1* to *NPHP5*) and at least two different loci for MCKD (*MCKD1* and *MCKD2*) and a large spectrum of phenotypes associated with these loci, the diseases should now be categorized according to the affected gene (see Table 8-1). This is even more important given that patients with other diseases such as Bardet-Biedl syndrome (BBS) may present with an NPH-like disorder.[14,15] BBS combines blindness, obesity, polydactyly, hypogenitalism, and cognitive impairment with NPH/MCKD, and at least eight different BBS genes have recently been described.[14] Several additional ones are waiting to be discovered.

There has been tremendous progress in the past few years in the understanding of the molecular pathogenesis of NPH. Several of the NPH genes have been identified using positional cloning strategies in affected families.[16–22] Many of the proteins that are encoded by these genes are evolutionary conserved, and functional studies in cells as well as model organisms have been of considerable help in deciphering critical steps in disease pathogenesis.[23–26]

In contrast to NPH, which typically presents as a tubulointerstitial nephropathy leading to ESRD in childhood and adolescence, MCKD leads to kidney failure later in life. Such cases are rare, with about 30 to 40 families reported. Two disease genes have been mapped on chromosome 1q21 (*MCKD1*)[27] and on chromosome 16p12 (*MCKD2*; see Table 8-1).[28] *MCKD2* displays features similar to the ones described in familial juvenile hyperuricemic nephropathy (FJHN), namely autosomal dominant inheritance of hyperuricemia and gout, and progressive renal failure. Common critical regions[29] raised the possibility that MCKD and FJHN could arise from mutations of the same gene. In fact, both diseases were found to be associated with uromodulin mutations.[30,31] Uromodulin, also referred to as Tamm-Horsfall protein, is exclusively expressed by epithelial cells of the thick ascending limb of the loop of Henle and by distal convoluted tubules and is the most abundant protein in urine. Uromodulin was initially characterized by Tamm and Horsfall in 1950,[32] but its function is still unclear.[33]

The understanding of the pathogenesis of cystic kidney disease has been transformed by the discovery that the products of autosomal dominant polycystic kidney disease (*ADPKD*), autosomal recessive polycystic kidney disease (*ARPKD*), and *NPH* genes localize to the primary cilium of tubular epithelial cells.

THE CILIARY HYPOTHESIS OF CYSTIC KIDNEY DISEASES

During renal development, more than a million nephrons have to assume a genetically predetermined three-dimensional structure that is maintained throughout the lifetime of the organism. Outgrowth of the ureteric bud, condensation of the metanephric mesenchyme, and its subsequent mesenchymal-to-epithelial conversion are developmental steps that are governed by the reciprocal interaction between the mesenchymal and epithelial tissues. Branching of the ureteric bud is an important step and controls the ultimate number of nephrons, but the principal programs that control and maintain the morphology of a mature nephron are poorly understood. Cystogenesis uniformly starts in late embryogenesis. For example, in mice deficient in PKD1, the initial cysts become detectable after embryonic day 15.[34] At this time, mature glomeruli are present at the cortical-medullary transition zone, while branching morphogenesis and formation of new glomeruli proceeds within the outer segments of the kidney. Thus, cyst formation seems to result from defective nephron

Table 8-1 Genetic Loci for Nephronopthisis and Medullary Cystic Kidney Disease

Disease	Gene	Locus	Mode of Inheritance	Renal Presentation	Extrarenal Manifestations	References
NPH1	NPHP1	2q13	AR	Juvenile NPH	Retinitis pigmentosa, Cogan syndrome, liver fibrosis, cone-shaped epiphysis, mental retardation	16, 19
NPH2	INVS (NPHP2)	9q31	AR	Infantile NPH	Situs inversus, cardiac ventricular septal defect	17
NPH3	NPHP3	3q22	AR	Juvenile NPH (may be adolescent)	Retinitis pigmentosa, liver fibrosis	18
NPH4	NPHP4	1p36	AR	Juvenile NPH	Retinitis pigmentosa, Cogan syndrome, liver fibrosis, cone-shaped epiphysis, mental retardation	21, 22
NPH5	IQCB1 (NPHP5)	3q13	AR	Juvenile NPH	Retinitis pigmentosa (=SLSN, Leber congenital amaurosis)	20
MCKD1	MCKD1	1q21	AD	Late adult	Hyperuricemia, gout	30, 31
MCKD2	MCKD2	16p12	AD	Early adult	Hyperuricemia, gout	28

AD, autosomal dominant; AR, autosomal recessive; MCKD, medullary cystic kidney disease; NPH, nephronophthisis.

maturation rather than defective nephrogenesis. Proliferation and migration of tubular epithelial cells are essential components of tubular elongation and maturation, but the signaling cascades defining the geometry of different nephron segments remain elusive. If cystic kidney disease is a disease of tubular maturation and/or maintenance, genes mutated in cystic kidney disease should represent excellent candidates of such cellular programs.

A novel concept of cystogenesis was pioneered by the identification of the *PKD1* and *PKD2* homologs *lov-1* and *pkd-2* in *Caenorhabditis elegans* (see also Chapter 6).[35] Both gene products are present in the cilia of male-specific mechanosensory neurons of male animals, and play an essential role in the male mating behavior.[36,37] Subsequently, several cystogenic proteins either involved in human cystic disease or mutated in animal models of cystic kidneys were localized in the monocilia of tubular epithelial cells.[38] These proteins participate in all aspects of ciliary homeostasis, including ciliogenesis, maintenance, and function. Mechan-ical bending of the cilium of Madin-Darby canine kidney (MDCK) cells triggers an increase in intracellular calcium[39] that requires an intact polycystin complex (see also Chapter 6).[40] These observations suggest that cilia act as mechanosensors to endow tubular epithelial cells with spatial information (that is, in addition to the typical apico-basolateral polarity of epithelial cells, every ciliated cell of a nephron should acquire a second, anterior-posterior polarity). Conceptually, cysts would arise from tubular epithelial cells that lost their orientation relative to the urine flow.

NPHP1 ENCODES THE MULTIFUNCTIONAL ADAPTOR PROTEIN NEPHROCYSTIN

The *NPHP1* gene on 2q13 was the first NPH gene to be identified.[16,19] NPH1 is by far the most common form of

NPH/MCKD and typically presents as juvenile NPH. In a study of 515 unrelated individuals with NPH, about 27% had NPH type I.[41] Juvenile NPH is a systemic disorder, and about 10% to 15% of individuals with NPH1 present with extrarenal findings. These include retinal dystrophy, which can be either severe (Leber amaurosis) with early blindness and a flat electroretinogram, or moderate with mild visual impairment and retinitis pigmentosa. The association of NPH and retinal involvement is referred to as Senior-Løken syndrome.[42] Other extrarenal anomalies have been described, in particular oculomotor apraxia (Cogan syndrome), hepatic fibrosis,[43] mental retardation,[44] and cone-shaped epiphysis.[45] In addition, brain stem and vermis hypoplasia were described in an individual with NPH type I,[46] revealing nephrocystin's role in normal cerebellar development. The initial symptoms of NPH type I occur before age 6 but are usually mild, consisting of polyuria and polydipsia.[8] Later, severe anemia, growth retardation, and development of end-stage renal failure at a mean age of 13 years are characteristic for *NPHP1* mutations. The histologic changes entail tubular basement membrane disruption, interstitial cell infiltration, tubular atrophy, and cyst formation at the corticomedullary junction. Although the glomeruli are not directly affected, a periglomerular fibrosis is evident at early stages of the disease. *NPHP1* encodes nephrocystin, a protein with 732 amino acids and a predicted molecular mass of 83 kDa. Most patients harbor a single homozygous deletion of about 290 kilobases (kb) on 2q13 resulting from an unequal recombination event between two 45-kb direct repeats flanking the *NPHP1* gene.[9,47] The C-terminal nephrocystin homology domain is highly conserved but does not reveal significant homology to other known proteins. In contrast, the N-terminus is modular, and contains a coiled-coil structure and an Src homology 3 (SH3) domain that is flanked by two highly charged acidic clusters. The domain architecture suggests that nephrocystin functions as a scaffold and/or adaptor protein. The typical thickening and disruption of the tubular basement membrane in NPH implicate nephrocystin in basement membrane homeostasis. Several nephrocystin-interacting proteins have been identified that support this hypothesis. Yeast two-hybrid screens with the SH3 domain of nephrocystin identified p130(Cas) as nephrocystin-interacting protein.[8,48] p130(Cas) is an essential component of focal adhesion complexes, and partially co-localizes with nephrocystin at the plasma membrane,[48] suggesting that nephrocystin is involved in the formation of cell-matrix contacts. Focal adhesions are formed through clustering of integrins, and assembly of large intracellular protein complexes that include tensin, talin, vinculin, α-actinin, paxillin, zyxin, vinexin, FA52, nexilin, and focal adhesion kinase (FAK).[49] Interestingly, nephrocystin interacts with Pyk2,[23] a non-receptor tyrosine kinase that shares with FAK the dependence of actin filament integrity for its function as well as the ability to interact with p130(Cas). Forming heteromeric complexes, nephrocystin may recruit Pyk2 to specialized cell matrix adhesions. Nephrocystin also interacts with tensin.[23] Because tensin-deficient mice develop cystic renal disease that closely resembles human NPH,[50] this animal model provides further evidence that nephrocystin is required for specific types of cell-matrix contacts.

Nephrocystin also localizes to the primary cilium of tubular epithelial cells.[17] Because nephrocystin interacts with the gene products of the NPHP2 (inversin) cells,[17] NPHP3 (nephrocystin-3)[18] and NPHP4 (nephrocystin-4),[22] it is conceivable that nephrocystin targets these proteins to distinct subcellular localizations, including the primary cilium. Interestingly, Pyk2 also localizes to the primary cilium of tubular epithelial cells. Thus, cystogenesis in NPH type I could result from either failure to recruit focal adhesion proteins to the sites of extracellular contacts, and/or failure to target other NPH proteins to the primary cilium. The C. elegans homologs of NPHP1 and NPHP4, nph-1 and nph-4, are both 23% identical to their human counterparts; there are no clear C. elegans orthologs of NPHP2 and NPHP3.[24] Although nph-1 and nph-4 are expressed more broadly during embryonic development, their expression pattern overlaps with PKD1 and PKD2 (lov-1, pkd-2) in the male-specific sensory cilia in adult animals.[24,51] Interestingly, nph-1 and nph-4 single and double mutants show normal embryonic development and sensory behaviors, including osmotic avoidance and nociception.[24] However, the double (but not the single) nph-1/nph-4 mutants demonstrate a decreased response after the initial contact with a potential mate; a similar defect has been observed in lov-1 or pkd-2 mutants. In addition, double nph-1/nph-4 mutants display turning defects during the mating process that have not been observed in lov-1 or pkd-2 mutants.[24] Taken together, these results indicate that in C. elegans the functions of nph-1 and nph-4 are redundant. Both proteins participate in the lov-1/pkd-2-dependent response pathway, but assume additional functions during the mating process not shared with lov-1/pkd-2.[24] In C. elegans, the function of nephrocystins seems to be confined to the cilium of mechanosensory neurons. NPH gene products are detectable in the connecting cilium of the photoreceptor (see Cloning of NPHP5 Suggests a Common Pathway for the Development of NPH and Retinitis Pigmentosa), an organelle necessary for transport processes between the inner and outer segment of the photoreceptor. Thus, the Senior-Løken syndrome in NPH can be viewed as a ciliary disease of the photoreceptor, intimately linking NPH gene products to the structural and functional integrity of cilia. So far, no correlation has been established between the presence and absence of extrarenal manifestations and mutations of certain NPH genes.

INVERSIN (NPHP2) IS A MOLECULAR SWITCH INVOLVED IN WNT SIGNALING

In contrast to the juvenile NPH type I, the infantile form (NPH type II) of the disease typically combines features of NPH with characteristics of autosomal dominant polycystic kidney disease (enlarged kidneys, cysts not limited to corticomedullary junction). Recently, INVS/NPHP2 was identified as the gene responsible for NPH type II.[17] INVS was originally identified in the OVE210 transgenic mouse with situs inversus, cystic kidney disease, liver abnormalities, and death due to renal failure shortly after birth.[52,53] Similarly to these mice, humans with this disorder can also present with hepatobiliary duct malformations and altered left-right asymmetry in addition to renal cystic disease.[17,54] INVS, the gene encoding inversin, consists of 17 exons located on chromosome 9q31 in humans. Full-length inversin contains 1,065 amino acids with 16 tandem ankyrin repeats, two nuclear localization signals, and a conserved lysine-rich central domain.[55] In MDCK cells, inversin has been localized to several cellular compartments, including the primary cilia, the plasma membrane, and the centrosome.[56,57] Although the full-length protein is predicted to encode a protein of 117 kDa, mass spectrometry and immunoblotting have detected five different species (90, 116, 125, 140, and 165 kDa) that seem to represent different inversin isoforms. In normal mouse kidney, four different transcripts can be detected by northern blot analysis, and reverse transcription–polymerase chain reaction reveals skipping of exon 5, 11, or 13, whereas exon 12 is deleted in MDCK. Inversin also contains two IQ domains that interact with calmodulin.[58,59] IQ2, encoded by exons 14 and 15, binds calmodulin in the absence of calcium and is required for inversin-mediated reversal of the left-right asymmetry in Xenopus embryos.[58] Skipping of exon 13 results in frameshift and loss of exons 14 and 15, suggesting that not every inversin isoform contains IQ2. The left-right axis in inv/inv mice is consistently reversed. In mouse embryos, the leftward flow of extraembryonic fluid at the ventral node is critical for the determination of the left-right axis of mouse embryos. This flow is generated by posteriorly tilted cilia. In inv/inv mice, cilia at the ventral node appear structurally normal, but nearly 20% of cilia are anteriorly tilted, suggesting that the inv mutation affects the alignment of modal pit cells along the anterior-posterior axis.[60] Inversin expression is detectable as early as the two-cell stage, and present in the 9+0 cilia of the ventral node, renal tubules, pituitary gland, and fibroblasts,[61] but can also be found in motile 9+2 cilia of tracheal epithelial cells (unpublished data). In immortalized renal epithelial cells (MDCK, IMCD), inversin can be detected in the nucleus and the plasma membrane, where it co-localizes with β-catenin and N-cadherin.[56,59] Inversin associates with the centrosome during early prophase and localizes to the spindle poles during mitosis,[59] a subcellular localization that inversin shares with polycystin-2.[62] The association of polycystin-2 with the spindle poles requires the mDia1, a member of the RhoA guanosine triphosphatase–binding formin homology protein family that participates in cytoskeletal organization, cytokinesis, and signal transduction. It will be interesting to test whether mDia1 recruits other cystoproteins to the spindle apparatus.

Inversin contains two destruction box (D-box) motifs that mediate ubiquitin-dependent degradation of many short-lived regulatory proteins. APC2, a subunit of the multimeric anaphase promoting complex/cyclosome (APC/C), binds to the first highly conserved D-box.[59] APC/C is an E3 ligase that mediates cell cycle–dependent degradation of cyclins; the interaction with APC2 provides further evidence that inversin is involved in cell cycle control.

Inversin interacts with disheveled, and co-localizes with this protein at the centrosome and at the plasma membrane of polarized epithelial cells.[26] Disheveled is a central component of the Wnt signaling cascades, located at the branch point between the canonical Wnt signaling pathway, and the non-canonical Wnt signaling pathway involved in cytoskeleton reorganization and planar cell polarity. Inversin targets disheveled for ubiquitin-dependent degradation, thereby inhibiting the canonical Wnt signaling pathway. However, inversin does not affect disheveled at the plasma membrane and is required for convergent-extension movements in *Xenopus laevis*. Deletion of inversin in zebrafish by antisense morpholino-oligonucleotides causes cystic kidney disease.[17] Interestingly, cystogenesis is almost completely reversed by diversin, an ankyrin-repeat protein with distant sequence similarities to inversin. The *Drosophila* homolog of diversin, Diego, belongs to a group of proteins that regulate planar polarity signaling pathways in the fly wing and eye.[63,64] Both proteins, inversin and diversin, share the capacity to inhibit canonical Wnt signaling and to promote noncanonical Wnt signaling. The overlapping functions of inversin and diversin in zebrafish[26] suggest that both inversin and diversin endow tubular epithelial cells with a second type of polarity that is oriented in the plane of the epithelial sheet (planar cell polarity). This type of polarity would orient each cell relative to the anterior-posterior axis (versus the typical apico-basolateral polarity). Because inversin is present at the cilium and releases calmodulin after an increase in intracellular calcium, it is tempting to postulate that cilial bending activates an inversin-dependent signaling cascade that ultimately helps to specify a spatial orientation in relationship to the urine flow. For tubular epithelial cells to form a tube of a genetically predetermined geometry, an orientation in relationship to neighboring cells seems mandatory, and inversin is the first member of a pathway that maintains these "neighborly relationships." A disruption of planar cell polarity signaling would prompt cells to redefine their position in relationship to neighboring cells, most likely through a process involving proliferation and migration. Both processes require dedifferentiation (e.g., epithelial-to-mesenchymal conversion), and this would explain why these phenomena are commonly seen in cystic kidney disease of different etiologies.

DOMAIN STRUCTURE OF THE *NPHP3* GENE PRODUCT SUGGESTS A ROLE IN REGULATING MICROTUBULE ORGANIZATION

Recently, the *NPHP3* gene was localized to chromosome 3q22[65] and subsequently identified by positional cloning.[18]

Patients carrying *NPHP3* mutations present with juvenile or adolescent NPH without or with extrarenal symptoms such as retinitis pigmentosa and liver fibrosis.[9,18] *NPHP3* encodes nephrocystin-3, a novel 1330–amino acid protein that interacts with nephrocystin-1.[18] The *pcy* mouse, a spontaneous mouse mutant with renal cystic disease similar to human NPH, was shown to harbor a homozygous missense mutation in the orthologous *Nphp3* gene. That this mouse model can be treated successfully with the vasopressin-2 receptor antagonist OPC31260 opens completely new prospects for potential therapeutic strategies in NPH in humans.[66] Nephrocystin-3 contains several putative protein interaction domains. A N-terminal coiled-coil domain is reminiscent of a similar region in nephrocystin-1.[23] This type of protein interaction module usually interacts with other coiled-coil domains, most frequently to allow homodimerization of proteins. α-helices wrap around each other to form a particularly stable structure. Each coiled-coil domain is composed of two or more α-helices that entwine to form a cable-like assembly.[67] In many proteins, these helical cables serve a mechanical role in forming stiff bundles of fibers. This structure can form when the two (or in some cases three) α-helices have most of their nonpolar (hydrophobic) side chains on one side, so that they can twist around each other with these side chains facing inward. Although it is conceivable that nephrocystin-3 dimerizes through coiled-coil domain interactions, thus far it is not clear if this is really the case and which additional protein may bind to this domain. In addition to the N-terminal coiled-coil domain, nephrocystin-3 contains eight C-terminal tetratrico peptide repeats (TPRs). TPR motifs have been identified in various organisms, ranging from bacteria to humans, and proteins containing TPRs are involved in a variety of biologic processes, such as cell cycle regulation, transcriptional control, mitochondrial and peroxisomal protein transport, neurogenesis, and protein folding.[68] These domains mediate protein-protein interactions and the assembly of multiprotein complexes. Classical examples are protein interactions that allow the assembly of the anaphase-promoting complex APC/C, a ubiquitin ligase complex that consists of at least 11 subunits and is required for cell cycle progression.[69] It is interesting to note that inversin, the product of the *NPHP2* gene, has been shown to associate with APC/C.[59] Though not tested experimentally, it may be conceivable that nephrocystin-3 also displays interactions with the APC/C. The typical TPR motif consists of tandem repeats of 34 amino acid residues.[68] Sequence alignment of the TPR domains reveals a consensus core sequence defined by a pattern of small and large amino acids.[70] Although binding partners of the nephrocystin-3 TPRs are still waiting to be discovered, it is interesting to note that several cilia-associated proteins such as BBS4 or the *TG737*-encoded protein Polaris contain these domains.[71,72] Polaris is the mammalian homolog of the intraflagellar transport protein IFT88 and required for ciliogenesis and sensory signaling from cilia.[73,74] Interestingly, deletion of the *Tg737* gene in mice results in cystic kidneys, situs inversus, and retinitis pigmentosa resembling features of human NPH.[72,74–76] However, whether nephrocystin-3 may be part of IFT complexes is not clear so far.[38]

In addition to these protein interaction modules, another domain in nephrocystin-3 suggests a function for the protein in regulating microtubule stability and dynamics. A putative tubulin tyrosine ligase (TTL) domain localizes to the center of the protein. The conserved amino acid exchange that probably causes cyst formation in the *pcy* mouse (I614S) lies in this domain,[18] supporting the critical role of the TTL domain for nephrocystin-3 function. TTLs are tubulin-modifying enzymes that catalyze the addition of tyrosine residues to the C terminus of tubulin.[77] The α/β tubulin dimer, the microtubule building block, is subject to a variety of specific post-translational modifications that principally affect the C termini of both subunits.[78] These C-terminal tails of α- and β-tubulin are essential for microtubule function. They lie on the outer surface of the microtubule, where they can influence the binding of associated proteins. The tyrosination cycle involves the enzymatic cyclic removal of the C-terminal tyrosine of tubulin by a thus-far-uncharacterized carboxypeptidase and the readdition of a tyrosine residue by the TTL. This tyrosination cycle is conserved among eukaryotes and generates two tubulin pools: intact tyrosinated tubulin and detyrosinated tubulin (glutamylated tubulin).[79] Although the biologic role of these different pools of tubulin is not clear, it has been demonstrated that TTL activity is essential for embryonic development. Gene disruption of a neuronal TTL in mice results in embryonic lethality due to the disorganization of neuronal networks, uncontrolled neurite outgrowth, and misguided axonal differentiation.[79] This is interesting in light of recent evidence that points to a role for nephrocystins in cerebellar and brain stem development.[9] NPH can be associated with oculomotor apraxia and cerebellar abnormalities, and recently, *NPHP1*-homozygous deletions—identical to the deletions observed in patients with isolated NPH—have been identified in a small percentage of patients with a mild neurologic form of Joubert syndrome that occurs in combination with NPH.[46,80,81] Joubert syndrome is characterized by a complex cerebellar and brain stem malformation, visible as the so-called "molar tooth sign" observed by magnetic resonance imaging.[82] This syndrome results in developmental delay, congenital hypotonia, ataxia, oculomotor apraxia, and abnormal breathing pattern. One could therefore speculate that nephrocystins have a role in modulating neurite outgrowth and neuron differentiation similarly to known TTLs.

In addition to their central role in serving as the skeleton for neurite outgrowth and building the mitotic spindle apparatus for cell division, microtubules form the axonemes of cilia. Thus, it is tempting to speculate that a tubulin-modifying function of nephrocystin-3 provides a common explanation for the renal cystic phenotype, the retinal abnormalities as well as the cerebellar defects that can be seen in NPH patients.

THE *NPHP4* GENE PRODUCT IS AN EVOLUTIONARILY CONSERVED COMPONENT OF CILIA AND CENTROSOMES

The *NPHP4* gene has also been recently identified by a positional cloning approach.[21,22] *NPHP4* mutations have been detected mainly in individuals with isolated NPH, but they also occur in individuals with NPH associated with Cogan syndrome or in Senior-Locken syndrome (SLNS), usually as NPH and late-onset retinitis pigmentosa.[9,41,83] Nephrocystin-4 (or nephroretinin),[21] the protein encoded by *NPHP4*,

interacts with nephrocystin-1.[22] It is a 1250–amino acid protein that does not contain predicted protein interaction modules or known functional domains. However, some light has been shed on a putative function of nephrocystin-4 by the recent demonstration that the protein is highly conserved from algae to humans and localized to basal bodies and centrioles.[84] Li et al took advantage of the idea that the ancestral eukaryote was ciliated and that organisms that have lost cilia and flagella (along with basal bodies) through evolution also lost most of the more than 400 to 500 genes that are predicted to be needed for forming and regulating the ciliary apparatus.[85] In a remarkable study, the authors subtracted the genome of *Arabidopsis* from the shared genome of the ciliated/flagellated organisms *Chlamydomonas* and human. They identified a flagellar and basal body (FABB) transcriptome that contains 688 genes. Incorporating into their analysis the genome of the nematode worm *C. elegans*, which has only nonmotile cilia, yielded a subset of the FABB transcriptome of 362 candidate proteins that would be sufficient to assemble a nonmotile cilium.[84] As measures of the success of their approach, 4 of 6 known *Chlamydomonas* basal body genes examined and 52 of 58 known *Chlamydomonas* flagellar proteins were present in the transcriptome.[84] In addition to established *Chlamydomonas* basal body and flagellar genes, the FABB proteome contained several known mammalian disease genes, including many of the BBS proteins as well as nephrocystin-4.[85] Proteomic analysis of isolated centrioles confirmed that the *Chlamydomonas* ortholog of nephrocystin-4 is a component of centrioles.[86] Subsequent studies in mammalian kidney epithelial cells also showed localization in basal bodies/centrioles and the ciliary axoneme of primary cilia.[25] Further insight into a potential function of nephrocystin-4 at cilia and basal bodies came from a recent study in the nematode *C. elegans*.[24] This worm has no kidney per se yet has proved to be an excellent model to study renal-related issues, including tubulogenesis of the excretory canal, membrane transport, and ion channel function, as well as human genetic diseases including ADPKD.[35] In the worm, ciliated sensory neurons located in the head and tail sense an extensive variety of environmental signals and mediate a wide spectrum of behaviors. For example, animals must locate food and males must find hermaphrodite mates. Of the 302 neurons in the hermaphrodite, 60 have dendritic endings that terminate in cilia.[35] The male possesses an additional 52 ciliated neurons primarily involved in male mating behavior. Interestingly, many of the genes required for the formation, maintenance, and function of *C. elegans* cilia have human counterparts that, when mutated, cause diseases with renal pathologies including ADPKD and BBS.[36,87–90] The *C. elegans* polycystins LOV-1 and PKD-2 localize to male-specific sensory cilia and are required specifically for male mating behaviors.[24] Thus, male mating behavior is a wonderful readout for sensory cilia function in the worm. Very recently, Jauregui and Barr demonstrated that the *C. elegans* homologs of *NPHP1* and *NPHP4* are expressed in these sensory cilia. *nphp-1;nphp-4* double, but not single, mutant males are response defective.[24,51] These data clearly indicate that nephrocystin and nephrocystin-4 play important and redundant roles in facilitating ciliary sensory signal transduction and suggest that one major function of nephrocystin-4 is in participating in sensory signaling in cilia.

CLONING OF *NPHP5* SUGGESTS A COMMON PATHWAY FOR THE DEVELOPMENT OF NPH AND RETINITIS PIGMENTOSA

Mutations in *IQCB1/NPHP5*, located on chromosome 3q13.33–q21.1, have been identified very recently in families with SLNS.[20] In contrast to all other known NPH genes, mutations in *IQCB1/NPHP5* seem to be always associated with retinal degenerative disease. In fact, this gene seems to be a major gene associated with SLNS, and a majority of SLNS patients harbor *IQCB1/NPHP5* mutations.[20] Nephrocystin-5, the encoded protein, shares IQ domains with the *NPHP2* gene product inversin and has been shown to interact with the retinitis pigmentosa guanosine phosphatase regulator (RPGR). RPGR is encoded by the X-linked *RP3* locus and has an essential role in maintaining photoreceptor viability.[91] Mutations in the human *RPGR* gene cause retinitis pigmentosa.[92,93] Targeted disruption of the mouse *Rpgr* gene and naturally occurring mutations in dogs also lead to photoreceptor degeneration.[94] However, the function of RPGR is elusive. The N-terminal sequence of RPGR is similar to that of RCC1, a nuclear protein that functions as a guanine nucleotide exchange factor for the small guanosine triphosphatase Ran. A guanine nucleotide exchange factor activity of RPGR toward any small GTPases has not been demonstrated directly.[91] However, protein mislocalization in photoreceptors in *Rpgr*-mutant mice suggests a role for RPGR in regulating protein trafficking.[95,96] Interestingly, RPGR has been shown to localize to the transition zone of cilia.[91] Although cilia and flagella are ostensibly open to the cytoplasm, it seems that only a subset of cytoplasmic proteins is admitted to the ciliary/flagellar compartment. In *Chlamydomonas reinhardtii,* the boundary between the cytoplasmic and flagellar compartments is demarcated by transition fibers, which extend from the distal end of the basal body and connect each of the nine basal-body triplet microtubules to the flagellar membrane.[97] Rosenbaum and Witman proposed that these transition fibers might be structural components of a flagellar pore complex that controls the movement of molecules and particles between the cytoplasmic and flagellar compartments, much as the nuclear pore controls movement between the cytoplasmic and nuclear compartments. Immunoelectron microscopy has shown that the transition fibers are docking sites for the intraflagellar transport particle proteins at the base of the flagellum.[97] Interestingly, in photoreceptors the transition zone is formed by the connecting cilium of rods and cones.[84,91] The outer segments of photoreceptors are built from modified cilia. During development of the outer segment, large amounts of lipid and protein are transported into the distal segment and assembled into the membranous disks.[98] In the mature photoreceptor, the distal portion of the outer segment is so highly modified that it no longer resembles a cilium. However, a short segment of the cilium, called the connecting cilium, remains to connect the outer segment to the inner segment. This connecting cilium is required for transport of proteins and lipids to reach their functionally active sites in the outer segments of the photoreceptor. Diseased protein transport in the connecting cilium of photoreceptors results in retinitis pigmentosa.[74,99] Thus, interaction of RPGR with nephrocystin-5, together with localization of RPGR to the transition zone suggests that nephrocystin-5 (or probably other nephrocystin proteins)

may serve a critical role at the transition zone of cilia. In fact, it has been recently shown that nephrocystin-1, in addition to its punctate pattern of staining in the ciliary axoneme, concentrates mainly at the transition zone (unpublished data). Thus, localization of nephrocystin at the transition zone may provide a common explanation for cystic kidney disease and retinitis pigmentosa in SLNS patients. What is the function of nephrocystin-5 at the transition zone? It is conceivable that nephrocystin-5 is involved in regulating access of proteins to intraflagellar transport (IFT). IFT has first been described by Rosenbaum and colleagues in the biflagellate alga *Chlamydomonas*. During IFT, non-membrane-bound particles are moved continuously along the axonemal doublet microtubules, just beneath the cilia membrane. IFT particles moving to the top of this organelle are driven by a kinesin II motor, whereas movement of IFT particles returning from the tip depends on dynein motors.[97] Disruption of IFT by *Cre-loxP* mutagenesis to remove the kinesin II subunit, KIF3A, specifically from photoreceptors resulted in retinitis pigmentosa.[100] The same approach was used to delete the *Kif3a* gene in kidney tubular cells which produced a renal cystic phenotype.[101]

In addition to a potential trafficking function, nephrocystin-5 may also be involved in transmitting signals from the ciliary axoneme to the cell body and vice versa. It has been shown that nephrocystin-1 is a signaling protein and mediates activation of tyrosine kinase signal transduction.[23] Because the transition zone is located precisely at the border between cilia and the cell body, it is conceivable that nephrocystins participate in signal transduction at the transition zone to transmit chemo- or mechanosensory signaling to the interior of the cell.

NPH—A CILIARY DISORDER?

The Ciliary Hypothesis of Cystic Kidney Disease

Nephrocystin and inversin are detectable in the ciliary axoneme and the transition zone adjacent to the basal body of the primary cilium projecting from tubular epithelial cells. During early prophase inversin associates with the centrosome; it localizes to the spindle poles at later phases of mitosis. Nephrocystin-3 shares structural features with Tg737, interacts with nephrocystin, and is highly expressed in the ventral node during mouse embryonic development. Nephrocystin-4 interacts with nephrocystin, and both proteins are found in the cilium of mechanosensory neurons of *C. elegans*. Nephrocystin-1, -2, -3, and -4 are present in the cilia of respiratory epithelial cells (unpublished data). With nephrocystin-5 present in the connecting cilium of the photoreceptor, all products of NPH genes have either been localized or predicted to localize to the primary cilium of tubular epithelial cells. These findings imply that perturbations of cilial integrity and/or functions lead to cyst formation and retinal degeneration in NPH. For many years, PKD researchers have tried to find such a unifying pathogenesis of renal cystic disease. Mutations of proteins that disrupt intraflagellary transport or function of cilia in both mouse models and human disease cause cyst formation.[38] These observations suggest that ciliary proteins are essential components of a cellular program that prevents cyst formation.

Mutations of PKD genes either disrupt the structural integrity of the primary cilium (e.g., *Tg737*),[102] or cause functional perturbations (e.g., polycystin-2).[40,103] Ciliogenesis is intimately linked to the IFT, a microtubular transport process that requires the presence of the motor proteins kinesin II and dynein for antegrade and retrograde transport, respectively.[74,97] These motor proteins propel cargo particles, termed IFT rafts, along the axonemal microtubes of the cilium. Both defective motor proteins (e.g., caused by mutation of the kinesin II subunit Kif3a[101]) and defective IFT particles compromise cilial homeostasis, resulting in structurally abnormal cilia and cystic kidney disease, often associated with disturbances of the left-to-right asymmetry.[104] Although the morphology of cilia has not been studied in detail in all types of NPH, mutations of *nph-1* and *nph-4* in *C. elegans* are apparently not associated with structural abnormalities. A careful analysis of the ventral node in *inv/inv* mice also revealed morphologically normal cilia,[60] although the ciliary dynamics was altered, causing a slowed, meandering flow at the ventral node. Taken together, these observations suggest that nephrocystins compromise the function rather than the structure of the cilium of tubular epithelial cells. Yet, it remains unclear what ciliary functions are altered, and whether ciliary dysfunction is directly responsible for cyst formation of tubular epithelial cells in NPH.

The Centrosomal Hypothesis

In nondividing cells the centrosome consists of two centrioles, the mother and daughter centriole. In polarized tubular epithelial cells, the two centrioles are separated and positioned just underneath the apical membrane.[105] The larger (mother) centriole gives rise to the basal body, which nucleates and anchors the microtubules of the ciliary axoneme. The microtubular network in polarized epithelial cells consists of an apical and basal web as well as longitudinal bundles along the apical-basal axis[106,107]; however, only a small subset of microtubules nucleates from the basal body/centriole during interphase (G_0/G_1).[108] In prophase the primary cilium is retracted, the basal body reverts into a centriole, and both centrioles move from the apical position to the nucleus, where they duplicate to organize the two spindle poles parallel to the plane of the epithelial cell layer. In other cells, the centrioles remain in close proximity to each other and form the microtubule-organizing center. The centrosome is positioned adjacent to the trans-Golgi network, and the basal body of some ciliated cells have been shown to form a physical link with parts of the Golgi apparatus.[109,110] Thus, the basal body together with the daughter centriole could not only serve as a docking site for vesicles destined for IFT but might also function as a more general sorting site in the secretory pathway. Many gene products involved in human hereditary disease have now been localized to the centrosome, thereby revealing the multifunctional properties of the centrosome. Although the importance of centrosomes in mitotic cell division has been appreciated for many years, their functions in proteolysis, cell migration, and vesicular transport in postmitotic cells have been uncovered by hereditary diseases such as autosomal recessive juvenile parkinsonism, lissencephaly, and Huntington disease.[111] The centrosome contains high concentrations of proteasomes as well as subunits of the APC/C.[112–114] Inversin interacts with APC2, a subunit of APC/C.[59] This interaction

appears to target disheveled for ubiquitin-dependent degradation. It is interesting to note that inversin is associated with the centrosomes and the mitotic spindle throughout the cell cycle, whereas disheveled disappears from the centrosome during mitosis (unpublished data), suggesting that inversin mediates the cell cycle–dependent degradation of disheveled at least in the proximity of the centrosome. Because the APC/C regulates axonal growth in the developing brain,[115] it is conceivable that the interaction of inversin with APC2 is required for normal cerebellar development. Several nephrocystins contain D-/KEN box motifs, and it will be interesting to test whether the centrosomal localization of nephrocystins is cell cycle dependent or whether they target other interacting proteins for degradation.

The Transport Hypothesis

The microtubular network guides the motor protein–powered transport of vesicles over long distances, for example in neuronal axons. Perturbation of microtubule-based transport has been implicated in diverse human disorders, including neurodegenerative disorders such as Alzheimer or Huntington disease.[116] Although it is unclear whether microtubule-based cargo transport plays a significant role in bulk protein trafficking of polarized epithelial cells, it is tempting to speculate that it assumes very specialized functions in epithelial cells and that the cerebral manifestations of NPH represent a disturbance of microtubule-based long-range protein transport. The domain architecture of both nephrocystin and nephrocystin-3 indicate that these two proteins may play a role in microtubule organization and/or microtubule-dependent transport processes. Although the importance of microtubule-dependent transport of IFT particles in ciliogenesis and ciliary function is clearly established, recent studies suggest that IFT-dependent transport processes play a role in cellular signaling events that are probably unrelated to the cilium. *Tg737*, the gene mutated in the oprk mouse model of cystic kidney disease, encodes Polaris, a mammalian homolog of the *Chlamydomonas* IFT88. Recently, IFT88 was found to play an important role in Hedgehog signaling.[73,117] IFT88 mediates the proteolytic cleavage of the transcriptional activator Gli3-190 to form the transcriptional repressor Gli3-83. Hypomorphic mutations of the gene encoding IFT88 fail to generate the Gli3 repressor, resulting in ventralization of the spinal cord and polydactyly similar to the phenotypic changes reported for mice deficient in Sonic Hedgehog. Although the precise molecular mechanism remains unknown, it seems plausible that IFT88 (and other IFTs) are required for the microtubule-dependent transport of Gli3 to a subcellular localization, responsible for the proteolytic cleavage of Gli3. Mutations of *Kif3a*, a kinesin II subunit responsible for microtubule-dependent transport, can cause similar phenotypic changes, providing further evidence for this hypothesis. Thus, cystogenic proteins, including the nephrocystins, could be involved in specialized cellular transport processes requiring IFTs and motor proteins. Mutations of these proteins can compromise ciliogenesis or ciliary function, but in this case the structurally abnormal cilium is solely an indicator of abnormal intracellular transport processes rather than the molecular basis for the disease-specific phenotypes.

IFT-dependent transport processes may not only be required to bridge long distances (e.g., the transport of cargo vesicles in neuronal axons or the connecting cilium of photo-receptors) but could also serve to establish cellular polarity and asymmetry.[118] Cellular asymmetry powered by IFT-dependent transport may be one of the fundamental programs involved in establishing pH or voltage gradients that determine body axis as well as tubular geometry. PKD researchers may ultimately get their unifying concept: the loss of asymmetry that forces tubular epithelial cells to assume their default value of symmetric, cystic structures. It is possible that the primary cilium of tubular epithelial cells will have to assume once again the role of a supporting actor, only to enter center stage during specialized cellular programs, such as reorientation of tubular epithelial cells after regeneration.

References

1. Cohen AH, Hoyer JR: Nephronophthisis. A primary tubular basement membrane defect. Lab Invest 55(5):564–572, 1986.
2. Waldherr R, Lennert T, Weber HP, et al: The nephronophthisis complex. A clinicopathologic study in children. Virchows Arch [Pathol Anat] 394(3):235–254, 1982.
3. Fanconi G, Hanhart E, Albertini A, et al: Die familiäre juvenile Nephronophthise. Helv Paediatr Acta 6:1–49, 1951.
4. Royer P, Habib R, Mathieu H, Courtecuisse V: [Chronic idiopathic tubulo-interstitial nephropathies in children.] Ann Pediatr (Paris) 10:620–633, 1963.
5. Mangos JA, Opitz JM, Lobeck CC, Cookson DU: Familial juvenile nephronophthisis: An unrecognized renal disease in the United States. Pediatrics 34:337–345, 1964.
6. Smith CH, Graham JB: Congenital medullary cysts of the kidneys with severe refractory anemia. Am J Dis Child 69:370–378, 1945.
7. Avasthi PS, Erickson DG, Gardner KD: Hereditary renal-retinal dysplasia and the medullary cystic disease–nephronophthisis complex. Ann Intern Med 84(2):157–161, 1976.
8. Hildebrandt F, Otto E: Molecular genetics of nephronophthisis and medullary cystic kidney disease. J Am Soc Nephrol 11(9):1753–1761, 2000.
9. Saunier S, Salomon R, Antignac C: Nephronophthisis. Curr Opin Genet Dev 15(3):324–331, 2005.
10. Salomon R, Gubler MC, Antignac C: Nephronophthisis. In Davidson AM, Cameron JS, Grünfeld JP, et al (editors): Oxford Textbook of Clinical Nephrology. New York, Oxford University Press, 2005, pp 2325–2334.
11. Omran H, Haffner K, Burth S, et al: Evidence for further genetic heterogeneity in nephronophthisis. Nephrol Dial Transplant 16(4):755–758, 2001.
12. Hildebrandt F, Waldherr R, Kutt R, Brandis M: The nephronophthisis complex: Clinical and genetic aspects. Clin Invest 70(9):802–808, 1992.
13. Hildebrandt F, Omram H: New insights: Nephronophthisis–medullary cystic kidney disease. Pediatr Nephrol 16(2):168–176, 2001.
14. Katsanis N: The oligogenic properties of Bardet-Biedl syndrome. Hum Mol Genet 13(Spec No 1):R65–R71, 2004.
15. Katsanis N, Lupski JR, Beales PL: Exploring the molecular basis of Bardet-Biedl syndrome. Hum Mol Genet 10(20):2293–2299, 2001.
16. Hildebrandt F, Otto E, Rensing C, et al: A novel gene encoding an SH3 domain protein is mutated in nephronophthisis type 1. Nat Genet 17(2):149–153, 1997.
17. Otto EA, Schermer B, Obara T, et al: Mutations in *INVS* encoding inversin cause nephronophthisis type 2, linking renal cystic disease to the function of primary cilia and left-right axis determination. Nat Genet 34(4):413–420, 2003.
18. Olbrich H, Fliegauf M, Hoefele J, et al: Mutations in a novel gene, *NPHP3*, cause adolescent nephronophthisis,

19. Saunier S, Calado J, Heilig R, et al: A novel gene that encodes a protein with a putative src homology 3 domain is a candidate gene for familial juvenile nephronophthisis. Hum Mol Genet 6(13):2317–2323, 1997.
20. Otto E, Loeys B, Khanna H, et al: A novel ciliary IQ domain protein, NPHP5, is mutated in Senior-Løken syndrome (nephronophthisis with retinitis pigmentosa), and interacts with RPGR and calmodulin. Nat Genet 37(3):282–288, 2005.
21. Otto E, Hoefele J, Ruf R, et al: A gene mutated in nephronophthisis and retinitis pigmentosa encodes a novel protein, nephroretinin, conserved in evolution. Am J Hum Genet 71(5):1161–1167, 2002.
22. Mollet G, Salomon R, Gribouval O, et al: The gene mutated in juvenile nephronophthisis type 4 encodes a novel protein that interacts with nephrocystin. Nat Genet 32(2):300–305, 2002.
23. Benzing T, Gerke P, Hopker K, et al: Nephrocystin interacts with Pyk2, p130(Cas), and tensin and triggers phosphorylation of Pyk2. Proc Natl Acad Sci U S A 98(17):9784–9789, 2001.
24. Jauregui AR, Barr MM: Functional characterization of the *C. elegans* nephrocystins NPHP-1 and NPHP-4 and their role in cilia and male sensory behaviors. Exp Cell Res 305(2):333–342, 2005.
25. Mollet G, Silbermann F, Delous M, et al. Characterization of the nephrocystin/nephrocystin-4 complex and subcellular localization of nephrocystin-4 to primary cilia and centrosomes. Hum Mol Genet 14(5):645–656, 2005.
26. Simons M, Gloy J, Ganner A, et al: Inversin, the gene product mutated in nephronophthisis type II, functions as a molecular switch between Wnt signaling pathways. Nat Genet 37(5):537–543, 2005.
27. Christodoulou K, Tsingis M, Stavrou C, et al: Chromosome 1 localization of a gene for autosomal dominant medullary cystic kidney disease. Hum Mol Genet 7(5):905–911, 1998.
28. Scolari F, Puzzer D, Amoroso A, et al: Identification of a new locus for medullary cystic disease, on chromosome 16p12. Am J Hum Genet 64(6):1655–1660, 1999.
29. Dahan K, Fuchshuber A, Adamis S, et al: Familial juvenile hyperuricemic nephropathy and autosomal dominant medullary cystic kidney disease type 2: Two facets of the same disease? J Am Soc Nephrol 12(11):2348–2357, 2001.
30. Turner JJ, Stacey JM, Harding B, et al: UROMODULIN mutations cause familial juvenile hyperuricemic nephropathy. J Clin Endocrinol Metab 88(3):1398–1401, 2003.
31. Hart TC, Gorry MC, Hart PS, et al: Mutations of the *UMOD* gene are responsible for medullary cystic kidney disease 2 and familial juvenile hyperuricaemic nephropathy. J Med Genet 39(12):882–892, 2002.
32. Tamm I, Horsfall FL, Jr: A mucoprotein derived from human urine which reacts with influenza, mumps, and Newcastle disease viruses. J Exp Med 95(1):71–97, 1952.
33. Rampoldi L, Caridi G, Santon D, et al: Allelism of MCKD, FJHN and GCKD caused by impairment of uromodulin export dynamics. Hum Mol Genet 12(24):3369–3384, 2003.
34. Lu W, Peissel B, Babakhanlou H, et al: Perinatal lethality with kidney and pancreas defects in mice with a targeted *Pkd1* mutation. Nat Genet 17(2)179–181, 1997.
35. Barr MM: *Caenorhabditis elegans* as a model to study renal development and disease: Sexy cilia. J Am Soc Nephrol 16(2):305–312, 2005.
36. Barr MM, DeModena J, Braun D, et al: The *Caenorhabditis elegans* autosomal dominant polycystic kidney disease gene homologs *lov-1* and *pkd-2* act in the same pathway. Curr Biol 11(17):1341–1346, 2001.
37. Barr MM, Sternberg PW: A polycystic kidney-disease gene homologue required for male mating behaviour in *C. elegans*. Nature 401(6751):386–389, 1999.

tapeto-retinal degeneration and hepatic fibrosis. Nat Genet 34(4):455–459, 2003.

38. Watnick T, Germino G: From cilia to cyst. Nat Genet 34(4):355–356, 2003.
39. Praetorius HA, Spring KR: Bending the MDCK cell primary cilium increases intracellular calcium. J Membr Biol 184(1):71–79, 2001.
40. Nauli SM, Alenghat FJ, Luo Y, et al: Polycystins 1 and 2 mediate mechanosensation in the primary cilium of kidney cells. Nat Genet 33(2):129–137, 2003.
41. Hoefele J, Sudbrak R, Reinhardt R, et al: Mutational analysis of the *NPHP4* gene in 250 patients with nephronophthisis. Hum Mutat 25(4):411, 2005.
42. Warady BA, Cibis G, Alon V, et al: Senior-Løken syndrome: revisited. Pediatrics 94(1):111–112, 1994.
43. Boichis H, Passwell J, David R, Miller H: Congenital hepatic fibrosis and nephronophthisis. A family study. Q J Med 42(165):221–233, 1973.
44. Steele BT, Lirenman DS, Beattie CW: Nephronophthisis. Am J Med 68(4):531–538, 1980.
45. Saldino RM, Mainzer F: Cone-shaped epiphyses (CSE) in siblings with hereditary renal disease and retinitis pigmentosa. Radiology 98(1):39–45, 1971.
46. Takano K, Nakamoto T, Okajima M, et al: Cerebellar and brainstem involvement in familial juvenile nephronophthisis type I. Pediatr Neurol 28(2):142–144, 2003.
47. Konrad M, Saunier S, Heidet L, et al: Large homozygous deletions of the 2q13 region are a major cause of juvenile nephronophthisis. Hum Mol Genet 5(3):367–371, 1996.
48. Donaldson JC, Dempsey PJ, Reddy S, et al: Crk-associated substrate p130(Cas) interacts with nephrocystin and both proteins localize to cell-cell contacts of polarized epithelial cells. Exp Cell Res 256(1):168–178, 2000.
49. Brugge JS: Casting light on focal adhesions. Nat Genet 19(4):309–311, 1998.
50. Lo SH, Yu QC, Degenstein L, et al: Progressive kidney degeneration in mice lacking tensin. J Cell Biol 136(6):1349–1361, 1997.
51. Wolf MT, Lee J, Panther F, et al: Expression and phenotype analysis of the nephrocystin-1 and nephrocystin-4 homologs in *Caenorhabditis elegans*. J Am Soc Nephrol 16(3):676–687, 2005.
52. Morgan D, Turnpenny L, Goodship J, et al: Inversin, a novel gene in the vertebrate left-right axis pathway, is partially deleted in the *inv* mouse. Nat Genet 20(2):149–156, 1998.
53. Mochizuki T, Saijoh Y, Tsuchiya K, et al: Cloning of *inv*, a gene that controls left/right asymmetry and kidney development. Nature 395(6698):177–181, 1998.
54. Mazziotti MV, Willis LK, Heuckeroth RO, et al: Anomalous development of the hepatobiliary system in the *inv* mouse. Hepatology 30(2):372–378, 1999.
55. Eley L, Turnpenny L, Yates LM, et al: A perspective on inversin. Cell Biol Int 28(2):119–124, 2004.
56. Nurnberger J, Bacallao RL, Phillips CL: Inversin forms a complex with catenins and N-cadherin in polarized epithelial cells. Mol Biol Cell 13(9):3096–3106, 2002.
57. Nurnberger J, Kribben A, Saez AO, et al: The *Invs* gene encodes a microtubule-associated protein. J Am Soc Nephrol 15(7):1700–1710, 2004.
58. Yasuhiko Y, Imai F, Ookubo K, et al: Calmodulin binds to *inv* protein: Implication for the regulation of *inv* function. Dev Growth Differ 43(6):671–681, 2001.
59. Morgan D, Eley L, Sayer J, et al: Expression analyses and interaction with the anaphase promoting complex protein APC2 suggest a role for inversin in primary cilia and involvement in the cell cycle. Hum Mol Genet 11(26):3345–3350, 2002.
60. Okada Y, Takeda S, Tanaka Y, et al: Mechanism of nodal flow: A conserved symmetry breaking event in left-right axis determination. Cell 121(4):633–644, 2005.
61. Watanabe D, Saijoh Y, Nonaka S, et al: The left-right determinant Inversin is a component of node monocilia and other 9+0 cilia. Development 130(9):1725–1734, 2003.
62. Rundle DR, Gorbsky G, Tsiokas L: PKD2 interacts and co-localizes with mDia1 to mitotic spindles of dividing cells: Role of mDia1 in PKD2 localization to mitotic spindles. J Biol Chem 279(28):29728–29739, 2004.
63. Schwarz-Romond T, Asbrand C, Bakkers J, et al: The ankyrin repeat protein Diversin recruits Casein kinase Iε to the β-catenin degradation complex and acts in both canonical Wnt and Wnt/JNK signaling. Genes Dev 16(16):2073–2084, 2002.
64. Feiguin F, Hannus M, Mlodzik M, Eaton S: The ankyrin repeat protein Diego mediates Frizzled-dependent planar polarization. Dev Cell 1(1):93–101, 2001.
65. Omran H, Fernandez C, Jung M, et al: Identification of a new gene locus for adolescent nephronophthisis, on chromosome 3q22 in a large Venezuelan pedigree. Am J Hum Genet 66(1):118–127, 2000.
66. Gattone VH, 2nd, Wang X, Harris PC, Torres VE: Inhibition of renal cystic disease development and progression by a vasopressin V2 receptor antagonist. Nat Med 9(10):1323–1326, 2003.
67. Woolfson DN: The design of coiled-coil structures and assemblies. Adv Protein Chem 70:79–112, 2005.
68. D'Andrea LD, Regan L: TPR proteins: The versatile helix. Trends Biochem Sci 28(12):655–662, 2003.
69. Vodermaier HC, Gieffers C, Maurer-Stroh S, et al: TPR subunits of the anaphase-promoting complex mediate binding to the activator protein CDH1. Curr Biol 13(17):1459–1468, 2003.
70. Das AK, Cohen PW, Barford D: The structure of the tetratricopeptide repeats of protein phosphatase 5: Implications for TPR-mediated protein-protein interactions. EMBO J 17(5):1192–1199, 1998.
71. Kim JC, Badano JL, Sibold S, et al: The Bardet-Biedl protein BBS4 targets cargo to the pericentriolar region and is required for microtubule anchoring and cell cycle progression. Nat Genet 36(5):462–470, 2004.
72. Yoder BK, Tousson A, Millican L, et al: Polaris, a protein disrupted in *orpk* mutant mice, is required for assembly of renal cilium. Am J Physiol Renal Physiol 282(3):F541–F552, 2002.
73. Huangfu D, Liu A, Rakeman AS, et al: Hedgehog signalling in the mouse requires intraflagellar transport proteins. Nature 426(6962):83–87, 2003.
74. Pazour GJ, Baker SA, Deane JA, et al: The intraflagellar transport protein, IFT88, is essential for vertebrate photoreceptor assembly and maintenance. J Cell Biol 157(1):103–113, 2002.
75. Haycraft CJ, Swoboda P, Taulman PD, et al: The *C. elegans* homolog of the murine cystic kidney disease gene *Tg737* functions in a ciliogenic pathway and is disrupted in *osm-5* mutant worms. Development 128(9):1493–1505, 2001.
76. Murcia NS, Richards WG, Yoder BK, et al:. The Oak Ridge Polycystic Kidney (*orpk*) disease gene is required for left-right axis determination. Development 127(11):2347–2355, 2000.
77. Janke C, Rogowski K, Wloga D, et al: Tubulin polyglutamylase enzymes are members of the TTL domain protein family. Science 308(5729):1758–1762, 2005.
78. Westermann S, Weber K. Post-translational modifications regulate microtubule function. Nat Rev Mol Cell Biol 4(12):938–947, 2003.
79. Erck C, Peris L, Andrieux A, et al: A vital role of tubulin-tyrosine-ligase for neuronal organization. Proc Natl Acad Sci U S A 102(22):7853–7858, 2005.
80. Parisi MA, Bennett CL, Eckert ML, et al: The *NPHP1* gene deletion associated with juvenile nephronophthisis is present in a subset of individuals with Joubert syndrome. Am J Hum Genet 75(1):82–91, 2004.

81. Castori M, Valente EM, Donati MA, et al: *NPHP1* gene deletion is a rare cause of Joubert syndrome–related disorders. J Med Genet 42(2):e9, 2005.

82. Maria BL, Quisling RG, Rosainz LC, et al: Molar tooth sign in Joubert syndrome: Clinical, radiologic, and pathologic significance. J Child Neurol 14(6):368–376, 1999.

83. Hoefele J, Otto E, Felten H, et al: Clinical and histological presentation of 3 siblings with mutations in the *NPHP4* gene. Am J Kidney Dis 43(2):358–364, 2004.

84. Snell WJ, Pan J, Wang Q: Cilia and flagella revealed: From flagellar assembly in *Chlamydomonas* to human obesity disorders. Cell 117(6):693–697, 2004.

85. Li JB, Gerdes JM, Haycraft CJ, et al: Comparative genomics identifies a flagellar and basal body proteome that includes the *BBS5* human disease gene. Cell 117(4):541–552, 2004.

86. Keller LC, Romijn EP, Zamora I, et al: Proteomic analysis of isolated *Chlamydomonas* centrioles reveals orthologs of ciliary-disease genes. Curr Biol 15(12):1090–1098, 2005.

87. Blacque OE, Reardon MJ, Li C, et al: Loss of *C. elegans* BBS-7 and BBS-8 protein function results in cilia defects and compromised intraflagellar transport. Genes Dev 18(13):1630–1642, 2004.

88. Ansley SJ, Badano JL, Blacque OE, et al: Basal body dysfunction is a likely cause of pleiotropic Bardet-Biedl syndrome. Nature 425(6958):628–633, 2003.

89. Fan Y, Esmail MA, Ansley SJ, et al: Mutations in a member of the Ras superfamily of small GTP-binding proteins causes Bardet-Biedl syndrome. Nat Genet 36(9):989–993, 2004.

90. Barr MM, Sternberg PW: A polycystic kidney-disease gene homologue required for male mating behaviour in *C. elegans* [See Comments]. Nature 401(6751):386–389, 1999.

91. Hong DH, Pawlyk B, Sokolov M, et al: RPGR isoforms in photoreceptor connecting cilia and the transitional zone of motile cilia. Invest Ophthalmol Vis Sci 44(6):2413–2421, 2003.

92. Roepman R, Bauer D, Rosenberg T, et al: Identification of a gene disrupted by a microdeletion in a patient with X-linked retinitis pigmentosa (XLRP). Hum Mol Genet 5(6):827–833, 1996.

93. Meindl A, Dry K, Herrmann K, et al: A gene (*RPGR*) with homology to the *RCC1* guanine nucleotide exchange factor is mutated in X-linked retinitis pigmentosa (RP3). Nat Genet 13(1):35–42, 1996.

94. Vervoort R, Wright AF: Mutations of *RPGR* in X-linked retinitis pigmentosa (RP3). Hum Mutat 19(5):486–500, 2002.

95. Hong DH, Pawlyk BS, Shang J, et al: A retinitis pigmentosa GTPase regulator (RPGR)–deficient mouse model for X-linked retinitis pigmentosa (RP3). Proc Natl Acad Sci U S A 97(7):3649–3654, 2000.

96. Zhao Y, Hong DH, Pawlyk B, et al: The retinitis pigmentosa GTPase regulator (RPGR)–interacting protein: Subserving RPGR function and participating in disk morphogenesis. Proc Natl Acad Sci U S A 100(7):3965–3970, 2003.

97. Rosenbaum JL, Witman GB: Intraflagellar transport. Nat Rev Mol Cell Biol 3(11):813–825, 2002.

98. Pazour GJ, Rosenbaum JL: Intraflagellar transport and cilia-dependent diseases. Trends Cell Biol 12(12):551–555, 2002.

99. Deretic D, Papermaster DS: Polarized sorting of rhodopsin on post-Golgi membranes in frog retinal photoreceptor cells. J Cell Biol 113(6):1281–1293, 1991.

100. Marszalek JR, Liu X, Roberts EA, et al: Genetic evidence for selective transport of opsin and arrestin by kinesin-II in mammalian photoreceptors. Cell 102(2):175–187, 2000.

101. Lin F, Hiesberger T, Cordes K, et al: Kidney-specific inactivation of the KIF3A subunit of kinesin-II inhibits renal ciliogenesis and produces polycystic kidney disease. Proc Natl Acad Sci U S A 100(9):5286–5291, 2003.

102. Pazour GJ, Dickert BL, Vucica Y, et al: *Chlamydomonas IFT88* and its mouse homologue, polycystic kidney disease gene *tg737*, are required for assembly of cilia and flagella. J Cell Biol 151(3):709–718, 2000.

103. Pazour GJ, San Agustin JT, Follit JA, et al: Polycystin-2 localizes to kidney cilia and the ciliary level is elevated in *orpk* mice with polycystic kidney disease. Curr Biol 12(11):R378–R380, 2002.

104. Pazour GJ: Intraflagellar transport and cilia-dependent renal disease: The ciliary hypothesis of polycystic kidney disease. J Am Soc Nephrol 15(10):2528–2536, 2004.

105. Reinsch S, Karsenti E: Orientation of spindle axis and distribution of plasma membrane proteins during cell division in polarized MDCKII cells. J Cell Biol 126(6):1509–1526, 1994.

106. Bacallao R, Antony C, Dotti C, et al: The subcellular organization of Madin-Darby canine kidney cells during the formation of a polarized epithelium. J Cell Biol 109(6 Pt 1):2817–2832, 1989.

107. Bacallao R, Fine LG: Molecular events in the organization of renal tubular epithelium: From nephrogenesis to regeneration. Am J Physiol 257(6 Pt 2):F913–F924, 1989.

108. Bre MH, Karsenti E: Effects of brain microtubule-associated proteins on microtubule dynamics and the nucleating activity of centrosomes. Cell Motil Cytoskeleton 15(2):88–98, 1990.

109. Tenkova T, Chaldakov GN: Golgi-cilium complex in rabbit ciliary process cells. Cell Struct Funct 13(5):455–458, 1988.

110. Poole CA, Jensen CG, Snyder JA, et al: Confocal analysis of primary cilia structure and colocalization with the Golgi apparatus in chondrocytes and aortic smooth muscle cells. Cell Biol Int 21(8):483–494, 1997.

111. Badano JL, Teslovich TM, Katsanis N: The centrosome in human genetic disease. Nat Rev Genet 6(3):194–205, 2005.

112. Harper JW: A phosphorylation-driven ubiquitination switch for cell-cycle control. Trends Cell Biol 12(3):104–107, 2002.

113. Harper JW, Burton JL, Solomon MJ. The anaphase-promoting complex: It's not just for mitosis any more. Genes Dev 16(17):2179–2206, 2002.

114. Wigley WC, Fabunmi RP, Lee MG, et al: Dynamic association of proteasomal machinery with the centrosome. J Cell Biol 145(3):481–490, 1999.

115. Konishi Y, Stegmuller J, Matsuda T, et al: Cdh1-APC controls axonal growth and patterning in the mammalian brain. Science 303(5660):1026–1030, 2004.

116. Gerdes JM, Katsanis N: Microtubule transport defects in neurological and ciliary disease. Cell Mol Life Sci 62:1556–1570, 2005.

117. Liu A, Wang B, Niswander LA: Mouse intraflagellar transport proteins regulate both the activator and repressor functions of Gli transcription factors. Development 132(13):3103–3111, 2005.

118. Levin M: The embryonic origins of left-right asymmetry. Crit Rev Oral Biol Med 15(4):197–206, 2004.

SECTION 3

Genetic Disorders of Renal Function

Chapter 9

Inherited Nephroses

Astrid Weins and Martin R. Pollak

Idiopathic nephrotic syndrome (NS) and focal segmental glomerulosclerosis (FSGS) represent a disparate but related group of clinical entities that account for as much as 5% of end-stage renal disease (ESRD) in adults and 15% to 20% in children. Despite substantial efforts of researchers, relatively little is known about the etiologic factors involved in the pathogenesis of the majority of these disorders. A significant percentage of idiopathic NS reflects an underlying genetic predisposition toward this condition. Through studies of mendelian forms of disease, it has become clear in recent years that a large percentage of cases are in fact caused by inherited genetic changes.

In the past decade, investigators have made substantial progress in further defining the genetic basis of familial forms of NS/FSGS. A growing number of genes have been identified that, when defective, lead to inherited forms of disease; many of their protein products play nonredundant roles in the podocyte, suggesting a central role of this cell type in the pathogenesis of NS/FSGS. This chapter will focus largely on the forms of NS/FSGS that belong to the subset of patients in whom the lesion is a downstream response to direct podocyte or slit-diaphragm injury. In addition, we will discuss other inherited forms of proteinuric disease that cannot be directly attributed to podocyte dysfunction (Table 9-1).

The podocyte, a unique, highly specialized, and terminally differentiated glomerular epithelial cell, exerts a wide range of functions in the glomerulus. It anchors the slit diaphragm and produces extracellular matrix proteins necessary for the maintenance of the glomerular basement membrane (GBM), both constituting essential parts of the filtration barrier. It also serves as a mechanical support system for the glomerular capillary wall, and provides numerous signaling platforms important for the dynamic adaptation to changes in its direct environment.

Mutations in different podocyte proteins can target the function of the podocyte through distinct pathologic mechanisms: by affecting the structure of the slit diaphragm, by directly or indirectly perturbing the intricate podocyte cytoskeleton, by breaking cell-matrix interactions, or by blocking important signaling pathways. All of these mechanisms result in a common final disease pathway characterized by podocyte foot process effacement, proteinuria, and ultimately disruption of the glomerular filter (Fig. 9-1).

Although mutations in many podocyte proteins have already been linked to a human disease phenotype, our knowledge is often based to a great extent on experimental animal models of disease. In the following, a subset of these proteins involved in the pathogenesis of podocyte injury will be discussed in more detail, including clinical course, genetic testing, and population genetics to the extent that data are available.

SLIT-DIAPHRAGM COMPLEX

NPHS1

Congenital nephrotic syndrome (CNS), also known to as CNS of the Finnish type, is characterized by autosomal recessive inheritance and onset at birth. The first CNS gene to be identified was NPHS1, encoding the nephrin protein. Mutations in NPHS1 lead to the most clinically severe of the inherited podocytopathies.[1] Disease begins in utero: abnormal glomerular filtration can be detected prenatally as an increase in maternal α-fetoprotein. The clinical and pathologic features of CNS were recognized several decades ago.[2] Proteinuria on the order of 20 g/day is not uncommon in these neonates with defects in both the maternally and paternally inherited nephrin alleles. Affected infants require intensive support to live. The clinical severity in the neonatal period is a result of the effects of nephrosis and hypoalbuminemia, rather than kidney failure. Treatment consists of aggressive supportive care until the child reaches a developmental stage at which nephrectomy and renal transplantation can be performed. In the absence of treatment, death typically occurs from the complications of severe nephrosis (infection, thrombosis, intravascular volume depletion). Bilateral nephrectomy is considered standard care, although clinicians are now increasingly performing unilateral nephrectomy before transplantation,

Table 9-1 Inherited Disorders of the Podocyte

Clinical Disorder	Gene	Locus	Inheritance	Gene Product	Age of Onset	OMIM No.*
Slit-diaphragm and podocyte-associated disease						
Congenital NS of the Finnish type	NPHS1	19q13.1	AR	Nephrin	Infancy	256300
Steroid-resistant NS/FSGS	NPHS2	1q25-31	AR	Podocin	3 months to adulthood	600995
FSGS	CD2AP	6p12	AD	CD2AP	Adult	604241
FSGS	TRPC6	11q21-22	AD	TRPC6	Adult	603965
FSGS	ACTN4	19q13	AD	α-actinin-4	Late	603278
DMS/FSGS	PLCE1	10Q23	AR	Phospholipase C epsilon	Childhood	608414
Syndromic podocyte disorders						
Denys-Drash syndrome	WT1	11p13	AD	WT1	Infancy	194080
Frasier syndrome						136680
Nail-patella syndrome	LMX1B	9q34	AD	LMX1B	Late	161200
Pierson syndrome	LAMB2	3p21	AR	Laminin-β2 chain	Infancy	609049
Fabry disease	GLA	Xq22	X-linked	α-galactosidase A	Adulthood	301500
Immuno-osseous dysplasia	SMARCAL1	2q34-36	AR	SMARCA-like protein 1	Childhood	242900
CD151 deficiency	CD151	11p15	AR	CD151	Adolescence	609057

AD, autosomal dominant; AR, autosomal recessive; DMS, diffuse mesangial sclerosis.
*OMIM: Online Mendelian Inheritance in Man[153]

reducing the degree of proteinuria while preserving some kidney function.[3–7]

The *NPHS1* gene was identified by positional cloning. The NPHS1 product nephrin is a transmembrane protein with a large extracellular domain, a single membrane-spanning segment, and a short intracellular tail that has roles in modulating a number of signaling pathways. It functions critically in maintaining the structure of the slit diaphragm.[8] Although low levels of nephrin have been reported outside of the kidney, expression is greatest in the podocyte.[9] Nephrin's function outside of the kidney is unclear.

CNS is significantly more common in Finland than most other locales, as are several other recessive diseases. Two different point mutations account for the majority of CNS, particularly in Finland. These mutations, named Fin-major and Fin-minor,[1] both cause premature termination of the translated nephrin protein. Fin-major is a deletion of nucleotides 121 and 122, leading to a frameshift. Fin-minor, the less common of these two Finnish alleles, is a premature stop codon at residue 1109. Though considered to be largely a Finnish disease, CNS is in fact seen worldwide. More than 70 mutations in *NPHS1* have been reported, including missense mutations, premature truncation mutations, and frameshift mutations.[10–15] In Old Order Mennonites in Pennsylvania there is also a high incidence of CNS (1 in 500 live births). Two distinct disease-associated *NPHS1* alleles have been observed in this population.[16]

In addition to truncation mutations, a large number of missense mutations in *NPHS1* have been described, several of which have been studied biochemically. Most of the mutations studied thus far alter proper targeting of nephrin to the slit diaphragm and lipid rafts.[17] In cell culture systems, chemical chaperone therapy restores proper targeting of several mutant forms of nephrin.[18,19]

Nephrin associates with other proteins with known roles in maintaining or modulating glomerular function. Nephrin-interacting proteins include CD2-associated protein (CD2AP) and podocin,[20] both of which are also encoded by disease-associated genes (see below). Several close nephrin homologs have been identified, named NEPH-1, NEPH-2, and NEPH-3.[21] Nephrin and NEPH-1 have been shown to interact directly.[22] Mice lacking the *Neph1* gene develop a CNS-like phenotype, as do nephrin "knockout" mice.[23–26] However, despite the existence of these close homologs, nephrin has a nonredundant function, as shown by the severe human and mouse "knockout" phenotypes. Nephrin-deficient mice, like humans with CNS, have severe nephrosis at birth.[24–26] In addition to confirming the essential and nonredundant role of nephrin in podocyte function, analysis of these several mouse models suggest that nephrin is not critical to glomerular development.

Proteinuria is observed in a significant percentage of children with CNS after renal transplantation. In general, this seems to be the result of the development of antibodies to nephrin in the recipient.[27,28] This may not always be the cause,

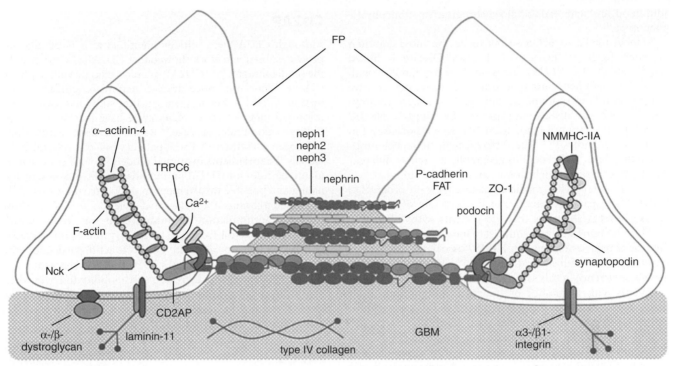

Figure 9-1 Schematic representation of podocyte foot processes (FP) and the interposed slit diaphragm (SD) covering the outer aspect of the glomerular basement membrane (GBM). Many of the indicated proteins have been shown to be mutated in human or murine forms of nephrotic syndrome and/or focal segmental glomerulosclerosis. (Modified from Moller CC, Pollak MR, Reiser J: The genetic basis of human glomerular disease. Adv Chronic Kidney Dis 13:166–173, 2006.)

as one recent report described a patient with recurrent proteinuria, absence of antibodies to nephrin, and a positive in vitro assay for serum glomerular permeability factor.[29] Studies on the nature and role of serum glomerular permeability factor in the development of proteinuria are currently continuing.

High concentrations of α-fetoprotein were often used for the prenatal diagnosis of CNS in Finland before the identification of *NPHS1*. Currently in Finland, where two mutations account for 95% of disease, antenatal genetic testing is readily available. This improves the specificity of such testing considerably, because heterozygosity for nephrin mutations in the fetus can also lead to in utero proteinuria and elevated α-fetoprotein, leading to potential false positives when this is used as a prenatal test.[30–33]

One recent report described muscular dystonia and athetosis in infants with NPHS1-mediated CNS. The neurologic disease was severe and persisted even among those patients receiving dialysis or kidney transplantation, indicating that these features may be a part of the spectrum of NPHS1-associated disease.[34] Additionally, a recent study examined the possible involvement of NPHS1 variation in minimal-change disease.[35] Resequencing of *NPHS1* in subjects with a documented history of childhood minimal-change disease showed a high frequency (about 20%) of heterozygous nonconservative amino acid changing variants, as compared with a control group. This small study suggests that nephrin mutations may also contribute to increased susceptibility to the development of minimal-change disease. Another recent study investigated the possible role of three common coding sequence missense variants in *NPHS1* on the degree of proteinuria and renal

function decline in IgA nephropathy. An association with one *NPHS1* variant (G349A) and heavier proteinuria and faster renal function decline was reported.[36] However, the nephrin locus on chromosome 19q does not seem to have a major role in the conferring susceptibility to diabetic nephropathy.[37]

Podocin

The podocin gene *NPHS2* was cloned by positional methods.[38] Through analysis of multiple families in which steroid-resistant nephrotic syndrome segregated as a recessive trait, a novel gene located at human chromosome 1p25-31, *NPHS2*, was identified. Prior to these studies, childhood steroid-resistant nephrotic syndrome was not generally recognized to be an inherited disease. Podocin, the gene product, is an integral membrane protein with a single hairpin-like transmembrane domain and intracellular C- and N-terminal tails. Podocin, a 42-kDa, 383–amino acid protein, localizes to the slit diaphragm and interacts directly with nephrin and CD2AP.[17]

Podocin-mediated disease is transmitted as an autosomal recessive trait. Affected individuals inherit one mutant *NPHS2* gene from each parent. More than 50 putative disease-causing mutations have been identified, including missense mutations as well as premature truncation mutants.[39–43] Some substitutions (e.g., R138Q) have been observed in several families without known common ancestors. However, unlike the case for *NPHS1*, there are no major *NPHS2* mutations accounting for the majority of disease cases. Rather, most mutations seem to be recent and independent. Most of the published studies of *NPHS2* genetics have focused on pediatric disease. However, podocin-mediated disease can also present in adolescence or adulthood, and may lead to a slowly progressive, subnephrotic phenotype.[44]

Podocin-mediated FSGS seems to be the most common inherited form of this set of diseases. Disease is linked genetically to the *NPHS2* locus in 50% of families with steroid-resistant nephrotic syndrome and autosomal recessive transmission.[45] In sporadic steroid-resistant disease (biopsy-proven FSGS or disease not proven by biopsy), *NPHS2* mutations are responsible for from 10% to 30% of disease in several large studies.[45,46] The differences in frequency probably reflect both differences in geography as well as different diagnostic criteria for inclusion in these various studies.

Patients with NPHS2-mediated disease typically progress to ESRD. These patients have a much lower rate of recurrent disease in renal allografts than do patients with "idiopathic FSGS".[45,47–49] One study, in contrast to most others, found that the rate of recurrent disease in NPHS2-associated disease was similar to those with idiopathic FSGS.[50] The mechanism for disease recurrence in this setting is not clear.[46]

Patients with frameshift or nonsense mutations in both alleles seem to have the most aggressive disease course. Patients with other variant alleles, particularly that causing an R229Q substitution, tend to have later onset disease.[44] This R229Q podocin variant is present in 7% of most populations (allele frequency 3.5%) and causes steroid-resistant nephrotic syndrome when inherited together with another, more deleterious allele. The R229Q change leads to a partial loss of function and altered association with nephrin.[44] In the heterozygous state, the presence of a R229Q variant increases the risk of microalbuminuria.[51]

The podocin and nephrin genes interact at a genetic level. In children, the presence of a single *NPHS2* mutation may increase the severity of NPHS1-associated disease.[12] Similarly, mouse genetic data suggest that heterozygous defects in multiple podocyte genes can act together to produce a disease phenotype.[52]

Patients with two mutant *NPHS2* alleles do not respond to steroid therapy.[47] There is no clear difference in clinical or pathologic phenotype that could help clinicians distinguish between podocin-mediated disease and "idiopathic" FSGS. Renal biopsy specimens in these patients show minimal-change disease or FSGS that is typical in its histologic appearance.[53] Given the effects of prolonged steroid treatment in children, a strong argument can be made for performing genetic testing for *NPHS2* mutations to help assess the risk that steroid therapy will fail.

There is large variability in the severity of disease from person to person with *NPHS2* mutations, suggesting that other factors, both genetic and nongenetic, are also important in modulating this disease. It is not clear how much of this variability derives from differences in the specific NPHS2 defects. Studies in a podocin-deficient mice have shown that strain-specific differences have a significant effect on the phenotype.[54] It seems probable that in humans, other genes also modify podocin-mediated disease.

Many of the identified podocin mutations lead to defective protein processing, folding, and/or localization, rather than an intrinsic defect in protein function.[55,56] Podocin defects can also alter the processing and localization of nephrin.[57] As with other membrane proteins, this has sparked interest in the possibility of using chaperone therapies to help correct the cellular defect.

CD2AP

Although CD2AP was initially identified as a T-cell adaptor protein, subsequent work showed that CD2AP also localizes to the slit diaphragm.[58–60] CD2AP interacts directly with nephrin. CD2AP "knockout" mice develop nephrosis, similar to that seen in NPHS1-deficient mice. Further study has shown that mice with one defective *Cd2ap* allele have increased susceptibility to glomerular damage.[61] Rare *CD2AP* splice mutations have been identified in FSGS patients but not control individuals.[61] Experiments in animal models and cell culture have identified roles for CD2AP in modulating slit-diaphragm signaling and possible involvement in podocyte endocytosis.[62,63] Mice heterozygous for a targeted deletion in *Cd2ap* show increased accumulation of immunoglobulins in the GBM, suggesting a role for Cd2ap in targeting proteins for degradation.[61] CD2AP associates with podocyte actin, particularly the dynamic actin in endosomes.[64–66] Mice heterozygous for Cd2ap deficiency show increased susceptibility to FSGS when bred to mice with other podocyte gene defects.[52] The role of CD2AP variants in human sporadic and familial disease has not yet been extensively evaluated.

TRPC6

TRPC6 is a member of a large family of ion channels, the transient receptor potential family. TRPC6 (for transient receptor potential canonical 6) is a nonselective cation channel. TRPC6 is activated by diacylglycerol in a protein kinase C–independent manner.[67] A *TRPC6* mutation was found to be responsible for FSGS in a large New Zealand kindred.[68] This P112Q substitution was found to increase channel activity. Several additional mutations have now been reported.[69] In all reported families, disease follows autosomal dominant inheritance. Affected individuals typically present with adult-onset proteinuria in their third or fourth decade of life. Approximately 60% of patients with FSGS-associated *TRPC6* mutations develop ESRD. Some, but not all, of the identified mutations increase TRPC6 activity in heterologous expression assays. TRPC6 localizes to the slit diaphragm and interacts directly with podocin and nephrin.[69] Although TRPC6 is a widely expressed protein, this form of disease seems to be limited to the kidney. Disease associated with *TRPC6* mutations is clinically similar to ACTN4-associated disease (see below), with kidney disease presenting in adolescence or adulthood. The variable expressivity of *TRPC6* mutations suggests that other factors, genetic or environmental, are required for full expression of the phenotype. Mice with *Trpc6* deleted show increased vascular smooth muscle contractility but no overt renal phenotype, consistent with the notion that human disease-associated mutations cause kidney disease via a gain-of-function mechanism.[70]

CYTOSKELETON

ACTN4

Mutations in the α-actinin-4 gene *ACTN4* cause a form of kidney disease characterized by subnephrotic proteinuria, the development of podocyte degeneration, and FSGS.[71,72] Thus far, five disease-causing mutations have been identified, all point mutations within the actin-binding domain of this protein. α-actinin-4 is a widely expressed homodimeric protein that bundles and cross-links filamentous actin. Its primary intrarenal localization is within the podocyte processes. ACTN4 also interacts with a large number of other proteins, including β-integrins, cell adhesion molecules, and signaling proteins.[73] ACTN4-mediated disease is transmitted in an autosomal dominant manner. In addition to increased affinity to F-actin, mutant α-actinin-4 is more rapidly degraded than the wild-type protein. Thus, the mechanism of disease may be a combination of loss-of-function and gain-of-function effects.[74]

Mice with a targeted deletion of the *Actn4* gene develop glomerular disease, confirming an essential and nonredundant role for α-actinin-4 in the glomerulus.[75] Transgenic mice expressing mutant-actinin in podocytes support a biologically dominant effect of human mutations.[76,77] Because disease-associated ACTN4 mutants increase the affinity of the encoded protein to actin, a biologically dominant perturbation in podocyte mechanics may be an important part of the disease mechanism.[71,72] The phenotype of this form of disease is late onset. Affected individuals do not develop nephrotic-range proteinuria or NS. Although data are limited, it seems that FSGS does not recur in kidneys transplanted into these patients.

STEROID-SENSITIVE DISEASE

Although most inherited forms of proteinuria and nephrosis are resistant to immunosuppressive therapy, this is not always the case. Ruf et al recently identified a locus on chromosome 2 that contains a gene responsible for steroid-sensitive nephrotic syndrome in a consanguineous family.[78] They also show that this locus is not responsible for disease in all steroid-sensitive nephrotic syndrome families, demonstrating that, like steroid-resistant disease, this phenotype is also genetically heterogeneous.

PLCE1

Hinkes et al used a positional approach to identify PLCE1, the phospholipase C epsilon 1 gene, as an NS-associated gene.[79] Mutations in PLCE1 cause an onset, recessive form of NS with diffuse mesangial sclerosis and/or FSGS. The mechanism of disease is unclear; in addition to its phospholipase C function, PLCε1 also functions as an effector protein in small G-protein signaling.[80] Some affected individuals responded to a course of immunosuppressive therapy, suggesting that PLCε1 plays a critical role in glomerular development, rather than glomerular physiology.

SYNDROMIC DISEASE

Podocyte dysfunction is also seen as a component of several inherited multi-organ syndromes. These include disorders in which the podocytopathy has been well studied as well as other disorders in which the nature and mechanism of the kidney lesion is obscure.

LMX1B

Individuals with nail-patella syndrome display dysplastic nails, hypoplastic patellae, and glomerular disease characterized by hematuria and proteinuria.[81] This disorder follows autosomal dominant inheritance. Affected patients show a highly variable renal phenotype. An altered GBM is a characteristic pathologic finding and may be associated with frank nephrosis. Nail-patella syndrome is caused by mutations in the *LMX1B* transcription factor.[82–84] LMX1B binds to the podocin promoter and seems to be critical to the transcription of several important podocyte-associated genes as well as genes encoding matrix proteins.[85–87] Mice with targeted deletion of the *Lmx1b* gene display a phenotype similar to the human disease.[84] Expression studies suggest that the disease is caused by Lmx1b haploinsufficiency, rather than a biologically dominant effect of mutant Lmx1b.[88]

WT1

The *WT1* transcription factor was cloned using positional methods on the basis of its role in the inheritance of Wilms' tumor.[89,90] WT1 has been extensively studied. Precise regulation of WT1 expression seems critical for kidney development as well as regulation of podocyte gene expression.[91–93]

Frasier syndrome and Denys-Drash syndrome are related disorders both caused by *WT1* mutations.[94–97] These related syndromes are characterized by glomerular disease as well as urogenital anomalies. Frasier syndrome is defined clinically by the presence of FSGS together with male pseudohermaphroditism and a high risk of gonadoblastoma. Control of alternative splicing of *WT1*, specifically the inclusion or omission of a three–amino acid (KTS) region, seems critical for normal glomerulogenesis and sex determination. Mice lacking the KTS-containing isoform show complete XY sex reversal.[98,99] *WT1* splice mutations that alter the regulation of the splicing of this KTS region cause Frasier syndrome.[97] XY individuals with such mutations may appear as phenotypic females, whereas XX individuals with the same mutations can rarely present with isolated glomerular disease.[100,101] Denys-Drash syndrome is defined by diffuse mesangial sclerosis, genitourinary tumors, and pseudohermaphroditism, and is most commonly caused by mutations in exon 9 of *WT1*. It is probably best to regard Frasier and Denys-Drash syndromes as parts of a spectrum of disorders resulting from *WT1* mutations. Although most reported mutations associated with Denys-Drash syndrome are missense point mutations, there is overlap in the spectrum of mutations associated with these disorders.

Recently, several non-coding variants (single-nucleotide polymorphisms) in the closely linked *WT1* and *WIT1* (Wilms' tumor upstream neighbor 1) genes were genotyped in African Americans with and without FSGS.[102] This study found a significant association between specific haplotypes in the *WT1/WIT1* gene locus and the risk of FSGS in this population.

Pierson Syndrome

Defects in the laminin-β2 gene *LAMB2* cause Pierson syndrome.[103] In addition to congenital nephrosis, affected neonates display a number of ocular abnormalities that typically include microcoria, extreme nonreactive narrowing of the pupils. Pierson syndrome is recessive. Affected neonates are homozygous or compound heterozygous for defects in LAMB2. Defects in LAMB2 can also cause congenital nephrosis with minimal eye abnormalities.[104] In addition to podocyte abnormalities, mesangial sclerosis is a frequent histologic feature. Mice deficient in Lamb2 show marked proteinuria before the onset of overt podocyte abnormalities, demonstrating the importance of GBM components as a barrier to protein filtration.[105] As with NPHS1-associated CNS, features of antenatal nephrosis can be detected antenatally by ultrasonography.[106]

Immuno-osseous Dysplasia

Immuno-osseous dysplasia is caused by mutations in the SMARCAL1 gene.[107,108] This rare autosomal recessive disorder presents with spondyloepiphyseal dysplasia, renal dysfunction, and T-cell immunodeficiency. The renal lesion has not been extensively characterized, but progressive renal insufficiency, FSGS, and proteinuria seem to be common features. SMARCAL1 encodes a widely expressed protein involved in chromatin remodeling, as indicated by the full name of the encoded protein, SWI/SNF related, matrix associated, actin-dependent regulator of chromatin, subfamily a–like 1.

CD151 Deficiency

A recent report described a pair of siblings with end-stage kidney disease, epidermolysis bullosa, and deafness in association with homozygosity for frameshift mutations in the CD151 gene.[109] CD151 is a member of the tetraspanin family of cell surface proteins. CD151 interacts with $\alpha\beta$-integrins to facilitate laminin binding.[110] Mice deficient in Cd151 develop proteinuria, FSGS, and kidney failure.[111]

Mitochondrial Disease

Mitochondrial disease can present with podocyte abnormalities.[112] The mitochondrial genome is a small circular extrachromosomal genome that is inherited maternally. Several reports have documented mutations in the tRNA(Leu(URR)) gene associated with podocyte abnormalities as well as various nonglomerular phenotypes.[113–116] A recent case report described a girl with FSGS in association with a mutation in the mitochondrial tRNA(Tyr) gene.[117] Even more recently, three infants were described who displayed nephrosis in association with a mitochondrial RC complex II+V deficiency.[118]

Animal Models

Several animal models that show podocyte abnormalities and significant proteinuria have been described. Although several genetically engineered mice have been generated with defects in human disease genes to help understand the biology of disease, defects in several genes without known involvement in human disease have been shown to cause podocyte disease in animal models. Fat1-deficient mice show a congenital nephrotic phenotype similar to nephrin deficiency.[119] Mice lacking the nephrin-interacting protein show a similar pheno-

type.[23] Several other spontaneous or genetically engineered mice show evidence of podocyte foot process effacement, proteinuria, and/or FSGS. Mice with a disrupted Mpv17 gene, which encodes a peroxisomal protein that regulates matrix metalloproteinase production, develop an FSGS-like lesion.[120] Mice deficient in RhoGDIα, a regulator of Rho activity, display massive proteinuria.[121] Mice homozygous for an N-ethyl-N-nitrosourea–induced mutation in the Kreisler gene, encoding a leucine zipper transcription factor, demonstrate proteinuria and podocyte foot process effacement.[122] This growing list of rodent models will inform studies of human disease. However, most of these genes have not been directly implicated in human podocytopathies.

The Buffalo/Mna rat strain is a particularly interesting model of FSGS.[123] "Normal" kidneys transplanted into these rats develop proteinuria, and lesions in Buffalo/Mna kidneys regress when transplanted into control rats.[124] In contrast to the FSGS/NS genes identified in humans, the gene or genes underlying this rat phenotype may encode a circulating molecule, rather than an intrinsic renal protein.

Genetic Heterogeneity/Other Loci

The known NS/FSGS-associated genes do not account for all inherited forms of these diseases. Mutations in the genes encoding NPHS2, NPHS1, ACTN4, CD2AP, and TRPC6 account for only a fraction of familial disease presenting after infancy. It is not clear what percentages of "sporadic" or "idiopathic" NS or FSGS reflect the effects of underlying gene defects. It seems likely that in addition to other mendelian forms of disease (in which very rare mutations cause a hugely increased disease risk), several genetic variants (in these and other genes) will be identified that increase the risk of disease but are not sufficient to cause disease. The approximately fourfold increased risk of FSGS in individuals of African descent is probably the result of such variants.

Other Forms of Inherited Proteinuric Disease

Several reports have described apparent familial aggregation of membranous nephropathy either alone or as part of inherited syndromes.[125–129] Responsible genes and loci have not been identified, and the genetic contribution to the development of membranous nephropathy is not well understood. Families with apparent inherited forms of membranoproliferative glomerulonephritis have also been described.[130] A locus responsible for membranoproliferative glomerulonephritis type III in a large Irish pedigree has been mapped to the long arm of chromosome 1.[131] Glomerulopathy with fibronectin deposits, an autosomal dominant disorder characterized by proteinuria, renal failure, and glomerular deposits of fibronectin, has been recently described.[132, 133] One report described the recurrence of disease in a renal transplant recipient, suggesting the possibility that responsible gene defect encodes a protein expressed outside the kidney.[134] A locus for glomerulopathy with fibronectin deposits has been mapped to chromosome 1q32.[135,136] This locus may reflect a shared genetic basis among the membranoproliferative glomerulonephritis type III family studied by Neary and colleagues[131] and glomerulopathy with fibronectin deposits.

Podocyte Protein Expression in Secondary Disease

Decreased nephrin protein expression has been seen in several rodent models of glomerular injury as well as in human primary and secondary glomerular disease, including diabetic nephropathy.[137,138] Loss of nephrin occurs at the protein rather than the transcriptional level, in that nephrin messenger RNA levels have been reported to be increased or unchanged in many of these disease states.[139–143] In some rodent models, angiotensin-converting enzyme inhibitor treatment has been reported to restore this decrease in nephrin expression.[144,145]

An increasing number of studies have examined the expression of disease-causing genes and the encoded proteins in sporadic and secondary forms of disease.[139,142,146–150] Increased transcript levels of several different podocyte markers together with a decrease in protein expression have been observed.[140] Podocin concentrations have been reported to decrease in childhood NS, as does nephrin expression.[146] Glomerular ACTN4 expression is increased in membranous glomerulopathy but decreased in minimal-change disease.[151] In all of these studies, it is difficult to determine which changes in gene and protein expression are proximal components of disease pathogenesis and which changes reflect a downstream response to the disease process.

GENETIC TESTING

Genetic testing is not yet a routine part of clinical care in the evaluation and management of patients with FSGS and/or NS. A reasonable case can be made for testing children with NS for *NPHS2* mutations, at least if there is no significant response to initial steroid therapy. It appears clear that NPHS2-mediated disease does not respond to immunosuppression. Early diagnosis could therefore spare children the adverse effects of prolonged immunosuppressive therapy. Mutations in *ACTN4*, *TRPC6*, and *CD2AP* are rare causes of disease. It is difficult to argue that mutational analysis of these genes should be a routine part of the evaluation of patients. When evaluating a patient with ESRD secondary to FSGS or NS for kidney transplant, however, physicians should be aware of the frequently familial nature of these diseases. Care should be taken so as not to transplant a living kidney from a presymptomatic but genetically affected family member. At present, several research laboratories and one commercial company perform mutational analysis of *NPHS2* and other NS/FSGS-associated genes. As noted earlier, prenatal genetic testing for *NPHS1* mutations is now routine in pregnancies in at-risk couples. This is straightforward in Finland, where two mutations account for 95% of disease. In other locales, where other variants explain a much larger fraction of disease, analysis is more complex.

TREATMENT

Immunosuppressive therapy is generally ineffective in individuals with FSGS or NS as a result of mutations in the known disease-associated podocyte genes. It has been clearly shown that children with podocin-mutant disease do not respond to glucocorticoids.[47] There have, however, been families reported in which disease does respond to steroids; the responsible

genes have not been identified.[78,152] Thus, a family history of NS/FSGS does not by itself rule out the possibility that the disease in that family may be treatment responsive. As the recent report identifying *PLCE1* as a gene underlying a treatment-responsive form of disease suggests, various genetic defects may lead to very different clinical presentations.[79] It is increasingly clear that the inherited podocytopathies form a genetically heterogeneous group of diseases, and it is likely that with a greater understanding of the underlying genetic alterations, we will be better able to predict response to therapy by genetic testing. At present, aggressive therapy with angiotensin-converting enzyme inhibitors and/or angiotensin receptor blockers seems to be the appropriate therapy for steroid-resistant inherited podocytopathies as with other nonfamilial proteinuric renal diseases, although the data in support of this are conjectural and anecdotal.

References

1. Kestila M, Lenkkeri U, Mannikko M, et al: Positionally cloned gene for a novel glomerular protein—nephrin—is mutated in congenital nephrotic syndrome. Mol Cell 1:575–582, 1998.
2. Norio R: Congenital nephrotic syndrome of Finnish type and other types of early familial nephrotic syndromes. Birth Defects Orig Artic Ser 10:69–72, 1974.
3. Mattoo TK, al-Sowailem AM, al-Harbi MS, et al: Nephrotic syndrome in 1st year of life and the role of unilateral nephrectomy. Pediatr Nephrol 6:16–18, 1992.
4. Licht C, Eifinger F, Gharib M, et al: A stepwise approach to the treatment of early onset nephrotic syndrome. Pediatr Nephrol 14:1077–1082, 2000.
5. Kovacevic L, Reid CJ, Rigden SP: Management of congenital nephrotic syndrome. Pediatr Nephrol 18:426–430, 2003.
6. Zuniga ZV, Ellis D, Moritz ML, Docimo SG: Bilateral laparoscopic transperitoneal nephrectomy with early peritoneal dialysis in an infant with the nephrotic syndrome. J Urol 170:1962, 2003.
7. Papez KE, Smoyer WE: Recent advances in congenital nephrotic syndrome. Curr Opin Pediatr 16:165–170, 2004.
8. Khoshnoodi J Sigmundsson K, Ofverstedt LG, et al: Nephrin promotes cell-cell adhesion through homophilic interactions. Am J Pathol 163:2337–2346, 2003.
9. Kuusniemi AM, Kestila M, Patrakka J, et al: Tissue expression of nephrin in human and pig. Pediatr Res 55:774–781, 2004.
10. Tryggvason K: Nephrin: role in normal kidney and in disease. Adv Nephrol Necker Hosp 31:221–234, 2001.
11. Beltcheva O, Martin P, Lenkkeri U, Tryggvason K: Mutation spectrum in the nephrin gene (*NPHS1*) in congenital nephrotic syndrome. Hum Mutat 17:368–373, 2001.
12. Koziell A, Grech V, Hussain S, et al: Genotype/phenotype correlations of *NPHS1* and *NPHS2* mutations in nephrotic syndrome advocate a functional inter-relationship in glomerular filtration. Hum Mol Genet 11:379–388, 2002.
13. Gigante M, Greco P, Defazio V, et al: Congenital nephrotic syndrome of the Finnish type in Italy: A molecular approach. J Nephrol 15:696–702, 2002.
14. Patrakka J, Kestila M, Wartiovaara J, et al: Congenital nephrotic syndrome (NPHS1): Features resulting from different mutations in Finnish patients. Kidney Int 58:972–980, 2000.
15. Schultheiss M, Ruf RG, Mucha BE, et al: No evidence for genotype/phenotype correlation in *NPHS1* and *NPHS2* mutations. Pediatr Nephrol 19:1340–1348, 2004.
16. Bolk S, Puffenberger EG, Hudson J, et al: Elevated frequency and allelic heterogeneity of congenital nephrotic syndrome, Finnish type, in the Old Order Mennonites. Am J Hum Genet 65:1785–1790, 1999.

17. Schwarz K, Simons M, Reiser J, et al: Podocin, a raft-associated component of the glomerular slit diaphragm, interacts with CD2AP and nephrin. J Clin Invest 108:1621–1629, 2001.
18. Liu XL, Done SC, Yan K, et al: Defective trafficking of nephrin missense mutants rescued by a chemical chaperone. J Am Soc Nephrol 15:1731–1738, 2004.
19. Shimizu J, Tanaka H, Aya K, et al: A missense mutation in the nephrin gene impairs membrane targeting. Am J Kidney Dis 40:697–703, 2002.
20. Huber TB, Kottgen M, Schilling B, et al: Interaction with podocin facilitates nephrin signaling. J Biol Chem 276:41543–41546, 2001.
21. Sellin L, Huber TB, Gerke P, et al: NEPH1 defines a novel family of podocin interacting proteins. FASEB J 17:115–117, 2003.
22. Gerke P, Huber TB, Sellin L, et al: Homodimerization and heterodimerization of the glomerular podocyte proteins nephrin and NEPH1. J Am Soc Nephrol 14:918–926, 2003.
23. Donoviel DB, Freed DD, Vogel H, et al: Proteinuria and perinatal lethality in mice lacking NEPH1, a novel protein with homology to nephrin. Mol Cell Biol 21:4829–4836, 2001.
24. Hamano Y, Grunkemeyer JA, Sudhakar A, et al: Determinants of vascular permeability in the kidney glomerulus. J Biol Chem 277:31154–31162, 2002.
25. Rantanen M, Palmen T, Patari A, et al: Nephrin TRAP mice lack slit diaphragms and show fibrotic glomeruli and cystic tubular lesions. J Am Soc Nephrol 13:1586–1594, 2002.
26. Putaala H, Soininen R, Kilpelainen P, et al: The murine nephrin gene is specifically expressed in kidney, brain and pancreas: Inactivation of the gene leads to massive proteinuria and neonatal death. Hum Mol Genet 10:1–8, 2001.
27. Patrakka J, Ruotsalainen V, Reponen P, et al: Recurrence of nephrotic syndrome in kidney grafts of patients with congenital nephrotic syndrome of the Finnish type: Role of nephrin. Transplantation 73:394–403, 2002.
28. Wang SX, Ahola H, Palmen T, et al: Recurrence of nephrotic syndrome after transplantation in CNF is due to autoantibodies to nephrin. Exp Nephrol 9:327–331, 2001.
29. Srivastava T, Garola RE, Kestila M, et al: Recurrence of proteinuria following renal transplantation in congenital nephrotic syndrome of the Finnish type. Pediatr Nephrol 21:711–718, 2006.
30. Kestila M, Jarvela I: Prenatal diagnosis of congenital nephrotic syndrome (CNF, NPHS1). Prenat Diagn 23:323–324.
31. Kallinen J, Heinonen S, Ryynanen M, et al: Antenatal genetic screening for congenital nephrosis. Prenat Diagn 21:81–84, 2001.
32. Mannikko M, Kestila M, Kenkkeri U, et al: Improved prenatal diagnosis of the congenital nephrotic syndrome of the Finnish type based on DNA analysis. Kidney Int 51:868–872, 1997.
33. Patrakka J, Martin P, Salonen R, et al: Proteinuria and prenatal diagnosis of congenital nephrosis in fetal carriers of nephrin gene mutations. Lancet 359:1575–1577, 2002.
34. Laakkonen H, Lonnqvist T, Uusimaa J, et al: Muscular dystonia and athetosis in six patients with congenital nephrotic syndrome of the Finnish type (NPHS1). Pediatr Nephrol 21:182–189, 2006.
35. Lahdenkari AT, Kestila M, Holmberg C, et al: Nephrin gene (NPHS1) in patients with minimal change nephrotic syndrome (MCNS). Kidney Int 65:1856–1863, 2004.
36. Narita I, Goto S, Saito N, et al: Genetic polymorphism of NPHS1 modifies the clinical manifestations of Ig A nephropathy. Lab Invest 83:1193–1200, 2003.
37. Iyengar SK, Fox KA, Schachere M, et al: Linkage analysis of candidate loci for end-stage renal disease due to diabetic nephropathy. J Am Soc Nephrol 14(7 Suppl 2):S195–S201, 2003.
38. Boute N, Gribouval O, Roselli S, et al: NPHS2, encoding the glomerular protein podocin, is mutated in autosomal recessive steroid-resistant nephrotic syndrome. Nat Genet 24:349–354, 2000.
39. Maruyama K, Iijima K, Ikeda M, et al: NPHS2 mutations in sporadic steroid-resistant nephrotic syndrome in Japanese children. Pediatr Nephrol 18:412–416, 2003.
40. Frishberg Y, et al: Mutations in NPHS2 encoding podocin are a prevalent cause of steroid-resistant nephrotic syndrome among Israeli-Arab children. J Am Soc Nephrol 13:400–405, 2002.
41. Caridi G, Perfumo F, Ghiggeri GM: NPHS2 (podocin) mutations in nephrotic syndrome. Clinical spectrum and fine mechanisms. Pediatr Res 57(5 Pt 2):54R–61R, 2005.
42. Caridi G, et al: Infantile steroid-resistant nephrotic syndrome associated with double homozygous mutations of podocin. Am J Kidney Dis 43:727–732, 2004.
43. Caridi G, et al: Broadening the spectrum of diseases related to podocin mutations. J Am Soc Nephrol 14:1278–1286, 2003.
44. Tsukaguchi H, et al: NPHS2 mutations in late-onset focal segmental glomerulosclerosis: R229Q is a common disease-associated allele. J Clin Invest 110:1659–1666, 2002.
45. Weber S, et al: NPHS2 mutation analysis shows genetic heterogeneity of steroid-resistant nephrotic syndrome and low post-transplant recurrence. Kidney Int 66:571–579, 2004.
46. Billing H, et al: NPHS2 mutation associated with recurrence of proteinuria after transplantation. Pediatr Nephrol 19:561–564, 2004.
47. Ruf RG, et al: Patients with mutations in NPHS2 (podocin) do not respond to standard steroid treatment of nephrotic syndrome. J Am Soc Nephrol 15:722–732, 2004.
48. Weber S, Tonshoff B: Recurrence of focal-segmental glomerulosclerosis in children after renal transplantation: clinical and genetic aspects. Transplantation 80(1 Suppl):S128–S134, 2005.
49. Karle SM, et al: Novel mutations in NPHS2 detected in both familial and sporadic steroid-resistant nephrotic syndrome. J Am Soc Nephrol 13:388–393, 2002.
50. Bertelli R, et al: Recurrence of focal segmental glomerulosclerosis after renal transplantation in patients with mutations of podocin. Am J Kidney Dis 41:1314–1321, 2003.
51. Pereira AC, et al: NPHS2 R229Q functional variant is associated with microalbuminuria in the general population. Kidney Int 65:1026–1030, 2004.
52. Huber TB, et al: Bigenic mouse models of focal segmental glomerulosclerosis involving pairwise interaction of CD2AP, Fyn, and synaptopodin. J Clin Invest 116:1337–1345, 2006.
53. Fuchshuber A, et al: Clinical and genetic evaluation of familial steroid-responsive nephrotic syndrome in childhood. J Am Soc Nephrol 12:374–378, 2001.
54. Roselli S, et al: Early glomerular filtration defect and severe renal disease in podocin-deficient mice. Mol Cell Biol 24:550–560, 2004.
55. Ohashi T, et al: Intracellular mislocalization of mutant podocin and correction by chemical chaperones. Histochem Cell Biol 119:257–264, 2003.
56. Roselli S, et al: Plasma membrane targeting of podocin through the classical exocytic pathway: Effect of NPHS2 mutations. Traffic 5:37–44, 2004.
57. Huber TB, et al: Molecular basis of the functional podocin-nephrin complex: Mutations in the NPHS2 gene disrupt nephrin targeting to lipid raft microdomains. Hum Mol Genet 12:3397–3405, 2003.
58. Dustin ML, et al: A novel adaptor protein orchestrates receptor patterning and cytoskeletal polarity in T-cell contacts. Cell 94:667–677, 1998.
59. Shih NY, et al: Congenital nephrotic syndrome in mice lacking CD2-associated protein. Science 286:312–315, 1999.
60. Shih NY, et al: CD2AP localizes to the slit diaphragm and binds to nephrin via a novel C-terminal domain. Am J Pathol 159:2303–2308, 2001.

61. Kim JM, et al: CD2-associated protein haploinsufficiency is linked to glomerular disease susceptibility. Science 300:1298–1300, 2003.

62. Cormont M, et al: CD2AP/CMS regulates endosome morphology and traffic to the degradative pathway through its interaction with Rab4 and c-Cbl. Traffic 4:97–112, 2003.

63. Huber TB, et al: Nephrin and CD2AP associate with phosphoinositide 3-OH kinase and stimulate AKT-dependent signaling. Mol Cell Biol 23:4917–4928, 2003.

64. Lehtonen S, Zhao F, Lehtonen E: CD2-associated protein directly interacts with the actin cytoskeleton. Am J Physiol Renal Physiol 283:F734–F743, 2002.

65. Welsch T, et al: CD2AP and p130Cas localize to different F-actin structures in podocytes. Am J Physiol Renal Physiol 281:F769–F777, 2001.

66. Welsch T, et al: Association of CD2AP with dynamic actin on vesicles in podocytes. Am J Physiol Renal Physiol 2005.

67. Dietrich A, et al: Cation channels of the transient receptor potential superfamily: Their role in physiological and pathophysiological processes of smooth muscle cells. Pharmacol Ther 11:744–760, 2006.

68. Winn MP, et al: Mutation in TRPC6 causes familial focal segmental glomerulosclerosis. J Am Soc Nephrol 15:33A, 2004.

69. Reiser J, et al: TRPC6 is a glomerular slit diaphragm–associated channel required for normal renal function. Nat Genet 37:739–744, 2005.

70. Dietrich A, et al: Increased vascular smooth muscle contractility in TRPC6$^{-/-}$ mice. Mol Cell Biol 25:6980–6989, 2005.

71. Kaplan JM, et al: Mutations in ACTN4, encoding α-actinin-4, cause familial focal segmental glomerulosclerosis. Nat Genet 24:251–256, 2000.

72. Weins A, et al: Mutational and biological analysis of α-actinin-4 in focal segmental glomerulosclerosis. J Am Soc Nephrol 16:3694–3701, 2005..

73. Otey CA, Carpen O: α-Actinin revisited: A fresh look at an old player. Cell Motil Cytoskeleton 58:104–111, 2004.

74. Yao J, et al: α-Actinin-4–mediated FSGS: an inherited kidney disease caused by an aggregated and rapidly degraded cytoskeletal protein. PLoS Biol 2:E167, 2004.

75. Kos CH, et al: Mice deficient in α-actinin-4 have severe glomerular disease. J Clin Invest 111:1683–1690, 2003.

76. Michaud JL, et al: FSGS-associated α-actinin-4 (K256E) impairs cytoskeletal dynamics in podocytes. Kidney Int 70:1054–1061, 2006.

77. Michaud JL, et al: Focal and segmental glomerulosclerosis in mice with podocyte-specific expression of mutant α-actinin-4. J Am Soc Nephrol 14:1200–1211, 2003.

78. Ruf RG, et al: Identification of the first gene locus (SSNS1) for steroid-sensitive nephrotic syndrome on chromosome 2p. J Am Soc Nephrol 14:1897–1900, 2003.

79. Hinkes B, et al: Positional cloning uncovers mutations in PLCE1 responsible for a nephrotic syndrome variant that may be reversible. Nat Genet, 2006.

80. Wing MR, Bourdon DM, Harden TK: PLC-ε: A shared effector protein in Ras-, Rho-, and G αβγ-mediated signaling. Mol Interv 3:273–280, 2003.

81. Sabnis SG, et al: Nail-patella syndrome. Clin Nephrol 14:148–153, 1980.

82. Dreyer SD, et al: Mutations in LMX1B cause abnormal skeletal patterning and renal dysplasia in nail-patella syndrome. Nat Genet 19:47–50, 1998.

83. McIntosh I, et al: Mutation analysis of LMX1B gene in nail-patella syndrome patients. Am J Hum Genet 63:1651–1658, 1998.

84. Chen H, et al: Limb and kidney defects in Lmx1b mutant mice suggest an involvement of LMX1B in human nail-patella syndrome. Nat Genet 19:51–55, 1998.

85. Morello R, Lee B: Insight into podocyte differentiation from the study of human genetic disease: Nail-patella syndrome and transcriptional regulation in podocytes. Pediatr Res 51:551–558, 2002.

86. Rohr C, et al: The LIM-homeodomain transcription factor Lmx1b plays a crucial role in podocytes. J Clin Invest 109:1073–1082, 2002.

87. Miner JH, et al: Transcriptional induction of slit diaphragm genes by Lmx1b is required in podocyte differentiation. J Clin Invest 109:1065–1072, 2002.

88. Heidet L, et al: In vivo expression of putative LMX1B targets in nail-patella syndrome kidneys. Am J Pathol 163:145–155, 2003.

89. Haber DA, et al: An internal deletion within an 11p13 zinc finger gene contributes to the development of Wilms' tumor. Cell 61:1257–1269, 1990.

90. Gessler M, et al: Homozygous deletion in Wilms' tumours of a zinc-finger gene identified by chromosome jumping. Nature 343:774–778, 1990.

91. Wagner N, et al: The major podocyte protein nephrin is transcriptionally activated by the Wilms' tumor suppressor WT1. J Am Soc Nephrol 15:3044–3051, 2004.

92. Guo G, et al: WT1 activates a glomerular-specific enhancer identified from the human nephrin gene. J Am Soc Nephrol 15:2851–2856, 2004.

93. Palmer RE, et al: WT1 regulates the expression of the major glomerular podocyte membrane protein podocalyxin. Curr Biol 11:1805–1809, 2001.

94. Coppes MJ, Huff V, Pelletier J: Denys-Drash syndrome: Relating a clinical disorder to genetic alterations in the tumor suppressor gene WT1. J Pediatr 123:673–678, 1993.

95. Schmitt K, et al: Nephropathy with Wilms' tumour or gonadal dysgenesis: Incomplete Denys-Drash syndrome or separate diseases? Eur J Pediatr 154:577–581, 1995.

96. Ghahremani M, et al: A novel mutation H373Y in the Wilms' tumor suppressor gene, WT1, associated with Denys-Drash syndrome. Hum Hered 46:336–338, 1996.

97. Barbaux S, et al: Donor splice-site mutations in WT1 are responsible for Frasier syndrome. Nat Genet 17:467–470, 1997.

98. Hammes A, et al: Two splice variants of the Wilms' tumor 1 gene have distinct functions during sex determination and nephron formation. Cell 106:319–329, 2001.

99. Lahiri D, et al: Nephropathy and defective spermatogenesis in mice transgenic for a single isoform of the Wilms' tumour suppressor protein, WT1-KTS, together with one disrupted Wt1 allele. Mol Reprod Dev 74:300–311, 2006.

100. Demmer L, et al: Frasier syndrome: A cause of focal segmental glomerulosclerosis in a 46,XX female. J Am Soc Nephrol 10:2215–2218, 1999.

101. Denamur E, et al: Mother-to-child transmitted WT1 splice-site mutation is responsible for distinct glomerular diseases. J Am Soc Nephrol 10:2219–2223, 1999.

102. Orloff MS, et al: Variants in the Wilms' tumor gene are associated with focal segmental glomerulosclerosis in the African American population. Physiol Genomics 21:212–221, 2005.

103. Zenker M, et al: Human laminin β2 deficiency causes congenital nephrosis with mesangial sclerosis and distinct eye abnormalities. Hum Mol Genet 13:2625–2632, 2004.

104. Hasselbacher K, et al: Recessive missense mutations in LAMB2 expand the clinical spectrum of LAMB2-associated disorders. Kidney Int 70:1008–1012, 2006.

105. Jarad G, et al: Proteinuria precedes podocyte abnormalities in Lamb2$^{-/-}$ mice, implicating the glomerular basement membrane as an albumin barrier. J Clin Invest 116:2272–2279, 2006.

106. Mark K, Reis A, Zenker M: Prenatal findings in four consecutive pregnancies with fetal Pierson syndrome, a newly defined congenital nephrosis syndrome. Prenat Diagn 26:262–266, 2006.

107. Clewing JM, et al: Schimke immuno-osseous dysplasia: A clinicopathological correlation. J Med Genet 44:122–130, 2006.

108. Boerkoel CF, et al: Mutant chromatin remodeling protein SMARCAL1 causes Schimke immuno-osseous dysplasia. Nat Genet 30:215–220, 2002.

109. Karamatic Crew V, et al: CD151, the first member of the tetraspanin (TM4) superfamily detected on erythrocytes, is essential for the correct assembly of human basement membranes in kidney and skin. Blood 104:2217–2223, 2004.

110. Yauch RL, et al: Direct extracellular contact between integrin α(3)β(1) and TM4SF protein CD151. J Biol Chem 275:9230–9238, 2000.

111. Sachs N, et al: Kidney failure in mice lacking the tetraspanin CD151. J Cell Biol 175:33–39, 2006.

112. Niaudet P, Rotig A: The kidney in mitochondrial cytopathies. Kidney Int 51:1000–1007, 1997.

113. Cheong HI, et al: Hereditary glomerulopathy associated with a mitochondrial tRNA(Leu) gene mutation. Pediatr Nephrol 13:477–480, 1999.

114. Doleris LM, et al: Focal segmental glomerulosclerosis associated with mitochondrial cytopathy. Kidney Int 58:1851–1858, 2000.

115. Lowik MM, et al: Mitochondrial tRNALeu(UUR) mutation in a patient with steroid-resistant nephrotic syndrome and focal segmental glomerulosclerosis. Nephrol Dial Transplant 20:336–341, 2005.

116. Jansen JJ, et al: Mutation in mitochondrial tRNA(Leu(UUR)) gene associated with progressive kidney disease. J Am Soc Nephrol 8:1118–1124, 1997.

117. Scaglia F, et al: Novel homoplasmic mutation in the mitochondrial tRNATyr gene associated with atypical mitochondrial cytopathy presenting with focal segmental glomerulosclerosis. Am J Med Genet 123A:172–178, 2003.

118. Goldenberg A, et al: Respiratory chain deficiency presenting as congenital nephrotic syndrome. Pediatr Nephrol 20:465–469, 2005.

119. Ciani L, et al: Mice lacking the giant protocadherin mFAT1 exhibit renal slit junction abnormalities and a partially penetrant cyclopia and anophthalmia phenotype. Mol Cell Biol 23:3575–3582, 2003.

120. Zwacka RM, et al: The glomerulosclerosis gene *Mpv17* encodes a peroxisomal protein producing reactive oxygen species. EMBO J 13:5129–5134, 1994.

121. Togawa A, et al: Progressive impairment of kidneys and reproductive organs in mice lacking Rho GDIα. Oncogene 18:5373–5380, 1999.

122. Sadl V, et al: The mouse Kreisler (*Krml1/MafB*) segmentation gene is required for differentiation of glomerular visceral epithelial cells. Dev Biol 249:16–29, 2002.

123. Nakamura T, et al: Sclerotic lesions in the glomeruli of Buffalo/Mna rats. Nephron 43:50–55, 1986.

124. Le Berre L, et al: Extrarenal effects on the pathogenesis and relapse of idiopathic nephrotic syndrome in Buffalo/Mna rats. J Clin Invest 109:491–498, 2002.

125. Short CD, et al: Familial membranous nephropathy. Br Med J (Clin Res Ed) 289:1500, 1984.

126. Meroni M, et al: Two brothers with idiopathic membranous nephropathy and familial sensorineural deafness. Am J Kidney Dis 15:269–272, 1990.

127. Guella A, Akhtar M, Ronco P: Idiopathic membranous nephropathy in identical twins. Am J Kidney Dis 29:115–118, 1997.

128. Tay AH, et al: Membranous nephropathy with anti-tubular basement membrane antibody may be X-linked. Pediatr Nephrol 14:747–753, 2000.

129. Vasmant D, et al: Familial idiopathic membranous glomerulonephritis. Int J Pediatr Nephrol 5:193–196, 1984.

130. Herrin JT, Bartsocas CS: Familial membranoproliferative glomerulonephritis type 2 (MPGN-2). Prog Clin Biol Res 305:161–166, 1989.

131. Neary JJ, et al: Linkage of a gene causing familial membranoproliferative glomerulonephritis type III to chromosome 1. J Am Soc Nephrol 13:2052–2057, 2002.

132. Strom EH, et al: Glomerulopathy associated with predominant fibronectin deposits: A newly recognized hereditary disease. Kidney Int 48:163–170, 1995.

133. Uesugi N, et al: [Clinicopathological and morphometrical analysis of 5 cases from 4 families of fibronectin glomerulopathy]. Nippon Jinzo Gakkai Shi 41:49–59, 1999.

134. Gemperle O, et al: Familial glomerulopathy with giant fibrillar (fibronectin-positive) deposits: 15-year follow-up in a large kindred. Am J Kidney Dis 28:668–675, 1996.

135. Vollmer M, et al: The gene for human fibronectin glomerulopathy maps to 1q32, in the region of the regulation of complement activation gene cluster. Am J Hum Genet 63:1724–1731, 1998.

136. Vollmer M, et al: Molecular cloning of the critical region for glomerulopathy with fibronectin deposits (GFND) and evaluation of candidate genes. Genomics 68:127–135, 2000.

137. Doublier S, et al: Nephrin expression is reduced in human diabetic nephropathy: Evidence for a distinct role for glycated albumin and angiotensin II. Diabetes 52:1023–1030, 2003.

138. Aaltonen P, et al: Changes in the expression of nephrin gene and protein in experimental diabetic nephropathy. Lab Invest 81:1185–1190, 2001.

139. Schmid H, et al: Gene expression profiles of podocyte-associated molecules as diagnostic markers in acquired proteinuric diseases. J Am Soc Nephrol 14:2958–2966, 2003.

140. Koop K, et al: Expression of podocyte-associated molecules in acquired human kidney diseases. J Am Soc Nephrol 14:2063–2071, 2003.

141. Baelde HJ, et al: Gene expression profiling in glomeruli from human kidneys with diabetic nephropathy. Am J Kidney Dis 43:636–650, 2004.

142. Kim BK, et al: Differential expression of nephrin in acquired human proteinuric diseases. Am J Kidney Dis 40:964–973, 2002.

143. Patrakka J, et al: Expression of nephrin in pediatric kidney diseases. J Am Soc Nephrol 12:289–296, 2001.

144. Benigni A, Gagliardini E, Remuzzi G: Changes in glomerular perm-selectivity induced by angiotensin II imply podocyte dysfunction and slit diaphragm protein rearrangement. Semin Nephrol 24:131–140, 2004.

145. Bonnet F, et al: Irbesartan normalises the deficiency in glomerular nephrin expression in a model of diabetes and hypertension. Diabetologia 44:874–877, 2001.

146. Guan N, et al: Expression of nephrin, podocin, α-actinin, and WT1 in children with nephrotic syndrome. Pediatr Nephrol 18:1122–1127, 2003.

147. Hingorani SR, et al: Expression of nephrin in acquired forms of nephrotic syndrome in childhood. Pediatr Nephrol 19:300–305, 2004.

148. Wernerson A, et al: Altered ultrastructural distribution of nephrin in minimal change nephrotic syndrome. Nephrol Dial Transplant 18:70–76, 2003.

149. Huh W, et al: Expression of nephrin in acquired human glomerular disease. Nephrol Dial Transplant 17:478–484, 2002.

150. Wang SX, et al: Patterns of nephrin and a new proteinuria-associated protein expression in human renal diseases. Kidney Int 61:141–147, 2002.

151. Goode NP, et al: Expression of α-actinin-4 in acquired human nephrotic syndrome: A quantitative immunoelectron microscopy study. Nephrol Dial Transplant 19:844–851, 2004.

152. Ruf RG, et al: A gene locus for steroid-resistant nephrotic syndrome with deafness maps to chromosome 14q24.2. J Am Soc Nephrol 14:1519–1522, 2003.

153. Hamosh A, et al: Online Mendelian Inheritance in Man (OMIM), a knowledge base of human genes and genetic disorders. Nucleic Acids Res 33 (Database issue):D514–D517, 2005.

Molecular and Genetic Basis of Alport Syndrome

Sai Ram Keithi-Reddy and Raghu Kalluri

Alport syndrome is an inhertied disease with diverse clinical presentations, arising from mutations in genes encoding polypeptide chains of type IV collagen.[1,2] Normal glomerular basement membrane (GBM) consists of assembled forms of α3-α4-α5 chains of type IV collagen. Studies in Alport mice (α3 chain of type IV collagen deficient mice) have unraveled the intricacies of this complex collagen network. Evidence suggests that *Col4A3/A4/A5* gene mutations prevent not only expression of the single α-chain that is mutated but also expression of all three chains in the GBM, namely, the α3, α4, and α5 chains of type IV collagen due to defective α3-α4-α5 assembly in the GBM. Renal involvement in Alport syndrome starts with alteration in thickness of GBM. Progressive chronic kidney disease then ensues, leading to end-stage renal disease (ESRD). It is often associated with neural hearing loss and ocular abnormalities.[1-4] The prevalence of the disease is estimated at approximately 1 in 50,000 live births.[5] In certain parts of the world, Alport syndrome accounts for nearly 2% of new cases of ESRD.[6] Although renal transplantation remains an important modality of renal replacement therapy once the ESRD develops, it is important to recognize that alloantibodies may develop against missing collagens (antigens) when a normal graft containing α3, α4, and α5 is implanted into an individual with Alport syndrome, conferring a risk for the development of post-transplant anti-GBM nephritis.[7-10] The role of stem cells in preventing progression of chronic kidney disease due to Alport disease is being explored.

TYPE IV COLLAGEN AND BASEMENT MEMBRANES

Biochemistry and Network of Type IV Collagen

Basement membranes are amorphous, dense, sheetlike structures that provide structural support, divide tissue into compartments, and regulate cell behavior.[11,12] Although by electron microscopy all basement membranes might appear similar, their molecular composition is unique in each tissue. Such molecular heterogeneity is obvious in renal basement membranes that contribute to functional specificity manifested in distinct nephron segments. Glomerular basement membrane structure reflects such a phenomenon in that it is important for anatomic integrity and filtration function. Most of our knowledge about basement membranes comes from studies using basement membrane–like material that is produced by the mouse Engelbrecht Holm-Swarm (EHS) sarcoma tumor.[13-17] EHS cells produce basement membrane components that accumulate within the tumor tissue and can be easily isolated. The major components of GBM are collagen IV, laminin, entactin/ nidogen, and sulfated proteoglycans similar to basement membranes in other parts of the body.[18] Collagen IV, which by weight forms the most abundant component of all basement membranes, in part determines GBM function.

Type IV collagen in mammals is derived from six genetically distinct chain polypeptides (α1–α6). The type IV collagen α-chains have similar domain structures and share between 50% and 70% homology at the amino acid level.[7,19] These chains have three major domains:

1. The N-terminal 7S domains play a key part in determining the specificity, affinity, and geometry of the tetramer formed through the connection of four protomers (7S box).[20,21] These interactions form the nucleus for a type IV collagen scaffold. The scaffold, which helps in deposition of matrix glycoproteins and attachment of cells, evolves into a type IV collagen suprastructure, with the help of end-to-end associations and also lateral associations between type IV collagen protomers.
2. The middle triple-helical domain contains the classical Gly-X-Y sequence motif, in which X and Y represent a variety of other amino acids, characteristic of collagens. This longest domain contains 1,400 amino acids (aa).
3. The C-terminal globular noncollagenous (NC1) domain of each chain is about 230 aa in length. The molecular recognition sequences encoded within the NC1 domains govern the selection of partner chains for both protomer formation and network assembly.

The assembly of a particular trimer begins when the three NC1 domains initiate an as-yet-unknown molecular interaction among three chains. Monomer trimerization proceeds similarly to a zipper from the C-terminal end, resulting in a fully assembled protomer (a trimer of α-chains). The assembled protomer is flexible and can bend at many triple-helical interruption points in the molecule. Two type IV collagen protomers associate via their C-terminal NC1 domains to form the type IV collagen dimer (an NC1 hexamer). The six type IV collagen chains self-assemble into three basic protomers (each a triple helix) with the composition α1-α1-α2, α5-α5-α6, and α3-α4-α5. These protomers then are organized into three distinct networks, α1/α2, α3/α4/α5, and α1/α2/α5/α6, through dimerization at the C terminal. The α3/α4/α5(IV)–α3/α4/α5(IV) network differs from the others in that it has a greater number of disulfide cross-links between triple-helical domains of 12 completely conserved cysteine residues of NC1 domains, which increase its resistance to proteolysis.

Distribution of Type IV Collagen in Basement Membranes

Expression of the various type IV collagen chains in human and animal tissues has been studied using monoclonal and affinity-purified polyclonal antibodies.[22–29] The $\alpha1(IV)$ and $\alpha2(IV)$ chains are normally present in all basement membranes; the $\alpha3(IV)$–$\alpha6(IV)$ chains exhibit a more restricted distribution. In the kidney the $\alpha1(IV)$ and $\alpha2(IV)$ chains are found in the glomerular mesangium, GBM, Bowman's capsule, all tubular basement membranes, and all vascular basement membranes. The $\alpha3(IV)$, $\alpha4(IV)$, and $\alpha5(IV)$ chains are present in GBM, Bowman's capsule, and the basement membranes of distal and collecting tubules, but absent from mesangium and vascular basement membranes, whereas the $\alpha6(IV)$ chain is found only in Bowman's capsule and distal and collecting tubule basement membranes. Analogous situations exist in other organs, such as the eye and the inner ear, in which the $\alpha1(IV)$ and $\alpha2(IV)$ chains are found in all basement membranes, whereas only selected basement membranes contain the $\alpha3(IV)$–$\alpha6(IV)$ chains. The distribution of type IV collagen is frequently altered in kidney disease, but the nature of the alteration varies according to the chain involved. For example, in diabetic nephropathy, the thickening GBM expresses increasing amounts of $\alpha3(IV)$, $\alpha4(IV)$, and $\alpha5(IV)$ chains, whereas the $\alpha1(IV)$ and $\alpha2(IV)$ chains disappear from the GBM.[30] The new GBM laid down by podocytes in membranous nephropathy contains $\alpha3(IV)$, $\alpha4(IV)$, and $\alpha5(IV)$ chains, but not $\alpha1(IV)$ and $\alpha2(IV)$ chains.[31,32] These findings, along with the changes observed in Alport syndrome (as discussed below), suggest that the $\alpha3(IV)$, $\alpha4(IV)$, and $\alpha5(IV)$ chains compose a basement membrane collagen network that is distinct from the network formed by $\alpha1(IV)$ and $\alpha2(IV)$ chains.[23,24,33]

Developmental Biology (Transitions) of GBM Complex

Basement membranes are dynamic because of developmentally regulated expression of isoforms of type IV collagen. This phenomenon of complex developmental transitions leading to varying expression of isoforms of type IV collagen with time course has been observed in glomerular and other basement membranes in humans as well other animals.[23,27,34–37] Basement membranes such as the seminiferous tubule basement membrane, epithelial basement membrane of the epididymis, and lens capsule of the eye contain all six isoforms of collagen and allow temporal study of basement membranes.[38,39] Studies on expression of collagen network in normal canine seminiferous tubular basement membrane at discrete time points suggested that the sequence of expression is the $\alpha1/\alpha2$ network appearing first, followed by the $\alpha1/\alpha2/\alpha5/\alpha6$ network, and finally the $\alpha3/\alpha4/\alpha5$ network. In this study $\alpha1$ and $\alpha2$ chains were strongly expressed by 11 days, the $\alpha5$ and $\alpha6$ chains by 1.5 months, and the $\alpha3$ and $\alpha4$ chains by 2 months of age. In the glomerulus the $\alpha1/\alpha2$ network is expressed from the earliest stages.[40] The $\alpha1/\alpha2/\alpha5/\alpha6$ network appears in developing glomeruli in the late S phase, shortly before there are defined capillary loops. The appearance of the $\alpha3/\alpha4/\alpha5$ network coincides with the time when capillary loops become apparent and the $\alpha1/\alpha2/\alpha5/\alpha6$ network comes to reside in Bowman's capsule.[27,34,35] In lens capsule the developmental shifts in networks are less well defined. Prenatal murine and human lens capsules contain the $\alpha1$, $\alpha2$, $\alpha5$, and $\alpha6$ chains, with the $\alpha3$ and $\alpha4$ chains appearing only postnatally.[16,38] Hence, expression of the $\alpha1/\alpha2/\alpha5/\alpha6$ network precedes that of the $\alpha3/\alpha4/\alpha5$ network, but there is no stage identified with the $\alpha1/\alpha2$ network only. Because the $\alpha1/\alpha2$ network is believed to be ubiquitous, the developmental shift involving the $\alpha5$ and $\alpha6$ chains probably occurs before the earliest time point yet examined. In the murine and canine inner ear, only the $\alpha1/\alpha2$ network is present at birth, with the $\alpha3/\alpha4/\alpha5$ network not detected until around 2 weeks in mice and 3 to 4 weeks in dogs.[23,36] The $\alpha1/\alpha2/\alpha5/\alpha6$ network is not expressed in this site except in vascular smooth muscle. In X-linked Alport syndrome the GBM usually contains only the $\alpha1/\alpha2$ network. In the canine model for Alport syndrome, the ultrastructure and function of the GBM are initially normal, although the $\alpha3/\alpha4/\alpha5$ network is absent. Deterioration of the GBM begins later in the course of the disease, leading to the conclusion that the $\alpha3/\alpha4/\alpha5$ network is necessary for long-term maintenance. The situation with the $\alpha1/\alpha2/\alpha5/\alpha6$ chains is much less clear. In X-linked Alport syndrome, the $\alpha1/\alpha2/\alpha5/\alpha6$ network is usually absent from the kidney and skin and smooth muscle of the bladder, arterioles, and the bronchial tree in canine X-linked Alport syndrome, without apparent clinical or pathologic consequences.[23,28,29,33,36] In normal mouse testis, the appearance of $\alpha3/\alpha4/\alpha5$ network coincides with the onset of spermatogenesis, prompting speculation that expression of this network might be required for normal function.

Interaction between GBM, Epithelial Cell, and Mesangial Matrix

Not only are basement membranes dynamic structures providing structural support, but they also contribute to the acquisition of cellular phenotype and behavior.[19,41] In fact, the $\alpha3$ chain of type IV collagen interacts with $\alpha_3\beta_1$ integrin and mediates the attachment of glomerular epithelial cells to GBM.[42] It was believed that a symbiotic relationship exists between podocyte and GBM. However, recent in vitro studies have refuted such a hypothesis. The podocyte cell line expressed various chains of type IV collagen at the messenger RNA (mRNA) level. However, immunohistologic studies are not conclusive with respect to their ability to export specific type IV collagen trimers into an extracellular matrix. There was no appreciable difference in expression between podocyte cells grown on type IV collagen that were extracted from normal or from Alport syndrome GBM. These findings suggest that the podocyte growth and differentiation are not influenced specifically by the $\alpha3/\alpha4/\alpha5$ network and further that the chain composition does not seem to affect the viability of the podocytes. This has implications for Alport syndrome, in which the GBM persistently lacks the $\alpha3/\alpha4/\alpha5$ network. These results suggest that missing collagen network is not accountable for the podocyte loss and eventual glomerulosclerosis that occurs in this disease. The pathogenesis in detail will be discussed later in this chapter.

MOLECULAR GENETICS OF ALPORT SYNDROME

The triple-helical type IV collagen molecules are coded by six distinct genes, namely the $\alpha1(IV)$ to $\alpha6(IV)$ chains, and these can be classified into three pairs: COL4A1/COL4A2, COL4A3/COL4A4, and COL4A5/COL4A6. The human $\alpha1$ and $\alpha2(IV)$ chains are encoded by the genes COL4A1 and COL4A2, respectively, on chromosome 13.[43] Similarly, COL4A3 and COL4A4 at the chromosome locus 2q36 encode the $\alpha3$ and $\alpha4$ chains, and the COL4A5 and COL4A6 genes on the long arm of the X chromosome of type IV collagen encode the $\alpha5$ and $\alpha6(IV)$ chains, respectively.[44–47] The five exons at the 3' end of each gene encode the C-terminal NC1 domain of the chain, whereas most of the remaining exons encode the collagenous portion. Interestingly, the 5' ends of each gene pair are adjacent to each other oriented head to head, separated by sequences of varying length containing motifs involved in the regulation of transcriptional activity (bifunctional promoters), and the genes are transcribed in opposite directions. Bifunctional promoters have been identified for all the six type IV collagen chain genes. The regulatory machinery controlling COL4A1/COL4A2 transcription consists of two promoters that overlap and operate in opposite directions. This region contains three functional protein binding sites: Sp1 site, CCAAT, and CTC boxes.[48,49] Activation regions in the area of the first exon-intron border of each gene are necessary for transcription of COL4A1 and COL4A2.[50] A sequence with inhibitory effects on COL4A1 and COL4A2 transcription, located within intron 3 of the COL4A2 gene, has been described.[51] The rate of COL4A1 and COL4A2 transcription in type IV collagen-producing cells may reflect the relative levels of promoter and silencer activity. Some information regarding the regulatory elements of the COL4A3/COL4A4 and COL4A5/COL4A6 gene pairs is available. The intergenic promoter region of the COL4A3 and COL4A4 genes also contains an Sp1 recognition site, a CCAAT box, as well as CTC boxes, and operates bidirectionally.[52] Both the COL4A3 and COL4A4 genes contain alternative transcription start sites. The intergenic region between COL4A5 and COL4A6 also contains a CTC box. The COL4A6 gene is transcribed from two alternative promoters, resulting in two distinct transcripts, in a tissue-specific manner.[47] It is also suggested that proximal promoter of this gene pair responds to growth factor in a cell type–specific manner. This unique plasticity explains the dichotomy in the localization of $\alpha5$ and $\alpha6$ chains in basement membranes.[53] Alternative splicing has been described for $\alpha3(IV)$ and $\alpha5(IV)$ chains.[54–56] Alternative splicing of $\alpha3(IV)$ pre-mRNA generates at least six transcripts predicting five distinct proteins, differing in the C-terminal domain. The functional significance of alternative splicing of $\alpha3(IV)$ mRNA is unclear. Sequences similar to the CTC box in the 5' flanking regions have not only been identified in genes coding for type IV collagen chains but also genes encoding other extracellular matrix proteins such as fibronectin and laminins, suggesting that regulation of extracellular matrix gene activity may be under the control of a common transcription factor or family of transcription factors.[57]

There are three genetic varieties of Alport syndrome: X-linked (XLAS), which results from mutations in the COL4A5 gene and accounts for about 80% of patients; autosomal recessive (ARAS), due to mutations in either COL4A3 or COL4A4 and responsible for about 15% of patients; and autosomal dominant, making up the remainder.

X-linked Alport Syndrome

An important clinical characteristic of the X-linked inheritance is that father-to-son transmission does not occur because the father passes on only the unaffected Y chromosome. Women with XLAS are heterozygous carriers of the disease mutation, most have some degree of microscopic hematuria, and a significant minority develops renal failure. Such a variable course is explained by the so-called Lyon hypothesis describing the pattern of X chromosome inactivation. More than 300 COL4A5 mutations have been identified thus far.

These mutations are distributed throughout the gene with no apparent mutational "hot spots." With few exceptions, each family carries a unique mutation. Approximately 10% to 15% of COL4A5 mutations are de novo, having occurred in the gamete of a parent. Although deletion of substantial portions of the gene contributes to 21% of the cases, major non-deletional rearrangement of the COL4A5 gene in XLAS families is seen in 5% to 15%. All families in which XLAS co-segregates with diffuse leiomyomatosis (see below) exhibit large deletions that span the adjacent 5' ends of the COL4A5 and COL4A6 genes.[63,64] These deletions involve varying lengths of COL4A5, but the COL4A6 breakpoint is always located in the second intron of the gene.[65,66] The X chromosome in general is rich in LINE-1 elements (mammal-specific retrotransposons). The disease-causing deletions seem to arise as a result of recombination events involving interspersed repetitive LINE-1 elements, at least in some cases.[49,67] Leiomyomatosis does not occur in XLAS patients with deletions of COL4A5 and COL4A6 that extend beyond intron 2 of COL4A6. Mutations of COL4A6 alone do not seem to cause XLAS, consistent with the absence of the $\alpha6(IV)$ chain from normal GBM.[64,68]

Other reported types of COL4A5 mutation include missense mutations causing amino acid substitutions (35%), mutations resulting in premature stop codons (nonsense mutations), small deletions or insertions, splice site mutations (39%), and small, in-frame deletions. The great majority of amino acid substitutions occur in the collagenous domain of $\alpha5(IV)$ and involve replacement of glycine residues.[59,60,69] Such mutations are thought to interfere with the normal folding of the mutant $\alpha5(IV)$ chain into triple helices with other type IV collagen α-chains. Glycine lacks a side chain, making it the least bulky of amino acids, and is small enough to allow three glycine residues to fit into the interior of a tightly wound triple helix.[70] The presence of a bulkier amino acid in a glycine position presumably creates a kink or an unfolding in the triple helix. Glycine substitutions in the $\alpha1$ chain of type I collagen account for the majority of mutations causing osteogenesis imperfecta. Abnormally folded collagen triple helices exhibit increased susceptibility to proteolytic degradation.[71,72] A minority of amino acid substitutions in the $\alpha5(IV)$ chain involve critical residues in the C-terminal NC1 domain, such as one of the 12 conserved cysteine moieties. The loss of these cysteines would eliminate a disulfide bond, which could interfere with the formation of triple helices, or with the construction of networks involving $\alpha5(IV)$ chains.

Autosomal Recessive Alport Syndrome

Autosomal recessive inheritance accounts for about 15% of patients with hereditary nephritis.[73] Mutations have been identified in the *COL4A3* gene in 6 patients and in the *COL4A4* gene in 12 patients. In this form of disease, females are as severely affected as males. The clinical manifestations are identical to those of classic X-linked hereditary nephritis.[43,62,74–78] Some of these patients are homozygous for these mutations, some are compound heterozygotes, and some are heterozygotes in whom only one of the mutant alleles has been identified. The *COL4A3* mutations include three amino acid substitutions that create premature stop codons (nonsense mutations) and three small frame-shifting deletions, as well as an intronic mutation that produces a frame shift. The *COL4A4* alterations consist of two nonsense mutations, three frame-shift mutations, one in-frame deletion, two splicing mutations, and two missense mutations. As with *COL4A5*, there seem to be no mutation hot spots in *COL4A3* or *COL4A4*.

Autosomal Dominant Alport Syndrome

About 5% of families have autosomal dominant disease, genetically linked to the *COL4A3* and *COL4A4* locus on chromosome 2.[79] A specific mutation of either gene is yet to be reported. The clinical and pathologic features of this form are similar to those of X-linked disease, although progression to renal failure is rare. It is unclear why some heterozygous mutations in the *COL4A3* or *COL4A4* gene region cause autosomal dominant Alport syndrome, a progressive renal disease, whereas others are associated with thin basement membrane nephropathy, which typically has a benign outcome with only microhematuria and absent proteinuria or renal function impairment.[80–84] Most evidence suggests that chain mutations produce a post-translational defect in protomer assembly. It has also been found that the *COL4A3* and *COL4A4* genes and genes that encode for nephrin, podocin, and CD2-associated protein, forming the glomerular slit-diaphragm and allowing filtration, are regulated by a transcription factor called LMX1B, which is mutated in patients with the nail-patella syndrome. Carriers of a mutant *LMX1B* gene have a renal lesion of variable severity, which is consistent with a reduction in the $\alpha3,\alpha4,\alpha5$(IV) network in GBM and loss of the glomerular filtration barrier.[85–88] Levels of Col4α3 and Col4α4 RNA and protein are reduced in *LMX1B*$^{-/-}$ glomeruli, and LMX1B binds to a site in their common regulatory region. Thus, reduced expression of COL4A3 and COL4A4 in individuals with nail-patella syndrome is a probable consequence of *LMX1B* haploinsufficiency. This reduction would contribute to the nephropathy that, like Alport syndrome, is characterized by the presence of distinct GBM abnormalities.

Benign Familial Hematuria or Thin GBM Disease

Benign familial hematuria or thin GBM disease are a set of genetically heterogeneous conditions. In some families, heterozygous missense mutations have been found in *COL4A4* in association with autosomal dominant transmission of hematuria in the absence of renal failure.[89] However, linkage to these genes has been excluded in other families with benign familial hematuria. The observation that carriers of a single mutant *COL4A4* allele may have hematuria provides further evidence that *COL4A4* defects are involved in at least some families with benign familial hematuria, although other alleles may be involved in other families.[90] Immunohistologic staining for type IV collagen chains reveals no abnormalities.

Contiguous Gene Syndromes Involving Alport Syndrome

Alport Syndrome–Diffuse Leiomyomatosis Complex

The association of Alport syndrome with leiomyomatosis of the esophagus and tracheobronchial tree has been reported in approximately 20 families.[91] Affected females in these kindreds typically exhibit genital leiomyomas as well, causing clitoral hypertrophy with variable involvement of the labia majora and uterus. Bilateral posterior subcapsular cataracts also occur frequently in affected individuals in these kindreds. Symptoms usually appear in late childhood and include dysphagia, postprandial vomiting, retrosternal or epigastric pain, recurrent bronchitis, dyspnea, cough, and stridor. Leiomyomatosis may be suspected by chest roentgenogram or barium swallow, and confirmed by computed tomography or magnetic resonance imaging. As noted above, all patients with the Alport syndrome–diffuse leiomyomatosis complex have been found to have deletions that encompass the 5' ends of the *COL4A5* and *COL4A6* genes and commonly associated with the juvenile form of Alport syndrome. In heterozygous females the penetrance of leiomyomatosis appears to be more than the penetrance of the Alport nephropathy.[92,93]

AMME Complex

A syndrome complex consisting of Alport nephropathy, mental retardation, midface hypoplasia, and elliptocytosis (AMME) has been described in two brothers who were shown to have a microdeletion involving the entire *COL4A5* gene and extending beyond its 3' end.[94] Thus far, two new genes have been identified in the deleted region downstream of the *COL4A5* gene: The gene responsible for the mental retardation, *ACSL4* (formerly *FACL4*), encodes an acyl-CoA synthetase with substrate preference for arachidonic acid and is highly expressed in the developing and adult brain. A rapid and sensitive enzymatic assay for this disorder that takes advantage of the expression of *ACSLR* in leukocytes has been developed [and *AMMECR1*, a gene that is evolutionarily conserved and encodes a protein with as yet unknown functions.] Other reports of the association of hereditary nephritis and mental retardation are rare.[95–97]

GENOTYPE-PHENOTYPE CORRELATIONS

The two major clinical features of the Alport phenotype are renal disease and deafness. Families with XLAS can be divided into two groups on the basis of the timing of ESRD in affected males. In families with the juvenile form of XLAS, the mean age of onset of ESRD in affected males is 30 years or younger, whereas in families with the adult form of the disease the mean age of onset of ESRD is older than 30 years. Mutations in *COL4A5* have been found in more than 300 families with XLAS throughout the world.[60] Major rearrangements, mainly deletions, are detected in 5% to 16% of the kindreds. These deletions are located throughout the gene, with no hot spots. Most deletions but also frame-shift mutations and stop codons leading to synthesis of a truncated α5(IV) chain in males are associated with a greater than 90% probability of developing ESRD before the age of 30, (with a 50% renal survival rate of 20 years), hearing loss (in 80%), and ocular changes (in 40%).[98]

As discussed earlier, small mutations in COL4A5, such as missense, splice site, and small in-frame deletions of a few base pairs are the most common lesions, and substitutions for glycine residues in the collagenous domain are a common type of missense mutation (25% of all mutations) and interfere with the normal folding of the α5 chain into triple helices with other α(IV) chains. The probability of developing ESRD before the age of 30 is 50% in patients with missense mutations; the median renal survival rate is 32 years.[60,99] However, the severity of the disease associated with such mutations is highly variable between families, with ESRD in some male individuals occurring as late as 70 years. The position of the substituted glycine, or the substituting amino acid itself, can influence the effect of the mutation on triple-helical folding, and ultimately the impact of the mutation on the severity of the clinical phenotype. Glycine-XY missense mutations of exons 21 to 47 (NC1 domain and collagenous domains proximal to the starting point of formation of the triple helix) are associated with the most severe form of the disease, unlike glycine-XY missense mutations of exons 1 to 20.[80] In general, phenotype severities and secondary structures are unpredictable in general from the analysis of genomic DNA or mRNA of the COL4A5 gene, because they depend also on the type of glycine substitutions.[100] Polymerase chain reaction (PCR) single-strand and conformation polymorphism analysis has been used to detect mutations in the COL4A5 gene, but this analysis is very laborious and has a sensitivity of only 30% to 50%. New methods (multiplex genomic amplification using a single PCR condition and primer set; nested reverse-transcription/PCR, denaturing high-performance liquid chromatography, or direct sequencing) have a higher sensitivity—between 79% and 90%. The genotype-phenotype correlations are described elsewhere. A more C-terminal position of the substituted glycine in the collagenous domain has in some studies been associated with a more severe phenotype.[61] The probability of developing hearing loss before the age of 30 in male patients was about 60% in patients with a missense mutation, whereas it reached 90% for the other types of mutations together. All patients with nonsense mutations developed hearing loss before 20 years. Lenticonus was more frequent in patients with large COL4A5 mutations or small mutations leading to a premature stop codon than in patients with missense or splice site mutations. In families with large or truncating mutations, intrafamilial homogeneity is frequent; furthermore, large intrafamilial variability (>20 years difference in age at onset of ESRD) can be observed, mainly associated with missense mutations, often involving glycine residues. In such a family with a proven mutation in the COL4A5 gene, ESRD in affected males was reached between 30 and 70 years of age. A strong genotype-phenotype correlation is observed in families with diffuse esophageal leiomyomatosis. In all cases, a deletion removing the 5′ end of COL4A5 and the first two exons of the adjacent COL4A6 has been identified. In affected males, the penetrance of nephritis and leiomyomatosis is 100%. However, in affected females the penetrance of leiomyomas is greater than the penetrance of nephritis. The precise consequence on the α6(IV) chain expression and its role in leiomyomatosis development remains unclear.[66] Detection of mutations may therefore have some utility for predicting prognosis in affected males with XLAS, in association with other clinical and familial features.

Among female patients who are heterozygous for a COL4A5 mutation, a small percentage develop renal insufficiency and deafness by middle age. The true incidence of renal failure in elderly heterozygotes is unknown. Fewer than 10% of heterozygotes are asymptomatic (i.e., cannot be shown to have hematuria or any hearing deficit). The majority of female carriers have asymptomatic microhematuria and normal hearing. In female carriers of XLAS, no significant correlation was found between the genotype and the severity of renal or hearing impairment.[98] Irrespective of the type of mutation, large intrafamilial variability of the phenotype is generally observed, due to the random inactivation of the X chromosome.

Linkage analysis using a polymorphism inside the COL4A5 gene may be useful to exclude a mutation at the X-located Alport syndrome locus. More decisively, mutations have been identified in COL4A3 or COL4A4 genes in several families. However, these are two large genes (each >50 exons), making mutation detection tedious. They can be nonsense, frame-shift, splicing, or missense mutations, the latter frequently affecting glycine residues, as in the α(IV) chain. Affected patients are true homozygotes or compound heterozygotes, having two different mutations on the two alleles of COL4A3 or COL4A4. The disease is severe, with a 50% renal survival at 22 years, but ESRD can be reached as late as 44 years. Heterozygous carriers of a COL4A3 or COL4A4 mutation usually present with no urinary abnormalities or microscopic hematuria.[81,101]

Some clinical features are highly suggestive of autosomal recessive inheritance of Alport syndrome in 10% to 15% of the families:

1. Appearance of the disease in the family after a consanguineous marriage;
2. Equally severe disease in males and females, or severe renal disease in females leading to ESRD before 35 years of age. Autosomal dominant AS caused by heterozygote mutations affecting only one allele of COL4A3 or COL4A4. It has been speculated that a dominant negative effect of the mutant is responsible for an intermediate phenotype. This form accounts for no more than 5% of Alport syndrome cases. On the basis of the few families described in the literature, it seems that the renal disease is less severe than in the autosomal recessive form.

It is perhaps not surprising that COL4A5 mutations that are associated with preservation of GBM expression of α3(IV), α4(IV), and α5(IV) chains often result in a less severe phenotype.[102–104] Information about the effects of individual COL4A5 mutations on basement membrane expression of these chains, and the relationship of chain expression to phenotype, is still being accumulated.

PATHOGENESIS

Renal Manifestations

An incidental observation helped elucidate the pathogenesis

of hereditary nephritis: the GBM of most affected patients did not bind antibodies from patients with anti-GBM antibody disease (including Goodpasture syndrome).[1,105] This finding suggested an abnormality in type IV collagen, against which the anti-GBM antibodies are directed. These studies helped to confirm the pathogenetic link between Alport syndrome and type IV collagen originally hypothesized.[106] The availability of monospecific antibodies against each of the six type IV collagen α-chains has made it possible to characterize the changes in type IV collagen expression that occur in patients with Alport syndrome.[4,29,33,47,107,108]

It is now clear that the tissue pathology of Alport syndrome results from abnormalities of basement membrane expression of the α3, α4, α5, and possibly α6 chains of type IV collagen. These chains are usually absent from or underexpressed in the basement membranes of individuals with Alport syndrome, so that the networks they form are absent or, if present, defective in structure and function. As discussed earlier, in the normal developing kidney, α1(IV) and α2(IV) chains predominate in the primordial GBM of immature glomeruli.[27,34,109] The formation of capillary loops within the maturing glomeruli is associated with the appearance of α3, α4, α5(IV) chains in the GBM. As glomerular maturation progresses the α3, α4, α5(IV) chains become the predominant type IV collagen chains in GBM. This process has been referred to as "isotype switching." Although this "isotype switch" does not occur in Alport syndrome, glomerular development otherwise proceeds normally, and the GBM of young animals and children with Alport syndrome exhibits a normal trilaminar appearance by electron microscopy. These glomeruli exhibit normal capacities for filtration and for selective permeability, as demonstrated by the normal glomerular filtration rates and absence of overt proteinuria that are characteristic of early Alport syndrome in both humans and animals. Therefore, it would appear that proteinuria and renal insufficiency, as well as sensorineural deafness, come about as the result of processes that are initiated by the absence of the α3/α4/α5(IV) network, rather than arising directly from the absence of this network.

The α3(IV), α4(IV), and α5(IV) chains are identically distributed within the glomerulus,[31] and there is evidence that they combine to form a type IV collagen network that is distinct from the network formed by the α1(IV) and α2(IV) chains.[4] An abnormality in the α5(IV) chain could limit formation of this network, thereby preventing incorporation of the α3(IV) and α4(IV) chains into GBM.[58,68,110] Similarly, formation of this network could be prevented by primary mutations in the α3(IV) or α4(IV) chain. Several observations tend to confirm this hypothesis. In most patients with α5(IV) mutations, the α3(IV) and α4(IV) chains, as well as α5(IV) chains, are absent from GBM.[58] Transcription of the α3(IV) and α4(IV) genes is not turned off in the renal cortex in patients with α5(IV) mutations, suggesting that failure of incorporation of these chains, rather than failure of synthesis, is responsible for the lack of glomerular expression.[111] In patients with ARAS, primary mutations in the α3(IV) chain prevent the expression of the α4(IV) and α5(IV) chains in GBM. Thus, an abnormality in any of these chains can impair the integrity of basement membranes in the glomerulus, eye, and cochlea, leading to the various clinical findings of Alport syndrome. Heterozygous mutations in the α3 and α4 chains are responsible for at least some cases of thin basement membrane disease, an autosomal dominant disorder that does not usually progress to renal failure. In severe forms of human Alport syndrome, mutations in any one of the collagen α3 to α5(IV) genes not only interfere with the assembly of the α3/α4/α5 network in the GBM but also arrest the normal developmental switch from the α1/α1/α2 network to the α3/α4/α5 network, leading to complete absence of all these three chains from the mature GBM, and retention of the α1 and α2(IV) chains at maturity.[29,63,107,111–114]

In Alport syndrome the GBM is able to function normally early in life, because the collagen α1 and α2(IV) chains substitute for the missing α3 to α5(IV) chains. However, there is a progressive thickening and splitting of Alport syndrome GBM that is associated with the onset of hematuria and eventual glomerular obsolescence. The reason for these typical abnormalities is not clear. Several hypotheses have been studied. First, intrinsic properties of the collagen α1/α2(IV) network in Alport syndrome GBM makes the GBM less structurally sound and more susceptible to mechanical strain caused by the pressure of ultrafiltration. Second, the collagen α1/α2(IV) network is more susceptible to proteolysis by endogenous proteases than is the normal α3/α4/α5(IV) network.[34] Third, replacement of the normal collagen IV network with the α1/α2(IV) network results in aberrant accumulation of noncollagenous extracellular matrix molecules, leading eventually to a disrupted ultrastructure.

In support of the first theory, the collagen α3 and α4(IV) chains contain significantly more cysteines than do the α1 and α2(IV) chains, so more extensive disulfide cross-linking, both within and between trimers, should occur.[115] This would be expected to impart increased mechanical stability to the collagen IV network. The most straightforward demonstration of the mechanical instability arising directly from the absence of the α3/α4/α5(IV) network from basement membranes is anterior lenticonus, in which the anterior lens capsule lacks the strength to maintain the normal conformation of the lens. Similarly, microhematuria, the first invariable renal manifestation of Alport syndrome, reflects GBM thinning and a tendency to develop focal ruptures.

Episodic gross hematuria precipitated by infections, which is not uncommon during the first two decades of life, may reflect increased susceptibility of the Alport syndrome GBM to proteolysis. Persistence of the fetal distribution of α1 and α2(IV) chains in Alport syndrome kidneys confers an increased susceptibility to proteolytic attack by collagenases and cathepsins in plasma traversing glomerular capillaries in vitro. Proteolytic injury over a prolonged period may be responsible for the progressive basement membrane splitting and eventual glomerulosclerosis that are characteristic of this disorder. It is possible that the cysteine-rich α3, α4, and α5(IV) chains confer a selective advantage by increasing the resistance of the GBM to proteolytic attack. Persistence of the fetal distribution of type IV collagen in glomeruli is also observed in canine models of hereditary nephritis.[109,116] Consistent with the hypothesis concerning an increased susceptibility to proteolytic injury, the persistent fetal GBM is associated with a decline in glomerular filtration rate only after several months of life. In a recent study α3(IV)α/α mice, the abnormal GBM composition was more susceptible to proteolytic degradation compared with wild-type mice. The initial disruption of GBM was associated with increased matrix metalloproteinase (MMP) levels from infiltrating monocytes augmenting GBM degradation in these mice.[117,118] Inhibition of basement membrane–degrading MMPs significantly delayed the onset of proteinuria in these mice when they were treated before proteinuria was observed (Fig. 10-1). Similarly, renal basement membrane isolated from human kidney samples with XLAS displays an increased susceptibility to proteolytic degradation by MMP-2, MMP-3, and MMP-9. Progression of renal disease in patients with XLAS is associated with increased expression of MMP-2, MMP-3, and MMP-9 as in the α3(IV)α/α mice. These results suggest that MMP-mediated degradation of GBM is a key event in the progression of renal disease in α3(IV)α/α mice and in individuals with XLAS. Such MMP upregulation is not unique to Alport disease. However, in the context of Alport disease, such MMP upregulation degrades the GBM faster as a result of defective type IV collagen composition, whereas the degradation kinetics are unaltered in other kidney diseases.

In support of the third theory, ectopic accumulation of the laminin α2 and α1 chains in the GBM occurs both in human Alport syndrome and in animal models of Alport syndrome.[119–121] In addition, ectopic accumulation of laminin α1 was found exclusively in mouse Alport syndrome GBM. Normally, laminin-11 (α5β2α1) is the only known laminin trimer present in the mature GBM.[122] Accumulation of the laminin α2, β1, and α1 chains could be pathogenic, perhaps leading to the typical lesions observed in Alport syndrome GBM and/or to aberrant behavior of the adjacent podocytes and subsequent foot process effacement and proteinuria. Expression of laminins α1 and α1 is particularly interesting, because these two chains are found in developing GBM yet are normally eliminated at maturity, when α1 is replaced by α5 and β1 is replaced by β2.[123] Studies have also shown that in still-developing kidneys, laminin α1 is eliminated on schedule at the capillary loop stage of glomerulogenesis, but it reappears

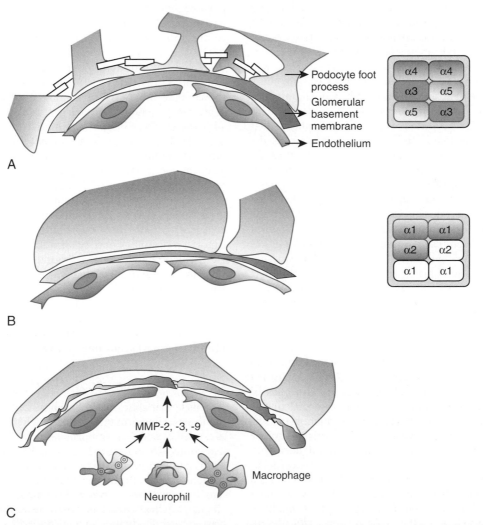

Figure 10-1 **A,** Podocyte foot process, glomerular basement membrane (GBM), slit-diaphragm, and endothelial cell constituting normal glomerular filtration apparatus. Inset shows collagen hexamer in normal mature GBM. **B,** Early manifestations of Alport syndrome are characterized by thinning of GBM, mild splitting, and podocyte effacement. Inset shows collagen hexamer in mature GBM of Alport syndrome. **C,** Delayed manifestations of Alport syndrome include effacement of foot process, irregular splitting and thinning of GBM; inflammatory cells release matrix metalloproteinases and other inflammatory mediators that further damage the GBM, and progressive glomerulosclerosis ensues.

in the mature GBM very soon thereafter. The sites of reappearance are those areas of GBM that exhibit the subepithelial thickening and delamination that is characteristic of Alport syndrome GBM. It has also been shown by immunoelectron microscopy that both podocytes and endothelial cells contribute laminin α1 to the affected GBM. Interestingly, no α1 or β1 was detected in ultrastructurally normal stretches of GBM, demonstrating a clear association between GBM lesions and deposition of ectopic laminins.[124]

Like all provocative findings, these lead to additional important questions that will hopefully be answered by future studies. First, do the GBM lesions elicit synthesis of the ectopic laminins by the adjacent glomerular cells, or does the aberrant type IV collagen complement present in Alport syndrome GBM elicit deposition of ectopic laminins, which then results in the observed lesions? If the latter is correct, then preventing ectopic expression of the laminin α1, β1, and α2 chains will perhaps improve GBM ultrastructure and slow disease progression. In fact, mutation of integrin α$_1$ in the same mouse model of Alport syndrome inhibited both accumulation of ectopic laminins (α2 and β1) and GBM delamination, and this was associated with slowed progression to renal failure.[120] (Whether α1 deposition was affected in this context was not studied.) Second, are the ectopic laminins themselves pathogenic, or are the GBM lesions alone sufficiently disruptive to either ultrafiltration or podocyte homeostasis so as to cause foot process effacement and disease? Whereas laminins α2 and β1 are widely expressed, laminin α1 is a relatively rare chain in tissues other than kidney,[125] and in nephrons it is normally confined primarily to basement membranes of the proximal tubule and loop of Henle. The restricted expression pattern of laminin α1 may suggest that it confers unique properties that are not compatible with some specialized basement membrane functions, such as those associated with glomerular ultrafiltration. This would be consistent with the abrupt elimination of laminin α1 from the developing GBM before the onset of significant glomerular capillary blood flow and ultrafiltration. A better understanding of both the mechanism of the reexpression of laminin α1 associated with Alport syndrome and its biologic consequences is certain to provide important new insights into diverse glomerulopathies and GBM homeostasis.

Using gene knockout mouse models, two different pathways, one mediated by transforming growth factor (TGF)-β1 and the other by integrin α1β1, have been demonstrated to affect Alport syndrome glomerular pathogenesis in distinct ways. In mice with Alport syndrome that are also null for integrin α1 expression, expansion of the mesangial matrix and podocyte foot process effacement are attenuated. The novel observation of non-native laminin isoforms (laminin-2 and/or laminin-4) accumulating in the GBM of mice with Alport syndrome is markedly reduced in the double knockouts. The second pathway, mediated by TGF-β1, was blocked using a soluble fusion protein comprising the extracellular domain of the TGF-β1 type II receptor. This inhibitor prevents focal thickening of the GBM but does not prevent effacement of the podocyte foot processes (Fig. 10-2). If both integrin α1β1 and TGF-β1 pathways are functionally inhibited, glomerular foot process and GBM morphology are primarily restored and renal function is markedly improved. These data suggest that integrin α1β1 and TGF-β1 play a significant role in the pathogenesis of progression in the glomerulonephritis of Alport syndrome. Absence of α1β1 integrin results in an inhibition of laminin α2 and β1 chain deposition in the GBM.[120,126] Before the onset of detectable renal dysfunction, multiple abnormalities in glomerular extracellular matrix production can be detected, including markedly elevated levels of fibronectin and perlecan (a heparan sulfate proteoglycan) in the basal laminae. Similar findings have been noted in X-linked hereditary nephritis in humans.[34]

The processes that bring about GBM thickening, proteinuria, and renal insufficiency in males with XLAS, and in both males and females with ARAS, remain undefined, although there are some clues to what may be occurring. Unlike other glomerulopathies, Alport syndrome is characterized by the accumulation of the α1(IV) and α2(IV) chains, along with types V and VI collagen, in the GBM. These proteins appear to spread from their normal subendothelial location, so that they come to occupy the full width of the GBM. As Alport syndrome glomeruli undergo sclerosis, the α1(IV) and α2(IV) chains disappear from the GBM, but type V and type VI collagen persist and, in fact, continue to accumulate. It is possible that the altered expression of the α1(IV) and α2(IV) chains, type V collagen, and type VI collagen represents a compensatory response to the loss of the α3(IV), α4(IV), and α5(IV) chains from the GBM, or may reflect altered gene expression resulting from changes in signaling from the extracellular matrix to the nucleus. For example, it has been shown that the α3β1 integrin, the predominant integrin expressed on visceral epithelial cells, interacts preferentially with the α3(IV) chain.[42] The absence of the α3(IV) chain could lead to changes in the activity or expression of this integrin, producing changes in intracellular signaling. In transgenic mice with ARAS due to partial deletion of COL4A3, renal mRNA levels for the α1(IV) and α2(IV) chains progressively increase, suggesting activation of these genes.[27] Whatever the underlying mechanism, the unrestrained deposition of certain collagens in GBM may contribute to glomerulosclerosis in Alport syndrome. Alport syndrome resembles other chronic glomerulopathies in that deterioration of glomerular filtration rate is closely correlated with fibrosis of the renal interstitium.[127] Measurable increases in cortical interstitial volume are unusual in males with XLAS under age 10 years, but progressive expansion of the interstitium frequently occurs during the second decade of life.[94] The processes driving interstitial fibrosis in Alport syndrome have yet to be characterized.

Extrarenal Manifestations

It is likely that abnormal collagen function is also responsible for the extrarenal manifestations of hereditary nephritis. As discussed above, lens abnormalities in the form of anterior lenticonus, which occurs in 20% to 30% of males with XLAS and is pathognomonic of the disease, results from thinning of the lens capsule, the basement membrane that surrounds the lens. The lens capsule normally contains α3, α4, and α5(IV) chains, but these chains are absent from the lens capsule in at least some individuals with lenticonus.[128]

The results indicate that isotype switching does not occur within the cochlea in Alport syndrome. The results are also consistent with the hypothesis that the sensorineural hearing loss in Alport syndrome may be due to alterations in cochlear micromechanics and/or dysfunction of the spiral ligament.[129,130] The pathogenetic relationship between partial

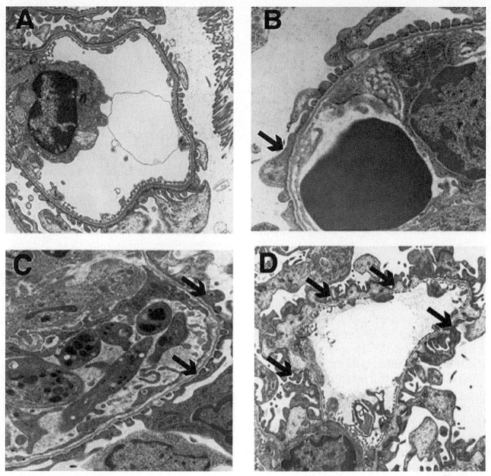

Figure 10-2 Ultrastructural analysis (transmission electron microscopy) of GBM from control mice and mice treated with MMP inhibitor. **A,** Control C57BL/6 mice at 14 weeks of age. **B,** Kidneys from 5-week-old α3(IV)$^{-/-}$ mice before the onset of proteinuria, displaying the beginning of splitting of the GBM and podocyte effacement (*arrow*). **C,** Kidneys from α3(IV) $^{-/-}$ mice at 14 weeks of age, which were treated from 5 weeks of age with MMP inhibitors for 9 weeks, displayed moderate GBM splitting and podocyte effacement (*arrows*). **D,** Kidneys from 12-week-old α3(IV)$^{-/-}$ mice without treatment showed severe lesions of the GBM associated with podocyte effacement (*arrows*). (From Zeisberg M, et al: Stage-specific action of matrix metalloproteinases influences progressive hereditary kidney disease. PLoS Med 3:e100, 2006.)

deletions of the 5′ end of the *COL4A6* gene and the formation of leiomyomas is not understood. Defects in the α6 chain gene alone do not appear to cause hereditary nephritis.

PATHOLOGY

There are no pathognomonic lesions in the kidney by light microscopy or direct immunofluorescence. Relatively more specific findings are seen in electron microscopy.

Light Microscopy

The light microscopic appearance of the glomerulus varies with the stage of the disease. Early in the disease course the glomeruli appear normal; with time, mesangial proliferation becomes evident, and eventually the glomeruli exhibit focal and global sclerosis. Similarly, the renal tubules and interstitium appear normal during childhood, with tubular atrophy and interstitial fibrosis developing over time. Direct immunofluorescence of kidney biopsy specimens is typically unremark-

able or reveals only nonspecific immunoprotein deposition. The changes on light microscopy are nonspecific and include focal increases in glomerular cellularity progressing to glomerulosclerosis, and an interstitial infiltrate containing lipid-laden foam cells of uncertain origin.

Indirect Immunofluorescence

Indirect immunofluorescence of type IV collagen α-chain expression in renal and/or skin basement membranes can be diagnostic. XLAS and ARAS cannot be differentiated by routine analysis of renal biopsy specimens, but in many cases the inheritance of Alport syndrome can be determined by analysis of type IV collagen α-chain expression.

Electron Microscopy

Electron microscopy of the kidney frequently reveals diagnostic abnormalities, which are seen regardless of the inheritance pattern or the presence or absence of sensorineural deafness or ocular abnormalities. The pathognomonic ultrastructural feature of the kidney in Alport syndrome is laminated appearance of basement membrane characterized by thickening of the GBM, with transformation of the lamina densa into a heterogeneous network of membranous strands, which enclose clear electron-lucent areas that may contain round granules of variable density measuring 20 to 90 nm in diameter. The origin of these granules is unknown, but they may represent degenerating islands of visceral epithelial cell cytoplasm. The altered capillary walls typically demonstrate epithelial foot process fusion, which may be extensive even in the absence of significant proteinuria. The epithelial aspect of the capillary wall is typically quite irregular. The pathognomonic GBM lesion occurs in most, but not all, individuals with Alport syndrome. Affected young males, heterozygous females at any age, and affected adult males on occasion, may have diffusely attenuated GBM measuring as little as 100 nm or less, rather than the pathognomonic lesion. Studies of males with human or canine Alport syndrome have shown that the earliest manifestation of the GBM lesion is attenuation, and that the extent and severity of thickening and multilamellation increase with age.[131] In males, the proportion of GBM showing splitting increases from about 30% by age 10 to over 90% by age 30. Heterozygous females may have normal-appearing GBM or, on the other end of the spectrum, diffuse GBM thickening and multilamellation, but most will display mild to moderate abnormalities.[132] Not all Alport syndrome kindreds demonstrate these characteristic ultrastructural features. Thick, thin, normal, and nonspecifically altered GBM have all been described. Although diffuse attenuation of GBM has been considered the hallmark of benign familial hematuria, some individuals with GBM attenuation have progressive renal disease and a COL4A5 mutation.[59] Correlation between the percentage of GBM showing splitting of the lamina densa and the degree of proteinuria in individuals with Alport syndrome, suggesting that increased permeability of the GBM to protein may be a functional consequence of the GBM alteration, was shown in earlier studies.[133] Morphometric parameters such as mesangial volume fraction, cortical interstitial volume fraction, and percentage of global glomerular sclerosis are inversely correlated with creatinine clearance in Alport syndrome. Similar relationships have been observed in other diseases, such as diabetic nephropathy and membranoproliferative glomerulonephritis. However, individuals with Alport syndrome show significantly greater impairment of filtration for any degree of structural change, in comparison with patients with diabetic nephropathy or membranoproliferative glomerulonephritis, suggesting that these morphologic abnormalities only partially account for reductions in creatinine clearance in Alport syndrome. Decreased conductivity of water across the altered glomerular capillary wall could contribute to the decrement in filtration. Expansion of the cortical interstitium, a measure of interstitial fibrosis, is rarely observed before the age of 10 years in males with Alport syndrome.

CLINICAL FEATURES

Several hundred unrelated kindreds with progressive hereditary nephritis, with or without deafness, representing all geographic and ethnic groups, have been reported in the medical literature. Alport syndrome accounts for about 3% of children with

ESRD in the United States, and the incidence of Alport syndrome among adults in the United States with ESRD is 0.2%, according to the United States Renal Data System. Alport syndrome was diagnosed in 11% of children undergoing renal biopsy for isolated hematuria.[134] In certain parts of the world, Alport syndrome accounts for nearly 2% of new cases of ESRD.[6]

Renal Involvement

The initial renal manifestation of Alport syndrome is asymptomatic microhematuria. Persistent microhematuria is a constant feature and is present from early in life in boys, but may not be diagnosed until adulthood unless the patient is screened because of an affected family member. Many also have episodic gross hematuria, precipitated by upper respiratory infections, during the first 2 decades of life. Males without hematuria by the age of 10 years are unlikely to have hereditary nephritis.[135] Female patients who are heterozygous for XLAS may have intermittent hematuria, and as many as 10% of obligate female heterozygotes never manifest hematuria. Hematuria seems to be persistent in both male and female patients with ARAS.

Proteinuria is usually absent during the first few years of life but develops eventually in males with XLAS and in both males and females with recessive disease. Proteinuria increases progressively with age and may culminate in the nephrotic syndrome. Significant proteinuria is relatively infrequent in females who are heterozygous for XLAS, but it may occur.

Hypertension also increases in incidence and severity with age. Like proteinuria, hypertension is much more likely to occur in affected males than in affected females in the X-linked form of the disease, but there do not seem to be gender differences in the autosomal recessive form.

The rate of progression to renal disease is fairly constant among affected males within a particular family, with ESRD developing in virtually all affected males with XLAS usually between the ages of 16 and 35, although significant intra-kindred variability has occasionally been reported.[136] The prognosis in affected females with XLAS is generally benign, with most surviving into old age with clinically mild renal disease. Approximately 15% of female heterozygotes develop renal insufficiency during adolescence and young adulthood. Many women with progressive nephritis maintain adequate renal function until late in life; the true risk of renal failure in elderly heterozygotes remains to be determined. Gross hematuria in childhood, nephrotic syndrome, and diffuse GBM thickening by electron microscopy are features suggestive of progressive nephritis in affected females.[137] As in women with other chronic nephritides, pregnancy does not seem to affect renal function adversely in those with mild disease, but it may be associated with accelerated loss of function in those with more severe disease. Both males and females with ARAS appear likely to progress to ESRD during the second or third decade of life.

Extrarenal Manifestations

A variety of extrarenal manifestations may be present in individuals with Alport syndrome. The most common are sensorineural hearing loss[138] (which begins in the high tones and progresses over time to frequencies in the range of conversational speech) and eye changes such as anterior lenticonus, white or yellow flecking of the perimacular region of the retina, and corneal lesions such as posterior polymorphous dystrophy and recurrent corneal erosions.[3] Anterior lenticonus, which occurs in 20% to 30% of males with XLAS, is pathognomonic of the disease. As previously mentioned, leiomyomas are seen in patients with deletions at the 5′ ends of both the *COL4A5* and *COL4A6* genes.[139] Sensorineural deafness and anterior lenticonus are also indicative of an unfavorable outcome in affected women.

Megathrombocytopenia (thrombocytopenia with large or giant platelets) has been described in some families with autosomal dominant hereditary nephritis and sensorineural deafness. This complex has been referred to as Epstein syndrome or, when associated with leukocyte cytoplasmic inclusions, Fechtner syndrome. These disorders have been mapped to chromosome 22, and result from mutations in the gene encoding nonmuscle myosin heavy chain 9 (MYH9).[140] Mutations in this gene can also cause Sebastian syndrome, another giant platelet disorder, and nonsyndromic hereditary deafness. Thus, Epstein and Fechtner syndromes represent distinct disorders arising from mutations in noncollagen genes, not variants of autosomal dominant Alport syndrome.

Carriers

As described above, females are usually carriers of X-linked disease and are much less likely than males to develop progressive renal injury. This was shown in the first study of the natural history of female carriers with proven *COL4A5* mutations.[141] Among female carriers followed in 195 affected families, the incidence of ESRD before age 40 was 12% (as compared with 50% to 90% in males).[98] However, older females are at increased risk of progressive renal disease, with a 30% probability of developing ESRD by the age of 60. This may represent an overestimate, because approximately one-third of women, probably those less severely affected, were lost to follow-up.

Risk factors for chronic renal insufficiency in female carriers include episodic gross hematuria in childhood, sensorineural deafness, heavy proteinuria, and extensive basket-weave GBM changes visible on renal biopsy specimens. By comparison, women carriers with only asymptomatic hematuria by the age of 30 to 40 years have a very small risk of eventually developing renal failure.

An interesting feature noted in the previous study is the large clinical heterogeneity observed among female carriers. As an example, there was little correlation between rapidly progressive disease in a particular young woman, and the severity of disease among related female carriers. A possible explanation is that the variability results from the random inactivation of the X chromosome within affected organs, with a large percentage of the wild-type allele being inactivated in the kidneys of severely affected women.

There seem to be similar clinical phenotype features among carriers of X-linked and autosomal recessive disease. As an example, among 47 carriers of X-linked disease, all had dysmorphic hematuria, but very few developed renal failure, clinical hearing loss, retinopathy, or lenticonus.[74] By comparison, 11 of 14 carriers (79%) from two families with autosomal recessive disease had dysmorphic hematuria, but none had renal failure, clinical hearing loss, retinopathy, or lenticonus.

DIAGNOSIS

Alport syndrome should be considered in the initial differential diagnosis of patients with persistent microscopic hematuria, once structural abnormalities of the kidneys or urinary tract have been excluded. It becomes a very important consideration in the presence of a significant family history and deafness. Persistent microscopic hematuria is also noted in other glomerular conditions such as IgA nephropathy, which can be ruled out with the absence of family history, and thin basement membrane disease with the absence of deafness and progressive renal failure. As many as 15% of the cases were diagnosed exclusively by biopsy, in the absence of family history. These cases usually represent autosomal recessive inheritance or are de novo in origin.[62]

Monoclonal antibody probes have helped to elucidate the tissue distribution of the α3, α4, and α5(IV) chains. These chains are normally located in the GBM, Bowman's capsule, the distal and collecting tubule basement membrane, and several basement membranes of the cochlea and eye.[33] The α5(IV) chain but not the α3 and α4(IV) chains is also present in the basement membrane underlying the epidermis.

IMMUNOHISTOCHEMISTRY

Skin Biopsy

Because the α5(IV) chain is expressed in the epidermal basement membrane, examination of skin biopsy samples by immunofluorescence for expression of α5(IV) is an important tool for making a diagnosis of Alport syndrome.[142,143] Incubation of skin biopsy specimens with a monoclonal antibody directed against the α5(IV) chain showed complete absence of staining of epidermal basement membranes in most males with XLAS, whereas female carriers had discontinuous (mosaic pattern) staining.[33] The latter observation is compatible with the Lyon hypothesis, in which it would be expected that one-half of cells would express a normal α5(IV) chain. Thus, in a male patient with clinical features and family history suggesting XLAS, examination of skin for α5(IV) expression may obviate the necessity for kidney biopsy. Although unambiguous mosaicism of α5(IV) expression is diagnostic of the carrier state, a normal result does not exclude heterozygosity. In other words, a female member of an Alport kindred who does not have hematuria may still be a carrier even in the absence of clearly defined mosaicism. About 20% of males with XLAS and an unknown percentage of heterozygous females exhibit normal staining of skin for the α5(IV) chain. In addition, all individuals with ARAS have normal skin reactivity for this chain. Thus, the presence of epidermal basement membrane staining for the α5(IV) chain does not exclude a diagnosis of Alport syndrome. Box 10-1 lists factors to take into account when considering a skin biopsy.

Renal Biopsy

Renal biopsy usually clinches the diagnosis of Alport syndrome. The indications for renal biopsy are:

1. Inconclusive family history and clinical features;
2. Skin biopsy equivocal;

Box 10-1 Advantages and Disadvantages of Skin Biopsy

Advantages

Early diagnosis possible, even in the absence of severe renal disease;
Less traumatic and less invasive;
Obviates need for renal biopsy;
Heterozygous females can be diagnosed.

Disadvantages

Normal staining of skin is exhibited in 20% of males with XLAS and an unknown percentage of heterozygous females;
Autosomal RAS will be associated with normal skin reactivity;
Not a good test for detecting asymptomatic carriers of COL4A5 mutations but only useful in the presence of other clinical findings;
A mutation in the COL4A5 gene that permits deposition of a functionally abnormal but antigenically normal α5(IV) chain gives misleading results.

3. Presence of features suggestive of progressive renal disease such as rise in creatinine, hypertension, and proteinuria.

Immunostaining of renal biopsy specimens for type IV collagen can also be useful in the evaluation of patients with suspected Alport syndrome.[108] Specimens from males with XLAS typically show complete absence of immunostaining for the α3, α4, and α5(IV) chains in their kidneys, whereas those from heterozygous females exhibit patchy loss of staining in GBM and tubular basement membranes. As with skin staining for the α5(IV) chain, approximately 20% of specimens from individuals with XLAS show normal staining of renal basement membranes for the α3, α4, and α5(IV) chains. At least some of these patients have missense mutations of COL4A5.[34]

Patients with ARAS show abnormalities of renal type IV collagen expression that differ from those of patients with X-linked disease. These patients typically exhibit complete absence of staining for the α3 and α4(IV) chains. However, whereas their GBM specimens show no staining for the α5(IV) chain, there is staining of Bowman's capsules and tubular basement membranes for the α5(IV) chain.[107] This observation makes sense if it is assumed that the α5(IV) chain must associate with α3 and α4(IV) chains to be incorporated into GBM, but can associate with the α6(IV) chain in tubular basement membranes, Bowman's capsules, and epidermal basement membranes. Hence, analysis of renal expression of type IV collagen α-chains can serve not only to confirm a diagnosis of Alport syndrome but also to distinguish between the X-linked and autosomal recessive forms of the disease. Biopsy specimens from patients with thin basement membrane nephropathy, who may present in a similar fashion to those with Alport syndrome, show normal renal basement membrane staining for type IV collagen chains. Thus, normal staining for these chains can be used to support a diagnosis of thin basement membrane disease, in the context of the appropriate clinical findings, family history, and histologic observations. However, normal staining for these chains does not exclude a diagnosis of Alport syndrome. Correlation of immunohistologic findings with pedigree information may help to clarify ambiguous results.[103]

Electron Microscopy

For many clinicians, electron microscopic examination of renal tissue remains the most readily available means for confirming a diagnosis of suspected Alport syndrome. The presence of diffuse thickening and multilamellation of the GBM predicts a progressive nephropathy, regardless of family history or the presence or absence of deafness.[144] This approach has some limitations, however. Ultrastructural information alone does not establish the mode of transmission in a particular family. Thus, in a patient with a negative family history, electron microscopy cannot distinguish de novo X-linked disease from autosomal recessive disease. In some individuals the biopsy findings may be ambiguous, particularly in females and young patients of either sex. Furthermore, families with progressive nephritis and COL4A5 mutations in association with thin GBMs have been described,[59] indicating that the classic GBM lesion is not present in all Alport kindreds. It is not unusual for the pediatric nephrologist to see a child with hematuria and discover that multiple relatives also have hematuria, none of whom has ever undergone kidney biopsy. Confirmation of Alport syndrome in one member of a kindred with familial hematuria virtually establishes the diagnosis for other affected members, so the person having the biopsy should ideally be the one person most likely to exhibit unambiguous renal lesions. The natural history of the renal lesion suggests that older male subjects are more likely to exhibit diagnostic ultrastructural abnormalities of GBM. In families in which a firm diagnosis of syndrome has been established, evaluation of individuals with newly recognized hematuria could be limited to ultrasonography of the kidneys and urinary tract in most instances. In the absence of tumor or structural anomalies of the urinary tract, a diagnosis other than Alport syndrome is unlikely.

Molecular Genetic Analysis

Molecular genetic testing may eventually become the diagnostic procedure of choice, because it is noninvasive and can be extremely accurate.[145,146] However, the use of single-strand conformational polymorphism analysis of PCR products may result in a relatively low mutation detection rate (37% to 50%), with some false negative results possibly arising from tandem duplications.[147] To improve accuracy, one future approach may be to detect mutations by sequencing of mRNA from cultured skin fibroblasts using reverse-transcriptase PCR.[148] Other approaches include multiplex genomic amplification and denaturing high-performance liquid chromatography. Molecular genetic testing, though laborious, has the potential to provide information essential for determining prognosis and guiding genetic counseling in the following settings[142]:

1. Prenatal diagnosis;
2. Provides the only means for reliably diagnosing the carrier state in asymptomatic female members of kindreds with XLAS and for making a prenatal diagnosis of Alport syndrome[73,148];
3. Clinical situations in which a firm diagnosis of Alport syndrome cannot be established by renal or skin biopsy;

4. Clinical situations in which it is not possible to determine the mode of transmission, despite careful evaluation of the pedigree and application of the immunohistologic methods.

In these situations, because reproductive decisions may be influenced by genetic counseling information, erroneous determination of the mode of inheritance of Alport syndrome can have profoundly unfortunate consequences.[149] The inheritance of Alport syndrome in a family can be determined by linkage analysis, which does not require identification of a particular mutation. Ideally, every individual with Alport syndrome would have the diagnosis and inheritance confirmed by molecular genetic analysis. At present, however, the clinical utility of molecular genetic analysis for diagnosis of Alport syndrome is limited. The sheer size of the type IV collagen loci (>50 exons), combined with the great variety of mutations, most of which are missense alterations of a single base pair, presents a formidable obstacle, even when automated sequencing is available. Consequently, screening for COL4A3, COL4A4, and COL4A5 mutations is time-consuming, expensive, and confined to a handful of research laboratories. Mutation screening utilizing single-strand conformational polymorphisms currently identifies only about 50% of COL4A5 mutations.[59] Complete sequencing of COL4A5 is a more sensitive method that is capable of detecting over 80% of COL4A5 mutations,[146] but this technique is expensive and not yet generally available to clinicians. As with other genetic disorders, presymptomatic identification of a mutation at one of the Alport-associated loci may have implications for health and life insurance.

INSIGHTS FROM ANIMAL MODELS

The existence of spontaneous and genetically engineered animal models of Alport syndrome provides excellent opportunities for investigating the pathogenesis of renal failure and deafness in this disease, for evaluating the effectiveness of potential interventions, and for understanding the roles of type IV collagen in basement membranes.

Canine Models

Samoyed Hereditary Glomerulopathy

Samoyed hereditary glomerulopathy (SHG), an X-linked dominant disease, was first described in 1977.[150,151] Both females and males develop proteinuria by 2 months of age. However, males tend to develop progressive decline in renal functions, and death ensues by 15 months of age. At birth, the GBM of affected males appears identical to that of normal dogs, but by 1 month of age splitting of the lamina densa is evident. With progressive splitting and irregular thickening, the GBM changes become indiscernible from those of human XLAS. Affected females have focal splitting of GBM. Immunochemical studies of SHG basement membranes have revealed changes in type IV collagen expression that are similar to those found in XLAS.[109,152,153] The identification of a mutation in COL4A5 resulting in a premature stop codon as the cause of SHG confirmed that it is a canine form of Alport syndrome.[154] When the seminiferous tubule basement membrane was examined in dogs with Alport syndrome, it was found to be thinner than in controls. However, spermatogenesis began at the same time as with normal dogs, although the number of mature sperm was significantly reduced in dogs with Alport syndrome. Thus, it would appear that $\alpha3/\alpha4/\alpha5$ and $\alpha1/\alpha2/\alpha5/\alpha6$ networks are not essential for the onset of spermatogenesis, but long-term function may be compromised by the loss of one or both networks. Although this situation could be analogous to the GBM in Alport syndrome, with testis serving as a model system to study the sequence of type IV collagen network expression, it is too preliminary to conclude this with certainty.[40]

Navasota Hereditary Nephritis

Lees et al[155] recently described an X-linked form of hereditary nephritis in a family of mixed-breed dogs centered in Navasota, Texas. The GBM of Navasota hereditary nephritis (NHN) males undergoes ultrastructural changes that are identical to those observed in Alport syndrome and in SHG, and NHN basement membranes exhibit alterations of $\alpha1(IV)$ through $\alpha6(IV)$ expression that mimic XLAS. Affected dogs do not carry the same COL4A5 mutation as SHG dogs, but the specific mutation causing NHN has yet to be identified.

Hereditary Nephritis in English Cocker Spaniels

The occurrence of a familial nephropathy in English cocker spaniels has been recognized for years.[156] Recently Lees and colleagues[118] reported that glomerular ultrastructural findings in affected dogs are identical to those of human Alport syndrome. Pedigree analysis suggests autosomal recessive inheritance, and immunohistochemical studies of type IV collagen expression have shown changes similar to those observed in ARAS.[157] The causative mutation has not been determined as yet.

Bull Terrier Nephritis

Hood et al described an autosomal dominant hereditary nephropathy in bull terriers that is associated with glomerular ultrastructural abnormalities characteristic of Alport syndrome. In these dogs, expression of the $\alpha3(IV)$ and $\alpha5(IV)$ chains in the GBM is preserved.[158]

Murine Models

ARAS models have been created in two transgenic mouse strains by introduction of Col4A3 mutations.[159,160] As with the spontaneous canine models, these mice develop glomerular ultrastructural changes that are characteristic of Alport syndrome, along with changes in the expression of type IV collagen chains that mimic those observed in the human ARAS. These mice lack the expression of $\alpha3$ chain at both the mRNA and protein levels. This mouse provided the opportunity to test the hypothesis of whether assembly of $\alpha3$ and $\alpha5$ chains is always regulated tightly in basement membranes in which they are both normally present. In an analysis of various basement membranes in the $\alpha3^{-/-}$ mice, it was found that in the kidney, a lack of $\alpha3$ was associated with the absence of $\alpha4$ and $\alpha5$, whereas in the anterior lens capsule and the strial capillary basement membrane of the cochlea, the expression of $\alpha5$ persisted despite the absence of $\alpha3$ chain in these basement membranes. It was also shown that $\alpha5$ NC1 co-localized with α1 chain in the same hexamer in the α3$^{-/-}$ and wild-type mice. These results suggest that α1 and α5 can be present in the same network in the absence of α3 chain. In the kidney, the expression of these two chains seems tightly coordinated and dependent on the expression of each other, but the study presents a possibility of tissue-specific type IV collagen assembly. Such tissue-specific α-chain assembly can be achieved presumably via factors such as chaperones. In this regard a heat shock protein (47 kDa) chaperone has been identified for collagen assembly, including the type IV collagen. It has been speculated that assembly of type IV collagen α-chains in the formation of organ basement membranes is potentially dependent on tissue-specific assembly factors that are yet to be discovered. Such structural differences among organ basement membranes potentially contribute to important functional diversity.[161]

Renal disease pathogenesis in the Alport mouse model seems to follow a two-step process that is divided by the onset of proteinuria. Before the onset of proteinuria the fundamental difference in the Alport syndrome glomerulus is the absence of the collagen α3(IV), α4(IV), and α5(IV) chains in the GBM. By 4 weeks of age (nearly 2 weeks before the onset of proteinuria), there are significant basement membrane changes, with focal thinning, thickening, and splitting. Also evident is a marked accumulation of extracellular matrix components in the GBM of affected animals. Alport mice have been very helpful animal models for the study of chronic renal disease in view of consistency in progression that disease.[162]

PREVENTION AND THERAPEUTIC MODALITIES

Pharmacotherapy

Angiotensin-Converting Enzyme Inhibitors

The availability of canine and murine models of Alport syndrome has allowed the testing of genetic or pharmacologic therapies, so as to select promising treatments for human trials. There is no specific treatment for Alport syndrome. If weakening of the GBM is important, then even normal intraglomerular pressures may be inappropriately high. As a result, it has been proposed (though not proven) that lowering the intraglomerular pressure with antihypertensive therapy—preferably with an angiotensin-converting enzyme (ACE) inhibitor—may diminish the rate of disease progression. Results from two animal models are compatible with this hypothesis.[163] In *COL4A3*-knockout mice, for example, the use of ramipril early in life substantially delayed the onset of renal failure and reduced renal fibrosis. The beneficial effect of ACE inhibition in murine Alport syndrome could reflect antifibrogenic and/or anti-inflammatory actions.

Clinically, there is preliminary evidence that ACE inhibitors can substantially reduce protein excretion at least in some patients with Alport syndrome, a possible marker for protection against long-term progression.[164–166] In the absence of more data, it is reasonable to treat any patient with hypertension with an ACE inhibitor, as well as normotensive males with evidence of progressive disease. As in other proteinuric states, the combination of an ACE inhibitor and an angiotensin II receptor blocker may be more effective in reducing urine protein excretion than either agent alone.

Cyclosporine

Preliminary evidence in affected patients suggests that cyclosporine may halt progressive disease in patients with poor prognostic signs (severe proteinuria).[167] After 8.4 years of therapy in one recent study, eight such patients had a stable creatinine clearance and a lower or equivalent degree of proteinuria as compared with baseline values. This result should be viewed with caution, given the small sample size and the lack of contemporaneous controls. These observations raise the possibility that proteinuria itself may be injurious to renal tubules and interstitium in Alport syndrome, and that effective suppression of proteinuria may retard progression to ESRD. The observation that mesangial expansion and interstitial fibrosis may correlate with progressive disease has led researchers to evaluate the effectiveness of cyclosporine. In a canine model of XLAS, cyclosporine treatment failed to diminish proteinuria but resulted in longer renal survival.[168] Knowledge of the proper role of this agent requires further study.

Matrix Metalloproteinase Inhibitor

Matrix metalloproteinases are upregulated in Alport syndrome.[169] Upregulation of MMPs is not unique to Alport disease. However, in the context of Alport disease such MMP upregulation degrades the GBM faster because of defective type IV collagen composition and consequent altered degradation kinetics. Considering that MMP-mediated degradation of GBM is the key event in the progression of renal disease in Alport syndrome, MMP inhibitors have been tried in mouse models of Alport syndrome. When used in the early phase, MMP inhibitors prevent progression of renal disease.[118]

Protein Restriction

Valli et al[201] found that feeding male dogs with SHG a diet restricted in protein, lipid, calcium, and phosphorus resulted in prolongation of survival and retardation of the progression of GBM splitting, although all eventually died.

Renal Transplantation

At present, renal transplantation is the only viable alternative to dialysis in Alport syndrome with ESRD. The data of the North American Pediatric Renal Transplant Cooperative Study (NAPRTCS) document equivalent allograft survival rates in patients with familial nephritis, as compared with patients with other diagnoses.[170] Recurrent disease does not occur in the transplant (because the donor GBM is normal), but approximately 3% to 4% of patients develop de novo anti-GBM antibody disease.[171,172] In one case report, acute vascular rejection occurred secondary to anti-GBM antibodies.[173]

Risk factors for development of post-transplant anti-GBM disease are male gender, presence of deafness, and ESRD before the age of 30.[174–176] In patients with X-linked disease, these antibodies are usually directed primarily against the α5(IV) chain, but antibodies against the α3(IV) chain are found in some patients. Anti-GBM antibody disease usually occurs in the first year after transplantation, but an interval of several years between transplantation and presentation with anti-GBM disease can occur. Affected patients typically have circulating anti-GBM antibodies and are at high risk (≤75%)

for crescentic glomerulonephritis and loss of the graft.[177,178] Treatment with plasmapheresis and cyclophosphamide, as used in patients with primary anti-GBM antibody disease, seems to be of limited benefit in this setting. High incidence of graft loss and recalcitrance to treatment have been attributed to the high affinity and avidity with which anti-GBM antibodies bind to the GBM.[179] Repeat transplantation in these patients is associated with a high risk of recurrence (seven of eight in one report).

Occurrence of a great majority of cases of post-transplant anti-GBM nephritis in Alport syndrome in males is consistent with the hypothesis that even a female heterozygote that developed ESRD has some cells synthesizing and secreting a normal $\alpha5(IV)$ chain. Alport syndrome patients who develop anti-GBM disease in the allograft presumably have failed to develop immunologic tolerance for the $\alpha5(IV)$ chain.[9] In patients with ARAS who develop post-transplant anti-GBM nephritis, the predominant target of anti-GBM antibodies is the $\alpha3(IV)$ chain, the Goodpasture epitope.[7,180] It is unclear why only some patients develop anti-GBM antibody disease after transplantation. One possibility is that the type of genetic defect in the COL4A5 gene plays an important role. The risk seems to be greatest in patients with COL4A5 mutations that prevent synthesis of the $\alpha5(IV)$ chain. A review of Alport syndrome patients with post-transplant anti-GBM disease found that 54% (7 of 13) had large deletions in the COL4A5 gene as compared with a deletion frequency of 16% in all patients with this disorder.[9] In comparison, less severe defects could allow critical parts of the $\alpha5(IV)$ chain to be expressed and therefore recognized as a self-antigen. The observation that glomeruli in some families with classic X-linked disease are able to bind anti-GBM antibodies is compatible with this hypothesis.[181] However, a COL4A5 gene deletion alone is not sufficient to cause anti-GBM disease in the renal transplant. In one study, only one of seven patients with a COL4A5 deletion and complete absence of the $\alpha5(IV)$ chain developed anti-GBM disease in the renal transplant. This observation indicates that variables other than exposure to a previously unseen antigen must be involved. This includes the complex interplay between the host's genetic complement and the way in which epitopes are presented to the immune system.[182] Differences in the ability to activate the cellular arm of the immune system may be another reason why only some patients develop post-transplant anti-GBM disease.[183,184] One study evaluated the variation in anti-GBM antibody formation in patients with Alport syndrome in whom post-transplant nephritis had or had not developed (12 and 10 patients, respectively). All patients displayed some combination of antibodies directed against the $\alpha3$, $\alpha4$, or $\alpha5$ chains of type IV collagen. The pattern of antibody expression did not differ between the two groups, suggesting that nonhumoral immune factors may contribute to the observed variation in incidence of nephritis. It has also been noted that some Alport syndrome patients develop linear IgG staining of the transplant GBM, without evidence of C3 deposition, glomerulonephritis, or allograft dysfunction.[178] It is clear that Alport syndrome patients with COL4A5 deletions can undergo renal transplantation without developing anti-GBM nephritis, indicating that other factors, presently unknown, must influence the initiation and elaboration of the immune response to the allograft. At this time, the only way to determine whether a previously untransplanted Alport syndrome patient will develop post-transplant anti-

GBM nephritis is to perform the transplant, although as noted above, certain patients are at very low risk. At the present time it is not possible to predict the outcome of a first renal transplant in any particular Alport syndrome patient, whether or not that patient's mutation has been characterized. Because individuals with Alport syndrome typically exhibit excellent graft survival rates, the use of the best functioning and matched kidney is recommended. The issue of whether a patient who has already lost an allograft to post-transplant anti-GBM nephritis should receive a second transplant is difficult, given the high likelihood of recurrent disease and subsequent graft failure. Should women who are heterozygous for COL4A5 mutations be allowed to serve as kidney donors? Clearly, those with proteinuria, hypertension, or renal insufficiency will not be allowed to donate, and the same should apply if any hearing loss is present. On the other hand, it may not be unreasonable to allow heterozygotes with hematuria but normal renal function and hearing to donate a kidney. There is no long-term follow-up information on the impact of uninephrectomy in such women, although there does not seem to be a drastic decline in renal function over the first several years after transplant.[185] The wishes of a heterozygous woman with asymptomatic microhematuria should be thoughtfully considered, but it must be assumed at this time that the risk to such an individual of ultimately developing significant renal insufficiency is substantially higher than it is for the usual kidney donor. The relatively low incidence of clinical anti-GBM antibody disease means that renal transplantation is not contraindicated in patients with Alport syndrome. However, the optimal management is uncertain in patients who lost their first graft to anti-GBM antibody disease. The recurrence rate is high in subsequent transplants, but isolated cases of successful repeat transplantation have been reported.

Gene Therapy

Kidney-targeted gene therapy could be an ideal treatment for renal diseases, because the effect of the therapeutic molecule is limited to the kidney. The harmful effects to other tissues can presumably be limited. The kidney is, however, a well-differentiated organ with specialized compartments, composed of glomerulus, tubule, vasculature, and interstitium. These anatomic compartments are separated by basement membranes and associated cells. The GBM separates the blood flow from the urine flow, and the tubular basement membrane separates urine flow from interstitial fluid. These membranes complicate gene transfection, because they act as anatomic barriers blocking passage of the vectors.[186]

Alport syndrome is not believed to be an attractive candidate for gene therapy, because it seems to be difficult to deliver the COL4A5 gene selectively to podocytes by passing the GBM. Heikkila et al developed a new gene transfer technique, that is, a perfusion of adenoviral vector for 2 to 12 hours, that allows gene transfer exclusively to glomerular cells.[187] They succeeded in the delivery of the $\alpha5(IV)$ collagen gene to the glomerular cells by renal perfusion of adenovirus vector. They further applied this technique to gene therapy in canine model Alport syndrome. The introduced gene for $\alpha5(IV)$ collagen expressed in the glomeruli and assembled triple-helical type IV collagen fiber composed of $\alpha3(IV)$, $\alpha4(IV)$, and $\alpha5(IV)$. A major issue remaining is how the

administration of the *COL4A5* gene can be repeated in the clinical situation. Generally, treatment of rare monogenic hereditary diseases is not so attractive from the viewpoint of industry and drug development. Gene therapy might be a less expensive alternative therapy for rare diseases.

Stem Cell Therapy

Transplantation of *Col4A3*$^{-/-}$ mice with wild-type bone marrow (*Col4A3*$^{+/+}$) cells was a revelation, in that not only did a successful engraftment of these cells into the damaged glomeruli as podocytes and mesangial cells occur, it also led to significant improvement in renal function recovery from glomerular architecture defects. The repair of GBM architecture and glomerular integrity is associated with expression of α3 chain of type IV collagen and restoration of α4 and α5 chain expression, with viable triple-helical molecules and network organization of type IV collagen in the renal basement membranes.[188] The use of stem cell therapy in human diseases remains a controversial issue because of ethical concerns of using human embryonic stem cells. Alternatively, in the last few years several reports have suggested the ability of bone marrow cells to implant and differentiate into different tissues, including the kidney.[189-191] Furthermore, bone marrow–derived cells localize to inflamed tissues of various organs. In this study, bone marrow transplantation was performed after kidney injury was established in the organ. This report showed how stem cells can be used to repair extracellular basement membrane defects. This study unequivocally demonstrated that soluble factors liberated by the putative stem cells cannot explain the therapeutic effect; instead, bone marrow–derived cells are required to become resident glomerular cells and provide the missing type IV collagen chain to enable repair and reversal of GBM defects and recovery of renal function. Alternatively, bone marrow–derived cells could fuse with the existing glomerular cells and provide therapeutic benefit or transfer their nuclei to damaged podocytes and enable repair. Further experiments are required to understand the specific mechanisms. The issue of immune cells and other cells from the bone marrow becoming trapped in the glomeruli and providing nonspecific benefit by liberating collagens does not arise, because immune cells do not produce matrix proteins. Transplantation of mice with bone marrow cells did not result in any immunoglobulin deposition along the GBM, suggesting a lack of humoral response toward the newly synthesized GBM at the time points evaluated (data not shown). Interestingly, this study demonstrated that inflamed and/or injured glomeruli recruit cells that are derived from bone marrow stem cell, suggesting that inflamed glomeruli (with respect to growth factors and other attractants) provide a molecular recognition sink for bone marrow–derived cells that is not provided by normal glomeruli. It is believed that such recruitment is caused by the special environment of the damaged glomeruli. Moreover, podocytes are present along the outer aspect of the GBM and, hence, recruitment of transplanted podocytes in this model could be specific to the nature of this disease with respect to GBM defects and breaks, providing significant gaps that enable the migration of bone marrow–derived cells to the outer aspects of the GBM. It was demonstrated that about 10% of the cells in *Col4A3*$^{-/-}$ mice with bone marrow transplant are transplanted cells, suggesting that, for therapeutic benefit, a small but significant number of cells is required versus total replacement of all damaged cells and complete repair of GBM. Finally, these results offer an opportunity for patients with Alport syndrome: a treatment of their inherited renal failure that is an alternative to lifelong dependence on hemodialysis or the prospect of repeated kidney transplantation starting at young adolescence.

SUMMARY

Understanding the complex structure of basement membranes has unveiled new paradigms in understanding of several genetic diseases including Alport syndrome. A genetically heterogeneous disease, Alport syndrome arises from mutations in genes coding for basement membrane type IV collagen. About 80% of Alport syndrome cases are X-linked, resulting from mutations in *COL4A5*, the gene encoding the α5 chain of type IV collagen. Most other patients have ARAS due to mutations in *COL4A3* or *COL4A4*, which encode the α3(IV) and α4(IV) chains, respectively. Autosomal dominant Alport syndrome has been mapped to chromosome 2 in the region of *COL4A3* and *COL4A4*. The primary pathologic event seems to be the loss from basement membranes of a type IV collagen network composed of α3, α4, and α5(IV) chains. Although this network is not critical for normal glomerulogenesis, its absence seems to trigger a complex interplay among several extracellular matrix proteins leading to destruction of basement membrane and additional glomerulosclerosis. A careful and diligent evaluation of family history and documentation of absence of epidermal basement membrane expression of α5(IV) through skin biopsy can obviate the need for kidney biopsy in the diagnosis of Alport syndrome. With the availability of molecular genetic tools, a simplified but mechanistic approach to the diagnosis of Alport syndrome is probable. There are no specific therapies for Alport syndrome. Renal transplantation for Alport syndrome with ESRD is usually very successful. Occasional patients develop anti-GBM nephritis of the allograft, almost always resulting in graft loss. Recent studies using stem cells to repair the collagen defects in Alport syndrome are promising. With advancements in basic science and new evidence from stem cell research, a pragmatic approach to management of Alport syndrome is evolving.

References

1. Kashtan CE: Familial hematuria due to type IV collagen mutations: Alport syndrome and thin basement membrane nephropathy. Curr Opin Pediatr 16:177–181, 2004.
2. Massella L, et al: Epidermal basement membrane α5(IV) expression in females with Alport syndrome and severity of renal disease. Kidney Int 64:1787–1791, 2003.
3. Grunfeld JP: The clinical spectrum of hereditary nephritis. Kidney Int 27:83–92, 1985.
4. Kashtan CE, Michael AF: Alport syndrome. Kidney Int 50:1445–1463, 1996.
5. Levy M, Feingold J: Estimating prevalence in single-gene kidney diseases progressing to renal failure. Kidney Int 58:925–943, 2000.
6. Persson U, Hertz JM, Wieslander J, Segelmark M: Alport syndrome in southern Sweden. Clin Nephrol 64:85–90, 2005.
7. Brainwood D, Kashtan C, Gubler MC, Turner AN: Targets of alloantibodies in Alport anti-glomerular basement membrane

disease after renal transplantation. Kidney Int 53:762–766, 1998.

8. Kalluri R, et al: Identification of α3, α4, and α5 chains of type IV collagen as alloantigens for Alport posttransplant anti-glomerular basement membrane antibodies. Transplantation 69:679–683, 2000.

9. Ding J, Zhou J, Tryggvason K, Kashtan CE: *COL4A5* deletions in three patients with Alport syndrome and posttransplant antiglomerular basement membrane nephritis. J Am Soc Nephrol 5:161–168, 1994.

10. Kalluri R, Gattone VH 2nd, Noelken ME, Hudson BG: The α3 chain of type IV collagen induces autoimmune Goodpasture syndrome. Proc Natl Acad Sci U S A 91:6201–6205, 1994.

11. Paulsson M: Basement membrane proteins: structure, assembly, and cellular interactions. Crit Rev Biochem Mol Biol 27:93–127, 1992.

12. Schittny JC, Yurchenco PD: Basement membranes: Molecular organization and function in development and disease. Curr Opin Cell Biol 1:983–988, 1989.

13. Orkin RW, et al: A murine tumor producing a matrix of basement membrane. J Exp Med 145:204–220, 1977.

14. Kleinman HK, et al: Basement membrane complexes with biological activity. Biochemistry 25:312–318, 1986.

15. Baron-Van Evercooren A, Gansmuller A, Gumpel M, et al: Schwann cell differentiation in vitro: Extracellular matrix deposition and interaction. Dev Neurosci 8:182–196, 1986.

16. Grant DS, et al: The basement-membrane-like matrix of the mouse EHS tumor: II. Immunohistochemical quantitation of six of its components. Am J Anat 174:387–398, 1985.

17. Hadley MA, Byers SW, Suarez-Quian CA, et al: Extracellular matrix regulates Sertoli cell differentiation, testicular cord formation, and germ cell development in vitro. J Cell Biol 101:1511–1522, 1985.

18. Kleinman HK, et al: Isolation and characterization of type IV procollagen, laminin, and heparan sulfate proteoglycan from the EHS sarcoma. Biochemistry 21:6188–6193, 1982.

19. Kalluri R: Basement membranes: Structure, assembly and role in tumour angiogenesis. Nat Rev Cancer 3:422–433, 2003.

20. Langeveld JP, et al: Bovine glomerular basement membrane. Location and structure of the asparagine-linked oligosaccharide units and their potential role in the assembly of the 7S collagen IV tetramer. J Biol Chem 266:2622–2631, 1991.

21. Nayak BR, Spiro RG: Localization and structure of the asparagine-linked oligosaccharides of type IV collagen from glomerular basement membrane and lens capsule. J Biol Chem 266:13978–13987, 1991.

22. Butkowski RJ, Wieslander J, Kleppel M, et al: Basement membrane collagen in the kidney: regional localization of novel chains related to collagen IV. Kidney Int 35:1195–1202, 1989.

23. Cosgrove D, Kornak JM, Samuelson G: Expression of basement membrane type IV collagen chains during postnatal development in the murine cochlea. Hear Res 100:21–32, 1996.

24. Kleppel MM, Kashtan C, Santi PA, et al: Distribution of familial nephritis antigen in normal tissue and renal basement membranes of patients with homozygous and heterozygous Alport familial nephritis. Relationship of familial nephritis and Goodpasture antigens to novel collagen chains and type IV collagen. Lab Invest 61:278–289, 1989.

25. Kleppel MM, Michael AF: Expression of novel basement membrane components in the developing human kidney and eye. Am J Anat 187:165–174, 1990.

26. Kleppel MM, Santi PA, Cameron JD, et al: Human tissue distribution of novel basement membrane collagen. Am J Pathol 134:813–825, 1989.

27. Miner JH, Sanes JR: Collagen IV α3, α4, and α5 chains in rodent basal laminae: sequence, distribution, association with laminins, and developmental switches. J Cell Biol 127:879–891, 1994.

28. Ninomiya Y, et al: Differential expression of two basement membrane collagen genes, *COL4A6* and *COL4A5*, demonstrated by immunofluorescence staining using peptide-specific monoclonal antibodies. J Cell Biol 130:1219–1229, 1995.

29. Peissel B, et al: Comparative distribution of the α1IV, α5IV, and α6IV collagen chains in normal human adult and fetal tissues and in kidneys from X-linked Alport syndrome patients. J Clin Invest 96:1948–1957, 1995.

30. Kim Y, et al: Differential expression of basement membrane collagen in membranous nephropathy. Am J Pathol 139:1381–1388, 1991.

31. Kim Y, et al: Differential expression of basement membrane collagen chains in diabetic nephropathy. Am J Pathol 138:413–420, 1991.

32. Minto AW, et al: Augmented expression of glomerular basement membrane specific type IV collagen isoforms α3–α5 in experimental membranous nephropathy. Proc Assoc Am Physicians 110:207–217, 1998.

33. Yoshioka K, et al: Type IV collagen α5 chain. Normal distribution and abnormalities in X-linked Alport syndrome revealed by monoclonal antibody. Am J Pathol 144:986–996, 1994.

34. Kalluri R, Shield CF, Todd P, et al: Isoform switching of type IV collagen is developmentally arrested in X-linked Alport syndrome leading to increased susceptibility of renal basement membranes to endoproteolysis. J Clin Invest 99:2470–2478, 1997.

35. Zheng K, et al: Absence of the α6(IV) chain of collagen type IV in Alport syndrome is related to a failure at the protein assembly level and does not result in diffuse leiomyomatosis. Am J Pathol 154:1883–1891, 1999.

36. Harvey SJ, et al: The inner ear of dogs with X-linked nephritis provides clues to the pathogenesis of hearing loss in X-linked Alport syndrome. Am J Pathol 159:1097–1104, 2001.

37. Kelley PB, Sado Y, Duncan MK: Collagen IV in the developing lens capsule. Matrix Biol 21:415–423, 2002.

38. Kahsai TZ, et al: Seminiferous tubule basement membrane. Composition and organization of type IV collagen chains, and the linkage of α3(IV) and α5(IV) chains. J Biol Chem 272:17023–17032, 1997.

39. Saito K, et al: Differential expression of mouse α5(IV) and α6(IV) collagen genes in epithelial basement membranes. J Biochem Tokyo 128:427–434, 2000.

40. Harvey SJ, et al: Sequential expression of type IV collagen networks: testis as a model and relevance to spermatogenesis. Am J Pathol 168:1587–1597, 2006.

41. Timpl R: Structure and biological activity of basement membrane proteins. Eur J Biochem 180:487–502, 1989.

42. Krishnamurti U, et al: Integrin-mediated interactions between primary/T-SV40 immortalized human glomerular epithelial cells and type IV collagen. Lab Invest 74:650–657, 1996.

43. Boyd CD, et al: The genes coding for human pro α1(IV) collagen and pro α2(IV) collagen are both located at the end of the long arm of chromosome 13. Am J Hum Genet 42:309–314, 1988.

44. Hostikka SL, et al: Identification of a distinct type IV collagen α-chain with restricted kidney distribution and assignment of its gene to the locus of X chromosome-linked Alport syndrome. Proc Natl Acad Sci U S A 87:1606–1610, 1990.

45. Mariyama M, Zheng K, Yang-Feng TL, Reeders ST: Colocalization of the genes for the α3(IV) and α4(IV) chains of type IV collagen to chromosome 2 bands q35–q37. Genomics 13:809–813, 1992.

46. Myers JC, et al: Molecular cloning of α5(IV) collagen and assignment of the gene to the region of the X chromosome containing the Alport syndrome locus. Am J Hum Genet 46:1024–1033, 1990.

47. Sugimoto M, Oohashi T, Ninomiya Y: The genes *COL4A5* and *COL4A6*, coding for basement membrane collagen chains

α5(IV) and α6(IV), are located head-to-head in close proximity on human chromosome Xq22 and COL4A6 is transcribed from two alternative promoters. Proc Natl Acad Sci U S A 91:11679–11683, 1994.

48. Fischer G, et al: Identification of a novel sequence element in the common promoter region of human collagen type IV genes, involved in the regulation of divergent transcription. Biochem J 292(Pt 3):687–695, 1993.

49. Segal Y, et al: LINE-1 elements at the sites of molecular rearrangements in Alport syndrome–diffuse leiomyomatosis. Am J Hum Genet 64:62–69 1999.

50. Poschl E, Pollner R, Kuhn K: The genes for the α1(IV) and α2(IV) chains of human basement membrane collagen type IV are arranged head-to-head and separated by a bidirectional promoter of unique structure. EMBO J 7:2687–2695, 1988.

51. Haniel A, Welge-Lussen U, Kuhn K, Poschl E: Identification and characterization of a novel transcriptional silencer in the human collagen type IV gene COL4A2. J Biol Chem 270:11209–11215, 1995.

52. Momota R, et al: Two genes, COL4A3 and COL4A4, coding for the human α3(IV) and α4(IV) collagen chains are arranged head-to-head on chromosome 2q36. FEBS Lett 424:11–16, 1998.

53. Sund M, Maeshima Y, Kalluri R: Bifunctional promoter of type IV collagen COL4A5 and COL4A6 genes regulates the expression of α5 and α6 chains in a distinct cell-specific fashion. Biochem J 387:755–761, 2005.

54. Guo C, et al: Differential splicing of COL4A5 mRNA in kidney and white blood cells: A complex mutation in the COL4A5 gene of an Alport patient deletes the NC1 domain. Kidney Int 44:1316–1321, 1993.

55. Penades JR, et al: Characterization and expression of multiple alternatively spliced transcripts of the Goodpasture antigen gene region. Goodpasture antibodies recognize recombinant proteins representing the autoantigen and one of its alternative forms. Eur J Biochem 229:754–760, 1995.

56. Saito A, Sakatsume M, Yamazaki H, Arakawa M: Alternative splicing in the α5(IV) collagen gene in human kidney and skin tissues. Nippon Jinzo Gakkai Shi 36:19–24, 1994.

57. Grodecki KM, et al: Treatment of X-linked hereditary nephritis in Samoyed dogs with angiotensin-converting enzyme ACE inhibitor. J Comp Pathol 117:209–225, 1997.

58. Antignac C, et al: Deletions in the COL4A5 collagen gene in X-linked Alport syndrome. Characterization of the pathological transcripts in nonrenal cells and correlation with disease expression. J Clin Invest 93:1195–1207, 1994.

59. Knebelmann B, et al: Spectrum of mutations in the COL4A5 collagen gene in X-linked Alport syndrome. Am J Hum Genet 59:1221–1232, 1996.

60. Lemmink HH, Schroder CH, Monnens LA, Smeets HJ: The clinical spectrum of type IV collagen mutations. Hum Mutat 9:477–499, 1997.

61. Renieri A, et al: X-linked Alport syndrome: An SSCP-based mutation survey over all 51 exons of the COL4A5 gene. Am J Hum Genet 58:1192–1204, 1996.

62. Tryggvason K, Zhou J, Hostikka SL, Shows TB: Molecular genetics of Alport syndrome. Kidney Int 43:38–44, 1993.

63. Antignac C, et al: Alport syndrome and diffuse leiomyomatosis: Deletions in the 5′ end of the COL4A5 collagen gene. Kidney Int 42:1178–1183, 1992.

64. Zhou J, et al: Deletion of the paired α5(IV) and α6(IV) collagen genes in inherited smooth muscle tumors. Science 261:1167–1169, 1993.

65. Heidet L, et al: Novel COL4A5/COL4A6 deletions and further characterization of the diffuse leiomyomatosis–Alport syndrome DL-AS locus define the DL critical region. Cytogenet Cell Genet 78:240–246, 1997.

66. Heidet L, et al: Deletions of both α5(IV) and α6(IV) collagen genes in Alport syndrome and in Alport syndrome associated with smooth muscle tumours. Hum Mol Genet 4:99–108, 1995.

67. Ueki Y, et al: Topoisomerase I and II consensus sequences in a 17-kb deletion junction of the COL4A5 and COL4A6 genes and immunohistochemical analysis of esophageal leiomyomatosis associated with Alport syndrome. Am J Hum Genet 62:253–261, 1998.

68. Heiskari N, et al: Identification of 17 mutations in ten exons in the COL4A5 collagen gene, but no mutations found in four exons in COL4A6: A study of 250 patients with hematuria and suspected of having Alport syndrome. J Am Soc Nephrol 7:702–709, 1996.

69. Kawai S, et al: The COL4A5 gene in Japanese Alport syndrome patients: Spectrum of mutations of all exons. The Japanese Alport Network. Kidney Int 49:814–822, 1996.

70. Piez K: Molecular and aggregate structures of the collagens. In Piez KR (ed): AH Extracellular Matrix Biochemistry. New York, Elsevier, 1984, pp 1–39.

71. Kuivaniemi H, Tromp G, Prockop DJ: Mutations in collagen genes: causes of rare and some common diseases in humans. FASEB J 5:2052–2060, 1991.

72. Prockop DJ: Seminars in medicine of the Beth Israel Hospital, Boston. Mutations in collagen genes as a cause of connective-tissue diseases. N Engl J Med 326:540–546, 1992.

73. Torra R, Tazon-Vega B, Ars E, Ballarin J: Collagen type IV α3-α4 nephropathy: From isolated haematuria to renal failure. Nephrol Dial Transplant 19:2429–2432, 2004.

74. Dagher H, et al: A comparison of the clinical, histopathologic, and ultrastructural phenotypes in carriers of X-linked and autosomal recessive Alport's syndrome. Am J Kidney Dis 38:1217–1228, 2001.

75. Mochizuki T, et al: Identification of mutations in the α3(IV) and α4(IV) collagen genes in autosomal recessive Alport syndrome. Nat Genet 8:77–81, 1994.

76. Ding J, Stitzel J, Berry P, et al: Autosomal recessive Alport syndrome: Mutation in the COL4A3 gene in a woman with Alport syndrome and posttransplant antiglomerular basement membrane nephritis. J Am Soc Nephrol 5:1714–1717, 1995.

77. Knebelmann B, et al: Splice-mediated insertion of an Alu sequence in the COL4A3 mRNA causing autosomal recessive Alport syndrome. Hum Mol Genet 4:675–679, 1995.

78. Lemmink HH, et al: Mutations in the type IV collagen α3 COL4A3 gene in autosomal recessive Alport syndrome. Hum Mol Genet 3:1269–1273, 1994.

79. Jefferson JA, et al: Autosomal dominant Alport syndrome linked to the type IV collagen α3 and α4 genes COL4A3 and COL4A4. Nephrol Dial Transplant 12:1595–1599, 1997.

80. Gross O, Netzer KO, Lambrecht R, et al: Novel COL4A4 splice defect and in-frame deletion in a large consanguine family as a genetic link between benign familial haematuria and autosomal Alport syndrome. Nephrol Dial Transplant 18:1122–1127, 2003.

81. Longo I, et al: COL4A3/COL4A4 mutations: From familial hematuria to autosomal-dominant or recessive Alport syndrome. Kidney Int 61:1947–1956, 2002.

82. Pescucci C, et al: Autosomal-dominant Alport syndrome: Natural history of a disease due to COL4A3 or COL4A4 gene. Kidney Int 65:1598–1603, 2004.

83. Pochet JM, Bobrie G, Landais P, et al: Renal prognosis in Alport's and related syndromes: influence of the mode of inheritance. Nephrol Dial Transplant 4:1016–1021, 1989.

84. van der Loop FT, et al: Autosomal dominant Alport syndrome caused by a COL4A3 splice site mutation. Kidney Int 58:1870–1875, 2000.

85. Hamano Y, et al: Determinants of vascular permeability in the kidney glomerulus. J Biol Chem 277:31154–31162, 2002.

86. McIntosh I, et al: Mutation analysis of *LMX1B* gene in nail-patella syndrome patients. Am J Hum Genet 63:1651–1658, 1998.
87. Miner JH, et al: Transcriptional induction of slit diaphragm genes by Lmx1b is required in podocyte differentiation. J Clin Invest 109:1065–1072, 2002.
88. Morello R, et al: Regulation of glomerular basement membrane collagen expression by LMX1B contributes to renal disease in nail-patella syndrome. Nat Genet 27:205–208, 2001.
89. Lemmink HH, et al: Benign familial hematuria due to mutation of the type IV collagen α4 gene. J Clin Invest 98:1114–1118, 1996.
90. Boye E, et al: Determination of the genomic structure of the *COL4A4* gene and of novel mutations causing autosomal recessive Alport syndrome. Am J Hum Genet 63:1329–1340, 1998.
91. Antignac C, Heidet L: Mutations in Alport syndrome associated with diffuse esophageal leiomyomatosis. Contrib Nephrol 117:172–182, 1996.
92. Cochat P, et al: Diffuse leiomyomatosis in Alport syndrome. J Pediatr 113:339–343, 1988.
93. Gobel J, et al: Kidney transplantation in Alport's syndrome: Long-term outcome and allograft anti-GBM nephritis. Clin Nephrol 38:299–304, 1992.
94. Vitelli F, et al: Identification and characterization of a highly conserved protein absent in the Alport syndrome A, mental retardation M, midface hypoplasia M, and elliptocytosis E contiguous gene deletion syndrome AMME. Genomics 55:335–340, 1999.
95. Jonsson JJ, et al: Alport syndrome, mental retardation, midface hypoplasia, and elliptocytosis: A new X linked contiguous gene deletion syndrome? J Med Genet 35:273–278, 1998.
96. Lane W, Robson M, Lowry RB, Leung AK: X-linked recessive nephritis with mental retardation, sensorineural hearing loss, and macrocephaly. Clin Genet 45:314–317, 1994.
97. Piccini M, et al: *FACL4*, a new gene encoding long-chain acyl-CoA synthetase 4, is deleted in a family with Alport syndrome, elliptocytosis, and mental retardation. Genomics 47:350–358, 1998.
98. Jais JP, et al: X-linked Alport syndrome: Natural history in 195 families and genotype- phenotype correlations in males. J Am Soc Nephrol 11:649–657, 2000.
99. Barker DF, et al: A mutation causing Alport syndrome with tardive hearing loss is common in the western United States. Am J Hum Genet 58:1157–1165, 1996.
100. Wang YF, Ding J, Wang F, Bu DF: Effect of glycine substitutions on α5(IV) chain structure and structure-phenotype correlations in Alport syndrome. Biochem Biophys Res Commun 316:1143–1149, 2004.
101. Heidet L, et al: Structure of the human type IV collagen gene *COL4A3* and mutations in autosomal Alport syndrome. J Am Soc Nephrol 12:97–106, 2001.
102. Mazzucco G, et al: Ultrastructural and immunohistochemical findings in Alport's syndrome: A study of 108 patients from 97 Italian families with particular emphasis on *COL4A5* gene mutation correlations. J Am Soc Nephrol 9:1023–1031, 1998.
103. Naito I, Kawai S, Nomura S, et al: Relationship between *COL4A5* gene mutation and distribution of type IV collagen in male X-linked Alport syndrome. Japanese Alport Network. Kidney Int 50:304–311, 1996.
104. Nakanishi K, et al: Immunohistochemical study of α1–5 chains of type IV collagen in hereditary nephritis. Kidney Int 46:1413–1421, 1994.
105. McCoy RC, Johnson HK, Stone WJ, Wilson CB: Absence of nephritogenic GBM antigens in some patients with hereditary nephritis. Kidney Int 21:642–652, 1982.
106. Spear GS: Editorial: Alport's syndrome: A consideration of pathogenesis. Clin Nephrol 1:336–337, 1973.
107. Gubler MC, et al: Autosomal recessive Alport syndrome: Immunohistochemical study of type IV collagen chain distribution. Kidney Int 47:1142–1147, 1995.
108. Kagawa M, et al: Epitope-defined monoclonal antibodies against type-IV collagen for diagnosis of Alport's syndrome. Nephrol Dial Transplant 12:1238–1241, 1997.
109. Harvey SJ, et al: Role of distinct type IV collagen networks in glomerular development and function. Kidney Int 54:1857–1866, 1998.
110. Hudson BG, et al: The pathogenesis of Alport syndrome involves type IV collagen molecules containing the α3(IV) chain: Evidence from anti-GBM nephritis after renal transplantation. Kidney Int 42:179–187 1992.
111. Nakanishi K, Yoskikawa N, Iijima K, Nakamura H: Expression of type IV collagen α3 and α4 chain mRNA in X-linked Alport syndrome. J Am Soc Nephrol 7:938–945, 1996.
112. Antignac C: Molecular genetics of basement membranes: The paradigm of Alport syndrome. Kidney Int Suppl 49:S29–S33, 1995.
113. Kashtan CE, Kim Y: Distribution of the α1 and α2 chains of collagen IV and of collagens V and VI in Alport syndrome. Kidney Int 42:115–126, 1992.
114. Tryggvason K: Mutations in type IV collagen genes and Alport phenotypes. Contrib Nephrol 117:154–171, 1996.
115. Zhou J, Reeders ST: The α chains of type IV collagen. Contrib Nephrol 117:80–104, 1996.
116. Kashtan CE: Animal models of Alport syndrome. Nephrol Dial Transplant 17:1359–1362, 2002.
117. Rodgers KD, et al: Monocytes may promote myofibroblast accumulation and apoptosis in Alport renal fibrosis. Kidney Int 63:1338–1355, 2003.
118. Zeisberg M, et al: Stage-specific action of matrix metalloproteinases influences progressive hereditary kidney disease. PLoS Med 3:e100, 2006.
119. Andrews KL, Mudd JL, Li C, Miner JH: Quantitative trait loci influence renal disease progression in a mouse model of Alport syndrome. Am J Pathol 160:721–730, 2002.
120. Cosgrove D, et al: Integrin α1β1 and transforming growth factor-β1 play distinct roles in Alport glomerular pathogenesis and serve as dual targets for metabolic therapy. Am J Pathol 157:1649–1659, 2000.
121. Kashtan CE, et al: Abnormal glomerular basement membrane laminins in murine, canine, and human Alport syndrome: Aberrant laminin α2 deposition is species independent. J Am Soc Nephrol 12:252–260, 2001.
122. Miner JH: Renal basement membrane components. Kidney Int 56:2016–2024, 1999.
123. Miner JH: Developmental biology of glomerular basement membrane components. Curr Opin Nephrol Hypertens 7:13–19, 1998.
124. Abrahamson DR, Prettyman AC, Robert B, St John PL: Laminin-1 reexpression in Alport mouse glomerular basement membranes. Kidney Int 63:826–834, 2003.
125. Virtanen I, et al: Laminin α1-chain shows a restricted distribution in epithelial basement membranes of fetal and adult human tissues. Exp Cell Res 257:298–309, 2000.
126. Sayers R, et al: Role for transforming growth factor-β1 in Alport renal disease progression. Kidney Int 56:1662–1673, 1999.
127. Kim KH, et al: Structural-functional relationships in Alport syndrome. J Am Soc Nephrol 5:1659–1668, 1995.
128. Cheong HI, Kashtan CE, Kim Y, et al: Immunohistologic studies of type IV collagen in anterior lens capsules of patients with Alport syndrome. Lab Invest 70:553–557, 1994.
129. Zehnder AF, et al: Distribution of type IV collagen in the cochlea in Alport syndrome. Arch Otolaryngol Head Neck Surg 131:1007–1013, 2005.

130. Kalluri R, Gattone VH 2nd, Hudson BG: Identification and localization of type IV collagen chains in the inner ear cochlea. Connect Tissue Res 37:143–150, 1998.

131. Jansen B, et al: Samoyed hereditary glomerulopathy SHG. Evolution of splitting of glomerular capillary basement membranes. Am J Pathol 125:536–545, 1986.

132. Meleg-Smith S, Magliato S, Cheles M, et al: X-linked Alport syndrome in females. Hum Pathol 29:404–408, 1998.

133. Rumpelt HJ: Hereditary nephropathy Alport syndrome: correlation of clinical data with glomerular basement membrane alterations. Clin Nephrol 13:203–207, 1980.

134. Trachtman H, Weiss RA, Bennett B, Greifer I: Isolated hematuria in children: Indications for a renal biopsy. Kidney Int 25:94–99, 1984.

135. Kashtan CE: Alport syndrome. An inherited disorder of renal, ocular, and cochlear basement membranes. Medicine (Baltimore) 78:338–360, 1999.

136. Hasstedt SJ, Atkin CL, San Juan AC Jr: Genetic heterogeneity among kindreds with Alport syndrome. Am J Hum Genet 38:940–953, 1986.

137. Grunfeld JP, Noel LH, Hafez S, Droz D: Renal prognosis in women with hereditary nephritis. Clin Nephrol 23:267–271, 1985.

138. Izzedine H, Tankere F, Launay-Vacher V, Deray G: Ear and kidney syndromes: Molecular versus clinical approach. Kidney Int 65:369–385, 2004.

139. Dahan K, et al: Smooth muscle tumors associated with X-linked Alport syndrome: Carrier detection in females. Kidney Int 48:1900–1906, 1995.

140. Seri M, et al: Mutations in MYH9 result in the May-Hegglin anomaly, and Fechtner and Sebastian syndromes. The May-Hegglin/Fechtner Syndrome Consortium. Nat Genet 26:103–105, 2000.

141. Jais JP, et al: X-linked Alport syndrome: Natural history and genotype-phenotype correlations in girls and women belonging to 195 families: A "European Community Alport Syndrome Concerted Action" study. J Am Soc Nephrol 14:2603–2610, 2003.

142. Kashtan CE: Alport syndrome: Is diagnosis only skin-deep? Kidney Int 55:1575–1576, 1999.

143. van der Loop FT, et al: Identification of COL4A5 defects in Alport's syndrome by immunohistochemistry of skin. Kidney Int 55:1217–1224, 1999.

144. Yoshikawa N, Matsuyama S, Ito H, et al: Nonfamilial hematuria associated with glomerular basement membrane alterations characteristic of hereditary nephritis: Comparison with hereditary nephritis. J Pediatr 111:519–524, 1987.

145. Inoue Y, et al: Detection of mutations in the COL4A5 gene in over 90% of male patients with X-linked Alport's syndrome by RT-PCR and direct sequencing. Am J Kidney Dis 34:854–862, 1999.

146. Martin P, et al: High mutation detection rate in the COL4A5 collagen gene in suspected Alport syndrome using PCR and direct DNA sequencing. J Am Soc Nephrol 9:2291–2301, 1998.

147. Arrondel C, et al: A large tandem duplication within the COL4A5 gene is responsible for the high prevalence of Alport syndrome in French Polynesia. Kidney Int 65:2030–2040, 2004.

148. Wang F, Wang Y, Ding J, Yang J: Detection of mutations in the COL4A5 gene by analyzing cDNA of skin fibroblasts. Kidney Int 67:1268–1274, 2005.

149. Turco AE, Rossetti S, Bresin E, Corra S: Erroneous genetic risk assessment of Alport syndrome. Lancet 346:1237, 1995.

150. Bernard MA, Valli VE: Familial renal disease in Samoyed dogs. Can Vet J 18:181–189, 1977.

151. Jansen B, et al: Mode of inheritance of Samoyed hereditary glomerulopathy: An animal model for hereditary nephritis in humans. J Lab Clin Med 107:551–555, 1986.

152. Thorner P, et al: Abnormalities in the NC1 domain of collagen type IV in GBM in canine hereditary nephritis. Kidney Int 35:843–850, 1989.

153. Thorner P, Jansen B, Baumal R, et al: Samoyed hereditary glomerulopathy. Immunohistochemical staining of basement membranes of kidney for laminin, collagen type IV, fibronectin, and Goodpasture antigen, and correlation with electron microscopy of glomerular capillary basement membranes. Lab Invest 56:435–443, 1987.

154. Zheng K, Thorner PS, Marrano P, et al: Canine X chromosome-linked hereditary nephritis: A genetic model for human X-linked hereditary nephritis resulting from a single base mutation in the gene encoding the α5 chain of collagen type IV. Proc Natl Acad Sci U S A 91:3989–3993, 1994.

155. Lees GE, et al: New form of X-linked dominant hereditary nephritis in dogs. Am J Vet Res 60:373–383, 1999.

156. Robinson WF, Huxtable CR, Gooding JP: Familial nephropathy in cocker spaniels. Aust Vet J 62:109–112, 1985.

157. Lees GE, et al: A model of autosomal recessive Alport syndrome in English cocker spaniel dogs. Kidney Int 54:706–719, 1998.

158. Hood JC, et al: Bull terrier hereditary nephritis: A model for autosomal dominant Alport syndrome. Kidney Int 47:758–765, 1995.

159. Cosgrove D, et al: Collagen COL4A3 knockout: A mouse model for autosomal Alport syndrome. Genes Dev 10:2981–2992, 1996.

160. Miner JH, Sanes JR: Molecular and functional defects in kidneys of mice lacking collagen α3(IV): Implications for Alport syndrome. J Cell Biol 135:1403–1413, 1996.

161. Kalluri R, Cosgrove D: Assembly of type IV collagen. Insights from α3(IV) collagen-deficient mice. J Biol Chem 275:12719–12724, 2000.

162. Zeisberg M, Soubasakos MA, Kalluri R: Animal models of renal fibrosis. Methods Mol Med 117:261–272, 2005.

163. Gross O, et al: Preemptive ramipril therapy delays renal failure and reduces renal fibrosis in COL4A3-knockout mice with Alport syndrome. Kidney Int 63:438–446, 2003.

164. Cohen EP, Lemann J Jr: In hereditary nephritis angiotensin-converting enzyme inhibition decreases proteinuria and may slow the rate of progression. Am J Kidney Dis 27:199–203, 1996.

165. Proesmans W, Knockaert H, Trouet D: Enalapril in paediatric patients with Alport syndrome: 2 years' experience. Eur J Pediatr 159:430–433, 2000.

166. Proesmans W, Van Dyck M: Enalapril in children with Alport syndrome. Pediatr Nephrol 19:271–275, 2004.

167. Callis L, Vila A, Carrera M, Nieto J: Long-term effects of cyclosporine A in Alport's syndrome. Kidney Int 55:1051–1056, 1999.

168. Chen D, et al: Cyclosporine a slows the progressive renal disease of Alport syndrome X-linked hereditary nephritis: Results from a canine model. J Am Soc Nephrol 14:690–698, 2003.

169. Rao VH, et al: Increased expression of MMP-2, MMP-9 type IV collagenases/gelatinases, and MT1-MMP in canine X-linked Alport syndrome XLAS. Kidney Int 63:1736–1748, 2003.

170. Kashtan CE, McEnery PT, Tejani A, Stablein DM: Renal allograft survival according to primary diagnosis: A report of the North American Pediatric Renal Transplant Cooperative Study. Pediatr Nephrol 9:679–684, 1995.

171. Byrne MC, Budisavljevic MN, Fan Z, et al: Renal transplant in patients with Alport's syndrome. Am J Kidney Dis 39:769–775, 2002.

172. Kalluri R, et al: COL4A5 gene deletion and production of post-transplant anti-α3(IV) collagen alloantibodies in Alport syndrome. Kidney Int 45:721–726, 1994.

173. Charytan D, et al: Allograft rejection and glomerular basement membrane antibodies in Alport's syndrome. J Nephrol 17:431–435, 2004.

174. Fleming SJ, et al: Anti-glomerular basement membrane antibody-mediated nephritis complicating transplantation in a patient with Alport's syndrome. Transplantation 46:857–859, 1988.

175. Milliner DS, Pierides AM, Holley KE: Renal transplantation in Alport's syndrome: anti-glomerular basement membrane glomerulonephritis in the allograft. Mayo Clin Proc 57:35–43, 1982.

176. Rassoul Z, al-Khader AA, al-Sulaiman M, et al: Recurrent allograft antiglomerular basement membrane glomerulonephritis in a patient with Alport's syndrome. Am J Nephrol 10:73–76, 1990.

177. Kashtan CE, Butkowski RJ, Kleppel MM, et al: Posttransplant anti-glomerular basement membrane nephritis in related males with Alport syndrome. J Lab Clin Med 116:508–515, 1990.

178. Querin S, et al: Linear glomerular IgG fixation in renal allografts: Incidence and significance in Alport's syndrome. Clin Nephrol 25:134–140, 1986.

179. Rutgers A, et al: High affinity of anti-GBM antibodies from Goodpasture and transplanted Alport patients to α3(IV)NC1 collagen. Kidney Int 58:115–122, 2000.

180. Kalluri R, et al: A COL4A3 gene mutation and post-transplant anti-α3(IV) collagen alloantibodies in Alport syndrome. Kidney Int 47:1199–1204, 1995.

181. Kashtan CE, Rich SS, Michael AF, de Martinville B: Gene mapping in Alport families with different basement membrane antigenic phenotypes. Kidney Int 38:925–930, 1990.

182. Wang XP, et al: Distinct epitopes for anti-glomerular basement membrane Alport alloantibodies and Goodpasture autoantibodies within the noncollagenous domain of α3(IV) collagen: A Janus-faced antigen. J Am Soc Nephrol 16:3563–3571, 2005.

183. Hopfer H, et al: The importance of cell-mediated immunity in the course and severity of autoimmune anti-glomerular basement membrane disease in mice. FASEB J 17:860–868, 2003.

184. Kalluri R, Danoff TM, Okada H, Neilson EG: Susceptibility to anti-glomerular basement membrane disease and Goodpasture syndrome is linked to MHC class II genes and the emergence of T cell-mediated immunity in mice. J Clin Invest 100:2263–2275, 1997.

185. Sessa A, et al: Renal transplantation from living donor parents in two brothers with Alport syndrome. Can asymptomatic female carriers of the Alport gene be accepted as kidney donors? Nephron 70:106–109, 1995.

186. Imai E, Takabatake Y, Mizui M, Isaka Y: Gene therapy in renal diseases. Kidney Int 65:1551–1555, 2004.

187. Heikkila P, Parpala T, Lukkarinen O, et al: Adenovirus-mediated gene transfer into kidney glomeruli using an ex vivo and in vivo kidney perfusion system—First steps towards gene therapy of Alport syndrome. Gene Ther 3:21–27, 1996.

188. Sugimoto H, et al: Bone-marrow-derived stem cells repair basement membrane collagen defects and reverse genetic kidney disease. Proc Natl Acad Sci U S A 103:7321–7326, 2006.

189. Bailey AS, et al: Transplanted adult hematopoietic stems cells differentiate into functional endothelial cells. Blood 103:13–19, 2004.

190. Krause DS, et al: Multi-organ, multi-lineage engraftment by a single bone marrow-derived stem cell. Cell 105:369–377, 2001.

191. Orlic D, et al: Bone marrow cells regenerate infarcted myocardium. Nature 410:701–705, 2001.

Chapter 11

Nail-Patella Syndrome

Ralph Witzgall

The development of the mammalian kidney from two interacting tissues, the metanephrogenic mesenchyme and the ureteric bud, is ultimately reflected by the presence of two distinct, yet connected systems, the nephrons and the collecting ducts, respectively. The nephrons consist of a filtration unit, the glomerulus, and a subsequent processing portion, the tubule, which empties into the collecting duct. Although it is clearly established that podocytes, like the rest of the nephron, originate from the metanephrogenic mesenchyme, it is far from understood what mechanisms underlie podocyte development, structure, and function. What signal tells parietal cells and podocytes to separate and form Bowman's space, how does the podocyte orchestrate the formation of primary and foot processes and the interdigitation of the latter, how is the formation of the slit diaphragm regulated, and what molecules mediate the communication between podocytes and glomerular endothelial cells? Fortunately, the identification of genes mutated in patients suffering from hereditary kidney diseases and the increasing data from genetically modified animals have begun to unravel parts of the puzzle.

PATHOLOGIC FEATURES OF PATIENTS WITH NAIL-PATELLA SYNDROME

This chapter will deal with the nail-patella syndrome, a complex of symptoms also known as hereditary osteo-onychodysplasia (HOOD syndrome), Turner-Kieser syndrome, Fong disease, and Österreicher syndrome. Nail-patella syndrome occurs only rarely; its prevalence has been repeatedly quoted at 1 in 50,000, although this author is not aware of a published epidemiologic study from which this figure has been derived. As already indicated by its name, the syndrome has been christened after the malformed fingernails and toenails and the hypoplastic or even absent kneecaps; however, it is the renal disease that determines the prognosis of individuals with this disorder. Despite being one of the first hereditary diseases for which linkage to a polymorphic marker, in this case the ABO blood group, was established,[1] more than 40 years passed before mutations in the *LMX1B* gene were found to be responsible for nail-patella syndrome.[2–4]

The *LMX1B* gene encodes a transcription factor with two zinc-binding LIM domains at the NH_2-terminus, a DNA-binding homeodomain in the middle, and a putative activation domain at the COOH-terminus. Orthologous genes were first cloned as *Lmx1* in the chick[5,6] and as *Lmx1.2* in the hamster[7]; only later were the human (then called *LMX1.2*),[8] the murine,[9] and the *Xenopus laevis*[10] genes identified. The protein is produced in a variety of tissues, and in actuality *Lmx1b* first gained prominence because it is necessary to specify the dorsoventral axis in the limb.[5,6] A lack of Lmx1b leads to dorsoventral axis defects, which explains the nail and patella symptoms in those suffering from the disorder. Nail changes of variable severity can be noted in 98% of patients, with the thumbnail usually being the most severely or only affected nail.[11] Patellar symptoms have been noticed in 74% of the patients, and again the severity was quite variable.[11] One other pathognomonic sign is the growth of bone spurs on the posterior face of the iliac bone, so-called iliac horns, which was detected in approximately two-thirds of the patients.[11] Nail-patella syndrome can be associated with several other symptoms, of which only one in addition to the renal involvement will be mentioned here.[11] A careful analysis of the expression pattern of the murine *Lmx1b* gene has demonstrated the existence of the Lmx1b messenger RNA in the anterior segment of the eye.[12] This correlates well with the observation that 10% of patients with nail-patella syndrome present with open-angle glaucoma.[11]

Renal involvement, the first evidence of which was published in 1950,[13] determines the prognosis of patients with nail-patella syndrome. Symptoms may range from light to severe proteinuria, through hematuria, and finally to chronic renal failure. Several studies have addressed this issue, so that the frequency of renal symptoms, which may start shortly after birth or only after several decades, can be estimated at close to 40%.[11] The morphologic changes are most telling on an ultrastructural level and affect the glomerular basement membrane (GBM) and podocytes (Fig. 11-1). In the original reports, a thickened GBM was described that contained both electron-lucent areas[14,15] and fibrillar deposits resembling collagen.[14] Indeed their periodicity of 64 to 66 nm[16] is consistent with that of fibrillar collagen, although in one publication a periodicity of 40 to 60 nm was reported.[17] Furthermore, foot process effacement was observed for some but not all podocytes.[14,15] These first descriptions have been confirmed several times and are important diagnostic criteria.[16–21]

GENETIC FINDINGS AND BIOCHEMISTRY OF LMX1B

Back-to-back reports in 1998 established that nail-patella syndrome was caused by mutations in the *LMX1B* gene on human chromosome 9q34,[2,9] and additional reports in the same year confirmed this initial finding.[3,4] The human *LMX1B* gene consists of 8 exons and encodes a ≈7-kb messenger RNA, which apparently can be alternatively spliced[22] and therefore gives rise to a 395–amino acid[23a] and a 402–amino acid

which corrects the enzymatic defect before development of renal failure. Given the recent demonstration of the association between complete to near complete pyridoxine responsiveness and c.508G>A homozygosity (see Fig. 12-6), routine genotyping may help stratify PH1 patients with this genotype to kidney-alone transplantation.[63]

In PH2, because expression of the deficient protein (GRHPR) has been documented in body tissues other than liver, orthotopic liver transplantation is currently not recommended for management of patients with this subtype of primary hyperoxaluria. Similarly, until a specific causative metabolic defect is identified in patients with unclassified forms of marked hyperoxaluria, definitive therapy in the form of organ transplantation cannot be recommended.

Clinical trials of hepatocyte transplantation, in lieu of orthotopic liver transplantation, for management of liver failure and hepatic-based inborn errors (ornithine transcarbamylase and α_1-antitrypsin deficiencies and Crigler-Najjar syndrome type 1) have appeared since the early to mid-1990s.[124,125] In contrast to orthotopic liver transplantation, which requires removal of a nonfunctional native organ and replacement with a donated functional counterpart, the technique of hepatocyte transplantation, whether autologous or allogenic, makes use of the inherent capacity of liver cells to proliferate in response to a mitogenic stimulus. Although a refinement of this method—particularly as it pertains to induction of preferential growth of the transplanted cells over host hepatocytes—is still needed, Guha and colleagues recently showed successful, progressive engraftment of ex vivo–implanted hepatocytes in a mouse model of type 1 primary hyperoxaluria.[126]

FUTURE PROSPECTS

Although all of the strategies so far described are useful and have largely resulted in long-term therapeutic benefit for patients with primary hyperoxaluria, none is entirely satisfying or free of potential adverse effects. As such, continued investigation into alternative therapeutic strategies is critical for future management of affected patients.

Identification of measurable markers of disease severity and of variables influencing phenotypic expression in primary hyperoxaluria will be of invaluable significance to the field in upcoming years. In addition to detection of as-yet-unrecognized genetic modifiers of these monogenic disorders, systematic evaluation of other potential inherent age-dependent differences between patients, such as excretion of inhibitors of calcium oxalate crystal formation, will be important. A shift from hepatic enzyme analysis as the gold standard for definitive diagnosis of the primary hyperoxalurias to a molecular-based approach is well underway.

Pharmacogenomics, in particular, may modify the current standard of care of primary hyperoxaluria patients in the next decade, facilitating selection of therapies (VB6 and kidney-only vs liver-kidney transplant procedures) based on genotyping. For PH1 patients with AGT protein mistargeting and/or residual immunoreactive material, alternative therapies such as pharmacoperones for correction of the metabolic defect may also become feasible. Innovative and improved molecular-based therapeutic techniques show early promise. Hepatocyte transplantation as a means of ex vivo gene therapy is an emerging science with potential application to primary hyperoxaluria.

References

1. Van Acker KJ, Eyskens FJ, Espeel MF, et al: Hyperoxaluria with hyperglycoluria not due to alanine:glyoxylate aminotransferase defect: A novel type of primary hyperoxaluria. Kidney Int 50:1747–1752, 1996.
2. Monico CG, Persson M, Ford GC, et al: Potential mechanisms of marked hyperoxaluria not due to primary hyperoxaluria I or II. Kidney Int 62:392–400, 2002.
3. Kopp N, Leumann E: Changing pattern of primary hyperoxaluria in Switzerland. Nephrol Dial Transplant 10:2224–2227, 1995.
4. Latta K, Brodehl J: Primary hyperoxaluria type I. Eur J Pediatr 149:518–522, 1990.
5. Van Woerden CS, Groothoff JW, Wanders RJA, et al: Primary hyperoxaluria type 1 in The Netherlands: Prevalence and outcome. Nephrol Dial Transplant 18:273–279, 2003.
6. Cochat P, Deloraine A, Rotily M, et al: Epidemiology of primary hyperoxaluria type 1. Nephrol Dial Transplant 10:3–7, 1995.
7. Broyer M, Brunner FP, Brynger H, et al: Kidney transplantation in primary oxalosis: Data from the EDTA Registry. Nephrol Dial Transplant 5:332–336, 1990.
8. Saborio P, Scheinman JI: Transplantation for primary hyperoxaluria in the United States. Kidney Int 56:1994–1100, 1999.
9. Helin I: Primary hyperoxaluria. An analysis of 17 Scandinavian patients. Scand J Urol Nephrol 14:61–64, 1980.
10. Rinat C, Wanders RJA, Drukker A, et al: Primary hyperoxaluria type I: A model for multiple mutations in a monogenic disease within a distinct ethnic group. J Am Soc Nephrol 10:2352–2358, 1999.
11. Santana A, Salido E, Torres A, Shapiro LJ: Primary hyperoxaluria type 1 in the Canary Islands: A conformational disease due to I244T mutation in the P11L-containing alanine:glyoxylate aminotransferase. Proc Natl Acad Sci U S A 100:7277–7282, 2003.
12. Van Woerden CS, Groothoff JW, Wijburg FA, et al: Clinical implications of mutation analysis in primary hyperoxaluria type 1. Kidney Int 66:746–752, 2004.
13. Wong PN, Tong GM, Lo KY, et al: Primary hyperoxaluria: A rare but important cause of nephrolithiasis. Hong Kong Med J 8:202–206, 2002.
14. Yuen YP, Lai CK, Tong GM, et al: Novel mutations of the *AGXT* gene causing primary hyperoxaluria type 1. J Nephrol 17:436–440, 2004.
15. Coulter-Mackie MB, Tung A, Henderson HE, et al: The *AGT* gene in Africa: A distinctive minor allele haplotype, a polymorphism (V326I) and a novel PH1 mutation (A112D) in black Africans. Molecular Genet Metab 78:44–50, 2003.
16. Milliner, D., D. Wilson, et al: Phenotypic expression of primary hyperoxaluria: Comparative features of types I and II. Kidney Int 59:31–36, 2001.
17. Lieske JC, Monico CG, Holmes WS, et al: International Registry for Primary Hyperoxaluria. Am J Nephrol 25:290–296, 2005.
18. Hockaday TDR, Clayton JE, Frederick EW, Smith LH: Primary hyperoxaluria. Medicine 43:315–345, 1964.
19. Donne MA: Tableau de differents depots de matieres salines et de substance organizes qui se font les urines, presentant les caracteres propre a les dintinguer entre eux et a reconnaitre leure nature. CR Acad Sci 6:419, 1838.
20. Lepoutre C: Calculs multiple chez un enfant. Infiltration du parenchyme renal par des cristaux. J Urol 20:424, 1925.
21. Archer HE, Dormer AE, Scowen EF, Watts RWE: Primary hyperoxaluria. Lancet 273:320–322, 1957.

22. Frederick EW, Rabkin MT, Richie RH, Smith LH: Studies on primary hyperoxaluria. In vivo demonstration of a defect in glyoxylate metabolism. N Engl J Med 269:821–829, 1963.

23. Hockaday TDR, Clayton JE, Smith LH: The metabolic error in primary hyperoxaluria. Arch Dis Child 40:485–491, 1965.

24. Koch J, Stokstad EL, Williams HE, et al: Deficiency of 2-oxo-glutarate:glyoxylate carboligase activity in primary hyperoxaluria. Proc Natl Acad Sci U S A 57:1123–1129, 1967.

25. Danpure CJ, Jennings PR: Peroxisomal alanine:glyoxylate aminotransferase deficiency in primary hyperoxaluria type I. FEBS Lett 201:20, 1986.

26. Danpure CJ: Primary hyperoxaluria. In Scriver CR, Beaudet AL, Sly WS, et al (eds): The Molecular and Metabolic Bases of Inherited Disease. New York, McGraw-Hill, 2001, pp 3323–3367.

27. Baker PRS, Cramer SD, Kennedy M, et al: Glycolate and glyoxylate metabolism in HepG2 cells. Am J Physiol Cell Physiol 287:C1359–C1365, 2004.

28. Danpure CJ, Guttridge KM, Fryer P, et al: Subcellular distribution of hepatic alanine:glyoxylate aminotransferase in various mammalian species. J Cell Sci 97:669–678, 1990.

29. Coulter-Mackie MB, Rumsby G: Genetic heterogeneity in primary hyperoxaluria type 1: Impact on diagnosis. Mol Genet Metab 83:38–46, 2004.

30. Lumb MJ, Danpure CJ: Functional synergism between the most common polymorphism in human alanine:glyoxylate aminotransferase and four of the most common disease-causing mutations. J Biol Chem 275:36415–36422, 2000.

31. Coulter-Mackie MB: Preliminary evidence for ethnic differences in primary hyperoxaluria type 1 genotype. Am J Nephrol 25:264–268, 2005.

32. Purdue PE, Lumb MJ, Fox M, et al: Characterization and chromosomal mapping of a genomic clone encoding human alanine:glyoxylate aminotransferase. Genomics 10:34, 1991.

33. Purdue PE, Takada Y, Danpure CJ: Identification of mutations associated with peroxisome-to-mitochondrion mistargeting of alanine/glyoxylate aminotransferase in primary hyperoxaluria type 1. J Cell Biol 11:2341–2351, 1990.

34. Danpure CJ, Birdsey GM, Rumsby G, et al: Molecular characterization and clinical use of a polymorphic tandem repeat in an intron of the human alanine:glyoxylate aminotransferase gene. Hum Genet 94:55, 1994.

35. Tarn AC, Von Schnakenburg C, Rumsby G: Primary hyperoxaluria type 1: Diagnostic relevance of mutations and polymorphisms in the alanine:glyoxylate aminotransferase gene (AGXT). J Inher Metab Dis 20:689–696, 1997.

36. Noguchi T, Takada Y: Peroxisomal localization of alanine:glyoxylate aminotransferase in human liver. Arch Biochem Biophys 196:645–647, 1979.

37. Yokota S, Oda T, Ichiyama A: Immunocytochemical localization of serine-pyruvate aminotransferase in peroxisomes of the human liver parenchymal cells. Histochemistry 87:601–606, 1987.

38. Cooper PJ, Danpure CJ, Wise PJ, Guttridge KM: Immunocytochemical localization of human hepatic alanine:glyoxylate aminotransferase in control subjects and patients with type 1 primary hyperoxaluria. J Histochem Cytochem 36:1285–1294, 1988.

39. Motley A, Lumb MJ, Oatey PB, et al: Mammalian alanine/glyoxylate aminotransferase 1 is imported into peroxisomes via the PTS1 translocation pathway. Increased degeneracy and context specificity of the mammalian PTS1 motif and implications for the peroxisome-to-mitochondrion mistargeting of AGT in primary hyperoxaluria type 1. J Cell Biol 131:95–109, 1995.

40. Leiper JM, Oatey PB, Danpure CJ: Inhibition of alanine:glyoxylate aminotransferase 1 dimerization is a prerequisite for its peroxisome-to-mitochondrion mistargeting in primary hyperoxaluria type 1. J Cell Biol 135:939–951, 1996.

41. Zhang X, Roe SM, Pearl LH, Danpure CJ: Crystallization and preliminary crystallographic analysis of human alanine:glyoxylate aminotransferase and its polymorphic variants. Acta Crystallogr D Biol Chrystallogr 57:1936–1937, 2001.

42. Zhang X, Roe SM, Hou Y, et al: Crystal structure of alanine:glyoxylate aminotransferase and the relationship between genotype and enzymatic phenotype in primary hyperoxaluria type 1. J Mol Biol 331:643–652, 2003.

43. Takada Y, Kaneko N, Esumi H, et al: Human peroxisomal L-alanine:glyoxylate aminotransferase. Evolutionary loss of a mitochondrial targeting signal by point mutation of the initiation codon. Biochem J 268:517–520, 1990.

44. Danpure CJ: Molecular and clinical heterogeneity in primary hyperoxaluria type 1. Am J Kidney Dis 17:366–369, 1991.

45. Danpure CJ, Jennings PR, Fryer P, et al: Primary hyperoxaluria type 1: Genotypic and phenotypic heterogeneity. J Inher Metab Dis 17:487–499, 1994.

46. Danpure CJ, Jennings PR: Further studies on the activity and subcellular distribution of alanine:glyoxylate aminotransferase in the livers of patients with type 1 primary hyperoxaluria. Clin Sci 75:315, 1988.

47. Danpure CJ, Rumsby G: Enzymology and molecular genetics of primary hyperoxaluria type 1. Consequences for clinical management. In Khan SR (ed): Calcium Oxalate in Biological Systems. Boca Raton, FL, CRC Press, 1995, p 189.

48. Wilson DM, Smith LH, Erickson SB, et al: Renal oxalate handling in normal subjects and patients with idiopathic renal lithiasis: Primary and secondary hyperoxaluria. In Walker VR, Sutton RAL, Cameron ECB, et al (eds): Urolithiasis. New York, Plenum Press, 1989, p 453.

49. Hatch M. Freel RW: Alterations in intestinal transport of Oxalate in disease states. Scanning Microsc 9:1121–1126, 1995.

50. Hatch M. Freel RW: Intestinal transport of an obdurate anion: Oxalate. Urol Res 33:1–16, 2005.

51. Zarembski PM: Elevation of the concentration of plasma oxalic acid in renal failure. Nature 212:511–512, 1966.

52. Worcester EM, Nakagawa Y, Bushinsky DA, Coe FL: Evidence that serum calcium oxalate supersaturation is a consequence of oxalate retention in patients with chronic renal failure. J Clin Invest 77:1888–1896, 1986.

53. Leumann EP, Niederwieser A, Fanconi A: New aspects of infantile oxalosis. Pediatr Nephrol 1:531–535, 1987.

54. Fielder AR, Garner A, Chambers TL: Ophthalmic manifestations of primary oxalosis. Br J Ophthalmol 64:782–788, 1980.

55. Dunn HG: Oxalosis. Report of a case with review of the literature. Am J Dis Child 90:58–80, 1955.

56. Morgan SH, Purkiss P, Watts RWE, Mansell MA: Oxalate dynamics in chronic renal failure. Nephron 46:253–257, 1987.

57. Constable AR, Joekes AM, Kasidas GP, et al: Plasma level and renal clearance of oxalate in normal subjects and in patients with primary hyperoxaluria or chronic renal failure or both. Clin Sci 56:299–304, 1979.

58. Hoppe B, Langman CB: A United States survey on diagnosis, treatment, and outcome of primary hyperoxaluria. Pediatr Nephrol 18:986–991, 2003.

59. Katz A, Freese D, Danpure CJ, et al: Success of kidney transplantation in oxalosis is unrelated to residual hepatic enzyme activity. Kidney Int 42:1408–1411, 1992.

60. Hoppe B, Danpure CJ, Rumsby G, et al: A vertical (pseudodominant) pattern of inheritance in the autosomal recessive disease primary hyperoxaluria type 1: Lack of relationship between genotype, enzymic phenotype, and disease severity. Am J Kidney Dis 29:36–44, 1997.

61. Von Schnakenburg C, Hulton SA, Milford DV, et al: Variable presentation of primary hyperoxaluria type 1 in 2 patients homozygous for a novel combined deletion and insertion mutation in exon 8 of the AGXT gene. Nephron 78:485–488, 1998.

62. Amoroso A, Pirulli D, Florian F, et al: *AGXT* gene mutations and their influence on clinical heterogeneity of type 1 primary hyperoxaluria. J Am Soc Nephrol 12:2072–2079, 2001.

63. Monico CG, Rossetti S, Olson JB, Milliner DS: Pyridoxine effect in type I primary hyperoxaluria is associated with the most common mutant allele. Kidney Int 67:1704–1709, 2005.

64. Monico CG, Olson JB, Milliner DS: Implications of genotype and enzyme phenotype in pyridoxine response of patients with type I primary hyperoxaluria. Am J Nephrol 311:183–188, 2005.

65. Williams H, Smith LJ: L-glyceric aciduria. A new genetic variant of primary hyperoxaluria. N Engl J Med 278:233–239, 1968.

66. Chalmers RAB, Tracey M, et al: L-glyceric aciduria (primary hyperoxaluria type 2) in siblings in two unrelated families. J Inherit Metab Dis 2:133–134, 1984.

67. Dawkins P, Dickens F: The oxidation of D- and L-glycerate by rat liver. Biochem J 94:353, 1965.

68. Willis JE, Sallach HJ: Evidence for a mammalian D-glyceric acid dehydrogenase. J Biol Chem 237:910–915, 1962.

69. Van Schaftingen E, Draye JP, et al: Coenzyme specificity of mammalian liver D-glycerate dehydrogenase. Eur J Biochem 186:355–359, 1989.

70. Cregeen D, Rumsby G: Recent developments in our understanding of primary hyperoxaluria type 2. J Am Soc Nephrol 10:S348–S350, 1999.

71. Giafi CF, Rumsby G: Kinetic analysis and tissue distribution of human D-glycerate dehydrogenase/glyoxylate reductase and its relevance to the diagnosis of primary hyperoxaluria type 2. Ann Clin Biochem 35:104–109, 1998.

72. Rumsby G, Sharma A, et al: Primary hyperoxaluria type 2 without L-glycericaciduria: Is the disease under-diagnosed? Nephrol Dial Transplant 16:1697–1699, 2001.

73. Mdluli K, Booth MPS, Brady RL, Rumsby G: A preliminary account of the properties of recombinant human glyoxylate reductase (GRHPR), LDHA and LDHB with glyoxylate, and their potential roles in its metabolism. Biochim Biophys Acta 1753:209–216, 2005.

74. Cramer SD, Ferree PM, et al: The gene encoding hydroxypyruvate reductase (*GRHPR*) is mutated in patients with primary hyperoxaluria type II. Hum Mol Genet 8:2063–2069, 1999.

75. Rumsby G, Cregeen D: Identification and expression of a cDNA for human hydroxypyruvate/glyoxylate reductase. Biochim Biophys Acta 1446:383–388, 1999.

76. Cregeen DP, Williams EL, et al: Molecular analysis of the glyoxylate reductase (*GRHPR*) gene and description of mutations underlying primary hyperoxaluria type 2. Hum Mutat: Mutation in Brief Online No. 671 (2003); doi: 10.1002/humu.9200.

77. Bhat S, Williams EL, Rumsby G: Tissue differences in the expression of mutations and polymorphisms in the *GRHPR* gene and implications for diagnosis of primary hyperoxaluria type 2. Clin Chem 51:2423–2424, 2005.

78. Rumsby G, Williams E, Coulter-Mackie M: Evaluation of mutation screening as a first line test for the diagnosis of the primary hyperoxalurias. Kidney Int 66:959–963, 2004.

79. Webster K, Ferree P, et al: Identification of missense, nonsense and deletion mutations in the *GRHPR* gene in patients with primary hyperoxaluria type II (PH2). Hum Genet 107:176–185, 2000.

80. Mistry J, Danpure CJ, et al: Hepatic D-glycerate dehydrogenase and glyoxylate reductase deficiency in primary hyperoxaluria type 2. Biochem Soc Trans 16:626–627, 1988.

81. Behnam JT, Williams EL, Brink S, et al: Reconstruction of human hepatocyte glyoxylate metabolic pathways in stably transformed Chinese-hamster ovary cells. Biochem J 394(Pt 2):409–416, 2006.

82. Chlebeck PT, Milliner DS, et al: Long-term prognosis in primary hyperoxaluria type II (L-glyceric aciduria). Am J Kidney Dis 23:255–259, 1994.

83. Johnson SA, Rumsby G, et al: Primary hyperoxaluria type 2 in children. Pediatri Nephrol 17:597–601, 2002.

84. Kemper MJ, Muller Wiefel DE: Nephrocalcinosis in a patient with primary hyperoxaluria type 2. Pediatr Nephrol 10:442–444, 1996.

85. Milliner DS: The primary hyperoxalurias: An algorithm for diagnosis. Am J Nephrol 25:154–160, 2005.

86. Van Woerden C, Groothoff J, et al: Primary hyperoxaluria type 1 in The Netherlands: Prevalence and outcome. Nephrol Dial Transplant 18:273–279, 2003.

87. Milliner DS, Eickholt JT, Bergstrahl, EJ, et al: Results of long-term treatment with orthophosphate and pyridoxine in patients with primary hyperoxaluria. N Engl J Med 331:1553–1558, 1994.

88. Gibbs DA, Watts RWE: The variation of urinary oxalate excretion with age. J Lab Clin Med 73:901–908, 1969.

89. Danpure CJ, Jennings PR, et al: Fetal liver alanine:glyoxylate aminotransferase and the prenatal diagnosis of primary hyperoxaluria type 1. Prenat Diagn 9:271–281, 1989.

90. Rumsby G, Uttley WS, et al: First trimester diagnosis of primary hyperoxaluria type I (Letter). Lancet 344:1018, 1994.

91. von Schnakenburg C, Weir T, et al: Linkage of microsatellites to the *AGXT* gene on chromosome 2q37.3 and their role in prenatal diagnosis of primary hyperoxaluria type 1. Ann Hum Genet 61:365–368, 1997.

92. Smith LH, Fromm H, Hofmann AF: Acquired hyperoxaluria, nephrolithiasis, and intestinal disease. N Engl J Med 286:1371–1375, 1972.

93. Cryer PE, Garber AJ, Hoffsten P, et al: Renal failure after small intestinal bypass for obesity. Arch Intern Med 135(12):1610–1612, 1975.

94. Hassan I, Juncos LA, Milliner DS, et al: Chronic renal failure secondary to oxalate nephropathy: A preventable complication after jejunoileal bypass. Mayo Clin Proc 76:758–760, 2001.

95. Mole DR, Tomson CRV, Mortensen N, Winearls CG: Renal complications of jejuno-ileal bypass for obesity. Q J Med 94:69–77, 2001.

96. Kumar S, Sigmon D, Miller T, et al: A new model of nephrolithiasis involving tubular dysfunction/injury. J Urol 146(5):1384–1389, 1991.

97. Khan SR: Role of renal epithelial cells in the initiation of calcium oxalate stones. Nephron Exp Nephrol 98(2):e55–e60, 2004.

98. Khan SR: Crystal-induced inflammation of the kidneys: Results from human studies, animal models, and tissue-culture studies. Clin Exp Nephrol 8(2):75–88, 2004.

99. Jonassen JA, Kohjimoto Y, Scheid CR, Schmidt M: Oxalate toxicity in renal cells. Urol Res 33(5):329–339, 2005. Epub 2005 Nov 13.

100. Toblli JE, Cao G, Casas G, et al: NF-κB and chemokine-cytokine expression in renal tubulointerstitium in experimental hyperoxaluria. Role of the renin-angiotensin system. Urol Res 33:358–367, 2005.

101. Khan SR: Hyperoxaluria-induced oxidative stress and antioxidants for renal protection. Urol Res 33:349–357, 2005.

102. Lieske JC, Swift HS, Martin T, et al: Renal epithelial cells rapidly bind and internalize calcium oxalate monohydrate crystals. Proc Natl Acad Sci U S A 91:6987–6991, 1994.

103. DeWater R, Noordermeer C, Van der Kwast TH, et al: Calcium oxalate nephrolithiasis: Effect of renal crystal deposition on the cellular composition of the renal interstitium. Am J Kidney Dis 33:761–771, 1999.

104. Scheid CR, Cao LC, Honeyman T, Jonassen JA: How elevated oxalate can promote kidney stone disease: Changes at the surface and in the cytosol of renal cells that promote crystal adherence and growth. Front Biosci 9:797–808, 2004.

105. Kohjimoto Y, Kennington L, Scheid CR, Honeyman TW. Role of phospholipase A2 in the cytotoxic effects of oxalate in cultured renal epithelial cells. Kidney Int 56(4):1432–1441, 1999.
106. Kohjimoto Y, Honeyman TW, Jonassen J, et al: Phospholipase A2 mediates immediate early genes in cultured renal epithelial cells: Possible role of lysophospholipid. Kidney Int 58(2):638–646, 2000.
107. Huang HS, Ma MC, Chen CF, Chen J: Lipid peroxidation and its correlations with urinary levels of oxalate, citric acid, and osteopontin in patients with renal calcium oxalate stones. Urology 62(6):1123–1128, 2003.
108. Toblli JE, Ferder L, Stella I, et al: Protective role of enalapril for chronic tubulointerstitial lesions of hyperoxaluria. J Urol 166:275–280, 2001.
109. Turan T, van Harten JG, de Water R, et al: Is enalapril adequate for the prevention of renal tissue damage caused by unilateral ureteral obstruction and/or hyperoxaluria? Urol Res 31:212–217, 2003.
110. Toussaint C: Pyridoxine-responsive PH1: Treatment. J Nephrol 1:49–50, 1998.
111. Dent CE, Stamp TCB: Treatment of primary hyperoxaluria. Arch Dis Child 45:735–745, 1970.
112. Holmes RP, Assimos DG, Wilson DM, Milliner DS: (L)-2-oxothiazolidine-4-carboxylate in the treatment of primary hyperoxaluria type 1. BJU Int 88:858–862, 2001.
113. Solomons CC, Goodman SI, Riley CM: Calcium carbimide in the treatment of primary hyperoxaluria. N Engl J Med 276:207–210, 1967.
114. Scheinman JI, Voziyan PA, Belmont JM, et al: Pyridoxamine lowers oxalate excretion and kidney crystals in experimental hyperoxaluria: A potential therapy for primary hyperoxaluria. Urol Res 33:368–371, 2005.
115. Chetyrkin SV, Kim D, Belmont JM, et al: Pyridoxamine lowers kidney crystals in experimental hyperoxaluria: A potential therapy for primary hyperoxaluria. Kidney Int 67(1):53–60, 2005.
116. Hoppe B, von Unruh G, Laube N, et al: Oxalate degrading bacteria: New treatment option for patients with primary and secondary hyperoxaluria? Urol Res 33(5):372–375, 2005. Epub 2005 Nov 13.
117. Leumann E, Hoppe B, Neuhaus T, Blau N: Efficacy of oral citrate administration in primary hyperoxaluria. Nephrol Dial Transplant 10:14–16, 1995.
118. Leumann E, Hoppe B, Neuhaus T: Management of primary hyperoxaluria: Efficacy of oral citrate administration. Pediatr Nephrol 7:207–211, 1993.
119. Byer K, Khan SR: Citrate provides protection against oxalate and calcium oxalate crystal induced oxidative damage to renal epithelium. J Urol 173(2):640–646, 2005.
120. Watts RWE, Rolles K, Morgan SH, et al: Successful treatment of primary hyperoxaluria type I by combined hepatic and renal transplantation. Lancet 2:474–475, 1987.
121. Jamieson NV: The results of combined liver/kidney transplantation for primary hyperoxaluria (PH1) 1984–1997. The European PH1 transplant registry report. European PH1 Transplantation Study Group. J Nephrol 11(Suppl 1):36–41, 1998.
122. Nolkemper D, Kemper MJ, Burdelski M, et al: Long-term results of pre-emptive liver transplantation in primary hyperoxaluria type 1. Pediatr Transplant 4(3):177–181, 2000.
123. Kemper MJ, Nolkemper D, Rogiers X, et al: Preemptive liver transplantation in primary hyperoxaluria type 1: Timing and preliminary results. J Nephrol 11(Suppl 1):46–48, 1998.
124. Mito M, Kusano M, Kawaura Y: Hepatocyte transplantation in man. Transplant Proc 24(6):3052–3053, 1992.
125. Strom SC, Fisher RA, Thompson MT, et al: Hepatocyte transplantation as a bridge to orthotopic liver transplantation in terminal liver failure. Transplantation 63(4):559–569, 1997.
126. Guha C, Yamanouchi K, Jiang J, et al: Feasibility of hepatocyte transplantation-based therapies for primary hyperoxalurias. Am J Nephrol 25:161–170, 2005.

Chapter 13

Fabry Disease

James A. Shayman and Paul D. Killen

α-Galactosidase A deficiency was independently described in 1898 by two dermatologists, Anderson and Fabry, based on the presence of a characteristic skin lesion termed angiokeratoma corporis diffusum.[1] Subsequent descriptions of additional individuals revealed the presence of other clinical manifestations including anhidrosis, acroparasthesias, corneal opacities, corneal and retinal vascular abnormalities, and renal failure. These reports established Fabry disease as a systemic disorder. In 1965 Fabry disease was reported to be heritable as an X-linked recessive trait.[2]

Sweeley and Klionsky characterized Fabry disease as a sphingolipidosis by isolating globotriaosylceramide (also known as Gb3 or GL-3) and galabiosylceramide from the kidney of a Fabry hemizygote.[3] Blood group B and B1 antigenic glycosphingolipids containing α-galactosyl groups were subsequently also shown to accumulate in Fabry disease.[4] Brady and co-workers established the defect as one associated with ceramide trihexosidase.[5] Kint demonstrated the defect to be in an α-galactosyl hydrolase.[6] Two lysosomal enzymes hydrolyze α-galactosyl linkages (α-galactosidase A and B), but only the α-galactosidase A is defective in patients with the clinical syndrome of Fabry disease.

Fabry disease is rare. The true frequency of the disease has not been established. However, it is estimated that the incidence ranges from 1 in 40,000 to 1 in 117,000.[7] Thus, there are probably in excess of 6,000 affected individuals in the United States. Although most of the reported patients are Caucasian, affected individuals representative of most geographic and ethnic groups have been identified. The clinical expression of Fabry disease is thought to result from the progressive deposition of Gb3 in a variety of tissues, particularly the vascular endothelium. Affected individuals die prematurely, usually from cardiovascular catastrophes. However, Fabry disease is of particular interest to nephrologists because it is one of only two lysosomal storage disorders recognized to result in renal failure. (Cystinosis is the other storage disease.) With the recent use of recombinant α-galactosidase A as a therapeutic for the treatment of patients with this disorder, there has been an upsurge in interest in Fabry disease. Yet although the genetic basis and biochemistry of Fabry disease are well characterized, the pathogenesis of the disease is poorly understood.

CLINICAL FEATURES

The classic presentation of Fabry disease involves clinical manifestations resulting from vascular deposition of glycolipid in skin, peripheral nerves, heart, brain, and kidney. The onset of symptoms typically occurs in childhood or adolescence, and a consistent natural history is typical of affected homozygous males. Diagnostic features that are common in male children with Fabry disease include pain or numbness of the fingers and toes, telangiectasias on the ears and conjunctiva, corneal opacities, edematous eyelids, blue or black angiomatous macules or papules, and Raynaud's phenomenon. By early adulthood, affected males may exhibit extensive telangiectasias and angiokeratomas, edema, fever or heat collapse in association with anhidrosis, lymphadenopathy, and urinary abnormalities. The latter include albuminuria, hematuria, and oval fat bodies by urinalysis. By 30 years of age, affected males may develop cardiac disease in the form of conduction defects, mitral insufficiency, ischemia, or left ventricular hypertrophy. They may also have renal insufficiency and suffer from strokes. Historically, the average age at death for hemizygous males with classic Fabry disease is 41 years.[8] This is reflective of major morbid complications associated with glycolipid deposition in the vasculature of heart, brain, and kidney.

Heterozygous females show more variable clinical signs and symptoms. These may range from the absence of any overt disease to the full-blown clinical manifestations seen in hemizygous males. The time of presentation with females may be more variable as well, with symptoms appearing early in childhood or later in life. The variable clinical expression in heterozygous females is presumably due to random X chromosome inactivation.

Cardiac Disease

Cardiac complications in Fabry disease include cardiomyopathy, valvular disease, and conduction system abnormalities. Coronary artery disease is often considered to be part of the clinical syndrome of Fabry disease. However, few data exist in support of the view that Fabry disease patients are at increased risk for ischemic heart disease. The cardiomyopathy of Fabry disease is most commonly associated with left ventricular hypertrophy and may be seen in upwards of 90% of affected male patients. Unlike other infiltrative diseases such as amyloidosis, the hypertrophy of Fabry disease is associated with increased voltage by electrocardiogram. An explanation for this difference is that amyloidosis results in the interstitial accumulation of amyloid protein; by contrast, Fabry disease results in the intracellular accumulation of Gb3. The ventricular hypertrophy of Fabry disease can be so great as to resemble hypertrophic cardiomyopathy. In the later stages of the disease, the left ventricular hypertrophy leads to decreased end-diastolic volume, impaired diastolic filling, and decreased cardiac output.

Valvular disease is thought to result from glycolipid deposition and fibrosis of the valvular tissues. Mitral valve thickening and prolapse are commonly observed in younger patients. More obvious mitral valve abnormalities are observed in older patients including papillary muscle thickening and

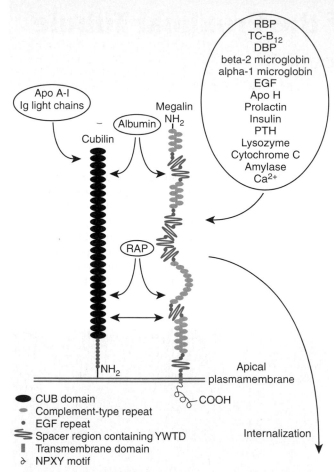

Figure 14-2 Cubilin and megalin are co-receptors for a number of filtered low molecular weight proteins. Cubilin is a peripheral membrane protein, whereas megalin is a transmembrane protein with 3 cytoplasmic NPXY motifs, directing the receptor into coated pits. A partial list of filtered ligands is shown, in addition to albumin and receptor-associated protein (RAP), which bind to both receptors. In addition, the binding of cubilin to megalin and the megalin-mediated internalization of the ligand-receptor-receptor complex are indicated. Apo, apolipoprotein; RBP, retinol-binding protein; TC, transcobalamin; DBP, vitamin D–binding protein; EGF, epidermal growth factor; PTH, parathyroid hormone. (From Christensen EI, Birn H: Megalin and cubilin: Synergistic endocytic receptors in renal proximal tubule. Am J Physiol Renal Physiol 280:F562–F573, 2001.)

nuclear factor 1a (HNF1a),[6] a transcription factor that functions in terminal differentiation of proximal tubule and other epithelial tissues. HNF1a plays a critical role in transcriptional activation of the Na^+-glucose cotransporter SGLT2,[7] with additional presumptive roles in the transcriptional regulation of other proximal tubular transport proteins.

At the posttranslational level, a number of scaffolding proteins play critical roles in the coordinated regulation of several apical and basolateral transport proteins. In particular, a family of scaffolding proteins that contain protein-protein interaction motifs known as PDZ domains, named for the *PSD95*, *Discs large* (Drosophila), and *ZO-1* proteins in which these domains were first discovered, functions in the regulated

clustering and trafficking of several critical transport proteins in the proximal nephron[8] (Fig. 14-3). The first of these proteins, NHE regulatory factor-1 (NHERF-1), was purified as a cellular factor required for the inhibition of NHE3 (Na^+-H^+ exchanger-3) by protein kinase A.[9] NHERF-2 was in turn cloned by yeast two-hybrid screens as a protein that interacts with the C terminus of the NHE3 protein; NHERF-1 and NHERF-2 have very similar effects on the regulation of NHE3 in cultured cells. The related protein PDZK1 interacts with NHE3 and a number of other epithelial transporters, including the apical urate exchanger URAT1.[10] A network of scaffolding proteins thus serves to coordinate the activity of multiple transporters at both the apical and basolateral membrane of the proximal tubule (see Fig. 14-3).

Aminoaciduria is a cardinal feature of Fanconi syndrome, and a critical regulatory factor for proximal tubular amino acid transport was recently identified.[11,12] Targeted deletion of the novel transmembrane protein collectrin thus results in profound overexcretion of multiple amino acids.[11,12] Collectrin is expressed at the apical membrane of proximal tubular cells, and brush border expression of several amino acid transporters is reduced in the kidneys of collectrin-deficient knockout mice. Moreover, co-expression of collectrin serves to activate amino acid transporters in heterologous expression systems. Notably, collectrin is a transcriptional target of HNF1a,[13] emphasizing the multitude of overlapping mechanisms whereby proximal tubular solute transport can be affected in Fanconi syndrome.

INHERITED CAUSES OF FANCONI SYNDROME

Cystinosis

Clinical Presentation and Diagnosis

Cystinosis is an autosomal-recessive disease characterized by the accumulation of cystine, the disulfide of cysteine, within lysosomes.[14] This disorder has an estimated incidence of 1 case per 100,000 to 200,000 live births,[15] and is the most common hereditary cause of Fanconi syndrome. Infantile or nephropathic cystinosis is the most common and severe form; patients typically present with renal tubular dysfunction within the first year of life.[15] "Juvenile" or "intermediate" cystinosis typically presents in adolescence and is characterized by lower intracellular cystine levels.[16] Renal impairment occurs much later and progresses more slowly; glomerular dysfunction predominates, and clinical manifestations of Fanconi syndrome are not a feature.[17] Patients with a third subtype, benign or ocular cystinosis, do not exhibit renal involvement, and present with photophobia in childhood or adulthood[18]; cystine crystals in these patients are restricted to the cornea, leukocytes, and bone marrow.[19]

Renal manifestations dominate the early clinical course of nephropathic cystinosis (Table 14-1). Common presenting symptoms include failure to thrive, polydipsia, and polyuria; initial evaluation can reveal a variety of electrolyte derangements (hypokalemia, hypouricemia, hypophosphatemia, etc.), in addition to a hyperchloremic metabolic acidosis from proximal tubular bicarbonate wasting. Patients with nephropathic cystinosis have a progressive, vasopressin-resistant renal concentrating defect,[20,21] with urine outputs of 2 to 6 L a day.[15]

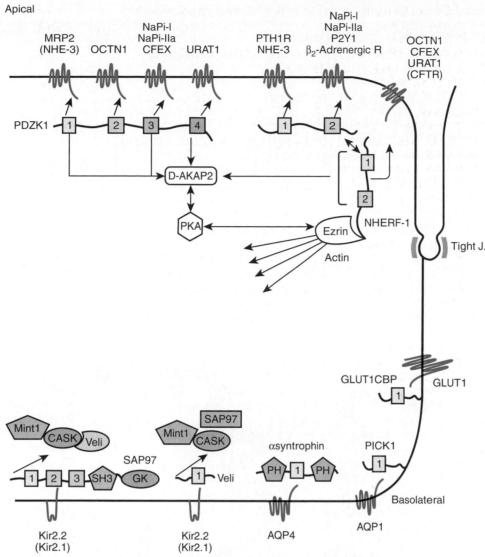

Figure 14-3 Interaction between apical and basolateral transporters expressed in proximal tubules with PDZ proteins. PDZ domains are represented as squares. Other protein-interacting domains are indicated as follows: SH3, Src homology 3 domain; GK, guanylate kinase-like domain; PH, pleckstrin homology domain; AQP, aquaporin; β_2-Adrenergic R, β_2-adrenergic receptor; CFEX, Slc26a6 anion exchanger; CFTR, cystic fibrosis transmembrane conductance regulator; D-AKAP2, dual kinase A anchoring protein 2; GLUT1CBP, GLUT1 C-terminal-binding protein; MRP, multidrug-resistance protein; NHE3, Na^+/H^+ exchanger 3; NHERF1, NHE3 regulatory factor-1; PICK1, protein that interacts with C-kinase; PKA, protein kinase A; PTH1R, parathyroid hormone receptor; SAP, synapse-associated protein; URAT, urate transporter. (From Hernando N, Wagner CA, Gisler SM, et al: PDZ proteins and proximal ion transport. Curr Opin Nephrol Hypertens 13:569–574, 2004.)

Several patients have been reported with hypokalemic alkalosis and marked increases in plasma renin activity and aldosterone, consistent with Bartter syndrome[22]; the concomitant Fanconi syndrome typically leads to the investigation and diagnosis of cystinosis.

Microdissected tubules from cystinotic kidneys classically demonstrate a "swan neck" lesion, due to atrophy of the early proximal tubule (Fig. 14-4). Serial biopsies in two young patients demonstrated the acquired nature of this lesion in cystinosis, which was preceded by lysosomal crystals and degenerative changes in the involved segment of the proximal tubule.[20] Development of the swan-neck lesion in these two patients coincided with marked worsening of the associated

Fanconi syndrome (Fig. 14-5). A more pathognomic finding is the presence of multinucleated podocytes in nephropathic cystinosis, which are exceedingly rare in other forms of renal disease.[23] Renal biopsy findings are otherwise relatively nonspecific, with varying degrees of tubulo-interstitial disease and glomerulosclerosis. Medullary nephrocalcinosis is relatively common[24]; however, only a few patients develop renal calculi, most likely due to their very dilute and alkaline urine.

Growth delay in nephropathic cystinosis is usually evident in the first year of life, prior to a decline in glomerular filtration rate (GFR).[25] This growth delay is attributed to multiple factors, including anorexia, chronic metabolic acidosis, and hypophosphatemic rickets secondary to phosphaturia. The

Table 14-1 Age-related Clinical Characteristics of Untreated Nephropathic Cystinosis

Age	Symptom or Sign	Prevalence in Affected Patients (%)
6–12 mo	Renal Fanconi syndrome (polyuria, polydipsia, electrolyte imbalance, dehydration, rickets, growth failure)	95
5–10 yr	Hypothyroidism	50
8–12 yr	Photophobia	50
8–12 yr	Chronic renal failure	95
12–40 yr	Myopathy, difficulty swallowing	20
13–40 yr	Retinal blindness	10–15
18–40 yr	Diabetes mellitus	5
18–40 yr	Male hypogonadism	70
21–40 yr	Pulmonary dysfunction	100
21–40 yr	Central nervous system calcifications	15
21–40 yr	Central nervous system symptomatic deterioration	2

From Gahl WA, Thoene JG, Schneider JA: Cystinosis. N Engl J Med 347:111–121, 2002.

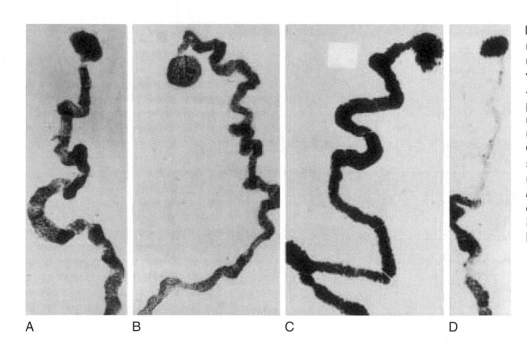

A   B   C   D

Figure 14-4 Microdissected nephrons from a healthy 5-month-old infant (**A**), a patient with nephropathic cystinosis at 5 months of age (**B**), a separate patient with nephropathic cystinosis at 6 months of age (**C**), and the patient from panel C, biopsied at age 14 months, showing the "swan-neck" deformity of cystinosis (**D**). (From Mahoney CP, Striker GE: Early development of the renal lesions in infantile cystinosis. Pediatr Nephrol 15:50–56, 2000.)

subsequent development of hypothyroidism and chronic renal disease further exacerbates growth failure in cystinosis.

Biochemical diagnosis of cystinosis can be accomplished by measuring leukocyte cystine content. Normal levels in leukocyte preparations are less than 0.2 nmol of half-cystine per milligram of protein; patients with nephropathic cystinosis exceed 2 nmol of half-cystine per milligram of protein.[26] Other clinical variants have intermediate levels of leukocyte or fibroblast cystine.[17] Notably, however, the use of purified polymorphonuclear leukocytes is required for the accurate detection of heterozygous carriers.[27] Cystine determinations from chorionic villus sampling can be exploited for diagnosis in utero[28]; alternatively, placental analysis at birth can make the diagnosis. Clinically, the presence of corneal crystals on slit-lamp examination is also diagnostic of cystinosis.[29]

In the absence of specific therapy for cystinosis (see Treatment section following), renal function will decline, with the development of end-stage renal disease occurring typically before 10 years of age.[30] Chronic dialysis is tolerated very well, and the disease does not recur in a transplanted kidney.[31,32] However, transplant recipients with cystinosis have progression of their primary disease in other organs affected by intralysosomal cystine accumulation. Corneal crystal deposits are absent at birth but develop very early in life, leading to photophobia and visual impairment. Deposits can also be found in the retina, with the development of a progressive retinopathy.[33] Other characteristic later complications include hypothyroidism from the destruction of the follicular cells of the thyroid[34,35]; a diffuse myopathy exhibited by distal skeletal muscle wasting,[36] a progressive dysphagia,[34,37] and restrictive

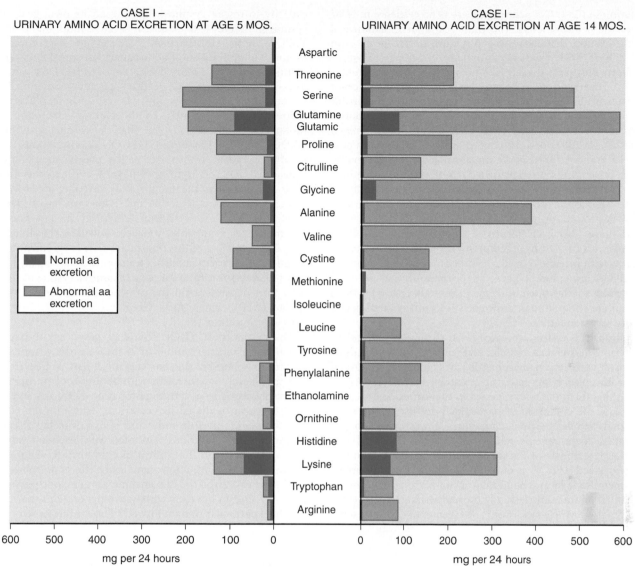

Figure 14-5 Progressive aminoaciduria in a patient with nephropathic cystinosis, measured at 5 months and 14 months of age. This is the same patient from panels B and D of Figure 14-4. (From Mahoney CP, Striker GE: Early development of the renal lesions in infantile cystinosis. Pediatr Nephrol 15:50–56, 2000.)

pulmonary disease[38]; primary hypogonadism in males[39]; pancreatic insufficiency, both endocrine and exocrine[40,41]; and cortical atrophy and central nervous system (CNS) deterioration.[42,43]

Cystine Transport and Cystinosin

Cystine accumulates within lysosomes of cystinotic leukocytes[14] and fibroblasts.[44] Chloroquine and other inhibitors of lysosomal protein degradation attenuate the re-accumulation of cystine in depleted cystinotic cells, indicating that intracellular protein degradation is the source of the excess cystine.[45] The cystine content of normal and cystinotic cells can also be increased by loading with cystine dimethyl ester[46] or cysteine-glutathione mixed disulfide[44]; notably, however, the egress of cystine from lysosomes is markedly impaired in cystine-loaded cystinotic cells.[44,46] Cystine efflux from cells derived from heterozygous carriers of the nephropathic cysti-

nosis gene is not significantly impaired when compared with wild-type cells.[44] However, measurement of cystine-cystine countertransport in lysosomal granules clearly demonstrates an absence in homozygous patients, with values for heterozygous carriers that are approximately one-half that of normal control cells[47]; defective lysosomal cystine transport is thus the causative defect in cystinosis.

The biochemical diagnosis of both patients[48] and heterozygous carriers[49] was critical to the fine mapping of the cystinosis gene on chromosome 17p13. A key breakthrough was the detection of genomic deletions for a linked microsatellite marker, followed by the identification of the CTNS gene within the minimum deletion interval.[50] The CTNS gene comprises 12 exons, encoding a 367–amino acid protein called cystinosin. Cystinosin consists of seven transmembrane domains, a 128–amino acid N terminus that contains seven glycosylation sites, and a 10–amino acid cytosolic C terminus. All patients with the various subtypes of cystinosis appear to have a mutation in the *CTNS* gene (i.e., there is no evidence thus far of genetic heterogeneity). The most common mutation is a 57-kb deletion that moves the 5′ region upstream of exon 10[51,52]; over 70% of patients with nephropathic cystinosis of northern European descent are homozygous for this mutation.[52–54] Bendavid and colleagues have developed fluorescence in situ hybridization probes for this large deletion, the first of its kind for a lysosomal storage disorder.[55] Separate putative founder effect mutations have been identified in French Canada[56] (W138X, of Irish origin) and in the Brittany province of France[57] (a splice-site mutation at the end of exon 8). One recurrent missense mutation (G339R) has been identified in two particular ethnic populations: two unrelated families of Amish-Mennonite descent and five unrelated families of Jewish-Moroccan origin.[58–61] An additional 50 mutations of *CTNS* have also been identified, including at least three patients with mutations in the promoter region of the gene.[62] Patients with juvenile or ocular cystinosis are homozygous for a "milder" mutation, typically a point mutation with no disruption to the open reading frame; alternatively, these patients are compound heterozygotes for a mild mutation and a more severe mutation.[17,59]

Cystinosin is widely expressed, with particularly abundant transcript in pancreas, muscle, and kidney.[50] Immunohistochemistry with anticystinosin antibodies[63] and transfection of cells with epitope-tagged complementary DNA (cDNA)[64,65] reveals that the protein is expressed in lysosomes. As expected, expression of cystinosin is particularly robust in the renal proximal tubule.[63] The localization of cystinosin to the lysosomal membrane is reliant on both a tyrosine-based GYDQL lysosomal sorting motif located on the C-terminal tail and on a YFPQA pentapeptide within the fifth intertransmembrane loop. The YFPQA motif is somewhat unique in that it is a rare example of a lysosomal sorting signal located outside the cytoplasmic tail.[64] It seems to exhibit some

capacity to rescue cystinosin sorting on its own, given that cystinosin mutant with an absent GYDQL motif but an intact YFPQA motif still partially localizes to lysosomes.[65] A minority of cystinosis mutations affect lysosomal targeting of cystinosin, due to primary disruption of the GYDQL motif or to as-yet-uncharacterized effects on secondary structure.[66]

Functional characterization of cystinosin exploited the redirection of the protein to the plasma membrane in a mutant, cystinosin-.GYDQL, that lacks the C-terminal GYDQL motif.[67] Cystinosin-.GYDQL thus functions as an H$^+$-driven cystine transporter at the plasma membrane of transfected cells. It is highly specific for L-cystine; other amino acids, in particular the monosulfide cysteine, are not substrates. Cystinosin is saturable and follows Michaelis-Menton kinetics, with a K_m for cystine of ~280 μM.[67] Inward transport is stimulated considerably by an acid-outside extracellular pH (Fig. 14-6); collapse of this transmembrane H$^+$ gradient by the addition of nigericin abolishes transport, consistent with H$^+$-cystine cotransport by cystinosin. Lysosomal cystine transport is in turn dependent on the presence of adenosine triphosphate (ATP), which fuels the lysosomal H$^+$-ATPase and drives cystine efflux (Fig. 14-7).[46,68,69]

The cystinosin-.GYDQL construct has been utilized for functional characterization of disease-associated missense mutations in cystinosin. For the most part, transport and clinical phenotypes correlate, with abolition of transport by mutations associated with nephropathic cystinosis and residual function mediated by constructs expressing mutations associated with juvenile and ocular subtypes of the disease.[66] However, some mutations associated with juvenile cystinosis abolish transport in the context of cystinosin-.GYDQL, suggesting that these mutations have lesser effects on full-length cystinosin expressed in lysosomal membranes; one possibility is that cystinosin interacts with lysosomal proteins that stabilize these particular mutant forms.[66] The converse also occurs,

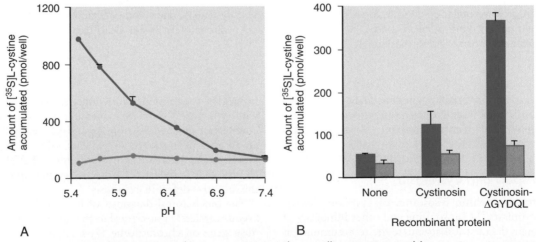

A

B

Figure 14-6 Effect of a transmembrane pH gradient on cystine uptake in cells expressing wild-type cystinosin protein or a mutant of cystinosin that traffics to the plasma membrane (cystinosin-.GYDQL, i.e., cystinosin-ΔGYDQL). **A,** [^{35}S]cystine uptake by mock-transfected (*light blue line*) and cystinosin-.GYDQL (*dark blue line*) expressing cells, as performed in uptake buffer adjusted to a pH ranging from 5.6 to 7.4. Cystinosin-mediated uptake increases with decreasing pH. **B,** Amount of [^{35}S]cystine accumulated by mock-transfected, cystinosin-expressing, and cystinosin-·GYDQL-expressing cells in an acidic extracellular medium (*dark blue*). The addition of 5 μM nigericin to the uptake media (*light blue*) abolishes [^{35}S]cystine uptake by cystinosin and cystinosin-.GYDQL, demonstrating the dependence of cystine transport on a proton gradient. (From Kalatzis V, Cherqui S, Antignac C, Gasnier B: Cystinosin, the protein defective in cystinosis, is a H(+)-driven lysosomal cystine transporter. EMBO J 20:5940–5949, 2001.)

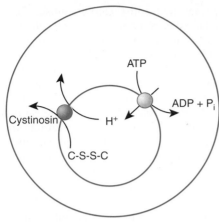

Figure 14-7 Chemiosmotic coupling between cystinosin and the lysosomal H+-ATPase. The interior of the lysosome (small grey circle) is acidified by a H+-ATPase present in its membrane. The efflux of cystine (C-S-S-C) from the lysosome by cystinosin, the lysosomal cystine transporter, is coupled to an efflux of H+; the influx of H+, mediated by the lysosomal H+-ATPase, drives cystinosin-mediated cystine transport to the cytoplasm. (From Kalatzis V, Cherqui S, Antignac C, Gasnier B: Cystinosin, the protein defective in cystinosis, is a H(+)-driven lysosomal cystine transporter. EMBO J 20:5940–5949, 2001.)

such that some nephropathic cystinosis mutations have minimal effect on transport mediated by cystinosin-.GYDQL.[66]

Targeted deletion of cystinosin in mice leads to cystine accumulation in multiple organs, including kidney.[70] Focal deposit of cystine crystals can be detected in several tissues, including within proximal tubule cells. However, these mice do not exhibit a proximal tubulopathy, which suggests that the accumulation of cystine crystals alone is not causative of disease.[70] However, ocular anomalies in cystinosin-deficient mice are very similar to patients with cystinosis. These animals thus develop corneal cystine crystal deposits and depigmented patches in their retina, indicative of a retinopathy.[70]

Cellular Pathophysiology

The proximal tubulopathy of nephropathic cystinosis dominates the early clinical manifestations of the disease. Notably, however, the pathophysiology of this cellular injury is not particularly clear, although it does not appear to directly involve or require cellular toxicity of cystine crystals. As noted above, for example, cystinosin-deficient knockout mice do not have a demonstrable renal phenotype, despite the presence of crystals within proximal tubular cells.[70] Several lines of evidence suggest that lysosomal accumulation of cystine is responsible for cell death and/or cellular dysfunction in the proximal tubule of patients with cystinosis. Intracellular cystine loading of perfused rabbit proximal tubules with cystine dimethyl ester (CME) reduces the tubular reabsorption of fluid, glucose, and bicarbonate.[71] Intraperitoneal injection of CME can also induce a Fanconi syndrome in rats, with marked polyuria, phosphaturia, and glucosuria.[72] Treatment with CME appears to induce respiratory dysfunction and reduced ATP generation in proximal tubular cells.[72–74]

However, despite a modest reduction in cellular ATP content, cystinotic fibroblasts do not have demonstrable defects in mitochondrial energy-generating capacity or Na+,K+-ATPase activity.[75] Cystinotic fibroblasts do, however, have an increased sensitivity to pro-apoptotic stimuli such as tumor necrosis factor-α (TNF-α); lysosomal loading of normal fibroblasts or proximal tubular epithelial cells with cystine (CME treatment) results in a comparable sensitivity.[76] Treatment of cystinotic cells with cysteamine reduces the observed sensitivity to pro-apoptotic stimuli, suggesting that lysosomal cystine accumulation is responsible for this cellular phenotype.[76] These findings have led to a re-appraisal of the role of lysosomes in apoptosis.[77] In particular, cystine accumulation appears to result in cysteinylation and activation of protein kinase Cδ (PKCδ), a pro-apoptic kinase; knockdown or pharmacologic inhibition of PKCδ attenuates apoptosis in cystinotic proximal tubular cells and fibroblasts.[78] A reduced sensitivity of murine PKCδ to cysteinylation has been speculated to underlie the lack of proximal tubulopathy in the cystinosin knockout mouse.[77]

Finally, cystinotic cells may have an increased sensitivity to oxidative injury. In particular, patients with nephropathic cystinosis excrete higher than usual amounts of pyroglutamic acid (5-oxoproline), suggesting depletion of glutathione, a major intracellular antioxidant.[79] Pyroglutamic acid and cysteine are major metabolites of the ATP-dependent γ-glutamyl cycle, which is reportedly more sensitive to ATP depletion and other stressors in cystinotic cells.[80] Modest reduction in cellular glutathione has been reported in some but not all studies of cystinotic cells.[81,82] However, increases in the ratio of oxidized glutathione disulfide (GSSG) to glutathione have been reported,[81] in addition to increases in the activity of superoxide dismutase[82]; both observations are consistent with increased oxidative stress in cystinotic cells.

Treatment

Supportive therapy is crucial in nephropathic cystinosis, particularly during infancy. The large fluid and electrolyte losses must be aggressively replenished. Treatment should thus include oral supplementation of bicarbonate and phosphate, along with oral vitamin D therapy. Indomethacin can be used in efforts to reduce high sodium and water losses.[83] Exogenous growth hormone can help restore normal growth rates.[84] Also, dysfunctions of other organ systems must be rectified, administering levothyroxine for hypothyroidism and testosterone for gonadal dysfunction. Patients with cystinosis often develop carnitine deficiency through the absence of carnitine reabsorption in the proximal tubule.[85] This is not unique to cystinosis; Fanconi syndrome of any etiology can lead to significant urinary carnitine loss.[86] Oral carnitine therapy can restore levels to normal in both serum and muscle.[87,88] Muscle lipid accumulation, characteristic of carnitine deficiency, also diminishes with therapy. Oral carnitine is very well tolerated. However, there is not yet any clear evidence demonstrating overt clinical improvements with such therapy.

Cysteamine is an aminothiol that facilitates depletion of lysosomal cystine.[89] It enters the lysosome through a specific transporter and reacts with cystine to form mixed disulfide cysteamine-cysteine molecules. These are then exported out of the lysosome through the lysosomal lysine transporter,[90]

Normal lysosome

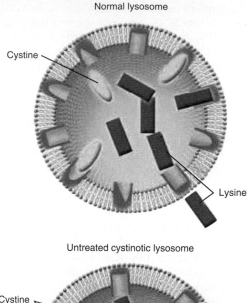

Untreated cystinotic lysosome

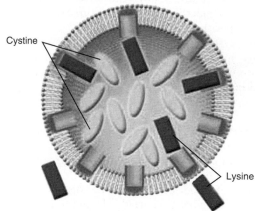

Cysteamine-treated cystinotic lysosome

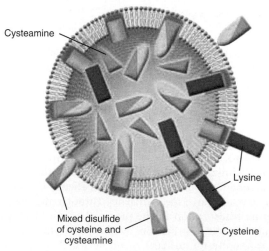

Figure 14-8 The mechanism of cystine depletion with cysteamine. **A,** In normal lysosomes, cystine and lysine are both transported across the lysosomal membrane. **B,** In cystinotic lysosomes, lysine is transported across the lysosomal membrane; cystine cannot cross the membrane, and accumulates inside the lysosome. **C,** In cysteamine-treated lysosomes, cysteamine combines with half-cystine (i.e., cysteine) to form the mixed disulfide cysteine-cysteamine, which exploits the lysine transporter to exit the lysosome. (From Gahl WA, Thoene JG, Schneider JA: Cystinosis. N Engl J Med 347:111–121, 2002.)

which is separate and distinct from cystinosin (Fig. 14-8). It is then reduced to cysteamine and cysteine by glutathione in the cytoplasm. The importance of early treatment with cysteamine cannot be emphasized enough; significant renal damage often has occurred by the time a diagnosis has been made, even at 1 year of age. Cysteamine therapy slows deterioration of renal function and improves linear growth. In a retrospective study by Markello and colleagues, cystinosis patients were divided according to the extent of cysteamine therapy they had received as children; early implementation and good compliance were strongly associated with a much slower rate of renal deterioration. More specifically, data from this study showed that each month of cysteamine therapy prior to 3 years of age preserved 14 months of subsequent renal function.[91] Compliance can be difficult, as cysteamine must be administered every 6 hours, and it has a distinct odor and taste. Capsules of cysteamine bitartrate are preferable to solutions, and the capsule contents can be dissolved for younger children. Corneal crystals do not respond to oral cysteamine therapy,[92] and necessitate the administration of cysteamine eye drops.[29,93] Again, with this and the many other extrarenal complications that these patients endure even after renal replacement therapy, life-long cysteamine administration is imperative.

Galactosemia

Galactosemia is an autosomal-recessive disorder caused by a deficiency in one of the primary enzymes involved in galactose metabolism. The most common subtype is the "transferase-deficient galactosemia," or "classic galactosemia," which is attributed to abnormal activity of the galactose-1-phosphate uridyl-transferase (GALT) enzyme, the second enzyme in the Leloir pathway. It has an approximate incidence of 1 in 60,000 live births. Infants consuming milk or formula containing lactose, the most common source of galactose (Fig. 14-9), accumulate galactose-1-phosphate and other metabolites,

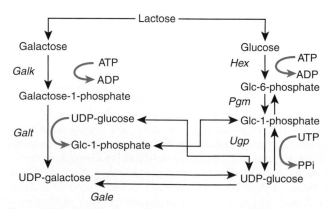

Figure 14-9 Metabolism of lactose; composite diagram of the Leloir pathway and uridine diphosphate (UDP)-glucose pyrophosphorylase pathway. *Galk,* galactokinase; *galt,* galactose-1-phosphate uridyltransferase; *Gale,* UDP-galactose 4-epimerase; *Hex,* hexokinase; *Pgm,* phosphoglucomutase; *Ugp,* UDP-glucose pyrophosphorylase. (From Leslie ND: Insights into the pathogenesis of galactosemia. Annu Rev Nutr 23:59–80, 2003.).

leading to cellular injury. The precise mechanisms of injury are still unclear.[94] Several pathways of carbohydrate metabolism are inhibited by galactose-1-phosphate, and defective protein and/or lipid galactosylation may also be a contributing factor.[95,96] Organs primarily affected include the liver, kidney (particularly the proximal tubule), ovaries, lens, and brain. The formation of galactitol from galactose, catalyzed by aldose reductase, appears to be responsible for cataract formation.[97] Proximal tubule dysfunction may be a direct effect of galactose itself.[98,99] However, galactokinase deficiency also disrupts galactose metabolism, without increasing levels of galactose-1-phosphate; notably, affected patients typically present only with cataracts, rarely pseudotumor cerebri, but not with renal disease.[100,101] Experimental galactosemia, induced by feeding rats a high-galactose diet, does lead to glomerular injury and proteinuria.[102] Ballooning of glomerular epithelial cells is observed in these models, along with glycation of the glomerular basement membrane.[102] Notably, glomerular filtration rates are elevated by experimental galactosuria, suggesting a hyperfiltration injury.[103]

Surprisingly, knockout mice deficient in GALT do not develop a phenotype. Tissues in these mice accumulate levels of galactose-1-phosphate, without much of an elevation in galactitol; combined elevation of both metabolites is conceivably required for organ damage in galactosemia due to GALT deficiency.[104]

Clinical Presentation and Diagnosis

Affected infants typically present with poor feeding, vomiting, diarrhea, and failure to thrive. If the diagnosis is not made early, many may quickly progress to develop jaundice, unconjugated hyperbilirubinemia, coagulopathy, and lethargy. Cataracts can appear within days of birth.[101] Continued lactose intake ultimately leads to hepatomegaly and cirrhosis, developmental delay, and mental retardation. Sepsis with *Escherichia coli* is classically associated with galactosemia[105]; this has been attributed to an inhibition of leukocyte bactericidal activity. Affected patients can develop aminoaciduria and proteinuria within days of birth. Of note, melituria in galactosemia is primarily a result of galactosuria, rather than glucosuria.

The presence of galactosuria is suggestive but not diagnostic of galactosemia; it can be seen in normal newborns or severe liver disease of any etiology. Erythrocyte transferase activity must be measured directly from erythrocytes to confirm the diagnosis.[106] Currently, most states include galactosemia testing as part of standard neonatal screening. The screening measures serum galactose-1-phosphate levels, and any anomalous results are confirmed by determining transferase enzyme activity.[107]

Molecular Genetics

The gene for GALT has been localized to chromosome 9p13.[108] Two common mutations have been identified, Q188R and K285N, accounting for approximately 60% to 70% of galactosemia mutants in patients of European descent.[109,110] Among black patients, a missense mutation, S135L, is prevalent.[111] To date, nearly 200 different mutations have been identified, making genetic confirmation testing difficult.

The Duarte variant, N314D, is a more benign mutation identified in 5% to 6% of the North American nongalac-tosemic population through newborn screening.[112] Homozygotes for this mutation have an approximate 50% reduction in GALT activity. These patients typically do not manifest any acute symptoms. However, Cramer and colleagues identified an increased risk for vaginal agenesis in women with the Duarte variant.[113] The mechanism of this effect is unclear, since more severe mutations do not produce a similar risk. In vitro studies show normal transcript levels for this mutation, with reduced stability and shortened half-life of the enzyme protein.[114] One other GALT enzyme, the Los Angeles (or D1) variant, has no effect on transcript levels, yet produces more GALT protein, resulting in increased enzyme activity.[115] This D1 variant has no associated phenotype.

Treatment

The elimination of galactose from the diet is essential for the resolution of acute symptoms. Hepatic and renal function improves, and cataracts will often regress. However, even with prompt and thorough dietary modifications, long-term sequelae, such as growth and developmental delay,[116] speech impairment,[117,118] and gonadal dysfunction (primarily in girls),[119,120] can develop.[121] These complications have been attributed to intrinsic galactose production or absent galactosylation of various lipids.[122,123] Hormone replacement therapy is often necessary to induce pubertal development and to prevent other complications of hypogonadism.[120,124] Growth hormone replacement can be effective; however, the hypogonadism must be addressed first.[120]

Tyrosinemia

Tyrosinemia (tyrosinemia type I, hepatorenal tyrosinemia) is an inborn error of metabolism affecting the liver, kidneys, and peripheral nerves. It has an estimated incidence of 1 in 100,000,[125] with clusters of increased incidence in Scandinavia and Quebec.[126] Notably, the name of this disorder is somewhat misleading. For one, the accumulation of tyrosine can be attributed to a variety of etiologies, including general liver dysfunction, hyperthyroidism, vitamin C deficiency, or even transiently in healthy newborns.[127–129] Additionally, tyrosine itself appears to have no direct hepatic or renal toxicity.

The primary defect in tyrosinemia is a deficiency in fumarylacetoacetate hydrolase (FAH), an enzyme expressed primarily in the liver and kidneys. This leads to the accumulation of several upstream metabolites, including fumarylacetoacetate (FAA), maleylacetoacetate (MAA), and their various derivatives, including succinylacetoacetate (SAA) (Fig. 14-10); these have been identified as the disease-causing agents in tyrosinemia. In particular, FAA has been shown to cause endoplasmic reticulum stress, genomic instability, and increased apoptosis.[130–132]

There are two other subtypes of genetic tyrosinemia.[125] Oculocutaneous tyrosinemia (tyrosinemia type II) presents with corneal thickening, developmental delay, and hyperkeratosis of the palms and soles.[133] Tyrosinemia type III, a primary deficiency of 4-hydroxy phenylpyruvate dioxygenase (HPD), an enzyme upstream of FAH, manifests with severe mental retardation and other neurologic disturbances.[134] Neither subtype is typically associated with hepatic or renal dysfunction. Finally, another variant is "transient tyrosinemia of the newborn"; not a true "metabolic error," this is caused by

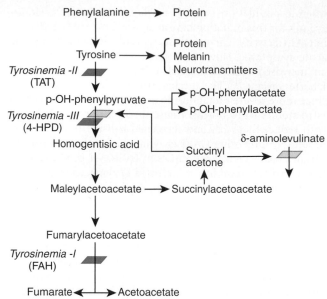

Figure 14-10 Tyrosine metabolism. The enzymes defective in different forms of tyrosinemia are indicated. TAT, tyrosine aminotransferase (tyrosinemia type II); 4-HPD, 4-hydroxyphenylpyruvic acid dioxygenase (tyrosinemia type III); FAH, fumarylacetoacetate hydrolase (tyrosinemia type I). (From Scott CR: The genetic tyrosinemias. Am J Med Genet C Semin Med Genet 142:121–126, 2006.)

a transient developmental deficiency in HPD. This was thought to be an entirely benign disorder since these children have no acute symptoms; however, on long-term follow-up, some of these children suffer from mild developmental delays and learning disorders.[135]

Clinical Features and Diagnosis

Symptoms of tyrosinemia can present in infancy, ranging from isolated clotting abnormalities with near-normal transaminases[136] to severe liver dysfunction; alternatively, the disease may be more chronic and indolent, with progressive cirrhosis and a high risk for the development of hepatocellular carcinoma. The malignancy risk has been attributed to the mutagenic properties of FAA.[130,132] Patients may also develop acute episodes of peripheral neuropathy and paresthesias, with eventual development of autonomic dysfunction. Renal involvement is almost universal. Proximal tubular function is most often affected, with resultant aminoaciduria, glycosuria, and hypophosphatemic rickets. However, these patients are also at risk for chronic kidney disease with progressive glomerulosclerosis, interstitial fibrosis, and eventual renal failure.[137–139] Bilateral nephromegaly and nephrocalcinosis are often observed on ultrasonography.[140]

Various other plasma biochemical markers are elevated in tyrosinemia, including tyrosine and methionine. Highly elevated levels of α-fetoprotein are often seen even prior to elevations of tyrosine,[141] but have a low specificity for diagnosis of tyrosinemia. However, the presence of succinylacetone (see Fig. 14-10) in the urine is diagnostic of tyrosinemia. FAH enzyme activity can also be directly measured in cultured skin fibroblasts to confirm the diagnosis.

Molecular Genetics and Renal Pathogenesis

FAH has been mapped to chromosome 15q23-q25.[142,143] Approximately 35 different mutations have been identified.[142–144] Prenatal diagnosis is possible through amniocentesis and genotyping of amniocytes or the measurement of FAH activity.[145] Amniotic succinylacetone levels may also be elevated. Notably, there is a considerable lack of a genotype to phenotype correlation in tyrosinemia. A wide range of clinical manifestations have been observed even within the same family. One possible explanation for this variance is the remarkable paradigm of spontaneous mutation reversion observed in tyrosinemia. Upon transplantation, livers of patients with tyrosinemia were found to have varying degrees of FAH activity. When stained for FAH, these livers were shown to be actual mosaics with patches positive for FAH.[146] Sequencing of these regions revealed them to be heterozygotic, with actual reversion of the original point mutation. The extent of this spontaneous reversion has been inversely correlated with the clinical severity of liver disease.[147]

Maleic acid, a derivative of MAA, and the structurally similar succinylacetone have been used to induce Fanconi syndrome in vivo.[148–150] Maleic acid has also been postulated to induce renin release through afferent arteriolar vasoconstriction, potentially resulting in chronic ischemic injury.[151] The use of knockout mice has provided elegant evidence for increased apoptosis of renal tubular cells in tyrosinemia. Targeted deletion of the murine FAH results in embryonic lethality, which is rescued by breeding with mice deficient in 4-hydroxy phenylpyruvate dioxygenase (HPD), the disease gene for type II tyrosinemia (see previous discussion of tyrosinemia subtypes). HPD catalyzes an earlier step in tyrosine metabolism (see Fig. 14-10), such that generation of FAA and other toxic metabolites is blocked in mice that are doubly deficient in FAH and HPD.[152] Renal tubular cells of these mice undergo rapid, massive apoptosis when treated with homogentisate, a precursor to FAA that is downstream of HPD (see Fig. 14-10). This is associated with development of renal impairment and a Fanconi syndrome.[152] Of interest, cellular evidence of apoptosis was blocked by caspase inhibitors, without an effect on renal tubular function.[152]

Treatment

Nutritional modifications with a low-phenylalanine and low-tyrosine diet have been shown to significantly improve renal tubule dysfunction in tyrosinemia.[153] However, the impact on hepatic function is less substantial. As a result, orthotopic liver transplantation was until recently the mainstay of long-term therapy for tyrosinemia, with good success.[140] Patients who undergo liver transplantation can show improvements in their renal function despite continued elevated urinary SA levels.[154,155] However, tubulopathy may still persist in other patients.[139] More recently, the use of nitisinone [2-(2nitro-4-trifluoromethylbenzoyl)-1,3cyclohexanedione] has diminished the need for transplantation. Its presumed mechanism is the inhibition of the 4-HPD, upstream of FAH, thereby reducing the accumulation of FAA and other toxic metabolites.[156,157]

Dent Disease

Mutations in the *CLCN5* gene, located on chromosome Xp11.22,[158] result in the clinical disease of X-linked hereditary nephrolithiasis. A total of four disease processes are caused by mutations in *CLCN5*: Dent disease, X-linked recessive nephrolithiasis (XRN), X-linked recessive hypophosphatemic rickets (XLRH), and idiopathic low-molecular-weight proteinuria of Japanese children (JILMWP). These disorders appear to reflect a phenotypic spectrum of one disease, grouped under the umbrella title of Dent disease. Common features include low-molecular-weight proteinuria, hypercalciuria, and nephrocalcinosis. In addition, patients with loss-of-function mutations in *CLCN5* all manifest some degree of proximal tubule dysfunction with aminoaciduria, phosphaturia, and glycosuria. Potassium wasting is also common. However, there are also distinct differences between these diseases: patients with Dent disease and XLRH develop rickets, not so with XRN and JILMWP. Renal failure is in turn a common finding only in Dent disease and XRN.

Genetic heterogeneity has recently been observed in Dent disease. In a study of 13 families whose male probands exhibited the clinical symptoms of Dent disease yet lacked mutations in *CLCN5*, five had mutations identified in the *ORCL1* gene (Xq25-Xq27.1). Mutations in *ORCL1* are typically associated with Lowe syndrome (see below). However, these patients did not exhibit any of the major clinical features of Lowe syndrome.[159] The identification of other disease-associated loci in Dent disease is sure to yield important insight into the pathophysiology of this intriguing disease.

Pathogenesis

CLCN5 encodes a chloride channel, ClC-5, part of a nine-member family of chloride channels involved in a wide variety of genetic diseases.[160] CLC-5 expression is renal-predominant,[161] with detectable protein in all subsegments of the proximal tubule, in thick ascending limb cells, and in type A intercalated cells of the collecting duct.[162–164] CLC-5 is predominantly an intracellular protein, as are the closely related paralogs CLC-3 and CLC-4.[165] However, there is sufficient expression at the plasma membrane to allow for functional characterization, in both *Xenopus* oocytes and HEK293 cells; CLC-4 and CLC-5 mediate outwardly rectifying anion currents in these cells, with a similar preference for $NO_3^- > Cl^- > I^-$.[166] A seminal observation in the biophysics of the CLC family was the demonstration that a bacterial paralog functions as an electrogenic $Cl-H^+$ exchanger, with an apparent stoichiometry of 2 Cl^- anions to 1 H^+.[167] Subsequent reports have revealed that CLC-4 and CLC-5 also function as electrogenic $Cl-H^+$ exchangers,[168,169] rather than as "pure" chloride channels. Regardless, genetic mutations associated with Dent disease significantly reduce or obliterate the chloride transport activity of CLC-5.[170–172]

Low-molecular-weight proteins pass through the glomerular filter and are reabsorbed by proximal tubule cells through endocytosis, followed by lysosomal degradation (Figs. 14-2 and 14-11). CLC-5 protein expression can be detected just

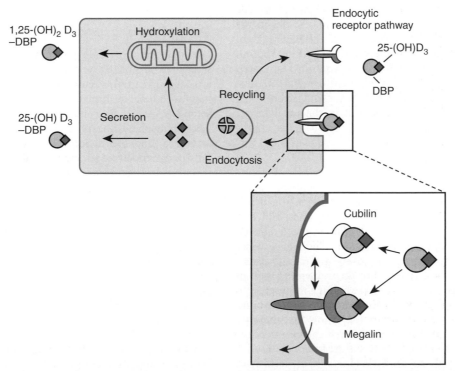

Figure 14-11 Megalin and cubilin function together in the proximal tubular uptake and activation of 25(OH)D₃ bound to vitamin D binding protein (DBP). Filtered 25(OH)D₃-DBP is endocytosed via the endocytic receptor pathway recognizing DBP. The complexes are delivered to lysosomes where DBP is degraded and 25(OH)D₃ is released to the cytosol; 25(OH)D₃ is either secreted or hydroxylated in the mitochandria to 1,25(OH)₂D₃, followed by release into the interstitial fluid and complex formation with DBP (*inset*). Cubilin facilitates the endocytic process by sequestering the steroid-carrier complex on the cell surface, prior to association with megalin and internalization of the cubilin-bound 25(OH)D₃-DBP. (From Nykjaer A, et al: Cubilin dysfunction causes abnormal metabolism of the steroid hormone 25(OH) vitamin D(3). Proc Natl Acad Sci U S A 98:13895–13900, 2001.)

below the apical brush border, where it colocalizes with H^+-ATPase in endosomal structures.[163] H^+-ATPase plays a key role in acidification of endosomes and lysosomes, and targeted deletion of mouse ClC-5 leads to an impairment in the acidification of early endosomes.[173] The chloride channel function of ClC-5 was initially thought to provide a charge dissipation to compensate for the buildup of H^+ in endosomes; however, this role is now considerably less clear, given that ClC-5 functions as a Cl—H^+ exchanger.[168,169] Regardless, it is clear that the endocytosis of low-molecular-weight proteins is reduced in the proximal tubule of ClC-5 knockout mice, with attenuation in the trafficking of both megalin and cubilin to the brush border.[5,174] This defect in endocytosis may be due to a loss of interactions between ClC-5 and cytoskeletal proteins such as cofilin,[175] and/or scaffolding proteins such as NHERF-1 and NHERF-2[176] (see Fig. 14-3).

The hypercalciuria and renal stones seen in Dent disease may also result from defective endocytosis, although in a more indirect manner. Parathyroid hormone (PTH) and vitamin D are filtered at the glomerulus and normally endocytosed in a megalin- and ClC-5-dependent manner. PTH is known to downregulate NaPi-2a, a proximal tubule transporter important for phosphate reabsorption. In ClC-5 knockout mice, urinary PTH concentrations are increased to about twice normal levels with normal serum levels and resultant hyperphosphaturia.[174] PTH also upregulates the enzymatic conversion of 25(OH)-vitamin D_3 to its active metabolite, 1,25(OH)$_2$-vitamin D_3, which can be elevated in patients with Dent disease.[177] The ensuing increase in intestinal calcium absorption potentially increases the calcium load filtered by the kidney, leading to hypercalciuria and stone formation. The two published strains of ClC-5 knockout mice differ in the presence[178] or absence[174] of hypercalciuria; the mouse strain with hypercalciuria has elevated levels of 1,25(OH)$_2$-vitamin D_3,[179] underlining the potential role of vitamin D–induced hypercalciuria. Moreover, the development of renal failure is unique to the hypercalciuric ClC-5 knockout strain,[178,179] emphasizing the role of hypercalciuria in the renal failure associated with Dent disease.

Clinical Presentation and Treatment

As described above, there is a considerable phenotypic spectrum in Dent disease (Table 14-2); however, all patients manifest some degree of proximal tubulopathy, and fluid and electrolyte loss can be significant. In addition to affected males, female carriers can develop proteinuria, albeit to a lesser degree.[180] Children may develop rickets and adults osteomalacia. Renal stone disease is a chronic problem, present in up to 50% of affected males and severe enough to progress to renal failure.[181] End-stage renal failure tends to occur around the fifth decade of life. Renal pathology shows a pattern of chronic interstitial nephritis, with scattered calcium deposits and prominent tubular atrophy with diffuse inflammation.[182]

Treatment is largely supportive. Fluids and electrolytes must be replenished, with generous intake of fluid to mitigate the high risk for stone disease. Thiazide diuretics can be used to reduce the hypercalciuria associated with Dent disease.[183] Notably, a high-citrate diet preserved renal function and slowed progression of renal disease in the hypercalciuric strain of ClC-5 knockout mice[179]; this intriguing strategy has yet to be extended to human patients.

Table 14-2 Clinical Features in 15 Patients with Dent Disease

Low-molecular-weight proteinuria	100%
Albuminuria	100%
Aminoaciduria	100%
Glucosuria*	8/15
Hypercalciuria†	12/13
Reduced clearance of creatinine or raised serum creatinine	11/15
Reduced concentrating capacity	9/9
Acidification defect	7/14
Nephrocalcinosis	11/15
Renal stones	8/15
Rickets	6/15
Hypokalemia (≤3.5) in patients with normal glomerular filtration rate	2/4

*No transport maximum performed, no high-performance liquid chromatography analysis.
†Excluding one patient with terminal renal failure.
From Ludwig M, Utsch B, Monnens LA: Recent advances in understanding the clinical and genetic heterogeneity of Dent's disease. Nephrol Dial Transplant 21:2708–2717, 2006.

Oculocerebrorenal Syndrome of Lowe

The oculocerebrorenal syndrome of Lowe (OCRL, Lowe syndrome) is an X-linked recessive syndrome characterized by a triad of symptoms: congenital cataracts, cognitive impairment, and renal dysfunction. It is linked to a gene on chromosome Xq24-q26, which encodes ORCL1, a phosphotidylinositol 4,5-bisphosphate phosphatase.[184,185] ORCL1 is ubiquitously expressed, and the molecular mechanism of disease is not fully understood (see review[186]). ORCL1 localizes to the Golgi complex and is thought to be involved with protein trafficking. This may lead to disruption of cell polarization, particularly important in renal tubules and the cornea, explaining perhaps the symptom cluster. Additionally, patients with Lowe syndrome often have lower urinary levels of megalin; this is attributed to defective recycling in a mechanism similar to Dent disease.[4]

Clinical Features

As its name indicates, symptoms in this syndrome are largely restricted to the eye, nervous system, and kidney. Cataracts are usually identified at birth,[187] and patients may also develop glaucoma and nystagmus. Mothers of patients with Lowe syndrome may also develop cataracts, in the absence of other symptoms of this disorder.[188] Although up to 25% of these patients may have low normal intelligence,[189] the large majority suffer from significant mental retardation and developmental delay. Infants will often present with areflexia and hypotonia and can develop a seizure disorder. Patients with loss-of-function mutations in ORCL1 have also been reported to exhibit features of Dent disease, without the major clinical features of Lowe syndrome.[159]

Renal function is typically normal at birth; however, by 1 year of age, proximal tubule dysfunction and proteinuria are nearly ubiquitous. Generalized aminoaciduria with sparing of branched-chain amino acids is characteristic of Lowe syndrome.[190] Glycosuria is variable and may be absent; phosphaturia typically progresses with age. Significant fluid and potassium losses are common in infancy. Proteinuria develops very early and may exceed 1 g/m^2 body surface area/day[190]; this is believed to cause progressive renal disease, with a falling GFR, glomerulosclerosis, and renal failure by the fourth decade of life. Linear growth delay is very common, with development of hypophosphatemic rickets and osteopenia. Though uncommon, hypercalciuria and nephrocalcinosis have been reported[191]; however, this is conceivably a complication of calcium and vitamin D therapy.

Histologic changes in the kidney can occur very early; dilatation and atrophy of proximal tubule cells have been seen in patients at just a few months of age.[192] Over time, patients develop thickening of the glomerular basement membranes and fusion of foot processes, glomerular hypercellularity, and glomerular and interstitial fibrosis.[193]

Diagnosis and Treatment

Although most patients have elevated creatine kinase, lactate dehydrogenase, and total serum protein,[190] no single laboratory evaluation or pattern is specific for the diagnosis of Lowe syndrome. Diagnosis is generally clinical, based on the patient's constellation of symptoms. Treatment is symptomatic and supportive. Electrolyte, bicarbonate, and vitamin D supplementation is required. Most children have their cataracts removed during infancy.[187] Antiepileptics are commonly administered, and developmental therapies should be implemented early. Progressive renal disease exerts the biggest influence on morbidity and mortality in this disorder.

Wilson's Disease

Wilson's disease (hepatolenticular degeneration) is a disorder of copper metabolism. It is caused by a mutation of the gene *ATP7B*, located on chromosome 13,[194,195] which encodes an ATPase copper-transporting polypeptide expressed primarily in the liver. The disease is inherited in an autosomal-recessive fashion with an estimated incidence of 1 in 30,000. It is present worldwide, with over 200 different mutations identified thus far. This, in addition to the large size of the *ATP7B* gene (80 kb with 21 exons), makes genetic screening and diagnosis difficult.

Pathogenesis

Ingested copper is absorbed and stored in intestinal cells. It is later moved into circulation by copper-transporting ATPase1 (*ATP7A*), expressed on the membrane of enterocytes. Bound to albumin, the copper is transported to hepatocytes where it is excreted into biliary canaliculi, which is regulated by *ATP7B*. *ATP7B* also facilitates the transfer of copper to apoceruloplasmin to form ceruloplasmin. In this form, copper is transported to peripheral organs. Mutations in *ATP7B* result in low ceruloplasmin levels and toxic accumulation of copper in hepatocytes. This leads to mitochondrial injury, cellular damage, and spillage of excess copper into the bloodstream, which overloads various end organs, such as the brain and kidney.

Clinical Features

The clinical presentation can be exceedingly varied, which presents a challenge to prompt and accurate diagnosis. Approximately 40% of patients present with hepatic disease, another 40% present with neuropsychiatric symptoms, and the remaining present with other organ system involvement. Liver involvement typically presents in adolescence.[196] It can show features of acute hepatitis, chronic liver disease, or fulminant hepatic failure. Symptoms can range from general malaise to jaundice and abdominal pain to hematemesis. Typically, the younger the age of presentation, the more progressive the liver disease, and orthotopic liver transplantation has been performed in patients with Wilson's disease during early childhood.[196]

Neurologic symptoms usually appear during the second or third decade of life but have been reported as late as 72 years of age.[197] As with liver involvement, presentation can be quite variable. A common presentation is with bulbar symptoms, including speech and swallowing difficulties and drooling. Cerebellar symptoms and parkinsonian features are also common. Psychiatric disturbances may be as mild as attention deficit/hyperactivity disorder and impulsivity, but may range to depression, paranoia, and psychosis.

Perhaps the most common sign of Wilson's disease is Kayser-Fleischer rings, seen around the periphery of the cornea, caused by copper deposition in Descernet's membrane. These rings are indicative of copper accumulation in the brain, so it follows that they are identified in nearly all patients with neuropsychiatric symptoms. However, they are present in only about 50% of patients without neurologic involvement.

Renal involvement is relatively common and usually precedes hepatic failure. Many patients exhibit signs of Fanconi syndrome with glycosuria, aminoaciduria, and hyperphosphaturia. Proteinuria and hematuria have been described but are less common.[198,199] Several cases of patients with Wilson's disease presenting with nephrolithiasis and hypercalciuria have been reported.[200–202]

Diagnosis

Laboratory confirmation of Wilson's disease can be elusive, leading to delayed diagnoses.[203] Ceruloplasmin is often described as a hallmark of Wilson's disease. However, it is an acute-phase reactant and therefore may be falsely elevated. Additionally, a low ceruloplasmin can be seen in Menkes' disease (a mutation in *ATP7A*), celiac disease, and significant liver disease of any etiology. A 24-hour urinary copper measurement can be very reliable if performed correctly.[204] It is typically quite elevated in Wilson's disease, often in excess of 100 µg per day, compared to 20 to 50 µg per day in normal individuals. Free copper in serum is also often elevated and can be helpful in cases where ceruloplasmin is falsely elevated. Copper content of hepatocytes can be measured directly after liver biopsy. However, patients often suffer from coagulation disturbances, contraindicating a biopsy, and the sensitivity of

Table 14-4 Uncharacterized and Specific Aminoacidurias

	Gene Defect	Locus	Amino Acids Affected	Inheritance	Clinical Manifestations	Organs Involved	References
Isolated cystinuria	Unknown	Unknown	Cystine	AR	Benign	Kidney	331
Hyperdibasic aminoaciduria type 1	Unknown	Unknown	Lysine, arginine, ornithine	AD	Mental retardation	Kidney, intestines	332,333
Isolated lysinuria	Unknown	Unknown	Lysine	AR	Failure to thrive, seizures, mental retardation	Kidney, intestines	334
Methioninuria	Unknown	Unknown	Methionine	AR	Edema, seizures, mental retardation	Kidney, intestine	335,336
Histidinuria	Unknown	Unknown	Histidine	AR	Mental retardation	Kidney, intestine	337–339
Iminoglycinuria	SLC6A20, SLC36A1, and SLC6A18(?)	3p21.3 5q33.1, 5p15(?)	Glycine, proline, hydroxyproline	AR	Benign	Kidney, intestine	340–343
Isolated glycinuria	Unknown	Unknown	Glycine	AR	Nephrolithiasis?	Kidney	344,345
Dicarboxylic aminoaciduria	EAAC1	9p24	Glutamate, aspartate	AR	Benign	Kidney, intestine	346,347

AR, autosomal recessive; AD, autosomal dominant; (?), unconfirmed candidate genes.

Cystinuria

Cystinuria is an inherited form of nephrolithiasis arising from the dysfunction of the proximal tubule reabsorption of cystine and other dibasic amino acids, such as ornithine, arginine, and lysine. Normally, only 1% of the filtered load of these amino acids is actually excreted in the urine; in classic cystinuria, the entire load filtered through the glomerulus is excreted, with no tubular reabsorption. As the cystine load moves to the acidic environment of the distal tubule, microcrystals can form and coalesce into larger stones.

Traditionally, cystinuria had been categorized into three subtypes. They all manifest the same phenotypes as homozygotes: very high levels of cystine in the urine with a very high risk of stone formation. However, the different subtypes can best be differentiated according to the phenotypes of their heterozygotes:

- Phenotype I (autosomal recessive): Ucystine less than 100 μmol/g creatinine
- Phenotype II (dominant): Ucystine greater than 1000 μmol/g creatinine
- Phenotype III (partially dominant): Ucystine = 100 to 1000 μmol/g creatinine

Two different genes have been identified as causative in cystinuria. In 1994, Pras and colleagues identified linkage between cystinuria type I and three genetic markers on chromosome 2p.[284] Later, Calonge and colleagues established SLC3A1 (rBAT) as the cystinuria gene.[285] They identified M467T as the most common causative mutation, preventing the trafficking of the protein to the plasma membrane. Although rBAT is expressed on the membrane surface, its topology of four transmembrane domains[286] made it an unlikely candidate for the primary amino acid transport protein.[287]

A few years later, a locus on chromosome 19q13 was also linked to cystinuria non-type I.[288,289] The gene SLC7A9 encodes a 12-transmembrane domain protein, part of a family of amino acid transporters.[290] Although their interaction is not entirely clear, rBAT appears to guide the transporter protein to the surface membrane and possibly activate it.[291] Therefore, SLC3A1 heterozygotes are able to maintain channel activity and normal tubular cystine uptake. In contrast, in cystinuria type II, even heterozygotes lose significant cystine transport function. The primary mutations here are in the SLC7A9 gene.[292,293] Type III heterozygotes have partial transport function; however, many similarly have defects in the SLC7A9 gene.[293] It is not clear why similar mutations cause different phenotypes. One proposal is a digenic mutation of both SLC3A1 and SLC7A9,[294,295] leading to a different classification system:

- Type A (type I): two mutations on SLC3A1
- Type B (type II): two mutations on SLC7A9
- Type AB (type III): one mutation on each SLC3A1 and SLC7A9

Notably, several haplotypes of SLC7A9 have been identified; the haplotype background of specific disease-associated mutations may influence the phenotype of SLC3A1 or SLC7A9 heterozygotes.[296] Scriver and colleagues have described a cohort of infants with elevated urinary cystine levels.[297] Within a year, the majority had reduced their cystine excretion to the level of their parents, many of whom were heterozygotes for cystinuria by phenotype. This entity has been termed transient neonatal cystinuria, and most of these infants are eventually classified as heterozygotes, most often for a mutant SLC7A9. Immaturity of rBAT expression limits cystine transport, exaggerating the cystinuria during early life in these patients.[298] In another clinical variant, a microdeletion of part of both the SLC3A1 and PREPL genes results in hypotonia-cystinuria syndrome. These patients present with generalized hypotonia at birth and go on to develop nephrolithiasis, growth hormone deficiency, and failure to thrive, followed by hyperphagia and rapid weight gain in later childhood. PREPL, or prolyl endopeptidase-like protein, although similar in structure to other serine peptidases, does not share any similar substrate specificity, and its precise function is yet unknown.[299]

Clinical Features and Diagnosis

The only clinical manifestation of cystinuria is nephrolithiasis and the complications thereof. Stones can first be seen in the first decade of life and account for up to 10% of stone disease in the pediatric population.[300,301] Although several amino acids are excreted in high concentrations, only cystine contributes to stone formation due to its insolubility, particularly in an acidic environment. Males tend to be more severely affected than females.[294] Renal biopsies of patients with cystine stones showed dilatation and blockage of the ducts of Bellini and inner medullary collecting ducts, which is associated with interstitial fibrosis and glomerular injury.[302]

The presence of hexagonal cystine crystals on urine microscopy is diagnostic of cystinuria. However, a more sensitive and definitive diagnostic evaluation is the direct measurement of urinary cystine, ideally from a 24-hour urine collection. Measurements of greater than 1,300 μmol/g creatinine are considered homozygous for a cystinuria mutation and mandate further evaluation.[303]

Treatment

The primary therapeutic goal is to minimize stone formation by promoting cystine solubility. First, patients are advised to adhere to a low-protein, low-sodium diet in efforts to diminish cystine production. Reduction in sodium excretion has been shown to reduce urinary cystine.[304] However, compliance can be difficult, and protein restriction is generally avoided in children due to concerns about their growth. Urine dilution and alkalinization are also crucial life-long interventions. Recommended fluid intake for an adult with cystinuria is 4 to 5 L per day, including nighttime intake to ensure continued diuresis overnight. Alkalizing beverages, such as herbal teas and citrus juices, are recommended. In addition, patients are often given potassium citrate to further promote urine alkalinization.

If these interventions are inadequate, chelating agents are recommended. D-Penicillamine and α-mercaptoproprionylglycine (MPG) are the two most widely used drugs. Both cleave cystine into two more soluble cysteine molecules, and both being sulfhydryl agents may cause frequent side effects,

including rash, thrombocytopenia, agranulocytosis, and significant proteinuria. MPG is generally better tolerated[305] and is perhaps the preferred drug for the treatment of cystinuria.

Even with good compliance with medical therapy in cystinuria, cystine stones may still form. Urologic intervention is commonly required; one study cited that by middle age, the average cystinuria patient will have undergone seven urologic procedures.[306] Shock-wave lithotripsy (SWL) can be effective if the stone is rather small, less than 1.5 cm.[307] Larger stones usually need more invasive procedures. Percutaneous nephrolithotomy (PNL) is still minimally invasive and is very effective.[308] Even larger, branched stones can very often be managed with a combination of PNL and SWL. With the introduction of smaller instruments, PNL has become an equally viable option in the treatment of children.[309] Whereas surgical intervention does not alter the rate of recurrence, if patients are free of stones after intervention, they do have a longer time before recurrence.[308]

Lysinuric Protein Intolerance

Lysinuric protein intolerance (LPI) is a rare autosomal-recessive disorder caused by defective transport of cationic dibasic amino acids, specifically lysine, arginine, and ornithine. Of note, cystine transport is normal. Abnormal basolateral efflux in intestinal, hepatic, and renal tubular cells results in poor amino acid absorption and urinary wasting. The low levels of amino acids impair urea cycle function, resulting in defective protein metabolism and postprandial hyperammonemia. Typically, infants remain asymptomatic until they are weaned and can present with vomiting, diarrhea, and coma. Over time, patients develop a strong aversion to high-protein diets, and chronically have a delay in bone growth with osteoporosis and muscle hypotonia. The majority of LPI patients develop asymptomatic pulmonary manifestations on radiograph with a few developing significant respiratory insufficiency[310] and showing pulmonary alveolar proteinosis on autopsy.[311] Immunologic anomalies have been seen with LPI,[312,313] with reported association with systemic lupus erythematosus.[314,315]

The gene responsible for LPI, SLC7A7, has been localized to chromosome 14q11.[316,317] It encodes y+LAT-1, a 12-transmembrane domain protein, which acts as a light-chain subunit bound to 4F2hc by a disulfide bridge to form a heteromeric amino acid transporter. It is expressed at the basolateral membrane of epithelial cells in the kidney, small intestines, and lungs.

Patients with LPI are maintained on a moderate protein restriction and supplemented with citrulline. As a neutral amino acid, citrulline is transported by a different pathway and is readily taken up by the liver. It is converted to ornithine and arginine, allowing the urea cycle to function.[318,319] Some investigation has been made into lysine supplementation; although patients are able to tolerate oral lysine supplements with good response in their serum levels, the impact of such therapy on the course of their disease is still unclear.[320,321]

Hartnup Disease

Named for the family in which this disorder was first described,[322] Hartnup disease is a condition of excessive urinary losses of neutral amino acids, including alanine, asparagine, glutamine, histidine, isoleucine, leucine, methionine, phenylalanine, serine, threonine, tryptophan, tyrosine, and valine. Of note, glycine, cystine, dibasic, and imino acids are excreted normally. Inheritance is autosomal recessive, with an estimated prevalence of 1 in 26,000.[323] At the time of its initial description, Hartnup disease was thought to be a rare syndrome, with a pellagra-like rash, cerebellar ataxia, mental retardation, and growth delay. However, this disorder is now known to be one of the most common forms of hyperaminoaciduria, with the majority of affected patients remaining largely asymptomatic.[324,325] Patients become symptomatic due to a cluster of factors[326,327]: diet, environment, and perhaps some host-specific variables. Patients can usually maintain normal serum amino acid levels through dietary replenishment, and lower plasma amino acid levels do seem to correlate with the onset and severity of symptoms.[327] Certainly in any patient with a pellagra-like rash and neurologic symptoms, Hartnup disease should be considered.

The gene responsible for Hartnup disease, *SLC6A19,* has been localized to chromosome 5p15.[328,329] The protein product of *SLC6A19* is a neutral amino acid transporter expressed primarily in the small intestines and in the kidney. To date, at least 10 different mutations have been identified in the *SLC6A19* gene, including one in the original Hartnup family.[330] Diagnosis is made from a urinary aminogram; normal excretion of proline and cystine serve to differentiate Hartnup disease from Fanconi syndrome. Treatment consists of the administration of nicotinamide; nicotinamide is derived from tryptophan, and deficiency results in the pellagra-like rash. It is unclear whether asymptomatic patients require nicotinamide supplementation; however, this treatment is relatively benign.

References

1. Igarashi T, et al: Mutations in *SLC4A4* cause permanent isolated proximal renal tubular acidosis with ocular abnormalities. Nat Genet 23:264–266, 1999.
2. Christensen EI, Gburek J: Protein reabsorption in renal proximal tubule-function and dysfunction in kidney pathophysiology. Pediatr Nephrol 19:714–721, 2004.
3. Leheste JR, et al: Megalin knockout mice as an animal model of low molecular weight proteinuria. Am J Pathol 155:1361–1370, 1999.
4. Norden AG, et al: Urinary megalin deficiency implicates abnormal tubular endocytic function in Fanconi syndrome. J Am Soc Nephrol 13:125–133, 2002.
5. Bacic D, et al: Impaired PTH-induced endocytotic down-regulation of the renal type IIa Na+/Pi-cotransporter in RAP-deficient mice with reduced megalin expression. Pflugers Arch 446:475–484, 2003.
6. Pontoglio M, et al: Hepatocyte nuclear factor 1 inactivation results in hepatic dysfunction, phenylketonuria, and renal Fanconi syndrome. Cell 84:575–585, 1996.
7. Pontoglio M, et al: HNF1alpha controls renal glucose reabsorption in mouse and man. EMBO Rep 1:359–365, 2000.
8. Hernando N, Wagner CA, Gisler SM, et al: PDZ proteins and proximal ion transport. Curr Opin Nephrol Hypertens 13:569–574, 2004.
9. Weinman EJ, Cunningham R, Shenolikar S: NHERF and regulation of the renal sodium-hydrogen exchanger NHE3. Pflugers Arch 450:137–144, 2005.
10. Anzai N, et al: The multivalent PDZ domain-containing protein PDZK1 regulates transport activity of renal urate-anion exchanger URAT1 via its C terminus. J Biol Chem 279:45942–45950, 2004.
11. Danilczyk U, et al: Essential role for collectrin in renal amino acid transport. Nature 444:1088–1091, 2006.
12. Malakauskas SM, et al: Aminoaciduria and altered renal expression of luminal amino acid transporters in mice lacking novel gene collectrin. Am J Physiol Renal Physiol 292:F533–F544, 2007.
13. Fukui K, et al: The HNF-1 target collectrin controls insulin exocytosis by SNARE complex formation. Cell Metab 2:373–384, 2005.
14. Schulman JD, Bradley KH, Seegmiller JE: Cystine: Compartmentalization within lysosomes in cystinotic leukocytes. Science 166:1152–1154, 1969.
15. Gahl WA, Thoene JG, Schneider JA: Cystinosis. N Engl J Med 347:111–121, 2002.
16. Goldman H, Scriver CR, Aaron K, et al: Adolescent cystinosis: Comparisons with infantile and adult forms. Pediatrics 47:979–988, 1971.
17. Thoene J, et al: Mutations of CTNS causing intermediate cystinosis. Mol Genet Metab 67:283–293, 1999.
18. Cogan DG, Kuwabara T, Kinoshita J, et al: Cystinosis in an adult. JAMA 164:394–396, 1957.
19. Anikster Y, et al: Ocular nonnephropathic cystinosis: Clinical, biochemical, and molecular correlations. Pediatr Res 47:17–23, 2000.
20. Mahoney CP, Striker GE: Early development of the renal lesions in infantile cystinosis. Pediatr Nephrol 15:50–56, 2000.
21. Holliday MA, Egan TJ, Morris CR, et al: Pitressin-resistant hyposthenuria in chronic renal disease. Am J Med 42:378–387, 1967.
22. Pennesi M, et al: A new mutation in two siblings with cystinosis presenting with Bartter syndrome. Pediatr Nephrol 20:217–219, 2005.
23. Bonsib SM, Horvath F Jr: Multinucleated podocytes in a child with nephrotic syndrome and Fanconi's syndrome: A unique clue to the diagnosis. Am J Kidney Dis 34:966–971, 1999.
24. Theodoropoulos DS, Shawker TH, Heinrichs C, Gahl WA: Medullary nephrocalcinosis in nephropathic cystinosis. Pediatr Nephrol 9:412–418, 1995.
25. Gahl WA, et al: Cysteamine therapy for children with nephropathic cystinosis. N Engl J Med 316:971–977, 1987.
26. Levtchenko E, et al: Comparison of cystine determination in mixed leukocytes vs polymorphonuclear leukocytes for diagnosis of cystinosis and monitoring of cysteamine therapy. Clin Chem 50:1686–1688, 2004.
27. Smolin LA, Clark KF, Schneider JA: An improved method for heterozygote detection of cystinosis, using polymorphonuclear leukocytes. Am J Hum Genet 41:266–275, 1987.
28. Jackson M, Young E: Prenatal diagnosis of cystinosis by quantitative measurement of cystine in chorionic villi and cultured cells. Prenat Diagn 25:1045–1047, 2005.
29. Gahl WA, Kuehl EM, Iwata F, et al: Corneal crystals in nephropathic cystinosis: Natural history and treatment with cysteamine eyedrops. Mol Genet Metab 71:100–120, 2000.
30. Gahl WA, Schneider JA, Thoene JG, Chesney R: Course of nephropathic cystinosis after age 10 years. J Pediatr 109:605–608, 1986.
31. Malekzadeh MH, et al: Cadaver renal transplantation in children with cystinosis. Am J Med 63:525–533, 1977.
32. Almond PS, et al: Renal transplantation for infantile cystinosis: Long-term follow-up. J Pediatr Surg 28:232–238, 1993.
33. Tsilou ET, et al: Nephropathic cystinosis: Posterior segment manifestations and effects of cysteamine therapy. Ophthalmology 113:1002–1009, 2006.
34. Geelen JM, Monnens LA, Levtchenko EN: Follow-up and treatment of adults with cystinosis in The Netherlands. Nephrol Dial Transplant 17:1766–1770, 2002.

35. Burke JR, El-Bishti MM, Maisey MN, Chantler C: Hypothyroidism in children with cystinosis. Arch Dis Child 53:947–951, 1978.

36. Vester U, Schubert M, Offner G, Brodehl J: Distal myopathy in nephropathic cystinosis. Pediatr Nephrol 14:36–38, 2000.

37. Sonies BC, Almajid P, Kleta R, et al: Swallowing dysfunction in 101 patients with nephropathic cystinosis: Benefit of long-term cysteamine therapy. Medicine (Baltimore) 84:137–146, 2005.

38. Anikster Y, et al: Pulmonary dysfunction in adults with nephropathic cystinosis. Chest 119:394–401, 2001.

39. Winkler L, Offner G, Krull F, Brodehl J: Growth and pubertal development in nephropathic cystinosis. Eur J Pediatr 152:244–249, 1993.

40. Fivush B, Flick JA, Gahl WA: Pancreatic exocrine insufficiency in a patient with nephropathic cystinosis. J Pediatr 112:49–51, 1988.

41. Fivush B, et al: Pancreatic endocrine insufficiency in posttransplant cystinosis. Am J Dis Child 141:1087–1089, 1987.

42. Vogel DG, et al: Central nervous system involvement in nephropathic cystinosis. J Neuropathol Exp Neurol 49:591–599, 1990.

43. Fink JK, et al: Neurologic complications in long-standing nephropathic cystinosis. Arch Neurol 46:543–548, 1989.

44. Jonas AJ, Greene AA, Smith ML, Schneider JA: Cystine accumulation and loss in normal, heterozygous, and cystinotic fibroblasts. Proc Natl Acad Sci U S A 79:4442–4445, 1982.

45. Thoene JG, Oshima RG, Ritchie DG, Schneider JA: Cystinotic fibroblasts accumulate cystine from intracellular protein degradation. Proc Natl Acad Sci U S A 74:4505–4507, 1977.

46. Gahl WA, Bashan N, Tietze F, et al: Cystine transport is defective in isolated leukocyte lysosomes from patients with cystinosis. Science 217:1263–1265, 1982.

47. Gahl WA, Bashan N, Tietze F, Schulman JD: Lysosomal cystine counter-transport in heterozygotes for cystinosis. Am J Hum Genet 36:277–282, 1984.

48. Cystinosis Collaborative Research Group: Linkage of the gene for cystinosis to markers on the short arm of chromosome 17. Nat Genet 10:246–248, 1995.

49. Jean G, et al: High-resolution mapping of the gene for cystinosis, using combined biochemical and linkage analysis. Am J Hum Genet 58:535–543, 1996.

50. Town M, et al: A novel gene encoding an integral membrane protein is mutated in nephropathic cystinosis. Nat Genet 18:319–324, 1998.

51. Touchman JW, et al: The genomic region encompassing the nephropathic cystinosis gene (CTNS): Complete sequencing of a 200-kb segment and discovery of a novel gene within the common cystinosis-causing deletion. Genome Res 10:165–173, 2000.

52. Forestier L, et al: Molecular characterization of CTNS deletions in nephropathic cystinosis: Development of a PCR-based detection assay. Am J Hum Genet 65:353–359, 1999.

53. Anikster Y, et al: Identification and detection of the common 65-kb deletion breakpoint in the nephropathic cystinosis gene (CTNS). Mol Genet Metab 66:111–116, 1999.

54. Heil SG, et al: The molecular basis of Dutch infantile nephropathic cystinosis. Nephron 89:50–55, 2001.

55. Bendavid C, et al: FISH diagnosis of the common 57-kb deletion in CTNS causing cystinosis. Hum Genet 115:510–514, 2004.

56. McGowan-Jordan J, et al: Molecular analysis of cystinosis: Probable Irish origin of the most common French Canadian mutation. Eur J Hum Genet 7:671–678, 1999.

57. Kalatzis V, et al: Characterization of a putative founder mutation that accounts for the high incidence of cystinosis in Brittany. J Am Soc Nephrol 12:2170–2174, 2001.

58. Shotelersuk V, et al: CTNS mutations in an American-based population of cystinosis patients. Am J Hum Genet 63:1352–1362, 1998.

59. Attard M, et al: Severity of phenotype in cystinosis varies with mutations in the CTNS gene: Predicted effect on the model of cystinosin. Hum Mol Genet 8:2507–2514, 1999.

60. Kalatzis V, et al: Identification of 14 novel CTNS mutations and characterization of seven splice site mutations associated with cystinosis. Hum Mutat 20:439–446, 2002.

61. Rupar CA, Matsell D, Surry S, Siu VA: G339R mutation in the CTNS gene is a common cause of nephropathic cystinosis in the south western Ontario Amish Mennonite population. J Med Genet 38:615–616, 2001.

62. Phornphutkul C, et al: The promoter of a lysosomal membrane transporter gene, CTNS, binds Sp-1, shares sequences with the promoter of an adjacent gene, CARKL, and causes cystinosis if mutated in a critical region. Am J Hum Genet 69:712–721, 2001.

63. Haq MR, et al: Immunolocalization of cystinosin, the protein defective in cystinosis. J Am Soc Nephrol 13:2046–2051, 2002.

64. Cherqui S, Kalatzis V, Trugnan G, Antignac C: The targeting of cystinosin to the lysosomal membrane requires a tyrosine-based signal and a novel sorting motif. J Biol Chem 276:13314–13321, 2001.

65. Helip-Wooley A, Park MA, Lemons RM, Thoene JG: Expression of CTNS alleles: Subcellular localization and aminoglycoside correction in vitro. Mol Genet Metab 75:128–133, 2002.

66. Kalatzis V, Nevo N, Cherqui S, et al: Molecular pathogenesis of cystinosis: Effect of CTNS mutations on the transport activity and subcellular localization of cystinosin. Hum Mol Genet 13:1361–1371, 2004.

67. Kalatzis V, Cherqui S, Antignac C, Gasnier B: Cystinosin, the protein defective in cystinosis, is a H(+)-driven lysosomal cystine transporter. EMBO J 20:5940–5949, 2001.

68. Greene AA, Clark KF, Smith ML, Schneider JA: Cystine exodus from normal leucocytes is stimulated by MgATP. Biochem J 246:547–549, 1987.

69. Jonas AJ, et al: Proton-translocating ATPase and lysosomal cystine transport. J Biol Chem 258:11727–11730, 1983.

70. Cherqui S, et al: Intralysosomal cystine accumulation in mice lacking cystinosin, the protein defective in cystinosis. Mol Cell Biol 22:7622–7632, 2002.

71. Salmon RF, Baum M: Intracellular cystine loading inhibits transport in the rabbit proximal convoluted tubule. J Clin Invest 85:340–344, 1990.

72. Ben-Nun A, Bashan N, Potashnik R, et al: Cystine loading induces Fanconi's syndrome in rats: In vivo and vesicle studies. Am J Physiol 265:F839–F844, 1993.

73. Coor C, Salmon RF, Quigley R, et al: Role of adenosine triphosphate (ATP) and NaK ATPase in the inhibition of proximal tubule transport with intracellular cystine loading. J Clin Invest 87:955–961, 1991.

74. Baum M: The Fanconi syndrome of cystinosis: Insights into the pathophysiology. Pediatr Nephrol 12:492–497, 1998.

75. Levtchenko EN, et al: Decreased intracellular ATP content and intact mitochondrial energy generating capacity in human cystinotic fibroblasts. Pediatr Res 59:287–292, 2006.

76. Park M, Helip-Wooley A, Thoene J: Lysosomal cystine storage augments apoptosis in cultured human fibroblasts and renal tubular epithelial cells. J Am Soc Nephrol 13:2878–2887, 2002.

77. Park MA, Thoene JG: Potential role of apoptosis in development of the cystinotic phenotype. Pediatr Nephrol 20:441–446, 2005.

78. Park MA, Pejovic V, Kerisit KG, et al: Increased apoptosis in cystinotic fibroblasts and renal proximal tubule epithelial cells results from cysteinylation of protein kinase Cdelta. J Am Soc Nephrol 17:3167–3175, 2006.

79. Rizzo C, et al: Pyroglutamic aciduria and nephropathic cystinosis. J Inherit Metab Dis 22:224–226, 1999.

80. Mannucci L, et al: Impaired activity of the gamma-glutamyl cycle in nephropathic cystinosis fibroblasts. Pediatr Res 59:332–335, 2006.

81. Levtchenko E, et al: Altered status of glutathione and its metabolites in cystinotic cells. Nephrol Dial Transplant 20:1828–1832, 2005.

82. Chol M, Nevo N, Cherqui S, et al: Glutathione precursors replenish decreased glutathione pool in cystinotic cell lines. Biochem Biophys Res Commun 324:231–235, 2004.

83. Haycock GB, Al-Dahhan J, Mak RH, Chantler C: Effect of indomethacin on clinical progress and renal function in cystinosis. Arch Dis Child 57:934–939, 1982.

84. Wuhl E, et al: Long-term treatment with growth hormone in short children with nephropathic cystinosis. J Pediatr 138:880–887, 2001.

85. Bernardini I, Rizzo WB, Dalakas M, et al: Plasma and muscle free carnitine deficiency due to renal Fanconi syndrome. J Clin Invest 75:1124–1130, 1985.

86. Steinmann B, Bachmann C, Colombo JP, Gitzelmann R: The renal handling of carnitine in patients with selective tubulopathy and with Fanconi syndrome. Pediatr Res 21:201–204, 1987.

87. Gahl WA, et al: Oral carnitine therapy in children with cystinosis and renal Fanconi syndrome. J Clin Invest 81:549–560, 1988.

88. Gahl WA, et al: Muscle carnitine repletion by long-term carnitine supplementation in nephropathic cystinosis. Pediatr Res 34:115–119, 1993.

89. Thoene JG, Oshima RG, Crawhall JC, et al: Cystinosis. Intracellular cystine depletion by aminothiols in vitro and in vivo. J Clin Invest 58:180–189, 1976.

90. Gahl WA, Tietze F, Butler JD, Schulman JD: Cysteamine depletes cystinotic leucocyte granular fractions of cystine by the mechanism of disulphide interchange. Biochem J 228:545–550, 1985.

91. Markello TC, Bernardini IM, Gahl WA: Improved renal function in children with cystinosis treated with cysteamine. N Engl J Med 328:1157–1162, 1993.

92. Cantani A, Giardini O, Ciarnella Cantani A: Nephropathic cystinosis: Ineffectiveness of cysteamine therapy for ocular changes. Am J Ophthalmol 95:713–714, 1983.

93. Bradbury JA, Danjoux JP, Voller J, et al: A randomised placebo-controlled trial of topical cysteamine therapy in patients with nephropathic cystinosis. Eye 5(Pt 6):755–760, 1991.

94. Fridovich-Keil JL: Galactosemia: The good, the bad, and the unknown. J Cell Physiol 209:701–705, 2006.

95. Charlwood J, Clayton P, Keir G, et al: Defective galactosylation of serum transferrin in galactosemia. Glycobiology 8:351–357, 1998.

96. Ornstein KS, McGuire EJ, Berry GT, et al: Abnormal galactosylation of complex carbohydrates in cultured fibroblasts from patients with galactose-1-phosphate uridyltransferase deficiency. Pediatr Res 31:508–511, 1992.

97. Ai Y, et al: A mouse model of galactose-induced cataracts. Hum Mol Genet 9:1821–1827, 2000.

98. Gitzelmann R, Curtius HC, Schneller I: Galactitol and galactose-1-phosphate in the lens of a galactosemic infant. Exp Eye Res 6:1–3, 1967.

99. Gabbay KH, Kinoshita JH: Mechanism of development and possible prevention of sugar cataracts. Isr J Med Sci 8:1557–1561, 1972.

100. Litman N, Kanter AI, Finberg L: Galactokinase deficiency presenting as pseudotumor cerebri. J Pediatr 86:410–412, 1975.

101. Colin J, Voyer M, Thomas D, et al: [Cataract due to galactokinase deficiency in a premature infant]. Arch Fr Pediatr 33:77–82, 1976.

102. Daniels BS, Hostetter TH: Functional and structural alterations of the glomerular permeability barrier in experimental galactosemia. Kidney Int 39:1104–1111, 1991.

103. Bank N, Coco M, Aynedjian HS: Galactose feeding causes glomerular hyperperfusion: Prevention by aldose reductase inhibition. Am J Physiol 256:F994–F999, 1989.

104. Ning C, et al: Galactose metabolism in mice with galactose-1-phosphate uridyltransferase deficiency: Sucklings and 7-week-old animals fed a high-galactose diet. Mol Genet Metab 72:306–315, 2001.

105. Levy HL, Sepe SJ, Shih VE, et al: Sepsis due to *Escherichia coli* in neonates with galactosemia. N Engl J Med 297:823–825, 1977.

106. Andersen MW, Williams VP, Helmer GR Jr, et al: Transferase-deficiency galactosemia: Evidence for the lack of a transferase protein in galactosemic red cells. Arch Biochem Biophys 222:326–331, 1983.

107. Levy HL, Cornier AS: Current approaches to genetic metabolic screening in newborns. Curr Opin Pediatr 6:707–711, 1994.

108. Shih LY, Suslak L, Rosin I, et al: Gene dosage studies supporting localization of the structural gene for galactose-1-phosphate uridyl transferase (GALT) to band p13 of chromosome 9. Am J Med Genet 19:539–543, 1984.

109. Leslie ND, et al: The human galactose-1-phosphate uridyltransferase gene. Genomics 14:474–480, 1992.

110. Tyfield L, et al: Classical galactosemia and mutations at the galactose-1-phosphate uridyl transferase (*GALT*) gene. Hum Mutat 13:417–430, 1999.

111. Lai K, Elsas LJ: Structure-function analyses of a common mutation in blacks with transferase-deficiency galactosemia. Mol Genet Metab 74:264–272, 2001.

112. Elsas LJ, et al: A common mutation associated with the Duarte galactosemia allele. Am J Hum Genet 54:1030–1036, 1994.

113. Menegazzi R, Busetto S, Dri P, et al: Chloride ion efflux regulates adherence, spreading, and respiratory burst of neutrophils stimulated by tumor necrosis factor-alpha (TNF) on biologic surfaces. J Cell Biol 135:511–522, 1996.

114. Fridovich-Keil JL, Quimby BB, Wells L, et al: Characterization of the N314D allele of human galactose-1-phosphate uridylyltransferase using a yeast expression system. Biochem Mol Med 56:121–130, 1995.

115. Langley SD, Lai K, Dembure PP, et al: Molecular basis for Duarte and Los Angeles variant galactosemia. Am J Hum Genet 60:366–372, 1997.

116. Panis B, Gerver WJ, Rubio-Gozalbo ME: Growth in treated classical galactosemia patients. Eur J Pediatr 166:443–446, 2006.

117. Webb AL, Singh RH, Kennedy MJ, Elsas LJ: Verbal dyspraxia and galactosemia. Pediatr Res 53:396–402, 2003.

118. Robertson A, Singh RH, Guerrero NV, et al: Outcomes analysis of verbal dyspraxia in classic galactosemia. Genet Med 2:142–148, 2000.

119. Kaufman FR, et al: Hypergonadotropic hypogonadism in female patients with galactosemia. N Engl J Med 304:994–998, 1981.

120. Zachmann M: Therapeutic indications for delayed puberty and hypogonadism in adolescent boys. Horm Res 36:141–146, 1991.

121. Schweitzer-Krantz S. Early diagnosis of inherited metabolic disorders towards improving outcome: The controversial issue of galactosaemia. Eur J Pediatr 162(Suppl 1):50–53, 2003.

122. Lebea PJ, Pretorius PJ: The molecular relationship between deficient UDP-galactose uridyl transferase (GALT) and ceramide galactosyltransferase (CGT) enzyme function: A possible cause for poor long-term prognosis in classic galactosemia. Med Hypotheses 65:1051–1057, 2005.

123. Petry K, et al: Characterization of a novel biochemical abnormality in galactosemia: Deficiency of glycolipids containing galactose or N-acetylgalactosamine and

accumulation of precursors in brain and lymphocytes. Biochem Med Metab Biol 46:93–104, 1991.

124. Forges T, Monnier-Barbarino P, Leheup B, Jouvet P: Pathophysiology of impaired ovarian function in galactosaemia. Hum Reprod Update 12:573–584, 2006.

125. Scott CR: The genetic tyrosinemias. Am J Med Genet C Semin Med Genet 142:121–126, 2006.

126. De Braekeleer M, Larochelle J: Genetic epidemiology of hereditary tyrosinemia in Quebec and in Saguenay-Lac-St-Jean. Am J Hum Genet 47:302–307, 1990.

127. Hou JW, Wang TR: Transient tyrosinemia presenting as lactic acidosis in a term baby: Report of one case. Zhonghua Min Guo Xiao Er Ke Yi Xue Hui Za Zhi 36:217–220, 1995.

128. Clow CL, Laberge C, Scriver CR: Neonatal hypertyrosinemia and evidence for deficiency of ascorbic acid in Arctic and subarctic peoples. Can Med Assoc J 113:624–626, 1975.

129. Kimura A, et al: Tyrosinemia type I–like disease: A possible manifestation of 3-oxo-delta 4-steroid 5 beta-reductase deficiency. Acta Paediatr Jpn 40:211–217, 1998.

130. Jorquera R, Tanguay RM: Fumarylacetoacetate, the metabolite accumulating in hereditary tyrosinemia, activates the ERK pathway and induces mitotic abnormalities and genomic instability. Hum Mol Genet 10:1741–1752, 2001.

131. Bergeron A, Jorquera R, Orejuela D, Tanguay RM: Involvement of endoplasmic reticulum stress in hereditary tyrosinemia type I. J Biol Chem 281:5329–5334, 2006.

132. Jorquera R, Tanguay RM: The mutagenicity of the tyrosine metabolite, fumarylacetoacetate, is enhanced by glutathione depletion. Biochem Biophys Res Commun 232:42–48, 1997.

133. Huhn R, et al: Novel and recurrent tyrosine aminotransferase gene mutations in tyrosinemia type II. Hum Genet 102:305–313, 1998.

134. Cerone R, et al: Tyrosinemia type III: Diagnosis and ten-year follow-up. Acta Paediatr 86:1013–1015, 1997.

135. Rice DN, et al: Transient neonatal tyrosinaemia. J Inherit Metab Dis 12:13–22, 1989.

136. Croffie JM, Gupta SK, Chong SK, Fitzgerald JF: Tyrosinemia type 1 should be suspected in infants with severe coagulopathy even in the absence of other signs of liver failure. Pediatrics 103:675–678, 1999.

137. Kvittingen EA, et al: Renal failure in adult patients with hereditary tyrosinaemia type I. J Inherit Metab Dis 14:53–62, 1991.

138. Russo P, O'Regan S: Visceral pathology of hereditary tyrosinemia type I. Am J Hum Genet 47:317–324, 1990.

139. Pierik LJ, van Spronsen FJ, Bijleveld CM, van Dael CM: Renal function in tyrosinaemia type I after liver transplantation: A long-term follow-up. J Inherit Metab Dis 28:871–876, 2005.

140. Paradis K, et al: Liver transplantation for hereditary tyrosinemia: The Quebec experience. Am J Hum Genet 47:338–342, 1990.

141. Pitkanen S, et al: Serum levels of oncofetal markers CA 125, CA 19-9, and alpha-fetoprotein in children with hereditary tyrosinemia type I. Pediatr Res 35:205–208, 1994.

142. Labelle Y, Phaneuf D, Leclerc B, Tanguay RM: Characterization of the human fumarylacetoacetate hydrolase gene and identification of a missense mutation abolishing enzymatic activity. Hum Mol Genet 2:941–946, 1993.

143. Phaneuf D, et al: Cloning and expression of the cDNA encoding human fumarylacetoacetate hydrolase, the enzyme deficient in hereditary tyrosinemia: Assignment of the gene to chromosome 15. Am J Hum Genet 48:525–535, 1991.

144. Awata H, et al: Structural organization and analysis of the human fumarylacetoacetate hydrolase gene in tyrosinemia type I. Biochim Biophys Acta 1226:168–172, 1994.

145. Kvittingen EA, et al: Prenatal diagnosis of hereditary tyrosinemia by determination of fumarylacetoacetase in cultured amniotic fluid cells. Pediatr Res 19:334–337, 1985.

146. Kvittingen EA, Rootwelt H, Berger R, Brandtzaeg P: Self-induced correction of the genetic defect in tyrosinemia type I. J Clin Invest 94:1657–1661, 1994.

147. Demers SI, Russo P, Lettre F, Tanguay RM: Frequent mutation reversion inversely correlates with clinical severity in a genetic liver disease, hereditary tyrosinemia. Hum Pathol 34:1313–1320, 2003.

148. Worthen HG: Renal toxicity of maleic acid in the rat: Enzymatic and morphologic observations. Lab Invest 12:791–801, 1963.

149. Roth KS, Carter BE, Higgins ES: Succinylacetone effects on renal tubular phosphate metabolism: A model for experimental renal Fanconi syndrome. Proc Soc Exp Biol Med 196:428–431, 1991.

150. Spencer PD, Roth KS: Effects of succinylacetone on amino acid uptake in the rat kidney. Biochem Med Metab Biol 37:101–109, 1987.

151. Arend LJ, Thompson CI, Brandt MA, Spielman WS: Elevation of intrarenal adenosine by maleic acid decreases GFR and renin release. Kidney Int 30:656–661, 1986.

152. Sun MS, et al: A mouse model of renal tubular injury of tyrosinemia type 1: Development of de Toni Fanconi syndrome and apoptosis of renal tubular cells in Fah/Hpd double mutant mice. J Am Soc Nephrol 11:291–300, 2000.

153. Fairney A, Francis D, Ersser RS, et al: Diagnosis and treatment of tyrosinosis. Arch Dis Child 43:540–547, 1968.

154. Tuchman M, et al: Contribution of extrahepatic tissues to biochemical abnormalities in hereditary tyrosinemia type I: Study of three patients after liver transplantation. J Pediatr 110:399–403, 1987.

155. Laine J, et al: The nephropathy of type I tyrosinemia after liver transplantation. Pediatr Res 37:640–645, 1995.

156. Barkaoui E, Debray D, Habes D, et al: [Favorable outcome of treatment with NTBC of acute liver insufficiency disclosing hereditary tyrosinemia type I]. Arch Pediatr 6:540–544, 1999.

157. Holme E, Lindstedt S: Tyrosinaemia type I and NTBC (2-(2-nitro-4-trifluoromethylbenzoyl)-1,3-cyclohexanedione). J Inherit Metab Dis 21:507–517, 1998.

158. Scheinman SJ, et al: Mapping the gene causing X-linked recessive nephrolithiasis to Xp11.22 by linkage studies. J Clin Invest 91:2351–2357, 1993.

159. Hoopes RR Jr, et al: Dent disease with mutations in OCRL1. Am J Hum Genet 76:260–267, 2005.

160. Jentsch TJ, Poet M, Fuhrmann JC, Zdebik AA: Physiological functions of ClC Cl- channels gleaned from human genetic disease and mouse models. Annu Rev Physiol 67:779–807, 2005.

161. Fisher SE, et al: Isolation and partial characterization of a chloride channel gene which is expressed in kidney and is a candidate for Dent's disease (an X-linked hereditary nephrolithiasis). Hum Mol Genet 3:2053–2059, 1994.

162. Luyckx VA, et al: Intrarenal and subcellular localization of rat CLC5. Am J Physiol 275:F761–F769, 1998.

163. Gunther W, Luchow A, Cluzeaud F, et al: ClC-5, the chloride channel mutated in Dent's disease, colocalizes with the proton pump in endocytotically active kidney cells. Proc Natl Acad Sci U S A 95:8075–8080, 1998.

164. Devuyst O, Christie PT, Courtoy PJ, et al: Intra-renal and subcellular distribution of the human chloride channel, CLC-5, reveals a pathophysiological basis for Dent's disease. Hum Mol Genet 8:247–257, 1999.

165. Jentsch TJ: Chloride and the endosomal-lysosomal pathway: Emerging roles of CLC chloride transporters. J Physiol 578:633–640, 2007.

166. Friedrich T, Breiderhoff T, Jentsch TJ: Mutational analysis demonstrates that CLC-4 and CLC-5 directly mediate plasma membrane currents. J Biol Chem 274:896–902, 1999.

167. Accardi A, Miller C: Secondary active transport mediated by a prokaryotic homologue of ClC Cl- channels. Nature 427:803–807, 2004.

258. Briggs WA, Kominami N, Wilson RE, Merrill JP: Kidney transplantation in Fanconi syndrome. N Engl J Med 286:25, 1972.

259. Oemar BS, Byrd DJ, Brodehl J: Complete absence of tubular glucose reabsorption: A new type of renal glucosuria (type 0). Clin Nephrol 27:156–160, 1987.

260. Santer R, et al: Molecular analysis of the SGLT2 gene in patients with renal glucosuria. J Am Soc Nephrol 14:2873–2882, 2003.

261. Calado J, et al: Familial renal glucosuria: SLC5A2 mutation analysis and evidence of salt-wasting. Kidney Int 69:852–855, 2006.

262. Kanai Y, Lee WS, You G, et al: The human kidney low affinity Na+/glucose cotransporter SGLT2. Delineation of the major renal reabsorptive mechanism for D-glucose. J Clin Invest 93:397–404, 1994.

263. Santer R, Schneppenheim R, Suter D, et al: Fanconi-Bickel syndrome—The original patient and his natural history, historical steps leading to the primary defect, and a review of the literature. Eur J Pediatr 157:783–797, 1998.

264. Manz F, et al: Fanconi-Bickel syndrome. Pediatr Nephrol 1:509–518, 1987.

265. Ichida K, et al: Clinical and molecular analysis of patients with renal hypouricemia in Japan-influence of URAT1 gene on urinary urate excretion. J Am Soc Nephrol 15:164–173, 2004.

266. Ohta T, Sakano T, Igarashi T, et al: Exercise-induced acute renal failure associated with renal hypouricaemia: Results of a questionnaire-based survey in Japan. Nephrol Dial Transplant 19:1447–1453, 2004.

267. Ames BN, Cathcart R, Schwiers E, Hochstein P: Uric acid provides an antioxidant defense in humans against oxidant- and radical-caused aging and cancer: A hypothesis. Proc Natl Acad Sci U S A 78:6858–6862, 1981.

268. Peden DB, et al: Uric acid is a major antioxidant in human nasal airway secretions. Proc Natl Acad Sci U S A 87:7638–7642, 1990.

269. Vollaard NB, Shearman JP, Cooper CE: Exercise-induced oxidative stress: Myths, realities and physiological relevance. Sports Med 35:1045–1062, 2005.

270. Kawabe K, Murayama T, Akaoka I: A case of uric acid renal stone with hypouricemia caused by tubular reabsorptive defect of uric acid. J Urol 116:690–692, 1976.

271. Cheong HI, et al: Mutational analysis of idiopathic renal hypouricemia in Korea. Pediatr Nephrol 20:886–890, 2005.

272. Kaneko K, et al: Analysis of urinary calculi obtained from a patient with idiopathic hypouricemia using micro area x-ray diffractometry and LC-MS. Urol Res 33:415–421, 2005.

273. Sorensen CM, Chandhoke PS: Hyperuricosuric calcium nephrolithiasis. Endocrinol Metab Clin North Am 31:915–925, 2002.

274. Pak CY, Poindexter JR, Peterson RD, et al: Biochemical distinction between hyperuricosuric calcium urolithiasis and gouty diathesis. Urology 60:789–794, 2002.

275. Maalouf NM, Cameron MA, Moe OW, Sakhaee K: Novel insights into the pathogenesis of uric acid nephrolithiasis. Curr Opin Nephrol Hypertens 13:181–189, 2004.

276. Sakhaee K, Adams-Huet B, Moe OW, Pak CY: Pathophysiologic basis for normouricosuric uric acid nephrolithiasis. Kidney Int 62:971–979, 2002.

277. Abate N, Chandalia M, Cabo-Chan AV Jr, et al: The metabolic syndrome and uric acid nephrolithiasis: Novel features of renal manifestation of insulin resistance. Kidney Int 65:386–392, 2004.

278. Grasbeck R: Imerslund-Grasbeck syndrome (selective vitamin B12 malabsorption with proteinuria). Orphanet J Rare Dis 1:17, 2006.

279. Aminoff M, et al: Mutations in CUBN, encoding the intrinsic factor-vitamin B12 receptor, cubilin, cause hereditary megaloblastic anaemia 1. Nat Genet 21:309–313, 1999.

280. Bouchlaka C, et al: Genetic heterogeneity of megaloblastic anaemia type 1 in Tunisian patients. J Hum Genet 52:262–270, 2007.

281. He Q, et al: Amnionless function is required for cubilin brush-border expression and intrinsic factor-cobalamin (vitamin B12) absorption in vivo. Blood 106:1447–1453, 2005.

282. Nykjaer A, et al: Cubilin dysfunction causes abnormal metabolism of the steroid hormone 25(OH) vitamin D(3). Proc Natl Acad Sci U S A 98:13895–13900, 2001.

283. Verrey F, et al: Novel renal amino acid transporters. Annu Rev Physiol 67:557–572, 2005.

284. Pras E, et al: Localization of a gene causing cystinuria to chromosome 2p. Nat Genet 6:415–419, 1994.

285. Calonge MJ, et al: Cystinuria caused by mutations in rBAT, a gene involved in the transport of cystine. Nat Genet 6:420–425, 1994.

286. Mosckovitz R, Udenfriend S, Felix A, et al: Membrane topology of the rat kidney neutral and basic amino acid transporter. FASEB J 8:1069–1074, 1994.

287. Broer S, Wagner CA: Structure-function relationships of heterodimeric amino acid transporters. Cell Biochem Biophys 36:155–168, 2002.

288. Wartenfeld R, et al: Molecular analysis of cystinuria in Libyan Jews: Exclusion of the SLC3A1 gene and mapping of a new locus on 19q. Am J Hum Genet 60:617–624, 1997.

289. Bisceglia L, et al: Localization, by linkage analysis, of the cystinuria type III gene to chromosome 19q13.1. Am J Hum Genet 60:611–616, 1997.

290. Feliubadalo L, et al: Non-type I cystinuria caused by mutations in SLC7A9, encoding a subunit (bo,+AT) of rBAT. Nat Genet 23:52–57, 1999.

291. Chillaron J, et al: An intracellular trafficking defect in type I cystinuria rBAT mutants M467T and M467K. J Biol Chem 272:9543–9549, 1997.

292. Stoller ML, et al: Linkage of type II and type III cystinuria to 19q13.1: Codominant inheritance of two cystinuric alleles at 19q13.1 produces an extreme stone-forming phenotype. Am J Med Genet 86:134–139, 1999.

293. Leclerc D, et al: SLC7A9 mutations in all three cystinuria subtypes. Kidney Int 62:1550–1559, 2002.

294. Dello Strologo L, et al: Comparison between SLC3A1 and SLC7A9 cystinuria patients and carriers: A need for a new classification. J Am Soc Nephrol 13:2547–2553, 2002.

295. Font-Llitjos M, et al: New insights into cystinuria: 40 new mutations, genotype-phenotype correlation, and digenic inheritance causing partial phenotype. J Med Genet 42:58–68, 2005.

296. Chatzikyriakidou A, Sofikitis N, Kalfakakou V, et al: Evidence for association of SLC7A9 gene haplotypes with cystinuria manifestation in SLC7A9 mutation carriers. Urol Res 34:299–303, 2006.

297. Scriver CR, et al: Ontogeny modifies manifestations of cystinuria genes: Implications for counseling. J Pediatr 106:411–416, 1985.

298. Boutros M, Vicanek C, Rozen R, Goodyer P: Transient neonatal cystinuria. Kidney Int 67:443–448, 2005.

299. Jaeken J, et al: Deletion of PREPL, a gene encoding a putative serine oligopeptidase, in patients with hypotonia-cystinuria syndrome. Am J Hum Genet 78:38–51, 2006.

300. Erbagci A, et al: Pediatric urolithiasis—Evaluation of risk factors in 95 children. Scand J Urol Nephrol 37:129–133, 2003.

301. Coward RJ, et al: Epidemiology of paediatric renal stone disease in the UK. Arch Dis Child 88:962–965, 2003.

302. Evan AP, et al: Renal crystal deposits and histopathology in patients with cystine stones. Kidney Int 69:2227–2235, 2006.

303. Guillen M, Corella D, Cabello ML, et al: Reference values of urinary excretion of cystine and dibasic aminoacids: Classification of patients with cystinuria in the Valencian Community, Spain. Clin Biochem 32:25–30, 1999.

304. Rodriguez LM, Santos F, Malaga S, Martinez V: Effect of a low sodium diet on urinary elimination of cystine in cystinuric children. Nephron 71:416–418, 1995.

305. Pak CY, Fuller C, Sakhaee K, et al: Management of cystine nephrolithiasis with alpha-mercaptopropionylglycine. J Urol 136:1003–1008, 1986.

306. Slavkovic A, Radovanovic M, Siric Z, et al: Extracorporeal shock wave lithotripsy for cystine urolithiasis in children: Outcome and complications. Int Urol Nephrol 34:457–461, 2002.

307. Kachel TA, Vijan SR, Dretler SP: Endourological experience with cystine calculi and a treatment algorithm. J Urol 145:25–28, 1991.

308. Chow GK, Streem SB: Contemporary urological intervention for cystinuric patients: Immediate and long-term impact and implications. J Urol 160:341–345, 1998.

309. Jackman SV, Hedican SP, Peters CA, Docimo SG: Percutaneous nephrolithotomy in infants and preschool age children: Experience with a new technique. Urology 52:697–701, 1998.

310. Parto K, Svedstrom E, Majurin ML, et al: Pulmonary manifestations in lysinuric protein intolerance. Chest 104:1176–1182, 1993.

311. Parto K, Kallajoki M, Aho H, Simell O: Pulmonary alveolar proteinosis and glomerulonephritis in lysinuric protein intolerance: Case reports and autopsy findings of four pediatric patients. Hum Pathol 25:400–407, 1994.

312. Nagata M, et al: Immunological abnormalities in a patient with lysinuric protein intolerance. Eur J Pediatr 146:427–428, 1987.

313. Lukkarinen M, et al: B and T cell immunity in patients with lysinuric protein intolerance. Clin Exp Immunol 116:430–434, 1999.

314. Parsons H, Snyder F, Bowen T, et al: Immune complex disease consistent with systemic lupus erythematosus in a patient with lysinuric protein intolerance. J Inherit Metab Dis 19:627–634, 1996.

315. Kamoda T, et al: Lysinuric protein intolerance and systemic lupus erythematosus. Eur J Pediatr 157:130–131, 1998.

316. Torrents D, et al: Identification of SLC7A7, encoding y+LAT-1, as the lysinuric protein intolerance gene. Nat Genet 21:293–296, 1999.

317. Lauteala T, et al: Lysinuric protein intolerance (LPI) gene maps to the long arm of chromosome 14. Am J Hum Genet 60:1479–1486, 1997.

318. Rajantie J, Simell O, Perheentupa J: Oral administration of urea cycle intermediates in lysinuric protein intolerance: Effect on plasma and urinary arginine and ornithine. Metabolism 32:49–51, 1983.

319. Rajantie J, Simell O, Rapola J, Perheentupa J: Lysinuric protein intolerance: A two-year trial of dietary supplementation therapy with citrulline and lysine. J Pediatr 97:927–932, 1980.

320. Lukkarinen M, Nanto-Salonen K, Pulkki K, et al: Oral supplementation corrects plasma lysine concentrations in lysinuric protein intolerance. Metabolism 52:935–938, 2003.

321. Lukkarinen M, Nanto-Salonen K, Pulkki K, et al: Effect of lysine infusion on urea cycle in lysinuric protein intolerance. Metabolism 49:621–625, 2000.

322. Baron DN, Dent CE, Harris H, et al: Hereditary pellagra-like skin rash with temporary cerebellar ataxia, constant renal amino-aciduria, and other bizarre biochemical features. Lancet 271:421–428, 1956.

323. Levy HL: Genetic screening. Adv Hum Genet 4:1–104, 1973.

324. Levy HL, Madigan PM, Shih VE: Massachusetts metabolic disorders screening program. I. Technics and results of urine screening. Pediatrics 49:825–836, 1972.

325. Wilcken B, Yu JS, Brown DA: Natural history of Hartnup disease. Arch Dis Child 52:38–40, 1977.

326. Scriver CR: Nutrient-gene interactions: The gene is not the disease and vice versa. Am J Clin Nutr 48:1505–1509, 1988.

327. Scriver CR, et al: The Hartnup phenotype: Mendelian transport disorder, multifactorial disease. Am J Hum Genet 40:401–412, 1987.

328. Seow HF, et al: Hartnup disorder is caused by mutations in the gene encoding the neutral amino acid transporter SLC6A19. Nat Genet 36:1003–1007, 2004.

329. Kleta R, et al: Mutations in SLC6A19, encoding B0AT1, cause Hartnup disorder. Nat Genet 36:999–1002, 2004.

330. Broer S, Cavanaugh JA, Rasko JE: Neutral amino acid transport in epithelial cells and its malfunction in Hartnup disorder. Biochem Soc Trans 33:233–236, 2005.

331. Brodehl J, Gellissen K, Kowalewski S: [Isolated cystinuria (without lysin-, ornithin and argininuria) in a family with hypocalcemic tetany]. Monatsschr Kinderheilkd 115:317–320, 1967.

332. Whelan DT, Scriver CR: Hyperdibasicaminoaciduria: An inherited disorder of amino acid transport. Pediatr Res 2:525–534, 1968.

333. Kihara H, Valente M, Porter MT, Fluharty AL: Hyperdibasicaminoaciduria in a mentally retarded homozygote with a peculiar response to phenothiazines. Pediatrics 51:223–229, 1973.

334. Omura K, Yamanaka N, Higami S, et al: Lysine malabsorption syndrome: A new type of transport defect. Pediatrics 57:102–105, 1976.

335. Smith AJ, Strang LB: An inborn error of metabolism with the urinary excretion of alpha-hydroxy-butyric acid and phenylpyruvic acid. Arch Dis Child 33:109–113, 1958.

336. Hooft C, et al: Methionine malabsorption syndrome. Ann Paediatr 205:73–104, 1965.

337. Sabater J, Ferre C, Puliol M, Maya A: Histidinuria: A renal and intestinal histidine transport deficiency found in two mentally retarded children. Clin Genet 9:117–124, 1976.

338. Holmgren G, Hambraeus L, de Chateau P: Histidinemia and "normohistidinemic histidinuria." Report of three cases and the effect of different protein intakes on urinary excretion of histidine. Acta Paediatr Scand 63:220–224, 1974.

339. Kamoun PP, Parvy P, Cathelineau L, Meyer B: Renal histidinuria. J Inherit Metab Dis 4:217–219, 1981.

340. Rosenberg LE, Durant JL, Elsas LJ: Familial iminoglycinuria. An inborn error of renal tubular transport. N Engl J Med 278:1407–1413, 1968.

341. Coskun T, Ozalp I, Tokatli A: Iminoglycinuria: A benign type of inherited aminoaciduria. Turk J Pediatr 35:121–125, 1993.

342. Broer A, Cavanaugh JA, Rasko JE, Broer S: The molecular basis of neutral aminoacidurias. Pflugers Arch 451:511–517, 2006.

343. Anderson CM, et al: H+/amino acid transporter 1 (PAT1) is the imino acid carrier: An intestinal nutrient/drug transporter in human and rat. Gastroenterology 127:1410–1422, 2004.

344. Greene ML, Lietman PS, Rosenberg LE, Seegmiller JE: Familial hyperglycinuria. New defect in renal tubular transport of glycine and imino acids. Am J Med 54:265–271, 1973.

345. De Vries A, Kochwa S, Lazebnik J, et al: Glycinuria, a hereditary disorder associated with nephrolithiasis. Am J Med 23:408–415, 1957.

346. Teijema HL, van Gelderen HH, Giesberts MA, Laurent de Angulo MS: Dicarboxylic aminoaciduria: An inborn error of glutamate and aspartate transport with metabolic implications, in combination with a hyperprolinemia. Metabolism 23:115–123, 1974.

347. Melancon SB, Dallaire L, Lemieux B, et al: Dicarboxylic aminoaciduria: An inborn error of amino acid conservation. J Pediatr 91:422–427, 1977.

from the above-mentioned hyperprostaglandin E syndrome by the presence of sensorineural deafness, absence of medullary nephrocalcinosis, and slowly deteriorating renal function.[13]

Taken together, renal salt-wasting syndromes associated with hypokalemia and hypochloremic metabolic alkalosis (frequently subsumed as "Bartter syndrome" in a broader sense) present with marked clinical variability (Table 15-1). Severe early-onset forms (the "antenatal Bartter syndrome" or "hyperprostaglandin E syndrome") with symptoms directly arising from profound saltwasting with extracellular volume depletion contrast with mild late-onset forms primarily characterized by the sequelae of secondary hyperaldosteronism (the "Gitelman syndrome"). In between these two extremes, the Bartter syndrome sensu stricto ("classic Bartter syndrome") presents as a disorder with intermediate severity. Variable extents of extracellular volume depletion and secondary electrolyte disturbances contribute to a variable disease phenotype, which in its extremes may mimic antenatal Bartter syndrome or Gitelman syndrome.

This classification based on clinical criteria was enriched by the decipherment of the underlying genetic defects (Table 15-2). As disclosed by molecular genetic analyses, antenatal Bartter syndrome results from disturbed salt reabsorption along the TAL due to defects in either NKCC2,[14] ROMK,[15] barttin,[16] or both ClC-Ka and ClC-Kb.[17] The classic Bartter syndrome is caused by dysfunction of ClC-Kb,[18] which impairs salt transport to some extent along the TAL and in particular along the DCT1. A pure defect of salt reabsorption along the DCT1 due to dysfunction of NCCT finally results in the Gitelman syndrome. Unfortunately, a frequently used classification merely based on molecular genetic criteria, which simply follows the chronology of the identification of the genetic defects, does not accommodate for a more perspicuous functional classification. According to this molecular genetic classification, Bartter syndrome type I refers to a defect of NKKC2 (gene name *SLC12A1*), Bartter syndrome type II to a defect of ROMK (*KCNJ1*), Bartter syndrome type III to a defect of ClC-Kb (*CLCNKB*), and Bartter syndrome type IV to a defect of barttin (*BSND*). Not included in this classification was Gitelman syndrome due to disturbed NCCT (*SLC12A3*) function, despite its apparent relatedness to this group of disorders. Instead, Bartter syndrome type V was suggested to refer to some gain-of-function mutations of the Ca^{2+},Mg^{2+}-sensing-receptor (CaSR), which, however, in the first instance cause autosomal dominant hypocalcemia with variable degrees of renal salt wasting explained by the inhibitory effect of CaSR activation on salt transport along the TAL.[19] The autosomal-dominant mode of inheritance and the clinically more relevant hypocalcemia are features not compatible with Bartter syndrome and make the designation Bartter syndrome type V rather impractical; therefore, we do not consider Bartter syndrome type V in the following sections.

Taken together, renal salt wasting with hypokalemia and hypochloremic metabolic alkalosis becomes manifest in three clinically defined syndromes: antenatal Bartter syndrome, classic Bartter syndrome, and Gitelman syndrome. From a functional point of view, antenatal Bartter syndrome arises from NaCl transport defects of the TAL. Classic Bartter

Table 15-1 Inherited Salt-Wasting Disorders with Secondary Hypokalemia

Disorder	OMIM No.	Inheritance	Gene Locus	Gene	Protein
Antenatal Bartter syndrome	601678	AR	15q15–21	*SLC12A1*	NKCC2, NaK2Cl co-transporter
	241200	AR	11q24	*KCNJ1*	ROMK, potassium channel
Antenatal Bartter syndrome with sensorineural deafness	602522	AR	1p31	*BSND*	Barttin, Cl⁻ channel subunit
	602522	AR (digenic)	1p36	*CLNKA/B*	renal Cl⁻ channels
Classic Bartter syndrome	607364	AR	1p36	*CLCNKB*	Renal Cl⁻ channel
Gitelman syndrome	263800	AR	16q13	*SLC12A3*	NCCT, NaCl co-transporter

AR, autosomal recessive.

Table 15-2 Clinical and Biochemical Characteristics

Disorder	Age at Onset	Polyhydramnios	Polyuria/ Polydipsia	Nephrocalcinosis	Urine Ca^{2+}	Urine Mg^{2+}	Blood pH	Serum K^+	Serum Mg^{2+}
Antenatal Bartter syndrome	Prenatal	Yes	Yes	Yes	↑↑↑	N	↑	↓	N
Antenatal Bartter syndrome with sensorineural deafness	Prenatal	Yes	Yes	Yes	↑↑↑	N	↑	↓	N
Classic Bartter syndrome	Infancy	Very rare	Yes	Very rare	↓ – ↑	↑	↑	↓	N or ↓
Gitelman syndrome	Adolescence	No	Rare	No	↓↓	↑↑	↑	↓	↓

syndrome combines features of weak TAL defects with disturbed DCT1 function, whereas Gitelman syndrome reflects pure DCT1 dysfunction. Accordingly, genetic defects associated with antenatal Bartter syndrome affect NKCC2, ROMK, barttin, and both ClC-K isoforms. Classic Bartter syndrome is caused by isolated ClC-Kb dysfunction, whereas Gitelman syndrome typically is caused by mutations affecting NCCT but may be mimicked by impaired ClC-Kb function.

Genetic Disorders of the TAL, the Antenatal Bartter Syndrome

Furosemide-Sensitive Na/K/2Cl Cotransporter (NKCC2)

Disruption of NaCl reabsorption in the TAL due to inactivating mutations in *NKCC2* causes a severe disorder with antenatal onset. Within the second trimenon, fetal polyuria leads to progressive maternal polyhydramnios. Cl⁻ concentration in the amniotic fluid is elevated to as high as 118 mmol/L.[20,21] Untreated, premature delivery occurs around 32 weeks of gestation. The most striking abnormality of the newborns is profound polyuria. With adequate fluid replacement, daily urinary outputs can easily exceed half of the body weight of the newborn (>20 mL/kg/h). Despite both extracellular fluid volume contraction and presence of high arginine vasopressin levels, urine osmolality hardly approaches that of plasma, indicating a severe renal concentrating defect. Salt reabsorption along the TAL segment is also critical for urine dilution, which explains that urine osmolality on the other hand typically does not decrease below 160 mOsmol/kg. Some preserved ability to dilute urine might be explained by an adaptive increase of DCT1 salt reabsorption, which functions as the most distal portion of the diluting segment. This moderate hyposthenuria clearly separates NKCC2-deficient patients from polyuric patients with nephrogenic diabetes insipidus, who typically display urine osmolalities below 100 mOsmol/kg.

Within the first months of life, nearly all patients develop medullary nephrocalcinosis in parallel with persistently high urinary Ca²⁺ excretion. Amazingly, conservation of Mg²⁺ is not affected to a similar extent, and NKCC2-deficient patients usually do not develop hypomagnesemia. This is even more surprising given that loss-of-function mutations in paracellin-1, which mediates paracellular transport of divalent cations in the TAL, invariably cause both hypercalciuria and hypermagnesiuria, leading to severe hypomagnesemia in paracellin-1-deficient patients.[22] With respect to Mg²⁺ transport, the difference between both disorders might be explained by an upregulation of Mg²⁺ reabsorption parallel to a compensatory increased NaCl reabsorption in DCT1 cells in case of a NKCC2 defect.[23]

Renal Outer-Medullary K⁺ Channel

ROMK-deficient patients similarly show a history of maternal polyhydramnios, prematurity with median age of gestation of 33 weeks, vasopressin-insensitive polyuria, isosthenuria, and hypercalciuria with secondary nephrocalcinosis. As in the case of NKCC2 dysfunction, the severity of the symptoms argues for a complete defect of NaCl reabsorption along the TAL. The mechanism of renin-angiotensin-aldosterone system activation

is virtually identical to that proposed for NKCC2-deficient patients. However, despite the presence of high plasma aldosterone levels, ROMK-deficient patients exhibit transient hyperkalemia in the first days of life.[24] The simultaneous appearance of hyperkalemia and hyponatremia resembles the clinical picture of mineralocorticoid deficiency (which, however, shows low aldosterone levels) or that of pseudohypoaldosteronism type I; high aldosterone levels). Indeed, several published cases of pseudohypoaldosteronism type I turned out to be misdiagnosed, and subsequent genetic analysis revealed ROMK mutations as the underlying defect.[25] The severity of initial hyperkalemia decreases with gestational age.[26] Hyperkalemia may be attributed to the additional role of ROMK in the CCD, where it participates in the process of K⁺ secretion (see Fig. 15-1). Though less pronounced as compared with NKCC2 deficiency, the majority of ROMK-deficient patients develop hypokalemia in the later course of the disease. The transient nature of hyperkalemia may be explained by the upregulation of alternative pathways for K⁺ secretion in the CCD. An attractive candidate for this alternative route would be a large-conductance K⁺ channel identified in the apical membrane of CCD principal cells.[27] Because of its low open probability this K⁺ channel provides no significant apical K⁺ release under normal conditions. Experimental data, however, suggest that its activity increases with enhanced fluid and solute delivery to the CCD.[28]

The Cl⁻ Channel (ClC-K) β-Subunit Barttin

Only recently a new player in the process of salt reabsorption along the TAL and DCT1 was identified—the ClC-K channel β-subunit barttin. Discovery of barttin was initiated by chromosomal linkage of a very rare variant of tubular salt wasting associated with sensorineural deafness. By a positional cloning strategy, a novel gene (*BSND*) was identified, and inactivating mutations were found in affected individuals.[16] Because the gene product, barttin, had no homology to any known protein, its physiologic function remained unclear until two groups independently described the role of barttin as an essential β-subunit of the ClC-K Cl⁻ channels.[29,30]

Two ClC-K isoforms of the CLC family of Cl⁻ channels are highly expressed along the distal nephron, with ClC-Ka being exclusively expressed in the thin ascending limb and decreasing expression levels along the adjacent distal nephron. Its homologue ClC-Kb is predominantly expressed in the DCT1. Along the TAL, both channel isoforms are equally expressed. Barttin, which is found in all ClC-K-expressing nephron segments, is essential for proper ClC-K channel function in that it facilitates the transport of ClC-K channels to the cell surface and modulates biophysical properties of the assembled channel complex.

In affected individuals, the barttin defect seems to completely disrupt Cl⁻ exit across the basolateral membrane in TAL as well as DCT1 cells. Accordingly, patients display the most severe salt-wasting kidney disorder described so far. As with defects of NKCC2 and ROMK, the first symptom of a barttin defect is maternal polyhydramnios due to fetal polyuria beginning at approximately 22 weeks of gestation. Again, polyhydramnios accounts for preterm labor and extreme prematurity. Postnatally, patients are at high risk of volume depletion. Plasma Cl⁻ levels fall to approximately 80 mmol/L; a further decrease usually can be avoided by close laboratory monitoring and rapid intervention on neonatal intensive care units. Polyuria again is resistant to vasopressin, and urine osmolalities range between 200 and 400 mOsmol/kg.

Unlike patients with loss-of-function mutations affecting ROMK and NKCC2, barttin-deficient patients exhibit only transitory hypercalciuria.[31] Medullary nephrocalcinosis is absent, yet progressive renal failure is common with histologic signs of pronounced tissue damage like glomerular sclerosis, tubular atrophy, and mononuclear infiltration. The mechanisms underlying the deterioration of renal function are not yet understood. The lack of hypercalciuria, however, may be explained by disturbed NaCl reabsorption along the DCT1. Isolated DCT1 dysfunction like in Gitelman syndrome (see below) or after long-term inhibition of NCCT-mediated transport by thiazides is known to induce hypocalciuria. This effect might counterbalance the hypercalciuric effect of TAL dysfunction in case of a combined impairment of salt reabsorption along the TAL and DCT1. In contrast to Ca^{2+}, the renal conservation of Mg^{2+} is severely impaired, leading to pronounced hypomagnesemia. This might be explained by the disruption of both Mg^{2+} reabsorption pathways, the paracellular one in the TAL and the transcellular one in the DCT1, respectively.

The barttin defect is invariably associated with sensorineurinal deafness. Clarification of the pathogenesis of this rare disorder has provided a deeper insight into the mechanisms of K^+-rich endolymph secretion in the inner ear: Marginal cells of the stria vascularis contribute to the endolymph formation by apical K^+ secretion. Transcellular K^+ transport is mediated by the furosemide-sensitive NaK2Cl cotransporter type 1 (NKCC1) ensuring basolateral K^+ entry into the marginal cells. Voltage-dependent K^+ channels mediate apical K^+ secretion into the endolymph. Proper function of NKCC1 requires basolateral recycling of Cl^-. Deafness associated with barttin deficiency suggests that this recycling is permitted by the ClC-K/barttin channel complex.

A Digenic Disorder: The ClC-Ka/b Phenotype

The concept of the physiologic role of barttin as a common β-subunit of ClC-K channels was substantiated by the recent description of an individual harboring inactivating mutations in both the ClC-Ka and ClC-Kb Cl^- channels, respectively.[17] The clinical symptoms associated with this digenic disease are indistinguishable from those of barttin-deficient patients. This observation not only proves the concept of the functional interaction of barttin with both ClC-K isoforms but also excludes important other functions of barttin not related to ClC-K channel interaction.

Disorders of the DCT1, the Classic Bartter Syndrome and the Gitelman Syndrome
The Basolateral Cl⁻ Channel ClC-Kb

In the context of a normal ClC-Ka function, an isolated defect of the gene encoding ClC-Kb leads to a more variable phenotype. Several studies have indicated that the clinical variability is not related to a certain type of mutation.[32,33] Even the most deleterious mutation, which implies the absence of the complete coding region of the gene encoding ClC-Kb and which affects nearly 50% of this patient cohort, can cause varying degrees of disease severity. Features of tubular dysfunction distal from the TAL predominate, suggesting a major role of ClC-Kb along the DCT1. Although TAL salt transport can be impaired to a variable extent, its function is never completely perturbed. Obviously, alternative routes of basolateral Cl^- exit can be recruited in the TAL segment, most likely via ClC-Ka.

With respect to renal function, the neonatal period in ClC-Kb-deficient patients usually passes without major problems. Maternal polyhydramnios is observed in only one-fourth of the patients and usually is mild. Accordingly, duration of pregnancy is not substantially decreased. More than half of the patients are diagnosed within the first year of life. Symptoms at initial presentation include failure to thrive, dehydration, muscular hypotonia, and lethargy. Laboratory examination typically reveals low plasma Cl^- concentrations (down to 60 mmol/L), decreased plasma Na^+ concentration, and severe hypokalemic alkalosis. At first presentation, electrolyte derangement is usually more pronounced as compared with the other groups, because renal salt wasting progresses slowly and is virtually not accompanied by polyuria, which might delay medical consultation. Plasma renin activity is strongly increased, whereas plasma aldosterone concentration is only slightly elevated. This discrepancy might be attributed to negative feedback regulation of aldosterone incretion by hypokalemia and alkalosis. Therefore, normal or slightly elevated aldosterone levels under conditions of profound hypokalemic alkalosis are in fact inadequately high.

Urinary concentrating ability is preserved at least to a certain extent. Indeed, some patients achieve urinary osmolalities above 700 mOsmol/kg in morning urine samples. Because renal medullary interstitial hypertonicity critically depends on NaCl reabsorption in the TAL, the ability to concentrate urine above 700 mOsmol/kg indicates nearly intact TAL function despite ClC-Kb deficiency. Moreover, the integrity of TAL function is also reflected by the finding that hypercalciuria is not a typical feature of ClC-Kb dysfunction and (if present) occurs only temporarily. The majority of patients exhibit normal or even low urinary Ca^{2+} excretion. Accordingly, medullary nephrocalcinosis—a hallmark of pure TAL dysfunction—is rare. The plasma Mg^{2+} concentration gradually decreases over time as a result of impaired renal Mg^{2+} conservation, as it is observed in other forms of derogated DCT1 function. Accordingly, several ClC-Kb-deficient patients exhibit both hypomagnesemia and hypocalciuria, a constellation that usually is thought to be highly indicative for an NCCT defect. ClC-Kb deficiency thus may mimic Gitelman syndrome.

The symptoms associated with malfunction of ClC-Kb largely parallel the features of Bartter's original description. The ethnic origin of Bartter's first patients supports this idea. Both were African Americans, and among this racial group only ClC-Kb mutations have been identified thus far. African Americans were also suggested to be affected from Bartter syndrome more frequently and to suffer from a more severe course of the disease. In a recent study in five African-American patients with ClC-Kb mutations, two of them had a history of polyhydramnios that elicited extreme prematurity.[34] Postnatal polyuria and electrolyte derangement led to diagnosis already in the early neonatal period. The incidence of chronic renal failure tends to be higher among African-American Bartter syndrome patients as compared with other ethnic groups.

Thiazide-Sensitive NaCl Cotransporter

DCT epithelia contain two cell types: DCT1 cells that express the NCCT as its predominant apical Na^+ entry pathway, and further distal residing DCT2 cells that express the epithelial Na channel as the main pathway for apical Na^+ reabsorption (Fig. 15-2). Both Na^+ entry pathways are inducible by aldosterone. DCT1 and DCT2 cells probably also differ with respect to their function in divalent cation transport.

NCCT deficiency results in only mild renal salt wasting. Initial presentation frequently occurs at school age or later, with the characteristic symptoms being muscular weakness, cramps, and fatigue. Not uncommonly, individuals with NCCT deficiency are diagnosed accidentally when they seek medical consultation because of growth retardation, constipation, or enuresis. A history of salt craving is common. Urinary concentrating ability typically is not affected. Laboratory examination shows a typical constellation of metabolic alkalosis, low normal Cl^- levels, hypokalemia, and hypomagnesemia; urine analysis shows hypocalciuria. Family studies revealed that electrolyte imbalances are present from infancy on, although the affected infants displayed no obvious clinical signs. Notably, the combination of hypokalemia and hypomagnesemia exerts an exceptionally unfavorable effect on cardiac excitability, which puts these patients at high risk for cardiac arrhythmias.

The pathognomonic feature of Gitelman syndrome is the dissociation of renal Ca^{2+} and Mg^{2+} handling, with low urinary Ca^{2+} and high urinary Mg^{2+} levels. Subsequent hypomagnesemia causes neuromuscular irritability and tetany. Decreased renal Ca^{2+} elimination together with Mg^{2+} deficiency favor deposition of mineral Ca^{2+} as demonstrated by increased bone density as well as chondrocalcinosis. Although the combination of hypomagnesemia and hypocalciuria is typical for NCCT deficiency, it is neither a specific nor universal finding. Clinical observations in NCCT-deficient patients disclosed intraindividual and interindividual variations in urinary Ca^{2+} concentrations; such results can be attributed to gender, age-related conditions of bone metabolism, intake of Mg^{2+} supplements, changes in diuresis and urinary osmolality, respectively. Likewise, hypomagnesemia might not be present from the beginning. Because less than 1% of total body Mg^{2+} is circulating in the blood, renal Mg^{2+} loss can be balanced temporarily by Mg^{2+} release from bone and muscle stores as well as by an increase of intestinal Mg^{2+} reabsorption. Accordingly, the strict definition of hypomagnesemia with coincident hypocalciuria so as to separate Gitelman (NCCT) syndrome from classic Bartter (ClC-Kb) syndrome seems arbitrary.

The mechanisms compromising distal Mg^{2+} reabsorption and favoring reabsorption of Ca^{2+} are not yet completely understood. The occasional coexistence of hypomagnesemia and hypocalciuria in ClC-Kb-deficient patients indicates that this phenomenon is not restricted to NCCT defects but is rather a consequence of impaired transcellular NaCl reabsorption along the DCT1. It is tempting to speculate that, in case of a functional defect of DCT1 cells, which in addition to NaCl reabsorb Mg^{2+} by apical TRPM6 Mg^{2+} channels, these

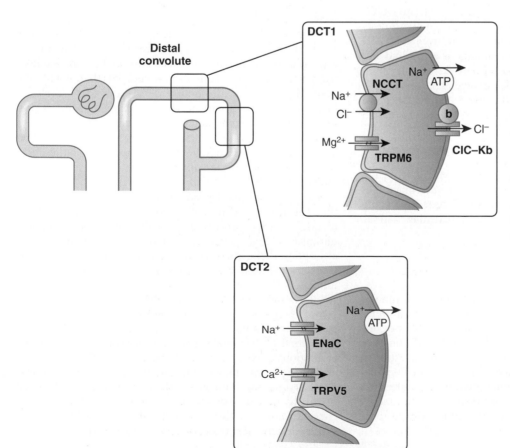

Figure 15-2 Divalent cation reabsorption along the distal convoluted tubule. DCT1 cells express an apical Mg^{2+} conductance (TRPM6), whereas DCT2 cells provide an apical Ca^{2+} conductance formed by the epithelial sodium channel (ECaC) (TRPV5). Impairment of DCT1 cell function by mutations of the genes encoding NCCT or ClC-Kb might shift the DCT1/DCT2 cell ratio in favor of DCT2 cells, which entails increased Mg and decreased Ca excretion.

cells are replaced by DCT2 cells, which reabsorb Na^+ via epithelial Na^+ channels and Ca^{2+} via epithelial Ca^{2+} channels (ECaC or TRPV5). Accordingly, reabsorption of Mg^{2+} would decrease and that of Ca^{2+} increase. Moreover, other phenomena such as the redistribution of renal tubular NaCl reabsorption to more proximal nephron segments (proximal tubule and TAL) might contribute to alterations in renal Ca^{2+} and Mg^{2+} handling.

Treatment

As with other hereditary diseases, the desirable correction of the primary genetic defects is not yet feasible. In the case of salt-wasting kidney disorders, however, the amendment of secondary phenomena such as increased renal prostaglandin synthesis or disturbed electrolyte homeostasis became part of their treatment virtually beginning from the first description of the diseases. Until recently the cornerstones in the treatment of renal salt wasting have been nonsteroidal anti-inflammatory drugs (NSAIDs) and long-term electrolyte substitution.

In the case of antenatal Bartter syndrome, inhibition of renal and systemic prostaglandin synthesis leads to reduced urinary PGE_2 excretion, markedly decreases polyuria, converts hyposthenuria to isosthenuria, reduces hypercalciuria, and stimulates catch-up growth. A convincing explanation for these unsurpassed effects of NSAIDs is still missing, albeit a reduction of glomerular filtration and blockage of an aberrant TGF certainly are important contributors. Despite these beneficial effects of NSAIDs, a lifelong substitution of KCl usually is required to prevent threatening extents of hypokalemia.

Consistent with the combined defect of the TAL and DCT1, NSAID treatment of antenatal Bartter syndrome with deafness proved clearly less effective. In addition to high NSAID doses, these patients need ample amounts of extra fluid and electrolytes (NaCl, KCl, Mg^{2+}) to prevent extracellular fluid volume contraction and electrolyte derangements.

In contrast to TAL defects, disturbed salt reabsorption along the DCT1 does not affect TGF and thus is not associated with increased renal prostaglandin synthesis.[35] Accordingly, NSAIDs are of little benefit in Gitelman syndrome. Substitution of KCl and Mg^{2+} is therefore central in the treatment of this disorder. As pointed out above, avoidance of factors that in addition to hypokalemia and hypomagnesemia might affect cardiac excitability (in particular QT-time prolonging drugs) is mandatory to prevent life-threatening cardiac arrhythmias.

Conclusion

Parallel loss of Na^+ and Cl^- by disturbed renal tubular function is the basis of several distinct diseases, which differ with respect to the degree of extracellular fluid volume contraction and secondary electrolyte derangements. Common features of all combined NaCl transport defects are extracellular fluid volume contraction, hypokalemia, hypochloremia, and metabolic alkalosis. The decipherment of the underlying genetic defects has contributed impressively to the understanding of the contribution of the affected proteins to renal salt transport.

INHERITED HYPOMAGNESEMIC DISORDERS

Mg^{2+} is the second most intracellular cation in the body. As a co-factor for many enzymes, it is involved in energy metabolism and protein and in nucleic acid synthesis. It also plays a critical role in the modulation of membrane transporters and in signal transduction. Under physiologic conditions, serum Mg^{2+} levels are maintained at almost constant values. Homeostasis depends on the balance between intestinal absorption and renal excretion. Mg^{2+} deficiency can result from reduced dietary intake, intestinal malabsorption, or renal loss. The control of body Mg^{2+} homeostasis primarily resides in the kidney tubules.

Several acquired and hereditary disorders of Mg^{2+} handling have been described, most of them due to renal Mg^{2+} loss and all of them being relatively rare. The phenotypic characterization of clinically affected individuals and experimental studies promoted the identification of various involved nephron segments. Together with the mode of inheritance, this led to a classification into different subtypes of inherited Mg^{2+}-wasting disorders.[36,37] During the past few years genetic studies in affected families were able to identify several genes involved in the pathogenesis of these diseases and provided a first insight into the physiology of epithelial Mg^{2+} transport at the molecular level. Depending on the genotype, the clinical course can be mild or even asymptomatic, so that the diagnosis is often delayed and the disease prevalences might be underestimated for some of these disorders.

Mg^{2+} Physiology

Mg^{2+} is the second most prevalent intracellular cation. The normal body Mg^{2+} content is approximately 24 g (1,000 mmol). Mg^{2+} is distributed mainly between bone and the intracellular compartments of muscle and soft tissues; less than 1% of total body Mg^{2+} circulates in the blood.[38] Serum Mg^{2+} levels are maintained within a narrow range. Circulating Mg^{2+} is present in three different states: dissociated/ionized, bound to albumin, or in complex with phosphate, citrate, or other anions. Ionized and complexed forms account for the ultrafiltrable fraction, the biologically active portion is the free, ionized Mg^{2+}.

Mg^{2+} homeostasis depends on the balance between intestinal absorption and renal excretion. The daily dietary intake of Mg^{2+} varies substantially. Within physiologic ranges, diminished Mg^{2+} intake is balanced by enhanced Mg^{2+} absorption in the intestine and reduced renal excretion. These transport processes are regulated by metabolic and hormonal influences.[39,40] The principal site of Mg^{2+} absorption is the small intestine, with smaller amounts being absorbed in the colon. Intestinal Mg^{2+} absorption occurs via two different pathways: a saturable active transcellular transport and a nonsaturable paracellular passive transport[39,41] (Fig. 15-3A). Saturation kinetics of the transcellular transport system are explained by the limited transport capacity of active transport. At low intraluminal concentrations Mg^{2+} is absorbed primarily via the active transcellular route and with rising concentrations via the paracellular pathway, yielding a curvilinear function for total absorption (Fig. 15-3B).

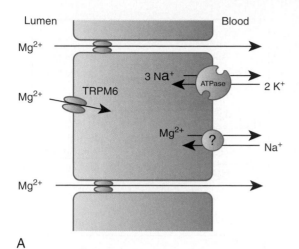

A

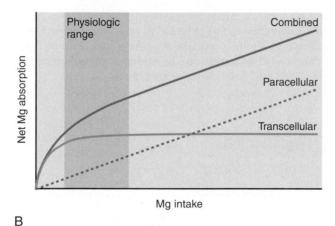

B

Figure 15-3 A, Schematic model of intestinal Mg^{2+} absorption via two independent pathways: passive absorption via the paracellular pathway and active, transcellular transport consisting of an apical entry through a putative Mg^{2+} channel and a basolateral exit mediated by a putative Na^+-coupled exchange. **B,** Kinetics of human intestinal Mg^{2+} absorption. Paracellular transport linearly rising with intraluminal concentrations (*dotted line*) and saturable active transcellular transport (*dashed line*) together yield a curvilinear function for net Mg^{2+} absorption (*solid line*).

In the kidney approximately 80% of total serum Mg^{2+} is filtered in the glomeruli. Of this amount, more than 95% is reabsorbed along the nephron. Mg^{2+} reabsorption differs in quantity and kinetics depending on the various nephron segments. Fifteen to twenty percent is reabsorbed in the proximal tubule of the adult kidney. Interestingly, the premature kidney of the newborn is able to reabsorb up to 70% of the filtered Mg^{2+} in this nephron segment.[42]

From early childhood onward, the majority of Mg^{2+} (~70%) is reabsorbed in the loop of Henle, especially in the cortical TAL. Transport in this segment is passive and paracellular, driven by the lumen-positive transepithelial voltage (Fig. 15-4A). Although only 5% to 10% of the filtered Mg^{2+} is reabsorbed in the DCT, this is the part of the nephron wherein the fine adjustment of renal excretion is accomplished. The reabsorption rate in the DCT defines the final urinary Mg^{2+} excretion, in that there is no significant reabsorption of Mg^{2+} in the collecting duct. Mg^{2+} transport in this part of the nephron is active and transcellular in nature (Fig. 15-4B). Physiologic studies indicate that apical entry into DCT cells is mediated by a specific and regulated Mg^{2+} channel driven by a favorable transmembrane voltage.[43] The mechanism of basolateral transport into the interstitium is unknown. Mg^{2+} has to be extruded against an unfavorable electrochemical gradient. Most physiologic studies favor a Na^+-dependent exchange mechanism.[44] Mg^{2+} entry into DCT cells seems to be the rate-limiting step and the site of regulation. Mg^{2+} transport in the distal tubule has been recently reviewed in detail by Dai et al.[43] Finally, 3% to 5% of the filtered Mg^{2+} is excreted in the urine.

Hereditary Disorders of Mg^{2+} Handling

Recent advances in molecular genetics of hereditary hypomagnesemia substantiated the role of a variety of genes and their encoded proteins in human epithelial Mg^{2+} transport (Table 15-3). The knowledge on underlying genetic defects helps to distinguish different clinical subtypes of hereditary disorders of Mg^{2+} homeostasis. However, careful clinical observation and additional biochemical parameters can in most cases distinguish among the different disease entities, even if there might be a considerable overlap in the phenotypic characteristics (Table 15-4).

Isolated Dominant Hypomagnesemia (OMIM 154020)

Isolated dominant hypomagnesemia (IDH) is caused by a mutation in the *FXYD2* gene on chromosome 11q23, which encodes a γ-subunit of the Na^+-ATPase.[45] Only two IDH families have been described so far.[46,47] The two index patients presented with seizures during childhood (at 7 and 13 years). Serum Mg^{2+} levels in the two patients at that time were approximately 0.4 mmol/L. One index patient was treated for seizures of unknown origin with antiepileptic drugs until serum Mg^{2+} levels were evaluated in adolescence. At that time severe mental retardation was evident. Systematic serum Mg^{2+} measurements performed in members of both families revealed low serum Mg^{2+} levels (~0.5 mmol/L) in numerous apparently healthy individuals. A 28 g–retention study in one index patient pointed to a primary renal defect.[46] The intestinal absorption of Mg^{2+} was preserved and even stimulated in compensation for the increased renal losses. Urinary Mg^{2+} measurements in affected family members revealed Mg^{2+} excretions of around 5 mmol per day despite profound hypomagnesemia.[46] In addition, urinary Ca^{2+} excretion rates were low in all hypomagnesemic family members, a finding reminiscent of patients presenting with Gitelman syndrome. However, in contrast to patients with Gitelman syndrome, no other associated biochemical abnormalities were reported, especially no hypokalemic alkalosis.

Pedigree analysis in the two families pointed to an autosomal dominant mode of inheritance. A genome-wide linkage study mapped the disease locus on chromosome 11q23.[48] Detailed haplotype analysis demonstrated a common haplotype segregating in the two families, suggesting a common ancestor. Indeed, subsequent mutational screening of the *FXYD2* gene demonstrated the identical mutation G41R in all affected individuals of both family branches.

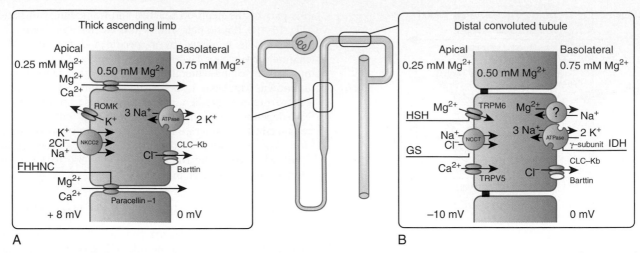

Figure 15-4 A, Mg^{2+} reabsorption in the thick ascending limb of Henle's loop. Paracellular reabsorption of Mg^{2+} and Ca^{2+} is driven by lumen-positive transcellular voltage generated by the transcellular reabsorption of NaCl. **B,** Mg^{2+} reabsorption in the distal convoluted tubule. In this nephron segment Mg^{2+} is reabsorbed actively via the transcellular pathway involving an apical entry step probably through a Mg^{2+}-selective ion channel and a basolateral exit, presumably mediated by a Na^+-coupled exchange mechanism. The molecular identity of basolateral exchange is unknown. GS, Gitelman syndrome.

Table 15-3 Inherited Disorders of Mg^{2+} Handling

Disorder	OMIM No.	Inheritance	Gene Locus	Gene	Protein
Isolated dominant hypomagnesemia	154020	AD	11q23	FXYD2	γ-subunit of the Na^+/K^+-ATPase
Isolated recessive hypomagnesemia	248250	AR	?	?	?
Autosomal dominant hypoparathyroidism	601198	AD	3q21	CASR	CaSR
Familial hypocalciuric hypercalcemia	145980	AD	3q21	CASR	CaSR
Neonatal severe hyperparathyroidism	239200	AR	3q21	CASR	CaSR
Familial hypomagnesemia with hypercalciuria/nephrocalcinosis	248250	AR	3q28	CLDN16	Paracellin-1, tight-junction protein
Hypomagnesemia with secondary hypocalcemia	602014	AR	9q22	TRPM6	TRPM6, putative ion channel
Hypomagnesemia/metabolic syndrome	500005	Maternal	mtDNA	MTTI	Mitochondrial tRNA (isoleucine)

CaSR, Ca^{2+}/Mg^{2+}-sensing receptor.

The γ-subunit encoded by *FXYD2* is a member of a family of small single transmembrane proteins which share the common amino acid motif F-X-Y-D. Out of the seven members, which differ in their tissue specificity, FXYD2 and FXYD4, also called channel-inducing factor, are highly expressed along the nephron, displaying an alternating expression pattern.[49] The γ-subunit comprises two isoforms (named γ-α and γ-β) that are differentially expressed in the kidney. The γ-α isoform is present predominantly in the proximal tubule, and expression of the γ-β isoform predominates in the distal nephron, especially in the DCT and connecting tubule.[50] The ubiquitous Na^+, K^+-ATPase is a dimeric enzyme invariably consisting of one α- and one β-subunit. FXYD proteins constitute a third or γ-subunit that represents a tissue-specific regulator of Na^+, K^+-ATPase. The FXYD2 γ-subunit increases the apparent affinity of Na^+, K^+-ATPase for ATP while decreasing its Na^+ affinity.[51] Thus, it might provide a mechanism for balancing energy utilization and maintaining appropriate salt gradients.

Expression studies of the mutant G41R γ-subunit in mammalian renal tubule cells revealed a dominant negative effect of the mutation leading to a retention of the γ-subunit within the cell. Whereas initial data pointed to a retention of the entire Na^+, K^+-ATPase complex in intracellular compartments, more recent data demonstrate an isolated trafficking defect of the mutant γ-subunit while trafficking of the α/β complex is preserved.[52] The mutant γ-subunit is obviously retarded in the Golgi complex, pointing to a disturbed post-translational processing. The assumption of a dominant negative effect is substantiated by the observation that individuals with a large heterozygous deletion of chromosome 11q including the *FXYD2* gene exhibit normal serum Mg^{2+} levels.[53]

Table 15-4 Clinical and Biochemical Characteristics

Disorder	Age at Onset	Serum Mg^{2+}	Serum Ca^{2+}	Serum K$^+$	Blood pH	Urine Mg^{2+}	Urine Ca^{2+}	Nephrocalcinosis	Renal Stones
Isolated dominant hypomagnesemia	Childhood	↓	N*	N	N	↑	↓	No	No
Isolated recessive hypomagnesemia	Childhood	↓	N	N	N	↑	N	No	No
Autosomal-dominant hypoparathyroidism	Infancy	↓	↓	N	N or ↓	↑	↑ to ↑↑	Yes*	Yes*
Familial hypocalciuric hypercalcemia	Often asymptomatic	N to ↑	↑	N	N	↓	↓	No	?
Neonatal severe hyperparathyroidism	Infancy	N to ↑	↑↑↑	N	N	↓	↓	No	?
Familial hypomagnesemia with hypercalciuria/ nephrocalcinosis	Childhood	↓	N	N	N or ↓	↑↑	↑↑	Yes	Yes
Hypomagnesemia with secondary hypocalcemia	Infancy	↓↓↓	↓	N	N	↑	N	No	No

*No change.
†Frequent complication under therapy with Ca^{2+} and vitamin D.

Urinary Mg^{2+} wasting together with the expression of the *FXYD2* gene indicate a defective transcellular Mg^{2+} reabsorption in the DCT in individuals with IDH. But how can a defect of Na$^+$, K$^+$-ATPase modulation lead to impaired renal Mg^{2+} conservation? One possible explanation is based on changes in intracellular Na$^+$ and K$^+$ levels. Meij and colleagues have suggested that diminished intracellular K$^+$ might depolarize the apical membrane, resulting in a decrease in Mg^{2+} uptake.[45] Alternatively, an increase in intracellular Na$^+$ could impair basolateral Mg^{2+} transport, which is presumably achieved by a Na$^+$-coupled exchange mechanism. Another explanation is that the γ-subunit is not only involved in Na$^+$, K$^+$-ATPase function but also an essential component of a yet unidentified ATP-dependent transport system specific for Mg^{2+}. As with Ca^{2+}, both a specific Mg^{2+}-ATPase and a Na$^+$-coupled exchanger might exist. Further studies are needed to clarify this issue.

An interesting feature of IDH is the finding of hypocalciuria, which is primarily observed in Gitelman syndrome (see above). Unfortunately, only one large family with IDH has been described, and an animal model for IDH is still lacking. Mice lacking the γ-subunit do not demonstrate any abnormalities in Mg^{2+} conservation or balance.[54] Therefore, data on the structural integrity of the DCT in IDH do not exist. One could speculate that, as in Gitelman syndrome, a defect in Na$^+$, K$^+$-ATPase function and energy metabolism might lead to an apoptotic breakdown of the early DCT responsible for Mg^{2+} reabsorption, whereas later parts of the distal nephron remain intact. In IDH there is no evidence for renal salt wasting and no stimulation of the renin-angiotensin-aldosterone system. The finding of hypocalciuria despite no apparent volume depletion apparently contradicts recent experimental data, which favor an increase in proximal tubular Ca^{2+} reabsorption due to volume depletion in Gitelman syndrome.[55]

Isolated Recessive Hypomagnesemia (OMIM 248250)

Geven et al reported a form of isolated hypomagnesemia in a consanguineous family, indicating autosomal recessive inheritance.[56] Two affected girls presented with generalized seizures during infancy. Unfortunately, late diagnosis resulted in neurodevelopmental deficits in both patients. A thorough clinical and laboratory workup at 4 and 8 years of age, respectively, revealed serum Mg^{2+} levels around 0.5 to 0.6 mmol/L with no other associated electrolyte abnormalities. A 28 g–retention study in one patient pointed to a primary renal defect, whereas intestinal Mg^{2+} uptake was preserved.[56] Both patients exhibited renal Mg^{2+} excretions of 3 to 6 mmol per day despite hypomagnesemia, confirming renal Mg^{2+} wasting. In contrast to IDH, renal Ca^{2+} excretion rates in isolated recessive hypomagnesemia are within the normal range. Haplotype analysis performed in this family excluded the gene loci involved in IDH, familial hypomagnesemia with hypercalciuria and nephrocalcinosis (FHHNC; see below), and Gitelman syndrome, indicating that isolated recessive hypomagnesemia is not allelic with these diseases.[53]

Disorders of the Ca^{2+},Mg^{2+}-Sensing Receptor

The extracellular Ca^{2+},Mg^{2+}-sensing receptor (CaSR) plays an essential role in Mg^{2+} and Ca^{2+} homeostasis by influencing not only parathyroid hormone (PTH) secretion in the parathyroid but also by directly regulating the rate of Mg^{2+} and Ca^{2+} reabsorption in the kidney. It was first cloned by Brown and colleagues in 1993.[57] Along the distal nephron, the CaSR is expressed basolaterally in TAL and DCT as well as at both the apical and basolateral membrane of the collecting duct.[58] Activation of the CaSR serves to coordinate changes in renal Ca^{2+} and Mg^{2+} excretion and in water diuresis.[59] The dilution of the urine by decreasing aquaporin expression in the collecting duct is thought to minimize the risk of stone formation in the face of an increase in Ca^{2+} and Mg^{2+} excretion. Several diseases associated with both activating and inactivating mutations in the *CASR* gene have been described. Because alterations in CaSR activity also affect renal Mg^{2+} handling, they are presented in this chapter with a special focus on Mg^{2+}.

Autosomal Dominant Hypoparathyroidism (OMIM 601198)

Activating mutations of the *CASR* result in autosomal dominant hypoparathyroidism. Patients typically manifest during childhood with seizures or carpopedal spasms. Laboratory evaluation reveals the typical combination of hypocalcemia and low PTH concentrations, but most patients also exhibit moderate hypomagnesemia with serum levels around 0.5 to 0.6 mmol/L.[60,61] Affected individuals are often given the diagnosis of primary hypoparathyroidism on the basis of inadequately low PTH levels despite their hypocalcemia. Serum Ca^{2+} levels are typically in a range of 6 to 7 mg/dL. The differentiation from primary hypoparathyroidism is of particular importance, because treatment with vitamin D can result in a marked increase in hypercalciuria and the occurrence of nephrocalcinosis and impairment of renal function in individuals with autosomal dominant hypoparathyroidism. Therefore, therapy with vitamin D or Ca^{2+} supplementation should be reserved for symptomatic patients with the aim to maintain serum Ca^{2+} levels just sufficient for the relief of symptoms.[61]

Activating *CASR* mutations lead to a lower setpoint of the receptor or an increased affinity for extracellular Ca^{2+} and Mg^{2+}. This inadequate activation by physiologic extracellular Ca^{2+} and Mg^{2+} levels then results in diminished PTH secretion and decreased reabsorption of both divalent cations mainly in the cTAL (cortical TAL). For Mg^{2+} the inhibition of PTH-stimulated reabsorption in the DCT may significantly contribute to an increased renal loss in addition to the effects observed in the TAL.[43,62] A pronounced hypomagnesemia is observed in patients with complete activation of the CaSR at physiologic serum Ca^{2+} and Mg^{2+} concentrations who also exhibit a Bartter-like phenotype.[19] In these patients, CaSR activation inhibits TAL-mediated salt and divalent cation reabsorption to an extent that cannot be compensated in later nephron segments.

Familial Hypocalciuric Hypercalcemia (OMIM 145980) and Neonatal Severe Hyperparathyroidism (OMIM 602014)

Familial hypocalciuric hypercalcemia and neonatal severe hyperparathyroidism result from inactivating mutations present in either the heterozygous or homozygous (or compound heterozygous) state, respectively.[60,63] Individuals with familial hypocalciuric hypercalcemia normally present with mild to moderate hypercalcemia accompanied by few if any symptoms and often do not require treatment. Urinary excretion rates for Ca^{2+} and Mg^{2+} are markedly reduced, and serum PTH levels are inappropriately high. In addition, affected individuals also show mild hypermagnesemia.[64] In contrast, patients with neonatal severe hyperparathyroidism with two CaSR mutations usually present in early infancy with polyuria and dehydration due to severe symptomatic hypercalcemia. Unrecognized and untreated, hyperparathyroidism and hypercalcemia result in skeletal deformities, extraosseous calcifications, muscle wasting, and a severe neurodevelopmental deficit. Early treatment with partial-to-total parathyroidectomy therefore seems to be essential for outcome.[65] Data on serum Mg^{2+} in neonatal severe hyperparathyroidism are sparse. However, elevations in PTH concentration to around 50% above normal have been reported.

Familial Hypomagnesemia with Hypercalciuria and Nephrocalcinosis (OMIM 248250)

Familial hypomagnesemia with hypercalciuria and nephrocalcinosis (FHHNC) is caused by mutations in the *CLDN16* gene encoding the tight-junction protein claudin-16 (paracellin-1).[22] Since its first description, at least 50 different kindreds have been reported, allowing a comprehensive characterization of the clinical spectrum of this disorder and discrimination from other Mg^{2+}-losing tubular diseases.[66–68] Due to excessive renal Mg^{2+} and Ca^{2+} wasting, patients develop the characteristic triad of hypomagnesemia, hypercalciuria, and nephrocalcinosis that gave the disease its name. Individuals with FHHNC usually present during early childhood with recurrent urinary tract infections, polyuria/polydipsia, nephrolithiasis, and/or failure to thrive. Signs of severe hypomagnesemia such as cerebral convulsions and muscular tetany are less common. Extrarenal manifestations, especially ocular involvement (including severe myopia, nystagmus, or chorioretinitis) have also been reported.[66–68] Additional laboratory findings include elevated serum PTH levels before the onset of chronic renal failure, incomplete distal tubule acidosis, hypocitraturia, and hyperuricemia present in most patients.[69] The clinical course of FHHNC patients is often complicated by the development of chronic renal failure early in life. A considerable number of patients exhibit a marked decline in glomerular filtration rate (<60 mL/min per 1.73 m²) already at the time of diagnosis, and about one-third of patients develop end-stage renal disease during adolescence. Hypomagnesemia may completely disappear with the decline of glomerular filtration rate due to a reduction in filtered Mg^{2+} limiting urinary Mg^{2+} excretion.

In addition to continuous Mg^{2+} supplementation, therapy aims at the reduction of Ca^{2+} excretion by using thiazides to prevent the progression of nephrocalcinosis and stone formation. The degree of renal calcification has been correlated with progression of chronic renal failure.[66] However, these therapeutic strategies do not seem to significantly influence the progression of renal failure. Supportive therapy is important for the protection of kidney function and should include provision of sufficient fluids and effective treatment of stone formation and bacterial colonization. As expected, renal transplantation is performed without evidence of recurrence, because the primary defect resides in the kidney.

Using a positional cloning approach, Simon et al could identify a new gene (*CLDN16*, formerly *PCLN1*), which is mutated in patients with FHHNC.[22] *CLDN16* codes for claudin-16, a member of the claudin family. More than 20 claudins identified so far compose a family of ≈22-kDa proteins with four transmembrane segments, two extracellular domains, and intracellular N and C termini. The individual composition of tight junctions strands with different claudins confers the characteristic properties of different epithelia regarding paracellular permeability and/or transepithelial resistance. In this context, a crucial role has been attributed to the first extracellular domain of the claudin protein, which is extremely variable in number and position of charged amino acid residues.[70] Individual charges have been shown to influence paracellular ion selectivity, suggesting that claudins positioned on opposing cells forming the paracellular pathway provide charge-selective pores within the tight-junction barrier.

The C terminus is remarkable for a consensus threonine-X-valine PDZ-binding domain, which is involved in protein-protein interactions and targeting of the paracellin-1 protein to tight-junction strands. The longest possible open reading frame of the human complementary DNA encodes a protein of 305 amino acids with a cytoplasmic N terminus of 73 amino acids. This structure contrasts with all other claudins, which share a very short N terminus of only 6 or 7 amino acids. Interestingly, there is a second in-frame start codon within a suitable Kozak consensus sequence at position Met71 that is analogous to the translation start site of all other claudins. Sequence comparison of the human complementary DNA with other species and the results of mutation analyses that identified a common insertion/deletion polymorphism (165_166delGGinsC) that would lead to a shift of the reading frame (R55fs71X) argue for the second translation initiation start site being used in vivo.[69,71] These observations are supported by in vitro data that show a much more robust expression of claudin-16 constructs lacking the first 70 amino acids.[72] Moreover, in the same study, the analysis of the subcellular localization of claudin-16 revealed that only the shorter protein is correctly expressed at cell-cell borders, whereas the full-length claudin-16 protein is mistargeted to endosomes or lysosomes.[72] It was speculated that in humans the native cellular environment contains regulatory factors to allow bypassing the first methionine (M1) in claudin-16 and ensure appropriate translation from the second methionine (M71).

The majority of mutations reported so far in FHHNC are simple missense mutations affecting the transmembrane domains and the extracellular loops with a particular clustering in the first extracellular loop containing the ion selectivity filter. Within this domain, patients originating from Germany and eastern European countries exhibit a common mutation (L151F) due to a founder effect.[69] Because this mutation is present in approximately 50% of mutant alleles, molecular diagnosis is greatly facilitated in patients originating from these countries. Defects in CLDN16 have also been shown to underlie the development of a chronic interstitial nephritis in Japanese cattle that rapidly develop chronic renal failure shortly after birth.[73] Interestingly, affected animals typically show hypocalcemia but no hypomagnesemia, which might be explained by advanced chronic renal failure present at the time of examination. The fact that, in contrast to the point mutations identified in human FHHNC, large deletions of CLDN16 are responsible for the disease in cattle might explain the more severe phenotype with early-onset renal failure. In FHHNC patients, progressive renal failure is more likely a consequence of massive urinary Ca^{2+} wasting and nephrocalcinosis. However, Cldn16-knockout

mice do not display renal failure during the first months of life.[74] Considering the ocular abnormalities observed in some individuals with FHHNC, it is interesting to note that cldn16 expression has been identified in bovine cornea and retinal pigment epithelia.[75] Further examination of the eyes of affected Japanese cattle and of Cldn16-knockout mice will hopefully provide an answer to the question whether myopia, nystagmus, and chorioretinitis observed in individuals with FHHNC are directly linked to CLDN16 mutations. Furthermore, there is evidence from family analyses that carriers of heterozygous CLDN16 mutations may also present with clinical symptoms. Two independent studies describe a high incidence of hypercalciuria, nephrolithiasis, and/or nephrocalcinosis in first-degree relatives of patients with FHHNC.[66,69] A subsequent study also found a tendency toward mild hypomagnesemia in family members with heterozygous CLDN16 mutations.[76] Thus, one might speculate that CLDN16 mutations could be involved in idiopathic hypercalciuric stone formation.

Recently, a homozygous CLDN16 mutation (T303R) affecting the C-terminal PDZ domain has been identified in two families with isolated hypercalciuria and nephrocalcinosis without disturbances in renal Mg^{2+} handling.[77] Interestingly, the hypercalciuria disappeared during follow-up, and urinary Ca^{2+} levels reached normal values beyond puberty. Transient transfection of MDCK cells with the CLDN16 (T303R) mutant revealed a mistargeting into lysosomes, whereas wild-type claudin-16 was correctly localized to tight junctions. It remains to be determined why this type of misrouting is associated with transient isolated hypercalciuria without increased Mg^{2+} excretion.

The exact physiologic role of claudin-16 is still not fully understood. From the FHHNC disease phenotype, it was concluded that claudin-16 might regulate the paracellular transport of Mg^{2+} and Ca^{2+} ions by contributing to a selective paracellular conductance through building a pore permitting paracellular fluxes of Mg^{2+} and Ca^{2+} down their electrochemical gradients.[22,78] However, recent functional studies in LLC-PK1 cells could show that the expression of claudin-16 selectively and significantly increased the permeability of Na^+ with a far less pronounced change of Mg^{2+} flux. From these observations it was hypothesized that in the TAL claudin-16 probably contributes to the generation of the lumen-positive potential (allowing the passive reabsorption of divalent cations) rather than to the formation of a paracellular channel selective for Ca^{2+} and Mg^{2+}.[72]

As mentioned above, many individuals with FHHNC develop chronic renal failure associated with progressive tubulointerstitial nephritis. The pathophysiology of this phenomenon, which is not regularly observed in other tubular disorders, is unclear. Traditionally, renal failure in FHHNC has been attributed to the concomitant hypercalciuria and nephrocalcinosis, but a true correlation could not be established. Therefore, it has been speculated that claudin-16 is involved not only in paracellular electrolyte reabsorption but also in tubular cell proliferation and differentiation.[79] This hypothesis is supported by the bovine cldn16-knockout phenotype observed in Japanese Black cattle, which exhibit early-onset renal failure due to interstitial nephritis with diffuse zonal fibrosis.[73,80] Tubular epithelial cells were reported as "immature" with loss of polarization and attachment to the basement membrane. A close association between fibrosis and abnormal tubules was noted, and the term "renal tubular dysplasia" was used to emphasize that the lesions initiate in the epithelial cells of the renal tubules.[81] These cattle have large homozygous deletions, whereas human FHHNC mutations are mainly missense mutations affecting the extracellular loops of claudin-16. From these observations it seems that the site and extent of the mutation determines the phenotypic manifestation, ranging from isolated alterations in channel conductance to an alteration in cell proliferation and and differentiation.

Hypomagnesemia with Secondary Hypocalcemia (OMIM 602014)

Hypomagnesemia with secondary hypocalcemia (HSH) is a rare autosomal recessive disorder that manifests in early infancy with generalized seizures or other symptoms of increased neuromuscular excitability as first described in 1968.[82] Delayed diagnosis or noncompliance with treatment can be fatal or result in permanent neurologic damage.

Biochemical abnormalities include extremely low serum Mg^{2+} and low serum Ca^{2+} levels. The mechanism leading to hypocalcemia is still not completely understood. Severe hypomagnesemia results in an impaired synthesis and/or release of PTH.[83] Consistently, PTH levels in individuals with HSH were found to be inappropriately low. The hypocalcemia observed in HSH is resistant to treatment with Ca^{2+} or vitamin D. Relief of clinical symptoms, normocalcemia, and normalization of PTH levels can only be achieved by administration of high doses of Mg^{2+}.[84]

Transport studies in HSH patients pointed to a primary defect in intestinal Mg^{2+} absorption.[85,86] However, in some patients an additional renal leak for Mg^{2+} was suspected.[87]

By linkage analysis, a gene locus (HOMG1) for HSH had been mapped to chromosome 9q22 in 1997.[88] Later, two independent groups identified TRPM6 at this locus and reported presumable loss-of-function mutations, mainly truncating mutations, as the underlying cause of HSH.[89,90] Thus far, in more than 20 families affected with HSH, mutations in TRPM6 have been identified.[91,92] TRPM6 encodes a member of the transient receptor potential (TRP) family of cation channels. TRPM6 protein is homologous to TRPM7, a Ca^{2+}- and Mg^{2+}-permeable ion channel regulated by Mg-ATP.[93] TRPM6 is expressed along the entire small intestine and colon but also in kidney in distal tubule cells. Immunofluorescence studies with an antibody generated against murine TRPM6 could localize TRPM6 to the apical membrane of the DCT.[94] The detection of TRPM6 expression in the DCT confirms the hypothesis of an additional role of renal Mg^{2+} wasting for the pathogenesis of HSH.[36] This was also supported by intravenous Mg^{2+}-loading tests in HSH patients, which disclosed a considerable renal Mg^{2+} leak, albeit still being hypomagnesemic.[90]

The observation that in HSH patients the substitution of high oral doses of Mg^{2+} achieves at least subnormal serum Mg^{2+} levels supports the theory of two independent intestinal transport systems for Mg^{2+}. TRPM6 probably represents a molecular component of active transcellular Mg^{2+} transport. An increased intraluminal Mg^{2+} concentration (by increased oral intake) permits compensation for the defect in active transcellular transport by increasing absorption via the passive paracellular pathway (see Fig. 15-3).

The TRP protein superfamily comprises more than 20 related cation channels playing important roles in various physiologic processes, including phototransduction, sensory physiology, and regulation of smooth muscle tone.[95] Drosophila flies carrying the trp mutation are inflicted with impaired vision because of the lack of a specific Ca^{2+} influx pathway in the photoreceptors.[96] The identification of the trp gene product as a cation channel and the rewarding search for TRP homologs in other species led to the discovery of a new family of cation channels.

TRP proteins are allocated to the structural superfamily of six-transmembrane ion channels encompassing most voltage-gated K^+ channels, the cyclic nucleotide-gated channel family, and single-transmembrane cassettes of voltage-activated Ca^{2+} and Na^+ channels. Both N and C termini of TRP proteins are thought to be located intracellularly, and a putative pore-forming region is bordered by transmembrane domains 5 and 6. Four TRP protein subunits assemble to form a functional channel complex.[97]

TRP proteins can be subdivided into three subfamilies: TRPC, TRPV, and TRPM. TRPM proteins display the structural hallmark of exceptionally long intracellular N and C termini. Within the TRPM family, three members (TRPM2, TRPM6, and TRPM7) are set apart because they harbor enzyme domains in their respective C termini and thus represent prototypes of an intriguing new protein family of enzyme-coupled ion channels. TRPM2 is C-terminally fused to an adenosine diphosphate–pyrophosphatase and has been found to be activated by one of the products of NAD hydrolysis, adenosine diphosphate–ribose.[98] TRPM6 as well as TRPM7 contain protein kinase domains in their C termini, which bear sequence similarity to elongation factor 2 serine/threonine kinases and other proteins that contain an α-kinase domain.[99] Despite the lack of detectable sequence homology to classical eukaryotic protein kinases, the crystal structure of TRPM7 kinase surprisingly revealed striking structural similarity to the catalytic core of eukaryotic protein kinases as well as to metabolic enzymes with ATP-grasp domains.[100] TRPM7 is widely expressed, and targeted disruption of the channel gene in cell lines proved to be lethal, underpinning a salient and nonredundant role in cell physiology.[93] Interestingly, TRPM7 exhibits significant Mg^{2+} permeation, a rather unusual feature of other cation channels, and is inhibited by cytosolic Mg^{2+} as well as Mg-ATP. A systematic analysis of the permeation properties of TRPM7 revealed that the latter channel has the unique property to conduct a wide range of divalent trace metal ions, some of these with detrimental consequences for the cell upon intoxication.[101] In light of its broad expression pattern and its constitutive activity, TRPM7 may provide a general mechanism for the entry of divalent cations into cells. However, recent data suggest that TRPM7 represents a primarily Mg^{2+}-permeable ion channel required for the cellular uptake of Mg^{2+}.[102] The Mg^{2+} permeability seems to be modulated by a functional coupling between TRPM7's ion channel and kinase domains indicated by coordinated changes in phosphotransferase activity and ion flow. By the phosphorylation of certain target proteins, the kinase domain might thus be involved in a negative-feedback mechanism that inhibits a further uptake of Mg^{2+} in the presence of rising intracellular Mg^{2+} concentrations.[102] Recently, annexin-1 has been identified as the first endogenous substrate of TRPM7 kinase.[103] Annexin-1 is a Ca^{2+}- and phospholipids-binding protein implicated in the regulation of cell growth and apoptosis.[104]

TRPM6 is closely related to TRPM7 and represents the second TRP protein being fused to a C-terminal α-kinase domain. The *TRPM6* gene is composed of 39 exons encoding a total of 2022 amino acid residues. *TRPM6* messenger RNA shows a more restricted expression pattern than TRPM7, with highest levels along the intestine (duodenum, jejunum, ileum, colon) and the DCT of the kidney.[89] Immunohistochemistry shows a complete colocalization with the Na^+/Cl^- cotransporter NCCT (also serving as a DCT marker) but also with parvalbumin and calbindin-D_{28K}, two cytosolic proteins that putatively act as intracellular (Ca^{2+} and) Mg^{2+} buffers.[94]

Biophysical characterization of TRPM6 is currently controversial. Voets et al could demonstrate striking parallels between TRPM6 and TRPM7 with respect to gating mechanisms and ion selectivity profiles, in that TRPM6 was shown to be regulated by intracellular Mg^{2+} levels and to be permeable for Mg^{2+} and Ca^{2+}.[94] Permeation characteristics with currents almost exclusively carried by divalent cations with a higher affinity for Mg^{2+} than Ca^{2+} support the role of TRPM6 as the apical Mg^{2+} influx pathway. Furthermore, TRPM6 (in analogy to TRPM7) exhibits a marked sensitivity to intracellular Mg^{2+}. Thus, one might postulate an inhibition of TRPM6-mediated Mg^{2+} uptake by rising intracellular Mg^{2+} concentrations as a possible mechanism of a regulated intestinal and renal Mg^{2+} (re)absorption. This inhibition might in part be mediated by intracellular Mg-ATP as shown for TRPM7.[93]

Using a similar expression model (but a different expression vector), Chubanov et al reported that TRPM6 is only present at the cell surface when associating with TRPM7.[105] Furthermore, fluorescence resonance energy transfer analyses showed a specific direct protein-protein interaction between both proteins. Electrophysiologic data in a *Xenopus* oocyte expression system indicated that co-expression of TRPM6 results in a significant amplification of TRPM7-induced currents.[105] The idea of heteromultimerization of TRPM7 with TRPM6 could be confirmed by Schmitz et al.[106] They could further demonstrate that TRPM6 and TRPM7 are not functionally redundant, but there is evidence that both proteins can influence each other's biologic activity. It has also been shown that TRPM6 can phosphorylate TRPM7 and that TRPM6 might modulate TRPM7 function in a Mg^{2+}-dependent manner.[106]

Mitochondrial Hypomagnesemia (OMIM 500005)

Recently, a mutation in the mitochondrial-coded isoleucine transfer RNA gene (*MTTI*), has been discovered in a large Caucasian kindred.[107] An extensive clinical evaluation of this family was prompted after the discovery of hypomagnesemia in the index patient. Pedigree analysis was compatible with mitochondrial inheritance, because the phenotype was exclusively transmitted by affected females. The phenotype includes hypomagnesemia, hypercholesterolemia, and hypertension. Of the adults on the maternal lineage, the majority of offspring exhibit at least one of the mentioned symptoms; approximately half of the individuals show a combination of two or more symptoms, and around one-sixth had all three features. Serum Mg^{2+} levels of family members on the maternal lineage greatly vary, ranging from about 0.8 to about 2.5 mg/dL (equivalent to ≈0.3 to ≈1.0 mmol/L), with approximately 50% of individuals being hypomagnesemic.

The hypomagnesemic individuals (serum Mg^{2+} <0.9 mmol/L) showed higher fractional excretions (median around 7.5%) than their normomagnesemic relatives on the maternal lineage (median ≈3%), clearly pointing to renal Mg^{2+} wasting as causative for hypomagnesemia. Interestingly, hypomagnesemia was accompanied by decreased urinary Ca^{2+} concentrations, a finding pointing to the DCT as the affected tubular segment.

The mitochondrial mutation observed in the examined family affects the isoleucine transfer RNA gene *MT-TI*. The observed nucleotide exchange occurs at the T nucleotide directly adjacent to the anticodon triplet. This position is highly conserved among species and critical for codon-anticodon recognition. The functional consequences of the transfer RNA defect in mitochondrial function remain to be elucidated in detail. Because ATP consumption along the tubule is highest in the DCT, the authors speculate on an impaired energy metabolism of DCT cells as a consequence of the mitochondrial defect, which could in turn lead to disturbed transcellular Mg^{2+} reabsorption. Further studies in these patients might help to better understand the mechanism of distal tubular Mg^{2+} wasting in these patients.

MEDULLARY CYSTIC KIDNEY DISEASE AND FAMILIAL JUVENILE HYPERURICEMIC NEPHROPATHY

Renal cystic diseases are an important group of inherited renal conditions and worldwide a leading genetic cause of end-stage renal disease. Autosomal dominant and recessive polycystic kidney disease represent the most frequent entities, but taken together, nephronophthisis (NPH), medullary cystic kidney disease/familial juvenile hyperuricemic nephropathy (MCKD/FJHN), autosomal dominant glomerulocystic kidney disease (GCKD), and Bardet-Biedl syndrome account for an important group of patients as well.

During recent decades, advances in molecular genetics have allowed the identification of responsible genes and provided information on the respective proteins and therefore insight into the pathobiology in many of the above-mentioned conditions. The genes associated with autosomal dominant (*PKD1*, *PKD2*) and autosomal recessive polycystic kidney disease (*PKHD1*),[108] nephronophthisis (*NPHS1-6*),[109] MCKD type 2 (*UMOD*),[110] FJHN (*UMOD*, *HNF1β*),[110,111] and Bardet-Biedl syndrome (*BBS1-11*)[112,113] have been identified.

The recent discovery of the above-mentioned genes and proteins puts forth a new classification of cystic kidney diseases, not exclusively based on clinical presentation but rather on a genetic and pathogenic basis.

This chapter focuses on MCKD/FJHN, especially on its genetics, and on uromodulin (the protein encoded by the gene that is mutated in many individuals with MCKD/FJHN), on the clinicopathologic presentation, as well as on diagnosis and treatment in MCKD/FJHN.

Genetics

The conditions referred to as MCKD/FJHN have been shown to be genetically heterogeneous, with linkage established to at least three distinct loci thus far. According to the linkage to different loci, investigators have classified occurrences of MCKD into two groups.

Although the responsible gene or genes have not yet been isolated, MCKD type 1 (MCKD1, OMIM 174000) has been localized to chromosome 1q21 and the locus further refined by several investigators.[114-118] In a recent study, Wolf et al[119] confirmed the haplotype-sharing hypothesis and detected three different haplotype subsets in several kindreds. By mutational analysis of all 37 positional candidates, the authors found sequence variations in three different genes, compatible with involvement of different genes within the MCKD1 critical region.

MCKD type 2 (MCKD2, OMIM 603860) was mapped to chromosome 16p12,[120] overlapping the locus subsequently identified for FJHN (OMIM 162000) in some families.[121,122] Dahan et al proposed MCKD2 and FJHN to be allelic disorders[123] and Hart et al[110] for the first time described mutations in the gene encoding uromodulin (*UMOD*), causing MCKD2 in one and FJHN in three families, findings that were confirmed by further investigations[110,124-129] in many affected pedigrees. Additionally, a *UMOD* mutation has been found in one family with autosomal dominant GCKD (OMIM 609886),[129] extending the allelism to MCKD2/FJHN/GCKD. Nevertheless, in some families inherited GCKD is associated with maturity-onset diabetes (*MODY5*), and in such patients mutations of the hepatocyte nuclear factor 1β (*HNF1β*) have been reported,[130] whereas a *HNF1β* mutation was also described in one family with FJHN and diabetes.[111] The significance of these findings in human disease has not been fully elucidated, but in at least one murine model, the role of the transcription factor HNF1β in regulating the terminal differentiation of renal tubular epithelial cells has been established: The expression of *Umod*, *Pkhd1*, *Pkd2*, *Nphp1*, and *Tg737*, all of them genes involved in cystic renal diseases, is reduced in conditionally, kidney-specific *HNF1β*-inactivated mice.[131]

Finally, in some families with typical MCKD, no linkage to either chromosome 1q21 or 16p12 could be established, suggesting the presence of another genetic locus.[115,132] The same applies for families with FJHN but without established linkage to *UMOD* mutations; in various studies linkage to chromosome 16p has been reported in 40% to 80% of them.[133]

Uromodulin

Uromodulin, also referred to as Tamm-Horsfall glycoprotein, is exclusively expressed by cells of the TAL of the loop of Henle, and in some species within the early DCT.[134] It was initially characterized by Tamm and Horsfall,[135] but despite intensive research during more than 50 years, the definite functions of uromodulin have remained mostly elusive. Given its gelling properties, it was originally thought to be mainly responsible in maintaining water impermeability within TAL. Additionally, uromodulin has been implicated with many physiologic functions and pathophysiologic conditions (see review[136]), such as protection against bacterial infection of the urinary tract, immunomodulation, nephrolithiasis and cast nephropathy, interstitial nephritis, and, most recently, MCKD2/FJHN/GCKD.

Uromodulin is a complex glycoprotein, inserted into the luminal surface of the cells by a glycosyl-phosphatidylinositol anchor. After proteolytic cleavage of the ectodomain by action of a yet-unidentified enzyme, uromodulin is excreted into the urine where it represents the most abundant protein in healthy individuals. The substantial amount of cysteine residues (7.5%), resulting in 24 potential disulfide bridges, suggests a complex structure of this protein. Mutations affecting the disulfide bonds or reducing the calcium-binding affinity are suspected to alter the tertiary structure of the protein and therefore to result in delayed maturation and hence intracellular accumulation of uromodulin.[129] This hypothesis is supported by experiments in vitro, through transient transfection of different cell lines with *UMOD*-mutant and wild-type constructs, respectively. Expression of mutant constructs results in delayed protein expression at the cell surface with a longer retention of uromodulin within the endoplasmic reticulum,[129] probably reflecting an abnormal folding of the protein. This fits very well with the following observations in humans: Many identified *UMOD* mutations in patients with MCKD2/FJHN affect cysteine residues and therefore are supposed to alter the tertiary structure of the protein. Accordingly, histopathology reveals patchy intracellular uromodulin deposits within the respective tubular segments associated with tubulointerstitial fibrosis and inflammation.[128,129,137] Electron microscopy demonstrates accumulation of dense fibrillar material, supposedly being uromodulin, within the endoplasmic reticulum. Finally, urinary uromodulin excretion in patients is significantly reduced;[128,129] that affected patients excrete less than the supposed 50% of wild-type uromodulin suggests a dominant-negative effect of the mutated protein on the wild-type allele. Some authors propose to combine these conditions into the entity of uromodulin storage disease. Most of *UMOD* mutations described thus far are missense mutations modifying cysteine or charged residues, located in exon 4 and some within exon 5 with evidence of significant ethnic differences.[128,129,138] It is notable that exon 4 contains a strongly conserved cysteine-rich sequence comprising three calcium-binding epidermal growth factor–like domains (cbEGF), linking mutations within these sequence with the supposed ultrastructural abnormalities of the protein as a consequence of misfolding.

Despite evidence that uromodulin deficiency in mice results in increased susceptibility to urinary tract infection[139,140] and increased renal formation of calcium crystals,[141] in patients with *UMOD*-associated MCKD2/FJHN the frequency of neither urinary tract infection nor nephrolithiasis is increased.[142] On the other hand, the above-mentioned individuals with MCKD2/FJHN unequivocally present with histologic renal lesions, whereas in uromodulin knockout mice the kidneys appear morphologically normal.[143,144] Therefore, it has been hypothesized that the characteristic renal histologic changes in humans might be the consequence of abnormal uromodulin processing and storage within tubular epithelial cells, with consecutive induction of inflammatory and profibrotic processes. The residual excretion of wild-type uromodulin—which has been shown to be the only form excreted in patients with FJHN[128]—could be sufficient to prevent them from increased susceptibility for urinary tract infection and crystal formation observed in mice completely lacking the expression of uromodulin.

Clinicopathologic Presentation

MCKD is a genetic tubulointerstitial disorder, mainly characterized by autosomal dominant transmission of defective urinary concentrating ability, frequent hyperuricemia/gout, tubular dilations/cysts (often located at the corticomedullary junction), and chronic renal failure progressing to end-stage kidney disease during adulthood in many patients. Given the similarities with respect to clinical presentation, macroscopic pathology, and renal histology, MCKD and NPH were thought to be the autosomal dominant and recessive counterparts of a unique disease complex, until recently referred to as NPH-MCKD complex.[145] In view of the recent advances in molecular genetics, however, NPH and MCKD should be distinguished and instead classified according to molecular genetics.[146]

Differentiation between MCKD1 and MCKD2 on clinical grounds alone is difficult and arbitrary; the designation of both types is primarily based on linkage to different loci as described above. However, the phenotype in MCKD2 is described to be more severe with respect to hyperuricemia/gout and earlier onset of end-stage renal disease (median 32 years in MCKD2 versus 62 years in MCKD1).[120]

The clinical presentation in families with FJHN is very similar to that for the above-mentioned description of MCKD, and most reports confirm, in addition to these overlapping symptoms between FJHN and MCKD2, an important intrafamilial and interfamilial heterogeneity of presentation in both. Even on the basis of the presence of corticomedullary cysts in presumed MCKD2 and hyperuricemia in individuals whose disease is classified as FJHN, no definite distinction between these two entities can be established. Therefore, differentiating these two seems artificial and probably not useful for clinical purposes.[146] Consequently, the designations MCKD2/FJHN complex or *UMOD*-related disorders for patients with proven mutations have been proposed. The most relevant features of MCKD/FJHN are discussed below.

Defective Urinary Concentrating Capacity

Given the characteristic pattern of expression, uromodulin was for a long time suspected to be involved in water impermeability of the TAL, the nephron segment crucial for the creation of the corticomedullary countercurrent and therefore for urine concentration. The exact mechanisms by which uromodulin is involved in tubular water impermeability and salt reabsorption have not been discovered until now. However, a vast majority of patients with *UMOD*-related disease present with a markedly reduced urinary concentrating capacity, reflected by early-morning urine osmolality below 600 mOsm/L.[146]

Hyperuricemia

Hyperuricemia is not only characteristic for FJHN but also often present in individuals with MCKD. When considering the two disease entities together, hyperuricemia can be found in at least two-thirds of patients with MCKD2/FJHN.[146] Bleyer et al described inappropriate fractional excretion of uric acid with an inverse correlation with creatinine clearance,[125] whereas Scolari et al found an inverse correlation between uric acid levels and urine osmolality.[146] The former observation suggests an effect of renal failure on the development of hyperuricemia; however, in general the degree of hyperuricemia is described as out of proportion to the degree of renal insufficiency. The inverse correlation between

hyperuricemia and urine osmolality, a supposed indirect marker for volume status, suggests an indirect effect through volume contraction and enhanced proximal sodium and water reabsorption. This hypothesis is supported by observations linking reduced sodium reabsorption in the TAL with elevated urate levels, as side effects of chronic administration of loop diuretics or in individuals with Bartter syndrome.[146]

Tubulointerstitial Fibrosis

Diffuse tubulointerstitial fibrosis, sometimes associated with thickening and splitting of tubular basement membrane, is an unequivocal feature in patients with typical MCKD/FJHN.[129] The exact mechanisms linking *UMOD* mutations with the characteristic histologic lesions remain to be detected. A immunomodulatory and proinflammatory effect of uromodulin has been shown by several investigators; that is, interstitial deposits of uromodulin and associated immune complexes frequently are surrounded by inflammatory cells (see review[134]); additionally, tubulointerstitial lesions can be induced in animals after injection with uromodulin, and interstitial uromodulin deposits have been shown in several human conditions associated with tubulointerstitial fibrosis, including MCKD.[146]

Tubular Dilation and Cysts

Despite the denomination, cystic tubular dilations/cysts are not as frequent as tubulointerstitial fibrosis and hyperuricemia in MCKD/FJHN. Medullary cysts are derived from progressively dilated collecting tubules, remaining connected to the afferent and efferent segments, comparable with the characteristic cystic dilations in autosomal recessive polycystic kidney disease. The exact pathogenic mechanisms leading to cystic dilations, notably with marked interfamilial and intrafamilial variations, remain elusive. Tubular obstructions—maybe through cellular protrusions—have been discussed as a possible explanation.[146]

Diagnosis and Treatment

The diagnosis of MCKD/FJHN should be considered in every individual presenting with a combination of the following symptoms and signs: chronic renal failure, hyperuricemia (especially if serum urate concentration is out of proportion as compared with the degree of renal insufficiency) and/or gout, hypertension, a normal urinalysis, and a family history of chronic renal failure. Genetic testing on a routine basis for *UMOD* mutations is available, facilitating the final diagnosis in suspected pedigrees. In contrast, because the gene or genes in MCKD1 have not yet been identified, confirming this diagnosis remains difficult, probably resulting in underestimation of the frequency and under-reporting of this entity.

No specific treatment for MCKD/FJHN has been available until now. Correction of water and electrolyte disturbances is necessary in some patients, and optimal antihypertensive treatment should be instituted in hypertensive ones. Recurrence of tubulointerstitial lesions in renal allograft of unaffected donors has not been observed. Given the excellent reported outcome,[147] renal transplantation is considered the preferred therapy. With regard to living-related donor transplantation, a challenge arises especially in small families without a family history suggestive for autosomal dominant MCKD.[148]

References

1. Jeck N, Schlingmann KP, Reinalter SC, et al: Salt handling in the distal nephron: Lessons learned from inherited human disorders. Am J Physiol Regul Integr Comp Physiol 288:R782–R795, 2005.
2. Rosenbaum P, Hughes M: Persistent, probably congenital hypokalemic metabolic alkalosis with hyaline degeneration of renal tubules and normal urinary aldosterone. Am J Dis Child 94:560, 1957.
3. Bartter F, Pronove P, Gill J, Jr, MacCardle R: Hyperplasia of the juxtaglomerular complex with hyperaldosteronism and hypokalemic alkalosis. A new syndrome. Am J Med 33:811–828, 1962.
4. Gitelman HJ, Graham JB, Welt LG: A new familial disorder characterized by hypokalemia and hypomagnesemia. Trans Assoc Am Physicians 79:221–235, 1966.
5. Rodriguez-Soriano J, Vallo A, Garcia-Fuentes M: Hypomagnesaemia of hereditary renal origin. Pediatr Nephrol 1:465–472, 1987.
6. Bettinelli A, Bianchetti MG, Girardin E, et al: Use of calcium excretion values to distinguish two forms of primary renal tubular hypokalemic alkalosis: Bartter and Gitelman syndromes. J Pediatr 120:38–43, 1992.
7. Bartter FC, Pronove P, Gill JR, Jr., MacCardle RC: Hyperplasia of the juxtaglomerular complex with hyperaldosteronism and hypokalemic alkalosis. A new syndrome. 1962. J Am Soc Nephrol 9:516–528, 1998.
8. Fanconi A, Schachenmann G, Nussli R, Prader A: Chronic hypokalaemia with growth retardation, normotensive hyperrenin-hyperaldosteronism ("Bartter's syndrome"), and hypercalciuria. Report of two cases with emphasis on natural history and on catch-up growth during treatment. Helv Paediatr Acta 26:144–163, 1971.
9. McCredie DA, Blair-West JR, Scoggins BA, Shipman R: Potassium-losing nephropathy of childhood. Med J Aust 1:129–135, 1971.
10. Ohlsson A, Sieck U, Cumming W, et al: A variant of Bartter's syndrome. Bartter's syndrome associated with hydramnios, prematurity, hypercalciuria and nephrocalcinosis. Acta Paediatr Scand 73:868–874, 1984.
11. Seyberth HW, Koniger SJ, Rascher W, et al: Role of prostaglandins in hyperprostaglandin E syndrome and in selected renal tubular disorders. Pediatr Nephrol 1:491–497, 1987.
12. Seyberth HW, Rascher W, Schweer H, et al: Congenital hypokalemia with hypercalciuria in preterm infants: A hyperprostaglandinuric tubular syndrome different from Bartter syndrome. J Pediatr 107:694–701, 1985.
13. Landau D, Shalev H, Ohaly M, Carmi R: Infantile variant of Bartter syndrome and sensorineural deafness: A new autosomal recessive disorder. Am J Med Genet 59:454–459, 1995.
14. Simon DB, Karet FE, Hamdan JM, et al: Bartter's syndrome, hypokalaemic alkalosis with hypercalciuria, is caused by mutations in the Na-K-2Cl cotransporter NKCC2. Nat Genet 13:183–188, 1996.
15. Simon DB, Karet FE, Rodriguez-Soriano J, et al: Genetic heterogeneity of Bartter's syndrome revealed by mutations in the K+ channel, ROMK. Nat Genet 14:152–156, 1996.
16. Birkenhager R, Otto E, Schurmann MJ, et al: Mutation of BSND causes Bartter syndrome with sensorineural deafness and kidney failure. Nat Genet 29:310–314., 2001.
17. Schlingmann KP, Konrad M, Jeck N, et al: Salt wasting and deafness resulting from mutations in two chloride channels. N Engl J Med 350:1314–1319, 2004.
18. Simon DB, Bindra RS, Mansfield TA, et al: Mutations in the chloride channel gene, CLCNKB, cause Bartter's syndrome type III. Nat Genet 17:171–178, 1997.
19. Watanabe S, Fukumoto S, Chang H, et al: Association between activating mutations of calcium-sensing receptor and Bartter's syndrome. Lancet 360:692–694., 2002.
20. Massa G, Proesmans W, Devlieger H, et al: Electrolyte composition of the amniotic fluid in Bartter syndrome. Eur J Obstet Gynecol Reprod Biol 24:335–340, 1987.
21. Proesmans W, Massa G, Vandenberghe K, Van Assche A: Prenatal diagnosis of Bartter syndrome. Lancet 1:394, 1987.
22. Simon DB, Lu Y, Choate KA, et al: Paracellin-1, a renal tight junction protein required for paracellular Mg^{2+} resorption. Science 285:103–106, 1999.
23. Kamel KS, Oh MS, Halperin ML: Bartter's, Gitelman's, and Gordon's syndromes. From physiology to molecular biology and back, yet still some unanswered questions. Nephron 92 Suppl 1:18–27, 2002.
24. Jeck N, Derst C, Wischmeyer E, et al: Functional heterogeneity of ROMK mutations linked to hyperprostaglandin E syndrome. Kidney Int 59:1803–1811, 2001.
25. Finer G, Shalev H, Birk OS, et al: Transient neonatal hyperkalemia in the antenatal (ROMK defective) Bartter syndrome. J Pediatr 142:318–323, 2003.
26. Peters M, Jeck N, Reinalter S, et al: Clinical presentation of genetically defined patients with hypokalemic salt-losing tubulopathies. Am J Med 112:183–190, 2002.
27. Schlatter E, Frobe U, Greger R: Ion conductances of isolated cortical collecting duct cells. Pflugers Arch 421:381–387, 1992.
28. Taniguchi J, Imai M: Flow-dependent activation of maxi K+ channels in apical membrane of rabbit connecting tubule. J Membr Biol 164:35–45, 1998.
29. Estevez R, Boettger T, Stein V, et al: Barttin is a Cl− channel β-subunit crucial for renal Cl− reabsorption and inner ear K+ secretion. Nature 414:558–561, 2001.
30. Waldegger S, Jeck N, Barth P, et al: Barttin increases surface expression and changes current properties of ClC-K channels. Pflugers Arch 444:411–418, 2002.
31. Jeck N, Reinalter SC, Henne T, et al: Hypokalemic salt-losing tubulopathy with chronic renal failure and sensorineural deafness. Pediatrics 108:E5, 2001.
32. Konrad M, Vollmer M, Lemmink HH, et al: Mutations in the chloride channel gene CLCNKB as a cause of classic Bartter syndrome. J Am Soc Nephrol 11:1449–1459, 2000.
33. Zelikovic I, Szargel R, Hawash A, et al: A novel mutation in the chloride channel gene, CLCNKB, as a cause of Gitelman and Bartter syndromes. Kidney Int 63:24–32, 2003.
34. Schurman SJ, Perlman SA, Sutphen R, et al: Genotype/phenotype observations in African Americans with Bartter syndrome. J Pediatr 139:105–110, 2001.
35. Luthy C, Bettinelli A, Iselin S, et al: Normal prostaglandinuria E2 in Gitelman's syndrome, the hypocalciuric variant of Bartter's syndrome. Am J Kidney Dis 25:824–828, 1995.
36. Cole DE, Quamme GA: Inherited disorders of renal magnesium handling. J Am Soc Nephrol 11:1937–1947, 2000.
37. Konrad M, Weber S: Recent advances in molecular genetics of hereditary magnesium-losing disorders. J Am Soc Nephrol 14:249–260., 2003.
38. Elin RJ: Magnesium: The fifth but forgotten electrolyte. Am J Clin Pathol 102:616–622, 1994.
39. Kerstan D, Quamme G: Physiology and pathophysiology of intestinal absorption of magnesium. In Massry SG, Morii H, Nishizawa Y (eds): Calcium in Internal Medicine. London, Springer-Verlag, 2002, pp 171–183.
40. Quamme GA, de Rouffignac C: Epithelial magnesium transport and regulation by the kidney. Front Biosci 5:D694–D711, 2000.

41. Fine KD, Santa Ana CA, Porter JL, Fordtran JS: Intestinal absorption of magnesium from food and supplements. J Clin Invest 88:396–402, 1991.

42. de Rouffignac C, Quamme G: Renal magnesium handling and its hormonal control. Physiol Rev 74:305–322, 1994.

43. Dai LJ, Ritchie G, Kerstan D, et al: Magnesium transport in the renal distal convoluted tubule. Physiol Rev 81:51–84., 2001.

44. Quamme GA: Renal magnesium handling: New insights in understanding old problems. Kidney Int 52:1180–1195, 1997.

45. Meij IC, Koenderink JB, van Bokhoven H, et al: Dominant isolated renal magnesium loss is caused by misrouting of the Na$^+$,K$^+$-ATPase γ-subunit. Nat Genet 26:265–266, 2000.

46. Geven WB, Monnens LA, Willems HL, et al: Renal magnesium wasting in two families with autosomal dominant inheritance. Kidney Int 31:1140–1144, 1987.

47. Meij IC, Koenderink JB, De Jong JC, et al: Dominant isolated renal magnesium loss is caused by misrouting of the Na$^+$, K$^+$-ATPase γ-subunit. Ann N Y Acad Sci 986:437–443, 2003.

48. Meij IC, Saar K, van den Heuvel LP, et al: Hereditary isolated renal magnesium loss maps to chromosome 11q23. Am J Hum Genet 64:180–188, 1999.

49. Sweadner KJ, Arystarkhova E, Donnet C, Wetzel RK: FXYD proteins as regulators of the Na,K-ATPase in the kidney. Ann N Y Acad Sci 986:382–387, 2003.

50. Arystarkhova E, Wetzel RK, Sweadner KJ: Distribution and oligomeric association of splice forms of (Na$^+$K$^+$ATPase) regulatory γ-subunit in rat kidney. Am J Physiol Renal Physiol 282:F393–F407, 2002.

51. Arystarkhova E, Donnet C, Asinovski NK, Sweadner KJ: Differential regulation of renal Na,K-ATPase by splice variants of the γ subunit. J Biol Chem 277:10162–10172, 2002.

52. Blostein R, Pu HX, Scanzano R, Zouzoulas A: Structure/function studies of the γ subunit of the Na, K-ATPase. Ann N Y Acad Sci 986:420–427, 2003.

53. Meij IC, Van Den Heuvel LP, Hemmes S, et al: Exclusion of mutations in FXYD2, CLDN16 and SLC12A3 in two families with primary renal Mg^{2+} loss. Nephrol Dial Transplant 18:512–516, 2003.

54. Jones DH, Li TY, Arystarkhova E, et al: Na,K-ATPase from mice lacking the γ subunit (FXYD2) exhibits altered Na$^+$ affinity and decreased thermal stability. J Biol Chem 280:19003–19011, 2005.

55. Nijenhuis T, Vallon V, van der Kemp AW, et al: Enhanced passive Ca^{2+} reabsorption and reduced Mg^{2+} channel abundance explains thiazide-induced hypocalciuria and hypomagnesemia. J Clin Invest 115:1651–1658, 2005.

56. Geven WB, Monnens LA, Willems JL, et al: Isolated autosomal recessive renal magnesium loss in two sisters. Clin Genet 32:398–402, 1987.

57. Brown EM, Gamba G, Riccardi D, et al: Cloning and characterization of an extracellular (Ca^{2+} sensing) receptor from bovine parathyroid. Nature 366:575–580, 1993.

58. Riccardi D, Lee WS, Lee K, et al: Localization of the extracellular (Ca^{2+} sensing) receptor and PTH/PTHrP receptor in rat kidney. Am J Physiol 271:F951–F956, 1996.

59. Hebert SC: Extracellular calcium-sensing receptor: Implications for calcium and magnesium handling in the kidney. Kidney Int 50:2129–2139, 1996.

60. Pollak MR, Brown EM, Estep HL, et al: Autosomal dominant hypocalcaemia caused by a (Ca^{2+} sensing) receptor gene mutation. Nat Genet 8:303–307, 1994.

61. Pearce SH, Williamson C, Kifor O, et al: A familial syndrome of hypocalcemia with hypercalciuria due to mutations in the calcium-sensing receptor [see Comments]. N Engl J Med 335:1115–1122, 1996.

62. Vargas-Poussou R, Huang C, Hulin P, et al: Functional characterization of a calcium-sensing receptor mutation in severe autosomal dominant hypocalcemia with a Bartter-like syndrome. J Am Soc Nephrol 13:2259–2266, 2002.

63. Pollak MR, Brown EM, Chou YH, et al: Mutations in the human (Ca^{2+} sensing) receptor gene cause familial hypocalciuric hypercalcemia and neonatal severe hyperparathyroidism. Cell 75:1297–1303, 1993.

64. Marx SJ, Attie MF, Levine MA, et al: The hypocalciuric or benign variant of familial hypercalcemia: Clinical and biochemical features in fifteen kindreds. Medicine (Baltimore) 60:397–412, 1981.

65. Cole DE, Janicic N, Salisbury SR, Hendy GN: Neonatal severe hyperparathyroidism, secondary hyperparathyroidism, and familial hypocalciuric hypercalcemia: Multiple different phenotypes associated with an inactivating Alu insertion mutation of the calcium-sensing receptor gene. Am J Med Genet 71:202–210, 1997.

66. Praga M, Vara J, Gonzalez-Parra E, et al: Familial hypomagnesemia with hypercalciuria and nephrocalcinosis. Kidney Int 47:1419–1425, 1995.

67. Rodriguez-Soriano J, Vallo A: Pathophysiology of the renal acidification defect present in the syndrome of familial hypomagnesaemia-hypercalciuria. Pediatr Nephrol 8:431–435, 1994.

68. Benigno V, Canonica CS, Bettinelli A, et al: Hypomagnesaemia-hypercalciuria-nephrocalcinosis: A report of nine cases and a review. Nephrol Dial Transplant 15:605–610, 2000.

69. Weber S, Schneider L, Peters M, et al: Novel paracellin-1 mutations in 25 families with familial hypomagnesemia with hypercalciuria and nephrocalcinosis. J Am Soc Nephrol 12:1872–1881, 2001.

70. Colegio OR, Van Itallie C, Rahner C, Anderson JM: Claudin extracellular domains determine paracellular charge selectivity and resistance but not tight junction fibril architecture. Am J Physiol Cell Physiol 284:C1346–C1354, 2003.

71. Weber S, Schlingmann KP, Peters M, et al: Primary gene structure and expression studies of rodent paracellin-1. J Am Soc Nephrol 12:2664–2672, 2001.

72. Hou J, Paul DL, Goodenough DA: Paracellin-1 and the modulation of ion selectivity of tight junctions. J Cell Sci 118:5109–5118, 2005.

73. Ohba Y, Kitagawa H, Kitoh K, et al: A deletion of the paracellin-1 gene is responsible for renal tubular dysplasia in cattle. Genomics 68:229–236, 2000.

74. Lu Y, Choate KA, Wang T, Lifton RP: Paracellin-1 knock-out mouse model of recessive renal hypomagnesemia, hypercalciuria and nephrocalcinosis (Abstract). J Am Soc Nephrol 12:, 2001.

75. Meij IC, van den Heuvel LP, Knoers NV: Genetic disorders of magnesium homeostasis. Biometals 15:297–307, 2002.

76. Blanchard A, Jeunemaitre X, Coudol P, et al: Paracellin-1 is critical for magnesium and calcium reabsorption in the human thick ascending limb of Henle. Kidney Int 59:2206–2215, 2001.

77. Muller D, Kausalya PJ, Claverie-Martin F, et al: A novel claudin 16 mutation associated with childhood hypercalciuria abolishes binding to ZO-1 and results in lysosomal mistargeting. Am J Hum Genet 73:1293–1301, 2003.

78. Wong V, Goodenough DA: Paracellular channels! Science 285:62, 1999.

79. Lee DB, Huang E, Ward HJ: Tight junction biology and kidney dysfunction. Am J Physiol Renal Physiol 290:F20–F34, 2006.

80. Hirano T, Kobayashi N, Itoh T, et al: Null mutation of PCLN-1/Claudin-16 results in bovine chronic interstitial nephritis. Genome Res 10:659–663, 2000.

81. Sasaki Y, Kitagawa H, Kitoh K, et al: Pathological changes of renal tubular dysplasia in Japanese black cattle. Vet Rec 150:628–632, 2002.

82. Paunier L, Radde IC, Kooh SW, et al: Primary hypomagnesemia with secondary hypocalcemia in an infant. Pediatrics 41:385–402, 1968.

83. Anast CS, Mohs JM, Kaplan SL, Burns TW: Evidence for parathyroid failure in magnesium deficiency. Science 177:606–608, 1972.

84. Shalev H, Phillip M, Galil A, et al: Clinical presentation and outcome in primary familial hypomagnesaemia. Arch Dis Child 78:127–130, 1998.

85. Lombeck I, Ritzl F, Schnippering HG, et al: Primary hypomagnesemia. I. Absorption Studies. Z Kinderheilkd 118:249–258, 1975.

86. Milla PJ, Aggett PJ, Wolff OH, Harries JT: Studies in primary hypomagnesaemia: Evidence for defective carrier-mediated small intestinal transport of magnesium. Gut 20:1028–1033, 1979.

87. Matzkin H, Lotan D, Boichis H: Primary hypomagnesemia with a probable double magnesium transport defect. Nephron 52:83–86, 1989.

88. Walder RY, Shalev H, Brennan TM, et al: Familial hypomagnesemia maps to chromosome 9q, not to the X chromosome: Genetic linkage mapping and analysis of a balanced translocation breakpoint. Hum Mol Genet 6:1491–1497, 1997.

89. Schlingmann KP, Weber S, Peters M, et al: Hypomagnesemia with secondary hypocalcemia is caused by mutations in *TRPM6*, a new member of the TRPM gene family. Nat Genet 31:166–170, 2002.

90. Walder RY, Landau D, Meyer P, et al: Mutation of *TRPM6* causes familial hypomagnesemia with secondary hypocalcemia. Nat Genet 31:171–174, 2002.

91. Schlingmann KP, Sassen MC, Weber S, et al: Novel *TRPM6* mutations in 21 families with primary hypomagnesemia and secondary hypocalcemia. J Am Soc Nephrol 16:3061–3069, 2005.

92. Jalkanen R, Pronicka E, Tyynismaa H, et al: Genetic background of HSH in three Polish families and a patient with an X;9 translocation. Eur J Hum Genet 14:55–62, 2006.

93. Nadler MJ, Hermosura MC, Inabe K, et al: LTRPC7 is a Mg-ATP-regulated divalent cation channel required for cell viability. Nature 411:590–595, 2001.

94. Voets T, Nilius B, Hoefs S, et al: TRPM6 forms the Mg^{2+} influx channel involved in intestinal and renal Mg^{2+} absorption. J Biol Chem 279:19–25, 2004.

95. Montell C, Birnbaumer L, Flockerzi V: The TRP channels, a remarkably functional family. Cell 108:595–598, 2002.

96. Hardie RC, Raghu P, Imoto K, Mori Y: Visual transduction in *Drosophila*. Nature 413:186–193, 2001.

97. Hofmann T, Schaefer M, Schultz G, Gudermann T: Subunit composition of mammalian transient receptor potential channels in living cells. Proc Natl Acad Sci U S A 99:7461–7466, 2002.

98. Perraud AL, Fleig A, Dunn CA, et al: ADP-ribose gating of the calcium-permeable LTRPC2 channel revealed by Nudix motif homology. Nature 411:595–599, 2001.

99. Runnels LW, Yue L, Clapham DE: TRP-PLIK, a bifunctional protein with kinase and ion channel activities. Science 291:1043-1047, 2001.

100. Yamaguchi H, Matsushita M, Nairn AC, Kuriyan J: Crystal structure of the atypical protein kinase domain of a TRP channel with phosphotransferase activity. Mol Cell 7:1047–1057, 2001.

101. Monteilh-Zoller MK, Hermosura MC, Nadler MJ, et al: TRPM7 provides an ion channel mechanism for cellular entry of trace metal ions. J Gen Physiol 121:49–60, 2003.

102. Schmitz C, Perraud AL, Johnson CO, et al: Regulation of vertebrate cellular Mg^{2+} homeostasis by TRPM7. Cell 114:191–200, 2003.

103. Dorovkov MV, Ryazanov AG: Phosphorylation of annexin I by TRPM7 channel-kinase. J Biol Chem 279:50643–50646, 2004.

104. Rescher U, Gerke V: Annexins—Unique membrane binding proteins with diverse functions. J Cell Sci 117:2631–2639, 2004.

105. Chubanov V, Waldegger S, Mederos y Schnitzler M, et al: Disruption of TRPM6/TRPM7 complex formation by a mutation in the *TRPM6* gene causes hypomagnesemia with secondary hypocalcemia. Proc Natl Acad Sci U S A 101:2894–2899, 2004.

106. Schmitz C, Dorovkov MV, Zhao X, et al: The channel kinases TRPM6 and TRPM7 are functionally nonredundant. J Biol Chem 280:37763–37771, 2005.

107. Wilson FH, Hariri A, Farhi A, et al: A cluster of metabolic defects caused by mutation in a mitochondrial tRNA. Science 306:1190–1194, 2004.

108. Bisceglia M, Galliani CA, Senger C, et al: Renal cystic diseases: A review. Adv Anat Pathol 13:26–56, 2006.

109. Sayer JA, Otto EA, O'Toole JF, et al: The centrosomal protein nephrocystin-6 is mutated in Joubert syndrome and activates transcription factor ATF4. Nat Genet 38:674–681, 2006.

110. Hart TC, Gorry MC, Hart PS, et al: Mutations of the *UMOD* gene are responsible for medullary cystic kidney disease 2 and familial juvenile hyperuricaemic nephropathy. J Med Genet 39:882–892, 2002.

111. Bingham C, Ellard S, van't Hoff WG, et al: Atypical familial juvenile hyperuricemic nephropathy associated with a hepatocyte nuclear factor-1β gene mutation. Kidney Int 63:1645–1651, 2003.

112. Stoetzel C, Laurier V, Davis EE, et al: *BBS10* encodes a vertebrate-specific chaperonin-like protein and is a major *BBS* locus. Nat Genet 38:521–524, 2006.

113. Chiang AP, Beck JS, Yen HJ, et al: Homozygosity mapping with SNP arrays identifies TRIM32, an E3 ubiquitin ligase, as a Bardet-Biedl syndrome gene (*BBS11*). Proc Natl Acad Sci U S A 103:6287–6292, 2006.

114. Christodoulou K, Tsingis M, Stavrou C, et al: Chromosome 1 localization of a gene for autosomal dominant medullary cystic kidney disease. Hum Mol Genet 7:905–911, 1998.

115. Auranen M, Ala-Mello S, Turunen JA, Jarvela I: Further evidence for linkage of autosomal-dominant medullary cystic kidney disease on chromosome 1q21. Kidney Int 60:1225–1232, 2001.

116. Wolf MT, Karle SM, Schwarz S, et al: Refinement of the critical region for *MCKD1* by detection of transcontinental haplotype sharing. Kidney Int 64:788–792, 2003.

117. Wolf MT, van Vlem B, Hennies HC, et al: Telomeric refinement of the *MCKD1* locus on chromosome 1q21. Kidney Int 66:580–585, 2004.

118. Fuchshuber A, Kroiss S, Karle S, et al: Refinement of the gene locus for autosomal dominant medullary cystic kidney disease type 1 (*MCKD1*) and construction of a physical and partial transcriptional map of the region. Genomics 72:278–284, 2001.

119. Wolf MT, Mucha BE, Hennies HC, et al: Medullary cystic kidney disease type 1: Mutational analysis in 37 genes based on haplotype sharing. Hum Genet 119:649–658, 2006.

120. Scolari F, Puzzer D, Amoroso A, et al: Identification of a new locus for medullary cystic disease, on chromosome 16p12. Am J Hum Genet 64:1655–1660, 1999.

121. Stiburkova B, Majewski J, Sebesta I, et al: Familial juvenile hyperuricemic nephropathy: Localization of the gene on chromosome 16p11.2-and evidence for genetic heterogeneity. Am J Hum Genet 66:1989–1994, 2000.

122. Kamatani N, Moritani M, Yamanaka H, et al: Localization of a gene for familial juvenile hyperuricemic nephropathy causing underexcretion-type gout to 16p12 by genome-wide linkage analysis of a large family. Arthritis Rheum 43:925–929, 2000.

123. Dahan K, Fuchshuber A, Adamis S, et al: Familial juvenile hyperuricemic nephropathy and autosomal dominant medullary cystic kidney disease type 2: Two facets of the same disease? J Am Soc Nephrol 12:2348–2357, 2001.

124. Turner JJ, Stacey JM, Harding B, et al: *UROMODULIN* mutations cause familial juvenile hyperuricemic nephropathy. J Clin Endocrinol Metab 88:1398–1401, 2003.

125. Bleyer AJ, Woodard AS, Shihabi Z, et al: Clinical characterization of a family with a mutation in the uromodulin (Tamm-Horsfall glycoprotein) gene. Kidney Int 64:36–42, 2003.

126. Bleyer AJ, Trachtman H, Sandhu J, et al: Renal manifestations of a mutation in the uromodulin (Tamm Horsfall protein) gene. Am J Kidney Dis 42:E20–E26, 2003.

127. Wolf MT, Mucha BE, Attanasio M, et al: Mutations of the uromodulin gene in MCKD type 2 patients cluster in exon 4, which encodes three EGF-like domains. Kidney Int 64:1580–1587, 2003.

128. Dahan K, Devuyst O, Smaers M, et al: A cluster of mutations in the *UMOD* gene causes familial juvenile hyperuricemic nephropathy with abnormal expression of uromodulin. J Am Soc Nephrol 14:2883–2893, 2003.

129. Rampoldi L, Caridi G, Santon D, et al: Allelism of MCKD, FJHN and GCKD caused by impairment of uromodulin export dynamics. Hum Mol Genet 12:3369–3384, 2003.

130. Bingham C, Bulman MP, Ellard S, et al: Mutations in the hepatocyte nuclear factor-1β gene are associated with familial hypoplastic glomerulocystic kidney disease. Am J Hum Genet 68:219–224, 2001.

131. Gresh L, Fischer E, Reimann A, et al: A transcriptional network in polycystic kidney disease. EMBO J 23:1657–1668, 2004.

132. Kroiss S, Huck K, Berthold S, et al: Evidence of further genetic heterogeneity in autosomal dominant medullary cystic kidney disease. Nephrol Dial Transplant 15:818–821, 2000.

133. Kudo E, Kamatani N, Tezuka O, et al: Familial juvenile hyperuricemic nephropathy: Detection of mutations in the uromodulin gene in five Japanese families. Kidney Int 65:1589–1597, 2004.

134. Serafini-Cessi F, Malagolini N, Cavallone D: Tamm-Horsfall glycoprotein: Biology and clinical relevance. Am J Kidney Dis 42:658–676, 2003.

135. Tamm I, Horsfall FL, Jr: Characterization and separation of an inhibitor of viral hemagglutination present in urine. Proc Soc Exp Biol Med 74:106–108, 1950.

136. Weichhart T, Zlabinger GJ, Saemann MD: The multiple functions of Tamm-Horsfall protein in human health and disease: A mystery clears up. Wien Klin Wochenschr 117:316–322, 2005.

137. Bleyer AJ, Hart TC, Willingham MC, et al: Clinico-pathologic findings in medullary cystic kidney disease type 2. Pediatr Nephrol 20:824–827, 2005.

138. Lens XM, Banet JF, Outeda P, Barrio-Lucia V: A novel pattern of mutation in uromodulin disorders: Autosomal dominant medullary cystic kidney disease type 2, familial juvenile hyperuricemic nephropathy, and autosomal dominant glomerulocystic kidney disease. Am J Kidney Dis 46:52–57, 2005.

139. Mo L, Zhu XH, Huang HY, et al: Ablation of the Tamm-Horsfall protein gene increases susceptibility of mice to bladder colonization by type 1-fimbriated *Escherichia coli*. Am J Physiol Renal Physiol 286:F795–F802, 2004.

140. Bates JM, Raffi HM, Prasadan K, et al: Tamm-Horsfall protein knockout mice are more prone to urinary tract infection: Rapid communication. Kidney Int 65:791–797, 2004.

141. Mo L, Huang HY, Zhu XH, et al: Tamm-Horsfall protein is a critical renal defense factor protecting against calcium oxalate crystal formation. Kidney Int 66:1159–1166, 2004.

142. Devuyst O, Dahan K, Pirson Y: Tamm-Horsfall protein or uromodulin: New ideas about an old molecule. Nephrol Dial Transplant 20:1290–1294, 2005.

143. Raffi H, Bates JM, Laszik Z, Kumar S: Tamm-Horsfall protein knockout mice do not develop medullary cystic kidney disease. Kidney Int 69:1914–1915, 2006.

144. Bachmann S, Mutig K, Bates J, et al: Renal effects of Tamm-Horsfall protein (uromodulin) deficiency in mice. Am J Physiol Renal Physiol 288:F559–F567, 2005.

145. Hildebrandt F, Otto E: Molecular genetics of nephronophthisis and medullary cystic kidney disease. J Am Soc Nephrol 11:1753–1761, 2000.

146. Scolari F, Caridi G, Rampoldi L, et al: Uromodulin storage diseases: Clinical aspects and mechanisms. Am J Kidney Dis 44:987–999, 2004.

147. Stavrou C, Deltas CC, Christophides TC, Pierides A: Outcome of kidney transplantation in autosomal dominant medullary cystic kidney disease type 1. Nephrol Dial Transplant 18:2165–2169, 2003.

148. Kiser RL, Wolf MT, Martin JL, Zalewski I, et al: Medullary cystic kidney disease type 1 in a large Native-American kindred. Am J Kidney Dis 44:611–617, 2004.

Chapter 16

Hereditary Disorders of Collecting Duct Sodium and Potassium Transport

David H. Ellison and Christie P. Thomas

This chapter will focus on inherited disorders of Na^+, K^+, and Cl^- that arise from mutations of transporters or regulatory molecules expressed in the aldosterone-sensitive distal nephron (ASDN). The ASDN comprises the late distal convoluted tubule (DCT2), the connecting tubule (CNT), and the cortical and medullary portions of the collecting duct (CCD and MCD). Morphologically and functionally there are three distinct cell types that make up the CNT and CCD: the principal cell and the α- and β-intercalated cells. The principal cell is involved in Na^+ reabsorption and K^+ secretion, and the intercalated cells are involved in K^+ reabsorption and in H^+ and HCO_3^- secretion. Cl^- is absorbed by the paracellular route in principal cells but may be absorbed transcellularly in intercalated cells. Na^+ is reabsorbed in the principal cell via the electrogenic amiloride-inhibitable epithelial Na^+ channel (ENaC), and K^+ is secreted via the K^+ channels, ROMK and Maxi-K (Fig. 16-1). ENaC and many of its regulatory systems are expressed throughout the ASDN (Fig. 16-2), and this chapter will be restricted to transport defects that relate to transcellular passage of Na^+ and K^+ and the paracellular

passage of Cl^- in the ASDN (Table 16-1). Disorders that arise from mutations in transport pathways expressed predominantly along the early distal convoluted tubule (DCT1), such as Gitelman syndrome, are discussed in Chapter 15.

ION TRANSPORT IN THE ALDOSTERONE-SENSITIVE DISTAL NEPHRON

Sodium

Although the filtered load of Na^+ is large, under normal conditions almost 95% of this load is absorbed by proximal nephron segments including the proximal convoluted tubule, the ascending limb of the loop of Henle, and DCT1. The remaining Na^+ in tubular fluid is reabsorbed variably in more distal nephron segments in response to dietary cues and to circulating hormones to precisely regulate volume homeostasis and the control of blood pressure. This reabsorption is

Table 16-1 Mendelian Disorders of Na^+, K^+ Transport in the Aldosterone-Sensitive Distal Nephron

Disorder	Site of Mutation	Inheritance	Serum K^+	Plasma Aldosterone
Hypertension				
Liddle syndrome	β- or γ-ENaC	AD	Low	Low
Syndrome of apparent mineralocorticoid excess (SAME)	HSD11B2	AR	Low	Low
Gordon syndrome (Pseudohypoaldosteronism type 2)	WNK1, WNK4, locus 3	AD	High	Variable
Autosomal dominant hypertension with severe exacerbation in pregnancy	NR3C2	AD	Low	Low
Glucocorticoid-remediable hyperaldosteronism*	Aldosterone synthase	AD	Low	High
Hypotension				
Pseudohypoaldosteronism type 1	α-, β-, or γ-ENaC	AR	High	Very high
Pseudohypoaldosteronism type 1	NR3C2	AD	High	High
Gitelman syndrome†	NCC	AR	Low	High
Bartter syndrome†	NKCC2, ROMK, ClC-Kb, Barttin	AR	Low	High

AD, autosomal dominant; AR, autosomal recessive.
*Disorder of aldosterone synthesis in the adrenal cortex.
†These disorders are discussed in chapter 15 on the thick ascending limb and distal convoluted tubule.

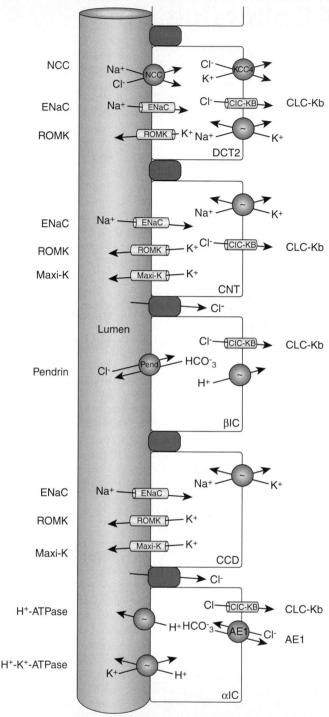

Figure 16-1 Schematic of tubular epithelial cells lining the aldosterone-sensitive distal nephron (ASDN). Transporters and ion channels relevant to this chapter are shown on the apical and basolateral aspects of the DCT2, CNT, CCD, α-intercalated cell (αIC), and β-intercalated cell (βIC).

more robust in the early portion of the ASDN, with a larger fraction of Na^+ reabsorption occurring in the DCT2 and the CNT, and a progressively smaller contribution from the CCD and MCD.[1] In fact, inactivation of ENaC in the collecting duct does not impair Na^+ or K^+ balance, reflecting the contributions of DCT2 and CNT to Na^+ and K^+ transport.[2]

Aldosterone is the principal hormone that regulates extracellular volume and renal K^+ excretion via its effects on Na^+ and K^+ transport in the ASDN. There are two principal stimuli for aldosterone release from the zona glomerulosa of the adrenal cell cortex: volume depletion and hyperkalemia. Volume depletion stimulates renin release, which increases circulating angiotensin II levels, which in turn stimulates aldosterone secretion. Hyperkalemia has a direct stimulatory effect on aldosterone release from the zona glomerulosa.[3,4] The major effects of aldosterone are genomic and mediated via its cytosolic receptor, the mineralocorticoid receptor (gene symbol *NR3C2*), which, when bound to its ligand, dimerizes and translocates to the nucleus to activate a set of target genes. Cortisol, the natural human glucocorticoid hormone, has equal affinity for the mineralocorticoid receptor, and its circulating levels are several-fold greater than that of aldosterone. In mineralocorticoid-responsive tissues such as the ASDN, an enzyme, 11β-hydroxysteroid dehydrogenase type 2 (gene symbol *HSD11B2*), metabolizes cortisol to the inactive cortisone allowing aldosterone unrestricted access to its cognate receptor (Fig. 16-3).[5,6]

The epithelial Na^+ channel is a heteromultimeric channel composed of α-, β-, and γ-ENaC subunits (gene symbols *SCNN1A*, *SCNN1B*, and *SCNN1G*) expressed in the apical plasma membrane of DCT2 and the principal cells of CNT, CCD, and MCD. Each of these subunits has an intracellular NH_2^+ and COO^- terminus, two transmembrane domains, and a single large extracellular domain.[7,8] Removal of the ENaC complex from the apical cell surface is mediated via conserved PPPXY (PY) motifs in the C termini of β- and or γ-ENaC subunits.[9] These PY motifs interact with E3-type ubiquitin ligases via their WW domains.[10–12] Ubiquitin ligases seem to regulate the endocytic retrieval, ubiquitination, and subsequent degradation of ENaC complexes and may serve to limit ENaC function.[13,14] Nedd4-2 is one such ubiquitin ligase that is expressed in the collecting duct, which can robustly inhibit ENaC function.[11,15,16]

The α-ENaC subunit when expressed alone in reconstituted cell systems has weak Na^+ transport activity, which is amplified several fold in the presence of β- and γ-ENaC subunits.[17] These three subunits are integral members of the transporting ENaC complex in the ASDN, although the exact stoichiometry is still under debate with the current evidence favoring either a tetramer composed of 2α:β:γ or a nonamer comprised of 3α:3β:3γ.[18–20] In the ASDN, β- and γ-ENaC are constitutively expressed and found within the cytosol, whereas the level of α-ENaC is low but exquisitely regulated in response to physiologic cues.

Two of the principal regulators of ENaC activity in the distal nephron are dietary Na^+ intake and circulating aldosterone. Under conditions of Na^+ depletion or an increase in aldosterone levels, there is the rapid induction of α-ENaC in the CNT and to a lesser extent in the CCD, which then appears to translocate together with β- and γ-ENaC to the apical plasma membrane.[21,22] Aldosterone binds to the mineralocorticoid receptor and induces the transcriptional expression of α-ENaC by activation of a hormone response element in the 5′ flanking region of the α-ENaC gene.[23] Aldosterone also increases the transcription of at least one other key regulatory molecule, the serum and glucocorticoid-regulated kinase, SGK1 (gene symbol *SGK*).[24,25] SGK1, in turn, can increase ENaC activity by at least two mechanisms (see Fig. 16-3). The

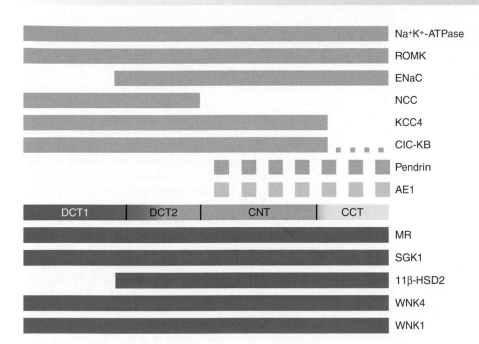

	Na⁺K⁺-ATPase
	ROMK
	ENaC
	NCC
	KCC4
	CIC-KB
	Pendrin
	AE1
DCT1	DCT2	CNT	CCT	
	MR
	SGK1
	11β-HSD2
	WNK4
	WNK1

Figure 16-2 Gene expression profile of transporters, channels, and regulatory molecules in the ASDN. Interrupted expression indicates that these proteins are expressed only in intercalated cells of the relevant segments. The expression of KS-WNK1 is not shown, but it is restricted to the cortex and is most evident in the DCT. AE1, a Cl⁻/HCO₃⁻ anion exchanger; MR, mineralocorticoid receptor. (From Delaloy C, Lu J, Houot AM, et al: Multiple promoters in the *WNK1* gene: One controls expression of a kidney-specific kinase-defective isoform. Mol Cell Biol 23:9208–9221, 2003.)

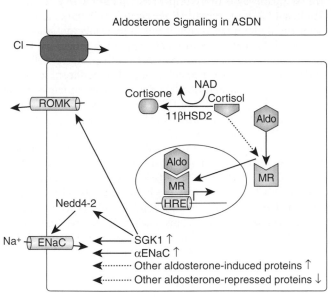

Figure 16-3 Aldosterone signaling in the ASDN. Cortisol is metabolized to inactive cortisone in the ASDN, allowing aldosterone (Aldo) unrestricted access to its cognate receptor, the mineralocorticoid receptor (MR). As a result a variety of aldosterone-sensitive genes are activated or repressed, leading to the stimulation of Na⁺ transport via ENaC. HRE, hormone response element; 11βHSD2, 11β-hydroxysteroid dehydrogenase type 2.

first involves the phosphorylation of Nedd4-2 at one or more consensus phosphorylation sites,[26,27] which facilitates its interaction with the 14-3-3 family of regulatory proteins.[28,29] This interaction then reduces the affinity of Nedd4-2 for the PY motifs of ENaC.[26,27] An inhibition of the ENaC–Nedd4-2 interaction leads to a reduction in the endocytic retrieval of ENaC, resulting in more Na⁺ channels at the apical cell surface. The second mechanism is a direct effect of SGK1 at a consensus phosphorylation site within the C terminus of

α-ENaC to increase ENaC activity.[30] This increase in activity seems to result from the conversion of silent channels to open channels or by an increase in channel insertion into the apical membrane. A third mechanism has recently been described: SGK1 can phosphorylate WNK4 and alleviate the inhibitory effect of WNK4 on ENaC.[30a]

SGK1 is a member of the AGC family of kinases and is an inducible serine threonine kinase that is widely expressed.[14] In addition to corticosteroids, SGK1 expression is induced by a variety of stimuli including growth factors such as transforming growth factor-β, fibroblast growth factor, platelet-derived growth factor, and granulocyte-macrophage colony-stimulating factor. SGK1 is activated by phosphorylation by a number of upstream kinases including PI-3 kinase, PDK-1, PKA, ERK5, p38-α, and WNK1.[14,31] Activated SGK1 can in turn directly or indirectly interact with Nedd4-2, WNK4, ENaC, and ROMK to stimulate collecting duct Na⁺ absorption and K⁺ secretion.

Although the canonical aldosterone-sensitive Na⁺ transport protein is ENaC, other Na⁺-transporting proteins, such as the thiazide-sensitive electroneutral NaCl cotransporter of the DCT2 (NCC; gene symbol *SLC12A3*), respond to aldosterone as well. The relation between increases in ENaC activity and changes in the activity of electroneutral transport proteins may determine the physiologic and pathophysiologic effects of the steroid hormone. Aldosterone increases the activity and abundance of NCC in vivo; changes in the abundance of this transport protein may contribute to the phenomenon of mineralocorticoid escape.[32–34] The nature of the overall response to aldosterone, whether electrogenic or electroneutral, may determine whether aldosterone functions primarily as a sodium Cl⁻ retaining hormone (as when stimulated by renin and angiotensin II) or as a K⁺ secretory hormone (as when stimulated by hyperkalemia).[35]

Potassium

The major site for K⁺ secretion in the kidney is the principal cells of the CNT and the CCD. The driving force for K⁺ secretion is the lumen-negative potential difference generated by the absorption of Na^+ via ENaC. K^+ secretion is mediated via at least two apical K^+ channels.[36] The first is the low-conductance K^+ channel, ROMK (SK, Kir 1.1; gene symbol *KCNJ1*), and the second is a large-conductance K^+ channel, BK (Maxi-K), composed of a pore-forming α-subunit (gene symbol *KCNMA1*) and a modulatory β-subunit (*KCNB1*) (see Fig. 16-1).

The renal outer medullary K^+ channel (ROMK) is expressed as one of three alternately spliced isoforms, and of these, ROMK1 is expressed exclusively in the CNT and CCD. An increase in dietary K^+ intake, which stimulates the secretion of aldosterone, increases the abundance of ROMK1 channels at the apical cell surface but does not seem to increase synthesis of ROMK1. One mechanism for this increase in ROMK1 is via the aldosterone-mediated activation of SGK1, which in turn can increase the apical abundance and activity of ROMK1.[37,38] K^+ secretion is increased by the enhanced activity of the apical Na^+ channel and the basolateral Na^+, K^+-ATPase, both of which are also stimulated by high plasma K^+. WNK1, a serine threonine kinase expressed in the CCD and CNT seems to inhibit ROMK1 by enhancing its endocytosis.[39,40] In preliminary studies, a kidney-specific truncated protein variant of WNK1, KS-WNK1, is increased with a high-K^+ diet and decreased on a low-K^+ diet.[40,41] KS-WNK1 antagonizes many of the effects of full-length WNK1; this may serve as an alternate pathway for increased surface expression of ROMK1 with hyperkalemia.

Low dietary K^+ intake, by contrast, stimulates the activity of protein tyrosine kinases like *c*-Src, which phosphorylates ROMK1 to facilitate its internalization from the apical cell surface.[42] WNK4, another serine threonine kinase expressed in the CCD and CNT, regulates ROMK activity by inhibiting its surface expression.[43] Whether changes in dietary or serum K^+ levels alter WNK4 abundance and/or function is not currently known.

The second apical K^+ channel in the principal cell of the CNT and CCD is the Ca^{2+}-activated, tetraethylammonium-sensitive Maxi-K channel, whose activity is increased by tubular fluid flow rates. An increase in distal nephron tubular flow may be sensed by the central cilium of the principal cell, stimulating a Ca^{2+} conductance, which in turn activates the Maxi-K channels to effect flow-dependent K^+ secretion.[44,45] An increase in plasma K^+ may also inhibit proximal tubular Na^+ and water reabsorption, which has also been postulated to lead to an increase in distal flow and increased K^+ secretion.[42]

K^+ is reabsorbed by the intercalated cells of the CCD and by the MCD via the apical H^+, K^+-ATPases, which include the SCH-28080-sensitive, ouabain-insensitive gastric isoform, the SCH-28080-insensitive, ouabain-sensitive colonic isoform, and a third as yet unidentified isoform that is insensitive to both SCH-28080 and ouabain.[46–48] A high-K^+ diet reduces the activity of H^+, K^+-ATPase and limits K^+ reabsorption in these circumstances. Conversely, a low-K^+ diet stimulates activity of the gastric H^+, K^+-ATPase with increased apical K^+ entry and its exit via basolateral K^+ channels.

Chloride Ion

Approximately 4% to 8% of filtered Cl^- is delivered to the distal tubule of hydropenic rats. Fractional Cl^- reabsorption amounts to 2% to 4% of filtered load along the superficial distal tubule. A similar amount is reabsorbed beyond the superficial distal tubule.[49] Volume expansion increases Cl^- delivery to the distal tubule and Cl^- reabsorption in that segment. The superficial distal tubule can reabsorb Cl^- actively, even though the transepithelial voltage favors passive Cl^- reabsorption.[50] The mechanisms by which Cl^- moves across DCT, CNT, and collecting duct epithelia remain incompletely defined.

Cl^- is believed to traverse DCT cells predominantly via a transcellular pathway (see Fig. 16-1). Cl^- enters the cell across the apical membrane, against an electrochemical gradient, largely via the thiazide-sensitive NCC, and driven by Na^+ entry. Cl^- exits DCT cells across the basolateral cell membrane via the Cl^- channel, ClC-Kb (gene symbol *CLCNKB*, which corresponds to *ClC-K2* in the rodent)[51] and via a KCl cotransporter, thought to be KCC4 (gene symbol *SLC12A4*).[52] The exit of Cl^- through ClC-Kb is driven by cell voltage, whereas that through the KCl cotransporter is driven by the chemical gradient for K^+. The Cl^- channel ClC-Kb seems to require a β-subunit, termed barttin (gene symbol *BSND*), which colocalizes with both CLC-K2 (ClC-Kb) and CLC-K1, and may enhance channel delivery to the plasma membrane.[53] Although deficiency of this Cl^- channel causes a form of Bartter syndrome, recent mathematical models of the DCT suggest that the KCl pathway is more important, quantitatively, for transepithelial Cl^- movement.[54,55] Paracellular Cl^- flux across this segment, under normal conditions, is probably minimal.[54,55]

Little information is available regarding routes of transepithelial Cl^- transport in the CNT. Both principal cells and intercalated cells are present along this nephron segment. CLC-K2 has been described at the basolateral membrane of the CNT,[56,57] but routes of Cl^- entry across the apical membrane have not been defined. Conversely, pendrin (gene symbol *SLC26A4*), a Na^+-independent Cl^-/HCO_3^- exchanger, is expressed at the apical surface of β-intercalated cells in the CNT and collecting duct (and occasionally along the DCT), where it may participate in HCO_3^- secretion (and Cl^- reabsorption). Cl^- enters across the basolateral membrane of α-intercalated cells via another Cl^-/HCO_3^- anion exchanger, AE1 (gene symbol *SLC4A1*). This exchanger seems to play an important role in maintaining acid/base balance.[58] Cl^- channels may also be present at the basolateral membrane of both α- and β-intercalated cells to allow exit of Cl^-. According to recently modeled parameters, significant transepithelial Cl^- transport would be expected to traverse β-intercalated cells via pendrin and the basolateral Cl^- channel.[54,55] Cl^- would largely recycle across the basolateral cell membrane of α-intercalated cells.

LIDDLE SYNDROME (PSEUDOALDOSTERONISM; OMIM 177200)

Historical Overview

Liddle syndrome is a rare autosomal dominant disorder with early-onset severe hypertension, variable hypokalemia, and metabolic alkalosis with suppressed renin and aldosterone levels. The first description of a large kindred with this disorder by Grant Liddle led to his eponymous association with this disease.[59] The proband, who presented at age 16 with severe hypertension and hypokalemic metabolic alkalosis, had a strong family history of early-onset hypertension with hypokalemia. The proband had very low basal aldosterone levels, and urinary aldosterone levels remained low despite correction of the hypokalemia and being placed on a low-Na$^+$ diet. Liddle and colleagues demonstrated that the salivary and sweat Na$^+$/K$^+$ ratio was high and found normal levels of glucocorticoid and mineralocorticoid metabolites in the urine, indicating that the syndrome was unlikely to be due to an excess of circulating corticosteroid-like compounds. Triamterene, a Na$^+$ channel blocker, but not spironolactone, a mineralocorticoid receptor blocker, improved blood pressure and corrected the hypokalemia The proband eventually developed renal failure, presumably from poorly controlled hypertension, and after undergoing a renal transplant had a reversal of the previously noted metabolic abnormalities.[60] The constellation of findings suggested that the abnormality in these patients were related to an intrinsic defect within the distal nephron leading to enhanced Na$^+$ absorption.

Genetic Basis

A genetic analysis of the original kindred demonstrated complete linkage of the disorder to the β-ENaC gene locus. Mutation analysis confirmed that affected members of the family had a nonsense mutation that truncated β-ENaC, removing the entire cytoplasmic C-terminal tail of β-ENaC. Additional studies in several kindred have shown nonsense or frameshift mutations in the C-terminal domain of either the β-ENaC or γ-ENaC subunit that deletes a conserved PY motif in these proteins.[61,62] Subsequently, three kindred with missense mutations that substituted one amino acid within the PY motif confirmed the importance of this motif in regulating channel activity.[63-65] Although a PY motif is also present in the α-ENaC subunit, thus far all mutations reported in Liddle syndrome have been heterozygous mutations in the C-terminal tail of the β- or γ-ENaC subunit (Table 16-2). Surprisingly, in one recently reported kindred, a missense mutation in the extracellular domain of γ-ENaC was identified.[66]

Clinical Features

Early-onset hypertension that is often severe in an individual with a strong family history of hypertension should prompt consideration of this disease. The classic laboratory features of the disease are hypokalemia with metabolic alkalosis.[67] In one instance the hypertension and metabolic abnormalities were evident in infancy.[68] Hypertension and the hypokalemia can be effectively treated with amiloride or triamterene but not by spironolactone or eplerenone, which is another feature that should increase the suspicion for Liddle syndrome.

If the hypertension is poorly treated or is not recognized, then end-organ damage including renal failure can occur early and be severe. Worsening renal function may mitigate the tendency to hypokalemia, and a clue to the diagnosis may be lost.

Pathophysiology

Mutations that disrupt or delete the PY motif of ENaC lead to an increase in the activity of the Na$^+$ channel. This has been demonstrated by expression of disease-causing mutant subunits in *Xenopus* oocytes and in Madin-Darby canine kidney cells.[69,70] The preponderance of evidence indicates that the increase in Na$^+$ transport with Liddle mutations comes about primarily from an increase in the number of channels at the

Table 16-2 Mutations That Cause Liddle Syndrome

Subunit	Codon Change*	Mutation	References
β	R566X	1696C→T	61,72
	A579fr	1735del1736	73
	Q591X	1770C→T	61
	T594fr	1907insC	61
	P596fr	1913delC	61
	T601Fr	1928insG	66
	E607X	1917insC	74
	P617S	1976C→T	65
	P618L	1980C→T	63,65,75,76
	P618R	1980C→G	77,78
	P618H	1980C→A	79
	P618S	1979C→T	80
	Y620H	1985T→C	64
γ	N530S	1589A→G	66
	W575X	1724G→A	62,76

*Numbering is based on NCBI reference sequence NP_000327 and NP_001030 as of 31 October 2005.

cell surface.[69,71] The PY motif normally binds to WW domain–containing proteins such as the E3-type ubiquitin ligase, Nedd4-2. The interaction between β- and/or γ-ENaC and Nedd4-2 targets the channel complex for ubiquitination, endocytosis, and possible degradation. In the absence of one of these PY motifs there is less retrieval of ENaC from the cell surface, which leads to an increase in the number of active channels at the apical membrane with resulting stimulation of Na$^+$ transport. The recent report of Liddle syndrome resulting from a mutation in the extracellular domain of γ-ENaC identified a second region of ENaC that when modified can lead to a gain of function. Although the precise mechanism for the increase in channel activity with this mutation is unknown, it is likely to regulate channel gating.[66]

Liddle syndrome is thus the consequence of an activating mutation in one copy of the β- or γ-ENaC subunit that leads to an increase in distal-nephron Na$^+$ transport. This primary increase in Na$^+$ transport increases the driving force for K$^+$ and H$^+$ loss from the collecting duct and explains the volume expansion, suppressed aldosterone levels, and hypokalemic alkalosis seen in this disease. The disease exhibits locus heterogeneity, in that mutations in either the β- or γ-ENaC subunit cause the same disease.

Animal Model

An animal model of Liddle syndrome has been generated by the creation of a mouse expressing one or two copies of the original Liddle mutation. These animals develop hypertension, hypokalemia, and metabolic alkalosis on a high-salt diet and recapitulate the cardinal features of the syndrome.[81,82] The Liddle mouse demonstrates increased Na$^+$

transport not only in the collecting duct of the kidney but also in the distal colon, suggesting that enhanced colonic Na$^+$ absorption may contribute to the phenotype in humans.

Laboratory Diagnosis

The classic laboratory features of Liddle syndrome are hypokalemia and metabolic alkalosis that occur in a young hypertensive with a strong family history of hypertension and hypokalemia. Hypokalemia can be especially severe in patients who have a high dietary salt intake. An extended pedigree analysis of the original Liddle kindred and several other kindred demonstrated that hypokalemia is not a universal finding.[60,64] Additional testing of affected individuals will demonstrate suppressed plasma renin activity (PRA) and reduced serum and urine aldosterone levels even on a low-salt diet.

An increase in amiloride-sensitive nasal potential difference has been described in one kindred with Liddle syndrome.[83] In another kindred an increase in amiloride-sensitive Na$^+$ transport was noted in peripheral blood lymphocytes.[84] The usefulness of these tests for screening or diagnosis of Liddle syndrome remains uncertain.

Differential Diagnosis

Other causes of hypokalemic alkalosis with hypertension include essential hypertension treated with thiazide or loop diuretics, primary hyperaldosteronism, Cushing syndrome and apparent mineralocorticoid excess (see Table 16-1). Primary hyperaldosteronism is the most common cause of secondary hypertension with hypokalemia and is distinguished from Liddle syndrome by the elevated serum and urine aldosterone levels that are not suppressible on a high-salt diet, and an elevated serum aldosterone-to-renin ratio. Cushing syndrome can be excluded by the absence of characteristic clinical features with a loss of diurnal variation of serum cortisol, and elevated serum, salivary, and urinary cortisol concentrations that are not suppressible by low-dose dexamethasone. The syndrome of apparent mineralocorticoid excess is an autosomal-recessive disease associated with growth retardation and an elevated urine tetrahydrocortisol-to-tetrahydrocortisone ratio (see below).

Genetic Testing

The diagnosis of Liddle syndrome can be confirmed by the identification of mutations within the C terminus of one allele of the β- or γ-ENaC subunit that result in disruption of the PY motif. Because the entire C terminus is contained within the terminal exon of β- and γ-ENaC, a single exon-specific polymerase chain reaction from genomic DNA obtained from a blood sample or buccal swab should be sufficient. This test is not commercially available.

Treatment

Because the defect is intrinsic to the epithelial Na$^+$ channel, the hypertension and hypokalemia should be readily treated with amiloride or triamterene, which are direct inhibitors of the channel. Published anecdotal reports on patients with Liddle syndrome indicate that this is generally true.[60] Renal transplantation in a few patients with Liddle syndrome has been reported in the pre-cyclosporine era, and, as expected, the hypertension and hypokalemia have resolved.

AUTOSOMAL RECESSIVE PSEUDOHYPOALDOSTERONISM TYPE 1 (OMIM 254350)

Historical Overview

Autosomal recessive pseudohypoaldosteronism type 1 (PHA1) is a rare disorder characterized by severe renal salt wasting associated with hyponatremia, hyperkalemia, and acidosis that begins early in life. The first description of a patient who may have had this disorder was in 1958.[85] In that report, a 3-month-old infant with lethargy and poor weight gain was noted to have renal salt wasting with mild hyponatremia and variable hyperkalemia and otherwise normal renal and adrenal function. The infant responded well to NaCl supplementation but was poorly responsive to deoxycorticosterone acetate, suggesting renal tubular resistance to aldosterone action.

Genetic Basis

The disease is caused by mutations in both copies of any of the three subunits (α-, β-, and γ-ENaC) that form the epithelial Na$^+$ channel.[86,87] Mutations are generally homozygous nonsense, frameshift, or splice site mutations within the coding region of the ENaC subunits and are predicted to lead to loss of Na$^+$ channel activity in the collecting duct and in other epithelia where ENaC is expressed and functional.[88,89] In one patient with severe disease, a large homozygous deletion in the promoter region of β-ENaC was identified.[90] In a few patients with a milder phenotype the disease arises from compound heterozygous mutations where at least one allele has a missense mutation.[89,91] The disease has been generally described in offspring of consanguineous unions, and in these matings heterozygous parents are asymptomatic carriers (see Edelheit et al[89] for a comprehensive list of mutations causing autosomal recessive PHA1).

Clinical Features

Occasionally autosomal-recessive PHA1 can present during pregnancy with polyhydramnios.[92,93] The disease classically presents with lethargy, failure to thrive, lack of growth, difficulty with feeding, vomiting, and volume depletion within the first week of life.[94,95] The infants manifest hypotension with hyperkalemia, hyponatremia, and metabolic acidosis. These infants require hospitalization, parenteral saline repletion, and emergent management of hyperkalemia during the hypotensive crises. Once stabilized, infants and children with the disorder generally respond to large doses of oral NaCl and can be maintained on salt supplementation and ion exchange resins. However, these children are prone to recurrent salt depletion crises that may require frequent hospitalizations. During these episodes there is excessive stimulation of the renin-angiotensin-aldosterone axis with massive elevations in PRA and aldosterone levels.

The disease is not limited to the kidney. There are elevated sweat and salivary electrolytes, and that may also contribute to the salt wasting. The excess salt in sweat during crises can predispose children to miliaria-like skin lesions on the face and trunk.[96,97] Newborns may also present with respiratory distress, although this seems to be unusual.[98,99] More commonly, pulmonary manifestations appear in the older child with increased airway secretions, chronic cough, and recurrent respiratory infections.[88,94,95] This disorder is thus also called systemic PHA1, in contrast to the autosomal-dominant form that is renal limited (see below).

Pathophysiology

A few of the ENaC mutations identified in autosomal-recessive PHA1 have been tested in *Xenopus* oocytes by co-expression with other subunits, and these studies demonstrate severely reduced Na$^+$ transport.[86,100] Mutations are generally homozygous nonsense, frameshift, or splice site mutations within the coding region of the ENaC subunits that are predicted to disrupt protein function. The disease is thus likely to be a result of loss of Na$^+$ transport from the inheritance of two hypomorphic or null alleles.

Na$^+$ absorption from the tubular lumen into the CNT and collecting duct of the kidney occurs through the epithelial Na$^+$ channel. Na$^+$ transport in this segment of the nephron can contribute to the reabsorption of 2% to 5% of the filtered Na$^+$ load. Loss-of-function mutations in ENaC subunits lead to failure of Na$^+$ reabsorption in the distal nephron with resulting urinary Na$^+$ loss, hypotension, and stimulation of aldosterone secretion. The failure to transport Na$^+$ directly leads to inhibition of apical membrane K$^+$ and H$^+$ secretion from the principal and α-interacalated cells of the CNT and collecting duct and account for the hyperkalemia and acidosis seen in this disease.

Na$^+$ transport via ENaC is seen throughout the airway epithelia from the nose to the terminal bronchioles as well as in alveolar epithelia. A reduction in Na$^+$ transport in the alveolar and airway epithelia leads to increased airway secretions that manifests as a runny nose with a chronic cough. Na$^+$ transport is also inhibited in sweat and salivary glands leading to high sweat and salivary gland electrolytes.

Animal Models

Each of the ENaC subunits has been deleted in mice and has provided information on the role of these subunits in renal and lung physiology. Inactivation of the α-ENaC subunit in mice leads to death within 2 to 4 days from respiratory distress, because the liquid filling the airway and alveolar spaces in utero is not reabsorbed after birth.[101] Transgenic expression of α-ENaC at a low level can rescue these mice from their lethal pulmonary phenotype, but they go on to manifest PHA1 with significant neonatal mortality, presumably because the renal expression of α-ENaC in the rescued animals is insufficient for ENaC function.[102]

Inactivation of the β- or γ-ENaC subunit leads to the PHA1 phenotype, and mice die within 2 days of birth with hyperkalemia.[103,104] There is little to no abnormality in lung tissues, indicating that the β- and γ-ENaC subunits are not critical for the transition to air breathing after birth, at least in mice. Despite the marked lung disease seen in the α-ENaC-knockout mouse, humans with homozygous loss-of-function mutations in α-ENaC do not generally present with neonatal respiratory distress. However, there are two clinical reports of newborns presenting with respiratory distress and PHA1.[98,99]

Laboratory Diagnosis

Individuals with autosomal-recessive PHA1 present with hyperkalemia, hyponatremia, and metabolic acidosis in infancy. An elevated PRA and high serum and urine aldosterone levels will be invariably found. The transtubular K$^+$ gradient is expected to be less than 5 in the presence of hyperkalemia, reflecting aldosterone resistance. Na$^+$ concentrations in the urine, sweat, and saliva will be high, reflecting the loss of ENaC-mediated Na$^+$ transport in these sites. Amiloride-sensitive nasal potential difference can be measured to demonstrate loss of Na$^+$ transport in airway epithelia.[88,105]

Differential Diagnosis

Other causes of salt wasting with hyperkalemic acidosis include congenital adrenal hyperplasia with mineralocorticoid deficiency, isolated hypoaldosteronism, and autosomal-dominant PHA1. Acquired hypoaldosteronism from adrenal insufficiency and drugs that interfere with aldosterone action may also manifest with hypotension and hyperkalemic metabolic acidosis.

Genetic Testing

Mutations that cause PHA1 are usually homozygous, although there are occasional reports of compound heterozygotes.[89,106] These mutations are nonsense, frameshift, or missense mutations that occur throughout the coding region (except in the C terminus) and have been more frequently reported for the α-ENaC subunit.[89] Mutations in the promoter of β-ENaC leading to near total loss of expression of β-ENaC have been described and add to the complexity of mutation screening.[90] A systematic search for mutations in all three subunits must be undertaken, and such testing is only available in research laboratories.

Treatment

Infants typically present early in life with severe and life-threatening symptoms, and the disease has been associated with a reported high mortality.[94,107] Emergent treatment of the volume depletion and hyponatremia requires parenteral saline repletion, and the management of hyperkalemia includes the use of ion exchange resins and in some cases temporary dialysis. Consistent with the pathophysiology, these patients do not respond to exogenous mineralocorticoids indicating an end-organ resistance to aldosterone. In the long term, children can be managed with large doses of oral NaCl together with chronic ion exchange resin therapy for those with resistant hyperkalemia. These children are prone to recurrent salt depletion crises that may require frequent hospitalizations.

AUTOSOMAL DOMINANT PSEUDOHYPOALDOSTERONISM TYPE 1 –(OMIM 177735)

Historical Overview

Patients with autosomal dominant PHA1 can present in infancy in a similar fashion to autosomal recessive PHA1 with failure to thrive, lethargy, vomiting, and volume depletion. The first description of autosomal dominant PHA1 was in 1991, where the proband presented with classic severe symptoms in infancy, whereas other affected family members had a milder phenotype.[95] Patients in this family were treated with a high-salt diet and responded well to this treatment.

Genetic Basis

Heterozygous mutations in the mineralocorticoid receptor have been identified in 75% of patients with autosomal dominant PHA1 and in some sporadic cases of autosomal recessive PHA1.[106] These mutations are found throughout the coding region and include nonsense, frameshift, and splice site mutations that lead to a truncated receptor and missense mutations that occur within a functional domain that is predicted to reduce or eliminate receptor function or trafficking (see Zennaro and Lombes[106] for a comprehensive list of mutations causing autosomal dominant PHA1). In some of the pedigrees with autosomal dominant PHA1, mutations in the mineralocorticoid receptor have not been identified, but linkage analysis was not performed to determine if the disease segregates with the mineralocorticoid receptor locus.[108] These patients may have mutations elsewhere in the gene, such as in untranslated regions or in regulatory regions. Alternatively this disease may exhibit genetic heterogeneity with a second, hitherto unknown locus that accounts for the remainder of cases.

Clinical Features

Autosomal dominant PHA1, like the autosomal-recessive form of PHA1, presents with failure to thrive, lethargy, vomiting, and volume depletion from salt wasting. This disorder, unlike the autosomal recessive form, has no pulmonary phenotype, because the airways are not a classic aldosterone-responsive tissue. Hyponatremia, hyperkalemia, and metabolic acidosis are prominent features, as are elevated PRA and plasma and urine aldosterone levels. Evidence of urinary Na^+ wasting despite hyperaldosteronemia and volume depletion is suggestive of end-organ resistance to mineralocorticoids. The disease usually presents with a family history, but sporadic cases have been well described.[106] Patients are treated with salt supplementation and with K^+ resins. Importantly, unlike autosomal recessive PHA1, the symptoms remit with age, and salt supplementation can be discontinued in many patients.

Pathophysiology

A few of the mineralocorticoid receptor mutations identified in autosomal dominant PHA1 have been tested in vitro and demonstrate impaired ligand binding, DNA binding, or diminished *trans*-activation function.[109–111] The disease is thus likely to be a result of haploinsufficiency from hypomorphic or null alleles, although as the active mineralocorticoid receptor is a dimer, some mutations may function in a dominant negative fashion.

Aldosterone acting via the mineralocorticoid receptor stimulates Na^+ transport in the CNT and the collecting duct. When there is a reduction in the number of functional mineralocorticoid receptors there is insufficient Na^+ reabsorption in the distal nephron, especially in the newborn and in early childhood, resulting in Na^+ wasting and an impairment in K^+ and H^+ secretion leading to the secondary effects of hyperkalemia and metabolic acidosis. The improvement in salt wasting and the impairment in K^+ and H^+ secretion with increasing age is not well understood. This suggests that in infancy and in early childhood there is a critical dependence on a full complement of functional mineralocorticoid receptors, and with increasing age there are pathways that can compensate for the hypomorphic allele.

Animal Models

The mineralocorticoid receptor–knockout mouse develops salt wasting with hyponatremia, hyperkalemia, and markedly elevated renin and aldosterone levels, and dies around 10 days of age unless rescued with a high-salt diet or with glucocorticoid therapy.[112–114] The heterozygous null mutation ($MR^{+/-}$) should more closely resemble the autosomal dominant PHA1 in humans. However, these mice develop normally and do not demonstrate electrolyte abnormalities, although there is an increase in urinary Na^+ loss and moderate elevation of renin and aldosterone levels.

Laboratory Diagnosis

Patients present in infancy with hyperkalemia, hyponatremia, and varying degrees of metabolic acidosis, although in later life the biochemical abnormalities may be mild. Patients are expected to have an elevated PRA and high serum and urine aldosterone levels. Unlike autosomal recessive PHA1, nasal potential difference should be normal, although this has not been formally validated.

Differential Diagnosis

Other causes of salt loss with hyperkalema and acidosis include autosomal recessive PHA1 and congenital adrenal hyperplasia with mineralocorticoid deficiency. Acquired aldosterone deficiency from adrenal insufficiency and aldosterone resistance from drugs that that interfere with aldosterone action may also manifest with variable hypotension and hyperkalemic acidosis. Patients with PHA2 (see below) have hyperkalemia and acidosis but are generally hypertensive and are unlikely to be confused with patients with PHA1.

Genetic Testing

Mutations in *NR3C2*, which encodes the mineralocorticoid receptor, have been found in 75% of patients with autosomal dominant PHA1 and in a few cases of sporadic PHA1. These mutations are spread throughout the coding region and in some cases are predicted to reduce its activity. Mutation testing is only available in research laboratories.

Treatment

Salt supplements should be provided enterally or parenterally in the newborn and in early childhood until symptoms remit. Hyperkalemia is managed by chronic ion exchange resin therapy. Children usually outgrow the syndrome, and in later life salt supplementation and resin therapy may not be required.

THE SYNDROME OF APPARENT MINERALOCORTICOID EXCESS (OMIM 218030)

Historical Overview

The genetic syndrome of apparent mineralocorticoid excess (SAME) is an autosomal recessive disorder with early onset severe hypertension, hypokalemia and metabolic alkalosis. It is also known as 11β-hydroxysteroid dehydrogenase II deficiency and as cortisol 11β-ketoreductase deficiency. The first reported case was a native American girl who had hypertension and hypokalemia with suppressed mineralocorticoid levels.[115] Adrenocorticotrophin administration worsened the hypertension and hypokalemia, whereas spironolactone or a low-salt diet corrected both.

Genetic Basis

The disorder arises from loss-of-function mutations in both copies of the gene encoding the enzyme 11β-hydroxysteroid dehydrogenase type 2 (*HSD11B2*). The disorder is typically reported in offspring of consanguineous families, and as expected in these cases, homozygous mutations in both alleles are found.[116] In a few patients compound heterozygous mutations are seen. The mutations are most often missense mutations in the C-terminal portion of the protein, but there are a few examples of frameshift and deletion mutations (see Quinkler and Stewart[6] for a comprehensive list of mutations that cause SAME).

Clinical Features

This is an autosomal-recessive disorder in which affected patients present with hypertension, hypokalemia, and metabolic alkalosis. The disease classically presents very early after birth with failure to thrive, growth retardation, and polyuria. Intrauterine growth retardation may be manifest by low birth weight, and hypertensive end-organ damage seems to occur early in severe forms of the disease.[117] Renal manifestations include nephrocalcinosis and chronic renal failure that is thought to be secondary to hypercalciuria. A smaller number of patients have milder hypertension with more modest biochemical defects and present later in life and have been labeled as AME type 2.[6] The disorder is characterized by suppressed renin and aldosterone activity and points to the presence of a circulating mineralocorticoid-like substance. The disease can be treated with spironolactone and amiloride and is exacerbated by adrenocorticotrophin administration.

Pathophysiology

Proteins containing these mutations have reduced enzymatic activity when tested in transfected cultured cells and explain the syndrome.[118,119] In one case, enzyme immunostaining and NAD-dependent enzyme activity was shown to be absent or severely reduced in the placenta from an affected pregnancy.[120]

The enzyme 11β-hydroxysteroid dehydrogenase type 2 is selectively expressed in certain mineralocorticoid-responsive tissues, including the CNT and collecting duct of the kidney. In these sites the enzyme converts cortisol to its inactive metabolite cortisone allowing aldosterone free access to its receptor. In the absence of this enzyme, cortisol, which is present in molar excess as compared with aldosterone and has equal affinity for the mineralocorticoid receptor, occupies this receptor and activates a mineralocorticoid-dependent gene profile in target tissues (see Fig. 16-3). This leads to an increase in Na^+ reabsorption via ENaC with enhanced K^+ and H^+ secretion by the principal and intercalated cells of the collecting duct. The resulting volume expansion suppresses PRA and aldosterone levels.

Animal Model

The 11β-hydroxysteroid dehydrogenase type 2–knockout mouse develops hypertension, hypokalemia, polyuria, and reduced urinary Na^+ excretion associated with suppressed aldosterone levels, thus recapitulating the clinical phenotype seen in humans. The knockout mice appeared weaker than their control littermates; they developed intestinal dilatation, and as many as 50% died within 48 hours, presumably from severe hypokalemia.[121] Some of the metabolic abnormalities could be reversed with spironolactone or with dexamethasone, although the effect on hypertension was not reported. As expected, the heterozygous mouse has no detectable clinical or metabolic abnormality.

Laboratory Diagnosis

The classic laboratory features of this syndrome are hypokalemia and metabolic alkalosis that occur in very young hypertensives with growth retardation. Suppressed PRA and low serum and urine aldoserone levels will be found on expanded testing. The deficiency in 11β-hydroxysteroid dehydrogenase type 2 can be detected by measuring the ratio of the metabolites of cortisol to the metabolities of cortisone in the urine (tetrahydrocortisol + allo-tetrahydrocortisol to tetrahydrocortisone).[122,123] Recent data suggest that the ratio of urinary free cortisol to cortisone is also a sensitive marker of 11β-hydroxysteroid dehydrogenase type 2 activity and can be used to identify patients with SAME.[124]

Differential Diagnosis

Other causes of severe early-onset hypertension should be considered in such patients. In those with a family history of early-onset hypertension, the differential diagnosis will include glucocorticoid-remediable hyperaldosteronism, Liddle syndrome, and Gordon syndrome. All of these have an autosomal dominant inheritance in contrast to SAME. The finding of a suppressed serum aldosterone would exclude glucocorticoid-remediable hyperaldosteronism, whereas the presence of hypokalemia would exclude Gordon syndrome. Acquired causes of hypokalemic alkalosis with hypertension include essential hypertension treated with thiazide or loop diuretics, primary hyperaldosteronism, and Cushing syndrome.

Genetic Testing

Homozygous or compound heterozygous mutations have been found in *HSD11B2* in type 1 and type 2 AME.[122,123] Mutation testing is available at the Molecular Hypertension Laboratory of the University of Berne, Switzerland (brigitte.frey@dkf.unibe.ch).

Treatment

Hypertension and the hypokalemia can be effectively treated with spironolactone, eplerenone, amiloride, or triamterene, although triamterene is best avoided in children. Thiazide diuretics have been reported to be useful when added to spironolactone to control hypertension and to reduce hypercalciuria with nephrocalcinosis.[119] Levels of the endogenous glucocorticoid cortisol can be suppressed by administration of a low-dose synthetic glucocorticoid-like dexamethasone that does not bind to the mineralocorticoid receptor and can be used as an alternative form of therapy.[116,125] There is one report of normalization of hypokalemia, improvement in blood pressure, and correction of the urinary cortisol-to-cortisone ratio following renal transplantation, suggesting that the disorder is primarily due to deficiency of renal 11β-hydroxysteroid dehydrogenase type 2.[124]

AUTOSOMAL-DOMINANT HYPERTENSION WITH EXACERBATION IN PREGNANCY (OMIM 60515)

Historical Overview

This disease has only been recognized in one kindred and was discovered by screening a large number of patients with early-onset severe hypertension for mutations in *NR3C2*, which encodes the mineralocorticoid receptor. Among 75 unrelated individuals, a 15-year-old boy with severe hypertension, suppressed PRA, and low serum aldosterone was identified with a novel mutation in *NR3C2*.[126]

Genetic Basis

A missense mutation in *NR3C2* results in a S810L substitution in the mineralocorticoid receptor, converting it into a constitutively active receptor.[126] The specificity of the receptor is altered, converting progesterone and spironolactone into potent agonists at the mineralocorticoid receptor. This is a gain-of-function mutation that leads to dominantly inherited hypertension at an early age. Because there is a large increase in circulating progesterone levels during pregnancy, there is also a marked increase in blood pressure during pregnancy resulting from overstimulation of mineralocorticoid receptors with Na^+ retention and hypokalemia.

Clinical Features and Pathophysiology

This is an exceedingly rare autosomal-dominant disorder that has so far been reported in only one kindred. An analysis of the kindred revealed that affected patients present with severe hypertension in their teens with suppressed PRA and low aldosterone levels.[126] Neither hypokalemia nor metabolic alkalosis seem to be prominent features of the syndrome. In the only pedigree examined, a missense mutation in *NR3C2* results in a S810L substitution in the mineralocorticoid receptor, converting it into a constitutively active receptor. Activation of the mineralocorticoid receptors in the connecting tubule and collecting duct leads to enhanced reabsorption of Na^+ with secondary K^+ secretion that leads to the clinical syndrome. The mutation described converts progesterone into a potent agonist for mineralocorticoid receptors.[126] This results in severe exacerbation of hypertension during pregnancy with hypokalemia but without other features of pre-eclampsia such as proteinuria or edema. Spironolactone, a classic mineralocorticoid receptor antagonist, also becomes a potent agonist of the abnormal mineralocorticoid receptors and should be avoided in patients known to carry this gene mutation. Exacerbation of hypertension with spironolactone in a young hypertensive with a strong family history may be a clue to this rare disorder.

Laboratory Diagnosis and Genetic Testing

Hypokalemia may be seen in the disorder but is not a common feature.[126] Evidence of low PRA and suppressed aldosterone levels may be found. History of pregnancy-related exacerbation of hypertension in affected family members may be an important clue to the disease. A definitive diagnosis can only be made by detection of a specific mutation in *NR3C2*. This test is not available commercially.

Treatment

Amiloride and triamterene should be effective in treating the hypertension in this disorder, but there is no published information on efficacy of any antihypertensive therapy in families with this disorder. Spironolactone should be avoided in patients known to carry this gene mutation, and in women pregnancy must be approached with caution.[126]

PSEUDOHYPOALDOSTERONISM TYPE 2 (GORDON SYNDROME, FAMILIAL HYPERKALEMIC HYPERTENSION, OMIM 145260)

Historical Overview

The first reported patient with this disorder was a 15-year-old with hypertension, hyperkalemia, and renal tubular acidosis (RTA) resulting from a specific renal tubular defect in K^+ secretion.[127] The patient had normal renal function, low PRA, a high-normal aldosterone level, and a remarkable response to low doses of a thiazide diuretic. Gordon reported a patient with additional features of short stature, mild mental retardation, and dental abnormalities.[128] Subsequent reports of "Gordon syndrome" emphasized the features of hypertensive hyperkalemia and RTA with normal renal function.[129–133] In 1981, Schambelan and colleagues reported a patient with hypertension, hyperkalemia, RTA, and normal renal function who responded dramatically to low-dose thiazide therapy.[134] They named this syndrome "type 2 pseudohypoaldosteronism" (PHA2) to differentiate it from type 1 pseudohypoaldosteronism, a previously reported disease of hyperkalemia and salt wasting. The patient reported by Schambelan and colleagues was clinically indistinguishable from the previously reported patients with Gordon syndrome, suggesting that these disorders are the same clinical entity. The term pseudohypoaldosteronism carries the connotation of salt wasting and peripheral aldosterone resistance, and has proved confusing because these patients are hypertensive and do not typically have elevated aldosterone levels. Some authors prefer the use of the more descriptive term, familial hyperkalemic hypertension, to designate this syndrome.

Genetic Basis

Most, if not all cases of PHA2 exhibit characteristics of an autosomal dominant disease with high penetrance.[135-141] The clinical phenotype of hypertension, hyperkalemia, and acidosis is the mirror image of Gitelman syndrome, which is known to be caused by loss-of-function mutations in the gene encoding the thiazide-sensitive NCC (gene symbol SLC12A3) in the DCT. Not surprisingly, patients with PHA2 were postulated to have a gain of function in NCC; however, a careful examination of this locus in PHA2 pedigrees excluded SLC12A3 as a candidate gene.[142,143]

PHA2 exhibits genetic heterogeneity, in that the disease maps to loci on chromosomes 1, 12, and 17 when examined in different kindred with this disease.[135,136,138,139,141] These three genetically distinct PHA2 subtypes have been classified as type A (linked to 1q), type B (linked to 17p), and type C (linked to 12p). In 2001 a new PHA2C family with a deletion in the linked interval on chromosome 12 was identified.[137] The deletion lies within the first intron of WNK1, a member of a novel kinase family, and leads to an increase in WNK1 expression, at least in leukocytes. The disease thus seems to be secondary to a gain of function of the mutant WNK1 allele. Separately, PHA2B pedigrees were shown to have missense mutations within the coding region of WNK4, a second member of the WNK kinase family that is expressed from the chromosome 17p locus.[137] These observations identify at least two forms of PHA2 as diseases of the WNK kinase pathway. The identity of the gene affected at the third locus, on chromosome 1, is unknown.

WNK kinases (representing with no lysine [K]) are recently described proteins.[144] WNK1 (gene symbol WNK1) is a large protein of 2,126 amino acids related to the MAP/extracellular signal regulated protein kinase (ERK) family. Although the open reading frame is predicted to encode a protein with a kinase domain, its structure is atypical. It lacks a lysine in subdomain 2, at a site that binds adenosine triphosphate, which is nearly invariant in all previously identified kinases. Instead, the lysine required for phosphoryl transfer lies in kinase subdomain 2. These proteins are, however, bona fide kinases: WNK1 can phosphorylate WNK4, synaptotagmin, SPAK, OSR1, and also themselves (autophosphorylation).[144-146] WNK4 (gene symbol WNK4) is homologous to WNK1 but is shorter, requires co-factors to exhibit kinase activity, and generally has substrates different from those of WNK1.[147-149]

Clinical Features

The most consistent feature of PHA2 is hyperkalemia. Serum K^+ concentrations range from 5.3 to 7.3 mEq, even in children.[138,150,151] Hypertension is commonly observed in PHA2, but its presence is more variable than is hyperkalemia. Blood pressure is dependent on age in affected individuals; frank hypertension is typical in adults but often absent in children, which may explain why some younger patients are not diagnosed with PHA2, despite hyperkalemia.[133,139,152] In a survey of the literature before 1993, hypertension was present in only 38 of 69 reported cases, although many of those who were not hypertensive were children.[153] More recently, a genetically characterized family with PHA2 resulting from mutations in WNK1 was studied. In this family with 17 affected individuals and 32 unaffected relatives, hyperkalemia was present universally among affected individuals, and blood pressure was only 7 (systolic) and 9 (diastolic) mmHg higher among affected than unaffected individuals.[139]

Despite the reported variability in blood pressure, some individuals with PHA2 have severe hypertension that is difficult to treat with combinations of antihypertensive drugs.[154] Most of these, however, can be treated with low doses of a thiazide diuretic.[151] Treatment with a thiazide diuretic also tends to normalize K^+ excretion and correct the RTA. The remarkable effectiveness of thiazide diuretics in this syndrome has been recently confirmed.[152] Thiazides reduce the systolic and diastolic pressures of PHA2 patients by 45 and 25 mmHg, respectively, compared with 13 and 10 mmHg in patients with essential hypertension. In contrast, loop diuretics do not reliably normalize the serum K^+ or blood pressure during prolonged follow-up.[155]

Hyperchloremia and metabolic acidosis are very common features of the disease. Serum Cl^- concentration typically varies from 105 to 116 mM and bicarbonate from 15 to 24 mM.[127,131,156-159] The causes of acidosis include both impaired ammonium excretion and a reduced bicarbonate-reabsorptive threshold. Reducing serum K^+ with oral cation exchange resins increased ammonium excretion but did not increase the bicarbonate threshold.[159] In contrast, dietary salt restriction led to correction of acidosis by increasing the bicarbonate threshold, without correcting hyperkalemia. Thus, PHA2 patients manifest two processes that limit proton excretion. First, they excrete reduced amounts of ammonium, secondary to hyperkalemia. Second, the bicarbonate threshold is low, which can be corrected by infusing non-Cl^- salts of Na^+ or by severe dietary salt restriction.

Many PHA2 patients waste calcium, a situation that can be worsened with furosemide administration.[152] In one kindred, whose disease resulted from WNK4 mutations, basal hypercalciuria was seen in all affected members, in comparison with their unaffected relatives. In these PHA2 patients bone mineral density was also reduced as compared with their unaffected relatives. In a kindred whose disease resulted from mutations in WNK1, hypercalciuria could not be detected.[139] Whether hypercalciuria is a feature of PHA2 resulting specifically from WNK4 mutations or whether other variables are responsible for the observed differences is not clear.

Several other features have been reported to occur in PHA2. Short stature and mental retardation were described in the earliest cases.[128,154,155,159] Most subsequent cases lack both features, although specific information about the height and intelligence of patients characterized genetically has been lacking (see below). Several reports indicate that when treated with thiazide diuretics, patients with Gordon syndrome grow and develop normally, suggesting that short stature and developmental delay are secondary to the electrolyte abnormalities and not a primary feature of the syndrome.

Pathophysiology

The clinical features of PHA2 are, in many respects, opposite to those observed in Gitelman syndrome, where hypokalemia, mild hypotension, hypocalciuria, and resistance to the effects of angiotensin II are seen.[128,160] This would suggest that the

PHA2 phenotype results from overactivity of the thiazide-sensitive NaCl cotransporter. Yet several features suggest that the phenotypic features reflect more complicated interactions. For example, patients with Gitelman syndrome nearly always manifest profound magnesium wasting and hypomagnesemia, yet abnormalities of magnesium balance do not appear prominent in PHA2.[150,152,160] Furthermore, some individuals with PHA2, perhaps primarily resulting from mutations in *WNK1*, do not waste calcium.[139]

WNK4 Mutations and PHA2

PHA2 is a disease of the distal nephron, both from functional studies and because the gene products affected in this disease are preferentially expressed along this nephron segment.[134,137] When co-expressed in *Xenopus* oocytes, WNK4 binds to the thiazide-sensitive NaCl cotransporter (NCC) and reduces its abundance at the plasma membrane by inhibiting exocytic insertion into the plasma membrane[137,161] (Fig. 16-4). Four missense mutations in *WNK4* have been associated with PHA2. At least one of the resulting substitutions, Q562E, is less active than wild-type WNK4 at inhibiting NCC activity.[161–163] Two other substitutions, E559K and D561A, were also initially thought to be inactive on NCC, although all three abnormal proteins bound normally to the NCC.[137] However, others have shown that E559K and D561A retain the ability to inhibit NCC in *Xenopus* oocytes and in the case of D561A reduce surface expression in MDCK II, an epithelial cell line.[161,164]

WNK4 is expressed along the lateral membrane of DCT2 and CNT cells, where it seems to play a role in increasing paracellular Cl⁻ conductivity (see Fig. 16-4). WNK4 was also shown to phosphorylate claudins, tight-junction proteins that play a central role in adjusting paracellular ion permeability.[165] PHA2-causing abnormal WNK4 was shown to increase Cl⁻ conductance, relative to Na⁺, across the paracellular pathway.[165,166]

Other ion transport proteins have been shown to be regulated by WNK4. WNK4 inhibits ROMK by enhancing endocytosis by a clathrin-coated pit-dependent pathway.[43] This effect is independent of WNK4 kinase activity and requires the C-terminal domain (see Fig. 16-4). In contrast to the effects of *WNK4* mutations on NCC activity, PHA2-causing mutations increase the suppression of ROMK. Thus, PHA2-causing mutations of *WNK4* may enhance NCC activity, enhance paracellular Cl⁻ permeability, and suppress ROMK activity; all these effects would enhance distal NaCl reabsorption and reduce distal K⁺ secretion.

WNK1 Mutations and PHA2

Mutations in *WNK1* also cause PHA2; the mutations reported thus far are large deletions within the first intron, which do not involve the coding sequence.[137] There are two principal transcripts for WNK1; the first encodes full-length WNK1 including a kinase domain, whereas the second arises from an alternative first exon (exon 4a) and is missing the N-terminal kinase domain. The predominant form of WNK1 expressed in the kidney is this truncated form, called KS-WNK1.[39,145,167] The effects of this intronic deletion on disease pathogenesis are not completely understood, but it seems to increase full-length WNK1 expression, at least in leukocytes.[137] Whether KS-WNK1 is also increased in PHA2 is currently unknown.

WNK1 can phosphorylate WNK4 and inhibit the WNK4 effect on NCC, an effect that requires an active WNK1 kinase domain[149,164] (see Fig. 16-4). Mutations that increase WNK1 expression would thus be expected to further release NCC from WNK4-mediated suppression, resulting in increases in

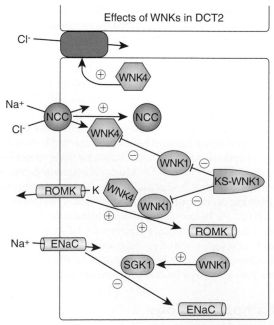
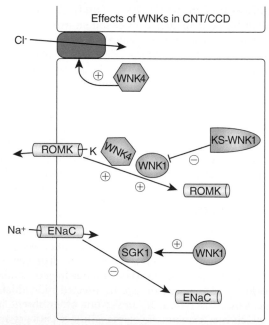

Figure 16-4 Schematic illustrating the normal effects of WNK4, WNK1, and KS-WNK1 in the ASDN. WNK4 inhibits transcellular Na⁺ and K⁺ transport by reducing NCC and ROMK expression and function. WNK4 stimulates paracellular Cl⁻ transport. WNK1 inhibits the effect of WNK4 on NCC. WNK1 stimulates ENaC activity via SGK1, whereas it inhibits ROMK activity. KS-WNK1 can inhibit the effect of WNK1 on ROMK and on WNK4.

NCC activity. KS-WNK1 exerts dominant negative effects on full-length WNK1, inhibiting both its kinase activity and its ability to inhibit WNK4.[168] If *WNK1* mutations were to increase the abundance of full-length WNK1 relative to KS-WNK1 in renal tissue, WNK4 activity would be inhibited, which is predicted to lead to an increase in NCC activity.

WNK1 has effects on other ion transport proteins. WNK1 binds to and activates SGK1 which can then stimulate ENaC-mediated Na^+ transport via phosphorylation of Nedd4-2 in *Xenopus* oocytes and in CHO cells[31] (see Fig. 16-4). Because mutations that cause PHA2 lead to increased expression of full-length WNK1, these mutations would be expected to increase ENaC expression and increase Na^+ reabsorption in the ASDN, thus contributing to the hypertension seen in PHA2. Whether KS-WNK1 can inhibit full-length WNK1 in its ability to activate SGK1 is not known. However, KS-WNK1 was recently shown to stimulate ENaC activity, and an increase in either isoform of WNK1 in PHA2 should lead to an increase in ENaC-mediated Na^+ absorption.[169]

WNK1 also inhibits ROMK1 by enhancing its endocytosis, and this effect can be suppressed by KS-WNK1[40] (see Fig. 16-4). Mutations that increase full-length WNK1 would be expected to reduce ROMK1 expression, thereby contributing to the hyperkalemia seen in PHA2. Thus, PHA2-causing mutations of *WNK1* may enhance NCC activity and increase ENaC activity, while simultaneously suppressing ROMK activity; all these effects would enhance distal NaCl reabsorption and reduce distal K^+ secretion. However, because the effect of PHA2 mutations on KS-WNK1 are unknown, a comprehensive mechanistic hypothesis relating the various effects of WNK kinases and their mutations to the clinical PHA2 phenotype requires more study.

Two other features of PHA2 are hypercalciuria and reduced bone density.[150,152,170] These features may also result from overactivity of the NCC. When the NCC is not active, as occurs during treatment with thiazide diuretics or with an NCC knockout (Gitelman syndrome), renal Ca^{2+} excretion is reduced. Activation of apical NaCl uptake activity in PHA2 would thus be expected to lead to hypercalciuria. However, hypercalciuria may not occur when PHA2 is caused by mutations in *WNK1*, a difference that requires further study.[139]

Animal Models

An animal model of PHA2 resulting from overexpression of WNK4 (Q562E) has been reported.[171] The animals displayed hypertension, hyperkalemia and hypercalciuria together with an increase in NCC abundance and marked hyperplasia of the DCT. The hypertension and the metabolic derangements were corrected in offspring carrying WNK4 (Q562E) and homozygous null mutation in NCC. A second animal model of PHA2 was generated by knockin of WNK4 (D561A/+).[171a] These animals developed hyperkalemia followed by hypertension and metabolic acidosis associated with increased apical expression of phosphorylated NCC. Although ENaC expression in the CCD was increased, thiazide treatment corrected the PHA2 phenotype. Together these mouse models indicate that PHA2 from WNK4 mutations arises from increased absorption of NaCl via NCC with reduced Na+ delivery to the CCD leading to diminished K+ secretion. The *WNK1* gene has been knocked out in mice and is embryonic lethal. Mice with heterozygous deletion survive normally but have a blood pressure that is 12 mmHg lower than wild-type animals.[172] Other phenotypic features of these mice have not been reported. Mice with gain-of-function mutations in *WNK1* akin to those that cause human disease have not yet been created.

Laboratory Diagnosis

The combination of hyperkalemia, hypertension, and normal anion gap metabolic acidosis in the absence of overt renal disease in a young patient with a family history of hyperkalemia is highly suggestive of the disorder. Although hyperkalemia is nearly universal in untreated patients, some patients may have hyperkalemia without hypertension; the diagnosis has been missed frequently when hypertension is absent. Hyperchloremic metabolic acidosis is frequently observed, as is hypercalciuria; this may be more prevalent in patients harboring *WNK4* mutations. Typically, PRA is suppressed, but plasma aldosterone is often normal, perhaps as a result of the hyperkalemia. No pathognomonic laboratory features have been described.

Differential Diagnosis

The differential diagnosis includes PHA1 and Addison disease, which are also associated with hyperkalemia and metabolic acidosis; yet those disorders are typically associated with frank salt wasting and a tendency toward hypotension. Other causes of hypertension with hyperkalemia include type 4 RTA from hyporeninemic hypoaldosteronism or aldosterone resistance; this syndrome most commonly results from early diabetic nephropathy or interstitial nephritis. The setting of diabetes or interstitial renal dysfunction and an older age of onset usually suggest that the hyperkalemia and hypertension are acquired phenomena. Calcineurin inhibitors, such as cyclosporine and tacrolimus, are a common iatrogenic cause of a syndrome that strongly resembles hyporeninemic hypoaldosteronism.[173] Any other process that leads to hyperkalemia that coexists with essential hypertension may also be confused with PHA2.

Genetic Testing

Commercial testing is not currently available.

Treatment

The most important features of PHA2 are hypertension and hyperkalemia. Various maneuvers have been used to increase urinary K^+ excretion and correct the hyperkalemia. These have included cation exchange resins, distal convoluted tubule (thiazide) diuretics, loop diuretics, carbonic anhydrase inhibitors, dietary salt restriction, exogenous mineralocorticoids, and infusions of non-Cl^- Na^+ salts.[151,154,159,174] The most consistently effective of these have been thiazide diuretics, dietary salt restriction, and infusions of non-Cl^- Na^+ salts.[131,150,155] Exogenous mineralocorticoids have been quite variable in their ability to enhance K^+ excretion, being most effective when combined with dietary salt restriction.[175] Dietary K^+ restriction is also useful. Thiazides may also improve bone density.[150,152] In fact, because the syndrome is often so thiazide-sensitive, overcorrection may occur with full doses. When thiazides fail to correct the syndrome fully, additional antihypertensives may be added.

References

1. Frindt G, Palmer LG: Na channels in the rat connecting tubule. Am J Physiol Renal Physiol 286:F669–F674, 2004.
2. Rubera I, Loffing J, Palmer LG, et al: Collecting duct-specific gene inactivation of α-ENaC in the mouse kidney does not impair sodium and potassium balance. J Clin Invest 112:554–565, 2003.
3. Quinn, SJ Williams GH: Regulation of aldosterone secretion. Annu Rev Physiol 50:409–426, 1988.
4. Spat A, Hunyady L: Control of aldosterone secretion: A model for convergence in cellular signaling pathways. Physiol Rev 84:489–539, 2004.
5. Funder J, Pearce P, Smith R, Smith A: Mineralocorticoid action: Target tissue specificity is enzyme, not receptor, mediated. Science 242:583–585, 1988.
6. Quinkler M, Stewart PM: Hypertension and the cortisol-cortisone shuttle. J Clin Endocrinol Metab 88:2384–2392, 2003.
7. de la Rosa DA, Canessa CM, Fyfe GK, Zhang P: Structure and regulation of amiloride-sensitive sodium channels. Annu Rev Physiol 62:573–594, 2000.
8. Kellenberger S, Schild L: Epithelial sodium channel/degenerin family of ion channels: A variety of functions for a shared structure. Physiol Rev 82:735–767, 2002.
9. Snyder PM: The epithelial Na$^+$ channel: Cell surface insertion and retrieval in Na$^+$ homeostasis and hypertension. Endocr Rev 23:258–275, 2002.
10. Kamynina E, Tauxe C, Staub O: Distinct characteristics of two human Nedd4 proteins with respect to epithelial Na$^+$ channel regulation. Am J Physiol Renal Physiol 281:F469–F477, 2001.
11. Fotia AB, Dinudom A, Shearwin KE, et al: The role of individual Nedd4-2 (KIAA0439) WW domains in binding and regulating epithelial sodium channels. FASEB J 17:70–72, 2003.
12. Itani OA, Campbell JR, Herrero J, et al: Alternate promoters and variable splicing lead to hNedd4-2 isoforms with a C2 domain and varying number of WW domains. Am J Physiol Renal Physiol 285:F916–F929, 2003.
13. Snyder PM: Minireview: regulation of epithelial Na$^+$ channel trafficking. Endocrinology 146:5079–5085, 2005.
14. Loffing J, Flores SY, Staub O: Sgk kinases and their role in epithelial transport. Annu Rev Physiol 68:16.11–16.30, 2006.
15. Kamynina E, Debonneville C, Bens M, et al: A novel mouse Nedd4 protein suppresses the activity of the epithelial Na$^+$ channel. FASEB J 15:204–214, 2001.
16. Itani OA, Stokes JB, Thomas CP: Nedd4-2 isoforms differentially associate with ENaC and regulate its activity. Am J Physiol Renal Physiol 289:F334–F446, 2005.
17. Garty H, Palmer LG: Epithelial sodium channels: function, structure, and regulation. Physiol Rev 77:359–396, 1997.
18. Firsov D, Gautschi I, Merillat AM, et al: The heterotetrameric architecture of the epithelial sodium channel (ENaC). EMBO J 17:344–352, 1998.
19. Snyder PM, Cheng C, Prince LS, et al: Electrophysiological and biochemical evidence that DEG/ENaC cation channels are composed of nine subunits. J Biol Chem 273:681–684, 1998.
20. Kosari F, Sheng S, Li J, et al: Subunit stoichiometry of the epithelial sodium channel. J Biol Chem 273:13469–13474, 1998.
21. Loffing J, Pietri L, Aregger F, et al: Differential subcellular localization of ENaC subunits in mouse kidney in response to high- and low-Na diets. Am J Physiol Renal Physiol 279:F252–F258, 2000.
22. Loffing J, Zecevic M, Feraille E, et al: Aldosterone induces rapid apical translocation of ENaC in early portion of renal collecting system: Possible role of SGK. Am J Physiol Renal Physiol 280:F675–F682, 2001.
23. Mick VE, Itani OA, Loftus RW, et al: The α-subunit of the epithelial sodium channel is an aldosterone-induced transcript in mammalian collecting ducts, and this transcriptional response is mediated via distinct cis-elements in the 5′ flanking region of the gene. Mol Endocrinol 15:575–588, 2001.
24. Webster MK, Goya L, Ge Y, et al: Characterization of sgk, a novel member of the serine/threonine protein kinase gene family which is transcriptionally induced by glucocorticoids and serum. Mol Cell Biol 13:2031–2040, 1993.
25. Itani OA, Liu KZ, Cornish KL, et al: Glucocorticoids stimulate human SGK1 gene expression by activation of a hormone response element in its 5′ flanking region. Am J Physiol Endocrinol Metab 283:E971–E979, 2002.
26. Debonneville C, Flores SY, Kamynina E, et al: Phosphorylation of Nedd4-2 by Sgk1 regulates epithelial Na$^+$ channel cell surface expression. EMBO J 20:7052–7059, 2001.
27. Snyder PM, Olson DR, Thomas BC: SGK modulates Nedd4-2-mediated inhibition of ENaC. J Biol Chem 277:5–8, 2002.
28. Ichimura T, Yamamura H, Sasamoto K, et al: 14-3-3 proteins modulate the expression of epithelial Na$^+$ channels by phosphorylation-dependent interaction with Nedd4-2 ubiquitin ligase. J Biol Chem 280:13187–13194, 2005.
29. Bhalla V, Daidie D, Li H, et al: SGK1 regulates ubiquitin ligase Nedd4-2 by inducing interaction with 14-3-3. Mol Endocrinol 19:3073–3084, 2005.
30. Diakov A, Korbmacher C: A novel pathway of ENaC activation involves an SGK1 consensus motif in the C terminus of the channel's α-subunit. J Biol Chem 279:38134–38142, 2004.
30a. Ring Am, Leng Q, Rinehart J, et al: An SGK1 site in WNK4 regulates Na+ channel and K+ channel activity and has implications for aldosterone signaling and K+ homeostasis. PNAS 104:4025–4029, 2007.
31. Xu BE, Stippec S, Chu PY, et al: WNK1 activates SGK1 to regulate the epithelial sodium channel. Proc Natl Acad Sci U S A 102:10315–10320, 2005.
32. Velazquez H, Bartiss A, Bernstein P, Ellison DH: Adrenal steroids stimulate thiazide-sensitive NaCl transport by rat renal distal tubules. Am J Physiol 270:F211–F219, 1996.
33. Kim GH, Masilamani S, Turner R, et al: The thiazide-sensitive Na-Cl cotransporter is an aldosterone-induced protein. Proc Natl Acad Sci U S A 95:14552–14557, 1998.
34. Wang XY, Masilamani S, Nielsen J, et al: The renal thiazide-sensitive Na-Cl cotransporter as mediator of the aldosterone-escape phenomenon. J Clin Invest 108:215–222, 2001.
35. Halperin ML, Kamel KS: Dynamic interactions between integrative physiology and molecular medicine: The key to understand the mechanism of action of aldosterone in the kidney. Can J Physiol Pharmacol 78:587–594, 2000.
36. Wang W: Renal potassium channels: Recent developments. Curr Opin Nephrol Hypertens 13:549–555, 2004.
37. Yun CC, Palmada M, Embark HM, et al: The serum and glucocorticoid-inducible kinase SGK1 and the Na$^+$H$^+$ exchange regulating factor NHERF2 synergize to stimulate the renal outer medullary K$^+$ channel ROMK1. J Am Soc Nephrol 13:2823–2830, 2002.
38. Yoo D, Kim BY, Campo C, et al: Cell surface expression of the ROMK (Kir 1.1) channel is regulated by the aldosterone-induced kinase, SGK1, and protein kinase A. J Biol Chem 278:23066–23075, 2003.
39. O'Reilly M, Marshall E, Speirs HJL, Brown RW: WNK1, a gene within a novel blood pressure control pathway, tissue-specifically generates radically different isoforms with and without a kinase domain. J Am Soc Nephrol 14:2447–2456, 2003.

40. Lazrak A, Liu Z, Huang C-L: Antagonistic regulation of ROMK by long and kidney specific isoforms. Proc Natl Acad Sci U S A 103:1615–1620, Epub 2006.
41. O'Reilly M, Marshall E, MacGillvray T, et al: Two WNKs on a changing diet. J Am Soc Nephrol 17:2402–2413, 2006.
42. Wang W: Regulation of renal K transport by dietary K intake. Annu Rev Physiol 66:547–569, 2004.
43. Kahle KT, Wilson FH, Leng Q, et al: WNK4 regulates the balance between renal NaCl reabsorption and K^+ secretion. Nat Genet 35:372–376, 2003.
44. Woda CB, Bragin A, Kleyman TR, Satlin LM: Flow-dependent K^+ secretion in the cortical collecting duct is mediated by a maxi-K channel. Am J Physiol Renal Physiol 280:F786–F793, 2001.
45. Liu W, Xu S, Woda C, Kim P, et al: Effect of flow and stretch on the $[Ca^{2+}]_i$ response of principal and intercalated cells in cortical collecting duct. Am J Physiol Renal Physiol 285:F998–F1012, 2003.
46. Wingo CS, Smolka AJ: Function and structure of H-K-ATPase in the kidney. Am J Physiol Renal Physiol 269:F1–F16, 1995.
47. Silver RB, Soleimani M: H^+-K^+-ATPases: Regulation and role in pathophysiological states. Am J Physiol Renal Physiol 276:F799–F811, 1999.
48. Petrovic S, Spicer Z, Greeley T, et al: Novel Schering and ouabain-insensitive potassium-dependent proton secretion in the mouse cortical collecting duct. Am J Physiol Renal Physiol 282:F133–F143, 2002.
49. DuBose TD, Jr, Seldin DW, Kokko JP: Segmental chloride reabsorption in the rat nephron as a function of load. Am J Physiol 234:F97–F105, 1978.
50. Rector FC, Jr, Clapp JR: Evidence for active chloride reabsorption in the distal renal tubule of the rat. J Clin Invest 41:101–107, 1962.
51. Uchida S, Sasaki S: Function of chloride channels in the kidney. Annu Rev Physiol 67:759–778, 2005.
52. Velazquez H, Silva T, Andujar E, et al: The distal convoluted tubule of rabbit kidney does not express a functional sodium channel. Am J Physiol Renal Physiol 280:F530–F539, 2001.
53. Hayama A, Rai T, Sasaki S, Uchida S: Molecular mechanisms of Bartter syndrome caused by mutations in the BSND gene. Histochem Cell Biol 119:485–493, 2003.
54. Weinstein AM: A mathematical model of rat distal convoluted tubule (I): Cotransporter function in early DCT. Am J Physiol Renal Physiol 289:F699–F720, 2005.
55. Weinstein AM: A mathematical model of rat distal convoluted tubule (II): Potassium secretion along the connecting segment. Am J Physiol Renal Physiol, 289:F721–F741, 2005.
56. Kobayashi K, Uchida S, Mizutani S, et al: Intrarenal and cellular localization of CLC-K2 protein in the mouse kidney. J Am Soc Nephrol 12:1327–1334, 2001.
57. Kobayashi K, Uchida S, Okamura HO, et al: Human CLC-KB gene promoter drives the EGFP expression in the specific distal nephron segments and inner ear. J Am Soc Nephrol 13:1992–1998, 2002.
58. Shayakul C, Alper SL: Defects in processing and trafficking of the AE1 Cl^-/$HCO3^-$ exchanger associated with inherited distal renal tubular acidosis. Clin Exp Nephrol 8:1–11, 2004.
59. Liddle GW, Bledsoe T, Coppage WS: A familial renal disorder simulating primary aldosteronism but with negligible aldosterone secretion. Transactions Assoc Am Physicians 76:199–213, 1963.
60. Botero-Velez M, Curtis JJ, Warnock DG: Liddle's syndrome revisited—A disorder of sodium reabsorption in the distal tubule. N Engl J Med 330:178–181, 1994.
61. Shimkets RA, Warnock DG, Bositis CM, et al.: Liddle's syndrome: Heritable human hypertension caused by mutations in the beta subunit of the epithelial sodium channel. Cell 79:407–414, 1994.
62. Hansson JH, Nelson-Williams C, Suzuki H, et al: Human hypertension caused by mutation in the gamma subunit of the epithelial sodium channel: Genetic heterogeneity of Liddle's syndrome. Nat Genet (Lond) 11:76–82, 1995.
63. Hansson JH, Schild L, Lu Y, et al: A de novo missense mutation of the beta subunit of the epithelial sodium channel causes hypertension and Liddle syndrome, identifying a proline-rich segment critical for regulation of channel activity. Proc Natl Acad Sci U S A 92:11495–11499, 1995.
64. Tamura H, Schild L, Enomoto N, et al: Liddle disease caused by a missense mutation of beta subunit of the epithelial sodium channel gene. J Clin Invest 97:1780–1784, 1996.
65. Inoue J, Iwaoka T, Tokunaga H, et al: A family with Liddle's syndrome caused by a new missense mutation in the beta subunit of the epithelial sodium channel. J Clin Endocrinol Metab 83:2210–2213, 1998.
66. Hiltunen TP, Hannila-Handelberg T, Petajaniemi N, et al: Liddle's syndrome associated with a point mutation in the extracellular domain of the epithelial sodium channel gamma subunit. J Hypertens 20:2383–2390, 2002.
67. Warnock DG: Liddle syndrome: An autosomal dominant form of human hypertension. Kidney Int 53:18–24, 1998.
68. Assadi F, Kimura R, Subramanian U, Patel S: Liddle syndrome in a newborn infant. Pediatr Nephrol 17:609, 2002.
69. Snyder PM, Price MP, McDonald FJ, et al: Mechanism by which Liddle's syndrome mutations increase activity of a human epithelial Na^+ channel. Cell 83:969–978, 1995.
70. Schild L, Lu Y, Gautschi I, et al: Identification of a PY motif in the epithelial Na channel subunits as a target sequence for mutations causing channel activation found in Liddle syndrome. EMBO J 15:2381–2387, 1996.
71. Firsov D, Schild L, Gautschi I, et al: Cell surface expression of the epithelial Na channel and a mutant causing Liddle syndrome: A quantitative approach. Proc Natl Acad Sci U S A 93:15370–15375, 1996.
72. Kyuma M, Ura N, Torii T, et al: A family with Liddle's syndrome caused by a mutation in the beta subunit of the epithelial sodium channel. Clin Exp Hypertens 23:471–478, 2001.
73. Jeunemaitre X, Bassilana F, Persu A, et al: Genotype-phenotype analysis of a newly discovered family with Liddle's syndrome. J Hypertens 15:1091–1100, 1997.
74. Nakano Y, Ishida T, Ozono R, et al: A frameshift mutation of beta subunit of epithelial sodium channel in a case of isolated Liddle syndrome. J Hypertens 20:2379–2382, 2002.
75. Gao PJ, Zhang KX, Zhu DL, et al: Diagnosis of Liddle syndrome by genetic analysis of beta and gamma subunits of epithelial sodium channel—A report of five affected family members. J Hypertens 19:885–889, 2001.
76. Yamashita Y, Koga M, Takeda Y, et al: Two sporadic cases of Liddle's syndrome caused by de novo ENaC mutations. Am J Kidney Dis 37:499–504, 2001.
77. Ciechanowicz A, Dolezel Z, Placha G, et al: Liddle syndrome caused by P616R mutation of the epithelial sodium channel beta subunit. Pediatr Nephrol 20:837–838, 2005.
78. Furuhashi M, Kitamura K, Adachi M, et al: Liddle's syndrome caused by a novel mutation in the proline-rich PY motif of the epithelial sodium channel β-subunit. J Clin Endocrinol Metab 90:340–344, 2005.
79. Freundlich M, Ludwig M: A novel epithelial sodium channel beta-subunit mutation associated with hypertensive Liddle syndrome. Pediatr Nephrol 20:512–515, 2005.
80. Uehara Y, Sasaguri M, Kinoshita A, et al.: Genetic analysis of the epithelial sodium channel in Liddle's syndrome. J Hypertens 16:1131–1135, 1998.
81. Pradervand S, Wang Q, Burnier M, et al: A mouse model for Liddle's syndrome. J Am Soc Nephrol 10:2527–2533, 1999.
82. Pradervand S, Vandewalle A, Bens M, et al: Dysfunction of the epithelial sodium channel expressed in the kidney of a mouse

model for Liddle's syndrome. J Am Soc Nephrol 14:2219–2228, 2003.

83. Baker E, Jeunemaitre X, James Portal A, et al: Abnormalities of nasal potential difference measurement in Liddle's syndrome. J Clin Invest 102:10–14, 1998.

84. Bubien JK, Ismailov II, Berdiev BK, et al: Liddle's disease: Abnormal regulation of amiloride-sensitive Na+ channels by beta-subunit mutation. Am J Physiol 270:C208–C213, 1996.

85. Cheek DB, Perry JW: A salt wasting syndrome in infancy. Arch Dis Child 33:252–256, 1958.

86. Chang SS, Grunder S, Hanukoglu A, et al: Mutations in subunits of the epithelial sodium channel cause salt wasting with hyperkalemic acidosis, pseudohypoaldosteronism type 1. Nat Genet 12:248–253, 1996.

87. Strautnieks SS, Thompson RJ, Gardiner RM, Chung E: A novel splice-site mutation in the gamma subunit of the epithelial sodium channel gene in three pseudohypoaldosteronism type 1 families. Nat Genet (Lond) 13:248–250, 1996.

88. Kerem E, Bistritzer T, Hanukoglu A, et al: Pulmonary epithelial sodium-channel dysfunction and excess airway liquid in pseudohypoaldosteronism. N Engl J Med 341:156–162, 1999.

89. Edelheit O, Hanukoglu I, Gizewska M, et al: Novel mutations in epithelial sodium channel (ENaC) subunit genes and phenotypic expression of multisystem pseudohypoaldosteronism. Clin Endocrinol (Oxf) 62:547–553, 2005.

90. Thomas CP, Zhou J, Liu KZ, et al: Systemic pseudohypoaldosteronism from deletion of the promoter region of the human bENaC subunit. Am J Respir Cell Mol Bio 27:314–319, 2002.

91. Schaedel C, Marthinsen L, Kristoffersson AC, et al: Lung symptoms in pseudohypoaldosteronism type 1 are associated with deficiency of the a-subunit of the epithelial sodium channel. J Pediatr 135:739–745, 1999.

92. Greenberg D, Abramson O, Phillip M: Fetal pseudohypoaldosteronism: Another cause of hydramnios. Acta Paediatr, Int J Paediatr 84:582, 1995.

93. Narchi H, Santos M, Kulaylat N: Polyhydramnios as a sign of fetal pseudohypoaldosteronism. Int J Gynecol Obstet 69:53, 2000.

94. Oberfield SE, Levine LS, Carey RM, et al: Pseudohypoaldosteronism: Multiple target organ unresponsiveness to mineralocorticoid hormones. J Clin Endocrinol Metab 48:228–234, 1979.

95. Hanukoglu A: Type I pseudohypoaldosteronism includes two clinically and genetically distinct entities with either renal or multiple target organ defects. J Clin Endocrinol Metab 73:936–944: 1991.

96. Urbatsch A, Paller AS: Pustular miliaria rubra: A specific cutaneous finding of type I pseudohypoaldosteronism. Pediatr Dermatol 19:317–319, 2002.

97. Martin JM, Calduch L, Monteagudo C, et al: Clinicopathological analysis of the cutaneous lesions of a patient with type I pseudohypoaldosteronism. J Eur Acad Dermatol Venereol 19:377–379, 2005.

98. Malagon-Rogers, M: A patient with pseudohypoaldosteronism type 1 and respiratory distress syndrome. Pediatr Nephrol 13:484–486, 1999.

99. Akcay A, Yavuz T, Semiz S, et al: Pseudohypoaldosteronism type 1 and respiratory distress syndrome. J Pediatr Endocrinol Metab 15:1557–1561, 2002.

100. Bonny O, Knoers N, Monnens L, Rossier BC: A novel mutation of the epithelial Na+ channel causes type 1 pseudohypoaldosteronism. Pediatr Nephrol 17:804–808, 2002.

101. Hummler E, Barker P, Gatzy J, et al: Early death due to defective neonatal lung liquid clearance in aENaC-deficient mice. Nat Genet 12:325–328, 1996.

102. Hummler E, Barker P, Talbot C, et al: A mouse model for the renal salt-wasting syndrome pseudohypoaldosteronism. Proc Nat Acad Sci USA 94:11710–11715, 1997.

103. McDonald F, Yang B, Hrstka R, et al: Disruption of the b subunit of the epithelial Na+ channel in mice: Hyperkalemia and neonatal death associated with pseudohypoaldosteronism phenotype. Proc Natl Acad Sci U S A 96:1727–1731, 1999.

104. Barker PM, Nguyen MS, Gatzy JT, et al: Role of gENaC subunit in lung liquid clearance and electrolyte balance in newborn mice. Insights into perinatal adaptation and pseudohypoaldosteronism. J Clin Invest 102:1634–1640, 1998.

105. Prince LS, Launspach JL, Geller DS, et al: Absence of amiloride-sensitive sodium absorption in the airway of an infant with pseudohypoaldosteronism. J Pediatr 135:786–789, 1999.

106. Zennaro MC, Lombes M: Mineralocorticoid resistance. Trends Endocrinol Metab15:264, 2004.

107. Rosler A: The natural history of salt-wasting disorders of adrenal and renal origin. J Clin Endocrinol Metab 59:689–700, 1984.

108. Viemann M, Peter M, Lopez-Siguero JP, et al: Evidence for genetic heterogeneity of pseudohypoaldosteronism type 1: Identification of a novel mutation in the human mineralocorticoid receptor in one sporadic case and no mutations in two autosomal dominant kindreds. J Clin Endocrinol Metab 86:2056–2059, 2001.

109. Tajima T, Kitagawa H, Yokoya S, et al: A novel missense mutation of mineralocorticoid receptor gene in one Japanese family with a renal form of pseudohypoaldosteronism type 1. J Clin Endocrinol Metab 85:4690–4694, 2000.

110. Sartorato P, Lapeyraque AL, Armanini D, et al.: Different inactivating mutations of the mineralocorticoid receptor in fourteen families affected by type I pseudohypoaldosteronism. J Clin Endocrinol Metab 88:2508–2517, 2003.

111. Sartorato P, Cluzeaud F, Fagart J, et al: New naturally occurring missense mutations of the human mineralocorticoid receptor disclose important residues involved in dynamic interactions with deoxyribonucleic acid, intracellular trafficking, ligand binding. Mol Endocrinol 18:2151–2165, 2004.

112. Berger S, Schmid W, Cole TJ, et al: Mineralocorticoid receptor knockout mice: Pathophysiology of Na+ metabolism. Proc Natl Acad Sci U S A 95:9424–9429, 1998.

113. Bleich M, Warth R, Schmidt-Hieber M, et al: Rescue of the mineralocorticoid receptor knock-out mouse. Pflugers Arch—Eur J Physiol 438:245–254, 1999.

114. Schulz-Baldes A, Berger S, Grahammer F, et al: Induction of the epithelial Na+ channel via glucocorticoids in mineralocorticoid receptor knockout mice. Pfluegers Arch—Eur J Physiol 443:297–305, 2001.

115. New MI, Levine LS, Biglieri EG, et al: Evidence for an unidentified steroid in a child with apparent mineralocorticoid hypertension. J Clin Endocrinol Metab 44:924–933, 1977.

116. Cooper M, Stewart P: The syndrome of apparent mineralocorticoid excess. QJM 91:453–455, 1998.

117. Wilson RC, Nimkarn S, New MI: Apparent mineralocorticoid excess. Trends Endocrinol Metabol 12:104–111, 2001.

118. White PC, Mune T, Rogerson FM, et al: Molecular analysis of 11[beta]-hydroxysteroid dehydrogenase and its role in the syndrome of apparent mineralocorticoid excess. Steroids 62:83–88, 1997.

119. Dave-Sharma S, Wilson RC, Harbison MD, et al: Examination of genotype and phenotype relationships in 14 patients with apparent mineralocorticoid excess. J Clin Endocrinol Metab 83:2244–2254, 1998.

120. Stewart PM, Krozowski ZS, Gupta A, et al: Hypertension in the syndrome of apparent mineralocorticoid excess due to

mutation of the 11 beta-hydroxysteroid dehydrogenase type 2 gene. Lancet 347:88–91, 1996.

121. Kotelevtsev Y, Brown RW, Fleming S, et al: Hypertension in mice lacking 11ß-hydroxysteroid dehydrogenase type 2. J Clin Invest 103:683–689, 1999.

122. Monder C, Shackleton CH, Bradlow HL, et al: The syndrome of apparent mineralocorticoid excess: Its association with 11 beta-dehydrogenase and 5 beta-reductase deficiency and some consequences for corticosteroid metabolism. J Clin Endocrinol Metab 63:550–557, 1986.

123. Shackleton CH, Rodriguez J, Arteaga E, et al: Congenital 11 beta-hydroxysteroid dehydrogenase deficiency associated with juvenile hypertension: Corticosteroid metabolite profiles of four patients and their families. Clin Endocrinol (Oxf) 22:701–712, 1985.

124. Palermo M, Delitala G, Mantero F, et al: Congenital deficiency of 11beta-hydroxysteroid dehydrogenase (apparent mineralocorticoid excess syndrome): Diagnostic value of urinary free cortisol and cortisone. J Endocrinol Invest 24:17–23, 2001.

125. Mantero F, Palermo M, Petrelli MD, et al: Apparent mineralocorticoid excess: Type I and type II. Steroids 61:193–196, 1996.

126. Geller DS, Farhi A, Pinkerton N, et al: Activating mineralocorticoid receptor mutation in hypertension exacerbated by pregnancy. Science 289:119–123, 2000.

127. Paver WK, Pauline, GJ: Hypertension and hyperpotassemia without renal disease in a young male. Med J Aust 2:305–306, 1964.

128. Gordon RD, Geddes RA, Pawsey CG, O'Halloran MW: Hypertension and severe hyperkalaemia associated with suppression of renin and aldosterone and completely reversed by dietary sodium restriction. Australas Ann Med 19:287–294, 1970.

129. Spitzer A, Edelmann C: Short stature, hyperkalemia and acidosis: A defect in renal transport of potassium. Kidney Int 3:251–257, 1973.

130. Weinstein SF, Allan DME, Mendoza SA: Hyperkalemia, acidosis, and short stature associated with a defect in renal potassium excretion. J Pediatr 85:355–358, 1974.

131. Lee MR, Ball SG, Thomas TH, Morgan DB: Hypertension and hyperkalaemia responding to bendrofluazide. Q J Med 48:245–258, 1979.

132. Grekin RJ, Nicholls MG, Padfield PL: Disorders of chloriuretic hormone secretion. Lancet 1:1116–1118, 1979.

133. Iitaka K, Watanabe N, Asakura A, et al: Familial hyperkalemia, metabolic acidosis and short stature with normal renin and aldosterone levels. Int J Ped Neph 28:782A, 1980.

134. Schambelan M, Sebastian A, Rector FC Jr: Mineralocorticoid-resistant renal hyperkalemia without salt wasting (type II pseudohypoaldosteronism): Role of increased renal chloride reabsorption. Kidney Int 19:716–727, 1981.

135. Disse-Nicodeme S, Achard JM, Desitter I, et al: A new locus on chromosome 12p13.3 for pseudohypoaldosteronism type II, an autosomal dominant form of hypertension. Am J Hum Genet 67:302–310, 2000.

136. Disse-Nicodeme S, Achard JM, Potier J, et al: Familial hyperkalemic hypertension (Gordon syndrome): Evidence for phenotypic variability in a study of 7 families. Adv Nephrol Necker Hosp 31:55–68, 2001.

137. Wilson FH, Disse-Nicodeme S, Choate KA, et al: Human hypertension caused by mutations in WNK kinases. Science 293:1107–1112, 2001.

138. Achard JM, Disse-Nicodeme S, Fiquet-Kempf B, Jeunemaitre X: Phenotypic and genetic heterogeneity of familial hyperkalaemic hypertension (Gordon syndrome). Clin Exp Pharmacol Physiol 28:1048–1052, 2001.

139. Achard JM, Warnock DG, Disse-Nicodeme S, et al: Familial hyperkalemic hypertension: Phenotypic analysis in a large family with the WNK1 deletion mutation. Am J Med 114:495–498, 2003.

140. Farfel Z, Iaina A, Rosenthal T, et al: Familial hyperpotassemia and hypertension accompanied by normal plasma aldosterone levels: Possible hereditary cell membrane defect. Arch Intern Med 138:1828–1832, 1978.

141. Mansfield TA, Simon DB, Farfel Z, et al: Multilocus linkage of familial hyperkalaemia and hypertension, pseudohypoaldosteronism type II, to chromosomes 1q31-42 and 17p11-q21. Nat Genet 16:202–205, 1997.

142. Simon DB, Farfel, Z, Ellison D, et al: Examination of the thiazide-sensitive Na-Cl cotransporter as a candidate gene in Gordon's syndrome. JASN 6:632, 1995.

143. Disse-Nicodeme S, Desitter I, Fiquet-Kempf B, et al: Genetic heterogeneity of familial hyperkalaemic hypertension. J Hypertens 19:1957–1964, 2001.

144. Xu B, English JM, Wilsbacher JL, et al: WNK1, a novel mammalian serine/threonine protein kinase lacking the catalytic lysine in subdomain II. J Biol Chem 275:16795–16801, 2000.

145. Xu BE, Min X, Stippec S, et al: Regulation of WNK1 by an autoinhibitory domain and autophosphorylation. J Biol Chem 277:48456–48462, 2002.

146. Moriguchi T, Urushiyama S, Hisamoto N, et al: WNK1 regulates phosphorylation of cation-chloride-coupled cotransporters via the STE20-related kinases, SPAK and OSR1. J Biol Chem 280:42685–42693, 2005.

147. Wang Z, Yang CL, Ellison DH: Comparison of WNK4 and WNK1 kinase and inhibiting activities. Biochem Biophys Res Commun 317:939–944, 2004.

148. Lee BH, Min X, Heise CJ, et al: WNK1 phosphorylates synaptotagmin 2 and modulates its membrane binding. Mol Cell 15:741–751, 2004.

149. Lenertz LY, Lee BH, Min X, et al: Properties of WNK1 and implications for other family members. J Biol Chem 280:26653–26658, 2005.

150. Mayan H, Vered I, Mouallem M, et al: Pseudohypoaldosteronism type II: Marked sensitivity to thiazides, hypercalciuria, normomagnesemia, and low bone mineral density. J Clin Endocrinol Metab 87:3248–3254, 2002.

151. Gordon RD: Syndrome of hypertension and hyperkalemia with normal glomerular filtration rate. Hypertension 8:93–102, 1986.

152. Mayan H, Munter G, Shaharabany M, et al: Hypercalciuria in familial hyperkalemia and hypertension accompanies hyperkalemia and precedes hypertension: Description of a large family with the Q565E WNK4 mutation. J Clin Endocrinol Metab 89:4025–4030, 2004.

153. Gordon RD, Klemm SA, Tunny TJ, Stowasser M: Gordon's syndrome: A sodium-volume dependent form of hypertension with a genetic basis. In Laragh JH, Brenner BM (eds): Hypertension: Pathophysiology, Diagnosis, and Management. New York, Raven Press, 1995, pp 211–2123.

154. Sanjad SA, Mansour FM, Hernandez RH, Hill LL: Severe hypertension, hyperkalemia, and renal tubular acidosis responding to dietary sodium restriction. Pediatrics 69:317–324, 1982.

155. Wayne VS, Stockigt JR, Jennings GL: Treatment of mineralocorticoid-resistant renal hyperkalemia with hypertension (type II pseudohypoaldosteronism). Aust NZ J Med 16:221–223, 1986.

156. Rodriguez-Soriano J, Vallo A, Dominguez MJ: 'Chloride-shunt' syndrome: An overlooked cause of renal hypercalciuria. Pediatr Nephrol 3:113–121, 1989.

157. Gereda JE, Bonilla–Felix M, Kalil B, Dewitt SJ: Neonatal presentation of Gordon syndrome. J Pediatr 129:615–617, 1996.

158. Tokunaga Y, Yoshida I, Endo F, Kato H: The effect of furosemide on a patient with hyperkalaemic hypertension and short stature. Eur J Pediatr 154:870, 1995.

159. Licht JH, Amundson D, Hsueh WA, Lombardo JV: Familiar hyperkalemic acidosis. Q J Med 54:161–176, 1985.

160. Ellison DH: Salt-wasting disorders. In DuBose T, Hamm LL (eds): Acid–Base and Electrolyte Disorders. Philadelphia, Saunders, 2002, pp 311–333.

161. Yang CL, Angell J, Mitchell R, Ellison DH: WNK kinases regulate thiazide-sensitive Na-Cl cotransport. J Clin Invest 111:1039–1045, 2003.

162. Choate KA, Kahle KT, Wilson FH, et al: WNK1, a kinase mutated in inherited hypertension with hyperkalemia, localizes to diverse Cl⁻-transporting epithelia. Proc Natl Acad Sci U S A 100:663–668, 2003.

163. Wilson FH, Kahle KT, Sabath E, et al: Molecular pathogenesis of inherited hypertension with hyperkalemia: The Na-Cl cotransporter is inhibited by wild-type but not mutant WNK4. Proc Natl Acad Sci U S A 100:680–684, 2003.

164. Yang CL, Zhu X, Wang Z, et al: Mechanisms of WNK1 and WNK4 interaction in the regulation of thiazide-sensitive NaCl cotransport. J Clin Invest 115:1379–1387, 2005.

165. Yamauchi K, Rai T, Kobayashi K, et al: Disease-causing mutant WNK4 increases paracellular chloride permeability and phosphorylates claudins. Proc Natl Acad Sci U S A 101:4690–4694, 2004.

166. Kahle KT, Macgregor GG, Wilson FH, et al: Paracellular Cl⁻ permeability is regulated by WNK4 kinase: Insight into normal physiology and hypertension. Proc Natl Acad Sci U S A 101:14877–14882, 2004.

167. Delaloy C, Lu J, Houot AM, et al: Multiple promoters in the WNK1 gene: One controls expression of a kidney-specific kinase–defective isoform. Mol Cell Biol 23:9208–9221, 2003.

168. Subramanya AR, Yang, CL, Zhu X, Ellison DH: Dominant-negative regulation of WNK1 by its kidney-specific kinase–defective isoform. Am J Physiol Renal Physiol 290:F617–F618, 2005.

169. Naray-Fejes-Toth A, Snyder PM, Fejes-Toth G: The kidney-specific WNK1 isoform is induced by aldosterone and stimulates epithelial sodium channel–mediated Na⁺ transport. Proc Natl Acad Sci U S A 101:17434–17439, 2004.

170. Stone RC, Vale P, Rosa FC: Effect of hydrochlorothiazide in pseudohypoaldosteronism with hypercalciuria and severe hyperkalemia. Pediatr Nephrol 10:501–503, 1996.

171. Lalioti MD, Kahle KT, Toka HR, et al: Mutant WNK4 in mouse reveals mechanisms of pseudohypoaldosteronism type II. Nat Genet 38:1124–1132, 2006.

171a. Yang S-S, Morimoto T, Rai T, et al: Molecular pathogenesis of pseudohypoaldosteronism type II: Generation and analysis of a Wnk4D561A/+ knockin mouse model. Cell Metabol 5:331–344, 2007.

172. Zambrowicz BP, Abuin A, Ramirez-Solis R, et al: Wnk1 kinase deficiency lowers blood pressure in mice: A gene-trap screen to identify potential targets for therapeutic intervention. Proc Natl Acad Sci U S A 100:14109–14114, 2003.

173. Olyaei AJ, de Mattos AM, Bennett WM: Immunosuppressant-induced nephropathy: Pathophysiology, incidence and management. Drug Saf 21:471–488, 1999.

174. Klemm SA, Gordon RD, Tunny TJ, Finn WL: Biochemical correction in the syndrome of hypertension and hyperkalaemia by severe dietary salt restriction suggests renin-aldosterone suppression critical in pathophysiology. Clin Exp Pharmacol Physiol 17:191–195, 1990.

175. Brautbar N, Levi J, Rosler A, et al: Familial hyperkalemia, hypertension, hyporeninemia with normal aldosterone levels. A tubular defect in potassium handling. Arch Intern Med 138:607–610, 1978.

Chapter 17

Hereditary Renal Tubular Acidosis

Christine E. Kurschat and Seth L. Alper

Renal tubular acidosis (RTA) is a failure of renal regulatory mechanisms to maintain systemic pH homeostasis. Patients present with hyperchloremic metabolic acidosis in the setting of an inappropriate inability to acidify urine pH below 5.5. The associated clinical syndrome can include any combination of hypokalemia, nephrocalcinosis, nephrolithiasis, growth retardation, rickets, osteomalacia, nausea, vomiting, polyuria, and dehydration. Hereditary RTA appears in autosomal dominant and recessive forms, and as four traditionally defined clinical types. Hereditary distal renal tubular acidosis (dRTA), or type 1 RTA, is associated with mutations impairing H^+ secretion by the intercalated cells of the distal nephron, resulting in metabolic acidosis without bicarbonaturia. "Complete" dRTA exhibits spontaneous metabolic acidosis. "Incomplete" dRTA exhibits no acidosis and requires either systemic acid loading with NH_4Cl or a modified furosemide test to elicit evidence for failure to lower urinary pH below the threshold level of 5.5. dRTA can be accompanied by deafness. Hereditary proximal renal tubular acidosis (pRTA), or type 2 RTA, is associated with mutations impairing HCO_3^- reabsorption in the proximal tubule, resulting in metabolic acidosis with bicarbonaturia. pRTA can be accompanied by ocular and cognitive abnormalities and by elevated circulating pancreatic enzymes. Hereditary mixed RTA, or type 3 RTA, results from mutations impairing both proximal tubular cell HCO_3^- reabsorption and distal nephron intercalated-cell H^+ secretion. Mixed RTA can be accompanied by osteopetrosis and cognitive abnormalities. Type 4 RTA is usually characterized by deficiency of, or distal nephron unresponsiveness to, aldosterone. The hyperkalemia often accompanying type 4 RTA contrasts with the hypokalemia seen in patients with type 1 dRTA, type 2 pRTA, or type 3 mixed RTA. RTA that is associated with autosomal dominant inheritance (hereafter referred to as dominant RTA) is usually milder and more slowly progressive than that associated with autosomal recessive inheritance (recessive RTA), which in early childhood may be associated with life-threatening dehydration.

This chapter will review recent advances in our understanding of the molecular defects and cell physiologic mechanisms underlying familial RTAs. Earlier reviews of this subject include the disease-focused articles of Rodriguez-Soriano,[1,2] Igarashi and colleagues[3] Quigley,[4] Toye,[5] Shayakul and Alper,[6] Nicoletta and Schwartz,[7] Wrong and associates,[8] Alper,[9] Karet,[10] Laing and Unwin,[11] among others. Additional molecule-oriented reviews with discussion of RTA include those of Aalkjaer et al,[12] Forgac,[13] Wagner and associates,[14] Beyenbach and Wieczorek,[15] Alper,[16] Pushkin and Kurtz,[17]

Romero,[18] Mount and Romero,[19] Romero and colleagues,[20] Alper,[21] Alper and colleagues,[22] and Schwartz.[23]

DIAGNOSIS, THERAPY, AND PROGNOSIS OF RTA

RTA should be considered in a patient with metabolic acidosis, hyperchloremia, and a normal plasma anion gap. Serum K^+ concentration, urine pH, urine NH_4^+ excretion, fractional HCO_3^- excretion, and urine anion gap ($Na^+ + K^+ - Cl^-$) are helpful parameters for diagnosis. Serum K^+ concentration is normal or reduced in patients with proximal (type 2) and distal (type 1) RTA but elevated in type 4 RTA. Urine pH can be reduced below 5.5 in proximal and type 4 RTA but not in distal RTA. Fractional NH_4^+ excretion is normal in proximal but decreased in distal and type 4 RTA. Fractional HCO_3^- excretion can be elevated above 5% to 10% in proximal (type 2) RTA and mixed (type 3) RTA. Nephrocalcinosis is often present in distal (type 1) RTA but absent in proximal (type 2) and type 4 RTA.

If spontaneous metabolic acidosis is not present or not pronounced, acid loading can be performed by administration of an acidifying salt such as NH_4Cl, $CaCl_2$, or arginine hydrochloride. Incomplete RTA can be present if metabolic acidosis becomes apparent only after systemic acid loading. Therapy of RTA consists of oral administration of alkali either as HCO_3^- or as citrate that is metabolized to HCO_3^- in the liver.[2] A mixture of Na^+ and K^+ salts, usually as the citrates, is recommended in split doses throughout the day. The amount of alkali per kilogram of body weight required to correct metabolic acidosis is higher in children and gradually decreases in adulthood. In pRTA and dRTA, therapy should be maintained throughout life to prevent the progression of nephrocalcinosis and the development of chronic renal failure. In some cases with sporadic pRTA the renal defect might improve over the years, and therapy can be gradually discontinued. In hyperkalemic RTA, hypoaldosteronism due to decreased adrenal aldosterone synthesis may be treated with fludrocortisone in combination with a loop diuretic to reduce potential extracellular volume overload. Patients with type 4 RTA may also require alkali supplements.

Prompt initiation of alkali therapy is crucial to prevent growth retardation, bone disease, and episodes of nausea, vomiting, and dehydration in infancy. Progression of nephrocalcinosis can also be slowed by alkali therapy. Without treatment, nephrocalcinosis may progress to chronic renal failure at any age.

dietary K^+ depletion specifically upregulates the colonic iso-form $HK_{\alpha 2}$, which mediates increased NH_4^+ secretion.[58,59]

The action of plasmalemmal H^+-ATPases increases intracellular $[OH^-]$, which is converted by cytosolic CA II into HCO_3^-. In the acid-secreting type A intercalated cell, HCO_3^- is transported across the basolateral membrane by the SLC4A1 electroneutral Cl^-/HCO_3^- exchanger, kidney AE1 (kAE1) (see Fig. 17-1). The *SLC4A1/AE1* gene transcribes mRNAs from two distinct promoters encoding, respectively, the major intrinsic protein of the erythrocyte, the eAE1 Cl^-/HCO_3^- exchanger, and the type A intercalated cell–specific kAE1. Human kAE1 differs from eAE1 in lacking 65 N-terminal amino acids present in eAE1[22] (Fig. 17-5, see also Fig 17-1). All SLC4 anion exchangers are characterized by a long N-terminal cytoplasmic domain followed by a transmembrane domain and a short C-terminal cytoplasmic tail. The N-terminal domain of eAE1 binds to cytoskeletal proteins such as the spectrin-binding protein ankyrin and actin-binding ezrin-radixin-moiesin family protein 4.1R, as well as to glycolytic enzymes. In contrast, the binding partners of the N-terminal domain of kAE1 are little understood. CA II can bind, at least in some assay formats, to the C-terminal tail of eAE1. Thus CA II and AE1 have been proposed to constitute a "metabolon," a metabolic unit that potentiates HCO_3^- transport activity by providing a physically linked enzyme to guarantee high local concentration of HCO_3^- for kAE1-mediated transport out of the cell.[23,60,61] kAE1 expression is increased in metabolic acidosis and decreased in metabolic alkalosis.[62,63]

Type A intercalated cells of the medullary but not cortical collecting duct have also been reported to express in their basolateral membranes the SLC26A7 Cl^-/HCO_3^- exchanger,[64] a member of the distinct SLC26 HCO_3^- transporter super-family.[19] SLC26A7 differs from kAE1 in that it is acutely activated by hypertonicity,[65] a response reinforced during prolonged hypertonic exposure by mobilization of intracellular vesicular protein to the plasma membrane.[66] mRNA expression of SLC26A7 is upregulated by increased medullary osmolality in water-deprived rats, whereas kAE1 mRNA is decreased.[67] Experiments in Brattleboro rats demonstrate that Slc26a7 expression can be controlled by vasopressin.[68] K^+ depletion in polarized Madin-Darby canine kidney (MDCK) cells also enhances basolateral membrane expression of heterologous SLC26A7,[66] and so SLC26A7 might assist apical H^+/K^+-ATPase in intercalated cell–mediated K^+ reabsorption. However, SLC26A7 has also been presented as an acid pH–activated Cl^- channel with minimal HCO_3^- permeability, rather than a Cl^-/HCO_3^- exchanger.[69] In addition, distinct antibodies have localized mouse Slc26a7 to the proximal tubular brush border rather than to medullary intercalated cells.[70] Thus, the specific roles played by SLC26A7 in medullary HCO_3^- homeostasis and cell volume regulation in different species remain uncertain.

Type B β-intercalated cells secrete HCO_3^- through an apical Cl^-/HCO_3^- exchanger. Immunocytochemistry has in most cases failed to demonstrate the presence of apical membrane kAE1 in these cells.[71,72] However, Royaux et al[73] identified pendrin/*SLC26A4*, the Pendred syndrome–associated gene, as the apical Cl^-/HCO_3^- exchanger in type B intercalated cells of the cortical collecting duct (see Fig. 17-1). Pendrin is also present apically in non-A, non-B intercalated cells.[74,75] In contrast, AE1 (in all recent studies) is absent from both type B

and non-A, non-B intercalated cells. Although the pendrin-knockout mouse is grossly normal and without alkalosis, HCO_3^- secretion by cortical collecting ducts isolated from mineralocorticoid-treated mice revealed decreased HCO_3^- secretion.[73] Pendrin expression in mouse and rat kidney is significantly reduced by acid loading.[76,77] Conversely, pendrin expression was modestly increased in response to alkali loading,[78] but a subsequent investigation suggested that pendrin is primarily regulated by systemic Cl^- balance.[79] Both aldosterone and Cl^- balance regulate pendrin primarily through subcellular protein redistribution.[50]

Tsuganezawa et al[80] cloned *SLC4A9/AE4* as a DIDS-insensitive Cl^-/HCO_3^- exchanger and demonstrated its presence in the apical membrane of rabbit type B intercalated cells. However, in rat and mouse cortical collecting duct, AE4 was present in the basolateral membrane of type A intercalated cells, and AE4-dependent Cl^-/HCO_3^- exchange was DIDS sensitive.[81] Moreover, others suggest that AE4 (more closely related by amino acid sequence to the Na^+/HCO_3^- cotransporters than to AE1 and other AE anion exchangers) is a Na^+-dependent transporter.[20] Thus, the function and physiologic role of AE4/SLC4A9 in intercalated cells remains in question. The electroneutral Na^+/HCO_3^- cotransporter NBCn1/SLC4A7 is also expressed in the apical membrane of intercalated cells, positioned where it might contribute to the luminal Na^+-stimulated component of collecting duct H^+ secretion.

Acid and base secretion in the connecting segment and cortical collecting duct take place in the environment of a mosaic epithelium, in which principal cell–mediated Na^+ reabsorption and K^+ secretion (see Fig. 17-1) influence acid-base balance. Epithelial Na^+ channel (ENaC)–mediated Na^+ reabsorption across the principal cell apical membrane generates a lumen-negative potential, thereby favoring coincident renal outer medullary K^+ channel–mediated K^+ secretion across the apical membrane, as well as paracellular Cl^- reabsorption. This lumen-negative potential also generates a favorable environment for H^+ secretion by α-intercalated cells (see Fig. 17-1). Aldosterone influences distal renal acidification through several mechanisms. It induces synthesis of new apical ENaCs in principal cells and may also prolong their residence in the apical membrane, thereby increasing Na^+ reabsorption in distal and cortical collecting tubules. This effect is potentiated by upregulation of the basolateral Na^+/K^+-ATPase. Aldosterone also increases vH^+-ATPase activity and NH_3 synthesis, additionally contributing to renal acid secretion.[82]

Familial loss of function of any of the molecular components discussed above must be considered as possible causes of hereditary RTA. The sections to follow will present familial syndromes of human RTA for which causative mutations have been defined. These mutations have been discovered by several paths of investigation. Some discoveries have come through investigation of candidate genes based on prior understanding of the renal physiology. Others have followed whole-genome linkage mapping of carefully selected family cohorts, at which point investigation of candidate genes could be restricted to genetically delimited regions within a single chromosome. Finally, some RTA-associated genes have been discovered by analysis of knockout mouse phenotypes and have yet to be proven relevant to human RTA. Examples of each will be described.

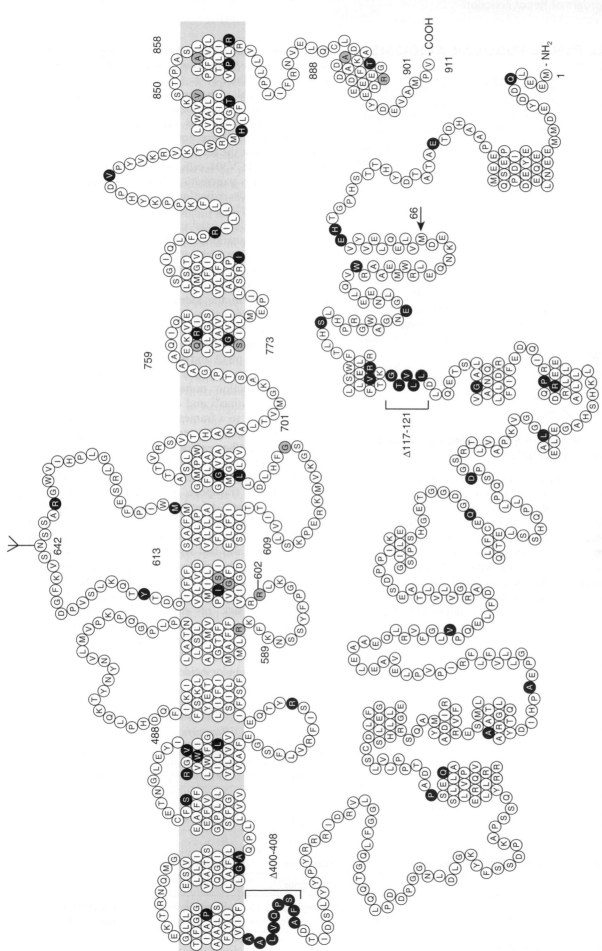

Figure 17-5 Mutations of the human AE1/SLC4A1 polypeptide associated with hereditary spherocytic anemia and altered erythroid shape are shaded in black, and include missense, nonsense, splicing, and deletion mutation. The sites of mutations associated with dominant and recessive dRTA (Table 17-3) are shaded in blue and are missense mutations except for A888/889X and R901X. eAE1 polypeptide begins with Met 1. kAE1 polypeptide begins with Met 66. (Modified from Shayakul C, Alper SL: Defects in processing and trafficking of the AE1 Cl^-/HCO_3^- exchanger associated with inherited distal renal tubular acidosis. Clin Exp Nephrol 8:1–11, 2004.)

and solute entry across the proximal tubular apical membrane. *Kcnk5$^{-/-}$* mice exhibit pRTA, with increased pre-weaning mortality, and volume depletion and hypotension in adults.[110] The pRTA is attributed to depolarization of the proximal tubular basolateral membrane, resulting in inadequate electrical driving force for NBCe1-mediated HCO_3^- efflux. As a homodimer, *TASK2* mutations might be dominant negative, allowing proposal of *TASK2* as a candidate gene for dominantly inherited pRTA. *TASK2* mutations might also cause mild recessive forms of pRTA, depending on the spectrum, regulation, and expression levels of other basolateral K$^+$ channels of the proximal tubular basolateral membrane.

Patients with sporadic isolated pRTA exhibit a transient, nonfamilial defect of both renal and intestinal HCO_3^- absorption.[2,111,112] They present with growth retardation and vomiting in early childhood without any obvious cause or other underlying disease. Treatment with alkali therapy completely reverses the clinical phenotype and can usually be discontinued safely after several years. The decreased HCO_3^- threshold observed in these patients, it has been speculated, might be due to continued immaturity of NHE3 function.[1]

DISTAL RENAL TUBULAR ACIDOSIS (dRTA TYPE 1)

Autosomal Dominant dRTA

Autosomal dominant dRTA is associated with mutations in the *SLC4A1* gene encoding the collecting duct type A intercalated cell Cl$^-$/HCO_3^- exchanger, kAE1.[113–115] (*AE1* mutations associated with recessive dRTA will be described in the following section.) The *AE1* gene on human chromosome 17q21–22 (Table 17-2) is transcribed under the control of two different promoters. An erythroid-specific promoter upstream of exon 1 regulates the transcription of the 911-aa human erythroid AE1 (eAE1). This Cl$^-$/HCO_3^- exchanger is the major intrinsic membrane protein of the red cell and is implicated in CO_2 transport in the blood. Numerous mutations in the *AE1* gene result in autosomal dominant hereditary spherocytosis with hemolytic anemia[21] or without anemia but with cation leak.[116] Renal transcription initiates from a distinct promoter within intron 3 of the *AE1* gene. The resultant kidney-specific kAE1 transcript is highly expressed in type A intercalated cells of the collecting duct and encodes a polypeptide that lacks the N-terminal 65 aa present in eAE1.[117] Although similar kidney-specific transcripts have been found in mice, rats, and all other mammals and birds examined, this promoter so highly specific for the type A intercalated cell has yet to be studied and mapped. Distinct mutations in the *AE1* gene result in RTA.

The *AE1* mutations found thus far in individuals with autosomal dominant dRTA are listed in Table 17-3. None of the dominant dRTA mutations have been found in homozygous state, suggesting embryonic or early postnatal lethality. Among the dominant mutations, R589 mutants have been reported in multiple unrelated families, and as a spontaneous mutation.[115] These dominant mutations have been found, with one exception (A858D) in Caucasian families. Remarkably, none of the eight dominant dRTA mutations of *AE1* express an erythroid phenotype. The same is true of four among the five recessive dRTA mutations of *AE1*. Conversely,

Table 17-2 Hereditary Syndromes of Renal Tubular Acidosis Attributed to Mutations in Defined Genetic Loci

Syndrome	MIM No.	Chromosomal Localization	Locus Symbol	Gene Product
Primary proximal RTA (type 2)				
Autosomal recessive with ocular abnormalities	603345, 604278	4q21	*SLC4A4*	NBCe1
Autosomal dominant?	179830	?	?	?
Primary distal RTA (type 1)				
Autosomal dominant	179800, 109270	17q21–22	*SLC4A1*	AE1
Autosomal recessive	602272, 109270	17q21–22	*SLC4A1*	AE1
Autosomal recessive with deafness	192132, 267300	2p13	*ATP6V1B1*	vH$^+$-ATPase B1 subunit
Autosomal recessive with variable deafness	602272, 605239	7q33–34	*ATP6V0A4*	vH$^+$-ATPase a4 subunit
Combined proximal and distal RTA (type 3)				
Autosomal recessive with osteopetrosis	259730	8q22	*CA2*	CA II
Dent disease*	300009	Xp11.22	*CLCN5*	CLC-5
Secondary hyperkalemic distal RTA (type 4)*				
Pseudohypoaldosteronism type 1*				
Autosomal dominant renal form*		4q31.1	*MR*	Mineralocorticoid receptor
Autosomal recessive multiple-organ form*		12p13.1	*SCNN1A*	ENaC α-subunit
		16p12–13.11	*SCNN1B*	ENaC β-subunit
		16p12–13.11	*SCNN1G*	ENaC γ-subunit
Pseudohypoaldosteronism type 2*	145260, 605232	12p13.3	*WNK1*	WNK1 kinase
Hyperkalemic hypertension* (Gordon syndrome)*	145260, 601844	17p11–q21	*WNK4*	WNK4 kinase

ENaC, epithelial Na$^+$ channel; RTA, renal tubular acidosis.
*Familial syndromes that are often but not necessarily accompanied by distal RTA.

none of the (at least) 48 distinct *AE1* mutations associated with autosomal dominant hereditary spherocytosis or ovalocytosis with anemia[21,114,118] express a renal acidification phenotype.[118–121] (The potential exceptions, AE1 S477fs[122] and AE1 Q203fs,[123] are reported to exhibit unexplained bicarbonaturia). *AE1*-associated hereditary spherocytosis mutations are nearly all loss-of-function mutations, most with nonsense-mediated decay of mRNA or with mutant protein instability. Also lacking a renal acidification phenotype are the five *AE1* mutations associated with nonanemic spherocytosis with cation leak, all of which exhibit normal red cell surface expression with reduced anion transport.[116] Southeast Asian ovalocytosis (SAO; AE1Δ400–408) has been recently reclassified in this category. Whereas *AE1* mutations of hereditary spherocytosis or ovalocytosis are found throughout the AE1 coding region, those associated with dRTA of either dominant or recessive form are found uniquely in the transmembrane domain or the C-terminal cytoplasmic tail (Fig. 17-6). With the single exception of V488M (to be discussed below), dRTA substitutions and hereditary spherocytosis mutations of the AE1 transmembrane domain are mutually exclusive subsets.

The erythrocytes of most patients with autosomal dominant hereditary spherocytosis express at least 50% of the wild-type membrane amount of eAE1 polypeptide. Assuming that the type A intercalated cells express a proportionally similar level of kAE1, this suggests that urinary acidification can tolerate haploinsufficiency of kAE1, whereas erythrocyte membrane stability cannot. Unfortunately, it has not been possible to maintain the type A intercalated cell in primary culture, and its phenotype has not been successfully immor-

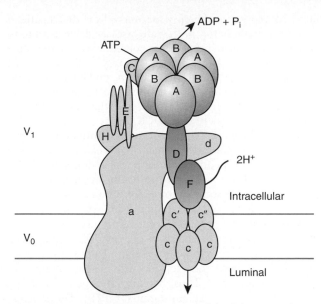

Figure 17-6 Simplified schematic model of the vacuolar H⁺-ATPase. The membrane-bound V_0 domain consists of subunits a through d, the cytosolic V_1 domain comprises subunits A through H. V_0 includes the proton translocation pathway, and V_1 hydrolyzes ATP, providing the energy to drive active H⁺ transport across the membrane bilayer.

Table 17-3 SLC4A1/AE1 Mutations Associated with Inherited Distal Renal Tubular Acidosis (MIM: 179800, 602272, 109270)

Mutation	Zygosity	Inheritance	References
V488M (Coimbra)	Homozygous	Recessive	Ribeiro et al[147]
R589H	Heterozygous	Dominant	Bruce et al[113] Jarolim et al[114] Karet et al[115]
R589C	Heterozygous	Dominant	Bruce et al[113]
R589S	Heterozygous	Dominant	Bruce et al[113]
R602H	Cmpd het	Recessive	Sritippayawan et al[140]
G609R	Heterozygous	Dominant	Rungroj et al[133]
S613F	Heterozygous	Dominant	Bruce et al[113]
G701D (Bangkok I)	Homozygote, Cmpd het	Recessive	Tanphaichitr et al[138] Bruce et al[141] Yenchitsomanus et al[241]
Q759H (Unimas)	Cmpd het	Recessive	Choo et al[143]
S773P	Cmpd het	Recessive	Kittanakom et al[142]
ΔV850	Homozygous, Cmpd het	Recessive	Bruce et al[141]
A858D	Heterozygous, Cmpd het	Dominant	Bruce et al[141]
A888L/889X	Heterozygous	Dominant	Cheidde et al[239]
R901X (Walton)	Heterozygous	Dominant	Karet et al[115]

Cmpd het, compound heterozygous; MIM, mendelian inheritance in man.

talized. Moreover, renal biopsy specimens from dRTA patients of known genetic status, in the rare cases available, tend to be complicated by scarring or other consequences of the other disease process(es) that justified the biopsy.[124] Therefore, AE1 dRTA mutant polypeptides have been studied in available human kidney cell lines, most often the nonpolarized but easily transfectable HEK 293 cells, and the polarizable but genetically more recalcitrant MDCK II cells.

Studies in these cells, complemented by studies in *Xenopus* oocytes, have revealed two principal mechanisms by which mutant kAE1 polypeptides probably cause dominant dRTA. The first is a dominant-negative trafficking mechanism, which can be seen only in some but not all heterologous expression systems. *Xenopus* oocyte studies have shown that the dominant-mutant polypeptides generally exhibit between 50% and 100% of wild-type transport activity. AE1 mutant with the R589H substitution functioned about half as well as wild-type AE1 in *Xenopus* oocytes and exhibited no dominant-negative phenotype.[114] Thus, haploinsufficiency of intrinsic AE1 function cannot explain dominant dRTA. The explanation was therefore sought in abnormalities of kAE1 polypeptide trafficking. Trafficking and oligomerization studies of AE1 polypeptides have been greatly aided by use of epitope-tagged constructs to facilitate surface biotinylation assays. Advances in the study of intracellular trafficking within compartments of the secretory pathway required conversion of the high-mannose, Endo H–resistant wild-type N-glycosylation site at N642 in the fourth extracellular loop of AE1 (Fig. 17-5) with an engineered artificial N-glycosylation site in the third extracellular loop in the triple mutant resulting from substitutions N642D/Y555N/V557T.[125] These mutations engineered to allow cell biologic study retained substantial, if not complete, transport activity in a wild-type background.

Expression of AE1 R589H in nonpolarized HEK 293 cells revealed isoform-specific trafficking, with normal surface expression of eAE1 R589H, but retention of most kAE1 R589H inside the cell, at least partially in endoplasmic reticulum. Co-expression of kAE1 R589H with wild-type kAE1 to mimic the heterozygous condition reduced surface expression of kAE1 with increased intracellular retention associated with, and thus most likely due to, hetero-oligomerization of mutant and wild-type polypeptides.[126]

Extension of these studies to polarized MDCK cells was initially troubled by low transient transfection efficiencies[10] and by instability of transgene expression in stably transfected populations and clonal cell lines.[127] Experiments have been advanced by use of recombinant, replication-deficient pseudotyped retrovirus[128] and of adenovirus vectors[129] for high-efficiency infection with moderate overexpression, boosting sensitivity of detection of recombinant AE1 polypeptide. Use of MDCK cells offered the added benefit over nonpolarized HEK 293 cells of the ability to process the complex N-glycan at N642 to a mature form, allowing study of the trafficking of protein with glycan in the native position. Nonpolarized MDCK cells retained dominant mutants kAE1 R589H and S613F inside the cell, largely in endoplasmic reticulum, but with some protein detected in late endosomes and lysosomes. This phenotype was replicated in polarized MDCK cells, in contrast to the basolateral localization of wild-type kAE1.[127,129] Co-expression of C-myc–tagged wild-type kAE1 with kAE1 R589H led to inhibition of surface delivery of the wild-type polypeptide, apparently accompanied by accelerated degradation.[129] Thus, retention in the endoplasmic reticulum of

hetero-oligomers of wild-type and mutant polypeptides is the probable mechanism of dominant dRTA caused by the *AE1* substitutions in residues R589 and S613.

A second mechanism by which *AE1* mutations lead to dominant dRTA is mistargeting to the apical membrane, resulting in apical HCO_3^- secretion that short-circuits apical H^+ secretion mediated by the vH$^+$-ATPase. This mechanism was first reported for AE1 901X, which truncates the final 11 aa from the C-terminal cytoplasmic tail,[115] without impairment of surface expression or function in *Xenopus* oocytes.[130,131] AE1 901X is retained in endoplasmic reticulum of transiently transfected HEK 293 cells[130] and, via hetero-oligomerization, can retain with it co-transfected wild-type kAE1, in a pre-medial Golgi compartment. kAE1 is also retained inside glass-grown MDCK cells[127] but exhibits a distinct phenotype in polarized MDCK monolayers grown on permeable-filter supports. In transiently transfected, polarized MDCK cells or rat IMCD cells, kAE1 901X was present in both apical and basolateral membranes, as well as with some intracellular retention.[132] In stably transfected cells, AE1 901X was present (within the limits of detection) exclusively in the apical membrane, in which conditions it seemed to have wild-type stability.[127]

Subsequent studies have revealed another *AE1* missense mutation associated with dominant dRTA by the same apparent mechanism. The mutant kAE1 polypeptide substituted at G609R exhibited normal anion transport function and surface expression in *Xenopus* oocytes. However, when expressed in polarized MDCK cells, the kAE1 mutant G609R accumulated to a greater degree at or near the apical membrane than in the basolateral membrane.[133] It remains to be determined whether the apical mis-sorting phenotype represents direct mistargeting or disordered retention of newly delivered protein due to altered stability in apical and basolateral membranes.

The polarized renal epithelial cell expression systems offered the opportunity to search for basolateral targeting signals in the human kAE1 amino acid sequence. CD8 fusion protein studies indicated the potential importance of a YXXΦ motif at AE1 aa 904–907. However, this motif did not appear to exert its influence via interaction with the μ1B subunit of AP-1B adaptin for sorting, as based on its continued importance in polarized LLC-PK1 cells, which lack μ1B.[132] Later studies indicated that the Y904F substitution in isolation sufficed to retain kAE1 inside polarized MDCK cells. A putative type II PDZ recognition motif in the four C-terminal amino acids of kAE1 was not crucial to its basolateral sorting in polarized MDCK cell monolayers.[127] However, removal of most of the long N-terminal cytoplasmic domain of kAE1 (resulting in a construct containing aa 361–911) led to its exclusively apical localization in MDCK cell monolayers, and to unimpaired surface expression in HEK 293 cells.[127] Thus, basolateral sorting determinants seem to be present in both the short C-terminal and the long N-terminal cytoplasmic tails of kAE1.

The potential role of Y904 phosphorylation in basolateral targeting of kAE1 is unknown. Also unknown are the identities of kAE1-interacting proteins of type A intercalated cells. Several candidate interacting proteins detected in preliminary yeast two-hybrid screens included kanadaptin, proposed to recognize selectively kAE1 but not eAE1,[134] and the PDZ domain proteins Pick-1 and syntenin, proposed to bind the putative C-terminal cytoplasmic tail type II PDZ recognition motif.[135]

However, subsequent conflicting data[136,137] have not supported these initial proposals, leading to a renewed search for interacting proteins that might control basolateral targeting.

An important proviso in interpretation of kAE1 expression studies in MDCK cells is the toxicity of kAE1 to host cells in which it is not normally expressed. Stable expression of wild-type kAE1 has not generally been possible to maintain for more than several months. In addition, stable overexpression was noted to increase paracellular permeability and to decrease transepithelial electrical resistance of MDCK monolayers.[127] MDCK cells are not type A intercalated cells. Achievement of a cell culture model of type A intercalated cells would greatly further progress in understanding the pathogenesis of RTA.

AE1 Mutations in Recessive dRTA

Five SLC4A1/AE1 mutations have been associated with recessive dRTA (see Tables 17-2 and 17-3). Four of these are unassociated with anemia, although all four can be found as compound heterozygotes with other dRTA mutations or with the SAO mutation.

Recessive dRTA associated with AE1 mutations has been found in Thailand (predominantly in the northeast), Malaysia, and Papua New Guinea.[138–143] The first described was AE1 G701D.[138] The patient had normal eAE1 abundance in red cells and normal red cell anion transport activity. However, expression of either eAE1 G701D or kAE1 G701D in Xenopus oocytes demonstrated loss of function secondary to failure of surface expression. An important difference between erythrocytes and type A intercalated cells is the erythroid-specific expression of the AE1-binding protein, glycophorin A. Glycophorin A–null erythrocytes have reduced AE1 activity,[144] and Ae1-null mouse erythrocytes lack glycophorin A.[145] Co-expression of glycophorin A with eAE1 in Xenopus oocytes can potentiate functional surface expression of AE1,[146] but glycophorin A is not expressed in the kidney. When glycophorin A was co-expressed with the recessive dRTA mutant kAE1 G701D in Xenopus oocytes, surface expression of polypeptide and anion transport were rescued to wild-type levels.[138]

Expression of kAE1 G701D in polarized MDCK cells similarly leads to its intracellular retention in the Golgi compartment,[129] and it can be rescued to the basolateral membrane surface by co-expression of glycophorin A (C. Shayakul and S.L. Alper, personal communication). Interestingly, the recessive mutant polypeptide kAE1 G701D can be partially rescued to the basolateral surface of MDCK cells by co-expressed wild-type kAE1, probably secondary to hetero-oligomer formation, and without decreasing surface expression of wild-type polypeptide.[129] Thus, the recessive dRTA-associated AE1 mutation G701D represents a conditional trafficking phenotype. The mutant traffics normally in the erythrocyte in the presence of its erythroid-specific subunit, glycophorin A, but is presumed to be retained intracellularly in the intercalated cell, which lacks glycophorin A. AE1 G701D heterozygotes are normal, probably because of normal traffic and function of the wild-type/G701D hetero-oligomer in type A intercalated cells, as in the laboratory models of Xenopus oocytes and MDCK cells.

Several additional recessive dRTA mutants of AE1 have since been described (see Table 17-3). In Xenopus oocytes, the loss-of-function recessive mutant ΔV850 and the less severe loss-of-function dominant mutant A858D are also potentiated in their anion transport activity by co-expressed glycophorin A, if to slightly lesser degrees than for G701D.[141] Thus, the glycophorin A–dependent conditional trafficking phenotype may be a general property of recessive dRTA-associated AE1 mutant polypeptides. However, glycophorin A rescue of the dominant AE1 mutant A858D in Xenopus oocytes was blocked by co-expression of AE1 SAO, mirroring the very low anion transport activity of red cells from the A858D/SAO compound heterozygote despite approximately half-normal red cell AE1 polypeptide content.[141]

Xenopus oocyte assays for glycophorin A–rescued transport activity of recessive dRTA-associated AE1 mutants R602H, Q759H, and S773P have not been reported. However, kAE1 S773P is nonfunctional in HEK 293 cells as a result of endoplasmic reticulum retention with reduced expression level and accelerated proteosomal degradation.[142] Interestingly, kAE1 S773P was targeted at only slightly reduced levels to the basolateral membrane of polarized MDCK cells. However, the patient harboring this mutation was a compound heterozygote with AE1 G701D. Co-expression in polarized MDCK monolayers of kAE1 mutants S773P and G701D impaired S773P expression at the basolateral membrane.[129] This observation, together with the abnormal biosynthetic folding of AE1 S773P,[142] probably explains recessive dRTA in this compound heterozygote.

dRTA with Complete Absence of AE1

AE1 mutations associated with isolated dominant dRTA have not been detected in the homozygous state. Similarly, the AE1 mutations encoding dominant spherocytic anemia and SSAO mutations[21] have not been detected in the homozygous state. Thus, the homozygous state for these loss-of-function mutations is probably embryonic lethal. Ribeiro et al[147] reported a newborn of two parents with mild hereditary spherocytosis due to AE1 heterozygous V488M. The homozygous infant was born with hydrops fetalis and severe hemolytic anemia with poikilocytosis. The erythrocytes were devoid of AE1 in the membrane. RTA was diagnosed at age 3 months, and nephrocalcinosis was detected soon afterwards. The patient survived early childhood with frequent blood transfusion and HCO_3^- supplementation.

The phenotype of hydrops fetalis with RTA is reproduced in spontaneous and engineered AE1-knockout models. The $Ae1^{-/-}$ mouse shows retarded growth, severe hemolytic anemia with spherocytosis and poikilocytosis, and most homozygous mice die before weaning.[148,149] Surviving homozygous $Ae1^{-/-}$ mice exhibit spontaneous metabolic acidosis exacerbated by an acid load that is tolerated by wild-type and heterozygous mice. The acidosis is not accompanied by proportionate acidification of the urine, but the pH difference between wild-type and knockout mouse urine increases after acid loading. Cl^-/HCO_3^- exchange in the $AE1^{-/-}$ outer medullary collecting duct is reduced. Intercalated cells remain present, though with reduced immunostaining for vH^+-ATPase and for pendrin. The dRTA is accompanied by a urinary concentrating defect associated with and possibly contributed to by nephrocalcinosis.[150]

Inaba et al[151] reported a bovine cohort with runted animals heterozygous for the nonsense mutation corresponding to human AE1 646X. Affected calves showed failure to thrive, with shortness of breath and hemolytic spherocytic anemia less severe than in $Ae1^{-/-}$ mice or in the hydropic patient homozygous for AE1 V488M, despite the surprising total absence of eAE1 red cells. Metabolic acidosis was notably unaccompanied by compensatory respiratory alkalosis. Three alleles of AE1 deficiency have been described in zebrafish with hematopoietic defects.[152] However, the zebrafish pronephric duct lacks the equivalent of the mammalian collecting duct, and zebrafish AE1 is not detectably expressed in pronephric duct epithelial cells.

Autosomal Recessive dRTA with Sensorineural Deafness

Genes encoding the subunits of vH+-ATPase have long been suspected to cause familial dRTA. However, the ubiquitous expression of vH+-ATPase activity initially decreased enthusiasm for searching for these mutations, because defects in so widely expressed a protein either would not be likely to give rise to isolated dRTA or might be incompatible with survival. The first clue that this need not be the case was the discovery of two B-subunit gene products of the V_1 domain expressed with distinct expression patterns. In contrast to the wide distribution of the B2 isoform, the B1 isoform was found mainly in kidney, and particularly in intercalated cells.[153–155] The lack of immunohistochemical staining for apical vH+-ATPase in intercalated cells of kidney biopsy samples from individuals with Sjögren's syndrome and acquired primary dRTA implicated diminished intercalated-cell expression of vH+-ATPase.[156–158]

Karet et al[159] followed a global genetic mapping strategy to identify a locus on chromosome 2p13 to which could be mapped the recessive dRTA phentoype in a subset of collected family cohorts. Using a candidate gene approach, they discovered 15 mutations within the ATP6V1B1 gene on chromosome 2p13 encoding the B1 subunit of vH+-ATPase (Table 17-4) in 31 kindreds with recessive dRTA, accompanied in many cases by hearing loss.[160] Additional mutations linked with recessive dRTA were reported by these and other authors. Although the cell biologic properties of the mutant B1 polypeptides have been little studied, in addition to the certainly inactive termination, frameshift, and splice site mutations, the missense mutations found are in evolutionarily conserved residues believed likely to interfere with B1 structure or assembly of the complex hetero-oligomeric vH+-ATPase.[159,161–164] Overexpression in rat inner medullary collecting duct (IMCD) cells of several GFP-fusion proteins of ATP6V1B1 containing dRTA-associated missense mutations showed that mutants failed to be incorporated into enzymatically active partial vH+-ATPase complexes, yet trafficked to the apical membrane in response to cellular acidification and inhibited microsomal proton pumping activity.[165] However, the relationship of this dominant-negative phenotype in cultured cells to the recessive disease phenotype in humans remains unclear.

dRTA in patients with mutations in the ATP6V1B1 gene can be successfully treated with dietary HCO_3^- supplementation. However, the accompanying progressive bilateral sensorineural hearing loss is not prevented by standard alkali replacement therapy. The inner ear is a unique site for pH homeostasis, and vH+-ATPase B1 subunit is expressed in cochlea and endolymphatic sac.[160] Cochlear endolymph, with its elevated K+ and low Na+, is highly electropositive such that equilibrium pH for endolymph is alkaline. However, active H+ secretion by the vH+-ATPase leads to physiologic pH values near 7.4 in cochlear endolymph and 6.6 in the endolymphatic sac.[166]

Inactivating mutations in the ATP6V1B1 gene are believed to irreversibly damage cochlear hair cells as a result of chronic stress associated with altered endolymph pH and ion gradients. In contrast to the progressive deafness in humans with dRTA secondary to ATP6V1B1 mutations, the $Atp6b1^{-/-}$ mouse is grossly normal, with normal inner ear development and normal hearing.[167] Normal hearing in $Atp6b1^{-/-}$ mice might be attributable to expression of the b2 subunit in the inner ear.

$Atp6b1^{-/-}$ mice, though not spontaneously acidotic, produce a significantly more alkaline urine as compared with their wild-type littermates. Upon oral challenge with an acid load, however, $Atp6b1^{-/-}$ mice exhibit metabolic acidosis. These mice thus present a model of incomplete dRTA without deafness.[168] Paunescu et al[169] have demonstrated that vH+-ATPase b2 subunit is coexpressed at low level with the b1 subunit in mouse and rat kidney collecting duct intercalated cells. Acetazolamide treatment increased apical localization of the b2 subunit in type A intercalated cells. b2-subunit expression was also increased in intercalated cells of the inner medullary collecting duct in $Atp6b1^{-/-}$ mice.[168] Thus, b2 expression probably compensates for the absence of b1 subunit in intercalated cells and may explain the incomplete dRTA of the mouse model in contrast to the severe complete dRTA of the corresponding genetic deficiency in the human.

Autosomal Recessive dRTA with Normal Hearing or Late-Onset Hearing Loss

Whole-genome genetic linkage and physical mapping analysis of 13 kindreds with recessive dRTA and normal hearing led to discovery of a novel dRTA gene, ATP6V0A4 (previously called ATP6N1B) on chromosome 7q33–34 (see Table 17-2). The gene comprises 23 exons and encodes an 840-aa, kidney-specific a4 isoform of the V_0 membrane-spanning sector of vH+-ATPase, with 61% identity to ATP6N1A-encoded a1 subunit.[159,170] Mutational analysis of the single a-subunit gene in yeast has shown important roles in proton translocation, targeting, dissociation and coupling of proton transport, and ATP hydrolysis.[171,172] The vH+-ATPase a4 subunit is expressed in the proximal tubule, loop of Henle, and distal tubule, as well as in collecting duct intercalated cells.[173] Dietary acid-base loading or K+ depletion in the mouse regulates a4 trafficking in intercalated cells without changing renal a4-subunit content.[173] dRTA-associated mutations in the ATP6V0A4 gene are listed in Table 17-5.

Although patients with recessive ATP6V0A4 mutations exhibited normal hearing when initially examined, long-term follow-up into young adulthood revealed mild, delayed-onset hearing impairment in some of the patients studied.[2,10,161] ATP6V0A4 is correspondingly expressed in both cochlea and vestibular epithelium of the human.[161]

Of the 13 kindreds examined by Smith et al,[170] 4 exhibited ATP6V1B1 or ATP6V0A4, indicating the presence of additional genes that cause recessive dRTA.[161] Genes encoding three additional vH+-ATPase subunits expressed mainly in the kidney (ATP6V1C2, ATP6V1G3, and ATP6V0D2) proved not to be disease-associated genes in eight otherwise unlinked kindreds studied.[174] The SLC4A2/AE2 Cl-/HCO_3^- exchanger of the inner ear was also excluded.[160]

It has been speculated that hypokalemic dRTA in a subset of patients in northeastern Thailand might be secondary to vanadium toxicity and subsequent inhibition of H+/K+-

Table 17-4 ATP6V1B1 Mutations Associated with Recessive Distal Renal Tubular Acidosis with Deafness (MIM No. 192132, 267300)

Mutation	Zygosity	Inheritance	References
R31X	Homozygous	Recessive	Karet et al[160]
(R74S)*	Cmpd het	Recessive	Hahn et al[164]
G78R†	Homozygous	Recessive	Borthwick et al[163]
L81P (L79)*	Homozygous, Cmpd het	Recessive	Karet et al[160] Ruf et al[162]
G123V (G121V)*	Homozygous Cmpd het	Recessive	Stover et al[161] Hahn et al[164]
R124W	Homozygous	Recessive	Karet et al[160]
R157C	Homozygous, Cmpd het	Recessive Recessive	Stover et al[161] Feldman et al[240]
T166fs (fsX174)	Homozygous Homozygous	Recessive Recessive	Karet et al[160] Ruf et al[162]
M174R	Homozygous	Recessive	Karet et al[160]
T275P	Homozygous	Recessive	Karet et al[160]
G316F	Cmpd het	Recessive	Karet et al[160]
P346R (P344R)	Homozygous, Cmpd het*	Recessive	Karet et al[160] Ruf et al[162]
G364S	Homozygous	Recessive	Karet et al[160]
P385fs	Homozygous	Recessive	Karet et al[160]
(R463H)*	Cmpd het	Recessive	Ruf et al[162]
and splice site mutations in introns 6,7,8,9.			

Cmpd het, compound heterozygous; MIM, Mendelian Inheritance in Man.
*Amino acid numbering in parentheses is that of Ruf et al[162] and Hahn et al[164] and is based on Genbank AAA36496. Amino acid numbering used by Karet et al,[160] Stover et al,[161] and Borthwick et al[163] is based on Genbank NP_001683, which is longer by two N-terminal residues. The two predicted polypeptides are encoded by two common polymorphic variants (Hahn et al[164] and HI Cheong, personal communication).
†In association with a second recessive mutation in TCIRG1/ATP6V0A3 causing osteopetrosis.

ATPase.[175] Thus far, however, evidence to support this proposal remains lacking. In addition, a report of a 21-month-old infant with failure to thrive, hypokalemia, and metabolic acidosis unaltered by alkali therapy led to the proposal of colonic H^+/K^+-ATPase deficiency,[176] but no data on H^+/K^+-ATPase regulation or expression was provided.

Mutations in a distinct tissue-specific isoform of the vH^+-ATPase is associated with an extrarenal disease. Recessive infantile osteopetrosis is associated with mutations in the osteoclast-specific a3 subunit of the V_0 sector of the vH^+-ATPase.[163] The disease is modeled by the *oc* osteosclerotic mouse, a spontaneous mutant that has a homozygous deletion spanning the translational initiation site of the a3 gene (see review[9]).

dRTA Due to Failure of Intercalated Cell Differentiation

The collecting duct arises from the ureteral bud, upon interaction with factors from the metanephric blastema. Intercalated cells expressing vH^+-ATPase and CA II are detectable in the E18 rat kidney, but AE1 expression lags.[177] However, the cellular and molecular origins of the three major cell types of the cortical collecting duct, and the identity of a possible precursor cell type, have remained controversial.[178] A new opportunity for understanding has arisen through study of dRTA in a mouse strain engineered for congenital systemic absence of the forkhead transcription factor Foxi1.[179] Foxi1 plays an important role during embryogenesis and is expressed in intercalated cells and in the inner ear. $Foxi1^{-/-}$ mice are deaf, with lack of pendrin expression and Cl^- absorption in the epithelium of the endolymphatic compartment. The gross development of the kidney proceeds normally in the $Foxi1^{-/-}$ mouse. However, the normal mosaic epithelium of the collecting duct is replaced by equal numbers of a uniform cell type exhibiting mixed characteristics of principal and intercalated cells, expressing both aquaporin 2 (AQP2) and CA II. This unusual cell type expresses no detectable AE1, vH^+-ATPase B1 subunit (ATPV1B1), AE4, or pendrin, whereas renal KCC4 K^+/Cl^- cotransporter mRNA expression is undiminished. $Foxi1^{-/-}$ mouse urine is alkaline on an acidic chow diet. The knockout mice are spontaneously hypokalemic and exhibit incomplete

organismic levels, but data at each level will contribute to our evolving understanding of acid-base disorders.

Not all identified families with heritable RTA have yet received molecular diagnoses. Among the candidate genes to explain RTA in these families are the K^+/Cl^- cotransporter KCC4 and the transcription factor Foxi1 whose congenital absences cause dRTA in the mouse. Additional candidate genes for which even mouse genetic evidence remains lacking are the proposed Cl^-/HCO_3^- exchanger SLC26A7, the carbonic anhydrases CA IV, CA XII, and CA XIV, the H^+, K^+-ATPases, and additional subunits of vH$^+$-ATPase with expression restricted largely to the kidney. Among the Rh class of NH_3/NH_4^+ channels, the basolateral RhBG protein of intercalated cells is dispensable for upregulation of urinary NH_4^+ excretion during metabolic acidosis in the mouse,[233] whereas the apical RhCG protein of intercalated cells (but not RhBG) is upregulated by metabolic acidosis in the rat.[234] Yet additional candidate genes include the putative Cl^-/HCO_3^- exchanger SLC26A11 and the unusual H^+-activated aquaporin Cl^- channel, AQP6, localized in intracellular vH$^+$-ATPase-containing vesicles of the type A intercalated cell.[235] Finally, still in its early stages is the study of regulators of acid-base and CO_2 sensing and the regulatory signals that coordinate transport at apical and basolateral membranes of epithelial cells, including general and specific trafficking and docking proteins. Molecular identification of these components may reveal additional RTA-associated genes but will certainly reveal important modifier genes for RTA that might explain the paucity of simple genotype-phenotype correlations among families with different mutations in the same RTA-associated gene. In addition, modifier genes should increase our understanding of clinical variability among family members with the same mutations.

Further progress in understanding dRTA will come with development of the long-elusive stable cell culture model of the type A intercalated cell. Achievement of that goal will be aided by progress in establishing in vivo markers of intercalated cell differentiation and development, and in greater understanding of the intercalated cell's requirements for specialized matrix components, growth factors presented within that matrix, and development of a molecular substitute for the apparently crucial influence of contact with neighboring principal cells in the unique mosaic epithelium of the collecting duct.

References

1. Rodriguez-Soriano J: New insights into the pathogenesis of renal tubular acidosis-from functional to molecular studies. Pediatr Nephrol 14:1121–1136, 2000.
2. Rodriguez-Soriano J: Renal tubular acidosis: The clinical entity. J Am Soc Nephrol 13:2160–2170, 2002.
3. Igarashi T, Sekine T, Inatomi J, Seki G: Unraveling the molecular pathogenesis of isolated proximal renal tubular acidosis. J Am Soc Nephrol 13:2171–2177, 2002.
4. Quigley R: Proximal renal tubular acidosis. J Nephrol 19(Suppl 9): S41–S45, 2006.
5. Toye AM: Defective kidney anion-exchanger 1 (AE1, Band 3) trafficking in dominant distal renal tubular acidosis (dRTA). Biochem Soc Symp X:47–63, 2005.
6. Shayakul C, Alper SL: Defects in processing and trafficking of the AE1 Cl^-/HCO_3^- exchanger associated with inherited distal renal tubular acidosis. Clin Exp Nephrol 8:1–11, 2004.
7. Nicoletta JA, Schwartz GJ: Distal renal tubular acidosis. Curr Opin Pediatr 16:194–198, 2004.
8. Wrong O, Bruce LJ, Unwin RJ, et al: Band 3 mutations, distal renal tubular acidosis, and Southeast Asian ovalocytosis. Kidney Int 62:10–19, 2002.
9. Alper SL: Genetic diseases of acid-base transporters. Annu Rev Physiol 64:899–923, 2002.
10. Karet FE: Inherited distal renal tubular acidosis. J Am Soc Nephrol 13:2178–2184, 2002.
11. Laing CM, Unwin RJ: Renal tubular acidosis. J Nephrol 19(Suppl 9):S46–S52, 2006.
12. Aalkjaer C, Frische S, Leipziger J, et al: Sodium coupled bicarbonate transporters in the kidney, an update. Acta Physiol Scand 181:505–512, 2004.
13. Forgac M: Structure, mechanism and regulation of the clathrin-coated vesicle and yeast vacuolar (H^+-ATPases). J Exp Biol 203:71–80, 2000.
14. Wagner CA, Finberg KE, Breton S, et al: Renal vacuolar H^+-ATPase. Physiol Rev 84:1263–1314, 2004.
15. Beyenbach KW, Wieczorek H: The V-type H^+ ATPase: Molecular structure and function, physiological roles and regulation. J Exp Biol 209:577–589, 2006.
16. Alper SL: Molecular physiology of SLC4 anion exchangers. Exp Physiol 91:153–161, 2006.
17. Pushkin A, Kurtz I: SLC4 base (HCO_3^-, CO_3^{2-}) transporters: Classification, function, structure, genetic diseases, and knockout models. Am J Physiol Renal Physiol 290:F580–F599, 2006.
18. Romero MF: Molecular pathophysiology of SLC4 bicarbonate transporters. Curr Opin Nephrol Hypertens 14:495–501, 2005.
19. Mount DB, Romero MF: The *SLC26* gene family of multifunctional anion exchangers. Pflugers Arch 447:710–721, 2004.
20. Romero MF, Fulton CM, Boron WF: The SLC4 family of HCO_3^- transporters. Pflugers Arch 447:495–509, 2004.
21. Alper SL: Diseases of mutations in the *SLC4A1/AE1* (band 3) Cl^-/HCO_3^- exchanger. In Broer S, Wagner CA (eds): Membrane Transporter Diseases. New York, Kluwer/Plenum, 2003, pp 39–63.
22. Alper SL, Darman RB, Chernova MN, Dahl NK: The *AE* gene family of Cl^-/HCO_3^- exchangers. J Nephrol 15(Suppl 5):S41–S53, 2002.
23. Schwartz GJ: Physiology and molecular biology of renal carbonic anhydrase. J Nephrol 15(Suppl 5):S61–S74, 2002.
24. Tsuruoka S, Kittelberger AM, Schwartz GJ: Carbonic anhydrase II and IV mRNA in rabbit nephron segments: Stimulation during metabolic acidosis. Am J Physiol 274:F259–F267, 1998.
25. Zhou Y, Bouyer P, Boron WF: Role of a tyrosine kinase in the CO_2-induced stimulation of HCO_3^- reabsorption by rabbit S2 proximal tubules. Am J Physiol Renal Physiol 291:F358–F367, 2006.
26. Karim Z, Szutkowska M, Vernimmen C, Bichara M: Renal handling of NH_3/NH_4^+: Recent concepts. Nephron Physiol 101:77–81, 2005.
27. Schroeder JM, Ibrahim H, Taylor L, Curthoys NP: Role of deadenylation and AUF1 binding in the pH-responsive stabilization of glutaminase mRNA. Am J Physiol Renal Physiol 290:F733–F740, 2006.
28. de Silva MG, Elliott K, Dahl HH, et al: Disruption of a novel member of a sodium/hydrogen exchanger family and DOCK3 is associated with an attention deficit hyperactivity disorder–like phenotype. J Med Genet 40:733–740, 2003.
29. Orlowski J, Grinstein S: Diversity of the mammalian sodium/proton exchanger *SLC9* gene family. Pflugers Arch 447:549–565, 2004.
30. Romero MF, Boron WF: Electrogenic Na^+/HCO_3^- cotransporters: Cloning and physiology. Annu Rev Physiol 61:699–723, 1999.
31. Boron WF, Boulpaep EL: Intracellular pH regulation in the renal proximal tubule of the salamander. Na-H exchange. J Gen Physiol 81:29–52, 1983.

32. Romero MF, Hediger MA, Boulpaep EL, Boron WF: Expression cloning and characterization of a renal electrogenic Na$^+$/HCO$_3^-$ cotransporter. Nature 387:409–413, 1997.

33. McAlear SD, Liu X, Williams JB, et al: Electrogenic Na$^+$/HCO$_3^-$ cotransporter (NBCe1) variants expressed in *Xenopus* oocytes: Functional comparison and roles of the amino and carboxy termini. J Gen Physiol 127:639–658, 2006.

34. Sciortino CM, Romero MF: Cation and voltage dependence of rat kidney electrogenic (Na$^+$HCO$_3^-$) cotransporter, rkNBC, expressed in oocytes. Am J Physiol 277:F611–F623, 1999.

35. Muller-Berger S, Ducoudret O, Diakov A, Fromter E: The renal Na$^+$/HCO$_3^-$ cotransporter expressed in *Xenopus laevis* oocytes: Change in stoichiometry in response to elevation of cytosolic Ca^{2+} concentration. Pflugers Arch 442:718–728, 2001.

36. Gross E, Hawkins K, Abuladze N, et al: The stoichiometry of the electrogenic sodium bicarbonate cotransporter NBC1 is cell-type dependent. J Physiol 531:597–603, 2001.

37. Gross E, Kurtz I: Structural determinants and significance of regulation of electrogenic (Na$^+$HCO$_3^-$) cotransporter stoichiometry. Am J Physiol Renal Physiol 283:F876–F887, 2002.

38. Pushkin A, Abuladze N, Gross E, et al: Molecular mechanism of kNBC1–carbonic anhydrase II interaction in proximal tubule cells. J Physiol 559:55–65, 2004.

39. Loiselle FB, Morgan PE, Alvarez BV, Casey JR: Regulation of the human NBC3 Na$^+$/HCO$_3^-$ cotransporter by carbonic anhydrase II and PKA. Am J Physiol Cell Physiol 286:C1423–C1433, 2004.

40. Lu J, Daly CM, Parker MD, et al: Effect of human carbonic anhydrase II on the activity of the human electrogenic Na$^+$/HCO$_3^-$ cotransporter NBCe1-A in *Xenopus* oocytes. J Biol Chem 281:19241–19250, 2006.

41. Kwon TH, Fulton C, Wang W, et al: Chronic metabolic acidosis upregulates rat kidney Na$^+$-HCO$_3^-$ cotransporters NBCn1 and NBC3 but not NBC1. Am J Physiol Renal Physiol 282:F341–F351, 2002.

42. Amlal H, Chen Q, Greeley T, et al: Coordinated down-regulation of NBC-1 and NHE-3 in sodium and bicarbonate loading. Kidney Int 60:1824–1836, 2001.

43. Watts BA, 3rd, Good DW: An apical (K$^+$-dependent) HCO$_3^-$ transport pathway opposes transepithelial HCO$_3^-$ absorption in rat medullary thick ascending limb. Am J Physiol Renal Physiol 287:F57–F63, 2004.

44. Quentin F, Eladari D, Frische S, et al: Regulation of the Cl$^-$/HCO$_3^-$ exchanger AE2 in rat thick ascending limb of Henle's loop in response to changes in acid-base and sodium balance. J Am Soc Nephrol 15:2988–2997, 2004.

45. Herrera M, Ortiz PA, Garvin JL: Regulation of thick ascending limb transport: Role of nitric oxide. Am J Physiol Renal Physiol 290:F1279–F1284, 2006.

46. Watts BA, 3rd, George T, Good DW: The basolateral NHE1 Na$^+$/H$^+$ exchanger regulates transepithelial HCO$_3^-$ absorption through actin cytoskeleton remodeling in renal thick ascending limb. J Biol Chem 280:11439–11447, 2005.

47. Burckhardt G, Di Sole F, Helmle-Kolb C: The Na$^+$/H$^+$ exchanger gene family. J Nephrol 15 (Suppl 5):S3–S21, 2002.

48. Batlle D, Ghanekar H, Jain S, Mitra A: Hereditary distal renal tubular acidosis: new understandings. Annu Rev Med 52:471–484, 2001.

49. Wagner CA, Geibel JP: Acid-base transport in the collecting duct. J Nephrol 15(Suppl 5):S112–S127, 2002.

50. Wall SM: Recent advances in our understanding of intercalated cells. Curr Opin Nephrol Hypertens 14:480–484, 2005.

51. Schwaderer AL, Vijayakumar S, Al-Awqati Q, Schwartz GJ: Galectin-3 expression is induced in renal β-intercalated cells during metabolic acidosis. Am J Physiol Renal Physiol 290:F148–F158, 2006.

52. Schwartz GJ, Tsuruoka S, Vijayakumar S, et al: Acid incubation reverses the polarity of intercalated cell transporters, an effect mediated by hensin. J Clin Invest 109:89–99, 2002.

53. Schwartz GJ, Barasch J, Al-Awqati Q: Plasticity of functional epithelial polarity. Nature 318:368–371, 1985.

54. Hurtado-Lorenzo A, Skinner M, El Annan J, et al: V-ATPase interacts with ARNO and Arf6 in early endosomes and regulates the protein degradative pathway. Nat Cell Biol 8:124–136, 2006.

55. Sautin YY, Lu M, Gaugler A, et al: Phosphatidylinositol 3-kinase-mediated effects of glucose on vacuolar H$^+$-ATPase assembly, translocation, and acidification of intracellular compartments in renal epithelial cells. Mol Cell Biol 25:575–589, 2005.

56. Lu M, Sautin YY, Holliday LS, Gluck SL: The glycolytic enzyme aldolase mediates assembly, expression, and activity of vacuolar H$^+$-ATPase. J Biol Chem 279:8732–8739, 2004.

57. Kraut JA, Helander KG, Helander HF, et al: Detection and localization of H$^+$-K$^+$-ATPase isoforms in human kidney. Am J Physiol Renal Physiol 281:F763–F768, 2001.

58. Nakamura S, Amlal H, Galla JH, Soleimani M: NH$_4^+$ secretion in inner medullary collecting duct in potassium deprivation: Role of colonic H$^+$-K$^+$-ATPase. Kidney Int 56:2160–2167, 1999.

59. Dherbecourt O, Cheval L, Bloch-Faure M, et al: Molecular identification of Sch28080-sensitive K$^+$-ATPase activities in the mouse kidney. Pflugers Arch 451:769–775, 2006.

60. Vince JW, Reithmeier RA: Carbonic anhydrase II binds to the carboxyl terminus of human band 3, the erythrocyte Cl$^-$/HCO$_3^-$ exchanger. J Biol Chem 273:28430–28437, 1998.

61. Sterling D, Reithmeier RA, Casey JR: A transport metabolon. Functional interaction of carbonic anhydrase II and chloride/bicarbonate exchangers. J Biol Chem 276:47886–47894, 2001.

62. Sabolic I, Brown D, Gluck SL, Alper SL: Regulation of AE1 anion exchanger and (H$^+$-ATPases) in rat cortex by acute metabolic acidosis and alkalosis. Kidney Int 51:125–137, 1997.

63. Huber S, Asan E, Jons T, et al: Expression of rat kidney anion exchanger 1 in type A intercalated cells in metabolic acidosis and alkalosis. Am J Physiol 277:F841–F849, 1999.

64. Lohi H, Kujala M, Makela S, et al: Functional characterization of three novel tissue-specific anion exchangers SLC26A7, -A8, and -A9. J Biol Chem 277:14246–14254, 2002.

65. Petrovic S, Barone S, Xu J, et al: SLC26A7: A basolateral Cl$^-$/HCO$_3^-$ exchanger specific to intercalated cells of the outer medullary collecting duct. Am J Physiol Renal Physiol 286:F161–F169, 2004.

66. Xu J, Worrell RT, Li HC, et al: Chloride/bicarbonate exchanger SLC26A7 is localized in endosomes in medullary collecting duct cells and is targeted to the basolateral membrane in hypertonicity and potassium depletion. J Am Soc Nephrol 17:956–967, 2006.

67. Barone S, Amlal H, Xu J, et al: Differential regulation of basolateral Cl$^-$/HCO$_3^-$ exchangers SLC26A7 and AE1 in kidney outer medullary collecting duct. J Am Soc Nephrol 15:2002–2011, 2004.

68. Petrovic S, Amlal H, Sun X, et al: Vasopressin induces expression of the Cl$^-$/HCO$_3^-$ exchanger SLC26A7 in kidney medullary collecting ducts of Brattleboro rats. Am J Physiol Renal Physiol 290:F1194–F1201, 2006.

69. Kim KH, Shcheynikov N, Wang Y, Muallem S: SLC26A7 is a Cl$^-$ channel regulated by intracellular pH. J Biol Chem 280:6463–6470, 2005.

70. Dudas PL, Mentone S, Greineder CF, et al: Immunolocalization of anion transporter Slc26a7 in mouse kidney. Am J Physiol Renal Physiol 290:F937–F945, 2006.

71. Alper SL, Natale J, Gluck S, et al: Subtypes of intercalated cells in rat kidney collecting duct defined by antibodies against erythroid band 3 and renal vacuolar H$^+$-ATPase. Proc Natl Acad Sci U S A 86:5429–5433, 1989.

72. van Adelsberg JS, Edwards JC, al-Awqati Q: The apical Cl$^-$/HCO$_3^-$ exchanger of β-intercalated cells. J Biol Chem 268:11283–11289, 1993.

73. Royaux IE, Wall SM, Karniski LP, et al: Pendrin, encoded by the Pendred syndrome gene, resides in the apical region of renal intercalated cells and mediates bicarbonate secretion. Proc Natl Acad Sci U S A 98:4221–4226, 2001.

74. Kim YH, Kwon TH, Frische S, et al: Immunocytochemical localization of pendrin in intercalated cell subtypes in rat and mouse kidney. Am J Physiol Renal Physiol 283:F744–F754, 2002.

75. Wall SM, Hassell KA, Royaux IE, et al: Localization of pendrin in mouse kidney. Am J Physiol Renal Physiol 284:F229–F241, 2003.

76. Wagner CA, Finberg KE, Stehberger PA, et al: Regulation of the expression of the Cl$^-$/anion exchanger pendrin in mouse kidney by acid-base status. Kidney Int 62:2109–2117, 2002.

77. Petrovic S, Wang Z, Ma L, Soleimani M: Regulation of the apical Cl$^-$/HCO$_3^-$ exchanger pendrin in rat cortical collecting duct in metabolic acidosis. Am J Physiol Renal Physiol 284:F103–F112, 2003.

78. Frische S, Kwon TH, Frokiaer J, et al: Regulated expression of pendrin in rat kidney in response to chronic NH$_4$Cl or NaHCO$_3$ loading. Am J Physiol Renal Physiol 284:F584–F593, 2003.

79. Quentin F, Chambrey R, Trinh-Trang-Tan MM, et al: The Cl$^-$/HCO$_3^-$ exchanger pendrin in the rat kidney is regulated in response to chronic alterations in chloride balance. Am J Physiol Renal Physiol 287:F1179–F1188, 2004.

80. Tsuganezawa H, Kobayashi K, Iyori M, et al: A new member of the HCO$_3^-$ transporter superfamily is an apical anion exchanger of β-intercalated cells in the kidney. J Biol Chem 276:8180–8189, 2001.

81. Ko SB, Luo X, Hager H, et al: AE4 is a DIDS-sensitive (Cl$^-$HCO$_3^-$) exchanger in the basolateral membrane of the renal CCD and the SMG duct. Am J Physiol Cell Physiol 283:C1206–C1218, 2002.

82. Tannen RL, Nissim I, Sahi A: Hormonal mediators of ammoniagenesis: Mechanism of action of PGF2α and the implications for other hormones. Kidney Int 50:15–25, 1996.

83. Lowe M: Structure and function of the Lowe syndrome protein OCRL1. Traffic 6:711–719, 2005.

84. Donckerwolcke RA, van Stekelenburg GJ, Tiddens HA: A case of bicarbonate-losing renal tubular acidosis with defective carboanhydrase activity. Arch Dis Child 45:769–773, 1970.

85. Igarashi T, Ishii T, Watanabe K, et al: Persistent isolated proximal renal tubular acidosis—A systemic disease with a distinct clinical entity. Pediatr Nephrol 8:70–71, 1994.

86. Winsnes A, Monn E, Stokke O, Feyling T: Congenital persistent proximal type renal tubular acidosis in two brothers. Acta Paediatr Scand 68:861–868, 1979.

87. Igarashi T, Inatomi J, Sekine T, et al: Mutations in SLC4A4 cause permanent isolated proximal renal tubular acidosis with ocular abnormalities. Nat Genet 23:264–266, 1999.

88. Satoh H, Moriyama N, Hara C, et al: Localization of Na$^+$-HCO$_3^-$ cotransporter (NBC-1) variants in rat and human pancreas. Am J Physiol Cell Physiol 284:C729–C737, 2003.

89. Horita S, Yamada H, Inatomi J, et al: Functional analysis of NBC1 mutants associated with proximal renal tubular acidosis and ocular abnormalities. J Am Soc Nephrol 16:2270–2278, 2005.

90. Igarashi T, Inatomi J, Sekine T, et al: Novel nonsense mutation in the Na$^+$/HCO$_3^-$ cotransporter gene (SLC4A4) in a patient with permanent isolated proximal renal tubular acidosis and bilateral glaucoma. J Am Soc Nephrol 12:713–718, 2001.

91. Dinour D, Chang MH, Satoh J, et al: A novel missense mutation in the sodium bicarbonate cotransporter (NBCe1/SLC4A4) causes proximal tubular acidosis and glaucoma through ion transport defects. J Biol Chem 279:52238–52246, 2004.

92. Inatomi J, Horita S, Braverman N, et al: Mutational and functional analysis of SLC4A4 in a patient with proximal renal tubular acidosis. Pflugers Arch 448:438–444, 2004.

93. Li HC, Szigligeti P, Worrell RT, et al: Missense mutations in Na$^+$:HCO$_3^-$ cotransporter NBC1 show abnormal trafficking in polarized kidney cells: A basis of proximal renal tubular acidosis. Am J Physiol Renal Physiol 289:F61–F71, 2005.

94. Demirci FY, Chang MH, Mah TS, et al: Proximal renal tubular acidosis and ocular pathology: A novel missense mutation in the gene (SLC4A4) for sodium bicarbonate cotransporter protein (NBCe1). Mol Vis 12:324–330, 2006.

95. Toye AM, Parker MD, Daly CM, et al: The human NBCe1-A mutant R881C, associated with proximal renal tubular acidosis, retains function but is mistargeted in polarized renal epithelia. Am J Physiol Cell Physiol 291:C788–801, 2006.

96. Quilty JA, Reithmeier RA: Trafficking and folding defects in hereditary spherocytosis mutants of the human red cell anion exchanger. Traffic 1:987–998, 2000.

97. Igarashi T, Inatomi J, Sekine T, et al: Mutational and functional analysis of the Na$^+$-HCO$_3^-$ cotransporter gene (SLC4A4) in patients with permanent isolated proximal renal tubular acidosis and ocular abnormalities (Abstract). J Am Soc Nephrol 14:302A, 2003.

98. Li HC, Worrell RT, Matthews JB, et al: Identification of a carboxyl-terminal motif essential for the targeting of Na$^+$-HCO$_3^-$ cotransporter NBC1 to the basolateral membrane. J Biol Chem 279:43190–43197, 2004.

99. Gawenis LR, Shull GE: Intestinal impactions and altered cAMP-stimulated anion secretion across murine proximal colon of NBC1 Na$^+$-HCO$_3^-$ cotransporter knockout mice (Abstract). Gastroenterology 130(S2):A-123, 2006.

100. Usui T, Hara M, Satoh H, et al: Molecular basis of ocular abnormalities associated with proximal renal tubular acidosis. J Clin Invest 108:107–115, 2001.

101. Bok D, Galbraith G, Lopez I, et al: Blindness and auditory impairment caused by loss of the sodium bicarbonate cotransporter NBC3. Nat Genet 34:313–319, 2003.

102. Reiners J, Nagel-Wolfrum K, Jurgens K, et al: Molecular basis of human Usher syndrome: Deciphering the meshes of the Usher protein network provides insights into the pathomechanisms of the Usher disease. Exp Eye Res 83:97–119, 2006.

103. Brenes LG, Brenes JN, Hernandez MM: Familial proximal renal tubular acidosis. A distinct clinical entity. Am J Med 63:244–252, 1977.

104. Lemann J, Jr, Adams ND, Wilz DR, Brenes LG: Acid and mineral balances and bone in familial proximal renal tubular acidosis. Kidney Int 58:1267–1277, 2000.

105. Schultheis PJ, Clarke LL, Meneton P, et al: Renal and intestinal absorptive defects in mice lacking the NHE3 Na$^+$/H$^+$ exchanger. Nat Genet 19:282–285, 1998.

106. Nakamura S, Amlal H, Schultheis PJ, et al: HCO$_3^-$ reabsorption in renal collecting duct of NHE-3-deficient mouse: A compensatory response. Am J Physiol 276:F914–F921, 1999.

107. Wang T, Yang CL, Abbiati T, et al: Mechanism of proximal tubule bicarbonate absorption in NHE3 null mice. Am J Physiol 277:F298–F302, 1999.

108. Lorenz JN, Schultheis PJ, Traynor T, et al: Micropuncture analysis of single-nephron function in NHE3-deficient mice. Am J Physiol 277:F447–F453, 1999.

109. Goyal S, Mentone S, Aronson PS: Immunolocalization of NHE8 in rat kidney. Am J Physiol Renal Physiol 288:F530–F538, 2005.

110. Warth R, Barriere H, Meneton P, et al: Proximal renal tubular acidosis in TASK2 K$^+$ channel-deficient mice reveals a mechanism for stabilizing bicarbonate transport. Proc Natl Acad Sci U S A 101:8215–8220, 2004.

111. Rodriguez-Soriano J, Boichis H, et al: Proximal renal tubular acidosis. A defect in bicarbonate reabsorption with normal urinary acidification. Pediatr Res 1:81–98, 1967.

112. Nash MA, Torrado AD, Greifer I, et al: Renal tubular acidosis in infants and children. Clinical course, response to treatment, and prognosis. J Pediatr 80:738–748, 1972.

113. Bruce LJ, Cope DL, Jones GK, et al: Familial distal renal tubular acidosis is associated with mutations in the red cell anion exchanger (Band 3, *AE1*) gene. J Clin Invest 100:1693–1707, 1997.

114. Jarolim P, Shayakul C, Prabakaran D, et al: Autosomal dominant distal renal tubular acidosis is associated in three families with heterozygosity for the R589H mutation in the AE1 (band 3) Cl^-/HCO_3^- exchanger. J Biol Chem 273:6380–6388, 1998.

115. Karet FE, Gainza FJ, Gyory AZ, et al: Mutations in the chloride-bicarbonate exchanger gene *AE1* cause autosomal dominant but not autosomal recessive distal renal tubular acidosis. Proc Natl Acad Sci U S A 95:6337–6342, 1998.

116. Bruce LJ, Robinson HC, Guizouarn H, et al: Monovalent cation leaks in human red cells caused by single amino-acid substitutions in the transport domain of the band 3 chloride-bicarbonate exchanger, AE1. Nat Genet 37:1258–1263, 2005.

117. Kollert-Jons A, Wagner S, Hubner S, et al: Anion exchanger 1 in human kidney and oncocytoma differs from erythroid AE1 in its NH_2 terminus. Am J Physiol 265:F813–F821, 1993.

118. Jarolim P, Murray JL, Rubin HL, et al: Characterization of 13 novel band 3 gene defects in hereditary spherocytosis with band 3 deficiency. Blood 88:4366–4374, 1996.

119. Baehner RL, Gilchrist GS, Anderson EJ: Hereditary elliptocytosis and primary renal tubular acidosis in a single family. Am J Dis Child 115:414–419, 1968.

120. Kaitwatcharachai C, Vasuvattakul S, Yenchitsomanus P, et al: Distal renal tubular acidosis and high urine carbon dioxide tension in a patient with southeast Asian ovalocytosis. Am J Kidney Dis 33:1147–1152, 1999.

121. Thong MK, Tan AA, Lin HP: Distal renal tubular acidosis and hereditary elliptocytosis in a single family. Singapore Med J 38:388–390, 1997.

122. Rysava R, Tesar V, Jirsa M, Jr, et al: Incomplete distal renal tubular acidosis coinherited with a mutation in the band 3 (*AE1*) gene. Nephrol Dial Transplant 12:1869–1873, 1997.

123. Lima PR, Gontijo JA, Lopes de Faria JB, et al: Band 3 Campinas: A novel splicing mutation in the band 3 gene (*AE1*) associated with hereditary spherocytosis, hyperactivity of Na^+/Li^+ countertransport and an abnormal renal bicarbonate handling. Blood 90:2810–2818, 1997.

124. Shayakul C, Jarolim P, Zachlederova M, et al: Characterization of a highly polymorphic marker adjacent to the *SLC4A1* gene and of kidney immunostaining in a family with distal renal tubular acidosis. Nephrol Dial Transplant 19:371–379, 2004.

125. Li J, Quilty J, Popov M, Reithmeier RA: Processing of N-linked oligosaccharide depends on its location in the anion exchanger, AE1, membrane glycoprotein. Biochem J 349:51–57, 2000.

126. Quilty JA, Cordat E, Reithmeier RA: Impaired trafficking of human kidney anion exchanger (kAE1) caused by hetero-oligomer formation with a truncated mutant associated with distal renal tubular acidosis. Biochem J 368:895–903, 2002.

127. Toye AM, Banting G, Tanner MJ: Regions of human kidney anion exchanger 1 (kAE1) required for basolateral targeting of kAE1 in polarised kidney cells: mis-targeting explains dominant renal tubular acidosis (dRTA). J Cell Sci 117:1399–1410, 2004.

128. Cheung JC, Cordat E, Reithmeier RA: Trafficking defects of the Southeast Asian ovalocytosis deletion mutant of anion exchanger 1 membrane proteins. Biochem J 392:425–434, 2005.

129. Cordat E, Kittanakom S, Yenchitsomanus PT, et al: Dominant and recessive distal renal tubular acidosis mutations of kidney anion exchanger 1 induce distinct trafficking defects in MDCK cells. Traffic 7:117--28, 2006.

130. Toye AM, Bruce LJ, Unwin RJ, et al: Band 3 Walton, a C-terminal deletion associated with distal renal tubular acidosis, is expressed in the red cell membrane but retained internally in kidney cells. Blood 99:342–347, 2002.

131. Quilty JA, Li J, Reithmeier RA: Impaired trafficking of distal renal tubular acidosis mutants of the human kidney anion exchanger kAE1. Am J Physiol Renal Physiol 282:F810–F820, 2002.

132. Devonald MA, Smith AN, Poon JP, et al: Non-polarized targeting of AE1 causes autosomal dominant distal renal tubular acidosis. Nat Genet 33:125–127, 2003.

133. Rungroj N, Devonald MA, Cuthbert AW, et al: A novel missense mutation in AE1 causing autosomal dominant distal renal tubular acidosis retains normal transport function but is mistargeted in polarized epithelial cells. J Biol Chem 279:13833–13838, 2004.

134. Chen J, Vijayakumar S, Li X, Al-Awqati Q: Kanadaptin is a protein that interacts with the kidney but not the erythroid form of band 3. J Biol Chem 273:1038–1043, 1998.

135. Cowan CA, Yokoyama N, Bianchi LM, et al: EphB2 guides axons at the midline and is necessary for normal vestibular function. Neuron 26:417–430, 2000.

136. Hubner S, Bahr C, Gossmann H, et al: Mitochondrial and nuclear localization of kanadaptin. Eur J Cell Biol 82:240–252, 2003.

137. Kittanakom S, Keskanokwong T, Akkarapatumwong V, et al: Human kanadaptin and kidney anion exchanger 1 (kAE1) do not interact in transfected HEK 293 cells. Mol Membr Biol 21:395–402, 2004.

138. Tanphaichitr VS, Sumboonnanonda A, Ideguchi H, et al: Novel *AE1* mutations in recessive distal renal tubular acidosis. Loss-of-function is rescued by glycophorin A. J Clin Invest 102:2173–2179, 1998.

139. Vasuvattakul S, Yenchitsomanus PT, Vachuanichsanong P, et al: Autosomal recessive distal renal tubular acidosis associated with Southeast Asian ovalocytosis. Kidney Int 56:1674–1682, 1999.

140. Sritippayawan S, Sumboonnanonda A, Vasuvattakul S, et al: Novel compound heterozygous *SLC4A1* mutations in Thai patients with autosomal recessive distal renal tubular acidosis. Am J Kidney Dis 44:64–70, 2004.

141. Bruce LJ, Wrong O, Toye AM, et al: Band 3 mutations, renal tubular acidosis and South-East Asian ovalocytosis in Malaysia and Papua New Guinea: Loss of up to 95% band 3 transport in red cells. Biochem J 350(Pt 1):41–51, 2000.

142. Kittanakom S, Cordat E, Akkarapatumwong V, et al: Trafficking defects of a novel autosomal recessive distal renal tubular acidosis mutant (S773P) of the human kidney anion exchanger (kAE1). J Biol Chem 279:40960–40971, 2004.

143. Choo KE, Nicoli TK, Bruce LJ, et al: Recessive distal renal tubular acidosis in Sarawak caused by AE1 mutations. Pediatr Nephrol 21:212–217, 2006.

144. Bruce LJ, Groves JD, Okubo Y, et al: Altered band 3 structure and function in glycophorin A- and B-deficient (MkMk) red blood cells. Blood 84:916–922, 1994.

145. Hassoun H, Hanada T, Lutchman M, et al: Complete deficiency of glycophorin A in red blood cells from mice with targeted inactivation of the band 3 (*AE1*) gene. Blood 91:2146–2151, 1998.

146. Groves JD, Tanner MJ: The effects of glycophorin A on the expression of the human red cell anion transporter (band 3) in *Xenopus* oocytes. J Membr Biol 140:81–88, 1994.

147. Ribeiro ML, Alloisio N, Almeida H, et al: Severe hereditary spherocytosis and distal renal tubular acidosis associated with the total absence of band 3. Blood 96:1602–1604, 2000.

148. Peters LL, Shivdasani RA, Liu SC, et al: Anion exchanger 1 (band 3) is required to prevent erythrocyte membrane surface loss but not to form the membrane skeleton. Cell 86:917–927, 1996.

149. Southgate CD, Chishti AH, Mitchell B, et al: Targeted disruption of the murine erythroid band 3 gene results in spherocytosis and severe haemolytic anaemia despite a normal membrane skeleton. Nat Genet 14:227–230, 1996.

150. Stehberger PA, Stuart-Tilley AK, Shmukler BE, et al: Impaired distal renal acidification in a mouse model for distal renal tubular acidosis lacking the AE1 (band 3) Cl⁻/HCO₃⁻ exchanger (Slc4a1) (Abstract). J Am Soc Nephrol 15:70A, 2004.

151. Inaba M, Yawata A, Koshino I, et al: Defective anion transport and marked spherocytosis with membrane instability caused by hereditary total deficiency of red cell band 3 in cattle due to a nonsense mutation. J Clin Invest 97:1804–1817, 1996.

152. Paw BH, Davidson AJ, Zhou Y, et al: Cell-specific mitotic defect and dyserythropoiesis associated with erythroid band 3 deficiency. Nat Genet 34:59–64, 2003.

153. Nelson RD, Guo XL, Masood K, et al: Selectively amplified expression of an isoform of the vacuolar (H⁺-ATPases) 56-kilodalton subunit in renal intercalated cells. Proc Natl Acad Sci U S A 89:3541–3545, 1992.

154. Puopolo K, Kumamoto C, Adachi I, et al: Differential expression of the "B" subunit of the vacuolar (H⁺-ATPases) in bovine tissues. J Biol Chem 267:3696–3706, 1992.

155. van Hille B, Richener H, Schmid P, et al: Heterogeneity of vacuolar (H⁺-ATPase): Differential expression of two human subunit B isoforms. Biochem J 303(Pt 1):191–198, 1994.

156. Cohen EP, Bastani B, Cohen MR, et al: Absence of (H⁺-ATPase) in cortical collecting tubules of a patient with Sjögren's syndrome and distal renal tubular acidosis. J Am Soc Nephrol 3:264–271, 1992.

157. Bastani B, Haragsim L, Gluck S, Siamopoulos KC: Lack of H⁺-ATPase in distal nephron causing hypokalaemic distal RTA in a patient with Sjögren's syndrome. Nephrol Dial Transplant 10:908–909, 1995.

158. Han JS, Kim GH, Kim J, et al: Secretory-defect distal renal tubular acidosis is associated with transporter defect in (H⁺-ATPase) and anion exchanger-1. J Am Soc Nephrol 13:1425–1432, 2002.

159. Karet FE, Finberg KE, Nayir A, et al: Localization of a gene for autosomal recessive distal renal tubular acidosis with normal hearing (rdRTA2) to 7q33–34. Am J Hum Genet 65:1656–1665, 1999.

160. Karet FE, Finberg KE, Nelson RD, et al: Mutations in the gene encoding B1 subunit of H⁺-ATPase cause renal tubular acidosis with sensorineural deafness. Nat Genet 21:84–90, 1999.

161. Stover EH, Borthwick KJ, Bavalia C, et al: Novel *ATP6V1B1* and *ATP6V0A4* mutations in autosomal recessive distal renal tubular acidosis with new evidence for hearing loss. J Med Genet 39:796–803, 2002.

162. Ruf R, Rensing C, Topaloglu R, et al: Confirmation of the *ATP6B1* gene as responsible for distal renal tubular acidosis. Pediatr Nephrol 18:105–109, 2003.

163. Borthwick KJ, Kandemir N, Topaloglu R, et al: A phenocopy of CAII deficiency: A novel genetic explanation for inherited infantile osteopetrosis with distal renal tubular acidosis. J Med Genet 40:115–121, 2003.

164. Hahn H, Kang HG, Ha IS, et al: *ATP6B1* gene mutations associated with distal renal tubular acidosis and deafness in a child. Am J Kidney Dis 41:238–243, 2003.

165. Yang Q, Li G, Singh SK, et al: Vacuolar H⁺-ATPase B1 subunit mutations that cause inherited distal renal tubular acidosis affect proton pump assembly and trafficking in inner medullary collecting duct cells. J Am Soc Nephrol 17:1858–1866, 2006.

166. Sterkers O, Saumon G, Tran Ba Huy P, et al: Electrochemical heterogeneity of the cochlear endolymph: Effect of acetazolamide. Am J Physiol 246:F47–F53, 1984.

167. Dou H, Finberg K, Cardell EL, et al: Mice lacking the B1 subunit of H⁺-ATPase have normal hearing. Hear Res 180:76–84, 2003.

168. Finberg KE, Wagner CA, Bailey MA, et al: The B1-subunit of the H⁺ATPase is required for maximal urinary acidification. Proc Natl Acad Sci U S A 102:13616–13621, 2005.

169. Paunescu TG, Da Silva N, Marshansky V, et al: Expression of the 56-kDa B2 subunit isoform of the vacuolar (H⁺-ATPase) in proton-secreting cells of the kidney and epididymis. Am J Physiol Cell Physiol 287:C149–C162, 2004.

170. Smith AN, Skaug J, Choate KA, et al: Mutations in *ATP6N1B*, encoding a new kidney vacuolar proton pump 116-kD subunit, cause recessive distal renal tubular acidosis with preserved hearing. Nat Genet 26:71–75, 2000.

171. Kawasaki-Nishi S, Bowers K, Nishi T, et al: The amino-terminal domain of the vacuolar proton-translocating ATPase a subunit controls targeting and in vivo dissociation, and the carboxyl-terminal domain affects coupling of proton transport and ATP hydrolysis. J Biol Chem 276:47411–47420, 2001.

172. Kawasaki-Nishi S, Nishi T, Forgac M: Arg-735 of the 100-kDa subunit a of the yeast V-ATPase is essential for proton translocation. Proc Natl Acad Sci U S A 98:12397–12402, 2001.

173. Stehberger PA, Schulz N, Finberg KE, et al: Localization and regulation of the ATP6V0A4 (a4) vacuolar H⁺-ATPase subunit defective in an inherited form of distal renal tubular acidosis. J Am Soc Nephrol 14:3027–3038, 2003.

174. Smith AN, Borthwick KJ, Karet FE: Molecular cloning and characterization of novel tissue-specific isoforms of the human vacuolar (H⁺-ATPase) C, G and d subunits, and their evaluation in autosomal recessive distal renal tubular acidosis. Gene 297:169–177, 2002.

175. Tosukhowong P, Tungsanga K, Eiam-Ong S, Sitprija V: Environmental distal renal tubular acidosis in Thailand: An enigma. Am J Kidney Dis 33:1180–1186, 1999.

176. Simpson AM, Schwartz GJ: Distal renal tubular acidosis with severe hypokalaemia, probably caused by colonic (H⁺K⁺ATPase) deficiency. Arch Dis Child 84:504–507, 2001.

177. Kim J, Tisher CC, Madsen KM: Differentiation of intercalated cells in developing rat kidney: An immunohistochemical study. Am J Physiol 266:F977–F990, 1994.

178. Fejes-Toth G, Naray-Fejes-Toth A: Differentiation of renal β-intercalated cells to α-intercalated and principal cells in culture. Proc Natl Acad Sci U S A 89:5487–5491, 1992.

179. Blomqvist SR, Vidarsson H, Fitzgerald S, et al: Distal renal tubular acidosis in mice that lack the forkhead transcription factor Foxi1. J Clin Invest 113:1560–1570, 2004.

180. Kurth I, Hentschke M, Hentschke S, et al: The forkhead transcription factor Foxi1 directly activates the AE4 promoter. Biochem J 393:277–283, 2006.

181. Schuster VL: Function and regulation of collecting duct intercalated cells. Annu Rev Physiol 55:267–288, 1993.

182. Boettger T, Hubner CA, Maier H, et al: Deafness and renal tubular acidosis in mice lacking the K-Cl co-transporter Kcc4. Nature 416:874–878, 2002.

183. Everett LA, Glaser B, Beck JC, et al: Pendred syndrome is caused by mutations in a putative sulphate transporter gene (PDS). Nat Genet 17:411–422, 1997.

184. Everett LA, Green ED: A family of mammalian anion transporters and their involvement in human genetic diseases. Hum Mol Genet 8:1883–1891, 1999.

185. Scott DA, Wang R, Kreman TM, et al: The Pendred syndrome gene encodes a chloride-iodide transport protein. Nat Genet 21:440–443, 1999.

186. Scott DA, Karniski LP: Human pendrin expressed in *Xenopus laevis* oocytes mediates chloride/formate exchange. Am J Physiol Cell Physiol 278:C207–C211, 2000.

187. Royaux IE, Suzuki K, Mori A, et al: Pendrin, the protein encoded by the Pendred syndrome gene (PDS), is an apical porter of iodide in the thyroid and is regulated by thyroglobulin in FRTL-5 cells. Endocrinology 141:839–845, 2000.

188. Verlander JW, Hassell KA, Royaux IE, et al: Deoxycorticosterone upregulates PDS (Slc26a4) in mouse

kidney: role of pendrin in mineralocorticoid-induced hypertension. Hypertension 42:356–362, 2003.

189. Sly WS, Whyte MP, Sundaram V, et al: Carbonic anhydrase II deficiency in 12 families with the autosomal recessive syndrome of osteopetrosis with renal tubular acidosis and cerebral calcification. N Engl J Med 313:139–145, 1985.

190. Hu PY, Lim EJ, Ciccolella J, et al: Seven novel mutations in carbonic anhydrase II deficiency syndrome identified by SSCP and direct sequencing analysis. Hum Mutat 9:383–387, 1997.

191. Fathallah DM, Bejaoui M, Lepaslier D, et al: Carbonic anhydrase II (CA II) deficiency in Maghrebian patients: Evidence for founder effect and genomic recombination at the CA II locus. Hum Genet 99:634–637, 1997.

192. Shah GN, Bonapace G, Hu PY, et al: Carbonic anhydrase II deficiency syndrome (osteopetrosis with renal tubular acidosis and brain calcification): Novel mutations in CA2 identified by direct sequencing expand the opportunity for genotype-phenotype correlation. Hum Mutat 24:272, 2004.

193. McMahon C, Will A, Hu P, et al: Bone marrow transplantation corrects osteopetrosis in the carbonic anhydrase II deficiency syndrome. Blood 97:1947–1950, 2001.

194. Sly WS, Hu PY: Human carbonic anhydrases and carbonic anhydrase deficiencies. Annu Rev Biochem 64:375–401, 1995.

195. Lewis SE, Erickson RP, Barnett LB, et al: N-ethyl-N-nitrosourea-induced null mutation at the mouse Car-2 locus: An animal model for human carbonic anhydrase II deficiency syndrome. Proc Natl Acad Sci U S A 85:1962–1966, 1988.

196. Brechue WF, Kinne-Saffran E, Kinne RK, Maren TH: Localization and activity of renal carbonic anhydrase (CA) in CA-II deficient mice. Biochim Biophys Acta 1066:201–207, 1991.

197. Breton S, Alper SL, Gluck SL, et al: Depletion of intercalated cells from collecting ducts of carbonic anhydrase II-deficient (CAR2 null) mice. Am J Physiol 269:F761–F774, 1995.

198. Bagnis C, Marshansky V, Breton S, Brown D: Remodeling the cellular profile of collecting ducts by chronic carbonic anhydrase inhibition. Am J Physiol Renal Physiol 280:F437–F448, 2001.

199. Lien YH, Lai LW: Respiratory acidosis in carbonic anhydrase II-deficient mice. Am J Physiol 274:L301–L304, 1998.

200. Lai LW, Chan DM, Erickson RP, et al: Correction of renal tubular acidosis in carbonic anhydrase II-deficient mice with gene therapy. J Clin Invest 101:1320–1325, 1998.

201. Lloyd SE, Pearce SH, Fisher SE, et al: A common molecular basis for three inherited kidney stone diseases. Nature 379:445–449, 1996.

202. Lloyd SE, Pearce SH, Gunther W, et al: Idiopathic low molecular weight proteinuria associated with hypercalciuric nephrocalcinosis in Japanese children is due to mutations of the renal chloride channel (CLCN5). J Clin Invest 99:967–974, 1997.

203. Lloyd SE, Gunther W, Pearce SH, et al: Characterisation of renal chloride channel, CLCN5, mutations in hypercalciuric nephrolithiasis (kidney stones) disorders. Hum Mol Genet 6:1233–1239, 1997.

204. Scheel O, Zdebik AA, Lourdel S, Jentsch TJ: Voltage-dependent electrogenic chloride/proton exchange by endosomal CLC proteins. Nature 436:424–427, 2005.

205. Devuyst O, Jouret F, Auzanneau C, Courtoy PJ: Chloride channels and endocytosis: New insights from Dent's disease and ClC-5 knockout mice. Nephron Physiol 99:69–73, 2005.

206. Devuyst O, Christie PT, Courtoy PJ, et al: Intra-renal and subcellular distribution of the human chloride channel, ClC-5, reveals a pathophysiological basis for Dent's disease. Hum Mol Genet 8:247–257, 1999.

207. Wrong OM, Norden AG, Feest TG: Dent's disease; a familial proximal renal tubular syndrome with low-molecular-weight proteinuria, hypercalciuria, nephrocalcinosis, metabolic bone

208. Gunther W, Luchow A, Cluzeaud F, et al: ClC-5, the chloride channel mutated in Dent's disease, colocalizes with the proton pump in endocytotically active kidney cells. Proc Natl Acad Sci U S A 95:8075–8080, 1998.

209. Luyckx VA, Goda FO, Mount DB, et al: Intrarenal and subcellular localization of rat CLC5. Am J Physiol 275:F761–F769, 1998.

210. Sakamoto H, Sado Y, Naito I, et al: Cellular and subcellular immunolocalization of ClC-5 channel in mouse kidney: Colocalization with H+-ATPase. Am J Physiol 277:F957–F965, 1999.

211. Moulin P, Igarashi T, Van der Smissen P, et al: Altered polarity and expression of H+-ATPase without ultrastructural changes in kidneys of Dent's disease patients. Kidney Int 63:1285–1295, 2003.

212. Piwon N, Gunther W, Schwake M, et al: ClC-5 Cl−-channel disruption impairs endocytosis in a mouse model for Dent's disease. Nature 408:369–373, 2000.

213. Hoopes RR, Jr, Shrimpton AE, Knohl SJ, et al: Dent disease with mutations in OCRL1. Am J Hum Genet 76:260–267, 2005.

214. DuBose TD, Jr: Hyperkalemic hyperchloremic metabolic acidosis: Pathophysiologic insights. Kidney Int 51:591–602, 1997.

215. Geller DS, Rodriguez-Soriano J, Vallo Boado A, et al: Mutations in the mineralocorticoid receptor gene cause autosomal dominant pseudohypoaldosteronism type I. Nat Genet 19:279–281, 1998.

216. Sartorato P, Lapeyraque AL, Armanini D, et al: Different inactivating mutations of the mineralocorticoid receptor in fourteen families affected by type I pseudohypoaldosteronism. J Clin Endocrinol Metab 88:2508–2517, 2003.

217. Zennaro MC, Lombes M: Mineralocorticoid resistance. Trends Endocrinol Metab 15:264–270, 2004.

218. Zennaro MC: Syndromes of glucocorticoid and mineralocorticoid resistance. Eur J Endocrinol 139:127–138, 1998.

219. Bonny O, Rossier BC: Disturbances of Na/K balance: Pseudohypoaldosteronism revisited. J Am Soc Nephrol 13:2399–2414, 2002.

220. O'Shaughnessy KM, Karet FE: Salt handling and hypertension. J Clin Invest 113:1075–1081, 2004.

221. Kerem E, Bistritzer T, Hanukoglu A, et al: Pulmonary epithelial sodium-channel dysfunction and excess airway liquid in pseudohypoaldosteronism. N Engl J Med 341:156–162, 1999.

222. Hogg RJ, Marks JF, Marver D, Frolich JC: Long-term observations in a patient with pseudohypoaldosteronism. Pediatr Nephrol 5:205–210, 1991.

223. Hanukoglu A, Bistritzer T, Rakover Y, Mandelberg A: Pseudohypoaldosteronism with increased sweat and saliva electrolyte values and frequent lower respiratory tract infections mimicking cystic fibrosis. J Pediatr 125:752–755, 1994.

224. Chang SS, Grunder S, Hanukoglu A, et al: Mutations in subunits of the epithelial sodium channel cause salt wasting with hyperkalaemic acidosis, pseudohypoaldosteronism type 1. Nat Genet 12:248–253, 1996.

225. Saxena A, Hanukoglu I, Saxena D, et al: Novel mutations responsible for autosomal recessive multisystem pseudohypoaldosteronism and sequence variants in epithelial sodium channel α-, β-, and γ-subunit genes. J Clin Endocrinol Metab 87:3344–3350, 2002.

226. Strautnieks SS, Thompson RJ, Gardiner RM, Chung E: A novel splice-site mutation in the γ subunit of the epithelial sodium channel gene in three pseudohypoaldosteronism type 1 families. Nat Genet 13:248–250, 1996.

227. Huey CL, Riepe FG, Sippell WG, Yu AS: Genetic heterogeneity in autosomal dominant pseudohypoaldosteronism type I:

Exclusion of claudin-8 as a candidate gene. Am J Nephrol 24:483–487, 2004.

228. Schambelan M, Sebastian A, Rector FC, Jr: Mineralocorticoid-resistant renal hyperkalemia without salt wasting (type II pseudohypoaldosteronism): Role of increased renal chloride reabsorption. Kidney Int 19:716–727, 1981.

229. Achard JM, Disse-Nicodeme S, Fiquet-Kempf B, Jeunemaitre X: Phenotypic and genetic heterogeneity of familial hyperkalaemic hypertension (Gordon syndrome). Clin Exp Pharmacol Physiol 28:1048–1052, 2001.

230. Gordon RD, Geddes RA, Pawsey CG, O'Halloran MW: Hypertension and severe hyperkalaemia associated with suppression of renin and aldosterone and completely reversed by dietary sodium restriction. Australas Ann Med 19:287–294, 1970.

231. Wilson FH, Disse-Nicodeme S, Choate KA, et al: Human hypertension caused by mutations in WNK kinases. Science 293:1107–1112, 2001.

232. Subramanya AR, Yang CL, McCormick JA, Ellison DH: WNK kinases regulate sodium chloride and potassium transport by the aldosterone-sensitive distal nephron. Kidney Int 70:630–634, 2006.

233. Chambrey R, Goossens D, Bourgeois S, et al: Genetic ablation of Rhbg in the mouse does not impair renal ammonium excretion. Am J Physiol Renal Physiol 289:F1281–F1290, 2005.

234. Seshadri RM, Klein JD, Kozlowski S, et al: Renal expression of the ammonia transporters, Rhbg and Rhcg, in response to chronic metabolic acidosis. Am J Physiol Renal Physiol 290:F397–F408, 2006.

235. Beitz E, Liu K, Ikeda M, et al: Determinants of AQP6 trafficking to intracellular sites versus the plasma membrane in transfected mammalian cells. Biol Cell 98:101–109, 2006.

236. Tatishchev S, Abuladze N, Pushkin A, et al: Identification of membrane topography of the electrogenic sodium bicarbonate cotransporter pNBC1 by in vitro transcription/translation. Biochemistry 42:755–765, 2003.

237. Zhu Q, Lee DW, Casey JR: Novel topology in C-terminal region of the human plasma membrane anion exchanger, AE1. J Biol Chem 278:3112–3120, 2003.

238. Wood PG: The anion exchange proteins: Homology and secondary structure. Prog Cell Res 2:325–352, 1992.

239. Cheidde L, Vieira TC, Lima PR, et al: A novel mutation in the anion exchanger 1 gene is associated with familial distal renal tubular acidosis and nephrocalcinosis. Pediatrics 112:1361–1367, 2003.

240. Feldman M, Prikis M, Athanasion Y, et al: Molecular investigation and long-term clinical progress in Greek Cypriot families with recessive distal renal tubular acidosis and sensorineural deafness due to mutations in the ATP6V1B1 gene. Clin Genet 69:135–144, 2006.

241. Yenchitsomanus PT, Sawasdee N, Paemanee A, et al: Anion exchanger 1 mutations associated with distal renal tubular acidosis in the Thai population. J Hum Genet 48:451–456, 2003.

Chapter 18

Hereditary Causes of Nephrogenic Diabetes Insipidus

Peter M.T. Deen, Joris H. Robben, and Nine V.A.M. Knoers

During the last decade our understanding of the vasopressin-mediated renal concentrating mechanisms has increased enormously through the identification of the molecular defects underlying congenital nephrogenic diabetes insipidus (NDI), a hereditary disorder characterized by renal insensitivity to the antidiuretic action of arginine vasopressin (AVP), resulting in a severe concentration defect. NDI was first described more than a century ago by McIlraith and for a long time was of interest for clinicians only. However, since the identification of the genes underlying the different genetic types of this disorder, a renewed interest in the physiologic and pathophysiologic regulation of renal water absorption from pro-urine by molecular biologists, physiologists, cell biologists, and physicians can be noticed.

In addition to providing new and surprising insight into the cellular mechanisms involved in diuresis and antidiuresis, the elucidation of the genetic and cellular defects in NDI has significantly improved the differential diagnosis of the disorder, and has allowed accurate genetic counseling of patients and their family members. Furthermore, new therapies for NDI, based on the understanding of the cellular defects in this disorder, are now being developed and seem promising, although their efficacy and safety still must be examined.

After a short review on the current knowledge of the normal physiology of the renal collecting duct water permeability, we will discuss the diagnosis of NDI and the molecular and cellular defects underlying the different types of NDI. Finally, we will discuss current therapeutic options and some potential new therapies.

PHYSIOLOGY OF WATER HOMEOSTASIS

The physiologic action of vasopressin in renal collecting duct cells has been one of the most intensively studied processes in the kidney. In response to high serum osmolality or reduced blood pressure, AVP is secreted by the posterior pituitary. In the collecting duct of the kidney, AVP binds to the vasopressin type 2 receptor (V2R) on the basolateral membrane of principal cells (Fig. 18-1). This interaction between AVP and its V2R initiates the activation of adenylate cyclase via the intermediacy of stimulatory G (Gs) protein, resulting in a transient increase in intracellular cyclic adenosine monophosphate (cAMP) concentration. The elevated cAMP levels stimulate protein kinase A (PKA), which in turn initiates a steady-state redistribution of aquaporin 2 (AQP2) water channels from intracellular vesicles to the apical plasma membrane, rendering this membrane water permeable. Phosphorylation by PKA of serine at position 256 in the cytoplasmic C terminus

of AQP2 is essential for this redistribution, because an AQP2 with a substitution at S256A (AQP2-S256A), which mimics nonphosphorylated AQP2, is impaired in its redistribution to the plasma membrane upon stimulation with AVP or the adenylate cyclase activator, forskolin.[1-4] Interesting in this respect is that in an unstimulated steady-state condition, phosphorylated AQP2 could be detected in intracellular vesicles.[5] However, AQP2 is expressed as a homotetramer,[3,6] and recent studies using oocytes as a model system indicated that plasma membrane localization requires that three out of four monomers in an AQP2 tetramer be phosphorylated.[7]

The increased permeability of the apical membrane subsequent to AQP2 insertion allows water to flow in a transcellular fashion from the tubule lumen to the hypertonic medullary interstitium, which is mediated via AQP2 in the apical membrane and AQP3 and AQP4 water channels in the basolateral membrane, ultimately leading to the formation of concentrated urine. As predicted by Wade et al in the "shuttle hypothesis" in the late 1980s,[8] withdrawal of vasopressin reverses this redistribution process of AQP2 and restores the water-impermeable state of the apical side of the cell.[9,10]

The localization of AQP2, however, is not only regulated by phosphorylation by PKA. With elegant osmotic flow measurements on dissected rat inner medullary collecting ducts and, later, immunocytochemical analyses, several hormones have been identified that counteract the action of AVP by reducing the apical membrane expression of AQP2. Some of these hormones (ATP/UTP, dopamine, endothelin) seemed to block the AVP-triggered increase of intracellular cAMP, which was thought to be conferred by activation of a counteracting protein kinase C (PKC; ATP/UTP),[11] coupling of the hormone receptor to an inhibitory G (Gi) protein (dopamine),[12] or both (endothelin).[13] Other hormones, such as carbachol and the epidermal growth factor, inhibited AVP- and cAMP-induced water permeability but did not impair the AVP-induced cAMP production.[14-18] Prostaglandin E_2 (PGE_2) seems to act in both ways. In the cortical collecting duct, PGE_2 seems to inhibit adenylate cyclase via a E-prostanoid-3 (EP-3) receptor–coupled Gi protein,[19,20] whereas in the inner medullary collecting duct PGE_2 seemed to have no effect on cAMP generation and was therefore suggested to act on the AQP2 shuttling process only.[14,18] This latter finding is supported by work of Zelenina and co-workers, who found that PGE_2 induced the internalization of AQP2 in collecting ducts without changing the level of AQP2 phosphorylation.[21]

In most cases where cAMP generation was not affected, the inhibitory effects were absent upon co-treatment of the ducts with PKC inhibitors.[14,18] Because phorbol myristate acetate, which activates several PKCs, also inhibits AVP-induced water

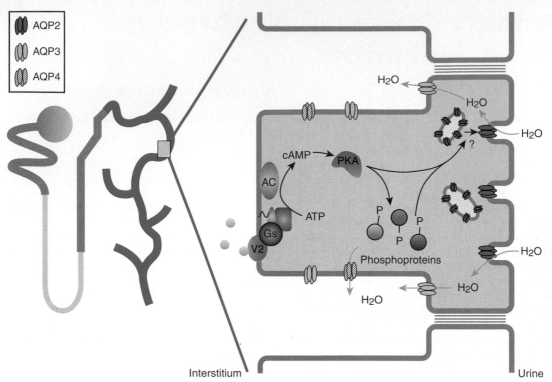

Figure 18-1 Regulation of the aquaporin-2 (AQP2)–mediated water transport by vasopressin. Vasopressin (AVP), vasopressin V2 receptor (V2), stimulatory guanosine triphosphate binding protein (Gs), adenylate cyclase (AC), adenosine triphosphate (ATP), cyclic adenosine monophosphate (cAMP), and phosphorylated proteins (O-P) are indicated. For details see text.

permeability,[15] these hormones were suggested to activate PKC isotypes that interfere shuttling of AQP2 to the apical membrane.

Recent data indicate that the action of these hormones is independent from AQP2 phosphorylation, because alteration of the three putative casein kinase II amino acid positions (S148, S229, T244) and one PKC position (S231) to alanines or aspartates, which are thought to mimic their constitutively nonphosphorylated or phosphorylated states, respectively, did not alter their subcellular localization, and neither did their translocation to the apical membrane with forskolin.[4] Only phosphorylation of the PKA site seemed to be relevant, because the AQP2-S256A resided in intracellular vesicles and AQP2-S256D was located in the apical membrane, independent of forskolin treatment. Also, activation of PKC enzymes by phorbol myristate acetate in the presence of forskolin resulted in the redistribution to intracellular vesicles of AQP2-S256D and all AQP2 kinase mutants, which were still phosphorylated at S256. These data indicated that, although phosphorylation of S256 is necessary for expression of AQP2 in the apical membrane, hormones that activate PKC enzymes can overcome the AVP-mediated phosphorylation and translocation of AQP2 to the apical membrane.

It is likely that the internalization of even phosphorylated AQP2 with these inhibitory hormones is mediated by the polymerization state of the actin cytoskeleton. In collecting ducts, vasopressin is known to induce a de- and repolymerization of the actin cytoskeleton,[22] and cytochalasins, which disrupt actin filaments, markedly inhibit the vasopressin response in target epithelia.[23] Indeed, Valenti, Rosenthal, and co-workers have shown recently in cultured cells that acti-

vated RhoA kinase, whether activated by PGE2 or other stimuli, induces F-actin polymerization and inhibits AQP2 translocation to the plasma membrane. In contrast, inactivation of RhoA kinase by phosphorylation with forskolin or with a specific RhoA kinase inhibitor allowed translocation of AQP2 to the plasma membrane.[24–27] Besides these general cellular mechanisms, several proteins have been found or suggested to have a role in AVP-induced AQP2 trafficking to and from the plasma membrane. However, the possible involvement of these proteins in AQP2 regulation has been well-covered in recent reviews[28–31] and will therefore not be further discussed here.

PATHOPHYSIOLOGY OF WATER HOMEOSTASIS

Clinical Phenotype

In congenital NDI the process above is disturbed, such that in this disease the distal renal nephron is unable to respond to AVP. As a consequence, the kidney loses its ability to concentrate urine, which may lead to severe dehydration and electrolyte imbalance (hypernatremia and hyperchloremia). The manifestations of NDI characteristically appear within the first weeks of life and include irritability, poor feeding, and poor weight gain.[32] Affected infants are eager to suck but may vomit during or shortly after the feeding. Dryness of the skin, loss of normal skin turgor, recessed eyeballs, depression of the anterior fontanelle, and a scaphoid abdomen are clinical signs of dehydration. Intermittent high fever is a frequent complication of the dehydrated state, particularly in very young patients; body temperature can be normalized by rehydration. Seizures have been reported in NDI patients, but these are rare and most often seen during therapy, particularly if rehydration proceeds too rapidly. Constipation is a common symptom in children with NDI. Nocturia and enuresis are frequent complaints emerging later in childhood.

Untreated, most patients fail to grow normally. In a retrospective study of 30 male NDI patients, most children grew below the 50th percentile and showed no clear catch-up growth after the first year of life. Weight-for-height standard deviation (SD) scores were initially low, followed by global normalization at school age.[33] The exact reasons for the failure to thrive in NDI remain to be explained. Feeding problems, the ingestion of large amounts of low-caloric fluid resulting in decreased appetite, and repeated episodes of dehydration may all play a role.[33–35]

Prolonged, unrecognized, or repeated episodes of hypernatremic dehydration may result in permanent brain damage, developmental delay, and mental retardation.[36,37] Additional evidence underscoring the assumption that NDI has adverse effects on the brain is provided by reports of NDI cases with intracerebral calcifications.[38,39] Such lesions are generally considered to be the result of hemorrhage or necrosis. Most of the patients with cerebral calcifications were mentally retarded. Mental retardation is currently rare because of earlier recognition and treatment of NDI. Exact estimates of the frequency of mental retardation under modern treatment are not available, but in the largest psychometric study of NDI patients ever reported, only 2 of the 17 male patients (aged 3–30 years) tested had a total intelligence quotient more than 2 SD below the norm. Fourteen patients scored within or above the normal range, and one patient had a general index score between −1 and −2 SD.[40]

As a result of a persistent desire for drinking and the need for frequent voiding, many NDI patients are characterized by hyperactivity, distractibility, short attention span, and restlessness. In the psychometric study mentioned above, the criteria for attention deficit hyperactivity disorder were met in 8 of 17 NDI patients.[40]

Although urologic complications are rare among NDI patients, megacystis, hydroureter, and hydronephrosis resulting from persistent polyuria and mimicking lower urinary tract obstruction, have been reported incidentally.[33,41–43] In order to monitor for these serious complications a renal ultrasound evaluation should be performed annually.

The clinical diagnosis of NDI depends upon demonstration of the inability to concentrate urine despite the presence of the antidiuretic hormone AVP. This is performed by a vasopressin test with 1-desamino-8-D-arginine vasopressin (dDAVP), a synthetic analog of AVP that produces a high and prolonged antidiuretic effect. After intranasal dDAVP administration NDI patients are unable to increase urinary osmolality, which remains below 200 mOsm/kg H_2O (normal ≥ 807 mOsm/kg H_2O) and cannot reduce urine volume or free-water clearance. Plasma vasopressin levels are normal or slightly increased in NDI patients.

Acquired and Congenital Forms of NDI

The primary congenital form of NDI must be differentiated from the secondary or acquired forms, which are much more common. A wide range of pathologic conditions and drug treatments can lead to acquired NDI (Table 18-1). In our experience, the urinary osmolality obtained after dDAVP administration in these disorders is always higher than in NDI. All these disease conditions have been shown to coincide with decreased expression of AQP2 in the collecting duct and in its apical membrane.[44]

The prevalence of congenital NDI is not exactly known, but the disease is assumed to be rare. Even in large pediatric and nephrology clinics it is observed infrequently. In the Netherlands population of approximately 16 million, 40 different families are known. Congenital NDI in humans is heterogeneous in that three different inheritance patterns of congenital NDI have been recognized in which two genes are involved. In most cases (≈90%) NDI is transmitted as an X-linked recessive trait (MIM No. 304800) caused by mutations in the V2R gene. A minority of patients (≈10%) shows an autosomal recessive (MIM No. 222000) or dominant trait (MIM No. 125800) as a result of mutations in the AQP2 water channel gene.

Differential Diagnosis between the X-linked and the Autosomal Forms of NDI

The X-linked and autosomal recessive forms of NDI do not differ with respect to the clinical symptoms of the disorder and, with a few exceptions, in the time of onset of the disease. Only in a minority of patients with X-linked NDI, namely in those individuals carrying mutations in the gene encoding V2R resulting in partial insensitivity to AVP, the disease onset is not directly after birth but later in childhood (Table 18-2). In general, the initial symptoms in most autosomal dominant cases also appear later, in some cases not before early adulthood (Table 18-3). Male patients with X-linked NDI can be distinguished from patients with autosomal recessive NDI on the basis of their extrarenal reaction to intravenous administration of dDAVP. Patients with autosomal NDI show normal increases in von Willebrand factor, factor VIII activity, and tissue-type plasminogen activator levels, whereas in patients with X-linked NDI these extrarenal responses are

Table 18-1 Common Causes of Acquired Nephrogenic Diabetes Insipidus

| Amyloidosis |
| Chronic pyelonephritis |
| Drug-side effect: Lithium Tetracyclines |
| Hypercalcemia/nephrocalcinosis |
| Hypokalemia |
| Juvenile nephronophthisis |
| Ureteral obstruction |
| Renal dysplasia |
| Sarcoidosis |
| Sickle-cell anemia |

absent as a result of a mutant extrarenal V2R.[42,45–48] In female patients, however, the interpretation of this dDAVP test with measurement of extrarenal responses is more complicated. Absence of extrarenal responses clearly points to the presence of a V2R defect in females. A normal extrarenal response to dDAVP administration, however, cannot be interpreted as indicative of an AQP2 defect.[49] Moses et al, for example, described a symptomatic female V2R mutation carrier with a twofold increase in factor VIII activity after intravenous dDAVP administration.[50] The discrepancy between renal and extrarenal responses to dDAVP in female carriers of a V2R mutation is assumed to be due to variability of the pattern of X-chromosome activation between different tissues.[51]

MOLECULAR BASIS OF CONGENITAL NDI

V2R Gene Mutations

The majority of NDI patients have mutations in the *AVPR2* gene, which encodes the vasopressin V2 receptor. The *AVPR2* gene maps to the X chromosome, locus q28, and is composed of three exons. The messenger RNA that is transcribed from this gene is 1.8 kb long and encodes a protein of 371 amino acids, with a predicted molecular weight of approximately 40 kDa.[52–54] The V2R is a member of the large superfamily of G protein–coupled receptors (GPCRs), which is characterized by seven transmembrane spanning domains, an extracellular N terminus, and an intracellular C terminus (Fig. 18-2). The N terminus of mature V2R proteins is heavily glycosylated, in that it is N-glycosylated at Asn22 and O-glycosylated at several serine and threonine residues, modification of which is suggested to be important in the processing, targeting, and stability of the V2R.[55,56] The C terminus is anchored to the plasma membrane by two palmitoyl groups that are covalently coupled to cysteine residues 341 and 342, which are suggested to be important for proper folding of the receptor[57] and in G protein activation.[58]

Besides inducing the translocation of AQP2, binding of AVP also regulates the fate of the V2R itself; upon binding of vasopressin, multiple serine residues in the V2R's C terminus are phosphorylated by a presently unknown GPCR kinase. The phosphorylated C terminus is subsequently bound by β-arrestin,[59] which leads to the internalization of the receptor, via clathrin-coated pits, early and late endosomes, to the lysosomes where it is degraded.[60] AVP binding decreases the half-life of the V2R approximately fourfold[60] and probably represents a cellular negative-feedback mechanism to prevent reabsorption of too much water from pro-urine.

Thus far, more than 180 mutations in the *AVPR2* gene have been described, of which most are documented at the Montreal Diabetes Insipidus Group (McGill University) website (http://www.medicine.mcgill.ca/nephros/), which was originally sponsored by the NDI foundation (http://www.ndif.org/). Several of these mutations are given in Table 18-2. *AVPR2* mutations are scattered throughout the gene.[31] Because a specific treatment of patients depends on the cellular fate of the mutant proteins conferred by the mutation, we recently adapted the classification used for the cystic fibrosis transmembrane conductance regulator (*CFTR*) gene to the cellular

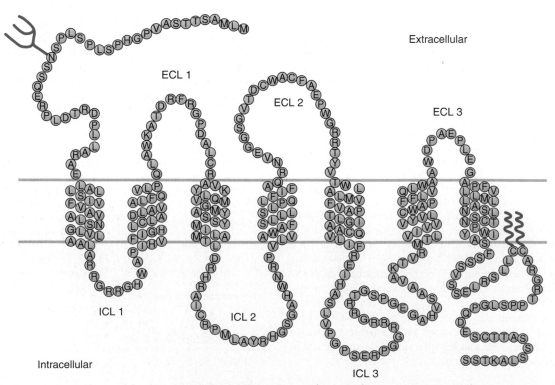

Figure 18-2 Proposed topology of human vasopressin V2 receptor. The V2R has seven transmembrane domains with its N terminus extracellular and its C terminus intracellular. The transmembrane domains are connected by three extracellular (ECL 1–3) and intracellular (ICL 1–3) loops. The N-glycosylation site (tree at N22) in its N terminus and the palmitoylated cysteines (C141–142) in its C terminus are indicated.

Table 18-2 V2R Mutations Involved in Nephrotic Diabetes Inspidus

Nucleotide	Amino Acid	References	Conserved/Location	Function	Class	Diagnosis	Treatment (Response)
492T→C	L44P	72, 137–140	Y (tmd1)	F	II	1 wk	dD (NR)
498T→A	I46K	71	N (tmd1)	F	II	5 yr	ndD (NR)
546T→C	L62P	139,141	Y (tmd1)	?	II ?	21,53 mo	dD (NR)
545–553del	Δ62-64	62, 69, 72	N (tmd1)	G	II	?	?
574G→A	W71X	63	N (ICL1)	–	I	?	dD (NR)
612C→A	A84D	67	N (tmd2)	A	II	?	?
614G→A	D85N	71, 132, 142	Y (tmd2)	F	III	32 mo	nD, dD-deh. (>400)
623G→A	V88M	33, 90, 139	Y (tmd2)	?	II	16 mo	ndD (NR), deh. (>500)
656T→C	W99R	67	Y (ECL1)	A	II, IV	?	?
671C→T	R104C	131, 143	Y (ECL1)	F	II	8 days	ndD (NR), dD (>300), thiaz., dD
674T→G	F105V	71	Y (ECL1)	A	IV	?	?
698C→T	R113W	70, 139	Y (tmd3)	F	II, IV	?	dD-deh. (NR)
749A→T	I130F	71, 72	N (tmd3)	F	II	1 mo	ndD (NR)
771G→A	R137H	63, 68, 73, 80, 131, 144–148	Y (ICL2)	G	II, III, V	?	dD-deh. (NR), dD (>400)
860T→A	S167T	72, 137, 138, 148	N (tmd4)	F	II	1 mo	dD (NR)
861C→T	S167L	72, 137–139, 148, 149	N (tmd4)	A	II	2 wk, 8 mo	ndD, dD (NR)
902C→T	R181C	62, 68, 77, 139, 150	N (tmd4)	A	IV	6 mo	ndD (NR)
914G→T	G185C	33, 53, 151	N (ECL3)	A	IV	7, 9, 108, 128, 204 mo	dD-deh. (>300)
963G→A	G201D	70, 72	Y (ECL3)	F	II, IV	?	dD-deh. (>400)
965C→T	R202C	67, 78, 141, 152, 153	N (ECL3)	A	IV	18 mo	?
965–967del	ΔR202	75	N (ECL3)	A	IV	?	dD (NR)
972C→A	T204N	140, 153, 154	N (ECL3)	A	II	15 mo	dD (NR), ndD* (>200)
975A→G	Y205C	33, 53, 90, 154, 155	Y (ECL3)	A	II	2 wk, 2.5 mo	dD (NR)
978T→A	V206D	72, 139, 154	N (tmd5)	A	II	?	dD (NR)
1431C→T	P322S	75, 90	Y (tmd7)	F	III, IV	10 mo, 9 yrs	dD-deh. (>400)
1476C→T	R337X	57, 58, 62, 136,139, 152, 155–157	N (C-tail)	A	I	4 mo	dD (NR)

Function: F, functional; A, disturbed AVP binding; G; disturbed Gs protein binding. Conserved (Y) or not (N) between human V1R, V2R, and V3R; tmd, transmembrane domain; ECL, extracellular loop; ICL, intracellular loop. Treatment: dD, infusion with dDAVP; ndD, nasal dDAVP; deh., dehydration. Response: NR, non-responsive; >200, urine > 200 mOsm/kg.
*Upon a double ndD dose.

Table 18-3 AQP2 Mutations Involved in Nephrogenic Diabetes Inspidus

Nucleotide	Amino Acid	Zygosity	R/D	Ref./Anal.	Function	Cons. (Loc.)	Class	Diagnosis	Treatment (Response)
64C→G	L22V	He3	R	98/86	P (60%)	N (tmd 1)	II	87	dD
83T→C	L28P	Ho	R	97/97	D	N (tmd 1)	II	1 mo	dD (NR)
140C→T	A47V	Ho	R	97/97	P (40%)	N (tmd 2)	II	?	dD-deh. (NR)
170A→C	Q57P	He5	R	92/92	D	N (tmd 2)	II	?	dD (NR)
190G→A	G64R	Ho	R	99/88, 89, 99	P (20%)	Y (b-loop)	II	1 mo	dD (NR)
293A→G	N68S	Ho	R	93/88	D	Y (b-loop)	II	1.5 mo	e:dD-deh. (>300), dD (NR)
211G→A	V71M	Ho	R	97/97	D	Y (b-loop)	II	?	ndD (NR)
253C→T	R85*	Ho	R	90/			I	2 mo	dD (NR)
299C→T	G100*	Ho	R	91/			I	?	dD (NR)
299G→T	G100V	He5	R	92/92	D	N (tmd 3)	II	?	dD (NR)
369delC	Out of frame	Ho	R	99/			I	?	?
374C→T	T125M	Ho, he8	R	95, 96/96, 97	P (25%)	N (c-loop)	II	?	?
377C→T	T126M	Ho	R	88/88, 93, 96	P (20%)	N (c-loop)	II	5 mo	dD-deh. (NR)
439G→A	A147T	Ho	R	93/88, 93	F	Y (d-loop)	II	3 mo	dD-deh. (NR)
450T→A	D150E	He7	R	100/100	D	Y (d-loop)	II	?	?
502G→A	V168M	He4, ho	R	90, 94/94	P (60%)	N (tmd 5)	II	?	He, ndD (NR), ho:dD (<200)
523G→A	G175R	Ho, he8	R	95, 96/96, 97	D	Y (tmd 5)	II	?	?
543C→G	C181W	He3	R	98/86, 87	D	N (e-loop)	II	87	?
553C→G	P185A	Ho	R	97/97	D	Y (e-loop)	II	1 wk	ndD (NR)

Table 18-3 AQP2 Mutations Involved in Nephrogenic Diabetes Inspidus—Cont'd

Nucleotide	Amino Acid	Zygosity	R/D	Ref./Anal.	Function	Cons. (Loc.)	Class	Diagnosis	Treatment (Response)
559C→T	R187C	Ho, he1	R	99, 102/88, 99	D	Y (e-loop)	II	2 wk, 5 mo	dD-deh. (NR)
568G→A	A190T	He2	R	85, 95/85, 95	D	N (e-loop)	II	?	dD (NR)
606G→T	W202C/splice	Ho	R	101/		Y (e-loop)	I	4–8 wk	dD (NR)
c606+1G→A	Splice	He6, all.2	R	97/		C (intr. 3)*	I	2 wk	dD (NR)
646T→C	S216P	He1, he4	R	102/88, 89	D	N (tmd 6)	II	3 mo	dD (NR)
652delC	Out of frame	He6, all.1	R	97/		N (tmd 6)	I	2 wk	dD (NR)
721delG	Out of frame	He	D	113/113	F	N (C-tail)	IV	12 mo	ndD (NR), deh. (>300)
727delG	Out of frame	He	D	108/108	F	N (C-tail)	IV	?	dD (NR)
761G→T	R254L	He	D	109/109	F	N (C-tail)	IV	<12 mo	?
763–772del	Out of frame	He	D	113/113	F	N (C-tail)	IV	36 mo	ndD (NR)
772G→A	E258K	He	D	111/111	F	N (C-tail)	IV	?	dD (>300)
779–780insA	Out of frame	He	D	112/112	F	N (C-tail)	IV	6–1 mo	dD (NR, 2, >300, 1)
785C→T	P262L	He2	R	85, 95/85, 95	F	N (C-tail)	IV	?	dD (NR)
812–818del	Out of frame	He	D	113/113	F	N (C-tail)	IV	16 mo	dD (incr.), deh. (>300)

Zygosity: He, heterozygous; ho, homozygous; all., allele; R, recessive; D, dominant. Function: F, functional; D, dead protein; P, partial functional (level in % between brackets). Conserved (Y) or not (N) between AQP proteins; tmd, transmembrane domain. Treatment: dD, infusion with dDAVP; ndD, nasal dDAVP; deh., dehydration; ind, indomethacin; NR, non-responsive; >200, etc., urine > 200 mOsm/kg thiaz, thiazide.
*C (intr. 3), C terminus, intron 3.

fate of GPCRs in general and the V2R in particular.[61] In the next section, V2R mutations belonging to the five different classes (Fig. 18-3A; see Table 18-2) will be discussed.

Class I mutations lead to defects in the synthesis of stable messenger RNA, resulting in absence of protein. Promoter alterations, exon skipping, aberrant splicing, and most frameshift and nonsense mutations fall into this category. In this class, the main research focus has been on nonsense mutations, which introduce a premature stop codon. Although they fail to produce full-length V2Rs, some stop codons encoded in individuals with NDI are in the C terminus of the receptor and may still lead to functional receptors. The mutations encoding V2R-W71X or -R337X, which have been identified in several related and unrelated NDI families, respectively, are probably the best characterized examples of class I mutations in the V2R gene.[62,63]

Class II mutations lead to fully translated proteins, but these mutant proteins are recognized as misfolded and retained by the quality control mechanism of the endoplasmic reticulum (ER). Subsequently, they are transported out of the ER and degraded by proteasomes.[64] Because of the high stringency of the ER quality control, more than 50% of the missense mutations (i.e., those causing the substitution of an amino acid) in the low-density lipoprotein receptor gene in familial hypercholesterolemia fall in this category.[65] Although many V2R mutations have not been functionally tested, this is probably similar for V2R missense mutants, in that L44P, I46K, L59P, Δ62–64, L83Q, A84D, R113W, I130F, R137H, S167T, S167L, G201D, T204N, V206D, and many others are ER retained.[66–72] Also, the marked overexpression of V2R

mutants, as is normal in the commonly used technique of transient transfection, will give plasma membrane expression of most V2R mutants, from which it has been deduced that some mutant V2Rs are impaired in their signal transduction (class III) or AVP binding (class IV). However, with stably transfected cells, in which expression levels are lower, plasma membrane expression of such mutants is often not observed.[72] Because GPCRs are usually expressed at low levels in vivo and class II mutants are often prone to extensive degradation, misfolding and degradation probably constitute the most important causal factor for NDI in individuals with V2R mutants that are found to be (partially) retained in the ER in in vitro studies. The extent of ER retention, however, does differ between V2R mutants. For example, the V2R mutants R113W, T204N, I130F, and G201D are ER-retained to a lower extent than other V2R mutants in stably transfected polarized renal cells.[72] Although such V2R mutants are then often also affected in other aspects of their functioning (classes III and IV), the partial expression of functional V2R mutants in the plasma membrane, such as V2R-T204N and anti-G201D, can explain their response to dDAVP in patients.

Class III mutants are normally transported to their site of action, where they exhibit a defect in activation or regulation. For the V2R, mutations that interfere with Gs-protein binding, thereby preventing intracellular signaling, fall into this category. The V2R mutants D85N, R137H, and P232S have been reported to fall into this class, although R137H is also a class II mutation.[73] The partial loss of Gs activation seen in these three mutants provides an explanation for the partial NDI phenotype in the affected patients.

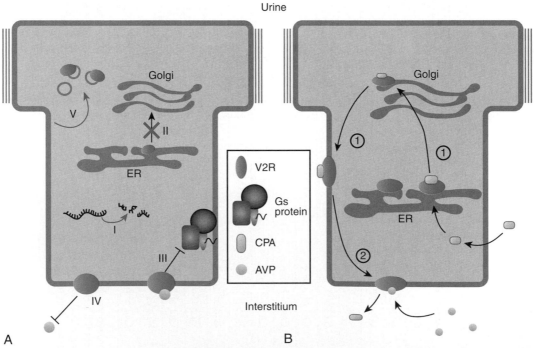

Figure 18-3 The cellular fate and rescue of vasopressin V2 receptor mutations in NDI. **A,** V2R mutation classes in NDI. The different classes of the cellular fate of V2R mutants are indicated in roman numbers. For details see text. **B,** Rescue of class II V2R mutants by pharmacologic chaperones. (1) Treatment of cells expressing class II V2R mutants with V1R or V2R cell-permeable antagonists (CPA) stabilize the structure of the V2R mutants in the ER, resulting in their further maturation and transport via the Golgi complex to the basolateral membrane. (2) Replacement of the inverse agonists for endogenous AVP (or exogenous dDAVP) at the basolateral membrane will initiate a V2R mutant–mediated cAMP signaling cascade. ER, endoplasmic reticulum.

Class IV mutations also do not affect protein trafficking but instead impair or decrease the receptor's ability to bind to vasopressin or one of its synthetic analogs. In many GPCRs, the first (P95–R113) and second extracellular (R181–T207) loops are thought to be involved in ligand binding, which is in the V2R stabilized by disulfide-bonded cysteines (C112, C192). V2R proteins with V88M, W99R, F105V, R113W, R181C, G185C, ΔR202, R202C, T204N, Y205C, or V206D substitutions showed reduced AVP binding, despite being expressed at the cell surface.[67,68,71,74–78] Lack of only AVP binding has been clearly established for V2R-ΔR202[75] and -R181C.[77] Unfortunately, the relevance of the lack of AVP binding in several of the other mutants as an explanation for their occurrence in NDI is doubtful, in that many of these mutants are also (partially) retained in the ER (e.g., R113W, R181C, T204N, V206D),[72] whereas this has not been studied for several others.

Finally, **class V** mutations lead to proteins that are not disturbed in any of the above, but are mis-sorted to another organelle in the cell. The R137H mutation, which is found in the highly conserved D$_{136}$RY/H motif of GPCRs, is a member of this class. As a consequence of this mutation, V2R-R137H proteins are constitutively internalized from the membrane and targeted for degradation, and are therefore only briefly present in the plasma membrane.[79] Because the R137H mutation also causes ER retention and interferes with G-protein binding,[80] it also falls into classes II and III.

AQP2 Gene Mutations: Autosomal Recessive NDI

Both the autosomal recessive and the autosomal dominant types of NDI are caused by mutations in the *AQP2* water channel gene (GenBank accession no. Z29491), which is located on chromosome 12q13.[81,82] The human *AQP2* gene is a small gene consisting of four exons, comprising 5 kb of genomic DNA. The 1.5-kb messenger RNA encodes a protein of 271 amino acids that has a predicted molecular weight of 29 kDa. Like other aquaporins, AQP2 is expressed in the membrane as a homotetramer in which each 29-kDa monomer, consisting of six membrane-spanning α-helical domains and intracellular N and C termini, is a functional water channel.[3,6,83] These six transmembrane domains are connected by five loops (A through E; Fig. 18-4) in which loops B and E fold back into the membrane, interact via their highly conserved motifs asparagine-proline-alanine (NPA boxes), and form the water pore.[83,84]

Thus far, 27 mutations in *AQP2* have reported in families with autosomal recessive NDI (see Table 18-3). These include 21 missense mutations, 2 nonsense mutations, two 1-bp deletions, and 2 splice site mutations.[85–102] Interestingly, all mutations in autosomal recessive NDI (except P262L; see later) are located in between the first and the last transmembrane domain. Although controversy exists for AQP2-T125M and AQP2-G175R, which were proposed by Goji et al to be

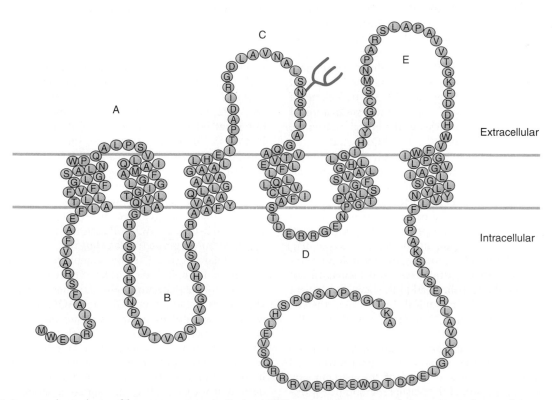

Figure 18-4 Proposed topology of human aquaporin 2. An AQP2 monomer consists of six transmembrane domains connected by five loops (A–E) and its N and C termini located intracellularly. Loops B and E meet each other with their characteristic NPA boxes in the membrane and form the water-selective pore. The N-glycosylation site (tree at N123) is indicated. NPA, asparagine-proline-alanine. (Redrawn from Heymann JB, Engel A: Structural clues in the sequences of the aquaporins. J Mol Biol 295:1039–1053, 2000.)

nonfunctional water channels, unaffected in their routing to the plasma membrane,[96] these and all other AQP2 missense mutants in recessive NDI seemed to be impaired in their export from the ER upon expression in cells (class II defect); as in the V2R, misfolding of these mutants leads to proteasomal degradation through the ER-associated degradation pathway. Indeed, the observed instability of several AQP2 mutants in recessive NDI could be reduced with proteasome inhibitors.[86,103,104] The low stability of these AQP2 mutants is in line with in vivo data, because mutant AQP2 proteins could not be detected in urine of patients suffering from autosomal recessive NDI, in contrast to wild-type AQP2 (wt-AQP2) in urine from healthy individuals.[105,106] Though retained in the ER, at higher expression levels in *Xenopus* oocytes, in which a proportion of the AQP2 mutant proteins escapes from the ER and is routed to the plasma membrane,[107] seven mutants (L22V, A47V, G64R, T125M, T126M, A147T, and V168M) seemed to be able to confer water permeability.[88,93,94,97,98]

AQP2 Gene Mutations: Autosomal Dominant NDI

At present, eight families have been described with autosomal dominant NDI, initially uncovered due to father-to-son transmission of the disease or the absence of mutations in the gene encoding V2R. In these families, subsequent sequencing revealed putative disease-causing mutations in the *AQP2* gene of one allele, which were missense mutations resulting in R254L, R254Q, and E258K substitutions, deletions of 1 (721delG, 727delG), 7 (812–818del), or 10 (763–772del) nucleotides resulting in a +1 frameshift, or a one-base insertion (779–780insA), resulting in a +2 frameshift. Interestingly, all of these mutations were found in the coding sequence of the C-terminal tail of AQP2, which is not a part of the water pore–forming segment. Indeed, all AQP2 proteins in dominant NDI were functional water channels. Instead, the C-terminal tail had been shown to be important in the trafficking of AQP2.[2,7] Indeed, whereas forskolin causes the translocation of wt-AQP2 from intracellular vesicles to the apical membrane when expressed in polarized cells, the AQP2 mutants in dominant NDI were mis-sorted to different destinations in the cell.[108–113] Importantly, because none of these mutants was misfolded, they were, in contrast to AQP2 mutants in recessive NDI, able to interact with and form heterotetramers with wt-AQP2.[3] In addition, in elegant microscopic studies on cells co-expressing wt and mutant AQP2 proteins, it appeared that, due to the wt-mutant interaction and dominancy of the mis-sorting signals in the mutant proteins, the wt-mutant complexes were also mis-sorted. Extrapolated to principal cells of the patients, this would probably lead to the lack of sufficient amounts of wt-AQP2 in the apical membrane, thereby explaining the dominant trait of NDI. As such, all these *AQP2* mutations are of class V.

Interestingly, six AQP2 mutants in dominant NDI are thought to be mis-sorted as a result of a signal introduced with the mutation. In oocytes, deletion of the segment surrounding E258 greatly restored the plasma membrane expression of AQP2-E258K, which indicated that the introduction of a lysine instead of the loss of E258 caused the dominant feature.[110] AQP2-insA, which has a +2 reading frameshift of the AQP2 C-tail, was targeted to the basolateral membrane, because of two introduced basolateral sorting signals in its

mutant C-terminal tail.[111] Though starting at different positions, the four mutations (721delG, 727delG, del763–772, and del812–818) that introduce a +1 reading frameshift result in a similar extended C-terminal tail. Studies in polarized cells revealed that AQP2-727delG accumulates in late endosomes/lysosomes and, to some extent, in the basolateral plasma membrane of polarized Madin-Darby canine kidney cells,[108] whereas the other three mutants have been reported to localize to the basolateral membrane. Because the extended tail in AQP2-del812–818 starts only at the stop codon of wt-AQP2 and the extended tails contain a di-leucine motif, which is a known basolateral membrane–targeting motif,[114] the dominance of these mutants in NDI is suggested to be due to this introduced basolateral sorting signal. Also, although AQP2-R254L cannot be phosphorylated at S256, because the mutation destroys the PKA phosphorylation consensus site in AQP2, the introduced leucine residue also appeared to introduce a basolateral sorting signal, such that AQP2-R254L-S256D, which mimics constitutively phosphorylated AQP2-R254L, was targeted to the apical and basolateral membrane in polarized cells.[109]

EXCEPTION TO THE RULE

As indicated previously, all mutations in recessive NDI were found in between the first and last transmembrane domains, except P262L (see Table 18-3). This substitution, which was found in two patients heterozygous for an R187C or A190T substitution, was located in the AQP2 C-terminal tail; on the basis of the AQP2 mutants studied above, this mutation would be expected to cause dominant NDI. Cell biologic studies provided the answer to this paradox.[85] Like mutants in dominant NDI, AQP2-P262L is a functional water channel, is retained in intracellular compartments different from the ER, and forms heteroligomers with wt-AQP2. Immunocytochemical analysis of cells co-expressing AQP2-P262L with wt-AQP2, however, revealed that, in contrast to mutants in dominant NDI, these wt-AQP2/AQP2-P262L complexes are located in the apical membrane, indicating that the apical sorting of wt-AQP2 is dominant over the mis-sorting signal of AQP2-P262L. On the basis of these data, the recessive inheritance of NDI in these families can be explained as follows: in the two patients involved, AQP2-R187C and AQP2-A190T mutants are retained in the ER, and do not interact with AQP2-P262L. AQP2-P262L is properly folded and assembles into homotetramers, but will be mainly retained in intracellular vesicles. The consequent lack of sufficient AQP2 proteins in the apical membrane of the collecting duct cells of the patients then explains their NDI phenotype. In the parents with alleles encoding wt-AQP2 and AQP2-R187C or -A190T, wt-AQP2 will not interact with either mutant but will form homotetrameric complexes, of which the insertion into the apical membrane in collecting duct cells will be properly regulated by vasopressin. Although the AQP2 expression levels in these humans might be reduced, because all AQP2 is derived from one allele, the apparent absence of an NDI phenotype indicates that AQP2 derived from one allele suffices for a healthy phenotype. In the proband's healthy relatives encoding wt-AQP2 and AQP2-P262L, both proteins are likely to assemble into heterotetramers. However, the dominancy of wt-AQP2 on the localization of AQP2-P262L will then result in a proper AVP-regulated trafficking of their heterotetrameric complexes to the apical membrane of their collecting duct cells.

TREATMENT OF NDI

Conventional Treatment of NDI

The most important component of treatment of NDI is replacement of urinary water losses by adequate supply of fluid. Most infants with NDI, however, cannot drink the required amounts of fluid. One approach to reduce urine output is provision of a low-solute diet to reduce the renal osmolar load and decrease obligatory water excretion. Initially, a diet low in sodium (1 mmol/kg/day) as well as protein (2 g/kg/day) was recommended. However, severe limitations of dietary protein may introduce serious nutritional deficiencies, and a dietary restriction of sodium only is therefore preferable.

Diuretics such as hydrochlorothiazide (2–4 mg/kg/day) were the first class of drugs shown to be effective in lowering urine volume in NDI.[115] When combined with low salt intake, hydrochlorothiazide reduces the urine volume by 20% to 50% of baseline values. However, thiazide-induced hypokalemia may cause further impairment or urinary concentrating ability in patients with NDI. Another potential risk associated with hypokalemia is cardiac arrhythmia. Simultaneous administration of potassium salt is therefore necessary in most cases.

The combined administration of hydrochlorothiazide with either a prostaglandin synthesis (or cyclooxygenase, or COX) inhibitor such as indomethacin (2 mg/kg/day), or the potassium-sparing diuretic amiloride, was shown to be much more effective in reducing urine volume than the thiazide diuretic alone.[47,116–121] Long-term use of prostaglandin-synthesis inhibitors, however, is often complicated by gastrointestinal and hematopoietic side effects. In addition, renal dysfunction has been described during indomethacin therapy, most often consisting of a reduction in glomerular filtration rate. Because of the known gastrointestinal safety of selective COX-2 inhibitors as compared with nonselective COX inhibitors, a potential role for these drugs in the treatment of NDI has been put forward. In one male infant with NDI, the effectiveness of a specific COX-2 inhibitor (rofecoxib) in decreasing urinary free-water losses was indeed demonstrated.[122] Nevertheless, in view of the recent discovery that prolonged use of that particular COX-2 inhibitor can cause severe cardiac side effects,[123] we believe that COX-2 inhibitors should not be used in the treatment of NDI until it has been strictly determined which of these specific inhibitors are completely safe.

Amiloride counterbalances the potassium loss from prolonged use of thiazides and thus prevents hypokalemia. Because amiloride seems to have only minor long-term side effects, the combination of hydrochlorothiazide (2–4 mg/kg/day) with amiloride (0.3 mg/kg/day) is the first choice of treatment. Our own experience of more than 14 years with the amiloride-hydrochlorothiazide combination, however, indicates that amiloride may cause persistent nausea in children younger than 4 to 6 years. For that reason we advise the temporary use of the combination of indomethacin-hydrochlorothiazide in these younger children.

For a long time the following mechanism for the paradoxical effect of thiazides in NDI has been suggested: thiazides decrease sodium reabsorption in the renal distal tubule by inhibition of the Na^+/Cl^- cotransporter. This in turn results in increased sodium excretion, extracellular volume contraction, decreased glomerular filtration rate, and increased proximal sodium and water reabsorption. As a consequence, less water and sodium are delivered to the collecting ducts and less water is excreted.[124,125] A few years ago this long-standing hypothesis was challenged by Magaldi's group; by microperfusion of isolated rat inner medullary collecting ducts, they showed that hydrochlorothiazide, when added to the luminal side and in the absence of vasopressin, increased osmotic and diffusional water permeabilities.[126,127] Increased permeability will facilitate water reabsorption in the collecting duct and thus reduce water excretion. When prostaglandins were added, the effect of thiazides decreased. This finding offers one explanation why indomethacin potentiates the effect of thiazides in NDI. Altogether, the results of these microperfusion studies indicate that thiazides act in nephron segments beyond the distal tubule. Because the effect of thiazides was only seen when they were applied to the luminal side of the rat inner medullary collecting ducts, it was concluded that these drugs do not interact with the basolaterally located V2R directly. Magaldi proposed the possibility that these drugs act at some point in the vasopressin cascade inside the cell, based on the observation that an inhibitor of PKA blocked the effect of thiazides.[127]

A recent study in lithium-induced NDI rats has given additional insight into the antidiuretic action of thiazides in NDI.[128] Using immunocytochemistry and immunoblotting, it was shown that hydrochlorothiazide treatment induces a significant increase in AQP2 abundance in the kidneys of these rats. In addition to the effect on AQP2, an upregulation of the Na^+/Cl^- cotransporter and the amiloride-sensitive epithelial sodium channel ENaC was found in these animals upon hydrochlorothiazide administration. The upregulation of sodium transporters and AQP2 was accompanied by a significant decrease in urinary output and an increase in urinary osmolality. Based on these findings, it is hypothesized that the antidiuretic action of hydrochlorothiazide in NDI may be the result of both an increase in sodium transport capacity in distal renal segments, leading to increased medullary tonicity, as well as an increase in the abundance of AQP2 proteins.

Tailored and Future Therapies in NDI

Although the conventional treatment described above generally relieves polyuria and polydipsia to a significant extent, the realization that V2R and AQP2 mutant proteins have different cellular fates suggests that "tailored therapy" might ultimately be successful. In patients carrying "milder" V2R mutations resulting in a partial response to AVP and dDAVP (partial NDI), a possible therapeutic benefit of high doses of dDAVP has been suggested. Indeed, in a 7-year-old boy, who encodes the partially ER-retained, but functional, V2R-R104C mutant and has a partial NDI, high doses of dDAVP resulted in a decrease in urinary volume and the disappearance of nocturia, but only when dDAVP was used in combination with a thiazide.[129,130] Because several patients with dominant NDI or partially functional V2Rs seemed to be able to transiently increase their urinary osmolality to 350 mOsm/kg

H_2O after dDAVP infusion (see Tables 18-1 and 18-2), many of these patients might also benefit from high doses of dDAVP. The response, however, might not necessarily be directly coupled to the V2R or AQP2 substitution, in that two brothers carrying the same V2R-R137H substitution and relatives encoding the same AQP2-insA mutant in dominant NDI responded quite differently to dDAVP infusion,[112,131] indicating that other factors than the V2R or AQP2 substitutions can influence the outcome of the therapy.

Besides these tailored treatments, different approaches have been undertaken to overcome the cellular problems of V2R mutants of the different classes, so as to develop alternative, "class-specific" treatments for NDI. If grown to full maturation, these therapies might best be used in combination with the conventional treatments.

For V2R mutants harboring premature stop codons or frameshift mutations in the C-terminal of the third intracellular loop (class I), it has been shown in vitro that functional rescue can be achieved when the mutant is co-expressed with a C-terminal V2R segment overlapping with the V2R segment containing the various mutations.[132] Because the complementing segment cannot function as a receptor on its own, general expression within cells of our body, mediated by gene therapy, would only lead to expression of functional V2Rs in those cells that express the class I mutant receptor. However, because of the difficulties in developing a safe and sustained gene transfer, the interest for gene therapy in NDI has waned during recent years. An alternative approach to provide a therapy for patients harboring stop codon mutations is based on the notion that, depending on surrounding nucleotides, aminoglycoside antibiotics allow the readthrough of termination signals, resulting in full-length proteins. Indeed, a gentamicin analog caused the readthrough of several stop codon V2R mutants in vitro.[133] However, considering the toxic effects of these antibiotics on the kidney, the application of such a therapy for NDI in the future is quite unlikely.

Much more promising are the approaches developed for the ER-retained V2R mutant proteins (class II). This is not only because several of these mutants have shown to be able to initiate a cAMP signaling cascade with AVP when expressed in the plasma membrane, but also because the majority of V2R gene mutations are of this class. An important step forward was the discovery that cell-permeable V2R[134] and V1R[135] inverse agonists are able to stabilize the conformation of several V2R mutants at the ER, which allowed their escape from the ER quality control mechanism, their maturation in the Golgi complex, and their further routing to the basolateral plasma membrane (see Fig. 18-3B([1])).[136] In an ideal situation, the antagonist would then dissociate from the receptor, allowing vasopressin to bind and activate the receptor (see Fig. 18-3B([2])) Because of their role in assisting protein folding, these cell-permeable antagonists are termed "pharmacologic chaperones." The main advantage of the use of pharmacologic chaperones is their high specificity, which is likely to result in a minimum of side effects. Even though clinical data involving pharmacologic chaperones are lacking at present, usage of this class of compounds is a promising approach in curing a large subset of NDI patients and may offer important insights for the treatment of other conformational diseases, i.e., those caused by protein misfolding.

Acknowledgments

The work of J.H. Robben is financed by the grant PC 104 of the Dutch Kidney Foundation to P.M.T. Deen and N.V.A.M. Knoers.

References

1. Fushimi K, Sasaki S, Marumo F: Phosphorylation of serine 256 is required for cAMP-dependent regulatory exocytosis of the aquaporin-2 water channel. J Biol Chem 272:14800–14804, 1997.
2. Katsura T, Gustafson CE, Ausiello DA, Brown D: Protein kinase A phosphorylation is involved in regulated exocytosis of aquaporin-2 in transfected LLC-PK1 cells. Am J Physiol 41:F816–F822, 1997.
3. Kamsteeg EJ, Wormhoudt TA, Rijss JPL, et al: An impaired routing of wild-type aquaporin-2 after tetramerization with an aquaporin-2 mutant explains dominant nephrogenic diabetes insipidus. EMBO J 18:2394–2400, 1999.
4. Van Balkom BWM, Savelkoul PJ, Markovich D, et al: The role of putative phosphorylation sites in the targeting and shuttling of the aquaporin-2 water channel. J Biol Chem 277:41473–41479, 2002.
5. Christensen BM, Zelenina M, Aperia A, Nielsen S: Localization and regulation of PKA-phosphorylated AQP2 in response to (V2 receptor) agonist/antagonist treatment. Am J Physiol Renal Physiol 278:F29–F42, 2000.
6. Werten PJ, Hasler L, Koenderink JB, et al: Large-scale purification of functional recombinant human aquaporin-2. FEBS Lett 504:200–205, 2001.
7. Kamsteeg EJ, Heijnen I, van Os CH, Deen PMT: The subcellular localization of an aquaporin-2 tetramer depends on the stoichiometry of phosphorylated and nonphosphorylated monomers. J Cell Biol 151:919–930, 2000.
8. Wade JB, Kachadorian WA: Cytochalasin B inhibition of toad bladder apical membrane responses to ADH. Am J Physiol 255:C526–C530, 1988.
9. Nielsen S, Digiovanni SR, Christensen EI, et al: Cellular and subcellular immunolocalization of vasopressin- regulated water channel in rat kidney. Proc Natl Acad Sci U S A 90:11663–11667, 1993.
10. Nielsen S, Chou CL, Marples D, et al: Vasopressin increases water permeability of kidney collecting duct by inducing translocation of aquaporin-CD water channels to plasma membrane. Proc Natl Acad Sci U S A 92:1013–1017, 1995.
11. Kishore BK, Chou CL, Knepper MA: Extracellular nucleotide receptor inhibits AVP-stimulated water permeability in inner medullary collecting duct. Am J Physiol 38:F863–F869, 1995.
12. Li L, Schafer JA: Dopamine inhibits vasopressin-dependent cAMP production in the rat cortical collecting duct. Am J Physiol 275:F62–F67, 1998.
13. Nadler SP, Zimpelmann JA, Hebert RL: Endothelin inhibits vasopressin-stimulated water permeability in rat terminal inner medullary collecting duct. J Clin Invest 90:1458–1466, 1992.
14. Nadler SP, Zimpelmann JA, Hebert RL: PGE2 inhibits water permeability at a post-cAMP site in rat terminal inner medullary collecting duct. Am J Physiol 262:F229–F235, 1992.
15. Han JS, Maeda Y, Ecelbarger C, Knepper MA: Vasopressin-independent regulation of collecting duct water permeability. Am J Physiol 266:F139–F146, 1994.
16. Breyer MD, Jacobson HR, Breyer JA: Epidermal growth factor inhibits the hydroosmotic effect of vasopressin in the isolated perfused rabbit cortical collecting tubule. J Clin Invest 82:1313–1320, 1988.
17. Ando Y, Jacobson HR, Breyer MD: Phorbol myristate acetate, dioctanoylglycerol, and phosphatidic acid inhibit the

hydroosmotic effect of vasopressin on rabbit cortical collecting tubule. J Clin Invest 80:590–593, 1987.

18. Maeda Y, Terada Y, Nonoguchi H, Knepper MA: Hormone and autacoid regulation of cAMP production in rat IMCD subsegments. Am J Physiol 263:F319–F327, 1992.

19. Fleming EF, Athirakul K, Oliverio MI, et al: Urinary concentrating function in mice lacking EP3 receptors for prostaglandin E2. Am J Physiol 275:F955–F961, 1998.

20. Breyer MD, Zhang Y, Guan YF, et al: Regulation of renal function by prostaglandin E receptors. Kidney Int Suppl 67:S88–S94, 1998.

21. Zelenina M, Christensen BM, Palmer J, et al: Prostaglandin E_2 interaction with AVP: Effects on AQP2 phosphorylation and distribution. Am J Physiol Renal Physiol 278:F388–F394, 2000.

22. Simon H, Gao Y, Franki N, Hays RM: Vasopressin depolymerizes apical F-actin in rat inner medullary. Am J Physiol 265:C757–C762, 1993.

23. Pearl M, Taylor A: Role of the cytoskeleton in the control of transcellular water flow by vasopressin in amphibian urinary bladder. Biol Cell 55:163–172, 1985.

24. Klussmann E, Tamma G, Lorenz D, et al: An inhibitory role of Rho in the vasopressin-mediated translocation of aquaporin-2 into cell membranes of renal principal cells. J Biol Chem 276:20451–20457, 2001.

25. Tamma G, Wiesner B, Furkert J, et al: The prostaglandin E2 analogue sulprostone antagonizes vasopressin-induced antidiuresis through activation of Rho. J Cell Sci 116:3285–3294, 2003.

26. Tamma G, Klussmann E, Procino G, et al: cAMP-induced AQP2 translocation is associated with RhoA inhibition through RhoA phosphorylation and interaction with RhoGDI. J Cell Sci 116:1519–1525, 2003.

27. Tamma G, Klussmann E, Maric K, et al: Rho inhibits cAMP-induced translocation of aquaporin-2 into the apical membrane of renal cells. Am J Physiol Renal Physiol 281:F1092–F1101, 2001.

28. Brown D: The ins and outs of aquaporin-2 trafficking. Am J Physiol Renal Physiol 284:F893–F901, 2003.

29. Nguyen MK, Nielsen S, Kurtz I: Molecular pathogenesis of nephrogenic diabetes insipidus. Clin Exp Nephrol 7:9–17, 2003.

30. Deen PMT, Brown D: Trafficking of native and mutant mammalian MIP proteins. In Hohmann S, Agre P, Nielsen S (eds): chap 6. San Diego, 2001, pp 235–276.

31. Knoers NVAM, Deen PMT: Molecular and cellular defects in nephrogenic diabetes insipidus. Pediatr Nephrol 16:1146–1152, 2001.

32. Kaplan SA: Nephrogenic diabetes insipidus. In Holliday MA, Barrat TM, Vernier RL (eds): Pediatric Nephrology. Baltimore, 1987, pp 623–625.

33. van Lieburg AF, Knoers NVAM, Monnens LA: Clinical presentation and follow-up of 30 patients with congenital nephrogenic diabetes insipidus. J Am Soc Nephrol 10:1958–1964, 1999.

34. Hillman DA, Neyzi O, Porter P, et al: Renal (vasopressin-resistant) diabetes insipidus; definition of the effects of a homeostatic limitation in capacity to conserve water on the physical, intellectual and emotional development of a child. Pediatrics 21:430–435, 1958.

35. Vest M, Talbot NB, Crawford JD: Hypocaloric dwarfism and hydronephrosis in diabetes insipidus. Am J Dis Child 105:175–181, 1963.

36. Forssman H: Is hereditary diabetes insipidus of nephrogenic type associated with mental deficiency? Acta Psychiatr Neurol Scand 30:577–587, 1955.

37. Macaulay D, Watson M: Hypernatraemia in infants as a cause of brain damage. Arch Dis Child 42:485–491, 1967.

38. Kanzaki S, Omura T, Miyake M, et al: Intracranial calcification in nephrogenic diabetes insipidus. JAMA 254:3349–3350, 1985.

39. Schofer O, Beetz R, Kruse K, et al: Nephrogenic diabetes insipidus and intracerebral calcification. Arch Dis Child 65:885–887, 1990.

40. Hoekstra JA, van Lieburg AF, Monnens LAH, et al: Cognitive and psychosocial functioning of patients with congenital nephrogenic diabetes insipidus. Am J Med Genet 61:81–88, 1996.

41. Uribarri J, Kaskas M: Hereditary nephrogenic diabetes insipidus and bilateral nonobstructive hydronephrosis. Nephron 65:346–349, 1993.

42. Miyakoshi M, Kamoi K, Uchida S, Sasaki S: A case of a novel mutant vasopressin receptor-dependent nephrogenic diabetes insipidus with bilateral non-obstructive hydronephrosis in a middle aged man: Differentiation from aquaporin-dependent nephrogenic diabetes insipidus by response of factor VII and von Willebrand factor to 1-diamino-8-arginine vasopressin administration. Endocr J 50:809–814, 2003.

43. Shalev H, Romanovsky I, Knoers NVAM, et al: Bladder function impairment in aquaporin-2 defective nephrogenic diabetes insipidus. Nephrol Dial Transplant 19:608–613, 2004.

44. Nielsen S, Frokiaer J, Marples D, et al: Aquaporins in the kidney: From molecules to medicine. Physiol Rev 82:205–244, 2002.

45. Kobrinsky NL, Doyle JJ, Israels ED, et al: Absent factor VIII response to synthetic vasopressin analogue (dDAVP) in nephrogenic diabetes insipidus. Lancet 1:1293–1294, 1985.

46. Bichet DG, Razi M, Lonergan M, et al: Hemodynamic and coagulation responses to 1-desamino [8-D-arginine] vasopressin in patients with congenital nephrogenic diabetes insipidus. N Engl J Med 318:881–887, 1988.

47. Knoers NVAM, Brommer EJ, Willems H, et al: Fibrinolytic responses to 1-desamino-8-D-arginine-vasopressin in patients with congenital nephrogenic diabetes insipidus [see comments]. Nephron 54:322–326, 1990.

48. van Lieburg AF, Knoers NVAM, Mallmann R, et al: Normal fibrinolytic responses to 1-desamino-8-D-arginine vasopressin in patients with nephrogenic diabetes insipidus caused by mutations in the aquaporin 2 gene. Nephron 72:544–546, 1996.

49. van Lieburg AF, Verdijk MAJ, Schoute F, et al: Clinical phenotype of nephrogenic diabetes insipidus in females heterozygous for a vasopressin type 2 receptor mutation. Hum Genet 96:70–78, 1995.

50. Moses AM, Sangani G, Miller JL: Proposed cause of marked vasopressin resistance in a female with an X-linked recessive V2 receptor abnormality. J Clin Endocrinol Metab 80:1184–1186, 1995.

51. Brown RM, Fraser NJ, Brown GK: Differential methylation of the hypervariable locus DXS255 on active and inactive X chromosomes correlates with the expression of a human X-linked gene. Genomics 7:215–221, 1990.

52. Rosenthal W, Seibold A, Antaramian A, et al: Molecular identification of the gene responsible for congenital nephrogenic diabetes insipidus. Nature 359:233–235, 1992.

53. van den Ouweland AM, Dreesen JC, Verdijk MAJ, Knoers NVAM: Mutations in the vasopressin type 2 receptor gene (AVPR2) associated with nephrogenic diabetes insipidus. Nat Genet 2:99–102, 1992.

54. Birnbaumer M, Seibold A, Gilbert S, et al: Molecular cloning of the receptor for human antidiuretic hormone. Nature 357:333–335, 1992.

55. Sadeghi H, Birnbaumer M: O-Glycosylation of the V2 vasopressin receptor. Glycobiology 9:731–737, 1999.

56. Innamorati G, Sadeghi H, Birnbaumer M: A fully active nonglycosylated V2 vasopressin receptor. Mol Pharmacol 50:467–473, 1996.

57. Oksche A, Dehe M, Schulein R, et al: Folding and cell surface expression of the vasopressin V2 receptor: Requirement of the intracellular C-terminus. FEBS Lett 424:57–62, 1998.

58. Sadeghi HM, Innamorati G, Birnbaumer M: An X-linked NDI mutation reveals a requirement for cell surface V2R expression. Mol Endocrinol 11:706–713, 1997.

59. Martin NP, Lefkowitz RJ, Shenoy SK: Regulation of V2 vasopressin receptor degradation by agonist-promoted ubiquitination. J Biol Chem 278:45954–45959, 2003.

60. Robben JH, Knoers NVAM, Deen PMT: Regulation of the vasopressin V2 receptor by vasopressin in polarized renal collecting duct cells. Mol Biol Cell 15:5693–5699, 2004.

61. Deen PMT, Marr N, Kamsteeg EJ, Van Balkom BWM: Nephrogenic diabetes insipidus. Curr Opin Nephrol Hypertens 9:591–595, 2000.

62. Bichet DG, Birnbaumer M, Lonergan M, et al: Nature and recurrence of *AVPR2* mutations in X-linked nephrogenic diabetes insipidus. Am J Hum Genet 55:278–286, 1994.

63. Bichet DG, Arthus M-F, Lonergan M, et al: X-linked nephrogenic diabetes insipidus mutations in North America and the Hopewell hypothesis. J Clin Invest 92:1262–1268, 1993.

64. Ellgaard L, Molinari M, Helenius A: Setting the standards: Quality control in the secretory pathway. Science 286:1882–1888, 1999.

65. Hobbs HH, Russell DW, Brown MS, Goldstein JL: The LDL receptor locus in familial hypercholesterolemia: Mutational analysis of a membrane protein. Annu Rev Genet 24:133–170, 1990.

66. Krause G, Hermosilla R, Oksche A, et al: Molecular and conformational features of a transport-relevant domain in the C-terminal tail of the vasopressin V$_2$ receptor. Mol Pharmacol 57:232–242, 2000.

67. Albertazzi E, Zanchetta D, Barbier P, et al: Nephrogenic diabetes insipidus: Functional analysis of new *AVPR2* mutations identified in Italian families. J Am Soc Nephrol 11:1033–1043, 2000.

68. Schoneberg T, Schulz A, Biebermann H, et al: V2 vasopressin receptor dysfunction in nephrogenic diabetes insipidus caused by different molecular mechanisms. Hum Mutat 12:196–205, 1998.

69. Morello JP, Salahpour A, Laperriere A, et al: Pharmacological chaperones rescue cell-surface expression and function of misfolded V2 vasopressin receptor mutants [see comments]. J Clin Invest 105:887–895, 2000.

70. Sadeghi H, Robertson GL, Bichet DG, et al: Biochemical basis of partial nephrogenic diabetes insipidus phenotypes. Mol Endocrinol 11:1806–1813, 1997.

71. Pasel K, Schulz A, Timmermann K, et al: Functional characterization of the molecular defects causing nephrogenic diabetes insipidus in eight families. J Clin Endocrinol Metab 85:1703–1710, 2000.

72. Robben JH, Knoers NVAM, Deen PM: Characterization of V2R mutants in nephrogenic diabetes insipidus in a polarized cell model. Am J Physiol Renal Physiol 289:F265–F272, 2005.

73. Rosenthal W, Antaramian A, Gilbert S, Birnbaumer M: Nephrogenic diabetes insipidus. A V2 vasopressin receptor unable to stimulate adenylyl cyclase. J Biol Chem 268:13030–13033, 1993.

74. Schulein R, Zuhlke K, Oksche A, et al: The role of conserved extracellular cysteine residues in vasopressin V2 receptor function and properties of two naturally occurring mutant receptors with additional extracellular cysteine residues [published erratum appears in FEBS Lett 473:24, 2000]. FEBS Lett 466:101–106, 2000.

75. Ala Y, Morin D, Mouillac B, et al: Functional studies of twelve mutant V2 vasopressin receptors related to nephrogenic diabetes insipidus: Molecular basis of a mild clinical phenotype. J Am Soc Nephrol 9:1861–1872, 1998.

76. Birnbaumer M, Gilbert S, Rosenthal W: An extracellular congenital nephrogenic diabetes insipidus mutation. Mol Endocrinol 8:886–894, 1994.

77. Pan Y, Wilson P, Gitschier J: The effect of eight V2 vasopressin receptor mutations on stimulation. J Biol Chem 269:31933–31937, 1994.

78. Tsukaguchi H, Matsubara H, Taketani S, et al: Binding-, intracellular transport-, and biosynthesis-defective mutants of vasopressin type 2 receptor in patients with X-linked nephrogenic diabetes insipidus. J Clin Invest 96:2043–2050, 1995.

79. Barak LS, Oakley RH, Laporte SA, Caron MG: Constitutive arrestin-mediated desensitization of a human vasopressin receptor mutant associated with nephrogenic diabetes insipidus. Proc Natl Acad Sci U S A 98:93–98, 2001.

80. Rosenthal W, Seibold A, Antaramian A, et al: Mutations in the vasopressin V2 receptor gene in families with nephrogenic diabetes insipidus and functional expression of the Q-2 mutant. Cell Mol Biol (Noisy-le-grand) 40:429–436, 1994.

81. Deen PMT, Weghuis DO, Sinke RJ, et al: Assignment of the human gene for the water channel of renal collecting duct aquaporin 2 (AQP2) to chromosome 12 region q12–q13. Cytogenet Cell Genet 66:260–262, 1994.

82. Sasaki S, Fushimi K, Saito H, et al: Cloning, characterization, and chromosomal mapping of human aquaporin of collecting duct. J Clin Invest 93:1250–1256, 1994.

83. Murata K, Mitsuoka K, Hirai T, et al: Structural determinants of water permeation through aquaporin-1. Nature 407:599–605, 2000.

84. Jung JS, Preston GM, Smith BL, et al: Molecular structure of the water channel through aquaporin CHIP. The hourglass model. J Biol Chem 269:14648–14654, 1994.

85. De Mattia F, Savelkoul PJ, Bichet DG, et al: A novel mechanism in recessive nephrogenic diabetes insipidus: Wild-type aquaporin-2 rescues the apical membrane expression of intracellularly retained AQP2-P262L. Hum Mol Genet 13:3045–3056, 2004.

86. Tamarappoo BK, Verkman AS: Defective aquaporin-2 trafficking in nephrogenic diabetes insipidus and correction by chemical chaperones. J Clin Invest 101:2257–2267, 1998.

87. Moses AM, Scheinman SJ, Oppenheim A: Marked hypotonic polyuria resulting from nephrogenic diabetes insipidus with partial sensitivity to vasopressin. J Clin Endocrinol Metab 59:1044–1049, 1984.

88. Marr N, Kamsteeg EJ, Van Raak M, et al: Functionality of aquaporin-2 missense mutants in recessive nephrogenic diabetes insipidus. Pflugers Arch 442:73–77, 2001.

89. Deen PMT, Croes H, van Aubel RA, et al: Water channels encoded by mutant aquaporin-2 genes in nephrogenic diabetes insipidus are impaired in their cellular routing. J Clin Invest 95:2291–2296, 1995.

90. Vargas-Poussou R, Forestier L, Dautzenberg MD, et al: Mutations in the vasopressin V2 receptor and aquaporin-2 genes in twelve families with congenital nephrogenic diabetes insipidus. Adv Exp Med Biol 449:387–390, 1998.

91. Hochberg Z, van Lieburg AF, Even L, et al: Autosomal recessive nephrogenic diabetes insipidus caused by an aquaporin-2 mutation. J Clin Endocrinol Metab 82:686–689, 1997.

92. Lin SH, Bichet DG, Sasaki S, et al: Two novel aquaporin-2 mutations responsible for congenital nephrogenic diabetes insipidus in Chinese families. J Clin Endocrinol Metab 87:2694–2700, 2002.

93. Mulders SM, Knoers NVAM, van Lieburg AF, et al: New mutations in the *AQP2* gene in nephrogenic diabetes insipidus resulting in functional but misrouted water channels. J Am Soc Nephrol 8:242–248, 1997.

94. Boccalandro C, De Mattia F, Guo DC, et al: Characterization of an aquaporin-2 water channel gene mutation causing partial nephrogenic diabetes insipidus in a Mexican family: Evidence of increased frequency of the mutation in the town of origin. J Am Soc Nephrol 15:1223–1231, 2004.

95. Kuwahara M: Aquaporin-2, a vasopressin-sensitive water channel, and nephrogenic diabetes insipidus. Intern Med 37:215–217, 1998.

96. Goji K, Kuwahara M, Gu Y, et al: Novel mutations in aquaporin-2 gene in female siblings with nephrogenic diabetes insipidus: Evidence of disrupted water channel function. J Clin Endocrinol Metab 83:3205–3209, 1998.

97. Marr N, Bichet DG, Hoefs S, et al: Cell-biologic and functional analyses of five new aquaporin-2 missense mutations that cause recessive nephrogenic diabetes insipidus. J Am Soc Nephrol 13:2267–2277, 2002.

98. Canfield MC, Tamarappoo BK, Moses AM, et al: Identification and characterization of aquaporin-2 water channel mutations causing nephrogenic diabetes insipidus with partial vasopressin response. Hum Mol Genet 6:1865–1871, 1997.

99. van Lieburg AF, Verdijk MAJ, Knoers NVAM, et al: Patients with autosomal nephrogenic diabetes insipidus homozygous for mutations in the aquaporin 2 water-channel gene. Am J Hum Genet 55:648–652, 1994.

100. Guyon C, Bissonnette P, Lussier Y, et al: Novel aquaporin-2 (AQP2) mutations responsible for autosomal recessive nephrogenic diabetes insipidus (Abstract). J Am Soc Nephrol 2004.

101. Oksche A, Moller A, Dickson J, et al: Two novel mutations in the aquaporin-2 and the vasopressin V2 receptor genes in patients with congenital nephrogenic diabetes insipidus. Hum Genet 98:587–589, 1996.

102. Deen PMT, Verdijk MAJ, Knoers NVAM, et al: Requirement of human renal water channel aquaporin-2 for vasopressin-dependent concentration of urine. Science 264:92–95, 1994.

103. Hirano K, Zuber C, Roth J, Ziak M: The proteasome is involved in the degradation of different aquaporin-2 mutants causing nephrogenic diabetes insipidus. Am J Pathol 163:111–120, 2003.

104. Buck TM, Eledge J, Skach WR: Evidence for stabilization of aquaporin-2 folding mutants by N-linked glycosylation in endoplasmic reticulum. Am J Physiol Cell Physiol 287:C1292–C1299, 2004.

105. Deen PMT, van Aubel RA, van Lieburg AF, van Os CH: Urinary content of aquaporin 1 and 2 in nephrogenic diabetes insipidus. J Am Soc Nephrol 7:836–841, 1996.

106. Kanno K, Sasaki S, Hirata Y, et al: Urinary excretion of aquaporin-2 in patients with diabetes insipidus. N Engl J Med 332:1540–1545, 1995.

107. Kamsteeg EJ, Deen PMT: Importance of aquaporin-2 expression levels in genotype -phenotype studies in nephrogenic diabetes insipidus. Am J Physiol Renal Physiol 279:F778-F784, 2000.

108. Marr N, Bichet DG, Lonergan M, et al: Heteroligomerization of an aquaporin-2 mutant with wild-type aquaporin-2 and their misrouting to late endosomes/lysosomes explains dominant nephrogenic diabetes insipidus. Hum Mol Genet 11:779–789, 2002.

109. De Mattia F, Savelkoul PJM, Kamsteeg EJ, et al: Lack of arginine vasopressin-induced phosphorylation of the aquaporin-2 mutant AQP2-R254L explains dominant nephrogenic diabetes insipidus. J Am Soc Nephrol 16:2872–2880, 2005.

110. Mulders SM, Bichet DG, Rijss JPL, et al: An aquaporin-2 water channel mutant which causes autosomal dominant nephrogenic diabetes insipidus is retained in the Golgi complex. J Clin Invest 102:57–66, 1998.

111. Kamsteeg EJ, Bichet DG, Konings IB, et al: Reversed polarized delivery of an aquaporin-2 mutant causes dominant nephrogenic diabetes insipidus. J Cell Biol 163:1099–1109, 2003.

112. Kuwahara M, Iwai K, Ooeda T, et al: Three families with autosomal dominant nephrogenic diabetes insipidus caused by aquaporin-2 mutations in the C-terminus. Am J Hum Genet 69:738–748, 2001.

113. Hirano K, Roth J, Zuber C, Ziak M: Expression of a mutant ER-retained polytope membrane protein in cultured rat hepatocytes results in Mallory body formation. Histochem Cell Biol 117:41–53, 2002.

114. Heilker R, Spiess M, Crottet P: Recognition of sorting signals by clathrin adaptors. Bioessays 21:558–567, 1999.

115. Crawford JD, Kennedy GC: Chlorothiazid in diabetes insipidus. Nature 183:891–892, 1959.

116. Monnens LAH, Jonkman A, Thomas C: Response to indomethacin and hydrochlorothiazide in nephrogenic. Clin Sci 66:709–715, 1984.

117. Alon U, Chan JC: Hydrochlorothiazide-amiloride in the treatment of congenital nephrogenic diabetes insipidus. Am J Nephrol 5:9–13, 1985.

118. Rascher W, Rosendahl W, Henrichs IA, et al: Congenital nephrogenic diabetes insipidus-vasopressin and prostaglandins in response to treatment with hydrochlorothiazide and indomethacin. Pediatr Nephrol 1:485–490, 1987.

119. Jakobsson B, Berg U: Effect of hydrochlorothiazide and indomethacin treatment on renal function in nephrogenic diabetes insipidus. Acta Paediatr 83:522–525, 1994.

120. Kirchlechner V, Koller DY, Seidl R, Waldhauser F: Treatment of nephrogenic diabetes insipidus with hydrochlorothiazide and amiloride. Arch Dis Child 80:548–552, 1999.

121. Konoshita T, Kuroda M, Kawane T, et al: Treatment of congenital nephrogenic diabetes insipidus with hydrochlorothiazide and amiloride in an adult patient. Horm Res 61:63–67, 2004.

122. Pattaragarn A, Alon US: Treatment of congenital nephrogenic diabetes insipidus by hydrochlorothiazide and cyclooxygenase-2 inhibitor. Pediatr Nephrol 18:1073–1076, 2003.

123. Singh D: Merck withdraws arthritis drug worldwide. BMJ 329:816, 2004.

124. Earley LE, Orloff J: The mechanism of antidiuresis associated with the administration of hydrochlorothiazide to patients with vasopressin-resistant diabetes insipidus. J Clin Invest 41:1988–1997, 1992.

125. Shirley DG, Walter SJ, Laycock JF: The antidiuretic effect of chronic hydrochlorothiazide treatment in rats with diabetes insipidus: Renal mechanisms. Clin Sci (Lond) 63:533–538, 1982.

126. Cesar KR, Magaldi AJ: Thiazide induces water absorption in the inner medullary collecting duct of normal and Brattleboro rats. Am J Physiol 277:F756–F760, 1999.

127. Magaldi AJ: New insights into the paradoxical effect of thiazides in diabetes insipidus therapy. Nephrol Dial Transplant 15:1903–1905, 2000.

128. Kim GH, Lee JW, Oh YK, et al: Antidiuretic effect of hydrochlorothiazide in lithium-induced nephrogenic diabetes insipidus is associated with upregulation of aquaporin-2, Na-Cl co-transporter, and epithelial sodium channel. J Am Soc Nephrol 15:2836–2843, 2004.

129. Mizuno H, Fujimoto S, Sugiyama Y, et al: Successful treatment of partial nephrogenic diabetes insipidus with thiazide and desmopressin. Horm Res 59:297–300, 2003.

130. Inaba S, Hatakeyama H, Taniguchi N, Miyamori I: The property of a novel V2 receptor mutant in a patient with nephrogenic diabetes insipidus. J Clin Endocrinol Metab 86:381–385, 2001.

131. Kalenga K, Persu A, Goffin E, et al: Intrafamilial phenotype variability in nephrogenic diabetes insipidus. Am J Kidney Dis 39:737–743, 2002.

132. Schoneberg T, Yun JN, Wenkert D, Wess J: Functional rescue of mutant V2 vasopressin receptors causing nephrogenic diabetes insipidus by a co-expressed receptor polypeptide. EMBO J 15:1283–1291, 1996.

133. Schulz A, Sangkuhl K, Lennert T, et al: Aminoglycoside pretreatment partially restores the function of truncated V^2

vasopressin receptors found in patients with nephrogenic diabetes insipidus. J Clin Endocrinol Metab 87:5247–5257, 2002.

134. Morello JP, Petaja-Repo UE, Bichet DG, Bouvier M: Pharmacological chaperones: A new twist on receptor folding. Trends Pharmacol Sci 21:466–469, 2000.

135. Bernier V, Lagace M, Lonergan M, et al: Functional rescue of the constitutively internalized V2 vasopressin receptor mutant R137H by the pharmacological chaperone action of SR49059. Mol Endocrinol 18:2074–2084, 2004.

136. Tan CM, Nickols HH, Limbird LE: Appropriate polarization following pharmacological rescue of V2 vasopressin receptors encoded by X-linked nephrogenic diabetes insipidus alleles involves a conformation of the receptor that also attains mature glycosylation. J Biol Chem 278:35678–35686, 2003.

137. Oksche A, Schulein R, Rutz C, et al: Vasopressin V2 receptor mutants that cause X-linked nephrogenic diabetes insipidus: Analysis of expression, processing, and function. Mol Pharmacol 50:820–828, 1996.

138. Oksche A, Dickson J, Schulein R, et al: Two novel mutations in the vasopressin V2 receptor gene in patients. Biochem Biophys Res Commun 205:552–557, 1994.

139. Knoers NV, van den Ouweland AM, Verdijk M, et al: Inheritance of mutations in the V2 receptor gene in thirteen families with nephrogenic diabetes insipidus. Kidney Int 46:170–176, 1994.

140. Andersen-Beckh B, Dehe M, Schulein R, et al: Polarized expression of the vasopressin V2 receptor in Madin-Darby canine kidney cells. Kidney Int 56:517–527, 1999.

141. Arthus MF, Lonergan M, Crumley MJ, et al: Report of 33 novel AVPR2 mutations and analysis of 117 families with X-linked nephrogenic diabetes insipidus. J Am Soc Nephrol 11:1044–1054, 2000.

142. Rocha JL, Friedman E, Boson W, et al: Molecular analyses of the vasopressin type 2 receptor and aquaporin-2 genes in Brazilian kindreds with nephrogenic diabetes insipidus. Hum Mutat 14:233–239, 1999.

143. Mizuno H, Sugiyama Y, Ohro Y, et al: Clinical characteristics of eight patients with congenital nephrogenic diabetes insipidus. Endocrine 24:55–59, 2004.

144. Innamorati G, Sadeghi H, Eberle AN, Birnbaumer M: Phosphorylation of the V2 vasopressin receptor. J Biol Chem 272:2486–2492, 1997.

145. Sadeghi HM, Innamorati G, Esqueda E, Birnbaumer M: Processing and ligand-induced modifications of the V2 vasopressin receptor. Adv Exp Med Biol 449:339–346, 1998.

146. Sadeghi HM, Innamorati G, Birnbaumer M: Maturation of receptor proteins in eukaryotic expression systems. J Rec Sign Transd Res 17:433–445, 1997.

147. Barak LS, Ferguson SSG, Zhang J, et al: Internal trafficking and surface mobility of a functionally intact (beta2adrenergic) receptor-green fluorescent protein conjugate. Mol Pharmacol 51:177–184, 1997.

148. Wuller S, Wiesner B, Loffler A, et al: Pharmacochaperones post-translationally enhance cell surface expression by increasing conformational stability of wild-type and mutant vasopressin V2 receptors. J Biol Chem 279:47254–47263, 2004.

149. Wildin RS, Cogdell DE, Valadez V: AVPR2 variants and V2 vasopressin receptor function in nephrogenic diabetes insipidus. Kidney Int 54:1909–1922, 1998.

150. Schulz A, Grosse R, Schultz G, et al: Structural implication for receptor oligomerization from functional reconstitution studies of mutant V2 vasopressin receptors. J Biol Chem 275:2381–2389, 2000.

151. Schulein R, Zuhlke K, Krause G, Rosenthal W: Functional rescue of the nephrogenic diabetes insipidus–causing vasopressin V2 receptor mutants G185C and R202C by a second site suppressor mutation. J Biol Chem 276:8384–8392, 2001.

152. Wenkert D, Schoneberg T, Merendino JJ, et al: Functional characterization of five V2 vasopressin receptor gene mutations. Mol Cell Endocrinol 124:43–50, 1996.

153. van Lieburg AF, Verdijk MAJ, Knoers NVAM, et al: In vitro expression of mutations in the V2 receptor gene-confirmation of their role in the pathogenesis of X-linked nephrogenic diabetes insipidus. Pediatr Nephrol 8:-c75, 1994.
Ref Type: Abstract

154. Postina R, Ufer E, Pfeiffer R, et al: Misfolded vasopressin V2 receptors caused by extracellular point mutations entail congential nephrogenic diabetes insipidus. Mol Cell Endocrinol 164:31–39, 2000.

155. Hermosilla R, Oueslati M, Donalies U, et al: Disease-causing vasopressin receptors are retained in different compartments of the early secretory pathway. Traffic 5:993–1005, 2004.

156. Chen CH, Chen WY, Liu HL, et al: Identification of mutations in the arginine vasopressin receptor 2 gene causing nephrogenic diabetes insipidus in Chinese patients. J Hum Genet 47:66–73, 2002.

157. Morello JP, Salahpour A, Petaja-Repo UE, et al: Association of calnexin with wild type and mutant AVPR2 that causes nephrogenic diabetes insipidus. Biochemistry 40:6766–6775, 2001.

Chapter 19

Genetic Disorders of Calcium and Phosphate Homeostasis

Harald W. Jüppner and Rajesh V. Thakker

Calcium and phosphate homeostasis is essential for bone integrity and involves several different hormonal regulators that act on kidney, intestine, and bone. For example, extracellular calcium ion concentration is tightly regulated through the actions of parathyroid hormone (PTH) on kidney and bone. The intact peptide is secreted by the parathyroid glands at a rate that is appropriate to, and dependent upon, the prevailing extracellular calcium ion concentration. Hypercalcemic or hypocalcemic disorders can be classified according to whether they arise from an excess or deficiency of PTH, a defect in the PTH receptor (i.e., the PTH/PTHrP receptor), or an insensitivity to PTH caused by defects downstream of the PTH/PTHrP receptor. Recent advances in understanding the biologic importance of key proteins involved in the regulation of PTH secretion and the responsiveness to PTH in target tissues have led to the identification of molecular defects in a variety of disorders and thus have permitted the characterization of some of the mechanisms involved in the regulation of parathyroid gland development, parathyroid cell proliferation, PTH secretion, and PTH-mediated actions in target tissues. Thus, mutations in the calcium-sensing receptor (CaSR) gene have been reported in patients with familial benign (hypocalciuric) hypercalcemia (FBH or FHH), neonatal severe hyperparathyroidism, and autosomal dominant hypocalcemia. Furthermore, the roles of the oncogene PRAD1, which encodes a novel cyclin, and of the multiple endocrine neoplasia type 1 (MEN1) and the hyperparathyroidism–jaw tumor (HPT-JT) genes, in the pathogenesis of some parathyroid tumors have been revealed (Fig. 19-1). In addition, mutations in the genes encoding PTH or GATA3, and in the mitochondrial genome have been demonstrated to be associated with some forms of hypoparathyroidism, and mutations in the PTH/PTHrP receptor gene have been identified in patients with two rare genetic disorders, Jansen's and Blomstrand's chondrodysplasia. Mutations in the GNAS gene, which encodes the stimulatory G protein (Gsα), have been found in individuals with McCune-Albright syndrome, pseudohypoparathyroidism type Ia (PHP-Ia), pseudopseudohypoparathyroidism (pPHP), and progressive osseous heteroplasia, and mutations in presumably regulatory regions upstream of or within GNAS were identified in pseudohypoparathyroidism type Ib (PHP-Ib). Furthermore, the gene associated with the DiGeorge syndrome (DGS) has been identified, and the chromosomal locations for the susceptibility genes that are responsible for the less frequent variants of FBH and Williams syndrome have been established.

Less is known about the hormonal factors involved in the regulation of extracellular phosphate concentration. However, considerable advances have recently led to the identification and characterization of several proteins that increase renal phosphate excretion (Fig. 19-2). These include fibroblast growth factor 23 (FGF23), which causes, when mutated, autosomal dominant hypophosphatemic rickets (ADHR) or an autosomal recessive form of tumoral calcinosis. Furthermore, patients with oncogenic osteomalacia (OOM) (also referred to as tumor-induced osteomalacia, TIO) and with X-linked hypophosphatemia (XLH) often have significantly increased plasma FGF23 concentrations, and the application of recombinant FGF23 leads to increased urinary phosphate excretion and hypophosphatemia in vivo, indicating that this protein is likely to be a major physiologic regulator of phosphate homeostasis. Other proteins like soluble frizzled-related protein (sFRP4), matrix extracellular phosphoglycoprotein (MEPE), and FGF7 also affect phosphate handling in vivo or in vitro, but their roles in regulating phosphate homeostasis require further exploration. In addition, mutations in PHEX (phosphate-regulating protein with homologies to endopeptidases encoded by a gene on the X chromosome) cause XLH; heterozygous mutations in SLC34A1, the gene encoding the Na/phosphate cotransporter NPT-2a, result in a form of nephrolithiasis that is associated with osteoporosis and hypophosphatemia; homozygous or compound heterozygous mutations in SLC34A3, the gene encoding the recently identified Na/phosphate cotransporter NPT-2c, seem to be a frequent cause of hereditary hypophosphatemic rickets with hypercalciuria (HHRH); mutations in GALNT3, which encodes a glycosyltransferase responsible for initiating mucin-type O-linked glycosylation, are the cause of the hyperphosphatemic, autosomal recessive form of tumoral calcinosis; and a mutation in the type 1 FGF receptor seems to be the cause of a distinct form of autosomal dominant hypophosphatemic rickets associated with craniofacial dysplasia (CFDH). Molecular genetic studies in particular have thus provided important new insights into the pathogenesis of rare disorders of calcium and phosphate homeostasis. These advances will be reviewed in this chapter.

REGULATORS OF CALCIUM AND PHOSPHATE HOMEOSTASIS

Parathyroid Hormone and PTH-Related Peptide

The PTH gene is located on chromosome 11p15 and consists of three exons that are separated by two introns.[1] Exon 1 of the PTH gene is 85 base pairs (bp) in length and is

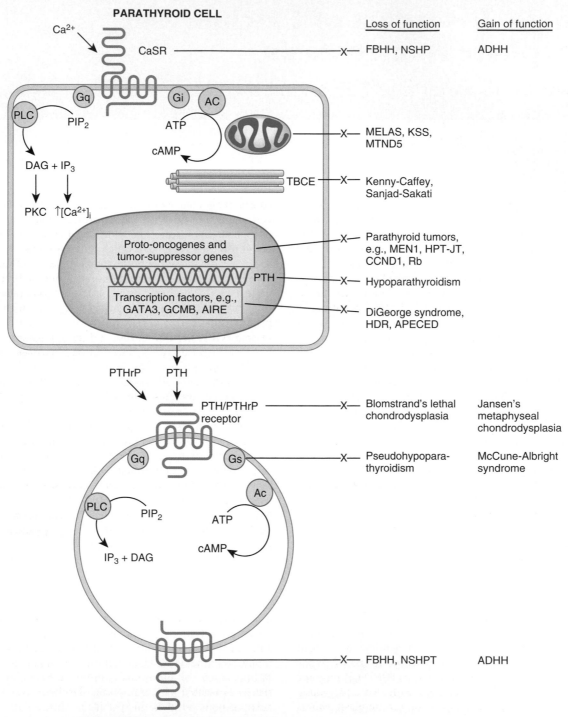

Figure 19-1 Schematic representation of some of the components involved in calcium homeostasis. Alterations in extracellular calcium are detected by the calcium-sensing receptor (CaSR), a G protein–coupled receptor. The PTH/PTHrP receptor, which mediates the actions of PTH and PTHrP, is also a G protein–coupled receptor. Thus, Ca^{2+}, PTH, and PTHrP involve G protein–coupled signaling pathways and activation of different α-subunits (i.e., Gs, Gi, and Gq, respectively). Gso stimulates adenylyl cyclase (AC), which catalyzes the formation of cAMP from ATP. Gi inhibits AC activity. cAMP stimulates protein kinase A which phosphorylates cell-specific substrates. Activation of Gq stimulates phospholipase C, which catalyzes the hydrolysis of the phosphoinositide (PIP_2) to inositol triphosphate (IP_3), which increases intracellular calcium, and diacylglycerol (DAG), which activates protein kinase C. These proximal signals modulate downstream pathways, which result in specific physiologic effects. Abnormalities in several genes, which lead to mutations in proteins in these pathways, have been identified in specific disorders of calcium homeostasis (see Table 19-1). (Adapted from Thakker R, Jüppner H: Genetics disorders of calcium homeostasis caused by abnormal regulation of parathyoid hormone secretion or responsiveness. In DeGroot L, Jameson J [eds]: Endocrinology. Philadelphia, WB Saunders, 2000, pp 1062–1074.)

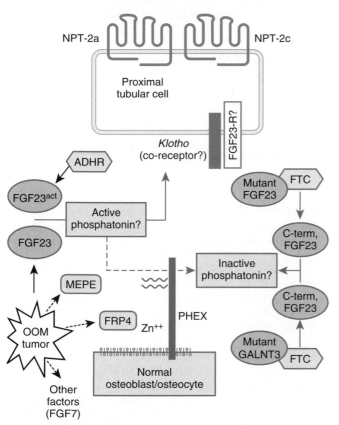

Figure 19-2 Roles of FGF23, PHEX, and other proteins in regulating phosphate homeostasis. Wild-type FGF23, possibly representing a putative "phosphatonin", is produced in abundant amounts by tumors that cause OOM. FGF23 seems to mediate its actions through one of the known FGF receptors, with Klotho being a plausible co-receptor.[34,35,35a] As a result of these actions NPT-2a and NPT-2c expression is diminished, thus reducing tubular phosphate reabsorption and leading to urinary phosphate wasting. Wild-type FGF23 seems to be cleaved into an inactive protein. This process may involve, directly or indirectly, PHEX, an endopeptidase that is most abundantly expressed on osteoblasts and osteocytes. Genetic mutations, rendering FGF23 resistant to cleavage (FGF23^{act}) lead to increased phosphaturic activity in renal tubules. Homozygous inactivating mutations in the genes encoding FGF23 or GALNT3, which have been identified in patients with familial forms of tumoral calcinosis and hyperostosis with hyperphosphatemia[264–266,270]; both mutations lead to the generation of excess amounts of C-terminal FGF23 fragments, which are likely to be biologically inactive. Note that other proteins produced by OOM tumors, such as MEPE or sFRP4, have also been implicated in renal phosphate wasting.[45,46] MEPE is a 525–amino acid protein that is a member of the short integrin-binding ligand N-linked glycoprotein (SIBLING) family, which includes also osteopontin and dentin matrix protein 1. Although MEPE administration to mice leads to hypophosphatemia and hyperphosphaturia,[46] it results also in a dose-dependent increase of serum 1,25(OH)$_2$ vitamin D and a decrease in serum alkaline phosphatase; these features are not observed in patients with XLH and OOM.[350,351] sFRPs, an extracellular inhibitor of Wnt signaling, inhibits sodium-dependent phosphate transport in OK cells, and sFRP4 infusion in rats results in hypophosphatemia and hyperphosphaturia, *continued*

untranslated (Fig. 19-3), whereas exons 2 and 3 encode the 115–amino acid pre-proPTH peptide. Exon 2 is 90 bp in length and encodes the initiation (ATG) codon, the pre-hormone sequence, and part of the prohormone sequence. Exon 3 is 612 bp in size and encodes the remainder of the prohormone sequence, the 84 amino acids composing the mature PTH peptide, and the 3′ untranslated region.[2] The 5′ regulatory sequence of the human PTH gene contains a vitamin D response element 125 bp upstream of the transcription start site, which downregulates PTH messenger RNA (mRNA) transcription in response to vitamin D receptor binding.[3,4] PTH gene transcription (as well as PTH peptide secretion) is also dependent on the extracellular calcium and phosphate[5,6] concentration, although the presence of specific upstream "calcium or phosphate response element(s)" has not yet been demonstrated.[7,8] The secretion of mature PTH from the parathyroid chief cell is regulated through a G protein–coupled CaSR, which is also expressed in renal tubules and in several other tissues, albeit at lower abundance. PTH mRNA is first translated into a pre-proPTH peptide. The "pre" sequence consists of a 25–amino acid signal peptide (leader sequence), which is responsible for directing the nascent peptide into the endoplasmic reticulum to be packaged for secretion from the cell.[9] The "pro" sequence is 6 amino acids in length and, although its function is less well defined than that of the "pre" sequence, it is also essential for correct PTH processing and secretion.[9] After the mature PTH peptide containing 84 amino acids is secreted from the parathyroid cell, it is cleared from the circulation with a short half-life of about 2 minutes, via nonsaturable hepatic and renal uptake.[10]

The PTH-related peptide (PTHrP; also known as PTHrH, PTH-related hormone), which was discovered and characterized almost two decades ago, most probably shares an evolutionary origin with PTH.[11–13] PTHrP has, at least in mammals, both chemical and functional overlaps with PTH. Thus, when secreted in large concentrations, for example, by certain tumors, PTHrP has PTH-like properties. Typically, however, it functions as an autocrine/paracrine rather than an endocrine factor.[14] PTHrP is a larger, more complex protein than PTH and is synthesized at multiple sites in different organs and tissues.[15,16] One of its most prominent functions is the regulation of chondrocyte proliferation and differentiation and, consequently, bone elongation and growth.[17] The human PTHrP gene is located on chromosome 12p12.1–p11.2, which has a region analogous to that containing the human PTH gene on chromosome 11p15.[15,16] Both the PTH and the PTHrP genes have a similar organization, including equivalent positions of the boundaries between some of the coding exons and the adjacent introns (see Fig. 19-3).[10,15,16] Like the PTH gene, the PTHrP gene contains a single exon that encodes most amino acid residues of the prepropeptide sequence, and both genes have an exon that encodes the remainder of the

without altering serum PTH or 1,25(OH)$_2$ vitamin D concentrations[45]; however, the putative role of sFRP4 in skeletal homeostasis remains to be established. Furthermore, FGF7 was recently shown to regulate phosphate uptake in vitro.[44] (Adapted from Holm IA, Econs MJ, Carpenter TO [eds]: Familial Hypophosphatemia and Related Disorders. San Diego, Academic Press, 2003, pp 603–631.)

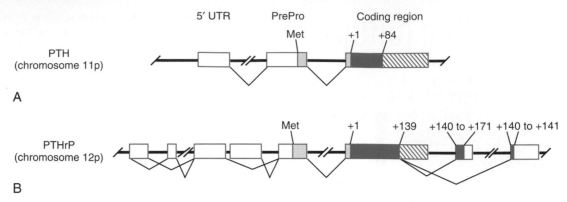

Figure 19-3 Schematic representation of the genes encoding PTH (**A**) and PTHrP (**B**). The introns are represented by a solid line; the coding and noncoding exons are shown. Met indicates the initiator methionine of the PrePro sequences. Numbers, representing amino acid positions, indicate the first and the last amino acid residue encoded by the different exons.

propeptide sequence, that is, two basic residues (lysine and arginine) that are required for endoproteolytic cleavage of the mature peptide. Overall, however, the PTHrP gene is more complex than the PTH gene, in that it uses at least three different promoters and alternative splice patterns that lead to the synthesis of several different mRNA species encoding peptides with different C-terminal ends.[10,16]

PTH and PTHrP both mediate their actions through a common receptor (see Fig. 19-1).[18,19] This PTH/PTHrP receptor is a member of a subgroup of G protein–coupled receptors; its gene is located on chromosome 3p21.3.[20,21] The PTH/PTHrP receptor is highly expressed in kidney and bone, where it mediates the endocrine actions of PTH. However, the most abundant expression of the PTH/PTHrP receptor occurs in chondrocytes of the metaphyseal growth plate where it mediates predominantly the autocrine/paracrine actions of PTHrP—in other words, it delays the hypertrophic differentiation of growth plate chondrocytes.[10,17,22] Mutations involving the genes that encode PTH, the CaSR, the PTH/PTHrP receptor, and Gsα all affect the regulation of calcium homeostasis and can thus be associated with genetic disorders characterized by hypercalcemia or hypocalcemia; mutations in PTHrP have not yet been described (Table 19-1).

Vitamin D and Its Metabolites

The biosynthesis, bioactivation, and physiologic actions of vitamin D involve several organs and regulatory steps. Despite fortification of foods with vitamin D, most of the vitamin D in healthy, active individuals is derived via the cutaneous synthesis pathway.[23,24] Thus, in the skin, 7-dehydrocholesterol is converted to cholecalciferol (vitamin D_3) by ultraviolet light (wavelength 290–310 nm).[23] Ergocalciferol (vitamin D_2) is the product of cutaneous ultraviolet irradiation of ergosterol, which is obtained from ingested animal or plant tissues or therapeutic supplements. Vitamin D should be regarded as a steroid hormone, not a nutrient, because it undergoes a series of bioactivation steps and binds to a nuclear receptor as follows. Vitamin D_2 and vitamin D_3 are prohormones that are transported by a high-affinity binding protein in the blood, to muscle or fat for storage, or to the liver and subsequently the kidney for bioactivation.[23,24] Vitamin D is hydroxylated in hepatocyte mitochondria by the enzyme P450c25, to form the

25-hydroxyvitamin D metabolite (25[OH]D), which is also called calcidiol. 25(OH)D is further hydroxylated in renal proximal convoluted tubular cells by the enzyme 25-hydroxyvitamin D, 1α-hydroxylase (1α-hydroxylase) to yield the potent, biologically active metabolite 1,25-dihydroxyvitamin D (1,25[OH]$_2$D), which is also called calcitriol.[23,24] The activity of 1α-hydroxylase is controlled by extracellular concentrations of ionized calcium, inorganic phosphate, PTH, and most likely FGF23. Calcitriol circulates to target organs (e.g., intestine, bones, kidneys, and parathyroids), where it binds to the intracellular vitamin D receptor (VDR).[25] The VDR activates the transcription of downstream genes in bone, kidney, and enterocytes to ensure adequate extracellular concentration of calcium and phosphate by increasing gut absorption of calcium, increased urinary calcium reclamation by the kidneys, increased bone resorption, and suppression of PTH synthesis.[24,25] Mutations in the genes encoding the 1α-hydroxylase and VDR are associated with some forms of rickets.[23,24]

Fibroblast Growth Factor 23 and Other Proteins with Phosphaturic Properties

FGF23 belongs to a large family of structurally related proteins. It was isolated through several independent approaches, including the homology-based search of genomic databases[26] and the sequence analysis of a large number of complementary DNAs (cDNAs) from tumors responsible for oncogenic osteomalacia.[27] However, it was primarily its identification through a positional cloning approach to determine the cause of ADHR[28] that provided first evidence for its involvement in the regulation of phosphate homeostasis. Consistent with such a biologic role, FGF23 mRNA and protein were found to be markedly overexpressed in tumors that cause oncogenic osteomalacia, suggesting that FGF23 promotes, either directly or indirectly, renal phosphate excretion.[29,30] The human FGF23 gene consists of three exons that span 10 kilobases (kb) of genomic sequence and encodes a 251–amino acid precursor protein comprising a hydrophobic amino acid sequence (residues 1–24), which probably serves as a leader sequence. Unlike most other FGFs, FGF23 thus appears to be efficiently secreted into the circulation.

FGF23 is most closely related to FGF21, FGF19, and FGF15 but shows limited homology also with other fibroblast growth

Table 19-1 Diseases of Calcium and Phosphorus Homeostasis and Their Chromosomal Locations

Primary Metabolic Abnormality	Disease	Inheritance	Gene Product	Chromosomal Location
Hypercalcemia	Multiple endocrine neoplasia type 1	Autosomal dominant	Menin	11q13
	Multiple endocrine neoplasia type 2	Autosomal dominant	Ret	10q11.2
	Hereditary hyperparathyroidism and jaw tumors (HPTJT)	Autosomal dominant	Parafibromin	1q31.1
	Hyperparathyroidism	Sporadic	PRAD1/CCND1	11q13
			Retinoblastoma	13q14
			Unknown	1p32-pter
	Parathyroid carcinoma	Sporadic	Parafibromin	1q25
	Familial benign hypercalcemia (FBH)			
	FBH1 FBH19p	Autosomal dominant	CaSR	3q21.1
	FBH2	Autosomal dominant	Unknown	19p13
	FBH3 (FBHOK)	Autosomal dominant	Unknown	19q13
	Neonatal severe hyperparathyroidism (NSHPT)	Autosomal recessive	CaSR	3q21.1
		Autosomal dominant		
	Jansen's disease	Autosomal dominant	PTHR/PTHrPR	3p21.3
	Williams syndrome	Autosomal dominant	Elastin, LIMK (and other genes)	7q11.23
	McCune-Albright syndrome	Somatic mutations during early embryonic development?	GNAS exon 8, R201	20q13.3
Hypocalcemia	Isolated hypoparathyroidism	Autosomal dominant	PTH	11p15*
		Autosomal recessive	PTH, GCMB	11p15*, 6p24.2
		X-linked recessive	SOX3	Xq26-27
	Hypocalcemic hypercalciuria	Autosomal dominant	CaSR	3q21.1
	Hypoparathyroidism associated with polyglandular autoimmune syndrome	Autosomal recessive	AIRE1	21q22.3
	Hypoparathyroidism associated with KSS, MELAS, and MTPDS	Maternal	Mitochondrial genome	
	Hypoparathyroidism associated with complex congenital syndromes			
	DiGeorge	Autosomal dominant	TBX1	22q11.2/10p
	HDR syndrome	Autosomal dominant	GATA3	10p14
	Blomstrand lethal chondrodysplasia	Autosomal recessive	PTHR/PTHrPR	3p21.3
	Kenney-Caffey, Sanjad-Sakati	Autosomal dominant/recessive†	TBCE	1q42.3
	Barakat	Autosomal recessive†	Unknown	?
	Lymphedema	Autosomal recessive	Unknown	?
	Nephropathy, nerve deafness	Autosomal dominant†	Unknown	?
	Nerve deafness without renal dysplasia	Autosomal dominant	Unknown	?
	Pseudohypoparathyroidism (type Ia)	Autosomal dominant, parentally imprinted	GNAS exons 1–13	20q13.3
	Pseudohypoparathyroidism (type Ib)	Autosomal dominant, parentally imprinted	Deletions within or upstream of GNAS locus	20q13.3

continued

Table 19-1 Diseases of Calcium and Phosphorus Homeostasis and Their Chromosomal Locations—Cont'd

Primary Metabolic Location	Disease	Inheritance	Gene Product	Chromosomal Abnormality
Hyperphosphatemia	Tumoral calcinosis	Autosomal recessive	GALNT3/FGF23	2q24-q31/12p13
	Hyperostosis with hyperphosphatemia	Autosomal recessive	GALNT3	2q24-q31
Hypophosphatemia	X-linked hypophosphatemia	X-linked, dominant	PHEX	Xp22.1
	Autosomal dominant hypophosphatemic rickets (ADHR)	Autosomal dominant	FGF23	12p13
	Craniofacial dysplasia with hypophosphatemia (CFDH)	Autosomal dominant	FGF receptor type I	8p11.2-p11.1
	Nephrolithiasis with osteoporosis and hypophosphatemia	Autosomal recessive	NPT-2a	5q35
	Hereditary hypophosphatemic rickets with hypercalciuria (HHRH)	Autosomal recessive	NPT-2c	9q34
	Lowe syndrome	X-linked, recessive	OCRL1	Xq25-q26
	Dent disease	X-linked, recessive	CLCN5	Xp11.22
	Vitamin D–independent rickets type I (VDDR I; pseudovitamin D deficiency)	Autosomal recessive	1α-hydroxylase, P450c1α	12q13
	Vitamin D–dependent rickets type II (VDDR II)	Autosomal recessive	Vitamin D receptor (VDR)	12q12-q14

HDR, hypoparathyroidism, deafness, renal dysplasia; KSS, Kearns-Sayre syndrome; MELAS, mitochondrial encephalopathy, strokelike episodes, and lactic acidosis; MTPDS, mitochondrial trifunctional protein deficiency syndrome.
*Mutations in the PTH gene identified only in some families with hypoparathyroidism.
†Most likely inheritance shown; location not known.

factors.[28,30] FGF23 mRNA could not be detected by Northern blot analysis in normal tissues, but it has been identified by reverse transcriptase–polymerase chain reaction in heart, liver, thymus, small intestine, brain, and osteoblasts, and by in situ hybridizations and through the use of *LacZ* fused to the endogenous mouse *Fgf23* promoter in bone cells.[28,30–32] A mutation in the type 1 FGF receptor (FGFR1) gene was recently shown to be the cause of a rare variant of ADHR associated with craniofacial dysplasia.[33] It furthermore appears that the type C splice variant of FGFR1, one of the other three FGF receptors, interacts with FGF23, possibly in conjunction with the Klotho gene product, which may be a co-receptor for FGF23.[34,35] In remains uncertain, however, whether additional, yet unknown receptors interact with FGF23.

Consistent with the hypothesis that FGF23 has phosphaturic properties (see Fig. 19-2), mice receiving the recombinant protein intraperitoneally and nude mice transplanted with cell lines stably expressing FGF23 develop hypophosphatemia due to increased urinary phosphate excretion.[30,36,37] Furthermore, these animals show increased alkaline phosphatase activity and low serum concentration of 1,25-dihydroxyvitamin D_3 ($1,25[OH]_2$ vitamin D_3), a marked increase of unmineralized osteoid, and significant widening of growth plates leading to deformities of weight-bearing bones. Similarly transgenic mice expressing FGF23 under the control of different promoters develop hypophosphatemia, renal phosphate wasting, and abnormal bone development.[38–40] Opposite findings were made in mice homozygous for the ablation of the *Fgf23* gene ($Fgf23^{-/-}$)—that is, these animals develop hyperphosphatemia and elevated serum $1,25(OH)_2$ vitamin D_3 concentration, and they die prematurely, partly because of renal failure secondary to calcifications of glomerular capillaries.[32,41] $Fgf23^{-/-}$ animals furthermore showed reduced bone turnover, an unexpected increased osteoid, and diminished osteoblast and osteoclast number and activity.[41]

Based on these findings, FGF23 is likely to be an important endocrine regulator of phosphate homeostasis (see Fig. 19-2). It remains uncertain, however, whether FGF23 acts directly or indirectly on renal tubular cells in vivo, because results from in vitro experiments with recombinant FGF23 using opossum kidney cells are inconsistent. Whereas one group showed an inhibitory effect of recombinant FGF23 on phosphate transport that was abolished by heparin,[42] another group showed that heparin was essential for the inhibitory effect of FGF23,[43] and a third group using a different opossum kidney cell subclone and experimental conditions without heparin failed to document an inhibition of phosphate uptake.[30] Furthermore, it remains uncertain whether the severe secondary hyperparathyroidism observed when FGF23 is expressed in transgenic animals contributes significantly to the changes in mineral ion homeostasis.[38,40]

Besides FGF23, MEPE, sFRP, and FGF7 were also shown to be over-represented in OOM tumor–derived cDNA libraries,[27,44] and all three affect phosphaturic handling in vivo and/or in vitro (see Fig. 19-2).[44–46] However, at least sFRP does not appear to circulate at elevated concentrations in patients with OOM,[45] making it less likely that sFRP has a major role in phosphate regulation. Furthermore, the mammalian homologs of stanniocalcin 1 and stanniocalcin 2 stimulate and inhibit renal phosphate reabsorption, respectively,[47–49] but their biologic importance remains unknown. Besides FGF23, several additional proteins may thus be

involved in the regulation of phosphate homeostasis (see Fig. 19-2), but the underlying regulatory pathways remain to be explored.

In summary, protein purification and molecular cloning techniques, and particularly the exploration of rare genetic disorders through positional cloning or candidate gene approaches, have provided important new insights and unique molecular tools, which will help in determining the pathogenesis of common and uncommon disorders associated with an abnormal regulation of calcium and phosphate.

HYPERCALCEMIA AND HYPOPHOSPHATEMIA DUE TO INCREASED PARATHYROID GLAND ACTIVITY

Similar to the findings in other tumor syndromes, the abnormal expression of an oncogene or the loss of a tumor suppressor gene can result in an abnormal proliferative activity of parathyroid cells, and the molecular exploration of these genes has provided important novel insights into the pathogenesis of different forms of hyperparathyroidism. Oncogenes are genes whose abnormal expression may transform a normal cell into a tumor cell. The normal form of the gene is referred to as a proto-oncogene, and a single mutant allele may affect the phenotype of the cell; these genes may also be referred to as dominant oncogenes (Fig. 19-4A). The mutant versions (i.e., the oncogenes), which are usually excessively or inappropriately active, may arise because of point mutations, gene amplifications, or chromosomal translocations. Tumor suppressor genes, also referred to as recessive oncogenes or anti-oncogenes, normally inhibit cell proliferation, whereas their mutant versions in cancer cells have lost their normal function. To transform a normal cell into a tumor cell, both alleles of the tumor suppressor gene must be inactivated. Inactivation arises by point mutations, or, alternatively, by small or larger intragenic deletions that can involve substantial genomic portions or a whole chromosome. Larger deletions may be detected by cytogenetic methods, by Southern blot analysis, or by analysis of polymorphic markers based on polymerase chain reaction. Typically, genomic DNA from the patient's tumor cells lack, in comparison to genomic DNA from other cells (e.g., leukocytes), certain chromosomal regions; this finding is therefore referred to as loss of heterozygosity (LOH) (Fig. 19-4B). Finding LOH therefore suggests an inactivating mutation or deletion in the other allele.

Parathyroid Tumors

Parathyroid tumors may occur as an isolated and sporadic endocrinopathy, or as part of inherited tumor syndromes[50] such as the multiple endocrine neoplasias (MEN) or hereditary hyperparathyroidism with jaw tumors (HPT-JT),[51] or in response to chronic overstimulation as in uremic hyperparathyroidism.[52] Genetic analyses of kindreds with MEN1 and MEN2A, and of tumor tissue from patients with single parathyroid adenomas have shown that some of the molecular mechanisms known to be involved in tumor genesis can also be responsible for the development of hyperparathyroidism.

Our current understanding indicates that sporadic parathyroid tumors are caused by single somatic mutations that lead

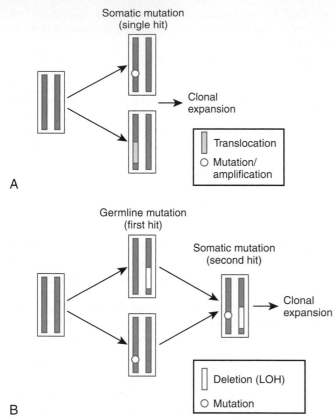

A

B

Figure 19-4 Schematic illustration of the molecular defects that can lead to the development of parathyroid tumors. **A,** A somatic mutation (point mutation or translocation) affecting a proto-oncogene (e.g., *PRAD1* or *RET*) results in a growth advantage of single parathyroid cell and thus its clonal expansion. **B,** An inherited single-point mutation or deletion affecting a tumor suppressor gene (first hit) makes the parathyroid cell susceptible to a second, somatic "hit" (point mutation or deletion, i.e., LOH), which then leads to the clonal expansion of a single cell.

to the activation or overexpression of proto-oncogenes such as *PRAD1* (parathyroid adenoma 1) or *RET* (see Fig. 19-4A). Furthermore, different tumor suppressor genes affecting the parathyroid glands are predicted to be located on several different chromosomes, and in a significant number of patients, LOH has been documented for one of these loci. For all these somatic mutations, a single-point mutation or a deletion provides a growth advantage of a single parathyroid cell and its progeny leading to their clonal expansion.

In hereditary forms of the disease, two distinct, sequentially occurring molecular defects are observed. The first "hit" (point mutation or deletion) is an inherited genetic defect, which affects only one allele that comprises a gene encoding an anti-oncogene (see Fig. 19-4B). Subsequently, a somatic mutation or deletion affecting the second allele occurs in a single parathyroid cell and this mutation leads, because of the resulting growth advantage, to its monoclonal expansion and thus the development of parathyroid tumors. Examples of this latter molecular mechanism in the development of hyperparathyroidism are the inactivation of tumor suppressor genes such as the multiple endocrine neoplasia type 1 (MEN1) gene, the hyperparathyroidism-jaw tumor (HPT-JT) gene, the

retinoblastoma (Rb) gene, and a yet unknown gene located on chromosome 1p (see Table 19-1).

PRAD1 Gene

Investigations of the PTH gene in sporadic parathyroid adenomas detected abnormally sized restriction fragment length polymorphisms (RFLPs) with a DNA probe for the 5′ part of the PTH gene in some adenomas,[53] indicating disruption of the gene. Further studies of the tumor DNA demonstrated that the first exon of the PTH gene (see Fig. 19-3) was separated from the fragments containing the second and third exons, and that a rearrangement had occurred juxtaposing the 5′ PTH regulatory elements with "new" non-PTH DNA.[54] This rearrangement was not found in the DNA from the peripheral leukocytes of the patients, thereby indicating that it represented a somatic event and not an inherited germline mutation. Investigation of this rearranged DNA sequence localized it to chromosome 11q13, and detailed analysis revealed that it was highly conserved in different species and expressed in normal parathyroids and in parathyroid adenomas. The protein expressed as a result of this rearrangement, which was designated PRAD1 (parathyroid adenoma 1), was demonstrated to encode a 295–amino acid member of the cyclin D family of cell cycle regulatory proteins. Cyclins were initially characterized in the dividing cells of budding yeast where they controlled the G_1 to S transition of the cell cycle and in marine mollusks where they regulated the mitotic phase (M phase) of the cell cycle.[55] Cyclins have also been identified in humans and have an important role in regulating many stages of cell cycle progression. Thus, PRAD1, which encodes a novel cyclin referred to as cyclin D1 (CCND1), is an important cell cycle regulator, and overexpression of PRAD1 may be an important event in the development of at least 15% of sporadic parathyroid adenomas.[56,57]

Interestingly, more than 66% of the transgenic mice overexpressing PRAD1 under the control of a mammary tissue–specific promoter were found to develop breast carcinoma in adult life,[58] and expression of this proto-oncogene under the control of the 5′ regulatory region of the PTH gene resulted in mild-to-moderate chronic hyperparathyroidism.[56,57] Taken together, these findings in transgenic animals provide further evidence for the conclusion that PRAD1 can be involved in the development of a significant number of parathyroid adenomas.

The MEN1 Gene

MEN1 is characterized by the combined occurrence of tumors of the parathyroids, pancreatic islet cells, and anterior pituitary (Table 19-2).[59,60] Parathyroid tumors occur in 95% of MEN1 patients, and the resulting hypercalcemia is the first manifestation of MEN1 in about 90% of patients. Pancreatic islet cell tumors occur in 40% of MEN1 patients and gastrinomas, leading to the Zollinger-Ellison syndrome, are the most common type and also the important cause of morbidity and mortality in MEN1 patients. Anterior pituitary tumors occur in 30% of MEN1 patients, with prolactinomas representing the most common type. Associated tumors, which may also occur in MEN1, include adrenal cortical tumors, carcinoid tumors, lipomas, angiofibromas, and collagenomas.[60,61] The gene linked to MEN1 was localized to a region smaller than 300 kb on chromosome 11q13 by genetic

Table 19-2 The Multiple Endocrine Neoplasia (MEN) Syndromes, Their Characteristic Tumors, and Associated Genetic Abnormalities*

Type (Chromosomal Location)	Tumors
MEN1 (11q13)	Parathyroids
	Pancreatic islets
	Gastrinoma
	Insulinoma
	Glucagonoma
	VIPoma
	Ppoma
	Pituitary (anterior)
	Prolactinoma
	Somatotrophinoma
	Corticotrophinoma
	Nonfunctioning
	Associated tumors
	Adrenal cortical
	Carcinoid
	Lipoma
	Angiofibromas
	Collagenomas
MEN2 (10cen–10q11.2)	
MEN2a	Medullary thyroid carcinoma
	Pheochromocytoma
	Parathyroid
MTC-only	Medullary thyroid carcinoma
MEN2b	Pheochromocytoma
	Medullary thyroid carcinoma
	Associated abnormalities
	Mucosal neuromas
	Marfanoid habitus
	Medullated corneal nerve fibers
	Megacolon

*Autosomal dominant inheritance of the MEN syndromes has been established.
VIPoma, vasoactive intestinal polypeptide tumor; Ppoma, pancreatic polypeptide tumor.

mapping studies that investigated MEN1-associated tumors for LOH and by segregation studies in MEN1 families.[62] The results of these studies, which were consistent with Knudson's model for tumor development, indicated that the *MEN1* gene represented a putative tumor suppressor gene (see Fig. 19-4B). Characterization of genes from this region led to the identification of the *MEN1* gene, which consists of 10 exons that encode a novel 610–amino acid protein, referred to as "Menin".[63,64] More than 600 germline *MEN1* mutations have been identified, and the majority (>80%) are inactivating and are consistent with its role as a tumor suppressor gene.[65] These mutations are diverse in their types; about 25% are nonsense, about 45% are deletions, about 15% are insertions, fewer than 5% are donor-splice mutations, and about 10% are missense mutations.[62,65,66] In addition, the *MEN1* mutations are scattered throughout the 1,830-bp coding region of the

gene with no evidence for clustering. Correlations between the *MEN1* germline mutations and the clinical manifestations of the disorder seem to be absent.[32,65–67] Tumors from MEN1 patients and non-MEN1 patients have been observed to harbor the germline mutation together with a somatic LOH involving chromosome 11q13, as expected from Knudson's model and the proposed role of the *MEN1* gene as a tumor suppressor.[68–78] The role of the *MEN1* gene in the etiology of familial isolated hyperparathyroidism (FIHP) has also been investigated, and germline *MEN1* mutations have been reported in fewer than 20 families with FIHP.[68,79,80] The sole occurrence of parathyroid tumors in these families is remarkable, and the mechanisms that determine the altered phenotypic expressions of these mutations remain to be authenticated.

Menin seems to have multiple functions in transcriptional regulation, genome stability, and cell division. Menin is predominantly a nuclear protein in nondividing cells, but in dividing cells it is found in the cytoplasm. Menin has been shown to interact with several proteins that are involved in transcriptional regulation, genome stability, and cell division. Thus, in transcriptional regulation, Menin has been shown to interact with: the activating protein-1 (AP1) and the transcription factors JunD and C-Jun to suppress Jun-mediated transcriptional activation[81]; certain members—for example, p50, p52, and p65—of the nuclear factor-κB (NFκB) family of regulators to repress NFκB-mediated transcriptional activation[82]; members of the Smad family, Smad3 and the Smad 1/5 complex, to inhibit the transforming growth factor (TGFβ) and the bone morphogenetic protein-2 (BMP-2) signaling pathways, respectively[83,84]; and to inhibit expression of the mouse placental embryonic (*Pem*) gene (current name *Rhox5*), which encodes a homeobox-containing protein.[85] A role for Menin in controlling genome stability has been proposed because of its interactions with: a subunit of replication protein (RPA2), which is a heterotrimeric protein required for DNA replication, recombination, and repair[86]; and the tumor metastases suppressor NM23-H1/nucleoside diphosphate kinase, which induces guanosine triphosphatase activity.[87] A role for Menin in cell division and the cytoskeleton has been proposed because of its interactions with the nonmuscle heavy chain IIA, the glial fibrillary acidic protein, and vimentin—all of which are involved in the intermediate-filament network.[88] Thus, Menin seems to have a large number of potential functions through its interactions with several different proteins. However, whether these alter cell proliferation mechanisms independently or act via a single pathway remains to be elucidated.

The MEN2 Gene (c-RET)

MEN2 describes the association of medullary thyroid carcinoma (MTC), pheochromocytomas, and parathyroid tumors.[59,62] Three clinical variants of MEN2 are recognized: MEN2a, MEN2b, and MTC-only (see Table 19-2). MEN2a is the most common variant, and the development of MTC is associated with pheochromocytomas (50% of patients), which may be bilateral, and parathyroid tumors (20% of patients). MEN2b, which represents 5% of all MEN2 cases, is characterized by the occurrence of MTC and pheochromocytoma in association with a Marfanoid habitus, mucosal neuromas, medullated corneal fibers, and intestinal autonomic ganglion dysfunction leading to multiple diverticulae and megacolon.

Parathyroid tumors do not usually occur in MEN2b. MTC-only is a variant in which medullary thyroid carcinoma is the sole manifestation of the syndrome. The gene causing all three MEN2 variants was mapped to chromosome 10cen–10q11.2, a region containing the *RET* proto-oncogene, which encodes a tyrosine kinase receptor with cadherin-like and cysteine-rich extracellular domains, and a tyrosine kinase intracellular domain.[89,90] Specific mutations of *RET* have been identified for each of the three MEN2 variants. Thus in 95% of patients, MEN2a is associated with mutations of the cysteine-rich extracellular domain, and mutations in codon 634 (Cys→Arg) account for 85% of MEN2a mutations. However, a search for *RET* mutations in sporadic non-MEN2a parathyroid adenomas revealed no codon 634 mutations.[91,92] MTC-only is also associated with missense mutations in the cysteine-rich extracellular domain, and most mutations are in codon 618. However, MEN2b is associated with mutations in codon 918 (Met→Thr) of the intracellular tyrosine kinase domain in 95% of patients. Interestingly, the *RET* proto-oncogene is also involved in the etiology of papillary thyroid carcinomas and in Hirschsprung's disease. Mutational analysis of *RET* to detect mutations in codons 609, 611, 618, 634, 768, and 804 in MEN2a and MTC-only, and codon 918 in MEN2b, has been used in the diagnosis and management of patients and families with these disorders.[90,93]

The Hyperparathyroidism–Jaw Tumor Syndrome Gene

The HPT-JT syndrome is an autosomal dominant disorder characterized by the development of parathyroid adenomas and carcinomas, and fibro-osseous jaw tumors.[94,95] In addition, some patients may also develop Wilms' tumors, renal cysts, renal hamartomas, renal cortical adenomas, papillary renal cell carcinomas, uterine tumors, pancreatic adenocarcinomas, testicular mixed germ cell tumors with a major seminoma component, and Hurthle cell thyroid adenomas.[51,96] It is important to note that the parathyroid tumors may occur in isolation and without any evidence of jaw tumors, and this may cause confusion with other hereditary hypercalcemic disorders such as MEN1, FBH (also referred to as familial hypocalciuric hypercalcemia, FHH), and FIHP.[97] HPT-JT can be distinguished from FBH, in that in FBH serum calcium levels are elevated during the early neonatal or infantile period whereas in HPT-JT such elevations are uncommon in the first decade. In addition, HPT-JT patients, unlike FBH patients, will have associated hypercalciuria. The distinction between HPT-JT patients and MEN1 patients, who have only developed the usual first manifestation of hypercalcemia (>90% of patients), is more difficult and is likely to be influenced by operative and histologic findings, and by the occurrence of other characteristic lesions in each disorder. It is important to note that HPT-JT patients will usually have single adenomas or a carcinoma, whereas MEN1 patients will often have multi-glandular parathyroid disease. The distinction between FIHP and HPT-JT in the absence of jaw tumors is difficult but important, because HPT-JT patients may be at a higher risk of developing parathyroid carcinomas.[98–100] These distinctions may be helped by the identification of additional features, and a search for jaw tumors, renal, pancreatic, thyroid, and testicular abnormalities may help to identify HPT-JT patients. The jaw tumors in HPT-JT are different from the brown tumors observed in some patients with primary hyperparathyroidism, and do not resolve after parathyroidectomy.[97] Indeed ossifying fibromas of the jaw are an important distinguishing feature of HPT-JT from FIHP, and the occurrence of these may occasionally precede the development of hypercalcemia in HPT-JT patients by several decades. The gene linked to HPT-JT is located on chromosome 1q31.1, and consists of 17 exons that encode a ubiquitously expressed 531–amino acid protein, designated parafibromin.[51,101] This gene is also referred to as *HRPT2* (i.e., hyperparathyroidism type 2). Germline mutations that predict truncated forms of parafibromin have been reported in HPT-JT families[101–103] and also in patients with nonfamilial isolated parathyroid carcinomas.[102] In addition, heterozygous somatic mutations have been reported in parathyroid carcinomas or atypical adenomas, and these all predict premature termination and truncated proteins.[102,103] These germline and somatic mutations are scattered throughout the coding region, and a genotype-phenotype correlation has not yet been established. In addition, the role of parafibromin in tumorigenesis and its normal function remain to be elucidated.

RB Gene

The *RB* gene, which is a tumor suppressor gene[104] located on chromosome 13q14, is involved in the pathogenesis of retinoblastomas, and a variety of common sporadic human malignancies including ductal breast, small-cell lung, and bladder carcinomas. Allelic deletion of the *RB* gene has been demonstrated in all parathyroid carcinomas and in 10% of parathyroid adenomas,[105,106] and was accompanied by abnormal staining patterns for the RB protein in 50% of the parathyroid carcinomas but in none of the parathyroid adenomas.[105] These results demonstrate an important role for the *RB* gene in the development of parathyroid carcinomas, and may be of help in the histologic distinction of parathyroid adenoma from carcinoma.[105] However, the findings of extensive deletions of the long arm of chromosome 13 (including the *RB* locus) in some parathyroid adenomas and carcinomas,[106] and similar findings in pituitary carcinomas[107] suggest that other tumor suppressor genes on chromosome 13q may also have a role in the development of such tumors.

Gene on Chromosome 1p

LOH studies have revealed allelic loss of chromosome 1p32-pter in 40% of sporadic parathyroid adenomas.[108] This region is estimated to be about 110 cM, equivalent to about 110 million base pairs (Mbp) of DNA, but additional studies have narrowed the interval containing this putative tumor suppressor gene(s) to an approximately 4 cM (~4 Mbp) region.[109]

Nonsyndromic Familial Isolated Hyperparathyroidism

FIHP may represent an incomplete manifestation of a syndromic form such as MEN1, FHH, or HPT-JT.[80,101,110] However, it is important to note that the genetic etiology of nonsyndromic FIHP in the majority of families remains to be elucidated.[111,112] Thus, studies of 32 kindreds with nonsyndromic FIHP for mutations of the MEN1, CaSR, and HPT-JT genes have revealed that only one family harbored a germline mutation, and this involved the HPT-JT gene that encodes parafibromin.[111,112] Thus, the genes and their underlying abnormalities that lead to nonsyndromic FIHP remain to be identified.

Hyperparathyroidism in Chronic Renal Failure

Chronic renal failure is often associated with a form of secondary hyperparathyroidism that may subsequently result in the hypercalcemic state of "tertiary" hyperparathyroidism. The parathyroid proliferative response in this condition led to the proposal that the autonomous parathyroid tissue might have undergone hyperplastic change and therefore be polyclonal in origin. However, studies of X-chromosome inactivation in parathyroids from patients on hemodialysis with refractory hyperparathyroidism have revealed at least one monoclonal parathyroid tumor in more than 60% of patients.[52] In addition, LOH involving several loci on chromosome Xp11 was detected in one of these parathyroid tumors, thereby suggesting the involvement of a tumor suppressor gene from this region in the pathogenesis of such tumors.[52] Interestingly, none of the parathyroid tumors from these patients with chronic renal failure had LOH involving loci from chromosome 11q13. This unexpected finding of monoclonal parathyroid tumors in the majority of patients with "tertiary" hyperparathyroidism suggests that an increased turnover of parathyroid cells in secondary hyperparathyroidism may possibly render the parathyroid glands more susceptible to mitotic nondisjunction or other mechanisms of somatic deletions, which may involve loci other than those (MEN1 and PRAD1) located on chromosome 11q13.

HYPERCALCEMIC DISORDERS WITH NORMAL PARATHYROID GLAND ACTIVITY

Disorders of the Calcium-Sensing Receptor

Three hypercalcemic disorders due to mutations of the calcium-sensing receptor (CaSR) have been reported.[110,113-118] These are FBH (also referred to as FHH, or familial hypocalciuric hypercalcemia) and neonatal severe hyperparathyroidism (NSHPT). Furthermore, an autoimmune hypocalciuric hypercalcemia (AHH) has been described (Table 19-3).

Familial Benign Hypercalcemia and Neonatal Severe Hyperparathyroidism

Mutational analyses of the human CaSR, which is a G protein–coupled receptor located on chromosome 3q21.1,[119] have revealed different mutations that result in a loss of function of the CaSR in patients with FBH and NSHPT[113-118] (see Fig. 19-1). Many of these mutations cluster around the aspartate- and glutamate-rich regions (codons 39–300) within the extracellular domain of the receptor, and this has been proposed to contain low-affinity calcium-binding sites, based on similarities to that of calsequestrin, in which the ligand-binding pockets also contain negatively charged amino acid

residues.[110,120] Approximately two-thirds of the FBH kindreds investigated have been found to have unique heterozygous mutations of the CaSR, and expression studies of these mutations have demonstrated a loss of CaSR function whereby there is an increase in the calcium ion–dependent set point for PTH release from the parathyroid cell.[113,118,121,122] NSHPT occurring in the offspring of consanguineous FBH families has been shown to be due to homozygous CaSR mutations.[113,114,116,123,124] However, some patients with sporadic neonatal hyperparathyroidism have been reported to be associated with de novo heterozygous CaSR mutations,[115] thereby suggesting that factors other than mutant gene dosage[123] (e.g., the degree of set-point abnormality, the bony sensitivity to PTH, and the maternal extracellular calcium concentration) may also all play a role in the phenotypic expression of a CaSR mutation in the neonate. The remaining one-third of FBH families in whom a mutation within the coding region of the CaSR has not been demonstrated may either have an abnormality in the promoter of the gene or a mutation at one of the two other FBH loci that have been revealed by genetic linkage studies. One of these FBH loci is located on chromosome 19p and is referred to as FBH$_{19p}$.[125] Studies of another FBH kindred from Oklahoma that also suffered from progressive elevations in PTH, hypophosphatemia, and osteomalacia[126,127] demonstrated that this variant, designated FBH$_{Ok}$, was linked to chromosome 19q13.[128] The three forms of FBH that are located on chromosomes 3q, 19p, and 19q have also been referred to as FBH (or FHH) types 1, 2, and 3, respectively.[128]

Autoimmune Hypocalciuric Hypercalcemia

Some patients who have the clinical features of FHH but not CaSR mutations may have autoimmune hypocalciuric hypercalcemia (AHH). Five patients from three unrelated families with AHH, who all had other autoimmune manifestations have been reported.[129,130] Thus, three patients had antibodies to thyroid, one had sprue with anti-gliadin and anti-endomyseal antibodies,[129] and one had antibodies to the hemidesmosome, a positive Coombs' test, and most likely immune hypophysitis.[130] All of these patients were shown to have circulating antibodies to the extracellular domain of the CaSR. Some of these antibodies stimulated PTH release from dispersed human parathyroid cells in vitro, probably by inhibiting the activation of the CaSR by extracellular calcium.[129] Antibody titers in another patient correlated well with the hypercalcemia and the elevation in PTH concentration.[130] Thus, AHH is a condition of extracellular calcium sensing that should be considered in FHH patients who do not have CaSR mutations.

Jansen's Disease

Jansen's disease (Figs. 19-5 and 19-6) is an autosomal dominant disease that is characterized by short-limbed dwarfism caused by an abnormal regulation of chondrocyte proliferation and differentiation in the metaphyseal growth plate, and it is usually associated with severe hypercalcemia and hypophosphatemia, despite normal or undetectable serum levels of PTH or PTHrP.[131] These abnormalities are caused by mutations in the PTH/PTHrP receptor that lead to constitutive,

Table 19-3 Diseases Associated with Abnormalities of the Extracellular Calcium-Sensing Receptor

CaSR Abnormality and Disease	CaSR Gene
Loss-of-function CaSR mutation	
Familial benign hypercalcemia (FBH1)	Heterozygous mutation
Neonatal severe primary hyperparathyroidism (NSHPT)	Homozygous (or heterozygous) mutation
Gain-of-function CaSR mutation	
Autosomal dominant hypocalcemic hypercalciuria (ADHH)	Heterozygous mutation
Bartter syndrome type V	Heterozygous mutation
CaSR autoantibodies	
Autoimmune hypocalciuric hypercalcemia (AHH)	Normal
Acquired hypoparathyroidism (AH)	Normal

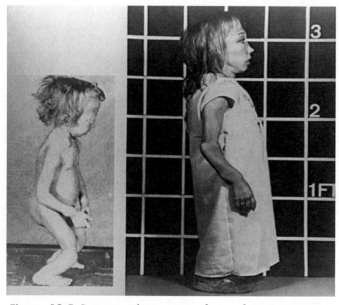

Figure 19-5 Patient with a severe form of Jansen's metaphyseal chondrodysplasia at ages 5 (left) and 22 years (right). (From Frame B, Poznanski AK: Conditions that may be confused with rickets. In DeLuca HF, Anast CS [eds]: Pediatric Diseases Related to Calcium. New York, Elsevier, 1980, pp 269–289.)

PTH- and PTHrP-independent receptor activation.[132–134] Three different, heterozygous mutations of the PTH/PTHrP receptor have been identified in the severe form of Jansen's disease, and these involve codon 223 (His→Arg), codon 410 (Thr→Pro), and codon 458 (Ile→Arg) (Fig. 19-7). Expression of the mutant receptors in COS-7 cells resulted in constitutive, ligand-independent accumulation of cyclic AMP (cAMP), whereas the basal accumulation of inositol phosphates was not measurably increased.[132–134] Because the PTH/PTHrP receptor is most abundantly expressed in kidney and bone and in the metaphyseal growth plate, these findings provide a probable explanation for the abnormalities observed in mineral homeostasis and growth plate development associated with this disorder. This conclusion is supported further by observations in mice that express the human PTH/PTHrP receptor with the His223Arg mutation under the control of the rat collagen type II(α) promoter.[135] This promoter targeted expression of the mutant receptor to the layer of proliferative chondrocytes, delayed their differentiation into hypertrophic cells, and led, at least in animals with multiple copies of the transgene, to a mild impairment in the growth of long bones. These observations are consistent with the conclusion that expression of a constitutively active human PTH/PTHrP receptor in growth plate chondrocytes causes the characteristic metaphyseal changes in patients with Jansen's disease.

Recently, a novel heterozygous PTH/PTHrP receptor mutation, Thr410Arg, was identified in several members of a small kindred with an apparently mild form of Jansen's disease (see Fig. 19-6).[136] Affected individuals had, as compared with patients carrying the previously identified activating PTH/PTHrP receptor mutations,[132–134] less severe growth plate abnormalities, relatively normal stature, high-normal plasma calcium concentration, yet significant hypercalciuria and normal or suppressed plasma PTH levels. When tested in vitro, the PTH/PTHrP receptor with the Thr410Arg mutation showed less constitutive activity than that observed with the previously described Thr410Pro mutant.[133,137] This less pronounced agonist-independent cAMP accumulation induced by the Thr410Arg mutation is consistent with the less severe skeletal and laboratory abnormalities observed in this milder form of Jansen's disease.

Williams Syndrome

Williams syndrome is an autosomal dominant disorder characterized by supravalvular aortic stenosis, elfin-like facies, psychomotor retardation, and infantile hypercalcemia. The underlying abnormality of calcium metabolism remains unknown, but abnormal $1,25(OH)_2$ vitamin D_3 metabolism or decreased calcitonin production have been implicated, although none have been consistently demonstrated. Studies have demonstrated hemizygosity at the elastin locus on chromosome 7q11.23 in more than 90% of patients with the classical Williams phenotype,[138–140] and only one patient had

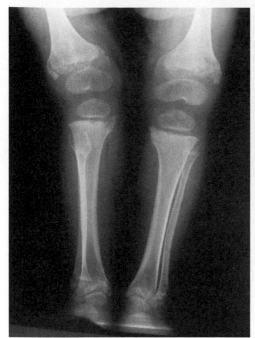

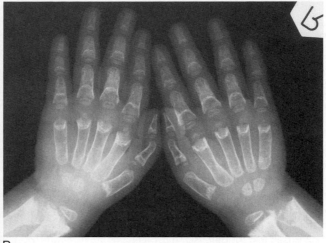

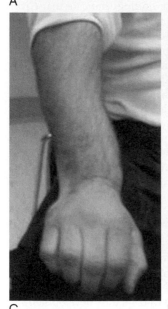

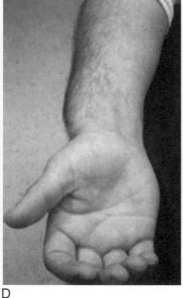

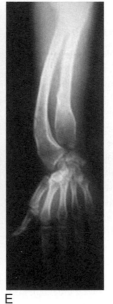

Figure 19-6 Radiographs and photographs of patients from a small family with a relatively mild form of Jansen's disease. Anterior-posterior radiographs of the knees (A) and hands (B) of one of two affected children showing the splayed and fragmented metaphyses and the mildly broadened diaphyses. Photographs of the right hands, wrist, and forearm of the affected father (C and D), and radiograph of his hand and arm (E) showing bowing of long bones. (From Bastepe M, Raas-Rothschild A, Silver J, et al: A form of Jansen's metaphyseal chondrodysplasia with limited metabolic and skeletal abnormalities is caused by a novel activating PTH/PTHrP receptor mutation. J Clin Endocrinol Metab 89:3595–3600, 2004.)

a cytogenetically identifiable deletion, thereby indicating that the syndrome is usually due to a microdeletion of 7q11.23.[140] Interestingly, ablation of the elastin gene in mice results in vascular abnormalities similar to those observed in patients with Williams syndrome.[141] However, the microdeletions that have been reported involve also another gene, designated LIM-kinase, that is expressed in the central nervous system.[142] The calcitonin receptor gene, which is located on chromosome 7q21, is not involved in the deletions found in Williams syndrome and is therefore unlikely to be implicated in the hypercalcemia of such children.[143] Whereas deletion of the elastin and LIM-kinase genes can explain the respective cardiovascular and neurologic features of Williams syndrome, it seems likely that another, as yet uncharacterized gene that is within this contiguously deleted region, is involved in this

disorder and could explain the abnormalities of calcium metabolism.

HYPOCALCEMIA AND HYPERPHOSPHATEMIA DUE TO REDUCED PARATHYROID GLAND ACTIVITY

Hypoparathyroidism

Hypoparathyroidism may occur as part of a pluriglandular autoimmune disorder or as a complex congenital defect, as for example in DGS. In addition, hypoparathyroidism may develop as a solitary endocrinopathy, and this has been called

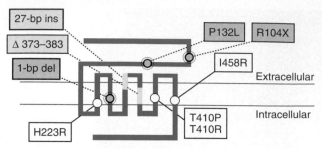

Figure 19-7 Schematic representation of the human PTH/PTHrP receptor. The approximate locations of heterozygous missense mutations, which lead in patients with Jansen's disease to constitutive receptor activation, are indicated by open circles. Loss-of-function mutations that were identified in patients with Blomstrand's disease are indicated by gray circles or stippled boxes (see text for details).

isolated or idiopathic hypoparathyroidism. Familial occurrences of isolated hypoparathyroidism with autosomal dominant, autosomal recessive, and X-linked recessive inheritances have been established.

Parathyroid Hormone Gene Abnormalities

DNA sequence analysis of the PTH gene (see Fig. 19-3) from one patient with autosomal dominant isolated hypoparathyroidism has revealed a single-base substitution (T→C) in exon 2,[144] which resulted in the substitution of arginine (**C**GT) for cysteine (**T**GT) in the signal peptide. The presence of this charged amino acid in the midst of the hydrophobic core of the signal peptide impeded the processing of the mutant preproPTH, as demonstrated by in vitro studies. These revealed that the mutation impaired the interaction with the nascent protein and the translocation machinery, and that cleavage of the mutant signal sequence by solubilized signal peptidase was ineffective.[144,145] In another family, with autosomal recessive hypoparathyroidism, a single-base substitution (T→C) involving codon 23 of exon 2 was detected. This resulted in the substitution of proline (**C**CG) for the normal serine (**T**CG) in the signal peptide.[146] This mutation alters the –3 position of the preproPTH protein cleavage site. Indeed, amino acid residues at the –3 and –1 positions of the signal peptidase recognition site have to conform to certain criteria for correct processing through the rough endoplasmic reticulum, and one of these is an absence of proline in the region –3 and +1 of the site. Thus, the presence of a proline, which is a strong helix-breaking residue, at the –3 position is likely to disrupt cleavage of the mutant preproPTH that would be subsequently degraded in the rough endoplasmic reticulum, and PTH would not be available.[146] Another abnormality of the PTH gene, involving a donor splice site at the exon 2/intron 2 boundary, has been identified in one family with autosomal recessive isolated hypoparathyroidism.[147] This mutation involved a single-base transition (g→c) at position 1 of intron 2, and an assessment of the effects of this alteration in the invariant gt dinucleotide of the 5′ donor splice site consensus on mRNA processing revealed that the mutation resulted in exon skipping, in which exon 2 of the PTH gene was lost and exon 1 was spliced to exon 3.

The lack of exon 2 would lead to a loss of the initiation codon (ATG) and the signal peptide sequence (see Fig. 19-3), which are required, respectively, for the commencement of PTH mRNA translation and for the translocation of the PTH peptide.

GCMB Abnormalities

GCMB (glial cells missing B), which is the human homolog of the *Drosophilia* gene *Gcm* and of the mouse *Gcm2* gene, is expressed exclusively in the parathyroid glands, suggesting that it may be a specific regulator of parathyroid gland development.[148] Mice that were homozygous for deletion of *Gcm2* lacked parathyroid glands and developed the hypocalcemia and hyperphosphatemia as observed in hypoparathyroidism.[148] However, despite their lack of parathyroid glands, *Gcm2*⁻/⁻ mice did not have undetectable serum PTH levels but instead had levels indistinguishable from those of normal (*Gcm2*⁺/⁺, wild type) and heterozygous (*Gcm2*⁺/⁻) mice. This endogenous level of PTH in the *Gcm2*⁻/⁻ mice was too low to correct the hypocalcemia, but exogenous continuous PTH infusion could correct the hypocalcemia.[148] Interestingly, there were no compensatory increases in PTHrP or 1,25(OH)₂ vitamin D₃. These findings indicate that *Gcm2* mice have a normal response (no resistance) to PTH, and that the PTH in the serum of *Gcm2*-deficient mice was active. The auxiliary source of PTH was identified to be a cluster of PTH-expressing cells under the thymic capsule. These thymic PTH-producing cells also expressed the CaSR, and long-term treatment of the *Gcm2*-deficient mice with 1,25(OH)₂ vitamin D₃ restored the serum calcium concentrations to normal and reduced the serum PTH levels, thereby indicating that the thymic production of PTH can be downregulated. Studies of a patient with isolated hypoparathyroidism have shown that a homozygous intragenic deletion of *GCMB* is associated with this apparently autosomal recessive disorder.[345]

X-Linked Recessive Hypoparathyroidism

X-linked recessive hypoparathyroidism has been reported in two multigenerational kindreds from the state of Missouri.[149,150] In this disorder only males are affected, and they suffer from infantile onset of epilepsy and hypocalcemia, which is due to an isolated defect in parathyroid gland development.[151] Relatedness of the two kindreds has been established by demonstrating an identical mitochondrial DNA sequence, which is inherited via the maternal lineage, in affected males from the two families.[152] Studies utilizing X-linked polymorphic markers in these families localized the mutant gene to chromosome Xq26–q27,[153] and a molecular deletional-insertion that involves chromosome 2p25 and Xq27 has been identified.[154] This complex deletion-insertion [del(X) (q27.1) inv ins (X;2) (q27.1; p25.3)] represents a novel abnormality causing hypoparathyroidism, and its location 67 kb downstream of the *SOX3* gene, which encodes a transcription factor with a role in vertebrate embryonic development, indicates that it may have a position effect on SOX3 expression. Indeed, SOX expression has been demonstrated to occur in the developing parathyroid tissue of mouse embryos, and these findings add SOX3 to the growing list of transcription factors, including GCMB, GATA3, TBX1, HOXA3, PAX1, and PAX9, that operate in parathyroid development.[154]

Pluriglandular Autoimmune Hypoparathyroidism

Hypoparathyroidism may occur in association with candidiasis and autoimmune Addison's disease, and the disorder has been referred to as either the autoimmune polyendocrinopathy-candidiasis-ectodermal dystrophy (APECED) syndrome or the autoimmune polyglandular syndrome type 1.[155] This disorder has a high incidence in Finland, and a genetic analysis of Finnish families indicated autosomal recessive inheritance of the disorder.[156] In addition, the disorder has been reported to have a high incidence among Iranian Jews, although the occurrence of candidiasis was less common in this population.[157] Linkage studies of Finnish families mapped the APECED gene to chromosome 21q22.3.[158] Further positional cloning approaches led to the isolation of a novel gene from chromosome 21q22.3. This gene, referred to as AIRE1 (autoimmune regulator type 1), encodes a 545–amino acid protein that contains motifs suggestive of a transcriptional factor and includes two zinc-finger motifs, a proline-rich region, and three LXXLL motifs.[159,160] Four AIRE1 mutations are commonly found in APECED families: Arg257Stop in Finnish, German, Swiss, British, and northern Italian families; Arg139Stop in Sardinian families; Tyr85Cys in Iranian Jewish families; and a 13-bp deletion in exon 8 in British, Dutch, German, and Finnish families.[159–164] AIRE1 has been shown to regulate the elimination of organ-specific T cells in the thymus, and thus APECED is likely to be caused by a failure of this specialized mechanism for deleting forbidden T cells and establishing immunologic tolerance.[165]

DiGeorge Syndrome

Patients with the DiGeorge syndrome (DGS) typically suffer from hypoparathyroidism, immunodeficiency, congenital heart defects, and deformities of the ear, nose, and mouth. The disorder arises from a congenital failure in the development of the derivatives of the third and fourth pharyngeal pouches with resulting absence or hypoplasia of the parathyroids and thymus. Most cases of DGS are sporadic, but an autosomal dominant inheritance of DGS has been observed and an association between the syndrome and an unbalanced translocation and deletions involving 22q11.2 have also been reported[166]; this is referred to as DGS type 1 (DGS1). In some patients, deletions of another locus on chromosome 10p have been observed in association with DGS,[167] and this is referred to as DGS type 2 (DGS2). Mapping studies of the DGS1 deleted region on chromosome 22q11.2 have defined a 250- to 3,000-kb critical region[168,169] that contains approximately 30 genes. Studies of DGS1 patients have reported deletions of several of the genes (e.g., rnex40 nex2.2–nex3, UDFIL, and TBX1) from the critical region,[166,170–172] and studies of transgenic mice deleted for such genes (e.g., Udf1l, Hira, and Tbx1) have revealed developmental abnormalities of the pharyngeal arches.[173–175] However, point mutations in DGS1 patients have only been detected in the TBX1 gene,[176] and TBX1 is now considered to be the gene linked to DGS1.[177] TBX1 is a DNA-binding transcriptional factor of the T-box family that is known to have an important role in vertebrate and invertebrate organogenesis and pattern formation. The TBX1 gene is deleted in about 96% of all DGS1 patients. Moreover, DNA sequence analysis of unrelated DGS1 patients who did not have deletions of chromosome 22q11.2 revealed the

occurrence of three heterozygous point mutations.[176] One of these mutations resulted in a frameshift with a premature truncation, whereas the other two were missense mutations (Phe148Tyr and Gly310Ser). All of these patients had the complete pharyngeal phenotype but did not have mental retardation or learning difficulties. Interestingly, transgenic mice with deletion of Tbx1 have a phenotype that is similar to that of DGS1 patients.[175] Thus, Tbx1-null mutant mice had all the developmental anomalies of DGS1 (i.e., thymic and parathyroid hypoplasia; abnormal facial structures and cleft palate; skeletal defects; and cardiac outflow tract abnormalities), whereas Tbx1 haploinsufficiency in mutant mice (i.e., heterozygous) was associated only with defects of the fourth branchial pouch (i.e., cardiac outflow tract abnormalities). The basis of the phenotypic differences between DGS1 patients, who are heterozygous, and the transgenic heterozygous mice remain to be elucidated. It is plausible that Tbx1 dosage, together with the downstream genes that are regulated by Tbx1, could provide an explanation, but the roles of these putative genes in DGS1 remains to be elucidated.

Some patients may have a late-onset DGS1, and these develop symptomatic hypocalcemia in childhood or during adolescence with only subtle phenotypic abnormalities.[178,179] These late-onset DGS1 patients have similar microdeletions in the 22q11 region. It is of interest to note that the age of diagnosis in the families of the three DGS1 patients with inactivating TBX1 mutations ranged from 7 to 46 years, which is in keeping with late-onset DGS1.[176]

Hypoparathyroidism, Deafness, and Renal Anomalies Syndrome

The combined inheritance of hypoparathyroidism, deafness, and renal dysplasia (HDR) as an autosomal dominant trait was reported in one family in 1992.[180] Patients had asymptomatic hypocalcemia with undetectable or inappropriately normal serum concentrations of PTH, and normal brisk increases in plasma cAMP in response to the infusion of PTH. The patients also had bilateral, symmetrical, sensorineural deafness involving all frequencies. The renal abnormalities consisted mainly of bilateral cysts that compressed the glomeruli and tubules, and led to renal impairment in some patients. Cytogenetic abnormalities were not detected, and abnormalities of the PTH gene were excluded.[180] However, cytogenetic abnormalities involving chromosome 10p14–10pter were identified in two unrelated patients with features that were consistent with HDR. These two patients suffered from hypoparathyroidism, deafness, and growth and mental retardation; one patient also had a solitary dysplastic kidney with vesicoureteric reflux and a uterus bicornis unicollis; the other patient, who had a complex reciprocal, insertional translocation of chromosomes 10p and 8q, had cartilaginous exostoses.[181] Neither of these patients had immunodeficiency or heart defects, which are key features of DGS2 (see above), and further studies defined two nonoverlapping regions; thus, the DGS2 region was located on 10p13–p14 and HDR on 10p14–10pter. Deletion mapping studies in two other HDR patients further defined a critical 200-kb region that contained GATA3,[181] which belongs to a family of zinc-finger transcription factors that are involved in vertebrae embryonic development. DNA sequence analysis in other HDR patients identified mutations that resulted in a haploinsufficiency and loss of *GATA3* function.[181–183] GATA3 has two zinc-fingers, and the C-terminal finger (ZnF2) binds DNA, whereas the N-terminal finger (ZnF1) stabilizes this DNA binding and interacts with other zinc-finger proteins, such as the "friends of GATA" (FOG).[184] HDR-associated mutations involving GATA3 ZnF2 or the adjacent basic amino acids were found to result in a loss of DNA binding, whereas those involving ZnF1 either lead to a loss of interaction with FOG2 ZnFs or altered DNA-binding affinity.[183] These findings are consistent with the proposed 3-dimensional model of GATA3 ZnF1, which has separate DNA- and protein-binding surfaces.[183,185]

The HDR phenotype is consistent with the expression pattern of GATA3 during human and mouse embryogenesis in the developing kidney, otic vesicle, and parathyroids. However, GATA3 is also expressed in the developing central nervous system and the hematopoietic organs in humans and mice, and this suggests that GATA3 may have a more complex role. Indeed, homozygous *GATA3*-knockout mice have defects of the central nervous system and a lack of T-cell development, although the heterozygous *GATA3*-knockout mice appear to have no abnormalities.[186] It is important to note that HDR patients with *GATA3* haploinsufficiency do not have immune deficiency, and this suggests that the immune abnormalities observed in some patients with 10p deletions are most likely to be caused by other genes on 10p. Similarly, the facial dysmorphism and growth and developmental delay, commonly seen in patients with larger 10p deletions, were absent in the HDR patients with *GATA3* mutations, further indicating that these features were probably due to other genes on 10p.[181] These studies of HDR patients clearly indicate an important role for GATA3 in parathyroid development and in the etiology of hypoparathyroidism.

Mitochondrial Disorders Associated with Hypoparathyroidism

Hypoparathyroidism has been reported to occur in three disorders associated with mitochondrial dysfunction: the Kearns-Sayre syndrome (KSS), the MELAS syndrome, and a mitochondrial trifunctional protein deficiency syndrome (MTPDS) (see below and Table 19-1). KSS is characterized by progressive external ophthalmoplegia and pigmentary retinopathy before the age of 20 years, and is often associated with heart block or cardiomyopathy. The MELAS syndrome consists of a childhood onset of mitochondrial encephalopathy, lactic acidosis, and stroke-like episodes. In addition, varying degrees of proximal myopathy can be seen in both conditions. Both the KSS and MELAS syndromes have been reported to occur with insulin-dependent diabetes mellitus and hypoparathyroidism.[187,188] A point mutation in the mitochondrial gene transfer RNA leucine (UUR) has been reported in one patient with the MELAS syndrome who also suffered from hypoparathyroidism and diabetes mellitus. Large deletions, consisting of 6,741 and 6,903 bp and involving more than 38% of the mitochondrial genome, have been reported in other patients who suffered from KSS, hypoparathyroidism, and sensorineural deafness.[189] Rearrangements and duplication of mitochondrial DNA have also been reported in KSS. MTPDS is a disorder of fatty-acid oxidation that is associated with peripheral neuropathy, pigmentary retinopathy, and acute fatty liver degeneration in pregnant women who carry an affected fetus. Hypoparathyroidism has been observed in one patient with MTPDS.[190] The role of these mitochondrial

mutations in the etiology of hypoparathyroidism remains to be further elucidated.

Kenny-Caffey and Sanjad-Sakati Syndromes

Hypoparathyroidism has been reported to occur in more than 50% of patients with the Kenny-Caffey syndrome, which is associated with short stature, osteosclerosis, and cortical thickening of the long bones, delayed closure of the anterior fontanel, basal ganglia calcification, nanophthalmos, and hyperopia.[191] Parathyroid tissue could not be found in a detailed postmortem examination of one patient,[192] and this suggests that hypoparathyroidism may be due to an embryologic defect of parathyroid development. In the Sanjad-Sakati syndrome hypoparathyroidism is associated with severe growth failure and dysmorphic features, and this has been reported in 12 patients from Saudi Arabia.[193] Consanguinity was noted in 11 of the 12 patients' families, the majority of which originated from the western province of Saudi Arabia. This syndrome, which is inherited as an autosomal recessive disorder, has also been identified in families of Bedouin origin, and homozygosity and linkage disequilibrium studies located this gene to chromosome 1q42–q43.[194] Molecular genetic investigations have identified that mutations of the tubulin-specific chaperone (*TBCE*) are associated with the Kenny-Caffey and Sanjad-Sakati syndromes.[195] *TBCE* encodes one of several chaperone proteins required for the proper folding of α-tubulin subunits and the formation of α/β-tubulin heterodimers (see Fig. 19-1).[195]

Additional Familial Syndromes

Single familial syndromes in which hypoparathyroidism is a component have been reported (see Table 19-1). The inheritance of the disorder in some instances has been established, and molecular genetic analysis of the PTH gene has revealed no abnormalities. Thus, an association of hypoparathyroidism, renal insufficiency, and developmental delay has been reported in one Asian family in whom autosomal recessive inheritance of the disorder was established.[196] An analysis of the PTH gene in this family revealed no abnormalities.[196] The occurrence of hypoparathyroidism, nerve deafness, and a steroid-resistant nephrosis leading to renal failure, which has been referred to as the Barakat syndrome,[197] has been reported in four brothers from one family, and an association of hypoparathyroidism with congenital lymphedema, nephropathy, mitral valve prolapse, and brachytelephalangy has been observed in two brothers from another family.[198] Molecular genetic studies have not been reported from these two families.

Calcium-Sensing Receptor Abnormalities

CaSR abnormalities are associated with three hypocalcemic disorders. These include autosomal dominant hypocalcemic hypercalciuria (ADHH), Bartter syndrome type V (i.e., ADHH with a Bartter-like syndrome), and a form of autoimmune hypoparathyroidism due to CaSR autoantibodies (see Table 19-3).

Autosomal Dominant Hypocalcemic Hypercalciuria

CASR mutations that result in a loss of function are associated with familial benign (hypocalciuric) hypercalcemia.[110,113–118]

It was therefore postulated that gain-of-function mutations in *CASR* lead to hypocalcemia with hypercalciuria, and the investigation of kindreds with autosomal dominant forms of hypocalcemia have indeed identified such *CASR* mutations.[110,199–203] The hypocalcemic individuals generally had normal serum intact PTH concentrations and hypomagnesemia, and treatment with vitamin D or its active metabolites to correct the hypocalcemia resulted in marked hypercalciuria, nephrocalcinosis, nephrolithiasis, and renal impairment. The majority (>80%) of *CASR* mutations that result in a functional gain are located within the extracellular domain,[110,199–203] which is different from the findings in other disorders that are the result of activating mutations in G protein–coupled receptors.

Bartter Syndrome Type V

Bartter syndrome is a heterozygous group of autosomal recessive disorders of electrolyte homeostasis characterized by hypokalemic alkalosis, renal salt wasting that may lead to hypotension, hyper-reninemic hyperaldosteronism, increased urinary prostaglandin excretion, and hypercalciuria with nephrocalcinosis.[204,205] Mutations of several ion transporters and channels have been associated with Bartter syndrome, and five types are now recognized.[205] Thus, type I is due to mutations involving the bumetamide-sensitive $Na^+/K^+/Cl^-$ cotransporter (NKCC2 or SLC12A2), type II is due to mutations affecting the outwardly rectifying renal potassium channel (ROMK), type III is due to mutations in the gene encoding the voltage-gated chloride channel (CLC-Kb), type IV is due to mutations affecting Barttin, which is a β-subunit that is required for trafficking of CLC-Kb and CLC-Ka (this form is also associated with deafness because Barttin, CLC-Ka, and CLC-Kb are also expressed in the marginal cells of the scala media of the inner ear that secrete potassium ion–rich endolymph), and type V is due to activating mutations of the *CASR*. Patients with Bartter syndrome type V have the classical features of the syndrome (i.e., hypokalemic metabolic alkalosis, hyper-reninemia, and hyperaldosteronism).[206,207] In addition, they develop hypocalcemia, which may be symptomatic and lead to carpo-pedal spasm, and an elevated fractional excretion of calcium that may be associated with nephrocalcinosis.[206,207] Such patients have been reported to have heterozygous gain-of-function *CASR* mutations, and in vitro functional expression of these mutations has revealed a more severe set-point abnormality for the receptor than that found in patients with ADHH.[206,207] This suggests that the additional features occurring in Bartter syndrome type V, but not in ADHH, are due to severe gain-of-function mutations of *CASR*.[205]

Autoimmune Acquired Hypoparathyroidism

Among patients who had acquired hypoparathyroidism (AH) in association with autoimmune hypothyroidism, 20% were found to have autoantibodies to the extracellular domain of the CaSR.[129,130,208] The CaSR autoantibodies did not persist for long; 72% of patients who had AH for less than 5 years had detectable CaSR autoantibodies, whereas only 14% of patients with AH for more than 5 years had such autoantibodies.[208] The majority of the patients who had CaSR autoantibodies were females, a finding that is similar to that found in other autoantibody-mediated diseases. Indeed, a few AH patients have also had features of autoimmune polyglandular syndrome type I. These findings establish that the CaSR is an autoantigen in AH.[129,208]

Pseudohypoparathyroidism

The term *pseudohypoparathyroidism* (PHP) was first introduced to describe patients with hypocalcemia and hyperphosphatemia due to PTH resistance rather than PTH deficiency.[209] Affected individuals show partial or complete resistance to biologically active, exogenous PTH as demonstrated by a lack of increase in urinary cAMP and urinary phosphate excretion; this condition is now referred to as PHP type I.[210–212] If associated with other endocrine deficiencies and characteristic physical stigmata, now collectively termed *Albright's hereditary osteodystrophy* (AHO), the condition is referred to as PHP type Ia. This latter syndrome is caused by heterozygous inactivating mutations within exons 1 through 13 of *GNAS* located on chromosome 20q13.3, which encode the stimulatory G protein (Gsα). These mutations were shown to lead to a 50% reduction in the activity of Gsα per protein in readily accessible tissues, like erythrocytes and fibroblasts, and explain at least partially the resistance against PTH and other hormones that mediate their actions through G protein–coupled receptors.[210–212] However, a similar reduction in Gsα activity is also found in patients with pseudopseudohypoparathyroidism (pPHP), who show the same physical appearance as individuals with PHP-Ia but lack endocrine abnormalities. Mutations in *GNAS* were thus thought to be necessary but not sufficient to fully explain either PHP-Ia or pPHP.[210,213–218]

Subsequent studies indicated that patients affected by PHP-Ia or pPHP are typically found within the same kindred, but not within the same sibship, and that hormonal resistance is parentally imprinted; in other words, PHP-Ia occurs only if the defective gene is inherited from a female affected by either PHP-Ia or pPHP, and pPHP occurs only if the defective gene is inherited from a male affected by either form of the two disorders.[219,220] Observations consistent with these findings in humans were made in mice that are heterozygous for the ablation of exon 2 of the *Gnas* gene. Animals that had inherited the mutant allele from a female showed undetectable Gsα protein in the renal cortex and decreased blood calcium concentration due to resistance against PTH. In contrast, offspring that had obtained the mutant allele lacking exon 2 from a male showed no evidence for endocrine abnormalities.[221] Tissue- or cell-specific Gsα expression is thus almost certainly involved in the pathogenesis of PHP-Ia and pPHP, and this provides also a reasonable explanation for the finding that heterozygous *GNAS* mutations result in a dominant phenotype.

Progressive osseous heteroplasia was recently shown to be caused also by heterozygous inactivating mutations in the *GNAS* exons encoding Gsα.[222–224] Interestingly, progressive osseous heteroplasia became only apparent when the Gsα mutation was inherited from a male, whereas inheritance from a female seems to have resulted in AHO, that is, pPHP. This aspect of the findings was surprising, because maternal inheritance of inactivating Gsα mutations usually leads to PHP-Ia, that is, AHO with hormonal resistance. However, PTH and thyroid-stimulating hormone levels were not reported,[224] and it is therefore conceivable that mild hormonal resistance may have been present in patients with maternally inherited Gsα mutations.

The *GNAS* locus is considerably more complex than previously thought. For example, alternative splicing results in several different mRNAs that are transcribed in the sense direction, and at least one mRNA is transcribed in the antisense direction.[210–212,225–227] Furthermore, some of these splice variants are derived only from either the paternal or the maternal allele, and it seems likely that this complexity of the *GNAS* locus contributes to the unique phenotypic abnormalities in patients with one of the different forms of PHP (Fig. 19-8). Gsα, which is encoded by exons 1 through 13 of *GNAS*, mediates the biologic functions of a large variety of G protein–coupled receptors, including the PTH/PTHrP receptor. A second transcript, XLαs, comprises a novel first exon (XL), which is spliced onto exons 2 through 13. The encoded protein (~92 kD) shares in the C-terminal portion complete amino acid sequence identity with Gsα,[228] and it was recently shown that XLαs can function as a stimulatory G protein, at least in the fibroblast-like cells that were used for these studies.[229] The mRNA encoding XLαs is found at numerous sites; particularly high concentrations were identified in endocrine and neuroendocrine cells,[228] and it is transcribed in all investigated tissues only from the paternal allele.[225–227] A third transcript, NESP55,[230] is transcribed only from the maternal allele[226,227] using yet another exon of the *GNAS* locus that is located upstream of exon XL and exons 1 through 13. NESP55, which is thought to act as a neuroendocrine secretory protein,[230] shares no amino acid sequence homology with either XLαs or Gsα, but its mRNA contains in its 3′ noncoding region a nucleotide sequence that is identical to that of the Gsα message. Additional recently identified transcripts include A/B (also referred to as exon 1A or 1′) and AS, which are both thought to be noncoding.[225–227,231,232] Because of the complexity of the *GNAS* locus and because of the use of different, allele- and strand-specific promoters, it seems plausible that mutations in the *GNAS* exons encoding Gsα (i.e., exons 1–13)[210,213–218] can affect not only the functional properties of Gsα but also those of XLαs, NESP55, A/B, and the antisense transcript AS.

Mutations in the gene encoding Gsα have not been detected in most patients with PHP-Ib, a disorder in which affected individuals show PTH-resistant hypocalcemia and hyperphosphatemia, but lack developmental defects. PHP-Ib patients seem also to have an increased incidence of thyroid-stimulating hormone resistance.[210–213,233,234] Furthermore, individuals with PHP-Ib frequently show a normal osseous response to

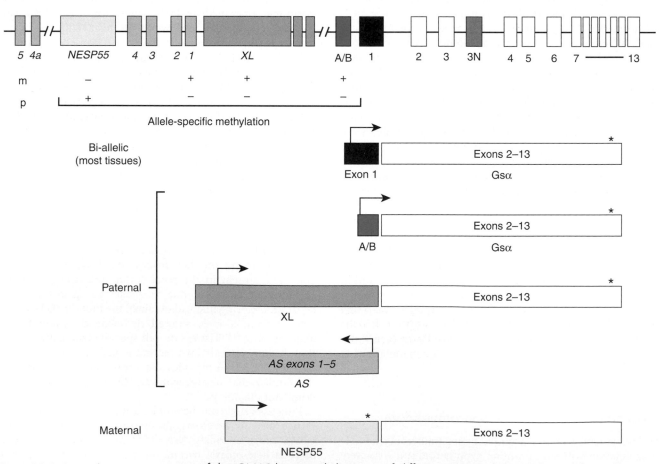

Figure 19-8 Intron/exon organization of the *GNAS* locus and depiction of different mRNAs that are derived from alternative splicing. The mRNA encoding Gsα is thought to be expressed in most tissues from both parental alleles; however, in the renal cortex transcripts seem to be derived predominantly or exclusively from the maternal allele; the mRNAs encoding the splice variants XLαs and NESP55 are derived from the paternal and maternal allele, respectively. A/B and AS, two presumably nontranslated messages, are transcribed from the paternal allele (see text for details).

PTH, or even biochemical and radiologic evidence for increased bone turnover and osteoclastic bone resorption, indicating that the PTH-dependent actions on osteoblasts are not impaired,[211–213,235–237] Moreover, PHP-Ib patients usually show no abnormalities in growth plate development and thus show normal longitudinal growth, indicating that the PTHrP-dependent regulation of chondrocyte growth and differentiation is normal. Particularly these latter findings made it unlikely that defects in the PTH/PTHrP receptor were the cause of PHP-Ib. Indeed studies of the PTH/PTHrP receptor gene and mRNA in PHP-Ib patients failed to identify disease-causing mutations.[238–241] A genome-wide search to identify the location of the "PHP-Ib gene" was therefore undertaken in four unrelated kindreds, and this mapped the PHP-Ib locus to chromosome 20q13.3, which contains the GNAS locus.[242] In this study it was furthermore shown that the genetic defect is parentally imprinted; in other words, it is inherited in the same mode as the PTH-resistant hypocalcemia in kindreds with PHP-Ia and/or pPHP.[219,220] Subsequently, it was shown that patients affected by PHP-Ib show a loss of methylation on the maternal allele, which is usually restricted to GNAS exon A/B.[243,244] Very recent studies revealed that most families with the autosomal dominant form of PHP-Ib with parental imprinting (AD-PHP-Ib) have a 3-kb deletion located between two 391-bp repeats about 220 kb upstream of exon A/B (Fig. 19-9).[237,245–247] Affected members of one additional AD-PHP-Ib kindred with loss of A/B methylation alone were recently shown to have a 4.4-kb deletion, which overlaps with the 3-kb deletion by 1286 bp.[248] In affected individuals with either mutation, the deletion is always found on the maternal allele, whereas it occurs on the paternal allele in unaffected healthy carriers. The affected members of two small families with broader methylation changes within the GNAS locus were recently shown to carry two distinct ~4-kb deletions on the maternal allele that remove NESP55 and the antisense exons 3 and 4.[249] Although indistinguishable broad methylation changes were observed in most patients with sporadic PHP-Ib, no deletions or point mutations have yet been identified in these individuals. Taken together these findings suggest that several different deletions upstream or within the GNAS locus lead to indistinguishable clinical and laboratory findings. However, it remains uncertain how the deletion affecting STX16 results in a loss of exon A/B methylation alone, whereas deletion of NESP55 results in a broader loss of methylation. Furthermore, it remains uncertain how the different deletions affect signaling through the PTH/PTHrP receptor in the proximal renal tubules, but not in most other tissues. Mice lacking the murine homolog of exon A/B were recently shown to have biallelic and thus increased Gsα transcription.[250] Loss of exon A/B methylation on the maternal allele, allowing active transcription from this promoter, seems therefore to have a prominent role in suppressing Gsα expression (see Fig. 19-9).

Blomstrand's Disease

Blomstrand's chondrodysplasia is an autosomal recessive human disorder characterized by early lethality, markedly advanced bone maturation, and accelerated chondrocyte differentiation.[251] Affected infants are typically born to consanguineous healthy parents (only in one instance did unrelated healthy parents have two affected offspring),[252–256] show

pronounced hyperdensity of the entire skeleton (Fig. 19-10) and markedly advanced ossification, and particularly the long bones are extremely short and poorly modeled. Recently, PTH/PTHrP receptor mutations that impair its functional properties were identified as the most likely cause of Blomstrand's disease (see Fig. 19-7). One of these defects is caused by a nucleotide exchange in exon M5 of the maternal PTH/PTHrP receptor allele, which introduces a novel splice acceptor site and thus leads to the synthesis of a receptor mutant that does not mediate, despite seemingly normal cell surface expression, the actions of PTH or PTHrP; the patient's paternal PTH/PTHrP receptor allele is, for yet unknown reasons, only poorly expressed.[257] In a second patient with Blomstrand's disease, the product of a consanguineous marriage, a nucleotide exchange was identified that changes proline at position 132 to leucine.[258,259] The resulting PTH/PTHrP receptor mutant showed, despite reasonable cell surface expression, severely impaired binding of radiolabeled PTH and PTHrP analogs, greatly reduced agonist-stimulated cAMP accumulation, and no measurable inositol phosphate response. Additional loss-of-function mutations involving the PTH/PTHrP receptor have recently been identified in three unrelated patients with Blomstrand's disease. Two of these mutations led to a frameshift and a truncated protein due either to a homozygous single-nucleotide deletion in exon EL2[260] or a 27-bp insertion between exon M4 and EL2.[261] The other defect was a nonsense mutation at residue 104 that resulted in a truncated receptor protein.[261] As in Jansen's disease, the identification of mutant PTH/PTHrP receptors provided a plausible explanation for the severe abnormalities in endochondral bone formation in patients with Blomstrand's disease. The disease is lethal and it is likely that affected infants show (in addition to the striking skeletal defects) abnormalities in other organs, including secondary hyperplasia of the parathyroid glands, presumably due to hypocalcemia. Indeed, analysis of fetuses with Blomstrand's disease have revealed abnormal breast development and tooth impaction, highlighting the involvement of the PTH/PTHrP receptor in the normal development of breast and tooth.[262]

HYPERPHOSPHATEMIC DISORDERS WITH NORMAL PARATHYROID GLAND ACTIVITY

Tumoral Calcinosis with/without Hyperphosphatemia

At least three variants of tumoral calcinosis have been described: an autosomal dominant form[263] and two apparently more common autosomal recessive forms that are caused by mutations in two different genes.[264] Patients affected by the autosomal dominant form usually have elevated serum 1,25(OH)$_2$ vitamin D levels, but classic findings of tumoral calcinosis may not always be present. The teeth are hypoplastic with short, bulbous roots and almost complete obliteration of pulp cavities, but they have fully developed enamel of normal color. The molecular defect of this autosomal dominant form of the disorder is not known.

The autosomal recessive forms of tumoral calcinosis are severe, sometimes fatal disorders, characterized by hyperphosphatemia and often massive calcium deposits in the skin and

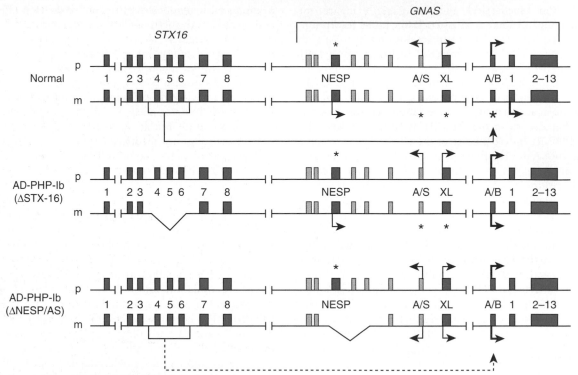

Figure 19-9 Location of microdeletions leading to autosomal dominant pseudohypoparathyroidism type Ib (AD-PHP-Ib) and possible molecular mechanism underlying the marked reduction of Gsα expression in the renal proximal tubules. *GNAS* gives rise to multiple transcripts, some of which show allele-specific methylation in their promoters (*asterisks*) and are expressed exclusively from the nonmethylated allele (*arrows*). The Gsα-specific promoter (exon 1) does not show differential methylation, and transcripts encoding the stimulatory G protein are therefore biallelically expressed in most tissues. However, Gsα expression seems to occur predominantly from the maternal (m) *GNAS* allele in the renal proximal tubules and a few other tissues. Exon A/B methylation is established in the female germline and maintained on the maternal allele through pre- and post-implantation development and is thus considered as an "imprint mark". In AD-PHP-Ib kindreds, maternal inheritance of microdeletions affecting *STX16* is associated with loss of methylation at exon A/B alone, whereas deletions affecting *NESP55* and two of the antisense exons lead to the loss of all maternal methylation imprints; paternal (p) inheritance of either deletion is not associated with imprinting defects, and individuals carrying these deletions on the paternal allele are healthy. It has been suggested that in the renal proximal tubules a lack of exon A/B methylation and thus active transcription of A/B mRNA, both of which are normally seen on the paternal *GNAS* allele, mediate, *in cis*, the silencing of Gsα transcription. The maternal loss of exon A/B methylation in AD-PHP-Ib is therefore predicted to cause a marked reduction in Gsα expression and consequently resistance to PTH (and perhaps to few other hormones). Black and gray boxes depict exons of *STX16* and *GNAS* that are transcribed in the sense or antisense direction, respectively. *Asterisk*, CpG methylation; *arrow*, active transcription.

subcutaneous tissues. Recently, Topaz and colleagues mapped the gene causing one form of the disease to 2q24–q31 and revealed homozygous or compound heterozygous mutations in GALNT3,[264] which encodes a glycosyltransferase responsible for initiating mucin-type O-glycosylation. Interestingly, the concentrations of C-terminal FGF23 were significantly elevated in affected individuals. These findings implied that defective post-translational modifications of FGF23 could be responsible for the abnormal regulation of phosphate homeostasis (see Fig. 19-2). Another form of tumoral calcinosis was shown to be caused by homozygous mutations in FGF23, and patients affected by this disorder also showed markedly elevated circulating concentration of C-terminal FGF23, whereas the concentration of the intact protein was within normal limits.[265–267] It remains uncertain whether forms of tumoral calcinosis without hyperphosphatemia are also caused by GALNT3 or FGF23 mutations.

Hyperostosis with Hyperphosphatemia

The combination of hyperostosis with hyperphosphatemia was first described in 1970.[268] Besides recurrent painful swelling of long bones, which can have features of tumoral calcinosis, affected patients present with elevated blood phosphate levels, yet normal renal function and usually normal serum calcium, $1,25(OH)_2$ vitamin D, and PTH concentrations.[269] Most cases seem to be sporadic, but consanguineous parents were described for some patients, implying that the disease can be recessive; the underlying molecular defect is not yet known. Recently, GALNT3 mutations were identified in the recessive form of this disease, indicating that one of the two forms of tumoral calcinosis and hyperostosis with hyperphosphatemia are allelic variants.[270] As in patients with the autosomal recessive forms of tumoral calcinosis, C-terminal FGF23 concentrations seem to be significantly elevated.[271]

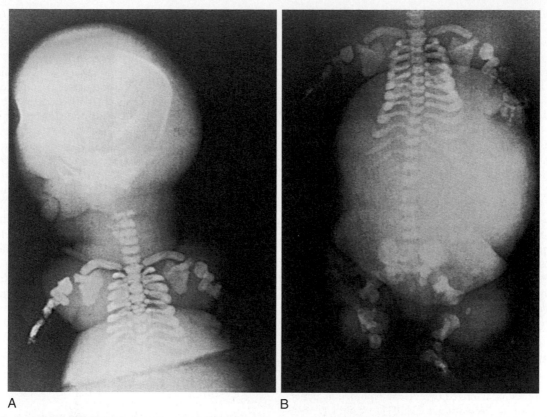

Figure 19-10 Radiologic findings in a patient with Blomstrand's disease. Note the markedly advanced ossification of all skeletal elements, and the extremely short limbs, despite the comparatively normal size and shape of hands and feet. Furthermore, note that the clavicles are relatively long and abnormally shaped. (From Leroy JG, Keersmaeckers G, Cooper M, et al: Blomstrand lethal chrondrodysplasia. Am Med Genet 63:84–89, 1996.)

HYPOPHOSPHATEMIC DISORDERS WITH NORMAL PARATHYROID GLAND ACTIVITY

The different forms of hypophosphatemia represent the commonest causes of hereditary rickets, which can be divided into two main groups according to the predominant metabolic abnormality.[272,273] In the first group, hypophosphatemia is the result of a renal tubular defect, which may consist of either a single (isolated) defect in renal phosphate handling, in that it occurs in the X-linked and autosomal dominant forms of hypophosphatemic rickets (XLH and ADHR, respectively), or of multiple tubular defects affecting phosphate, amino acids, glucose, bicarbonate, and potassium handling as occurs in the Fanconi syndromes of Lowe syndrome and Dent's disease. In the second group vitamin D metabolism is abnormal, either because of a defect in the 1α-hydroxylase enzyme or because of defects in the 1,25(OH)$_2$ vitamin D$_3$ receptor (VDR) leading to end-organ resistance. The application of molecular genetic approaches has helped to elucidate some of the mechanisms underlying these disorders of hereditary hypophosphatemic rickets. Thus, XLH has been shown to be due to inactivating mutations of *PHEX* (phosphate-regulating gene with homologies to endopeptidases on the X chromosome);[274,275] Lowe syndrome (oculocerebrorenal syndrome; X-linked recessive) is caused by mutations that result in a deficiency of a lipid phosphatase, which most likely controls cellular levels of the metabolite, phosphatidylinositol 4,5-bisphosphate (PIP$_2$) 5-phosphatase[276,277]; Dent's disease (X-linked recessive) results from loss-of-function mutations affecting a member of the voltage-gated chloride channel family, CLC-5[278]; vitamin D–dependent rickets type (VDDR type I; autosomal recessive) results from a deficiency of the renal 1α-hydroxylase enzyme,[279,280] which is a cytochrome P-450 enzyme that forms part of the superfamily of heme-containing proteins that are bound to the membranes of microsomes and mitochondria and serve as oxidation-reduction components of the mixed-function oxidase system; and VDDR type II (autosomal recessive) is caused by mutations involving the VDR, which is closely related to the thyroid hormone receptors and represents another member of the *trans*-acting transcriptional factors that include the family of steroid hormone receptors. Recent studies have furthermore identified the molecular basis of ADHR[28] and elucidated a role for this novel member of the FGF family in normal phosphate homeostasis (see Fig. 19-2), and acquired and inherited disorders of affecting the regulation of blood phosphate concentration.[30,36,281]

Autosomal Dominant Hypophosphatemic Rickets

ADHR is characterized by low serum phosphate concentrations, bone pain, rickets that can result in deformities of the legs, osteomalacia, and dental caries (clinical and laboratory findings can be variable). ADHR and XLH (see below) thus have marked clinical similarities but differ in their modes of inheritance. Genetic linkage studies mapped the *ADHR* locus to chromosome 12p13.3[282] and defined a 1.5-Mb critical region that contained 12 genes. Mutational analyses of 6 of these 12 genes revealed the occurrence of missense mutations involving a new member of the FGF family.[28] Three missense mutations of FGF23 (see Fig. 19-2) have been identified in four unrelated ADHR families affecting codons 176 and 179. Two unrelated ADHR families have an identical mutation involving codon 176, in which the normal positively charged arginine residue is replaced by a polar but uncharged glutamine residue (Arg176Gln). The other two mutations involve codon 179, and in one ADHR family the normal arginine residue is replaced by a nonpolar tryptophan (Trp) residue (Arg179Trp) and in the other ADHR family, it is replaced by a glutamine residue (Arg179Gln). The clustering of these ADHR missense mutations that alter arginine residues has led to the speculation that they may cause a gain of function. Mutational analysis of FGF23 in 18 patients, who had hypophosphatemic rickets but did not have *PHEX* mutations, revealed no abnormalities, suggesting a role(s) for other genes in these hereditary disorders of hypophosphatemic rickets.

Oncogenic Osteomalacia

OOM (also referred to as tumor-induced osteomalacia, TIO) is a rare disorder characterized by hypophosphatemia, hyperphosphaturia, a low circulating $1,25(OH)_2$ vitamin D_3 concentration, and osteomalacia that develops in previously unaffected individuals.[283] Thus, there are considerable similarities among OOM, XLH, and ADHR. OOM is caused by usually small, often difficult to locate tumors, most frequently hemangiopericytomas. The clinical and biochemical abnormalities resolve rapidly after the removal of the tumor, whereas in XLH and ADHR these abnormalities are lifelong. However, the similarities among OOM, ADHR, and XLH suggest that they may involve the same phosphate-regulating pathway, and it is important to note that OOM tumors do express PHEX,[284,285] which is mutated in XLH (see below). The possibility that FGF23, which is mutated in ADHR, may also be expressed in OOM tumors and that FGF23 may be a secreted protein was therefore explored.[27,29,286,287] Indeed, OOM tumors were found by Northern blot analysis to contain high levels of FGF23 mRNA and protein. Consistent with this finding, FGF23 plasma concentrations can be increased considerably in OOM patients, until the tumors are successfully removed.[287,288]

Tumors responsible for oncogenic osteomalacia produce two molecular forms of FGF23 (~32 and ~12 kD), and both variants were also observed when assessing conditioned medium from cell lines, such as OK-E, COS-7, and HEK 293 cells, expressing full-length, wild-type FGF23.[29] Thus, OOM tumors abundantly express FGF23, and these findings suggest that FGF23 may be the phosphaturic factor referred to as "phosphatonin" (see Fig. 19-2). When conditioned medium from cells expressing R176Q-FGF23 or R179Q-FGF23 was investigated by Western blot analysis, only the larger protein band was observed.[29,36,37] This implies that the known mutations in ADHR, which affect a consensus cleavage site for furin-type enzymes, impair FGF23 degradation thus enhancing and/or prolonging its biologic activity. In addition to furin-type enzymes, one recent in vitro study indicates that wild-type FGF23, but not the R179Q mutant, may also represent a substrate for PHEX[42] (see below).

X-Linked Hypophosphatemia

XLH is the most frequently inherited phosphate-wasting disorder. Just like ADHR, it is characterized by hypophosphatemia, hyperphosphaturia, low circulating $1,25(OH)_2$ vitamin D_3 concentration, and osteomalacia (Table 19-4). This disorder is caused by inactivating mutations in *PHEX*, a gene located on Xp22.1.[274,275] PHEX, which is expressed in kidney, bone, and other tissues, shows significant amino acid sequence homology to the M13 family of zinc metallopeptidases, which include neutral endopeptidase neprilysin, endothelin-converting

Table 19-4 Biochemical Features of Some Disorders Associated with Hypophosphatemic Rickets

Type	Serum				Urine				
	Ca^{2+}	PO_4^{3-}	$1,25(OH)_2D_3$	PTH	PO_4^{3-}	Ca^{2+}	Aminoaciduria	Glucose	pH <5.5
Renal Tubular Defect									
Hypophosphatemic rickets	N	↓	↓/N	N	↑	↓/N	–	–	Yes
Lowe syndrome	N/↓	↓	↓/N	N/↑	↑	↑/N	+	+	Yes
Dent's disease	N	↓	↑/N	N	↑	↑	+	+	Yes
Vitamin D Metabolism Defect									
Vitamin D–dependent rickets type I (VDDR I)	↓	↓/N	↓	↑	↑	↓	+	–	Yes
Vitamin D–dependent rickets type II (VDDR II)	↓	↓/N	↑↑	↑	↑	↓	+	–	Yes

N, normal; ↓ decreased; ↑ increased; + present; – absent. In these disorders, the serum 25-hydroxyvitamin D_3 concentrations are normal and the serum alkaline phosphatase is usually elevated. Urine pH <5.5 refers to that found during a severe metabolic acidosis or an ammonium chloride loading test.

enzyme 1, and 2, and the Kell antigen. All of these are type II integral membrane glycoproteins that have endopeptidase activity and consist of a short N-terminal cytoplasmic domain, a single transmembrane hydrophobic region, and a large extracellular domain. Thus, neutral endopeptidase neprilysin functions as a membrane-bound ectoenzyme that proteolytically inactivates a number of peptides that include atrial natruretic peptide, enkephalin, substance P, and bradykinin, whereas endothelin-converting enzyme proteolytically activates endothelin. The substrate(s) for PHEX remains to be established, but three possible candidates (see Fig. 19-2) can be considered. These are FGF23 (see above), matrix extracellular phosphoglycoprotein (MEPE),[46,289] and secreted frizzled related protein 4 (sFRP4).[27,45] Among these proteins, FGF23 seems the most likely substrate for PHEX and hence the candidate for being phosphatonin. Consistent with this conclusion, serum FGF23 concentrations are elevated in about two-thirds of patients with XLH,[234,288] and they are unequivocally elevated in all *Hyp* mice (the murine homolog of XLH).[290,291]

However, PHEX-dependent cleavage of FGF23 could not yet be demonstrated in vivo, and FGF23 cleavage in vitro has been documented thus far only in one study. If FGF23 cleavage by PHEX can be confirmed, it is conceivable that the different inactivating *PHEX* mutations identified in patients with XLH and the large *Phex* deletions in *Hyp* and *Gy* mice adversely affect not only osteoblast-specific functions but may result also in impaired degradation of FGF23. Different molecular mechanisms (e.g., overexpression/production of FGF23 by the tumors responsible for oncogenic osteomalacia, generation of a mutant FGF23 that is resistant to cleavage in patients with ADHR, and failure of FGF23 degradation due to loss or reduction in PHEX activity in patients with XLH) may thus lead to elevated FGF23 concentrations, and consequently to renal phosphate wasting and possibly impaired functional properties of osteoblasts. In OOM, on the other hand, overproduction of FGF23 may exceed the capacity of PHEX to inactivate FGF23, thus leading to an excess of phosphatonin. Attractive as this hypothesis may be, one still needs to prove that FGF23 is really a substrate for PHEX. Interestingly, preliminary studies revealed that *Hyp* mice, which were injected with inactivating antibodies to FGF23, normalized their blood phosphate concentration and furthermore healed their rachitic changes, thus supporting the conclusion that Phex is directly or indirectly involved in the metabolism of FGF23.[290] Furthermore, genetic ablation of *Fgf23* in male *Hyp* mice (i.e., animals that are null for *Fgf23* and *Phex*) leads to blood phosphate levels that are indistinguishable from those in mice lacking *Fgf23* alone,[32,292] thereby suggesting that *Fgf23* resides genetically upstream of *Phex*.

Nephrolithasis or Osteoporosis Associated with Hypophosphatemia

Two different heterozygous mutations (A48P and V147M) in *NPT2a*, the gene encoding a sodium-dependent phosphate transporter, have been reported in patients with urolithiasis or osteoporosis and persistent idiopathic hypophosphatemia due to decreased tubular phosphate reabsorption.[293] When expressed in *Xenopus laevis* oocytes, the mutant NPT2a showed impaired function and, when co-injected, dominant negative properties. However, these in vitro findings were not confirmed in another study using oocytes and OK cells,

raising the concern that the identified *NPT2a* mutation alone cannot explain the findings in the described patients.[294] On the other hand, additional new mutations were recently identified in other patients with a similar clinical phenotype.

Hereditary Hypophosphatemic Rickets with Hypercalciuria

The homozygous ablation of *Npt2a* in mice (*Npt2a*$^{-/-}$) results, as expected, in increased urinary phosphate excretion leading to hypophosphatemia. As a result of the hypophosphatemia, *Npt2a*$^{-/-}$ mice show an appropriate elevation in the serum levels of 1,25(OH)$_2$ vitamin D leading to hypercalcemia, hypercalciuria, and decreased serum PTH levels, and increased serum alkaline phosphatase activity.[295] These biochemical features are typically observed in patients with hereditary hypophosphatemic rickets with hypercalciuria (HHRH), a presumably autosomal recessive disorder affecting renal tubular phosphate reabsorption.[296] HHRH patients develop rickets, have short stature, and increased renal phosphate clearance (tubular maximum for phosphate corrected for glomerular filtration rate [TmP/GFR] is usually 2–4 standard deviations below the age-related normal range), hypercalciuria despite normal serum calcium levels, increased gastrointestinal absorption of calcium and phosphorus due to an elevated serum concentration of 1,25(OH)$_2$ vitamin D, suppressed parathyroid function, and normal urinary cAMP excretion. Long-term phosphate supplementation as the sole therapy leads, with the exception of persistently decreased TmP/GFR, to reversal of the clinical and biochemical abnormalities.[296] Unlike HHRH patients, *Npt2a*$^{-/-}$ mice do not have rickets or osteomalacia. Instead, they have poorly developed trabecular bone and retarded secondary ossification, and in older animals there is a marked reversal and eventual overcompensation of the skeletal phenotype. Consistent with these phenotypic differences, mutations in *SLC34A1*, the gene encoding the Na/phosphate cotransporter NPT2a were excluded in several kindreds, including the one in whom this syndrome was first described.[296,297] However, recent studies have led to the identification of homozygous or compound heterozygous mutations in *SLC34A3*, the gene encoding the Na/phosphate cotransporter NPT2c, in patients affected by HHRH.[298,299] These findings indicate that NPT2c has a more important role in phosphate homeostasis than previously thought.[300]

Dent Disease

Dent disease is an X-linked recessive renal tubular disorder characterized by a low-molecular-weight proteinuria, hypercalciuria, nephrocalcinosis, nephrolithiasis, and eventual renal failure.[278] Dent's disease is also associated with the other multiple proximal tubular defects of the renal Fanconi syndrome, which include aminoaciduria, phosphaturia, glycosuria, kaliuresis, uricosuria, and impaired urinary acidification (see Table 19-4). With the exception of rickets, which occurs in a minority of patients, there appear to be no extrarenal manifestations in Dent disease. The gene linked to Dent disease, *CLCN5*, encodes the voltage-gated chloride channel, ClC-5.[301] Members of the voltage-gated chloride channel (CLC) family conduct chloride currents that are outwardly rectifying and with a conductivity sequence that prefers chloride to iodide. These CLCs have important diverse functions that include the control of membrane excitability, transepithelial transport, and regulation of cell volume.[302] CLC-5, which is predominantly expressed in the kidney, particularly the proximal tubule, thick ascending limb of Henle, and the α-intercalated cells of the collecting duct, has been reported to be critical for acidification in the endosomes that participate in solute reabsorption and membrane recycling in the proximal tubule.[303,304] CLC-5 is also known to alter membrane trafficking via the receptor-mediated endocytic pathway that involves megalin and cubulin.[305] *CLCN5* mutations associated with Dent disease impair chloride flow through ClC-5 and probably lead to impaired acidification of the endosomal lumen, and thereby also disrupt trafficking of endosomes back to the apical surface.[303–306] This will result in impairment of solute reabsorption by the renal tubule and in the defects observed in Dent disease. Mice that are deficient in Clc5 develop the phenotypic abnormalities associated with Dent disease.[304,306] Mutations of the gene encoding PIP_2 5-phosphatase, which are linked to Lowe syndrome (see below), also may be associated with Dent disease.[307]

The Oculo-Cerebro-Renal Syndrome of Lowe

The oculo-cerebro-renal syndrome of Lowe (OCRL) is an X-linked recessive disorder that is characterized by congenital cataracts, mental retardation, muscular hypotonia, rickets, and defective proximal tubular reabsorption of bicarbonate, phosphate, and amino acids (see Table 19-4).[308] The disease is nearly always confined to males, who develop renal dysfunction in the first year of life, have delayed bone age and reduced height, and may die in childhood. Female carriers who have normal neurologic and renal function, can be identified in 80% of cases by micropunctate cortical lens opacities.[309] The Lowe syndrome gene, *OCRL1*, is located on Xq25–q26.[310] Point mutations and deletions were demonstrated in affected individuals, thereby providing conclusive evidence that the *OCRL1* gene is the cause of Lowe syndrome.[311] OCRL1 consists of 23 exons that encode a member of the type II family of inositol polyphosphate-5-phosphatases.[312] These enzymes hydrolyze the 5-phosphate of 1,4,5-inositol triphosphate and of 1,3,4,5-inositol tetrakisphosphate, phosphatidylinositol-4,5,-bisphosphonate, and phosphatidylinositol-3,4,5 -trisphosphate, thereby presumably inactivating them as second messengers in the phosphatidylinositol signaling pathway. The preferred substrate of OCRL1 is phosphatidylinositol-4,5-bisphosphate, and this lipid accumulates in renal proximal tubule cells from patients with Lowe syndrome.[277] OCRL1 has been localized to lysosomes in renal proximal tubular cells and to the trans-Golgi network in fibroblasts.[276,313] This localization is consistent with the role for OCRL1 in lysosomal enzyme trafficking from the trans-Golgi network to lysosomes, and the activities of several lysosomal hydrolases are found to be elevated in plasma from affected patients. OCRL1 has also been shown to interact with clathrin and indeed colocalizes with clathrin on endosomal membranes that contain transferrin and mannose 6-phosphate receptors.[314] Mannose 6-phosphate receptor-bound lysosomal enymes are recruited by appendage subunits and Golgi-localized binding proteins into clathrin-coated vesicles that transport them from the trans-Golgi network to endosomes.[314] Thus, it seems likely the *OCRL1* mutations in Lowe syndrome patients result

in OCRL1 protein deficiency, which leads to disruptions in lysosomal trafficking and endosomal sorting.[314] This abnormality is similar to that observed in Dent disease, and it is of interest to note that some patients with the latter disease, who had no demonstrable *CLCN5* mutations, were found instead to have *OCRL1* mutations.[307] The absence of cataracts in patients with Dent disease due to *OCRL1* mutations was the major phenotypic difference when compared with patients with Lowe syndrome.[307] The molecular and cellular basis of these phenotypic differences still remains to be elucidated.

Vitamin D–Dependent Rickets

Patients with VDDR type I show clinical and laboratory findings that are similar to those observed in patients with vitamin D–deficient rickets. However, unlike in vitamin D deficiency, patients with VDDR type I do not respond to treatment with vitamin D and instead require treatment with $1,25(OH)_2$ vitamin D. VDDR type I was therefore named pseudovitamin D deficiency rickets.[315] Clarification of the abnormal vitamin D metabolism[316] led to the recognition that VDDR type I was due to a defect in the renal 1α-hydroxylase enzyme; consequently serum $1,25(OH)_2$ vitamin D concentration is low. Subsequently another condition was recognized and called VDDR type II. In this condition, which is due to end-organ resistance to $1,25(OH)_2$ vitamin D, the serum $1,25(OH)_2$ vitamin D concentration is markedly elevated. This condition does not respond to vitamin D therapy, including calcitriol, and so the term *vitamin D dependency* is not satisfactory and it may be better to refer to this condition as "end organ–resistant rickets".

1α-Hydroxylase Deficiency

Patients affected by VDDR type I (autosomal recessive) show almost all the clinical and biochemical features of VDDR. Typically, the child is well at birth and within the next 2 years develops hypotonia, muscle weakness, an inability to stand or walk, growth retardation, convulsions, frontal bossing, and the clinical and radiographic signs of rickets: rachitic rosary, thickened wrists and ankles, bowed legs, and fractures. A history of an adequate intake of vitamin D is usually obtained. Trousseau's and Chvostek's signs may be present. The permanent teeth show marked enamel hypoplasia, a feature not seen in X-linked hypophosphatemic rickets.[317] Laboratory investigations (see Table 19-4) reveal hypocalcemia with secondary hyperparathyroidism and associated increased urinary cAMP, phosphate, and amino acid excretion, elevated serum alkaline phosphatase activity, either normal or low serum phosphate levels, a low urinary calcium excretion, and decreased intestinal absorption of calcium. VDDR type I is an autosomal recessive disorder.

The pathogenesis of VDDR type I was first elucidated by studying vitamin D metabolism in affected patients, and it was shown that massive doses of vitamin D_3 and high doses of 25(OH) vitamin D_3, but only small doses of $1,25(OH)_2$ vitamin D_3 were required to correct the clinical and biochemical abnormalities.[316] This provided indirect evidence that the condition was due to an inborn error of vitamin D metabolism, that is, a defect in the renal 1α-hydroxylase enzyme, the enzyme that converts 25(OH) vitamin D_3 to $1,25(OH)_2$ vitamin D_3. Studies of circulating vitamin D metabolites in patients provided further support for this hypothesis. The serum 25(OH) vitamin D_3 concentration was normal in untreated patients and high in patients treated with vitamin D, whereas the serum concentration of $1,25(OH)_2$ vitamin D_3 was low in untreated patients[318] and remained low or low-normal in patients treated with vitamin D_3.[319] The low serum concentrations of $1,25(OH)_2$ vitamin D_3 despite the normal or high serum 25(OH) vitamin D_3 can be explained by a deficiency in the renal 1α-hydroxylase[319–321] and molecular genetic studies have later confirmed this conclusion. Indeed, genetic linkage studies in affected French-Canadian families mapped VDDR type I to a region on chromosome 12q13.3,[322] which comprises the gene encoding the 25(OH) vitamin D 1α-hydroxylase. DNA sequence analysis of patients affected by VDDR type I have identified more than 20 different mutations of the 25(OH) 1α-hydroxylase gene[279,323–326] in 26 kindreds. All patients with VDDR type I were found to carry homozygous or compound heterozygous mutations, whereas the obligate carriers are heterozygous in having the mutant and normal alleles.

End-Organ Resistance (VDR Mutations, VDDR Type II)

Vitamin D–dependent rickets type II (VDDR type II; autosomal recessive) is an autosomal recessive disorder caused by end-organ resistance to $1,25(OH)_2$ vitamin D_3.[327–329] The laboratory and radiographic features of VDDR type II are similar to those found in VDDR type I (see Table 19-4), with one major exception; patients with VDDR type II have markedly elevated circulating concentrations of $1,25(OH)_2$ vitamin D_3. The disease varies in its clinical and biochemical manifestations, which suggested heterogeneity in the underlying molecular defects.[329] Most of the patients have early-onset rickets, but the first reported patient was a 22-year-old woman who had skeletal pain for 7 years,[327] and another patient presented at the age of 50 years after being symptomatic for 5 years.[330] Alopecia totalis occurs in some patients, and it was suggested that the therapeutic response to the 1α-hydroxylated derivative of vitamin D_3 in patients with normal hair growth was better than in those with alopecia totalis,[331] but this was not found to be a constant predictive sign.[332] The severity of resistance to $1,25(OH)_2$ vitamin D_3 is variable, and some patients have improved following therapy with very large doses of vitamin D[333] or $1,25(OH)_2$ vitamin D_3.[334–336] In patients who are refractory to vitamin D therapy, alternative treatments with oral calcium supplements have been tried with limited success. However, long-term nocturnal intravenous calcium infusions followed by oral calcium supplementation have successfully healed rickets and promoted bone mineralization in VDDR II patients,[337] although there are considerable practical difficulties with this therapy.

The elevated serum concentrations of $1,25(OH)_2$ vitamin D_3 in patients with VDDR II suggested an abnormality in the mode of action of $1,25(OH)_2$ vitamin D_3 within target tissues. The functions of $1,25(OH)_2$ vitamin D_3 are mediated by an intracellular receptor that binds DNA and concentrates the hormone in the nucleus,[338] analogous to the classical steroid hormones.[339] The interactions between $1,25(OH)_2$ vitamin D_3 and its intracellular receptor have been studied using cultured skin fibroblasts from control subjects and patients with VDDR II.[340,341] Several defects were identified, including absent receptors, a decreased number of receptors with normal affinity, a normal receptor-hormone binding but a subsequent failure to translocate the hormone to the nucleus, and a post-receptor defect, in which normal receptors are present but there is a deficiency in the induction of the 25(OH) vitamin D-24 hydroxylase enzyme in response to $1,25(OH)_2$ vitamin D. Thus, the heterogeneity suggested from clinical observations in VDDR II patients could be demonstrated at the cellular level with various combinations of defective receptor-hormone binding and expression. The $1,25(OH)_2$ vitamin D_3 receptor (VDR), which is closely related to the thyroid hormone receptors and represents another member of the *trans*-acting transcriptional factors including the steroid and thyroid hormone receptors, is an intracellular protein with a molecular weight of 60,000 daltons. The binding site for $1,25(OH)_2$ vitamin D_3 resides in the C-terminal part of the protein whereas the N-terminal part of the molecule possesses the DNA-binding domain.[342] Zinc and other divalent cations are important in maintaining the DNA-binding function of the receptor, possibly by determining the conformation of the protein and giving rise to processes that can interdigitate between the helices of DNA. This hormone-receptor complex binds to a DNA region, which is located upstream of the promoter of genes encoding calcium-binding proteins and other proteins.

The availability of cDNAs encoding the avian and human VDR[343] helped to clarify the molecular basis of VDDR type II.[344] Nucleotide sequence analysis of genomic DNA revealed that the human VDR gene consists of 9 exons; exons 2 and 3 encode the DNA-binding domain, whereas exons 7, 8, and 9 encode the vitamin D–binding domain. The gene is located on chromosome 12q12–q14 in humans,[322] that is, in a region that comprises the gene encoding the 1α-hydroxylase. Mutational analysis of the VDR gene in VDDR II patients demonstrated the presence of nonsense and missense mutations affecting different parts of the receptor. Expression of these mutations in COS-1 monkey kidney cells demonstrated that these mutations result in a reduction or a loss of VDR function similar to the heterogeneous effects observed in cultured fibroblasts from VDDR II patients. Furthermore, VDR-null mutant (knockout) mice produced by targeted gene disruption[345,346] were found to have growth retardation, skeletal deformities, and an earlier mortality, and adult mice developed alopecia. In addition, biochemical investigations revealed that the VDR-knockout mice were hypocalcemic and hypophosphatemic, with markedly elevated serum $1,25(OH)_2$ vitamin D_3 concentrations. Thus, the VDR-null mutant mice have the features consistent with those observed in patients with VDDR type II.

Hypophosphatasia

Hypophosphatasia is a rare inherited form of rickets[347] that is characterized by a deficient activity of the tissue-nonspecific (i.e., liver, bone, and kidney) isoenzyme of alkaline phosphatase (TNSALP). Although TNSALP is ubiquitous in tissues and especially abundant in liver, kidney, cartilage, and bone, hypophosphatasia seems to affect only hard tissues. Moreover, the severity of hypophosphatasia is remarkably variable, ranging from premature loss of teeth, to intrauterine death because of profound skeletal hypomineralization. Thus, six clinical types of hypophosphatasia are recognized depending on the age of onset and the extent of the skeletal disease.[347]

Perinatal, infantile, childhood, and adult hypophosphatasia cause skeletal and dental disease. Odontohypophosphatasia, which refers to the occurrence of premature tooth loss without skeletal disease, may also occur in childhood or adulthood. The major biochemical abnormality is a serum alkaline phosphatase activity that is subnormal for age and sex (i.e., hypophosphatasemia).[347] Serum calcium and phosphate are not low, and hypercalcemia with hypercalciuria often accompany the infantile form. Serum levels of PTH, 25(OH) vitamin D, and 1,25(OH)$_2$ vitamin D are usually normal. Three phosphocompounds accumulate endogenously in hypophatasia. These are phosphoethanolamine, inorganic pyrophosphate, and pyridoxal 5′-phosphate. Urinary phosphoethanolamine and plasma pyridoxal 5′-phosphate may be measured, and an increased plasma pyridoxal 5′-phosphate concentration is a sensitive and specific marker for hypophosphatasia.[347] Defective skeletal mineralization occurs in all clinical forms of hypophosphatasia but not odontohypophosphatasia. The radiologic and histologic findings are similar to those of other forms of rickets or osteomalacia without secondary hyperparathyroidism.[347] The perinatal and infantile forms are inherited as autosomal recessive traits. The inheritance of the childhood, adult, and odonto-forms of hypophosphatasia is often not clear, although some patients seem to show autosomal recessive inheritance. The gene encoding TNSALP is located on chromosome 1p36.1–p34 and consists of 12 exons.[347] Patients with perinatal and infantile hypophosphatasia are either homozygotes or compound heterozygotes for the mutations. Conventional treatments for rickets or osteomalacia are best avoided in patients with hypophosphatasia, because this may provoke or exacerbate hypercalcemia and hypercalciuria. Enzyme replacement by intravenous infusion of various forms of alkaline phosphatase has been disappointing, but improvement following bone marrow cell transplantation has been reported to result in an improvement.[347,348]

CONCLUSION

Remarkable advances have been made in identifying key proteins that are involved, either directly or indirectly, in the regulation of calcium and phosphate homeostasis, the hormones that are involved in these mechanisms, and receptors that mediate these hormonal actions in the different target tissues. Furthermore, the identification of mutations in several of these proteins provided a plausible molecular explanation for a variety of familial and sporadic disorders of mineral ion homeostasis and/or bone development. In addition to advances in further defining the biologic role(s) of known proteins, genetic loci and/or candidate genes have been identified for many of the inherited disorders associated with an abnormal regulation of calcium and phosphate homeostasis. It is likely that the definition of these familial disorders at the molecular level, which is greatly aided by the rapid progress in the Human Genome Project, and the exploration of the underlying cellular mechanisms will provide further important insights into the regulation of calcium and phosphate.

Acknowledgments

R.V.T. is grateful to the Medical Research Council (UK) and Wellcome Trust for support, and H.J. is supported by grants from the National Institutes of Health, NIDDK (DK-46718 and DK-50708). The authors would like to thank Mrs. Tracey Walker and Mrs. Latanya Turner for typing the manuscript and expert secretarial assistance.

References

1. Naylor SL, Sakaguchi AU, Szoka P, et al: Human parathyroid hormone gene (PTH) is on short arm of chromosome 11. Somat Cell Gene 9:609–616, 1983.
2. Vasicek T, McDevitt BE, Freeman MW, et al: Nucleotide sequence of genomic DNA encoding human parathyroid hormone. Proc Natl Acad Sci U S A 80:2127–2131, 1983.
3. Okazaki T, Igarashi T, Kronenberg HM: 5′-Flanking region of the parathyroid hormone gene mediates negative regulation by 1,25(OH)$_2$ vitamin D$_3$. J Biol Chem 263:2203–2208, 1989.
4. Demay MB, Kiernan MS, DeLuca HF, Kronenberg HM: Sequences in the human parathyroid hormone gene that bind the 1,25-dihydroxyvitamin D$_3$ receptor and mediate transcriptional repression in response to 1,25-dihydroxyvitamin D$_3$. Proc Natl Acad Sci U S A 89:8097–8101, 1992.
5. Naveh-Many T, Rahaminov R, Livini N, Silver J: Parathyroid cell proliferation in normal and chronic renal failure in rats. The effects of calcium, phosphate, and vitamin D. J Clin Invest 96:1786–1793, 1995.
6. Almaden Y, Canalejo A, Hernandez A, et al: Direct effect of phosphorus on PTH secretion from whole rat parathyroid glands in vitro. J Bone Miner Res 970–976, 1996.
7. Russell J, Lettieri D, Sherwood LM: Direct regulation by calcium of cytoplasmic messenger ribonucleic acid coding for pre-proparathyroid hormone in isolated bovine parathyroid cells. J Clin Invest 72:1851–1855, 1983.
8. Naveh-Many T, Friedlaender MM, Mayer H, Silver J: Calcium regulates parathyroid hormone messenger ribonucleic acid (mRNA), but not calcitonin mRNA in vivo in the rat. Dominant role of 1,25-dihydroxyvitamin D. Endocrinology 125:275–280, 1989.
9. Kemper B, Habener JF, Mulligan RC, et al: Preproparathyroid hormone: A direct translation product of parathyroid messenger RNA. Proc Natl Acad Sci U S A 71:3731–3735, 1974.
10. Jüppner H, Gardella T, Brown E, et al: Parathyroid hormone and parathyroid hormone–related peptide in the regulation of calcium homeostasis and bone development. In DeGroot L, Jameson J (eds): Endocrinology. Philadelphia, WB Saunders, 2000, pp 969–998.
11. Suva LJ, Winslow GA, Wettenhall RE, et al: A parathyroid hormone–related protein implicated in malignant hypercalcemia: Cloning and expression. Science 237:893–896, 1987.
12. Mangin M, Webb AC, Dreyer BE, et al: Identification of a cDNA encoding a parathyroid hormone–like peptide from a human tumor associated with humoral hypercalcemia of malignancy. Proc Natl Acad Sci U S A 85:597–601, 1988.
13. Strewler GJ, Stern PH, Jacobs JW, et al: Parathyroid hormone–like protein from human renal carcinoma cells. Structural and functional homology with parathyroid hormone. J Clin Invest 80:1803–1807, 1987.
14. Strewler GJ: Mechanisms of disease: The physiology of parathyroid hormone-related protein. N Engl J Med 342:177–185, 2000.
15. Broadus AE, Stewart AF: Parathyroid hormone–related protein: Structure, processing, and physiological actions. In Bilezikian JP, Levine MA, Marcus R (eds): The Parathyroids: Basic and Clinical Concepts. New York, Raven Press, 1994, pp 259–294.
16. Yang KH, Stewart AF: Parathyroid hormone-related protein: The gene, its mRNA species, and protein products. In

Bilezikian JP, Raisz LG, Rodan RA (eds): Principles of Bone Biology. New York, Academic Press, 1996, pp 347–362.

17. Kronenberg H: Developmental regulation of the growth plate. Nature 423:332–336, 2003.

18. Jüppner H, Abou-Samra AB, Freeman MW, et al: A G protein–linked receptor for parathyroid hormone and parathyroid hormone–related peptide. Science 254:1024–1026, 1991.

19. Abou-Samra AB, Jüppner H, Force T, et al: Expression cloning of a common receptor for parathyroid hormone and parathyroid hormone–related peptide from rat osteoblast-like cells: A single receptor stimulates intracellular accumulation of both cAMP and inositol triphosphates and increases intracellular free calcium. Proc Natl Acad Sci U S A 89:2732–2736, 1992.

20. Gelbert L, Schipani E, Jüppner H, et al: Chromosomal location of the parathyroid hormone/parathyroid hormone–related protein receptor gene to human chromosome 3p21.2–p24.2. J Clin Endocrinol Metab 79:1046–1048, 1994.

21. Pausova Z, Bourdon J, Clayton D, et al: Cloning of a parathyroid hormone/parathyroid hormone related peptide receptor (PTHR) cDNA from a rat osteosarcoma (UMR106) cell line: Chromosomal assignment of the gene in the human, mouse, and rat genomes. Genomics 20:20–26, 1994.

22. Lee K, Deeds JD, Segre GV: Expression of parathyroid hormone–related peptide and its receptor messenger ribonucleic acid during fetal development of rats. Endocrinology 136:453–463, 1995.

23. Whyte MP: Rickets and osteomalacia. In Wass J, Shalet S (eds): Oxford Textbook of Endocrinology. New York, Oxford University Press, 2002, pp 697–715.

24. Liberman U, Marx SJ: Vitamin D and other calciferols. In Scriver C, Beaudlt A, Sly W, Valle D (eds): The Metabolic and Molecular Bases of Inherited Disease. New York, McGraw-Hill, 2001, pp 4223–4240.

25. Haussler MR, Haussler CA, Jurutka PW, et al: The vitamin D hormone and its nuclear receptor: Molecular actions and disease states. J Endocrinol 154(Suppl):S57–S73, 1997.

26. Yamashita T, Yoshioka M, Itoh N: Identification of a novel fibroblast growth factor, FGF-23, preferentially expressed in the ventrolateral thalamic nucleus of the brain. Biochem Biophys Res Commun 277:494–498, 2000.

27. Jan De Beur S, Finnegan R, Vassiliadis J, et al: Tumors associated with oncogenic osteomalacia express genes important in bone and mineral metabolism. J Bone Miner Res 17:1102–1110, 2002.

28. ADHR Consortium; White KE, Evans WE, O'Riordan JLH, et al: Autosomal dominant hypophosphataemic rickets is associated with mutations in FGF23. Nat Genet 26:345–348, 2000.

29. White K, Jonsson K, Carn G, et al: The autosomal dominant hypophosphatemic rickets (ADHR) gene is a secreted polypeptide overexpressed by tumors that cause phosphate wasting. J Clin Endocrinol Metab 86:497–500, 2001.

30. Shimada T, Mizutani S, Muto T, et al: Cloning and characterization of FGF23 as a causative factor of tumor-induced osteomalacia. Proc Natl Acad Sci U S A 98:6500–6505, 2001.

31. Riminucci M, Collins M, Fedarko N, et al: FGF-23 in fibrous dysplasia of bone and its relationship to renal phosphate wasting. J Clin Invest 112:683–692, 2003.

32. Sitara D, Razzaque MS, Hesse M, et al: Homozygous ablation of fibroblast growth factor-23 results in hyperphosphatemia and impaired skeletogenesis, and reverses hypophosphatemia in Phex-deficient mice. Matrix Biol 23:421–432, 2004.

33. White K, Cabral J, Evans W, et al: A missense mutation in FGFR1 causes a novel syndrome: craniofacial dysplasia with hypophosphatemia (CFDH). Am J Hum Genet 76:361–367, 2005.

34. Yu X, Ibrahimi O, Goetz R, et al: Analysis of the biochemical mechanisms for the endocrine actions of FGF23. Endocrinology 146:4648–4656, 2005.

35. Urakawa I, Yamazaki Y, Shimada T, et al: Klotho converts canonical FGF receptor into a specific receptor for FGF23. Nature 444:770–774, 2006.

35a. Kurosu H, Ogawa Y, Miyoshi M, et al: Regulation of fibroblast growth factor–23 signaling by Klotho. J Biol Chem 281:6120–6123, 2006.

36. Shimada T, Muto T, Urakawa I, et al: Mutant FGF-23 responsible for autosomal dominant hypophosphatemic rickets is resistant to proteolytic cleavage and causes hypophosphatemia in vivo. Endocrinology 143:3179–3182, 2002.

37. Bai XY, Miao D, Goltzman D, Karaplis AC: The autosomal dominant hypophosphatemic rickets R176Q mutation in FGF23 resists proteolytic cleavage and enhances in vivo biological potency. J Biol Chem 278:9843–9849, 2003.

38. Bai X, Miao D, Li J, et al: Transgenic mice overexpressing human fibroblast growth factor 23(R176Q) delineate a putative role for parathyroid hormone in renal phosphate wasting disorders. Endocrinology 145:5269, 2004.

39. Shimada T, Urakawa I, Yamazaki Y, et al: FGF-23 transgenic mice demonstrate hypophosphatemic rickets with reduced expression of sodium phosphate cotransporter type IIa. Biochem Biophys Res Commun 314:409–414, 2004.

40. Larsson T, Marsell R, Schipani E, et al: Transgenic mice expressing fibroblast growth factor 23 under the control of the a1(I) collagen promoter exhibit growth retardation, osteomalacia and disturbed phosphate homeostasis. Endocrinology 145:3087–3094, 2004.

41. Shimada T, Kakitani M, Yamazaki Y, et al: Targeted ablation of Fgf23 demonstrates an essential physiological role of FGF23 in phosphate and vitamin D metabolism. J Clin Invest 113:561–568, 2004.

42. Bowe A, Finnegan R, Jan de Beur S, et al: FGF-23 inhibits renal tubular phosphate transport and is a PHEX substrate. Biochem Biophys Res Commun 284:977–981, 2001.

43. Yamashita T, Konishi M, Miyake A, et al: Fibroblast growth factor (FGF)-23 inhibits renal phosphate reabsorption by activation of the mitogen-activated protein kinase pathway. J Biol Chem 277:28265–28270, 2002.

44. Carpenter T, Ellis B, Insogna K, et al: FGF7—An inhibitor of phosphate transport derived from oncogenic osteomalacia-causing tumors. J Clin Endocrinol Metab 90:1012–1020, 2005.

45. Berndt T, Craig T, Bowe A, et al: Secreted frizzled-related protein 4 is a potent tumor-derived phosphaturic agent. J Clin Invest 112:785–794, 2003.

46. Rowe P, Kumagai Y, Gutierrez G, et al: MEPE has the properties of an osteoblastic phosphatonin and minhibin. Bone 34:303–319, 2004.

47. Olsen H, Cepeda M, Zhang Q, et al: Human stanniocalcin: A possible hormonal regulator of mineral metabolism. Proc Natl Acad Sci U S A 93:1792–1796, 1996.

48. Ishibashi K, Miyamoto K, Taketani Y, et al: Molecular cloning of a second human stanniocalcin homologue (STC2). Biochem Biophys Res Commun 250:252–258, 1998.

49. Chang A, Reddel R: Identification of a second stanniocalcin cDNA in mouse and human: Stanniocalcin 2. Mol Cell Endocrinol 141:95–99, 1998.

50. Thakker RV: Molecular genetics of parathyroid disease. Curr Opin Endocrinol Diabetes 3:521–528, 1996.

51. Szabo J, Heath B, Hill VM, et al: Hereditary hyperparathyroidism-jaw tumor syndrome: The endocrine tumor gene HRPT2 maps to chromosome 1q21–q31. Am J Hum Genet 56:944–950, 1995.

52. Arnold A, Brown MF, Urena P, et al: Monoclonality of parathyroid tumors in chronic renal failure and in primary parathyroid hyperplasia. J Clin Invest 95:2047–2053, 1995.

53. Arnold A, Kim HG, Gaz RD, et al: Molecular cloning and chromosomal mapping of DNA rearranged with the parathyroid hormone gene in a parathyroid adenoma. J Clin Invest 83:2034–2040, 1989.

54. Motokura T, Bloom T, Kim HG, et al: A BCL1-linked candidate oncogene which is rearranged in parathyroid tumors encodes a novel cyclin. Nature 350:512–515, 1991.

55. Nurse P: Universal control mechanism regulating onset of M-phase. Nature 344:503–508, 1990.

56. Hosokawa Y, Yoshimoto K, Bronson R, et al: Chronic hyperparathyroidism in transgenic mice with parathyroid-targeted overexpression of cyclin D1/PRAD1. J Bone Miner Res 12(Suppl 1):S110, 1997.

57. Imanishi Y, Hosokawa Y, Yoshimoto K, et al: Primary hyperparathyroidism caused by parathyroid-targeted overexpression of cyclin D1 in transgenic mice. J Clin Invest 107:1093–1102, 2001.

58. Wang TC, Cardiff RD, Zukerberg L, et al: Mammary hyperplasia and carcinoma in MMTV-cyclin D1 transgenic mice. Nature 369:669–671, 1994.

59. Thakker RV: The molecular genetics of the multiple endocrine neoplasia syndromes. Clin Endocrinol (Oxf) 38:1–14, 1993.

60. Trump D, Farren B, Wooding C, et al: Clinical studies of multiple endocrine neoplasia type 1 (MEN1). QJM 89:653–669, 1996.

61. Marx S: Multiple endocrine neoplasia type 1. In Vogelstein B, Kinzler K (eds): Genetic Basis of Human Cancer. New York, McGraw-Hill, 1998, pp 489–506.

62. Thakker RV: Multiple endocrine neoplasia—Syndromes of the twentieth century. J Clin Endocrinol Metab 83:2617–2620, 1998.

63. Chandrasekharappa SC, Guru SC, Manickam P, et al: Positional cloning of the gene for multiple endocrine neoplasia-type 1. Science 276:404–407, 1997.

64. Lemmens I, Van de Ven WJ, Kas K, et al: Identification of the multiple endocrine neoplasia type 1 (MEN1) gene. The European Consortium on MEN1. Hum Mol Genet 6:1177–1183, 1997.

65. Pannett AA, Thakker RV: Multiple endocrine neoplasia type 1. Endocr Relat Cancer 6:449–473, 1999.

66. Turner JJ, Leotlela PD, Pannett AA, et al: Frequent occurrence of an intron 4 mutation in multiple endocrine neoplasia type 1. J Clin Endocrinol Metab 87:2688–2693, 2002.

67. Bassett JH, Forbes SA, Pannett AA, et al: Characterization of mutations in patients with multiple endocrine neoplasia type 1. Am J Hum Genet 62:232–244, 1998.

68. Teh BT, Kytola S, Farnebo F, et al: Mutation analysis of the MEN1 gene in multiple endocrine neoplasia type 1, familial acromegaly and familial isolated hyperparathyroidism. J Clin Endocrinol Metab 83:2621–2626, 1998.

69. Heppner C, Kester MB, Agarwal SK, et al: Somatic mutation of the MEN1 gene in parathyroid tumours. Nat Genet 16:375–378, 1997.

70. Zhuang Z, Vortmeyer AO, Pack S, et al: Somatic mutations of the MEN1 tumor suppressor gene in sporadic gastrinomas and insulinomas. Cancer Res 57:4682–4686, 1997.

71. Zhuang Z, Ezzat SZ, Vortmeyer AO, et al: Mutations of the MEN1 tumor suppressor gene in pituitary tumors. Cancer Res 57:5446–5451, 1997.

72. Prezant TR, Levine J, Melmed S: Molecular characterization of the MEN1 tumor suppressor gene in sporadic pituitary tumors. J Clin Endocrinol Metab 83:1388–1391, 1998.

73. Debelenko LV, Brambilla E, Agarwal SK, et al: Identification of MEN1 gene mutations in sporadic carcinoid tumors of the lung. Hum Mol Genet 6:2285–2290, 1997.

74. Vortmeyer AO, Boni R, Pak E, et al: Multiple endocrine neoplasia 1 gene alterations in MEN1-associated and sporadic lipomas. J Natl Cancer Inst 90:398–399, 1998.

75. Farnebo F, Teh BT, Kytola S, et al: Alterations of the MEN1 gene in sporadic parathyroid tumors. J Clin Endocrinol Metab 83:2627–2630, 1998.

76. Carling T, Correa P, Hessman O, et al: Parathyroid MEN1 gene mutations in relation to clinical characteristics of nonfamilial primary hyperparathyroidism. J Clin Endocrinol Metab 83:2960–2963, 1998.

77. Tanaka C, Kimura T, Yang P, et al: Analysis of loss of heterozygosity on chromosome 11 and infrequent inactivation of the MEN1 gene in sporadic pituitary adenomas. J Clin Endocrinol Metab 83:2631–2634, 1998.

78. Pannett AA, Thakker RV: Somatic mutations in MEN type 1 tumors, consistent with the Knudson "two-hit" hypothesis. J Clin Endocrinol Metab 86:4371–4374, 2001.

79. Teh BT, Esapa CT, Houlston R, et al: A family with isolated hyperparathyroidism segregating a missense MEN1 mutation and showing loss of the wild-type alleles in the parathyroid tumors. Am J Hum Genet 63:1544–1549, 1998.

80. Pannett AA, Kennedy AM, Turner JJ, et al: Multiple endocrine neoplasia type 1 (MEN1) germline mutations in familial isolated primary hyperparathyroidism. Clin Endocrinol (Oxf) 58:639–646, 2003.

81. Agarwal SK, Guru SC, Heppner C, et al: Menin interacts with the AP1 transcription factor JunD and represses JunD-activated transcription. Cell 96:143–152, 1999.

82. Heppner C, Bilimoria KY, Agarwal SK, et al: The tumor suppressor protein menin interacts with NF-κB proteins and inhibits NF-κB-mediated transactivation. Oncogene 20:4917–4925, 2001.

83. Kaji H, Canaff L, Lebrun JJ, et al: Inactivation of menin, a Smad3-interacting protein, blocks transforming growth factor type β signaling. Proc Natl Acad Sci U S A 98:3837–3842, 2001.

84. Sowa H, Kaji H, Canaff L, et al: Inactivation of Menin, the product of the multiple endocrine neoplasia type 1 gene, inhibits the commitment of multipotential mesenchymal stem cells into the osteoblast lineage. J Biol Chem 278:21058–21069, 2003.

85. Lemmens IH, Forsberg L, Pannett AA, et al: Menin interacts directly with the homeobox-containing protein Pem. Biochem Biophys Res Commun 286:426–431, 2001.

86. Sukhodolets KE, Hickman AB, Agarwal SK, et al: The 32-kilodalton subunit of replication protein A interacts with menin, the product of the MEN1 tumor suppressor gene. Mol Cell Biol 23:493–509, 2003.

87. Ohkura N, Kishi M, Tsukada T, Yamaguchi K: Menin, a gene product responsible for multiple endocrine neoplasia type 1, interacts with the putative tumor metastasis suppressor nm23. Biochem Biophys Res Commun 282:1206–1210, 2001.

88. Lopez-Egido J, Cunningham J, Berg M, et al: Menin's interaction with glial fibrillary acidic protein and vimentin suggests a role for the intermediate filament network in regulating menin activity. Exp Cell Res 278:175–183, 2002.

89. Mulligan LM, Kwok JBJ, Healey CS, et al: Germ-line mutations of the RET proto-oncogene in multiple endocrine neoplasia type 2A. Nature 363:458–460, 1993.

90. Mulligan LM, Ponder BA: Genetic basis of endocrine disease: Multiple endocrine neoplasia type 2. J Clin Endocrinol Metab 80:1989–1995, 1995.

91. Pausova E, Janicic N, Konrad EM, et al: Analysis of the RET proto-oncogene in sporadic parathyroid tumors. J Bone Miner Res 9:S151, 1994.

92. Padberg BC, Schroder S, Jochum W, et al: Absence of RET proto-oncogene point mutations in sporadic hyperplastic and neoplastic lesions of the parathyroid gland. Am J Pathol 147:1600–1607, 1995.

93. Heshmati HM, Gharib H, Khosla S, et al: Genetic testing in medullary thyroid carcinoma syndromes: Mutation types and clinical significance. Mayo Clin Proc 72:430–436, 1997.

94. Kennett S, Pollick H: Jaw lesions in familial hyperparathyroidism. Oral Surg Oral Med Oral Pathol 31:502–510, 1971.

95. Jackson CE, Norum RA, Boyd SB, et al: Hereditary hyperparathyroidism and multiple ossifying jaw fibromas: A clinically and genetically distinct syndrome. Surgery 108:1006–1012; discussion 1012–1003, 1990.

96. Bradley KJ, Hobbs MR, Buley ID, et al: Uterine tumours are a phenotypic manifestation of the hyperparathyroidism–jaw tumour syndrome. J Intern Med 257:18–26, 2005.

97. Cavaco BM, Barros L, Pannett AA, et al: The hyperparathyroidism–jaw tumour syndrome in a Portuguese kindred. QJM 94:213–222, 2001.

98. Wassif WS, Moniz CF, Friedman E, et al: Familial isolated hyperparathyroidism: A distinct genetic entity with an increased risk of parathyroid cancer. J Clin Endocrinol Metab 77:1485–1489, 1993.

99. Williamson C, Cavaco BM, Jauch A, et al: Mapping the gene causing hereditary primary hyperparathyroidism in a Portuguese kindred to chromosome 1q22–q31. J Bone Miner Res 14:230–239, 1999.

100. Weinstein LS, Simonds WF: HRPT2, a marker of parathyroid cancer. N Engl J Med 349:1691–1692, 2003.

101. Carpten JD, Robbins CM, Villablanca A, et al: *HRPT2*, encoding parafibromin, is mutated in hyperparathyroidism–jaw tumor syndrome. Nat Genet 32:676–680, 2002.

102. Shattuck TM, Valimaki S, Obara T, et al: Somatic and germ-line mutations of the *HRPT2* gene in sporadic parathyroid carcinoma. N Engl J Med 349:1722–1729, 2003.

103. Howell VM, Haven CJ, Kahnoski K, et al: *HRPT2* mutations are associated with malignancy in sporadic parathyroid tumours. J Med Genet 40:657–663, 2003.

104. Weinberg RA: Tumor suppressor genes. Science 254:1138–1146, 1991.

105. Cryns VL, Thor A, Xu HJ, et al: Loss of the retinoblastoma tumor suppressor gene in parathryoid carcinoma. N Engl J Med 330:757–761, 1994.

106. Pearce SH, Trump D, Wooding C, et al: Loss of heterozygosity studies at the retinoblastoma and breast cancer susceptibility (*BRCA2*) loci in pituitary, parathyroid, pancreatic and carcinoid tumours. Clin Endocrinol (Oxf) 45:195–200, 1996.

107. Pei L, Melmed S, Scheithauer B, et al: Frequent loss of heterozygosity at the retinoblastoma susceptibility gene (*RB*) locus in aggressive pituitary tumors: Evidence for a chromosome 13 tumor suppressor gene other than *RB*. Cancer Res 55:1613–1616, 1995.

108. Cryns VL, Yi SM, Tahara H, et al: Frequent loss of chromosomes arm 1p DNA in parathyroid adenomas. Genes Chromosomes Cancer 13:9–17, 1995.

109. Williamson C, Pannett AA, Pang JT, et al: Localisation of a gene causing endocrine neoplasia to a 4 cM region on chromosome 1p35–p36. J Med Genet 34:617–619, 1997.

110. Brown EM, MacLeod RJ: Extracellular calcium sensing and extracellular calcium signaling. Physiol Rev 81:239–297, 2001.

111. Simonds WF, James-Newton LA, Agarwal SK, et al: Familial isolated hyperparathyroidism: Clinical and genetic characteristics of 36 kindreds. Medicine (Baltimore) 81:1–26, 2002.

112. Simonds WF, Robbins CM, Agarwal SK, et al: Familial isolated hyperparathyroidism is rarely caused by germline mutation in *HRPT2*, the gene for the hyperparathyroidism–jaw tumor syndrome. J Clin Endocrinol Metab 89:96–102, 2004.

113. Pollak MR, Brown EM, WuChou YH, et al: Mutations in the human Ca^{2+} sensing receptor gene cause familial hypocalciuric hypercalcemia and neonatal severe hyperparathyroidism. Cell 75:1297–1303, 1993.

114. Chou YH, Pollak MR, Brandi ML, et al: Mutations in the human Ca^{2+} sensing-receptor gene that cause familial hypocalciuric hypercalcemia. Am J Hum Genet 56:1075–1079, 1995.

115. Pearce S, Trump D, Wooding C, et al: Calcium-sensing receptor mutations in familial benign hypercalcaemia and neonatal hyperparathyroidism. J Clin Invest 96:2683–2692, 1995.

116. Janicic N, Pausova Z, Cole DE, Hendy GN: Insertion of an Alu sequence in the Ca^{2+} sensing receptor gene in familial hypocalciuric hypercalcemia and neonatal severe hyperparathyroidism. Am J Hum Genet 56:880–886, 1995.

117. Aida K, Koishi S, Inoue M, et al: Familial hypocalciuric hypercalcemia associated with mutation in the human Ca^{2+} sensing receptor gene. J Clin Endocrinol Metab 80:2594–2598, 1995.

118. Heath H, Odelberg S, Jackson CE, et al: Clustered inactivating mutations and benign polymorphisms of the calcium receptor gene in familial benign hypocalciuric hypercalcemia suggest receptor functional domains. J Clin Endocrinol Metab 81:1312–1317, 1996.

119. Janicic N, Soliman E, Pausova Z, et al: Mapping of the calcium-sensing receptor gene (*CASR*) to human chromosome 3q13.3–q21 by fluorescence in situ hybridization, and localization to rat chromosome 11 and mouse chromosome 16. Mamm Genome 6:798–801, 1994.

120. Morten KJ, Cooper JM, Brown GK, et al: A new point mutation associated with mitochondrial encephalomyopathy. Hum Mol Genet 2:2081–2087, 1993.

121. Pearce SH, Bai M, Quinn SJ, et al: Functional characterization of calcium-sensing receptor mutations expressed in human embryonic kidney cells. J Clin Invest 98:1860–1866, 1996.

122. Bai M, Quinn S, Trivedi S, et al: Expression and characterization of inactivating and activating mutations in the human Ca^{2+}-sensing receptor. J Biol Chem 271:19537–19545, 1996.

123. Pollak MR, Chou YH, Marx SJ, et al: Familial hypocalciuric hypercalcemia and neonatal severe hyperparathyroidism. Effects of mutant gene dosage on phenotype. J Clin Invest 93:1108–1112, 1994.

124. Bai M, Pearce SH, Kifor O, et al: In vivo and in vitro characterization of neonatal hyperparathyroidism resulting from a de novo, heterozygous mutation in the Ca^{2+}-sensing receptor gene: Normal maternal calcium homeostasis as a cause of secondary hyperparathyroidism in familial benign hypocalciuric hypercalcemia. J Clin Invest 99:88–96, 1997.

125. Heath H, Jackson CE, Otterrud B, Leppert MF: Genetic linkage analysis in familial benign (hypocalciuric) hypercalcemia: Evidence for locus heterogeneity. Am J Hum Genet 53:193–200, 1993.

126. McMurtry CT, Schranck FW, Walkenhorst DA, et al: Significant developmental elevation in serum parathyroid hormone levels in a large kindred with familial benign (hypocalciuric) hypercalcemia. Am J Med 93:247–258, 1992.

127. Trump D, Whyte MP, Wooding C, et al: Linkage studies in a kindred from Oklahoma, with familial benign (hypocalciuric) hypercalcaemia (FBH) and developmental elevations in serum parathyroid hormone levels, indicate a third locus for FBH. Hum Genet 96:183–187, 1995.

128. Lloyd SE, Pannett AA, Dixon PH, et al: Localization of familial benign hypercalcemia, Oklahoma variant (FBH$_{Ok}$), to chromosome 19q13. Am J Hum Genet 64:189–195, 1999.

129. Kifor O, Moore FD Jr, Delaney M, et al: A syndrome of hypocalciuric hypercalcemia caused by autoantibodies directed at the calcium-sensing receptor. J Clin Endocrinol Metab 88:60–72, 2003.

130. Pallais J Kifor O, Chen Y, et al: Acquired hypocalciuric hypercalcemia due to autoantibodies against the calcium-sensing receptor. N Engl J Med 351:362–369, 2004.

131. Jüppner H, Schipani E, Silve C: Jansen's metaphyseal chondrodysplasia and Blomstrand's lethal chondrodysplasia: two genetic disorders caused by PTH/PTHrP receptor mutations. In Bilezikian J, Raisz L, Rodan G (eds): Principles of Bone Biology. San Diego, Academic Press, 2002, pp 1117–1135.

132. Schipani E, Kruse K, Jüppner H: A constitutively active mutant PTH-PTHrP receptor in Jansen-type metaphyseal chondrodysplasia. Science 268:98–100, 1995.

133. Schipani E, Langman CB, Parfitt AM, et al: Constitutively activated receptors for parathyroid hormone and parathyroid hormone-related peptide in Jansen's metaphyseal chondrodysplasia. N Engl J Med 335:708–714, 1996.

134. Schipani E, Langman CB, Hunzelman J, et al: A novel PTH/PTHrP receptor mutation in Jansen's metaphyseal chondrodysplasia. J Clin. Endocrinol Metab 84:3052–3057, 1999.

135. Schipani E, Lanske B, Hunzelman J, et al: Targeted expression of constitutively active PTH/PTHrP receptors delays endochondral bone formation and rescues PTHrP-less mice. Proc Natl Acad Sci U S A 94:13689–13694, 1997.

136. Bastepe M, Raas-Rothschild A, Silver J, et al: A form of Jansen's metaphyseal chondrodysplasia with limited metabolic and skeletal abnormalities is caused by a novel activating PTH/PTHrP receptor mutation. J Clin Endocrinol Metab 89:3595–3600, 2004.

137. Schipani E, Jensen GS, Pincus J, et al: Constitutive activation of the cAMP signaling pathway by parathyroid hormone (PTH)/PTH-related peptide (PTHrP) receptors mutated at the two loci for Jansen's metaphyseal chondrodysplasia. Mol Endocrinol 11:851–858, 1997.

138. Ewart AK, Morris CA, Atkinson DL, et al: Hemizygosity at the elastin locus in a developmental disorder, Williams syndrome. Nat Genet 5:11–16, 1993.

139. Nickerson E, Greenberg F, Keating MT, et al: Deletions of the elastin gene at 7q11.23 occur in approximately 90% of patients with Williams syndrome. Am J Hum Genet 56:1156–1161, 1995.

140. Lowery MC, Morris CA, Ewart A, et al: Strong correlation of elastin deletions, detected by FISH, with Williams syndrome: Evaluation of 235 patients. Am J Hum Genet 57:49–53, 1995.

141. Li D, Brooke B, Davis E, et al: Elastin is an essential determinant of arterial morphogenesis. Nature 393:276–280, 1998.

142. Tassabehji M, Metcalfe K, Fergusson WD, et al: LIM-kinase deleted in Williams syndrome. Nat Genet 13:272–273, 1996.

143. Perez Jurado LA, Li X, Francke U: The human calcitonin receptor gene (CALCR) at 7q21.3 is outside the deletion associated with the Williams syndrome. Cytogenet Cell Genet 70:246–249, 1995.

144. Arnold A, Horst SA, Gardella TJ, et al: Mutation of the signal peptide-encoding region of the preproparathyroid hormone gene in familial isolated hypoparathyroidism. J Clin Invest 86:1084–1087, 1990.

145. Karaplis AC, Lim SK, Baba H, et al: Inefficient membrane targeting, translocation, and proteolytic processing by signal peptidase of a mutant preproparathyroid hormone protein. J Biol Chem 270:1629–1635, 1995.

146. Sunthornthepvarakul T, Churesigaew S, Ngowngarmratana S: A novel mutation of the signal peptide of the preproparathyroid hormone gene associated with autosomal recessive familial isolated hypoparathyroidism. J Clin Endocrinol Metab 84:3792–3796, 1999.

147. Parkinson D, Thakker R: A donor splice site mutation in the parathyroid hormone gene is associated with autosomal recessive hypoparathyroidism. Nat Genet 1:149–153, 1992.

148. Günther T, Chen ZF, Kim J, et al: Genetic ablation of parathyroid glands reveals another source of parathyroid hormone. Nature 406:199–203, 2000.

149. Peden V: True idiopathic hypoparathyroidism as a sex–linked recessive trait. Am J Human Genet 12:323–337, 1960.

150. Whyte MP, Weldon VV: Idiopathic hypoparathyroidism presenting with seizures during infancy: X-linked recessive inheritance in a large Missouri kindred. J Pediatr 99:608–611, 1981.

151. Whyte M, Kim G, Kosanovich M: Absence of parathyroid tissue in sex-linked recessive hypoparathyroidism. J Paediatr 109:915, 1986.

152. Mumm S, Whyte MP, Thakker RV, et al: mtDNA analysis shows common ancestry in two kindreds with X-linked recessive hypoparathyroidism and reveals a heteroplasmic silent mutation. Am J Hum Genet 60:153–159, 1997.

153. Thakker RV, Davies KE, Whyte MP, et al: Mapping the gene causing X-linked recessive idiopathic hypoparathyroidism to Xq26–Xq27 by linkage studies. J Clin Invest 86:40–45, 1990.

154. Bowl M, Nesbit M, Harding B, et al: An interstitial deletion-insertion involving chromosomes 2p25.3 and Xq27.1, near SOX3, causes X-linked recessive hypoparathyroidism. J Clin Invest 115:2822–2831, 2005.

155. Ahonen P, Myllarniemi S, Sipila I, Perheentupa J: Clinical variation of autoimmune polyendocrinopathy-candidiasis-ectodermal dystrophy (APECED) in a series of 68 patients. N Engl J Med 322:1829–1836, 1990.

156. Ahonen P: Autoimmune polyendocrinopathy-candidosis-ectodermal dystrophy (APECED): autosomal recessive inheritance. Clin Genet 27:535–542, 1985.

157. Zlotogora J, Shapiro MS: Polyglandular autoimmune syndrome type I among Iranian Jews. J Med Genet 29:824–826, 1992.

158. Aaltonen J, Bjorses P, Sandkuijl L, et al: An autosomal locus causing autoimmune disease: autoimmune polyglandular disease type I assigned to chromosome 21. Nat Genet 8:83–87, 1994.

159. Nagamine K, Peterson P, Scott HS, et al: Positional cloning of the APECED gene. Nat Genet 17:393–398, 1997.

160. The Finnish-German APECED Consortium: Autoimmune polyendocrinopathy-candidiasis-ectodermal dystrophy. an autoimmune disease, APECED, caused by mutations in a novel gene featuring two PHD-type zinc-finger domains. Nat Genet 17:399–403, 1997.

161. Pearce SH, Cheetham T, Imrie H, et al: A common and recurrent 13-bp deletion in the autoimmune regulator gene in British kindreds with autoimmune polyendocrinopathy type 1. Am J Hum Genet 63:1675–1684, 1998.

162. Scott HS, Heino M, Peterson P, et al: Common mutations in autoimmune polyendocrinopathy-candidiasis-ectodermal dystrophy patients of different origins. Mol Endocrinol 12:1112–1119, 1998.

163. Rosatelli MC, Meloni A, Devoto M, et al: A common mutation in Sardinian autoimmune polyendocrinopathy-candidiasis-ectodermal dystrophy patients. Hum Genet 103:428–434, 1998.

164. Bjorses P, Halonen M, Palvimo JJ, et al: Mutations in the AIRE gene: Effects on subcellular location and transactivation function of the autoimmune polyendocrinopathy-candidiasis-ectodermal dystrophy protein. Am J Hum Genet 66:378–392, 2000.

165. Liston A, Lesage S, Wilson J, et al: Aire regulates negative selection of organ-specific T cells. Nat Immunol 4:350–354, 2003.

166. Scambler PJ, Carey AH, Wyse RK, et al: Microdeletions within 22q11 associated with sporadic and familial DiGeorge syndrome. Genomics 10:201–206, 1991.

167. Monaco G, Pignata C, Rossi E, et al: DiGeorge anomaly associated with 10p deletion. Am J Med Genet 39:215–216, 1991.

168. Gong W, Emanuel BS, Collins J, et al: A transcription map of the DiGeorge and velo-cardio-facial syndrome minimal critical region on 22q11. Hum Mol Genet 5:789–800, 1996.

169. Scambler PJ: The 22q11 deletion syndromes. Hum Mol Genet 9:2421–2426, 2000.

170. Augusseau S, Jouk S, Jalbert P, Prieur M: DiGeorge syndrome and 22q11 rearrangements. Hum Genet 74:206, 1986.

171. Budarf ML, Collins J, Gong W, et al: Cloning a balanced translocation associated with DiGeorge syndrome and

identification of a disrupted candidate gene. Nat Genet
10:269–278, 1995.

172. Yamagishi H, Garg V, Matsuoka R, et al: A molecular pathway
revealing a genetic basis for human cardiac and craniofacial
defects. Science 283:1158–1161, 1999.

173. Lindsay EA, Botta A, Jurecic V, et al: Congenital heart disease
in mice deficient for the DiGeorge syndrome region. Nature
401:379–383, 1999.

174. Magnaghi P, Roberts C, Lorain S, et al: *HIRA*, a mammalian
homologue of *Saccharomyces cerevisiae* transcriptional
co-repressors, interacts with *Pax3*. Nat Genet 20:74–77, 1998.

175. Jerome LA, Papaioannou VE: DiGeorge syndrome phenotype
in mice mutant for the T-box gene, *Tbx1*. Nat Genet
27:286–291, 2001.

176. Yagi H, Furutani Y, Hamada H, et al: Role of *TBX1* in human
del22q11.2 syndrome. Lancet 362:1366–1373, 2003.

177. Baldini A: DiGeorge's syndrome: A gene at last. Lancet
362:1342–1343, 2003.

178. Scire G, Dallapiccola B, Iannetti P, et al: Hypoparathyroidism
as the major manifestation in two patients with 22q11
deletions. Am J Med Genet 52:478–482, 1994.

179. Sykes K, Bachrach L, Siegel-Bartelt J, et al: Velocardiofacial
syndrome presenting as hypocalcemia in early adolescence.
Arch Pediatr Adolesc Med 151:745–747,1997.

180. Bilous R, Murty G, Parkinson D, et al: Autosomal dominant
familial hypoparathyroidism, sensineural deafness and renal
dysplasia. N Engl J Med 327:1069–1084, 1992.

181. Van Esch H, Groenen P, Nesbit MA, et al: *GATA3*
haplo-insufficiency causes human HDR syndrome.
Nature 406:419–422, 2000.

182. Muroya K, Hasegawa T, Ito Y, et al: *GATA3* abnormalities and
the phenotypic spectrum of HDR syndrome. J Med Genet
38:374–380, 2001.

183. Nesbit MA, Bowl MR, Harding B, et al: Characterization of
GATA3 mutations in the hypoparathyroidism, deafness, and
renal dysplasia (HDR) syndrome. J Biol Chem
279:22624–22634, 2004.

184. Tsang AP, Visvader JE, Turner CA, et al: FOG, a multitype zinc
finger protein, acts as a cofactor for transcription factor
GATA-1 in erythroid and megakaryocytic differentiation. Cell
90:109–119, 1997.

185. Dai YS, Markham BE: p300 functions as a coactivator of
transcription factor GATA-4. J Biol Chem 276:37178–37185,
2001.

186. Pandolfi PP, Roth ME, Karis A, et al: Targeted disruption of
the *GATA3* gene causes severe abnormalities in the nervous
system and in fetal liver haematopoiesis. Nat Genet 11:40–44,
1995.

187. Moraes CT, DiMauro S, Zeviani M, et al: Mitochondrial DNA
deletions in progressive external ophthalmoplegia and
Kearns-Sayre syndrome. N Engl J Med 320:1293–1299, 1989.

188. Zupanc ML, Moraes CT, Shanske S, et al: Deletion of
mitochondrial DNA in patients with combined features of
Kearns-Sayre and MELAS syndromes. Ann Neurol
29:680–683, 1991.

189. Isotani H, Fukumoto Y, Kawamura H, et al: Hypoparathyroidism
and insulin-dependent diabetes mellitus in a patient with
Kearns-Sayre syndrome harbouring a mitochondrial DNA
deletion. Clin Endocrinol (Oxf) 45:637–641, 1996.

190. Dionisi-Vici C, Garavaglia B, Burlina AB, et al:
Hypoparathyroidism in mitochondrial trifunctional protein
deficiency. J Pediatr 129:159–162, 1996.

191. Franceschini P, Testa A, Bogetti G, et al: Kenny-Caffey
syndrome in two sibs born to consanguineous parents:
Evidence for an autosomal recessive variant. Am J Med Genet
42:112–116, 1992.

192. Boynton JR, Pheasant TR, Johnson BL, et al: Ocular findings
in Kenny's syndrome. Arch Ophthalmol 97:896–900, 1979.

193. Sanjad SA, Sakati NA, Abu-Osba YK, et al: A new syndrome of
congenital hypoparathyroidism, severe growth failure, and
dysmorphic features. Arch Dis Child 66:193–196, 1991.

194. Parvari R, Hershkovitz E, Kanis A, et al: Homozygosity and
linkage-disequilibrium mapping of the syndrome of
congenital hypoparathyroidism, growth and mental
retardation, and dysmorphism to a 1-cM interval on
chromosome 1q42–q43. Am J Hum Genet 63:163–169, 1998.

195. Parvari R, Hershkovitz E, Grossman N, et al: Mutation of
TBCE causes hypoparathyroidism-retardation-dysmorphism
and autosomal recessive Kenny-Caffey syndrome. Nat Genet
32:448–452, 2002.

196. Parkinson D, Shaw N, Himsworth R, Thakker R: Parathyroid
hormone gene analysis in autosomal hypoparathyroidism
using an intragenic tetranucleotide $(AAAT)_n$ polymorphism.
Hum Genet 91:281–284, 1993.

197. Barakat AY, D'Albora JB, Martin MM, Jose PA: Familial
nephrosis, nerve deafness, and hypoparathyroidism. J Pediatr
91:61–64, 1977.

198. Dahlberg PJ, Borer WZ, Newcomer KL, Yutuc WR: Autosomal
or X-linked recessive syndrome of congenital lymphedema,
hypoparathyroidism, nephropathy, prolapsing mitral valve,
and brachytelephalangy. Am J Med Genet 16:99–104, 1983.

199. Pollak MR, Brown EM, Estep HL, ct al: Autosomal dominant
hypocalcaemia caused by a Ca^{2+} sensing receptor gene
mutation. Nat Genet 8:303–307, 1994.

200. Finegold DN, Armitage MM, Galiani M, et al: Preliminary
localization of a gene for autosomal dominant
hypoparathyroidism to chromosome 3q13. Pediatr Res
36:414–417, 1994.

201. Pearce SH, Williamson C, Kifor O, et al: A familial syndrome
of hypocalcemia with hypercalciuria due to mutations in the
calcium-sensing receptor. N Engl J Med 335:1115–1122, 1996.

202. Baron J, Winer K, Yanovski J, et al: Mutations in the Ca^{2+}
sensing receptor gene cause autosomal dominant and
sporadic hypoparathyroidism. Hum Mol Genet 5:601–606,
1996.

203. Okazaki R, Chikatsu N, Nakatsu M, et al: A novel activating
mutation in calcium-sensing receptor gene associated with a
family of autosomal dominant hypocalcemia. J Clin
Endocrinol Metab 84:363–366, 1999.

204. Thakker RV: Molecular pathology of renal chloride channels
in Dent's disease and Bartter's syndrome. Exp Nephrol
8:351–360, 2000.

205. Hebert SC: Bartter syndrome. Curr Opin Nephrol Hypertens
12:527–532, 2003.

206. Watanabe S, Fukumoto S, Chang H, et al: Association between
activating mutations of calcium-sensing receptor and Bartter's
syndrome. Lancet 360:692–694, 2002.

207. Vargas-Poussou R, Huang C, Hulin P, et al: Functional
characterization of a calcium-sensing receptor mutation in
severe autosomal dominant hypocalcemia with a Bartter-like
syndrome. J Am Soc Nephrol 13:2259–2266, 2002.

208. Li Y, Song YH, Rais N, et al: Autoantibodies to the extracellular
domain of the calcium sensing receptor in patients with
acquired hypoparathyroidism. J Clin Invest 97:910–914, 1996.

209. Albright F, Burnett CH, Smith PH, ParsonW:
Pseudohypoparathyroidism—An example of "Seabright-
Bantam syndrome." Endocrinology 30:922–932, 1942.

210. Weinstein LS: Albright hereditary osteodystrophy,
pseudohypoparathyroidism, and G_s deficiency. In Spiegel AM
(ed): G Proteins, Receptors, and Disease. Totowa, NJ, Humana
Press, 1998, pp 3–56.

211. Bastepe M, Jüppner H: Pseudohypoparathyroidism: New
insights into an old disease. In Strewler GJ (ed):
Endocrinology and Metabolism Clinics of North America:
Hormones and Disorders of Mineral Metabolism.
Philadelphia, WB Saunders, 2000, pp 569–589.

212. Jan de Beur SM, Levine MA: Pseudohypoparathyroidism: Clinical, biochemical, and molecular features. In Bilezikian JP, Markus R, Levine MA (eds): The Parathyroids: Basic and Clinical Concepts. New York, Academic Press, 2001, pp 807–825.

213. Levine MA: Pseudohypoparathyroidism. In Bilezikian JP, Raisz LG, Rodan GA (eds): Principles of Bone Biology. New York, Academic Press, 1996, pp 853–876.

214. Schuster V, Eschenhagen T, Kruse K, et al: Endocrine and molecular biological studies in a German family with Albright hereditary osteodystrophy. Eur J Pediatr 152:185–189, 1993.

215. Miric A, Vechio JD, Levine MA: Heterogeneous mutations in the gene encoding the α-subunit of the stimulatory G protein of adenylyl cyclase in Albright hereditary osteodystrophy. J Clin Endocrinol Metab 76:1560–1568, 1993.

216. Weinstein LS, Gejman PV, Friedman E, et al: Mutations of the Gs α-subunit gene in Albright hereditary osteodystrophy detected by denaturing gradient gel electrophoresis. Proc Natl Acad Sci U S A 87:8287–8290, 1990.

217. Ahrens W, Hiort O, Staedt P, et al: Analysis of the GNAS1 gene in Albright's hereditary osteodystrophy. J Clin Endocrinol Metab 86:4630–4634, 2001.

218. Linglart A, Carel J, Garabédian M, et al: GNAS1 lesions in pseudohypoparathyroidism Ia and Ic: Genotype phenotype relationship and evidence of the maternal transmission of the hormonal resistance. J Clin Endocrinol Metab 87:189–197, 2002.

219. Davies AJ, Hughes HE: Imprinting in Albright's hereditary osteodystrophy. J Med Genet 30:101–103, 1993.

220. Wilson LC, Oude-Luttikhuis MEM, Clayton PT, et al: Parental origin of Gsα gene mutations in Albright's hereditary osteodystrophy. J Med Genet 31:835–839, 1998.

221. Yu S, Yu D, Lee E, et al: Variable and tissue-specific hormone resistance in heterotrimeric Gs protein α-subunit (Gsα) knockout mice is due to tissue-specific imprinting of the Gsα gene. Proc Natl Acad Sci U S A 95:8715–8720, 1998.

222. Eddy MC, De Beur SM, Yandow SM, et al: Deficiency of the α-subunit of the stimulatory G protein and severe extraskeletal ossification. J Bone Miner Res 15:2074–2083, 2000.

223. Yeh GL, Mathur S, Wivel A, et al: GNAS1 mutation and Cbfa1 misexpression in a child with severe congenital platelike osteoma cutis. J Bone Miner Res 15:2063–2073, 2000.

224. Shore E, Ahn J, Jan de Beur S, et al: Paternally inherited inactivating mutations of the GNAS1 gene in progressive osseous heteroplasia. N Engl J Med 346:99–106, 2002.

225. Hayward B, Kamiya M, Strain L, et al: The human GNAS1 gene is imprinted and encodes distinct paternally and biallelically expressed G proteins. Proc Natl Acad Sci U S A 95:10038–10043, 1998.

226. Hayward BE, Moran V, Strain L, Bonthron DT: Bidirectional imprinting of a single gene: GNAS1 encodes maternally, paternally, and biallelically derived proteins. Proc Natl Acad Sci U S A 95:15475–15480, 1998.

227. Peters J, Wroe SF, Wells CA, et al: A cluster of oppositely imprinted transcripts at the Gnas locus in the distal imprinting region of mouse chromosome 2. Proc Natl Acad Sci U S A 96:3830–3835, 1999.

228. Kehlenbach RH, Matthey J, Huttner WB: XLas is a new type of G protein. Nature 372:804–809, 1994.

229. Bastepe M, Gunes Y, Perez-Villamil B, et al: Receptor-mediated adenylyl cyclase activation through XLas, the extra-large variant of the stimulatory G protein α-subunit. Mol Endocrinol 16:1912–1919, 2002.

230. Ischia R, Lovisetti-Scamihorn P, Hogue-Angeletti R, et al: Molecular cloning and characterization of NESP55, a novel chromogranin-like precursor of a peptide with 5-HT1B receptor antagonist activity. J Biol Chem 272:11657–11662, 1997.

231. Hayward B, Bonthron D: An imprinted antisense transcript at the human GNAS1 locus. Hum Mol Genet 9:835–841, 2000.

232. Liu J, Yu S, Litman D, et al: Identification of a methylation imprint mark within the mouse Gnas locus. Mol Cell Biol 20:5808–5817, 2000.

233. Bastepe M, Lane AH, Jüppner H: Paternal uniparental isodisomy of chromosome 20q (patUPD20q)—and the resulting changes in GNAS1 methylation—as a plausible cause of pseudohypoparathyroidism. Am J Hum Genet 68:1283–1289, 2001.

234. Weber T, Liu S, Indridason O, Quarles L: Serum FGF23 levels in normal and disordered phosphorus homeostasis. J Bone Miner Res 18:1227–1234, 2003.

235. Murray T, Gomez Rao E, Wong MM, et al: Pseudohypoparathyroidism with osteitis fibrosa cystica: Direct demonstration of skeletal responsiveness to parathyroid hormone in cells cultured from bone. J Bone Miner Res 8:83–91, 1993.

236. Farfel Z: Pseudohypohyperparathyroidism-pseudohypoparathyroidism type Ib. J Bone Miner Res 14:1016, 1999.

237. Mahmud F, Linglart A, Bastepe M, et al: Molecular diagnosis of pseudohypoparathyroidism type Ib in a family with presumed paroxysmal dyskinesia. Pediatrics 115:e242–e244, 2005.

238. Schipani E, Weinstein LS, Bergwitz C, et al: Pseudohypoparathyroidism type Ib is not caused by mutations in the coding exons of the human parathyroid hormone (PTH)/PTH-related peptide receptor gene. J Clin Endocrinol Metab 80:1611–1621, 1995.

239. Bettoun JD, Minagawa M, Kwan MY, et al: Cloning and characterization of the promoter regions of the human parathyroid hormone (PTH)/PTH-related peptide receptor gene: Analysis of deoxyribonucleic acid from normal subjects and patients with pseudohypoparathyroidism type Ib. J Clin Endocrinol Metab 82:1031–1040, 1997.

240. Suarez F, Lebrun JJ, Lecossier D, et al: Expression and modulation of the parathyroid hormone (PTH)/PTH-related peptide receptor messenger ribonucleic acid in skin fibroblasts from patients with type Ib pseudohypoparathyroidism. J Clin Endocrinol Metab 80:965–970, 1995

241. Fukumoto S, Suzawa M, Takeuchi Y, et al: Absence of mutations in parathyroid hormone (PTH)/PTH-related protein receptor complementary deoxyribonucleic acid in patients with pseudohypoparathyroidism type Ib. J Clin Endocrinol Metab 81:2554–2558, 1996.

242. Jüppner H, Schipani E, Bastepe M, et al: The gene responsible for pseudohypoparathyroidism type Ib is paternally imprinted and maps in four unrelated kindreds to chromosome 20q13.3. Proc Natl Acad Sci U S A 95:11798–11803, 1998.

243. Liu J, Litman D, Rosenberg M, et al: A GNAS1 imprinting defect in pseudohypoparathyroidism type IB. J Clin Invest 106:1167–1174, 2000.

244. Bastepe M, Pincus JE, Sugimoto T, et al: Positional dissociation between the genetic mutation responsible for pseudohypoparathyroidism type Ib and the associated methylation defect at exon A/B: Evidence for a long-range regulatory element within the imprinted GNAS1 locus. Hum Mol Genet 10:1231–1241, 2001.

245. Bastepe M, Fröhlich L, Hendy G, et al: Autosomal dominant pseudohypoparathyroidism type-Ib is associated with a heterozygous microdeletion that likely disrupts a putative imprinting control element of GNAS. J Clin Invest 112:1255–1263, 2003.

246. Laspa E, Bastepe M, Jüppner H, Tsatsoulis A: Phenotypic and molecular genetic aspects of pseudohypoparathyroidism type Ib in a Greek kindred: Evidence for enhanced uric acid excretion due to parathyroid hormone resistance. J Clin Endocrinol Metab 89:5942–5947, 2004.

247. Liu J, Nealon J, Weinstein L: Distinct patterns of abnormal *GNAS* imprinting in familial and sporadic pseudohypoparathyroidism type IB. Hum Mol Genet 14:95–102, 2005.

248. Linglart A, Gensure R, Olney R, et al: A novel *STX16* deletion in autosomal dominant pseudohypoparathyroidism type Ib delineates a *cis*-acting imprinting control element of *GNAS*. Am J Hum Genet 76:804–814, 2005.

249. Bastepe M, Fröhlich L, Linglart A, et al: Deletion of the *NESP55* differentially methylated region causes loss of maternal *GNAS* imprints and pseudohypoparathyroidism type Ib. Nat Genet 37:25–27, 2005.

250. Williamson C, Ball S, Nottingham W, et al: A *cis*-acting control region is required exclusively for the tissue-specific imprinting of *Gnas*. Nat Genet 36:793–795, 2004.

251. Blomstrand S, Claësson I, Säve-Söderbergh J: A case of lethal congenital dwarfism with accelerated skeletal maturation. Pediatr Radiol 15:141–143, 1985.

252. Young ID, Zuccollo JM, Broderick NJ: A lethal skeletal dysplasia with generalised sclerosis and advanced skeletal maturation: Blomstrand chondrodysplasia. J Med Genet 30:155–157, 1993.

253. Leroy JG, Keersmaeckers G, Coppens M, et al: Blomstrand lethal chondrodysplasia. Am J Med Genet 63:84–89, 1996.

254. Loshkajian A, Roume J, Stanescu V, et al: Familial Blomstrand chondrodysplasia with advanced skeletal maturation: Further delineation. Am J Med Genet 71:283–288, 1997.

255. den Hollander NS, van der Harten HJ, Vermeij-Keers C, et al: First-trimester diagnosis of Blomstrand lethal osteochondrodysplasia. Am J Med Genet 73:345–350, 1997.

256. Oostra RJ, Baljet B, Dijkstra PF, Hennekam RCM: Congenital anomalies in the teratological collection of museum Vrolik in Amsterdam, The Netherlands. II: Skeletal dysplasia. Am J Med Genet 77:116–134, 1998.

257. Jobert AS, Zhang P, Couvineau A, et al: Absence of functional receptors parathyroid hormone and parathyroid hormone-related peptide in Blomstrand chondrodysplasia. J Clin Invest 102:34–40, 1998.

258. Zhang P, Jobert AS, Couvineau A, Silve C: A homozygous inactivating mutation in the parathyroid hormone/parathyroid hormone-related peptide receptor causing Blomstrand chondrodysplasia. J Clin Endocrinol Metab 83:3365–3368, 1998.

259. Karaplis AC, Bin He MT, Nguyen A, et al: Inactivating mutation in the human parathyroid hormone receptor type 1 gene in Blomstrand chondrodysplasia. Endocrinology 139:5255–5258, 1998.

260. Karperien MC, van der Harten HJ, van Schooten R, et al: A frame-shift mutation in the type I parathyroid hormone/parathyroid hormone-related peptide receptor causing Blomstrand lethal osteochondrodysplasia. J Clin Endocrinol Metab 84:3713–3720, 1999.

261. Karperien M, Sips H, van der Harten H, et al: Novel mutations in the type I PTH/PTHrP receptor causing Blomstrand lethal osteochondrodysplasia (Abstract). J Bone Miner Res 16(Suppl 1):S549, 2001.

262. Wysolmerski JJ, Cormier S, Philbrick W, et al: Absence of functional type 1 PTH/PTHrP receptors in humans is associated with abnormal breast development and tooth impactation. J Clin Endocrinol Metab 86:1788–1794, 2001.

263. Lyles K, Burkes E, Ellis G, et al: Genetic transmission of tumoral calcinosis: autosomal dominant with variable clinical expressivity. J Clin Endocrinol Metab 60:1093–1096, 1985.

264. Topaz O, Shurman D, Bergman R, et al: Mutations in *GALNT3*, encoding a protein involved in O-linked glycosylation, cause familial tumoral calcinosis. Nat Genet 36:579–581, 2004.

265. Benet-Pages A, Orlik P, Strom T, Lorenz-DepiereuxB: An *FGF23* missense mutation causes familial tumoral calcinosis with hyperphosphatemia. Hum Mol Genet 14:385–390, 2005.

266. Larsson T, Davis S, Garringer H, et al: Fibroblast growth factor-23 mutants causing familial tumoral calcinosis are differentially processed. J Clin Endocrinol Metab 146:3883–38912005.

267. Araya K, Fukumoto S, Backenroth R, et al: A novel mutation in fibroblast growth factor (FGF)23 gene as a cause of tumoral calcinosis. J Clin Endocrinol Metab 90:5523–5527, 2005.

268. Melhem R, Najjar S, Khachadurian A: Cortical hyperostosis with hyperphosphatemia: A new syndrome? J Pediatr 77:986–990, 1970.

269. Narchi H: Hyperostosis with hyperphosphatemia: Evidence of familial occurrence and association with tumoral calcinosis. Pediatrics 99:745–748, 1997.

270. Frishberg Y, Topaz O, Bergman R, et al: Identification of a recurrent mutation in *GALNT3* demonstrates that hyperostosis-hyperphosphatemia syndrome and familial tumoral calcinosis are allelic disorders. J Mol Med 83:33–38, 2005 [erratum published in J Mol Med 83:240, 2005].

271. Frishberg Y, Araya K, Rinat C, et al: Hyperostosis-hyperphosphatemia syndrome caused by mutations in *GALNT3* and associated with augmented processing of FGF-23. Meeting of the American Society of Nephrology. Philadelphia, 2004. F-P0937.

272. Trump D, Thakker R: Inherited hypophosphataemic rickets. In Thakker R (ed): Molecular Genetics of Endocrine Disorders. London, Chapman and Hall, 1997, pp 123–151.

273. Glorieux F, Karsenty G, Thakker R: Metabolic bone disease in children. In Avioli LV, Krane SM (eds): Metabolic Bone Disease. New York, Academic Press, 1997, pp 759–783.

274. The HYP Consortium: A gene (*PEX*) with homologies to endopeptidases is mutated in patients with X-linked hypophosphatemic rickets. Nat Genet 11:130–136, 1995.

275. Holm IA, Huang X, Kunkel LM: Mutational analysis of the *PEX* gene in patients with X-linked hypophosphatemic rickets. Am J Hum Genet 60:790–797, 1997.

276. Suchy SF, Olivos-Glander IM, Nussabaum RL: Lowe syndrome, a deficiency of phosphatidylinositol 4,5-bisphosphate 5-phosphatase in the Golgi apparatus. Hum Mol Genet 4:2245–2250, 1995.

277. Zhang X, Jefferson AB, Auethavekiat V, Majerus PW: The protein deficient in Lowe syndrome is a phosphatidylinositol-4,5-bisphosphate 5-phosphatase. Proc Natl Acad Sci U S A 92:4853–4856, 1995.

278. Scheinman SJ, Guay-Woodford LM, Thakker RV, Warnock DG: Genetic disorders of renal electrolyte transport. N Engl J Med 340:1177–1187, 1999.

279. Fu GK, Lin D, Zhang MY, et al: Cloning of human 25-hydroxyvitamin D–1α-hydroxylase and mutations causing vitamin D–dependent rickets type 1. Mol Endocrinol 11:1961–1970, 1997.

280. St. Arnaud R, Messerlian S, Moir JM, et al: The 25-hydroxyvitamin D 1α-hydroxylase gene maps to the pseudovitamin D–deficiency rickets (*PDDR*) disease locus. J Bone Miner Res 12:1552–1559, 1997

281. White K, Carn G, Lorenz-Depiereux B, et al: Autosomal-dominant hypophosphatemic rickets (ADHR) mutations stabilize FGF-23. Kidney Int 60:2079–2086, 2001.

282. Econs M, McEnery P, Lennon F, Speer M: Autosomal dominant hypophosphatemic rickets is linked to chromosome 12p13. J Clin Invest 100:2653–2657, 1997.

283. Drezner MK: Phosphorus homeostasis and related disorders. In Bilezikian JP, Raisz LG, Rodan GA (eds): Principles in Bone Biology. New York, Academic Press, 2002, pp 321–338.

284. Lipman M, Panda D, Bennett H, et al: Cloning of human PEX cDNA. Expression, subcellular localization, and endopeptidase activity. J Biol Chem 273:13729–13737, 1998.

285. John M, Wickert H, Zaar K, et al: A case of neuroendocrine oncogenic osteomalacia associated with a PHEX and fibroblast growth factor-23 expressing sinusidal malignant schwannoma. Bone 29:393–402, 2001.

286. Seufert J, Ebert K, Müller J, et al: Octreotide therapy for tumor-induced osteomalacia. N Engl J Med 345:1883–1888, 2001.

287. Yamazaki Y, Okazaki R, Shibata M, et al: Increased circulatory level of biologically active full-length FGF-23 in patients with hypophosphatemic rickets/osteomalacia. J Clin Endocrinol Metab 87:4957–4960, 2002.

288. Jonsson K, Zahradnik R, Larsson T, et al: Fibroblast growth factor 23 in oncogenic osteomalacia and X-linked hypophosphatemia. N Engl J Med 348:1656–1662, 2003.

289. Rowe P, de Zoysa P, Dong R, et al: MEPE, a new gene expressed in bone marrow and tumors causing osteomalacia. Genomics 67:54–68, 2000.

290. Aono Y, Shimada T, Yamazaki Y, et al: The neutralization of FGF-23 ameliorates hypophosphatemia and rickets in Hyp mice. Paper presented at the 25th Meeting of the American Society for Bone and Mineral Research, Minneapolis, MN, date, 2003, p 1056.

291. Liu S, Brown T, Zhou J, et al: Role of matrix extracellular phosphoglycoprotein in the pathogenesis of X-linked hypophosphatemia. J Am Soc Nephrol 16:1645–1653, 2005.

292. Liu S, Zhou J, Tang W, et al: Pathogenic role of FGF23 in Hyp mice. Am J Physiol Endocrinol Metab 291:E38–E49, 2006.

293. Prié D, Huart V, Bakouh N, et al: Nephrolithiasis and osteoporosis associated with hypophosphatemia caused by mutations in the type 2a sodium-phosphate cotransporter. N Engl J Med 347:983–991, 2002.

294. Virkki L, Forster I, Hernando N, et al: Functional characterization of two naturally occurring mutations in the human sodium-phosphate cotransporter type IIa. J Bone Miner Res 18:2135–2141, 2003.

295. Beck L, Karaplis AC, Amizuka N, et al: Targeted inactivation of Ntp2 in mice leads to severe renal phosphate wasting, hypercalciuria, and skeletal abnormalities. Proc Natl Acad Sci U S A 95:5372–5377, 1998.

296. Tieder M, Modai D, Samuel R, et al: Hereditary hypophosphatemic rickets with hypercalciuria. N Engl J Med 312:611–617, 1985

297. Jones A, Tzenova J, Frappier D, et al: Hereditary hypophosphatemic rickets with hypercalciuria is not caused by mutations in the Na/Pi cotransporter NPT2 gene. J Am Soc Nephrol 12:507–514, 2001.

298. Bergwitz C, Roslin N, Tieder M, et al: SLC34A3 mutations in patients with hereditary hypophosphatemic rickets with hypercalciuria (HHRH) predict a key role for the sodium-phosphate co-transporter NaPi-IIc in maintaining phosphate homeostasis and skeletal function. Am J Hum Genet 78:179–192, 2006.

299. Lorenz-Depiereux B, Benet-Pages A, Eckstein G, et al: Hereditary hypophosphatemic rickets with hypercalciuria is caused by mutations in the sodium/phosphate cotransporter gene SLC34A3. Am J Hum Genet 78:193–201, 2006.

300. Segawa H, Kaneko I, Takahashi A, et al: Growth-related renal type II Na/Pi cotransporter. J Biol Chem 277:19665–19672, 2002.

301. Lloyd SE, Pearce SH, Fisher SE, et al: A common molecular basis for three inherited kidney stone diseases. Nature 379:445–449, 1996.

302. Jentsch TJ, Gunther W, Pusch M, Schwappach B: Properties of voltage-gated chloride channels of the CLC gene family. J Physiol 482:19S–25S, 1995.

303. Devuyst O, Christie PT, Courtoy PJ, et al: Intra-renal and subcellular distribution of the human chloride channel, ClC-5, reveals a pathophysiological basis for Dent's disease. Hum Mol Genet 8:247–257, 1999.

304. Piwon N, Gunther W, Schwake M, et al: ClC-5 Cl⁻-channel disruption impairs endocytosis in a mouse model for Dent's disease. Nature 408:369–373, 2000.

305. Christensen EI, Devuyst O, Dom G, et al: Loss of chloride channel ClC-5 impairs endocytosis by defective trafficking of megalin and cubilin in kidney proximal tubules. Proc Natl Acad Sci U S A 100:8472–8477, 2003.

306. Wang SS, Devuyst O, Courtoy PJ, et al: Mice lacking renal chloride channel, ClC-5, are a model for Dent's disease, a nephrolithiasis disorder associated with defective receptor-mediated endocytosis. Hum Mol Genet 9:2937–2945, 2000.

307. Hoopes RR, Jr, Shrimpton AE, Knohl SJ, et al: Dent disease with mutations in OCRL1. Am J Hum Genet 76:260–267, 2005.

308. Lowe CU, Terrey M, Mac LE: Organic-aciduria, decreased renal ammonia production, hydrophthalmos, and mental retardation; a clinical entity. Am J Dis Child 83:164–184, 1952.

309. Johnston SS, Nevin NC: Ocular manifestations in patients and female relatives of families with the oculocerebrorenal syndrome of Lowe. Birth Defects Orig Artic Ser 12:569–577, 1976.

310. Silver DN, Lewis RA, Nussbaum RL: Mapping the Lowe oculocerebrorenal syndrome to Xq24–q26 by use of restriction fragment length polymorphisms. J Clin Invest 79:282–285, 1987.

311. Leahey AM, Charnas LR, Nussbaum RL: Nonsense mutations in the OCRL-1 gene in patients with the oculocerebrorenal syndrome of Lowe. Hum Mol Genet 2:461–463, 1993.

312. Attree O, Olivos IM, Okabe I, et al: The Lowe's oculocerebrorenal syndrome gene encodes a protein highly homologous to inositol polyphosphate-5-phosphatase. Nature 358:239–242, 1992.

313. Zhang X, Hartz PA, Philip E, et al: Cell lines from kidney proximal tubules of a patient with Lowe syndrome lack OCRL inositol polyphosphate 5-phosphatase and accumulate phosphatidylinositol 4,5-bisphosphate. J Biol Chem 273:1574–1582, 1998.

314. Ungewickell A, Ward ME, Ungewickell E, Majerus PW: The inositol polyphosphate 5-phosphatase Ocrl associates with endosomes that are partially coated with clathrin. Proc Natl Acad Sci U S A 101:13501–13506, 2004.

315. Prader A, Illig R, Heierli E: An unusual form of primary vitamin D–resistant rickets with hypocalcemia and autosomal-dominant hereditary transmission: Hereditary pseudo-deficiency rickets. Helv Paediatr Acta 16:452–468, 1961.

316. Fraser D, Kooh SW, Kind HP, et al: Pathogenesis of hereditary vitamin-D-dependent rickets. An inborn error of vitamin D metabolism involving defective conversion of 25-hydroxyvitamin D to 1α-25-dihydroxyvitamin D. N Engl J Med 289:817–822, 1973.

317. Scriver CR: Vitamin D dependency. Pediatrics 45:361–363, 1970.

318. Delvin EE, Glorieux FH, Marie PJ, Pettifor JM: Vitamin D dependency: Replacement therapy with calcitriol? J Pediatr 99:26–34, 1981.

319. Scriver CR, Reade TM, DeLuca HF, Hamstra AJ: Serum 1,25-dihydroxyvitamin D levels in normal subjects and in patients with hereditary rickets or bone disease. N Engl J Med 299:976–979, 1978.

320. DeLuca HF: Vitamin D metabolism and function. Arch Intern Med 138(Spec No):836–847, 1978.

321. Chesney RW, Rosen JF, Hamstra AJ, DeLuca HF: Serum 1,25-dihydroxyvitamin D levels in normal children and in vitamin D disorders. Am J Dis Child 134:135–139, 1980.

322. Labuda M, Morgan K, Glorieux FH: Mapping autosomal recessive vitamin D dependency type I to chromosome 12q14 by linkage analysis. Am J Hum Genet 47:28–36, 1990.

323. St-Arnaud R, Messerlian S, Moir JM, et al: The 25-hydroxyvitamin D 1α-hydroxylase gene maps to the pseudovitamin D–deficiency rickets (PDDR) disease locus. J Bone Miner Res 12:1552–1559, 1997.

324. Kitanaka S, Takeyama K, Murayama A, et al: Inactivating mutations in the 25-hydroxyvitamin D$_3$ 1α-hydroxylase gene in patients with pseudovitamin D–deficiency rickets. N Engl J Med 338:653–661, 1998.

325. Yoshida T, Monkawa T, Tenenhouse HS, et al: Two novel 1α-hydroxylase mutations in French-Canadians with vitamin D dependency rickets type I. Kidney Int 54:1437–1443, 1998.

326. Wang JT, Lin CJ, Burridge SM, et al: Genetics of vitamin D 1α-hydroxylase deficiency in 17 families. Am J Hum Genet 63:1694–1702, 1998.

327. Brooks MH, Bell NH, Love L, et al: Vitamin-D-dependent rickets type II. Resistance of target organs to 1,25-dihydroxyvitamin D. N Engl J Med 298:996–999, 1978.

328. Marx SJ, Spiegel AM, Brown EM, et al: A familial syndrome of decrease in sensitivity to 1,25-dihydroxyvitamin D. J Clin Endocrinol Metab 47:1303–1310, 1978.

329. Liberman UA, Samuel R, Halabe A, et al: End-organ resistance to 1,25-dihydroxycholecalciferol. Lancet 1:504–506, 1980.

330. Fujita T, Nomura M, Okajima S, Furuya H: Adult-onset vitamin D–resistant osteomalacia with the unresponsiveness to parathyroid hormone. J Clin Endocrinol Metab 50:927–931, 1980.

331. Liberman UA, Eil C, Marx SJ: Resistance to vitamin D. In Cohn DV, Fujita T, Potts JT Jr, Talmage RV (eds): Endocrine Control of Bone and Calcium Metabolism. Amsterdam, Exerpta Medica, 1984, pp 32–40.

332. Fraher LJ, Karmali R, Hinde FR, et al: Vitamin D–dependent rickets type II: Extreme end organ resistance to 1,25-dihydroxy vitamin D$_3$ in a patient without alopecia. Eur J Pediatr 145:389–395, 1986.

333. Tsuchiya Y, Matsuo N, Cho H, et al: An unusual form of vitamin D–dependent rickets in a child: Alopecia and marked end-organ hyposensitivity to biologically active vitamin D. J Clin Endocrinol Metab 51:685–690, 1980.

334. Rosen JF, Fleischman AR, Finberg L, et al: Rickets with alopecia: An inborn error of vitamin D metabolism. J Pediatr 94:729–735, 1979.

335. Liberman UA, Eil C, Marx SJ: Resistance to 1,25-dihydroxyvitamin D. Association with heterogeneous defects in cultured skin fibroblasts. J Clin Invest 71:192–200, 1983.

336. Castells G, Greig F, Fusi L, et al: Vitamin D–dependent rickets type II (VDDRII) with alopecia. Treatment with mega doses of 1,25(OH)$_2$D$_3$ overcomes affinity defect in receptor for 1,25(OH)$_2$D$_3$. Pediatr Res 18:1174, 1984.

337. Balsan S, Garabédian M, Larchet M, et al: Long-term nocturnal calcium infusions can cure rickets and promote normal mineralization in hereditary resistance to 1,25-dihydroxyvitamin D. J Clin Invest 77:1661–1667, 1986.

338. Haussler MR, Manolagas SC, Deftos LJ: Evidence for a 1,25-dihydroxyvitamin D$_3$ receptor-like macromolecule in rat pituitary. J Biol Chem 255:5007–5010, 1980.

339. O'Malley BW: Steroid hormone action in eucaryotic cells. J Clin Invest 74:307–312, 1984.

340. EilC, Liberman UA, Rosen JF, Marx SJ: A cellular defect in hereditary vitamin-D-dependent rickets type II: Defective nuclear uptake of 1,25-dihydroxyvitamin D in cultured skin fibroblasts. N Engl J Med 304:1588–1591, 1981.

341. Eil C, Marx SJ: Nuclear uptake of 1,25-dihydroxy[^{3}H]cholecalciferol in dispersed fibroblasts cultured from normal human skin. Proc Natl Acad Sci U S A 78:2562–2566, 1981.

342. Haussler MR, Mangelsdorf DJ, Komm BS, et al: Molecular biology of the vitamin D hormone. In Cohn DV, Martin TJ, Mennier PJ (eds): Calcium Regulation and Bone Metabolism: Basic and Clinic Aspects. Amsterdam, Elsevier, 1987, pp 465–474.

343. McDonnell DP, Mangelsdorf DJ, Pike JW, et al: Molecular cloning of complementary DNA encoding the avian receptor for vitamin D. Science 235:1214–1217, 1987.

344. Hughes MR, Malloy PJ, Kieback DG, et al: Point mutations in the human vitamin D receptor gene associated with hypocalcemic rickets. Science 242:1702–1705, 1988.

345. Yoshizawa T, Handa Y, Uematsu Y, et al: Disruption of the vitamin D receptor (VDR) in the mouse. J Bone Miner Res 11:S119, 1996.

346. Li YC, Amling M, Pirro AE, et al: Normalization of mineral ion homeostasis by dietary means prevents hyperparathyroidism, rickets, and osteomalacia, but not alopecia in vitamin D receptor–ablated mice. Endocrinology 139:4391–4396, 1998.

347. Whyte MP: Hypophosphatasia. In Scriver C, Beaudet A, Sly W, Valle D (eds): Metabolic and Molecular Bases of Inherited Disease. New York, McGraw-Hill, 2001, pp 5313–5329.

348. Whyte MP, et al: Marked clinical and radiographic improvement in infantile hypophosphatasia transiently after haploidentical bone marrow transplantation. Bone 5:5191, 1998.

349. Thakker R, Jüppner H: Genetics disorders of calcium homeostasis caused by abnormal regulation of parathyoid hormone secretion or responsiveness. In DeGroot L, Jameson J (eds): Endocrinology. Philadelphia, WB Saunders, 2000, pp 1062–1074.

350. Argiro L, Desbarats M, Glorieux F, Ecarot B: *Mepe*, the gene encoding a tumor-secreted protein in oncogenic hypophosphatemic osteomalacia, is expressed in bone. Genomics 74:342–351, 2001.

351. Bielesz B, Klaushofer K, Oberbauer R: Renal phosphate loss in hereditary and acquired disorders of bone mineralization. Bone 35:1229–1239, 2004.

352. Holm IA, Econs MJ, Carpenter TO (eds): Familial Hypophosphatemia and Related Disorders. San Diego, Academic Press, 2003, pp 603–631.

353. Frame B, Poznanski AK: Conditions that may be confused with rickets. In DeLuca HF, Anast CS (eds): Pediatric Diseases Related to Calcium. New York, Elsevier, 1980, pp 269–289.

354. Ding C, Buckingham B, Levine M: Familial isolated hypoparathyroidism caused by a mutation in the gene for the transcription factor GCMB. J Clin Invest 108:1215–1220, 2001.

355. Lapointe JY, Tessier J, Paquette Y, et al: NPT2a gene variations in calcium nephrolithiasis with renal phosphate leak. Kidney 69:2261–2267, 2006.

Chapter 20

Genetics and Renal Pathophysiology of Essential Hypertension

Pedro A. Jose, John E. Jones, Scott M. Williams, Gilbert M. Eisner and Robin A. Felder

Hypertension is a major contributor to the number one cause of death, cardiovascular disease.[1] In the United States, from 1999 to 2000, the death rate from high blood pressure increased almost 4% over the previous study (NHANES 1988–1991). Overall, 28.7% of Americans have hypertension, but the prevalence is higher in those 60 years and older (65.4%), and in non-Hispanic Blacks (33.5%). An increasing number of women has developed hypertension (30.1%) after 1999.[2]

HERITABILITY OF BLOOD PRESSURE

Blood pressure is distributed continuously; however, the distribution is skewed to the higher end of the curve.[3] There is a direct and quantitative relationship between higher blood pressure and mortality. The lack of a definable bimodal distribution of blood pressure suggests that it is regulated by a complex group of interacting genes. This is reinforced by the lack of a clear-cut mode of inheritance; in other words, there is no evidence that essential hypertension is a dominant or a recessive trait. About half of blood pressure variability is thought to be genetically determined, but the variation of blood pressure is the result of interactions among genes and environmental factors.[4–7] Genetic studies of essential hypertension have used two approaches: family-based linkage studies and the study of the association of candidate genes in a population-based design. Several loci have been linked to hypertension, and variants of many genes have been reported to be associated with hypertension, albeit inconsistently.[7] Harrap has suggested that, instead of searching for every allele that controls blood pressure, an effort should be made to search for molecular clues to the common physiologic mechanisms underlying disease.[4]

PATHOPHYSIOLOGY OF ESSENTIAL HYPERTENSION

Primary Role of the Kidney

Because the kidney is important in the long-term regulation of blood pressure, many studies have focused on abnormal renal handling of sodium in the pathogenesis of essential hypertension.[8–10] Both direct and indirect measurements (e.g., lithium clearance) have shown increased sodium and fluid transport in the renal proximal tubule and thick ascending limb of Henle in rodent models of essential hypertension (e.g.,

spontaneously hypertensive rat [SHR], Dahl salt-sensitive rat, Milan hypertensive rat, Sabra hypertensive rat).[11–13] Essential hypertension in humans is also associated with increased sodium transport in the renal proximal tubule and medullary thick ascending limb, although increased distal tubular transport has also been reported.[11,12,14–16] In contrast, monogenic hypertension is caused by increased sodium transport that is limited to the distal nephron.[11,12,17]

The impaired renal sodium handling in essential hypertension[8–10] may be the result of abnormal regulation of natriuretic and antinatriuretic pathways.[18–28] The sympathetic nervous system[29–34] and the renin-angiotensin system[8–10,34–41] are antinatriuretic pathways. Products of arachidonic acid metabolism, dopamine, and nitric oxide (NO), among others, provide important counter-regulatory natriuretic pathways (Table 20-1).[22–28,42–46]

Essential hypertension has been attributed to increased extracellular fluid (ECF) volume, caused by a failure of the kidneys to eliminate sodium chloride and water. However, in cross-sectional studies an increased ECF volume has not been as consistently detected in hypertensive individuals as one might expect. In fact, total blood volume is usually normal in mild hypertension and tends to be decreased in more severe forms.[4] This apparent paradox can be explained by the temporal development of hypertension. Initially, hypertension develops slowly and there is a relatively brief stage in which ECF volume is elevated. This stage is followed by an elevation of total peripheral resistance.[9] This can be demonstrated in rodent models where ECF volume is greater in the SHRs as compared with their normotensive control, the Wistar-Kyoto (WKY) rat, but only in the young.[47,48]

Evidence from Rodent Models of Essential Hypertension

Direct proof of the importance of the kidney in the long-term regulation of blood pressure comes from renal transplantation studies. Several studies have shown that the transplantation of WKY kidneys into first-generation (F1) offspring from a cross of WKY rats and SHRs reduces or prevents the increase in blood pressure with age; conversely, transplantation of SHR kidneys results in an increase in blood pressure. Cross-transplantation experiments in Dahl salt-sensitive rats have also demonstrated the importance of the kidney and the contribution of extrarenal factors to the long-term regulation of blood pressure.[49–52] The high blood pressure is associated with sodium retention,[53] and an elevated sensitivity of the

Table 20-1 Natriuretic and Antinatriuretic Humoral/Hormonal Agents and Receptors Acting in the Proximal Tubule and/or Thick Ascending Limb of Henle

Antinatriuretic Agents (Receptors)	Natriuretic Agents (Receptors)
Adenosine (A_1)	Adenosine (A_2)
Angiotensin II (AT_1)	Angiotensin II (AT_2, AT_4)
Carbon monoxide	Angiotensin 1–7
Endothelin (ETA)	Arachidonic acid metabolites (e.g., 20- hydroxyeicosatetraenoic acid)
Insulin	Calcium-sensing receptor
Norepinephrine (α_1, α_2, β_2)	Dopamine (D_1, D_3)
Neuropeptide Y	Endothelin (ETB)
Serotonin ($5\text{-}HT_{1A}$, $5\text{-}HT_2$)	Natriuretic peptides (NPRA, NPRB)
Vasopressin (V_2)—thick ascending limb	Nitric oxide Parathyroid hormone
Reactive oxygen species—thick ascending limb	Reactive oxygen species (e.g., hydrogen peroxide)—proximal tubule Uroguanylin and guanylin

blood pressure of SHRs to sodium intake has been previously documented.[54,55] However, that transplantation of WKY kidneys into SHRs does not always normalize blood pressure supports the notion that extrarenal mechanisms may also contribute to the long-term regulation of blood pressure.[56] Subsequent experiments have shown that the contribution of the kidneys to hypertension, even in SHRs, is modified by extrarenal factors.[57] One example of extrarenal contribution to blood pressure regulation is the reduction of the sensitivity of blood pressure to sodium intake with neonatal sympathectomy.[58]

Evidence from Humans with Essential Hypertension

The importance of the kidney in the long-term regulation of blood pressure in humans was first supported by the report of Curtis et al.[59] They reported the normalization of blood pressure in six African Americans with malignant hypertension after renal transplantation. Subsequently, Guidi et al reported that the ability of a transplanted (hypertensive) kidney to transmit hypertension is found only in those recipients without a family history of hypertension.[60] Surprisingly, this did not occur in renal transplant recipients with a positive family history of hypertension. The authors suggested that recipients with a family history of hypertension may have developed extrarenal mechanisms that counteract the renal pressor effect of the transplanted kidney.

Nonrenal Mechanisms: Secondary Role of the Kidney

Several reports have documented a primary role of neuroendocrine and cardiac mechanisms in the pathogenesis of hypertension, whereas a secondary role is played by vasoconstrictor and vasodilatory agents from the endothelial cells.[22,29–34,61–65] For example, there is an increase in activity of Na^+Ca^{2+}-exchanger type 1 in vascular smooth muscles in salt-sensitive hypertension, but only during renally mediated sodium retention.[66]

The renin-angiotensin system also regulates blood pressure by renal and nonrenal mechanisms. Disrupting or silencing genes in the renin-angiotensin system, such as angiotensinogen, angiotensin-converting enzyme type I (ACEI), and angiotensin type 1A (AT_{1A}) receptor, in mice and rats decreases blood pressure.[67–72] However, the contribution of renal and extrarenal mechanisms could not be determined from these reports. To determine the contribution of renal AT_1 receptors in the regulation of blood pressure, Crowley et al studied the effect of transplanting kidneys from $AT_{1A}^{-/-}$ mice into bilaterally nephrectomized wild-type nontransgenic mice, and vice versa. These investigators estimated that under basal conditions, 42% of blood pressure control resides in AT_1 receptors in the kidney and 58% outside the kidney.[73] However, the hypertension induced by angiotensin II infusion requires only the presence of renal AT1A receptors.

The sympathetic nervous system,[29–32,34,57,58] like the renin-angiotensin system,[5,8,10,28,33–40,67–74] is important in the pathogenesis of essential hypertension and may regulate blood pressure by extrarenal mechanisms. Humans with essential hypertension[75,76] and rodent models of genetic hypertension (e.g., SHR)[29–32,34,57,58,77–79] have increased sympathetic nervous activity outside the kidney. However, the high blood pressure that develops in the F1 generation of WKY and SHR recipients of SHR kidneys is apparently not caused by abnormalities of the renin-angiotensin or sympathetic nervous system. Sodium and fluid retention, or renal interlobar and mesenteric vascular smooth muscle reactivity (vasoconstrictor response to vasopressin and norepinephrine, vasodilator response to acetylcholine and nitroprusside) could not be demonstrated in these hypertensive rats, either.[80] Therefore, other vasoactive agents, especially those that exert their effects independent of the vascular endothelium, must play a role in the development of hypertension. One such vasodepressor agent is dopamine. In the SHR (and in some subjects with essential hypertension), the renal and mesenteric vasodilator response to D_1-like receptor stimulation is impaired, independently of the endothelium.[81–84]

Role of Reactive Oxygen and Nitrogen Species

Reactive oxygen species (ROS) were first discovered in phagocytes; the stimulated production of ROS is named after the respiratory burst due to the transient consumption of oxygen.[85,86] ROS encompass a series of oxygen intermediates, including superoxide anion (O_2^-), hydrogen peroxide (H_2O_2), hydroxyl radical (OH), and hypochlorous acid.[85–87] The mitochondria are a major site of generation of ROS, whereas nonmitochondrial, membrane-associated NADH/NADPH oxidase seems to be the most important source of O_2^- in nonphagocytic cells, including vascular smooth muscle and renal epithelial cells.[88,89] In nonphagocytic cells, ROS, acting as intracellular and extracellular second messengers, play a physiologic role in vascular tone and cell growth, and a pathophysiologic role in inflammation, ischemia, hypertension, and other diseases.[20,87–96] Oxidative stress may be an important mechanism that contributes to the maintenance of the high blood pressure initiated by other primary processes. In the SHR, the increase in ROS activity occurs after the development of hypertension.[97] Thus, whether increased ROS production is causal or secondary to hypertension or to activation of receptors that increase blood pressure remains to be determined.

ROS can regulate the expression and/or activity of G protein–coupled receptors (which have been associated with hypertension) and vice versa. For example, oxytocin, which has been implicated in the regulation of blood pressure,[98] increases NADPH-dependent H_2O_2 generation,[99] and H_2O_2 can increase the activity of oxytocin.[100] Vasopressin, which has also been implicated in hypertension,[101,102] can also increase O_2^- production.[103] The ability of angiotensin II to increase ROS production is well known,[20,22,65,87–96] but ROS have also been reported to decrease AT_1 receptor expression.[104] In contrast to the pro-oxidant properties of many G protein–coupled receptors, physiologic concentrations of dopamine, via all five dopamine receptor subtypes, have antioxidant properties.[105–111]

Reactive nitrogen species, including nitrosonium cation (NO^+), nitroxyl anion (NO^-), and peroxynitrite ($ONOO^-$), are generated by reaction of ROS with NO or NO-related products.[112,113] NO can increase sodium excretion by increasing renal blood flow and by inhibition of sodium transport in many segments (proximal tubule, thick ascending limb of Henle, cortical collecting duct, inner medullary collecting duct) of the kidney[24,112–120]; NO and $ONOO^-$ can decrease ion transport by inhibition of Na^+/K^+-ATPase activity[116] and by increasing paracellular permeability.[117] O_2^- has also been reported to increase ion transport in the thick ascending limb of Henle.[42] ROS can also increase sodium transport by decreasing the availability of NO.[113]

SUBTYPES OF ESSENTIAL HYPERTENSION

Salt-Sensitive and Salt-Resistant Hypertension

Salt sensitivity is defined as an increase in blood pressure (>10%) following an increase or decrease in sodium load,

respectively.[121–125] The most reliable diagnostic method necessitates putting the patient on a diet with normal sodium intake for 5 to 7 days, followed by a reduction of sodium intake for 5 to 7 days, and then followed by a high-sodium diet intake for 5 to 7 days.[121,123,125] Although a shorter 2-week protocol has been suggested, there is only a 0.69 correlation coefficient between blood pressure obtained in the shorter protocol[126] and the definitive method of strict dietary regimen.[121,123,125]

The incidence of salt sensitivity with or without hypertension varies among ethnic groups.[2,127] Salt sensitivity, independent of hypertension, is a risk factor for cardiovascular morbidity and mortality.[128–133] Indeed, the morbidity and mortality of salt-sensitive normotensive subjects are the same as that of hypertensive subjects.[128]

Salt sensitivity depends on the intake of sodium as halide salts.[134] Sodium bicarbonate and other nonchloride salts of sodium do not elevate blood pressure in humans[134–136] and rodents.[137–139] The differential effect of chloride and nonchloride salts of sodium may[140] be related to differences in sodium balance or body weight.[137–139]

Low-Renin, Normal-Renin, and High-Renin Essential Hypertension

High plasma renin has been considered as an independent risk factor in hypertension.[141,142] Low-renin hypertension has been defined as an impaired response (≤2.4 ng/mL/hr) to upright posture.[143,144] Low-renin hypertension has also been defined as plasma renin activity less than 1 ng/mL/hr in the recumbent position while on a normal sodium diet.[145] Low plasma renin activity is associated with salt-sensitive hypertension and has been used as a surrogate marker for salt sensitivity.[143,144,146] However, plasma renin activity may not predict the salt-sensitive phenotype and therefore cannot be used to diagnose salt sensitivity,[147,148] especially in those individuals who are normotensive.

Modulating and Nonmodulating Hypertension

The expected response to a low-salt diet is an increase in plasma aldosterone levels and a decrease in the renal vascular response to infused angiotensin II. During a high salt intake, the expected response is a decrease in plasma aldosterone and an increase in renal vascular response to infused angiotensin II. Those who fail to respond in this way are termed nonmodulators and represent 40% to 50% of patients with normal- and high-renin essential hypertension.[146] Nonmodulators do not excrete a salt load appropriately. Plasma renin activity has been reported to be higher in nonmodulating than modulating hypertension.[148–150] Interestingly, nonmodulators do not increase urinary dopamine in response to a high sodium intake.[151] Impaired renal production of dopamine in response to a sodium load has also been reported in essential hypertension.[152–155]

Dipper and Nondipper Hypertension

Ambulatory blood pressure monitoring has made possible the characterization of the circadian patterns of blood pressure. Nocturnal blood pressure is usually 10% lower than daytime blood pressure. The absence of a decline in blood pressure at night or less than a 10% decline from the daytime value (nondipper) in both hypertensive and normotensive subjects has been associated with increased cardiovascular morbidity and mortality and renal insufficiency.[156,157] The reproducibility of nondipping has been questioned.[157] Nevertheless, some investigators have suggested that nondippers may have abnormalities in NO[158] and melatonin production,[159] and sympathetic/parasympathetic regulation of blood pressure.[160] Nondipping does not seem to be related to salt sensitivity,[161] or to deficient suppression of the renin-angiotensin system at night.[162,163]

GENETIC CAUSE(S) OF ESSENTIAL HYPERTENSION

Several chromosomal loci have been linked to hypertension, and many gene variants have been reported to be associated with increased risk for essential hypertension (Table 20-2). In addition to gene variants, telomere dysfunction has also been suggested to be important in the pathogenesis of hypertension and its complications.[164–166]

Determination of the Gene or Groups of Genes Responsible for Hypertension

Glazier et al have suggested criteria that should be used in determining whether a gene or groups of genes are responsible for the causation of complex diseases (Table 20-3).[167]

Linkage of Gene Loci and Association of Gene Variants with Essential Hypertension

The first required criterion for evidence of a genetic basis of a complex disease (see Table 20-3) is the demonstration of a (statistically sound genome-wide association in a single or multiple studies.[167] Genome-wide mapping studies have linked loci in several chromosomes to essential hypertension,[168–171] but these studies have not yet led to the identification of specific gene variants that may be causal. Although linkage studies have been successful in the identification of rare and highly penetrant alleles,[172] as in the case of monogenic hypertension,[17] such studies lack power to detect alleles conferring moderate risks that are likely to be the norm in complex disease states,[172] such as essential hypertension. Even if a disease risk locus is identified by linkage, the power of linkage disequilibrium to detect an association with a specific variant may be limited if multiple variants at each locus confer disease susceptibility. As can be gleaned from Table 20-2, many loci and/or alleles, by themselves or in combination, have been associated with essential hypertension.

Association studies have made use of case control design (population-based) and/or transmission disequilibrium tests (family-based).[172,173] The former tests for different frequencies of a variant in cases and controls, whereas the latter tests for a nonrandom transmission of a specific allele to affected individuals. The success of association studies of hypertension has been limited, with many association findings replicating in some but not all reports.[7] The failures to replicate include studies that use the same ethnic group, but especially those using different ethnic groups. One possible reason for these inconsistent results is that some sample sizes are not large enough to detect and confirm genetic variants that confer small risks. False-positive and false-negative results can occur with small sample sizes and when minor allele frequency is low.[172] It has been suggested that success can be improved by increasing the sample size and by careful selection of candidate genes and gene variants. However, large sample sizes may result in the samples representing stratified populations, which can lead to spurious associations.[172,174] One way to avoid the potential confounder of population stratification is to study populations that have had recent founders and have been relatively isolated from their source populations. The use of founder populations has been quite successful for mapping monogenic diseases and rare variants of recent origin but may not confer any advantage over outbred populations in the study of complex disease.[172] An alternative reason for the lack of replication is that risk is dependent on other, unmeasured variants that interact with the variants being studied.[7] If the interacting loci differ in frequency in the different populations, then detectable effects will be variable, leading to an inability to replicate single site associations.

After the identification of disease susceptibility alleles in complex diseases such as hypertension, gene-gene interactions have to be assessed. Parametric tests to determine gene-gene interaction, such as logistic regression, can be confounded by large numbers of disease loci, significantly decreasing the power to detect effects. Multivariate effects may be identified in relatively small samples with nonparametric methods (cluster analysis, linear discriminant analysis, recursive partitioning, and multifactorial dimensionality reduction [MDR]). The MDR approach uses data reduction to collapse genotypes from multiple loci into just two phenotypic classes that best define high risk and low risk of disease.[175,176,176a] A single best genetic model is selected from different combinations of loci using 10-fold cross-validation and permutation testing. The advantages of MDR are that it: (1) is capable of identifying specific multilocus genotypes that predict high and low risk of disease in relatively small case-control data sets; (2) has reduced sensitivity to multiple testing issues due to the cross-validation and permutation approach used; (3) is free of an assumed genetic model (i.e., model-free); (4) is nonparametric (i.e., no parameters are estimated); and (5) has the ability to estimate the prediction error of disease risk. Using MDR, the G protein–coupled receptor kinase 4 (GRK4) variant R65L, which impairs the inhibitory effect of dopamine receptors on sodium transport in the renal proximal tubule and thick ascending limb of Henle[177–179] and insertion/deletion variants of the angiotensin-converting enzyme, ACEI/D, have been shown to associate with essential hypertension with a predictive accuracy of 70% in a Ghanaian population,[180] confirming an earlier study, using a multilocus disequilibrium analysis.[181] Another GRK4 gene variant, GRK4 A486V, has also shown association with salt-sensitive hypertension.[182] Interestingly, both α-adducin, whose gene variant G460W is associated with salt-sensitive essential hypertension and abnormal renal proximal sodium transport[183–185] and GRK4 are mapped to chromosome 4p16.3, less than 50 kilobases apart.[186,187]

Text continued on p. 366

Table 20-2 Essential Hypertension-Related Genes

Gene	Allele or Amino Acid Substitution	Chromosomal Location	Association with Essential Hypertension	Population	Reference
Acyl-CoA dehydrogenase, short/branched chain (ACADSB)	rs2277249, G-512A rs2277250, G-254A	10q25-q26	Yes Yes	Japanese females Japanese females	Kamide et al (2007) Kamide et al (2007)
Adenosine A₂ receptor (ADORA2, RDC8)	T1083C	22q11.2	No	Japanese	Soma et al (1998)
α-adducin	A386G	10q24.2-q24.3	No	Hani & Yi Chinese	Zhou et al (2006)
α-adducin	Gly460Trp	4p16.3	Yes	Caucasian	Cusi et al (1997)
	Gly460Trp		No	Japanese	Ishikawa et al (1998)
	Gly460Trp		No	Caucasian	Wang et al (1999)
	Gly460Trp		No	Caucasian	Clark et al (2000)
	Gly460Trp		Yes	Chinese (northern)	Ju et al (2003)
	Gly460Trp		No	Chinese	Niu et al (1999)
Linkage analysis	D4S432		No	Chinese	Chu et al (2002)
	Gly460Trp		No	Caucasian (Hispanic)	Castejon et al (2003)
β-adducin	C1797T	2p14-p13	Yes	Caucasian females	Wang et al (2002)
α₂ᵦ-adrenergic receptor (ADRA2B); α₂-adrenergic receptor-like 1 (ADRA2L1)	Indel polymorphism	Chr. 2	Yes	Caucasian	von Wowern et al (2004)
β₂-adrenergic receptor (ADRB2)	Arg16Gly	5q32-q34	No	Caucasian	Tomaszewski et al (2002)
	Gln27Glu		No	Caucasian	Tomaszewski et al (2002)
	Thr164Ile		No	Caucasian	Tomaszewski et al (2002)
	Arg16Gly		No	Caucasian	Galletti et al (2004)
	Gln27Glu		No	Caucasian	Galletti et al (2004)
Aldosterone synthase (CYP11B2)	T-344C	8q21	Yes	Japanese	Tsukada et al (2002)
	T-344C		Yes	African, Asian, Caucasian	Barbato et al (2004)
	344C		Yes	Caucasian	Kumar et al (2003)
	T4986C		No	Caucasian	Kumar et al (2003)
	A6547G		Yes	Caucasian	Kumar et al (2003)
Angiotensinogen (AGT)	G-217A	1q42-q43	Yes	African-American	Jain et al (2002)
	G-217A		No	Chinese	Liu et al (2004)
			No	African-American	Zhu et al (2003)
			No	European American	
			Yes	Chinese	Wu et al (2004)
	G-152A		Yes, via haplotype	Chinese	Liu et al (2004)
	A-20C		Yes, via haplotype	Chinese	Liu et al (2004)

Continued

Table 20-2 Essential Hypertension-Related Genes—Cont'd

Gene	Allele or Amino Acid Substitution	Chromosomal Location	Association with Essential Hypertension	Population	Reference
CC-Chemokine receptor 5 (CCR5)	CCR5Δ32	3p21	Yes	Caucasian	Mettimano et al (2003)
Cold-induced auto-inflammatory syndrome 1 (CIAS1)	VNTR 12x Intron 4	1q44	Yes	Japanese	Omi et al (2006)
Connexin 37 (gap junction protein)	C1019T, Pro319Ser	1p35.1	No	Japanese	Izawa et al (2003)
Connexin 40, gap junction protein (CX40)	A-44G	1q21.1	Yes	Caucasian males	Firouzi et al (2006)
	A+71G		Yes	Caucasian males	Firouzi et al (2006)
CYP2J2*7	G-50 T	1p31.3–p31.2	Yes	Caucasian males	King et al (2005)
CYP2C8*3	R139K, K399R	10q23.33	No	Caucasian males	King et al (2005)
(CYP4A11) 20-HETE synthase	T8590C	1p33	Yes	Caucasians, None in Blacks	Gainer et al (2005)
			Yes	Germans	Mayer B et al (2005)
Cytochrome b(-245), α subunit (CYBA), p22phox	G-930A	16q24	Yes	Caucasian	Moreno et al (2003)
	G-930A		Yes	Japanese males	Kokubo et al (2005)
	H72Y		Yes	Caucasian	Moreno et al (2006)
Cytotoxic T lymphocyte-associated 4 (CTLA4)	rs231775, A17T	2q33	Yes	Japanese males	Kokubo et al (2006)
Dopamine D1 receptor	TaqI RFLP	11q23	Yes	Chinese	Fang et al (2005)
Dopamine D2 receptor	A-48G	5q35.2	Yes	Japanese	Sato et al (2000)
Dopamine D3 receptor	Ser9Gly	3q13.3	No	Japanese	Soma et al (2002)
E-selectin	Ser128Arg	1q23–q25	No	Japanese	Izawa et al (2003)
Epithelial sodium channel, β and γ (ENaC)	β, γENaC D16S403	16p13–p12	Yes	Caucasian	Wong et al (1999)
	β, γENaC D16S420		Yes	Caucasian	Wong et al (1999)
	β, γENaC D16S420		No	Black Caribbean	Munroe et al (1998)
	β, γENaC D16S420		No	Chinese	Niu et al (1999)
	β, γENaC D16S403		No	Chinese	Niu et al (1999)
Endothelial nitric oxide synthase (eNOS)	T-786C	7q36	No	Han Chinese (northern)	Zhao et al (2006)
	Intron 4b/a		No	Han Chinese (northern)	Zhao et al (2006)
	G894T		No	Han Chinese (northern)	Zhao et al (2006)
	G894T		No	Pakistani Pathans	Khawaja et al (2007)
Endothelin 1 (EDN1)	K198N	6p24–p23	Yes (interaction with BMI)	Caucasian	Tiret et al (1999)
	K198N		Yes (interaction with BMI)	Japanese	Jin et al (2003)

Continued

Table 20-2 Essential Hypertension-Related Genes—Cont'd

Gene	Allele or Amino Acid Substitution	Chromosomal Location	Association with Essential Hypertension	Population	Reference
Endothelin 2 (EDN2)	A985G	1p34	Yes	Caucasian	Sharma et al (1999)
Endothelin receptor type A (EDNRA)	5' UTR G→A; Exon 8 C→T	Chr. 4	Yes; Yes (weak)	Caucasian; Caucasian	Benjafield et al (2003); Benjafield et al (2003)
Factor V deficiency (F5)	rs6020, K513R	1q23	Yes	Japanese females	Kokubo et al (2006)
FK506-binding protein 1B (FKBP1B)	Exon 4 T→C	Chr. 2	No	Caucasian	Benjafield et al (2003)
Gα subunit 2 (GNAI2)	C-318G	3p21	Yes	Caucasian	Menzaghi et al (2006)
G protein–dependent receptor kinase 4 (GRK4)	Arg65Leu; Arg65Leu; Ala142Val; Ala486Val	4p16.3	No; Yes (Strongly when associated with ACE polymorphism); Yes; Yes	Caucasian; African (Ghana); Caucasian; Caucasian	Bengra et al (2002); Williams et al (2004); Speirs et al (2004); Bengra et al (2002)
Glucocorticoid receptor	Asn363Ser	5q31	No	Caucasian	Lin et al (2003)
Glucagon receptor (GCGR)	Gly40Ser; Gly40Ser; Gly40Ser	17q25	Yes; No; Yes	Caucasian; Caucasian; Caucasian (male only study)	Morris and Chambers (1996); Brand et al (1999); Strazzullo et al (2001)
Glycogen synthase 1 (GYS1)	XbaI RFLP; XbaI RFLP	19q13.3	Yes; Yes	Caucasian; Caucasian	Gharavi et al (1996); Schalin-Jantti et al (1996)
Group-specific component, vitamin D-binding protein (GC)	rs9016, R445C	4q12	Yes	Japanese females	Kokubo et al (2006)
Growth hormone receptor (GHR)	rs6180, L544I	5p13-p12	Yes	Japanese females	Kokubo et al (2006)
Guanine nucleotide binding protein, β3 subunit (GNB3)	C825T (splice variant)	12p13	Yes	Japanese	Izawa et al (2003)
Heme oxygenase-1 (HMOX-1)	T-413A	22q12	Yes	Japanese females (association not observed in males)	Ono et al (2003c)
Hepatic lipase (LIPC)	rs6078, V95M	15q21-q23	Yes	Japanese males	Kokubo et al (2006)

Continued

Table 20-2 Essential Hypertension-Related Genes—Cont'd

Gene	Allele or Amino Acid Substitution	Chromosomal Location	Association with Essential Hypertension	Population	Reference
11β-Hydroxysteroid dehydrogenase type 2 (HSD11B2, 11βHSD2) Linkage analysis	D16S503	16q22	No	Chinese	Chu et al (2002)
	G534A (high-salt association)		Yes	Caucasian	Poch et al (2001)
Hypertension-associated SA Linkage analysis	Pst RFLP	16p13.11	Yes	Japanese	Iwai et al (1994)
	D16S412		No	Chinese	Chu et al (2002)
Insulin receptor (INSR)	BglI RFLP	19p13.2	No	Caucasian	Ying et al (1991)
	R1 (RsaI) RFLP		Yes	Caucasian	Ying et al (1991)
	Insertion polymorphism		Yes	Caucasian	Morris et al (1993)
	CA repeat (intron 9)		Yes	Caucasian	Zee et al (1994)
	RsaI RFLP		No	Caucasian	Munroe et al (1995)
	SstI RFLP		No	Caucasian	Munroe et al (1995)
	GAG-1040-GAA (SSCP)		Yes	Chinese	Qiu et al (1995)
	NsiI RFLP (exon 8)		Yes	Caucasian	Schrader et al (1996)
Interleukin 6 (IL-6)	G-174C	1q21.3	No	Caucasian	Pola et al (2002)
	C-634G		No	Japanese	Izawa et al (2003)
Interleukin 10 (IL-10)	T-819C	1q31–q32	No	Japanese	Izawa et al (2003)
	A-592C		No	Japanese	Izawa et al (2003)
Lamin A/C	Arg482Gln	1q21.2	Yes	Caucasian	Hegele et al (2000)
Lipoprotein lipase (LPL)	IVS4-214C→T	8p22	Yes, via haplotype	Chinese	Li et al (2004)
	7754C→A				
	S447X				
12-lipoxygenase (12-LOX, ALOX12)	rs4987104, K259E	17p13.1	ND (not determined)	Caucasian	Quintana et al (2006)
	rs1126667, R261Q		Yes	Caucasian	Quintana et al (2006)
	rs434473, S322N		ND	Caucasian	Quintana et al (2006)
	rs11571342, H430R		ND	Caucasian	Quintana et al (2006)
	rs2070589, C1559T (Intron 2)		No	Caucasian	Quintana et al (2006)
	rs438444, G12185C (Intron 12)		No	Caucasian	Quintana et al (2006)
Methylentetrahydrofolate reductase (MTHFR)	C677T	1p36.3	Yes	Caucasian	Heux et al (2004)
Mineralocorticoid receptor (MLR) Linkage analysis	D4S1604	4q31	No	Chinese	Chu et al (2002)

Continued

Table 20-2 Essential Hypertension-Related Genes—Cont'd

Gene	Allele or Amino Acid Substitution	Chromosomal Location	Association with Essential Hypertension	Population	Reference
Mineralocorticoid receptor, aldosterone receptor (MCR)	F826Y	4q31.1	Yes	Japanese	Kamide et al (2005)
NADH/NADPH oxidase p22 phox (CYBA)	C242T His72Tyr	16q24	No	Japanese	Izawa et al (2003)
Natriuretic peptide receptor, type A (NPRA, atrial natriuretic peptide receptor, type A)	Met341Ile Indel 15,129 (3' UTR)	1q21–q22	No Yes	Japanese Caucasian	Nakayama et al (2002a) Lucarelli et al (2002)
Natriuretic peptide, type C (CNP)	G733A G1612C G2347T G2628A	2q24–qter	No No No Yes	Japanese Japanese Japanese Japanese	Ono et al (2002) Ono et al (2002) Ono et al (2002) Ono et al (2002)
Nitric oxide synthase 3 (NOS3), Endothelial NO (eNOS)	(CA)ₙ repeat, intron 13 A27C, intron 18 G10T, intron 23 G10T, intron 23 T-786C T-786C G894T G894T	7q36	No No No Yes (low BP) Yes No Yes (low BP) No	Caucasian Caucasian Caucasian Caucasian/African American Caucasian Japanese Caucasian/African American Chinese	Bonnardeaux et al (1995) Bonnardeaux et al (1995) Bonnardeaux et al (1995) Chen et al (2004) Hyndman et al (2002) Izawa et al (2003) Chen et al (2004) Tan et al (2004)
Paraoxonase (PON1)	G584A, Gln192Arg	7q21.3	No	Japanese	Izawa et al (2003)
Phenylethanolamine N-methyltransferase (PNMT)	G-148A G-353A G-353A	17q21	No Yes No	Caucasian/African American African American Caucasian	Cui et al (2003) Cui et al (2003) Cui et al (2003)
Phospholipase A2, group VII (PLA2G7)	rs1805018, I198T	6p21.2–p12	Yes	Japanese females	Kokubo et al (2006)
Plasma membrane calcium ATPase 2 (ATP2B2) Linkage analysis	D3S1263	3p24	No	Chinese	Chu et al (2002)
Plasminogen-activator inhibitor 1	-668/4G → 5G	7q21.3–q22	No	Japanese	Izawa et al (2003)

Continued

Table 20-2 Essential Hypertension-Related Genes—Cont'd

Gene	Allele or Amino Acid Substitution	Chromosomal Location	Association with Essential Hypertension	Population	Reference
Platelet-activating factor acetyl hydrolase phospholipase A$_2$, Group VII (PLA2G7)	G994T, Val279Phe G994T, Val279Phe	6p21.2–p12	No No	Japanese Japanese	Yoshida et al (1998) Izawa et al (2003)
Potassium channel, calcium activated, large conductance, subfamily M, Beta 1 (KCNMB1)	E65K E65K	5q34	Yes No	Caucasian Japanese	Fernández-Fernández et al (2004) Kokubo et al (2005)
Prostacyclin synthase, Prostaglandin I2 synthase (PTGIS), CYP8A1	T-192G	20q13.11–q13.13	Yes	Japanese	Nakayama et al (2002b)
Protein kinase, lysine-deficient 4 (WNK4)	G1662A G/A intron 10, bp 1156666 G/A intron 10, bp 1156666 Exon 8 A589S Exon 10 R665W Exon 14 P813L Exon 14 T879M Exon 10 tetranucleotide repeat	17q21–q22	Yes Yes No No No No No	Chinese Caucasian Caucasian African American African American African American African American Caucasian	Sun et al (2003) Erlich et al (2003) Speirs and Morris (2004) Erlich et al (2003) Erlich et al (2003) Erlich et al (2003) Erlich et al (2003) Benjafield et al (2003)
Protein tyrosine phosphatase (PTP1B)	1484insG	20q13.1–q13.2	No	Caucasian	Speirs et al (2004)
Regulator of G protein signaling 2 (RGS2)	A-638G T1026A 1891-1892 del.TC	1q31	No Yes Yes	Japanese Japanese females Japanese females	Yang et al (2005) Yang et al (2005) Yang et al (2005)
Regulator of G protein signalling 5 (RGS5)	rs1056514 rs3806366 rs15049 rs1354939 rs2255642 rs2815287 rs2456899 rs4620514 rs4657247 rs4657251 rs7513108 rs2999967 rs1553695	1q23	Yes Yes (strongest) Yes Yes Yes Yes Yes Yes Yes Yes Yes Yes (strongest) Yes	African American African American African American African American African American African American African American African American African American European American European American European American European American	Chang et al (2007) Chang et al (2007) Chang et al (2007) Chang et al (2007) Chang et al (2007) Chang et al (2007) Chang et al (2007) Chang et al (2007) Chang et al (2007) Chang et al (2007) Chang et al (2007) Chang et al (2007) Chang et al (2007)

Continued

Table 20-2 Essential Hypertension-Related Genes—Cont'd

Gene	Allele or Amino Acid Substitution	Chromosomal Location	Association with Essential Hypertension	Population	Reference
Renin	HindIII RFLP	1q32	No	Caucasian	Zee et al (1991)
	HindIII RFLP		Yes	Chinese	Chiang et al (1997)
	MboI RFLP		Yes	Caucasian	Frossard et al (1998)
	BglI RFLP		Yes	Caucasian	Frossard et al (2001)
	Intron 4 T+17int4G		No	Japanese	Hasimu et al (2003b)
	Intron 7 VNTR		No	Japanese	Hasimu et al (2003a)
	Exon 9 G1051A		Yes	Japanese	Hasimu et al (2003b)
	C-4021T		Yes	European American, African American	Zhu et al (2003)
Resistin (RETN, RSTN)	G+62A 3'-UTR	19p13.2	Yes	Caucasian	Gouni-Berthold et al (2005)
RGS2	Insertion/deletion		Yes	African American	Riddle et al (2006)
Selectin E (SELE)	rs2076059	1q23-q25	Yes	African American	Chang et al (2007)
	rs5359, rs5368, rs2076059 (haplotype)		Yes (strongest)	African American	Chang et al (2007)
Sodium channel, nonvoltage-gated-1 α-subunit (SCNN1A)	A2139G	12p13.3	Yes	Japanese	Iwai et al (2002)
	D12S889		No	Caribbean Africans	Munroe et al (1998)
Sodium channel, nonvoltage-gated-1 β-subunit (SCNN1B)	Gly589Ser	16p13-p12	No	Caucasians/Afro-Caribbeans	Persu et al (1998)
	Thr594Met		No	Caucasians/Afro-Caribbeans	Persu et al (1998)
	Arg597His		No	Caucasians/Afro-Caribbeans	Persu et al (1998)
	Arg624Cys		No	Caucasians/Afro-Caribbeans	Persu et al (1998)
	Glu632Gly		No	Caucasians/Afro-Caribbeans	Persu et al (1998)
	Gly442Val		No	Caucasians/Afro-Caribbeans	Persu et al (1998)
	Val434Met		No	Caucasians/Afro-Caribbeans	Persu et al (1998)
			No	Chinese	Niu et al (1999)
	G589S and a novel intronic i12–17CT substitution		Yes (but no effect on Finnish ENaC function)		Hannila-Handelberg et al (2005)
Sodium channel, nonvoltage-gated-1 γ-subunit (SCNN1G)	594ins Pro	16p13-p12	No	Caucasians/Afro-Caribbeans	Persu et al (1999)
	Arg631His		No	Caucasians/Afro-Caribbeans	Persu et al (1999)
	G-173A		Yes	Japanese	Iwai et al (2001)
	C649G		No (salt sensitive)	Caucasian	Poch et al (2000)
Linkage analysis	D16S412		No	Chinese	Chu et al (2002)

Continued

Table 20-2 Essential Hypertension-Related Genes—Cont'd

Gene	Allele or Amino Acid Substitution	Chromosomal Location	Association with Essential Hypertension	Population	Reference
Serum- and Glucocorticoid-regulated kinase (SGK1)	Intron 6 TT/CT	6q23	Yes	Caucasians	Busjahn et al (2002)
	Exon 8 CT/CC		Yes	Caucasians	Busjahn et al (2002)
	Intron 6 and Exon 8		No	Caucasians (97%)	Trochen et al (2004)
			Yes	Swedish	von Wowern et al (2005)
Sodium bicarbonate exchanger (SLC4A5)	hcv1137534	Chr. 2	Yes		Hunt et al (2006)
Sodium calcium exchanger 1 (SLC8A1) Linkage analysis	D2S119	2p21–p23	No	Chinese	Chu et al (2002)
Sodium hydrogen exchanger 3, NHE3, (SLC9A3) Linkage analysis	D5S392	5p15.3	No	Chinese	Chu et al (2002)
	G1579A		No	Caucasian/African/Afro-Caribbean	Zhu et al (2004)
	G1709A		No	Caucasian/African/Afro-Caribbean	Zhu et al (2004)
	G1867A		No	Caucasian/African/Afro-Caribbean	Zhu et al (2004)
	C1945T		No	Caucasian/African/Afro-Caribbean	Zhu et al (2004)
	A2041G		No	Caucasian/African/Afro-Caribbean	Zhu et al (2004)
	C2405T		No	Caucasian/African/Afro-Caribbean	Zhu et al (2004)
Sodium hydrogen exchanger 5 (SLC9A5) Linkage analysis	D16S512	16q21–16q22.1	No	Chinese	Chu et al (2002)
Solute carrier family 4, member 1 (SLC4A1)	rs5036, K56E	17q21–q22	Yes	Japanese males	Kokubo et al (2006)
Solute carrier family 6, member 2 (SLC6A2)	Promoter 3 A→G	16q12.2	Yes	Japanese	Ono et al (2003a)
Solute carrier family 6, member 18 (SLC6A18)	Y319X	5p15.33	No	Japanese	Eslami et al (2006)
	rs1390938, I136T		Yes	Japanese females	Kokubo et al (2006)
Solute carrier family 8, member A1 sodium calcium exchanger 1 (SLC8A1, NCX1)	T-23200C	2p23–p22	Yes	Japanese males	Kokubo et al (2004)
	T-23181C		Yes	Japanese males	Kokubo et al (2004)
	T-23181C		Yes	Japanese females	Kokubo et al (2004)
Stromelysin 1	−1171/5A→6A	22q13.3	No	Japanese	Izawa et al (2003)

Continued

Table 20-2 Essential Hypertension-Related Genes—*Cont'd*

Gene	Allele or Amino Acid Substitution	Chromosomal Location	Association with Essential Hypertension	Population	Reference
Sulfonylurea receptor regulatory subunit (Sur2)	rs12366938	12p12.1	No	Japanese	Sato et al (2006)
	rs704217		No	Japanese	Sato et al (2006)
	rs4148666		No		
	rs3782668		No		
	rs704187		No		
	rs2307024		No		
	rs704178		No		
			Yes, via haplotype		
Thrombomodulin (*THBD*)	C2136T, Ala455Val	20p11.2	No	Japanese	Izawa et al (2003)
Thrombopoietin (*THPO*)	A5713G	3q26.3–q27	No	Japanese	Izawa et al (2003)
Thrombospondin 4 (*THBS4*)	G1186C Ala378Pro	Chr. 5	No	Japanese	Izawa et al (2003)
Thyrotropin-releasing hormone (TRH)	rs5658, V8L	3q13.3–q21	Yes	Japanese females	Kokubo et al (2006)
Transforming growth factor β1 (*TGFB1*)	T869C Leu10Pro	19q13.1	No	Japanese	Izawa et al (2003)
Tumor necrosis factor-α (*TNFα*)	C-863A	6p21.3	No	Japanese	Izawa et al (2003)
	C-850T		Yes	Japanese females	Izawa et al (2003)
	G-238A		No	Japanese	Izawa et al (2003)
Tumor necrosis factor receptor 2 (TNFRSF1B)	T-1710A	1p36.3–p36.2	No	Caucasian	Speirs et al (2005)
	A257G		No	Caucasian	Speirs et al (2005)
	Exon 4 CA repeat		No	Caucasian	Speirs et al (2005)
	E232K		No	Caucasian	Speirs et al (2005)
	M196R		No	Caucasian	Speirs et al (2005)
	T1668G 3′ Untranslated		No	Caucasian	Speirs et al (2005)
	T1690C 3′ Untranslated		No	Caucasian	Speirs et al (2005)
Uncoupling protein 2 (*UCP2*)	G-866A	11q13	Yes	Japanese	Ji et al (2004)
Vasopressin receptor 1A (*V1AR*) Linkage analysis	D12S398	12q14–q15	Yes	Chinese	Chu et al (2002)
Von Willebrand Factor (vWF)	rs1063856, T769A	12p13.3	Yes	Japanese females	Kokubo et al (2006)
WNK4 (See Protein kinase, lysine-deficient 4)					

ACE, angiotensin-converting enzyme; BMI, body mass index; BP, blood pressure; ENaC, epithelial sodium channel; RFLP, restriction fragment length polymorphism; UTR, untranslated region; VNTR, variable number tandem repeated.

Table 20-2 Essential Hypertension-Related Genes—Cont'd

References for Table 20-2

Barbato A, Russo P, Siani A, et al. 2004. Aldosterone synthase gene (CYP11B2) C-344T polymorphism, plasma aldosterone, renin activity and blood pressure in a multi-ethnic population. J Hypertens 22:1895–1901.

Barley J, Blackwood A, Miller M, et al. 1996. Angiotensin-converting enzyme gene I/D polymorphism, blood pressure and the renin-angiotensin system in Caucasian and Afro-Caribbean peoples. J Hum Hypertens 10:31–35.

Bengra C, Mifflin TE, Khripin Y, et al. 2002. Genotyping of essential hypertension single-nucleotide polymorphisms by a homogeneous PCR method with universal energy transfer primers. Clin Chem 48:2131–2140.

Benjafield AV, Katyk K, Morris BJ. 2003. Association of EDNRA, but not WNK4 or FKBP1B, polymorphisms with essentqq1ial hypertension. Clin Genet 64:433–438.

Benjafield AV, Wang WY, Morris BJ. 2004. No association of angiotensin-converting enzyme 2 gene (ACE2) polymorphisms with essential hypertension. Am J Hypertens 17:624–628.

Bonnardeaux A, Nadaud S, Charru A, et al. 1995. Lack of evidence for linkage of the endothelial cell nitric oxide synthase gene to essential hypertension. Circulation 91:96–102.

Brand E, Bankir L, Plouin PF, Soubrier F. 1999. Glucagon receptor gene mutation (Gly40Ser) in human essential hypertension: the PEGASE study. Hypertension 34:15–17.

Busjahn A, Aydin A, Uhlmann R, et al. 2002. Serum- and glucocorticoid-regulated kinase (SGK1) gene and blood pressure. Hypertension 40:256–260.

Castejon AM, Alfieri AB, Hoffmann IS, et al. 2003. α-adducin polymorphism, salt sensitivity, nitric oxide excretion, and cardiovascular risk factors in normotensive Hispanics. Am J Hypertens 16:1018–1024.

Chang YP, Liu X, Kim JD, et al. 2007. Multiple genes for essential-hypertension susceptibility on chromosome 1q. Am J Hum Genet 80:253–264.

Chen W, Srinivasan SR, Li S, et al. 2004. Gender-specific influence of NO synthase gene on blood pressure since childhood: the Bogalusa Heart Study. Hypertension 44:668–673.

Chiang FT, Hsu KL, Tseng CD, et al. 1997. Association of the renin gene polymorphism with essential hypertension in a Chinese population. Clin Genet 51:370–374.

Chu SL, Zhu DL, Xiong MM, et al. 2002. Linkage analysis of twelve candidate gene loci regulating water and sodium metabolism and membrane ion transport in essential hypertension. Hypertens Res 25:635–639.

Clark CJ, Davies E, Anderson NH, et al. 2000. α-adducin and angiotensin I-converting enzyme polymorphisms in essential hypertension. Hypertension 36:990–994.

Cui J, Zhou X, Chazaro I, et al. 2003. Association of polymorphisms in the promoter region of the PNMT gene with essential hypertension in African Americans but not in whites. Am J Hypertens 16:859–863.

Cusi D, Barlassina C, Azzani T, et al. 1997. Polymorphisms of α-adducin and salt sensitivity in patients with essential hypertension. Lancet 349:1353–1357.

Duru K, Farrow S, Wang JM, et al. 1994. Frequency of a deletion polymorphism in the gene for angiotensin-converting enzyme is increased in African-Americans with hypertension. Am J Hypertens 7:759–762.

Erlich PM, Cui J, Chazaro I, et al. 2003. Genetic variants of WNK4 in whites and African Americans with hypertension. Hypertension 41:1191–1195.

Eslami B, Kinboshi M, Inoue S, et al. 2006. A nonsense polymorphism (Y319X) of the solute carrier family 6 member 18 (SLC6A18) gene is not associated with hypertension and blood pressure in Japanese. Tohoku J Exp Med 208:25–31.

Fernandez-Fernandez JM, Tomas M, Vazquez E, et al. 2004. Gain-of-function mutation in the KCNMB1 potassium channel subunit is associated with low prevalence of diastolic hypertension. J Clin Invest 113:1032–1039.

Firouzi M, Kok B, Spiering W, et al. 2006. Polymorphisms in human connexin40 gene promoter are associated with increased risk of hypertension in men. J Hypertens 24:325–330.

Frossard PM, Lestringant GG, Elshahat YI, et al. 1998. An MboI two-allele polymorphism may implicate the human renin gene in primary hypertension. Hypertens Res 21:221–225.

Frossard PM, Malloy MJ, Lestringant GG, Kane JP. 2001. Haplotypes of the human renin gene associated with essential hypertension and stroke. J Hum Hypertens 15:49–55.

Gainer JV, Brown NJ, Bachvarova M, et al. 2000. Altered frequency of a promoter polymorphism of the kinin B2 receptor gene in hypertensive African-Americans. Am J Hypertens 13:1268–1273.

Gainer JV, Bellamine A, Dawson EP, et al. 2005. Functional variant of CYP4A11 20-hydroxyeicosatetraenoic acid synthase is associated with essential hypertension. Circulation 111:63–69.

Galletti F, Iacone R, Ragone E, et al. 2004. Lack of association between polymorphism in the β2-adrenergic receptor gene, hypertension, and obesity in the Olivetti heart study. Am J Hypertens17:718–720.

Gesang L, Liu G, Cen W, et al. 2002. Angiotensin-converting enzyme gene polymorphism and its association with essential hypertension in a Tibetan population. Hypertens Res 25:481–485.

Gharavi AG, Phillips RA, Finegood DT, Lipkowitz MS. 1996. Glycogen synthase polymorphism, insulin resistance and hypertension. Blood Press 5:86–90.

Gouni-Berthold I, Giannakidou E, Faust M, et al. 2005. Resistin gene 3′-untranslated region +62G→A polymorphism is associated with hypertension but not diabetes mellitus type 2 in a German population. J Intern Med 258:518–526.

Hannila-Handelberg T, Kontula K, Tikkanen I, et al. 2005. Common variants of the β and γ-subunits of the epithelial sodium channel and their relation to plasma renin and aldosterone levels in essential hypertension. BMC Med Genet 6:4.

Hasimu B, Nakayama T, Mizutani Y, et al. 2003a. A novel variable number of tandem repeat polymorphism of the renin gene and essential hypertension. Hypertens Res 26:473–477.

Hasimu B, Nakayama T, Mizutani Y, et al. 2003b. Haplotype analysis of the human renin gene and essential hypertension. Hypertension 41:308–312.

Hegele RA, Anderson CM, Wang J, et al. 2000. Association between nuclear lamin A/C R482Q mutation and partial lipodystrophy with hyperinsulinemia, dyslipidemia, hypertension, and diabetes. Genome Res 10:652–658.

Heux S, Morin F, Lea RA, et al. 2004. The methylentetrahydrofolate reductase gene variant (C677T) as a risk factor for essential hypertension in Caucasians. Hypertens Res 27:663–667.

Hingorani AD, Jia H, Stevens PA, et al. 1995. Renin-angiotensin system gene polymorphisms influence blood pressure and the response to angiotensin-converting enzyme inhibition. J Hypertens 13:1602–1609.

Continued

Table 20-2 Essential Hypertension-Related Genes—Cont'd

Hunt SC, Xin Y, Wu LL, et al. 2006. Sodium bicarbonate cotransporter polymorphisms are associated with baseline and 10-year follow-up blood pressures. Hypertension 47:532–536.

Hyndman ME, Parsons HG, Verma S, et al. 2002. The T-786→C mutation in endothelial nitric oxide synthase is associated with hypertension. Hypertension 39:919–922.

Inoue I, Nakajima T, Williams CS, et al. 1997. A nucleotide substitution in the promoter of human angiotensinogen is associated with essential hypertension and affects basal transcription in vitro. J Clin Invest 99:1786–1797.

Ishigami T, Tamura K, Fujita T, et al. 1999. Angiotensinogen gene polymorphism near transcription start site and blood pressure: Role of a T-to-C transition at intron I. Hypertension 34:430–434.

Ishikawa K, Baba S, Katsuya T, et al. 2001. T+31C polymorphism of angiotensinogen gene and essential hypertension. Hypertension 37:281–285.

Ishikawa K, Katsuya T, Sato N, et al. 1998. No association between α-adducin 460 polymorphism and essential hypertension in a Japanese population. Am J Hypertens 11:502–506.

Iwai N, Baba S, Mannami T, et al. 2001. Association of sodium channel γ-subunit promoter variant with blood pressure. Hypertension 38:86–89.

Iwai N, Baba S, Mannami T, et al. 2002. Association of a sodium channel α-subunit promoter variant with blood pressure. J Am Soc Nephrol 13:80–85.

Iwai N, Ohmichi N, Hanai K, et al. 1994. Human SA gene locus as a candidate locus for essential hypertension. Hypertension 23:375–380.

Izawa H, Yamada Y, Okada T, et al. 2003. Prediction of genetic risk for hypertension. Hypertension 41:1035–1040.

Jain S, Tang X, Narayanan CS, et al. 2002. Angiotensinogen gene polymorphism at −217 affects basal promoter activity and is associated with hypertension in African-Americans. J Biol Chem 277:36889–36896.

Jeck N, Waldegger S, Lampert A, et al. 2004. Activating mutation of the renal epithelial chloride channel ClC-Kb predisposing to hypertension. Hypertension 43:1175–1181.

Jeng JR, Harn HJ, Jeng CY, et al. 1997. Angiotensin I converting enzyme gene polymorphism in Chinese patients with hypertension. Am J Hypertens 10:558–561.

Ji Q, Ikegami H, Fujisawa T, et al. 2004. A common polymorphism of uncoupling protein 2 gene is associated with hypertension. J Hypertens 22:97–102.

Jin JJ, Nakura J, Wu Z, et al. 2003. Association of endothelin-1 gene variant with hypertension. Hypertension 41:163–167.

Ju Z, Zhang H, Sun K, et al. 2003. α-adducin gene polymorphism is associated with essential hypertension in Chinese: A case-control and family-based study J Hypertens 21:1861–1868.

Kamide K, Yang J, Kokubo Y, et al. 2005. A novel missense mutation, F826Y, in the mineralocorticoid receptor gene in Japanese hypertensives: Its implications for clinical phenotypes. Hypertens Res 28:703–709.

Kamide K, Kokubo Y, Yang J, et al. 2007. Association of genetic polymorphisms of ACADSB and COMT with human hypertension. J Hypertens 25:103–110.

Khawaja MR, Taj F, Ahmad U, et al. 2007. Association of endothelial nitric oxide synthase gene G894T polymorphism with essential hypertension in an adult Pakistani Pathan population. Int J Cardiol 116:113–115.

King LM, Gainer JV, David GL, et al. 2005. Single nucleotide polymorphisms in the CYP2J2 and CYP2C8 genes and the risk of hypertension. Pharmacogenet Genomics 15:7–13.

Kokubo Y, Iwai N, Tago N, et al. 2005. Association analysis between hypertension and CYBA, CLCNKB, and KCNMB1 functional polymorphisms in the Japanese population—the Suita Study. Circ J 69:138–142.

Kokubo Y, Inamoto N, Tomoike H, et al. 2004. Association of genetic polymorphisms of sodium-calcium exchanger 1 gene, NCX1, with hypertension in a Japanese general population. Hypertens Res 27:697–702.

Kokubo Y, Tomoike H, Tanaka C, et al. 2006. Association of sixty-one non-synonymous polymorphisms in forty-one hypertension candidate genes with blood pressure variation and hypertension. Hypertens Res 29:611–619. Erratum in: Hypertens Res 2006 29:833–834.

Kumar NN, Benjafield AV, Lin RC, et al. 2003. Haplotype analysis of aldosterone synthase gene (CYP11B2) polymorphisms shows association with essential hypertension. J Hypertens 21:1331–1337.

Li B, Ge D, Wang Y, Zhao W, et al. 2004. Lipoprotein lipase gene polymorphisms and blood pressure levels in the Northern Chinese Han population. Hypertens Res 27:373–378.

Lin RC, Wang XL, Dalziel B, et al. 2003. Association of obesity, but not diabetes or hypertension, with glucocorticoid receptor N363S variant. Obes Res 11:802–808.

Liu Y, Qin W, Hou S, et al. 2001. A-6G variant of the angiotensinogen gene and essential hypertension in Han, Tibetan, and Yi populations. Hypertens Res 24:159–163.

Liu Y, Jin W, Jiang ZW, et al. 2004. [Relationship between six single nucleotide polymorphisms of angiotensinogen gene and essential hypertension] Chinese. Zhonghua Yi Xue Yi Chuan Xue Za Zhi 21:116–119.

Lucarelli K, Iacoviello M, Dessi-Fulgheri P, et al. 2002. [Natriuretic peptides and essential arterial hypertension] Italian. Ital Heart J 3(Suppl):1085–1091.

Mastana S, Nunn J. 1997. Angiotensin-converting enzyme deletion polymorphism is associated with hypertension in a Sikh population. Hum Hered 47:250–253.

Mayer B, Lieb W, Gotz A, et al. 2005. Association of the T8590C polymorphism of CYP4A11 with hypertension in the MONICA Augsburg echocardiographic substudy. Hypertension 46:766–771.

Menzaghi C, Paroni G, De Bonis C, et al. 2006. The -318 C>G single-nucleotide polymorphism in GNAI2 gene promoter region impairs transcriptional activity through specific binding of Sp1 transcription factor and is associated with high blood pressure in Caucasians from Italy. J Am Soc Nephrol 17(Suppl 2):S115–119.

Mettimano M, Specchia ML, Ianni A, et al. 2003. CCR5 and CCR2 gene polymorphisms in hypertensive patients. Br J Biomed Sci 60:19–21

Mondorf UF, Russ A, Wiesemann A, et al. 1998. Contribution of angiotensin I converting enzyme gene polymorphism and angiotensinogen gene polymorphism to blood pressure regulation in essential hypertension. Am J Hypertens 11:174–183.

Moreno MU, San Jose G, Orbe J, et al. 2003. Preliminary characterisation of the promoter of the human p22(phox) gene: Identification of a new polymorphism associated with hypertension. FEBS Lett 542:27–31.

Moreno MU, Jose GS, Fortuno A, et al. 2006. The C242T CYBA polymorphism of NADPH oxidase is associated with essential hypertension. J Hypertens 24:1299–1306.

Continued

Table 20-2 Essential Hypertension-Related Genes—Cont'd

Morris BJ, Chambers SM. 1996. Hypothesis: glucagon receptor glycine to serine missense mutation contributes to one in 20 cases of essential hypertension. Clin Exp Pharmacol Physiol 23:1035–1037.

Morris BJ, Zee RY, Ying LH, Griffiths LR. 1993. Independent, marked associations of alleles of the insulin receptor and dipeptidyl carboxypeptidase-I genes with essential hypertension. Clin Sci (Lond). 85:189–195.

Munroe PB, Daniel HI, Farrall M, et al. 1995. Absence of genetic linkage between polymorphisms of the insulin receptor gene and essential hypertension. J Hum Hypertens 9:669–670.

Munroe PB, Straunieks SS, Farrall M, et al. 1998. Absence of linkage to the epithelial sodium channel to hypertension in black Caribbeans. Am J Hypertens 11:942–945.

Nakayama T, Soma M, Mizutani Y, et al. 2002a. A novel missense mutation of exon 3 in the type A human natriuretic peptide receptor gene: Possible association with essential hypertension. Hypertens Res 25:395–401

Nakayama T, Soma M, Rahmutula D, et al. 2002b. Association study between a novel single nucleotide polymorphism of the promoter region of the prostacyclin synthase gene and essential hypertension. Hypertens Res 25:65–68.

Niu T, Xu X, Cordell HJ, et al. 1999. Linkage analysis of candidate genes and gene-gene interactions in Chinese hypertensive sib pairs. Hypertension 33:1332–1337.

Omi T, Kumada M, Kamesaki T, et al. 2006. An intronic variable number of tandem repeat polymorphisms of the cold-induced autoinflammatory syndrome 1 (CIAS1) gene modifies gene expression and is associated with essential hypertension. Eur J Hum Genet 14:1295–1305.

Ono K, Mannami T, Baba S, et al. 2002. A single-nucleotide polymorphism in C-type natriuretic peptide gene may be associated with hypertension. Hypertens Res 25:727–730

Ono K, Iwanaga Y, Mannami T, et al. 2003a. Epidemiological evidence of an association between SLC6A2 gene polymorphism and hypertension. Hypertens Res 26:685–689.

Ono K, Mannami T, Baba S, et al. 2003b. Lack of association between angiotensin II type 1 receptor gene polymorphism and hypertension in Japanese. Hypertens Res 26:131–134

Ono K, Mannami T, Iwai N. 2003c. Association of a promoter variant of the haeme oxygenase-1 gene with hypertension in women. J Hypertens 21:1497–1503.

Persu A, Barbry P, Bassilana F, et al. 1998. Genetic analysis of the β-subunit of the epithelial Na+ channel in essential hypertension. Hypertension 32:129–137.

Persu A, Coscoy S, Houot AM, et al. 1999. Polymorphisms of the γ-subunit of the epithelial Na+ channel in essential hypertension. J Hypertens 17:639–645.

Poch E, Gonzalez D, Giner V, et al. 2001. Molecular basis of salt sensitivity in human hypertension. Evaluation of renin-angiotensin-aldosterone system gene polymorphisms. Hypertension 38:1204–1209.

Poch E, Gonzalez D, de la Sierra A, et al. 2000. Genetic variation of the γ-subunit of the epithelial Na+ channel and essential hypertension. Relationship with salt sensitivity. Am J Hypertens 13(Pt 1):648–653.

Pola R, Flex A, Gaetani E, et al. 2002. The −174 G/C polymorphism of the interleukin-6 gene promoter and essential hypertension in an elderly Italian population. J Hum Hypertens 16:637–640.

Qiu C, Zheng Y, Cen W, et al. 2000. [Analyses on the association of CA-repeat polymorphism and A1166→C variant in the 3'-flanking region of AT(1)R gene with

essential hypertension in Tibetans] Chinese. Zhonghua Yi Xue Yi Chuan Xue Za Zhi 17:381–385.

Qiu C, Zhu X, Ji T, et al. 1995. [Detection of mutation in insulin receptor gene in patients with essential hypertension] Chinese. Zhongguo Yi Xue Ke Xue Yuan Xue Bao 17:81–85.

Quintana LF, Guzman B, Collado S, et al. 2006. A coding polymorphism in the 12-lipoxygenase gene is associated to essential hypertension and urinary 12(S)-HETE. Kidney Int 69:526–530.

Rahmutula D, Nakayama T, Soma M, et al. 2001. Association study between the variants of the human ANP gene and essential hypertension. Hypertens Res 24:291–294.

Riddle EL, Rana BK, Murthy KK, et al. 2006. Polymorphisms and haplotypes of the regulator of G protein signaling–2 gene in normotensives and hypertensives. Hypertension 47:415–420

Sato N, Nakayama T, Asai S, et al. 2006. A haplotype in the human Sur2 gene is associated with essential hypertension. J Hum Hypertens 20:87–90.

Sato M, Soma M, Nakayama T, Kanmatsuse K. 2000. Dopamine D1 receptor gene polymorphism is associated with essential hypertension. Hypertension 36:183–186

Schalin-Jantti C, Nikula-Ijas P, Huang X, et al. 1996. Polymorphism of the glycogen synthase gene in hypertensive and normotensive subjects. Hypertension 27:67–71.

Schrader AP, Zee RY, Morris BJ. 1996. Association analyses of NsiI RFLP of human insulin receptor gene in hypertensives. Clin Genet 49:74–78.

Sharma P, Hingorani A, Jia H, et al. 1999. Quantitative association between a newly identified molecular variant in the endothelin-2 gene and human essential hypertension. J Hypertens 17:1281–1287.

Soma M, Nakayama T, Satoh M, et al. 1998. A T1083C polymorphism in the human adenosine A2a receptor gene is not associated with essential hypertension. Am J Hypertens 11:1492–1494.

Soma M, Nakayama K, Rahmutula D, et al. 2002. Ser9Gly polymorphism in the dopamine D3 receptor gene is not associated with essential hypertension in the Japanese. Med Sci Monit 8:CR1–CR4.

Speirs HJ, Katyk K, Kumar NN, et al. 2004. Association of G-protein-coupled receptor kinase 4 haplotypes, but not HSD3B1 or PTP1B polymorphisms, with essential hypertension. J Hypertens 22:931–936.

Speirs HJ, Morris BJ. 2004. WNK4 intron 10 polymorphism is not associated with hypertension. Hypertension 43:766–768

Speirs HJ, Wang WY, Benjafield AV, Morris BJ. 2005. No association with hypertension of CLCNKB and TNFRSF1B polymorphisms at a hypertension locus on chromosome 1p36. J Hypertens 23:1491–1496.

Stankovic A, Zivkovic M, Glisic S, Alavantic D. 2003. Angiotensin II type 1 receptor gene polymorphism and essential hypertension in Serbian population. Clin Chim Acta 327:181–185.

Stankovic A, Zivkovic M, Alavantic D. 2002. Angiotensin I-converting enzyme gene polymorphism in a Serbian population: A gender-specific association with hypertension. Scand J Clin Lab Invest 62:469–475.

Strazzullo P, Iacone R, Siani A, et al. 2001. Altered renal sodium handling and hypertension in men carrying the glucagon receptor gene (Gly40Ser) variant. J Mol Med 79:574–580.

Continued

Table 20-2 Essential Hypertension-Related Genes—*Cont'd*

Sun ZJ, Wang XN, Lu JY, et al. 2003. [Correlation analysis between *WNK4* gene and essential hypertension] Chinese. Zhongguo Yi Xue Ke Xue Yuan Xue Bao 25:145–148

Tan JC, Zhu ZM, Zhu SJ, et al. 2004. [Study on the relationship between nitric oxide synthase gene G894T polymorphism and hypertension related risk factors in patients with essential hypertension in Chongqing city] Chinese. Zhonghua Liu Xing Bing Xue Za Zhi 25:158–161.

Tiret L, Poirier O, Hallet V, et al. 1999. The Lys198Asn polymorphism in the endothelin-1 gene is associated with blood pressure in overweight people. Hypertension 33:1169–1174.

Tomaszewski M, Brain NJ, Charchar FJ, et al. 2002. Essential hypertension and β_2-adrenergic receptor gene: Linkage and association analysis. Hypertension 40:286–291.

Trochen N, Ganapathipillai S, Ferrari P, et al. 2004. Low prevalence of nonconservative mutations of serum and glucocorticoid-regulated kinase (*SGK1*) gene in hypertensive and renal patients. Nephrol Dial Transplant 19:2499–2504.

Tsukada K, Ishimitsu T, Teranishi M, et al. 2002. Positive association of *CYP11B2* gene polymorphism with genetic predisposition to essential hypertension. J Hum Hypertens 16:789–793

von Wowern F, Bengtsson K, Lindblad U, et al. 2004. Functional variant in the α_{2B} adrenoceptor gene, a positional candidate on chromosome 2, associates with hypertension. Hypertension 43:592–597.

von Wowern F, Berglund G, Carlson J, et al. 2005. Genetic variance of SGK-1 is associated with blood pressure, blood pressure change over time and strength of the insulin-diastolic blood pressure relationship. Kidney Int 68:2164–2172.

Wang WY, Adams DJ, Glenn CL, Morris BJ. 1999. The Gly460Trp variant of α-adducin is not associated with hypertension in white Anglo-Australians. Am J Hypertens 12:632–636.

Wang JG, Staessen JA, Barlassina C, et al. 2002. Association between hypertension and variation in the α- and β-adducin genes in a white population. Kidney Int 62:2152–2159.

Williams SM, Ritchie MD, Phillips JA, Et al. 2004. Multilocus analysis of hypertension: a hierarchical approach. Hum Hered 57:28–38.

Wu SJ, Chiang FT, Chen WJ, et al. 2004. Three single-nucleotide polymorphisms of the angiotensinogen gene and susceptibility to hypertension: Single locus genotype vs. haplotype analysis. Physiol Genomics 17:79–86.

Wu X, Luke A, Rieder M, et al. 2003. An association study of angiotensinogen polymorphisms with serum level and hypertension in an African-American population. J Hypertens 21:1847–1852.

Yang J, Kamide K, Kokubo Y, et al. 2005. Genetic variations of regulator of G-protein signaling 2 in hypertensive patients and in the general population. J Hypertens 23:1497–1505.

Ying LH, Zee RY, Griffiths LR, Morris BJ. 1991 Association of a RFLP for the insulin receptor gene, but not insulin, with essential hypertension. Biochem Biophys Res Commun 181:486–492.

Yoshida H, Imaizumi T, Fujimoto K, et al. 1998. A mutation in plasma platelet-activating factor acetylhydrolase (Val279Phe) is a genetic risk factor for cerebral hemorrhage but not for hypertension. Thromb Haemost 80:372–375.

Zee RY, Lou YK, Griffiths LR, Morris BJ. 1992. Association of a polymorphism of the angiotensin I–converting enzyme gene with essential hypertension. Biochem Biophys Res Commun. 184:9–15.

Zee RY, Lou YK, Morris BJ. 1994. Insertion variant in intron 9, but not microsatellite in intron 2, of the insulin receptor gene is associated with essential hypertension. J Hypertens 12(Suppl):S13–S22.

Zee RY, Ying LH, Morris BJ, Griffiths LR. 1991. Association and linkage analyses of restriction fragment length polymorphisms for the human renin and antithrombin III genes in essential hypertension. J Hypertens 9:825–830.

Zhao Q, Su SY, Chen SF, et al. 2006. Association study of the endothelial nitric oxide synthase gene polymorphisms with essential hypertension in northern Han Chinese. Chin Med J (Engl) 119:1065–1071.

Zhou X, Tang W, Wu H, et al. 2006. Are the beta-adducin C1797T polymorphism and gamma-adducin A386G polymorphism associated with essential hypertension in Yi and Hani populations? Clinica Chimica Acta 374:153–154.

Zhu H, Sagnella GA, Dong Y, et al. 2004. Molecular variants of the sodium/hydrogen exchanger type 3 gene and essential hypertension. J Hypertens 22:1269–1275.

Zhu X, Chang YP, Yan D, et al. 2003. Associations between hypertension and genes in the renin-angiotensin system. Hypertension 41:1027–1034.

Table 20-3 Criteria for the Determination of Genetic Cause(s) of Heritable Complex Disease*

Linkage or Association Study
Demonstrate a statistically sound genome-wide association in a single or multiple studies.
Quantitative trait locus should map to < 30 cM.
Fine mapping
Demonstrate linkage disequilibrium to < 1 cM.
Sequence analysis
Perform sequence analysis to identify specific single-nucleotide polymorphisms.
Circumstantial Evidence
Comparison of wild-type and variant biochemistry and physiology
Tissue location
Engineered mutations
Transfected cell models
Regulatory Elements
3'–Untranslated regions can have a profound influence on gene expression and function.
Promoter or intergenic variants can influence protein expression.
Complicating factors
Functional Tests for Candidate Genes (Definitive Test)
Knockout
Transgenic complementation

*Criteria are among those suggested by Glazier et al[167] for use in determining whether a gene or group of genes is responsible for the causation of complex diseases.

CIRCUMSTANTIAL EVIDENCE OF THE INVOLVEMENT OF GENE VARIANTS IN ESSENTIAL HYPERTENSION

Organ/tissue expression of the putative gene(s) and their concomitant function(s) should make physiologic sense. Because the kidney is responsible for at least 50% of the increase in blood pressure in essential hypertension, and because the increase in sodium reabsorption in essential hypertension occurs mainly in the proximal tubule and thick ascending limb of Henle, genes that regulate transport in these nephron segments are prime candidates to play a significant role in the pathogenesis of this disease (see Table 20-1). Because the distal nephron can contribute to sodium retention in essential hypertension, genes that regulate transport in the cortical collecting duct, such as those encoding aldosterone synthase and 11β-hydroxysteroid dehydrogenase, can be accessory genes.

The mechanism by which sodium chloride transport is regulated is an important consideration in the determination of candidate genes in hypertension. Gene products that increase sodium transport primarily by increasing Na^+/K^+-ATPase activity is prohypertensive. However, the stimulatory effect on sodium transport may not be confined to the proximal tubule and thick ascending limb of Henle, the nephron segments of increased sodium transport in essential hypertension.[11,12,14-16] So far, only the dopaminergic system has

been implicated in the increased Cl^-/HCO_3^- exchanger activity in renal proximal tubules in the SHR.[188] Increased Na^+/K^+-ATPase activity does not explain the important role of chloride in the pathogenesis of hypertension.[188] Further, increased Na^+/K^+-ATPase activity in resistance vessels would be vasodilatory.

A generalized inhibition of Na^+/K^+-ATPase activity is antihypertensive by increasing sodium excretion but would cause increased vascular smooth muscle cell reactivity, unless other mechanisms exist to inhibit smooth muscle cell contraction, for example, protein kinase A, inhibition of calcium channels or sodium/calcium exchanger, or activation of potassium channels.[19,66,188a,189] In addition to being able to alter renal sodium and/or chloride transport, such genes should also be able to regulate or modulate the formation of ROS (e.g., renin angiotensin II genes, dopamine receptor genes). These genes should also be able to influence the neurogenic control of blood pressure.

Renal blood flow is decreased and renal vascular resistance is increased in subjects with established hypertension. However, genes with products that regulate vascular resistance by themselves are probably not good candidate genes, because resting renal blood flow is not decreased in borderline hypertension and normotensive offspring of hypertensive parents.[190] In contrast, prehypertensive subjects[191] and offspring of hypertensive parents may have a higher proximal tubule sodium reabsorption than offspring of normotensive parents.[192,193] Simultaneous homozygosities for *AGT M235*, *AT1R A1166*, and *CYP11B2 C-344*, in the presence of the D allele at *ACE D* were associated with increased proximal tubule sodium transport in male hypertensive Italians.[194] The α-adducin G460W allele[6,183,184,195] and *GRK4 A486V*[182] with *AGT M235T* or *ACEI/D* have also been linked to salt sensitivity among Italians. Salt-sensitive hypertension is associated with the presence of *GRK4 R65L*, *A142V*, and *A486V* in Japanese, with a 94% predictive accuracy.[196] As mentioned above, both α-adducin and *GRK4* are located on chromosome 4p16.3.[186,187] Genes that have widespread expression are also not good candidates for hypertension because vascular resistance should be similarly increased in all vascular beds. However, borderline essential hypertension is not associated with an increase in vascular resistance in skeletal muscle or hepatic bed.[190]

Conclusive Evidence That Gene Variants Cause Hypertension

According to Glazier et al, the most conclusive evidence that gene variants are causal of complex disease is the demonstration that replacement of the variant nucleotide results in switching one phenotype for another.[167] The polymorphism of α-adducin has been found in the Milan hypertensive rat,[197] and expression of α-adducin G460W increases Na⁺/K⁺-ATPase activity.[198] However, this polymorphism has not been shown to cause hypertension in transgenic mice, although disruption of β-adducin gene in mice increases blood pressure.[199] Expression of GRK4-γ variants (R65L, A142V, or A486V) in Chinese hamster ovary cells impairs D$_1$ receptor function and produces hypertension in transgenic mice.[177] Inhibition of the expression of GRK4 in renal proximal tubule cells from hypertensive subjects normalizes D$_1$ receptor function,[177] and renal inhibition of GRK4 expression ameliorates the hypertension in spontaneously hypertensive rats.[200]

In summary, a characteristic of essential hypertension is a failure of the kidneys to eliminate sodium chloride and water. This defect can be primary to the kidney or to neural, endocrine, vascular, and cardiac mechanisms, with the kidney serving a secondary role. The proximal tubule and thick ascending limb of Henle are the nephron segments with enhanced sodium chloride transport in essential hypertension, whereas more distal nephron segments are involved in monogenic hypertension. Because hypertension is a complex disease, interactions of variants in a single gene or several genes are probably needed. The putative gene variants in essential hypertension should make physiologic sense. However, the definitive proof of causality in transgenic studies is the demonstration that overexpression in mice of the wild-type gene is associated with normal blood pressure, whereas expression of the variant gene results in hypertension.

References

1. World Health Organization. The World Health Report 2002. Reducing Risks, Promoting Healthy Life. Geneva, Switzerland, World Health Organization, 2002, p 58.
2. Hajjar I, Kotchen TA: Trends in prevalence, awareness, treatment, and control of hypertension in the United States, 1988–2000. JAMA 290:199–206, 2003.
3. Pickering TG: Modern definitions and clinical expressions of hypertension. In Laragh JH, Brenner BM (eds): Hypertension: Pathophysiology, Diagnosis, and Management, 2nd ed. New York, Raven Press, 1995, pp 17–21.
4. Harrap SB: Where are all the blood-pressure genes? Lancet 361:2149–2151, 2003.
5. Luft FC: Geneticism of essential hypertension. Hypertension 43:1155–1159, 2004.
6. Kardia SL, Turner ST, Schwartz GL, Moore JH: Linear dynamic features of ambulatory blood pressure in a population-based study. Blood Press Monit 9:259–267, 2004.
7. Williams SM, Haines JL, Moore JH: The use of animal models in the study of complex disease: All else is never equal or why do so many human studies fail to replicate animal findings? Bioessays 26:170–179, 2004.
8. Hall JE, Brands MW, Henegar JR: Angiotensin II and long-term arterial pressure regulation: The overriding dominance of the kidney. J Am Soc Nephrol 10(Suppl 12):S258–S265, 1999.
9. Guyton AC, Hall JE, Coleman TG, et al: The dominant role of the kidneys in long-term arterial pressure regulation in normal and hypertensive states. In Laragh JH, Brenner BM (eds): Hypertension: Pathophysiology, Diagnosis, and Management, 2nd ed. New York, Raven Press, 1995, pp 1311–1333.
10. Navar LG, Harrison-Bernard LM, Nishiyama A, Kobori H: Regulation of intrarenal angiotensin II in hypertension. Hypertension 39:316–322, 2002.
11. Doris PA: Renal proximal tubule sodium transport and genetic mechanisms of essential hypertension. J Hypertens 18:509–519, 2000.
12. Ortiz PA, Garvin JL: Intrarenal transport and vasoactive substances in hypertension. Hypertension 38:621–624, 2001.
13. Ferrandi M, Salardi S, Parenti P, et al: Na⁺K⁺Cl⁻ cotransporter-mediated Rb⁺ fluxes in membrane vesicles from kidneys of normotensive and hypertensive rats. Biochim Biophys Acta 1021:13–20, 1990.
14. Aviv A, Hollenberg NK, Weder A: Urinary potassium excretion and sodium sensitivity in blacks. Hypertension 43:707–713, 2004.
15. Chiolero A, Maillard M, Nussberger J, et al: Proximal sodium reabsorption: An independent determinant of blood pressure response to salt. Hypertension 36:631–637, 2000.
16. Strazzullo P, Galletti F, Barba G: Altered renal handling of sodium in human hypertension: Short review of the evidence. Hypertension 41:1000–1005, 2003.
17. Lifton RP, Wilson FH, Choate KA, Geller DS: Salt and blood pressure: New insight from human genetic studies. Cold Spring Harb Symp Quant Biol 67:445–450, 2002.
18. Huang WC, Bell PD, Harvey D, et al: Angiotensin influences on tubuloglomerular feedback mechanism in hypertensive rats. Kidney Int 34:631–637, 1988.
19. Unlap MT, Bates E, Williams C, et al: Na⁺/Ca²⁺ exchanger: Target for oxidative stress in salt-sensitive hypertension. Hypertension 42:363–368, 2003.
20. Wilcox CS: Reactive oxygen species: Roles in blood pressure and kidney function. Curr Hypertens Rep 4:160–166, 2002.
21. Loberg RD, Northcott CA, Watts SW, Brosius FC: PI3-kinase–induced hyperreactivity in DOCA-salt hypertension is independent of GSK-3 activity. Hypertension 41:898–902, 2003.
22. Savoia C, Schiffrin EL: Significance of recently identified peptides in hypertension: endothelin, natriuretic peptides, adrenomedullin, leptin. Med Clin North Am 88:39–62, 2004.
23. Granger JP, Alexander BT, Llinas M: Mechanisms of pressure natriuresis. Curr Hypertens Rep 4:152–159, 2001.
24. Cowley AW Jr, Mori T, Mattson D, Zou AP: Role of renal NO production in the regulation of medullary blood flow. Am J Physiol Regul Integr Comp Physiol 284:R1355–R1369, 2003.

25. Pollock DM: Chronic studies on the interaction between nitric oxide and endothelin in cardiovascular and renal function. Clin Exp Pharmacol Physiol 26:258–261, 1999.

26. Roman RJ: P-450 metabolites of arachidonic acid in the control of cardiovascular function. Physiol Rev 82:131–185, 2002.

27. McGiff JC, Quilley J: 20-hydroxyeicosatetraenoic acid and epoxyeicosatrienoic acids and blood pressure. Curr Opin Nephrol Hypertens 10:231–237, 2001.

28. Nasjletti A, Arthur C: Corcoran Memorial Lecture. The role of eicosanoids in angiotensin-dependent hypertension. Hypertension 31:194–200, 1998.

29. Luo M, Hess MC, Fink GD, et al: Differential alterations in sympathetic neurotransmission in mesenteric arteries and veins in DOCA-salt hypertensive rats. Auton Neurosci 104:47–57, 2003.

30. Hinojosa-Laborde C, Chapa I, Lange D, Haywood JR: Gender differences in sympathetic nervous system regulation. Clin Exp Pharmacol Physiol 26:122–126, 1999.

31. Sved AF, Ito S, Sved JC: Brainstem mechanisms of hypertension: Role of the rostral ventrolateral medulla. Curr Hypertens Rep 5:262–268, 2003.

32. Zimmerman MC, Davisson RL: Redox signaling in central neural regulation of cardiovascular function. Prog Biophys Mol Biol 84:125–149, 2004.

33. Veerasingham SJ, Sellers KW, Raizada MK: Functional genomics as an emerging strategy for the investigation of central mechanisms in experimental hypertension. Prog Biophys Mol Biol 84:107–123, 2004.

34. DiBona GF: Sympathetic nervous system and the kidney in hypertension. Curr Opin Nephrol Hypertens 11:197–200, 2002.

35. Reckelhoff JF, Fortepiani LA: Novel mechanisms responsible for postmenopausal hypertension. Hypertension 43:918–923, 2004.

36. Fuchs S, Frenzel K, Xiao HD, et al: Newly recognized physiologic and pathophysiologic actions of the angiotensin-converting enzyme. Curr Hypertens Rep 6:124–128, 2004.

37. Luft FC: Present status of genetic mechanisms in hypertension. Med Clin North Am 88:1–18, 2004.

38. Gurley SB, Le TH, Coffman TM: Gene-targeting studies of the renin-angiotensin system: Mechanisms of hypertension and cardiovascular disease. Cold Spring Harb Symp Quant Biol 67:451–457, 2002.

39. Ferrario CM, Chappell MC, Tallant EA, et al: Counterregulatory actions of angiotensin-1–7. Hypertension 30:535–541, 1997.

40. Lavoie JL, Sigmund CD: Minireview: Overview of the renin-angiotensin system—An endocrine and paracrine system. Endocrinology 144:2179–2183, 2003.

41. Davy KP, Hall JE: Obesity and hypertension: Two epidemics or one? Am J Physiol Regul Integr Comp Physiol 286:R803–R813, 2004.

42. Ortiz PA, Garvin JL: Superoxide stimulates NaCl absorption by the thick ascending limb. Am J Physiol Renal Physiol 283:5957–5962, 2002.

43. Bek MJ, Reinhardt HC, Fischer KG, et al: Up-regulation of early growth response gene-1 via the CXCR3 receptor induces reactive oxygen species and inhibits Na$^+$/K$^+$-ATPase activity in an immortalized human proximal tubule cell line. J Immunol 170:931–940, 2003.

44. Han HJ, Yoon BC, Park SH, et al: Ginsenosides protect apical transporters of cultured proximal tubule cells from dysfunctions induced by H$_2$O$_2$. Kidney Blood Press Res 25:308–314, 2002.

45. McDonough AA, Biemesderfer D: Does membrane trafficking play a role in regulating the sodium/hydrogen exchanger isoform 3 in the proximal tubule? Curr Opin Nephrol Hypertens 12:533–541, 2003.

46. Khundmiri SJ, Rane MJ, Lederer ED: Parathyroid hormone regulation of type II sodium-phosphate cotransporters is dependent on an A kinase anchoring protein. J Biol Chem 278:10134–10141, 2003.

47. Beierwaltes WH, Arendshorst WJ, Klemmer PJ: Electrolyte and water balance in young spontaneously hypertensive rats. Hypertension 4:908–915, 1982.

48. Harrap SB: Genetic analysis of blood pressure and sodium balance in spontaneously hypertensive rats. 8:572–582, 1986.

49. Morgan DA, DiBona GF, Mark AL: Effects of interstrain renal transplantation on NaCl-induced hypertension in Dahl rats. Hypertension 15:436–442, 1990.

50. Churchill PC, Churchill MC, Bidani AK, Kurtz TW: Kidney-specific chromosome transfer in genetic hypertension: The Dahl hypothesis revisited. Kidney Int 60:705–714, 2001.

51. Dahl LK, Heine M, Thompson K: Genetic influence of the kidneys on blood pressure. Evidence from chronic renal homografts in rats with opposite predispositions to hypertension. Circ Res 40:94–101, 1974.

52. Bianchi G, Fox U, Di Francesco GF, et al: Blood pressure changes produced by kidney cross-transplantation between spontaneously hypertensive rats and normotensive rats. Clin Sci Mol Med 47:435–448, 1974.

53. Frey BA, Grisk O, Bandelow N, et al: Sodium homeostasis in transplanted rats with a spontaneously hypertensive rat kidney. Am J Physiol Regul Integr Comp Physiol 279:31099–31104, 2000.

54. Calhoun DA, Zhu S, Wyss JM, Oparil S: Diurnal blood pressure variation and dietary salt in spontaneously hypertensive rats. Hypertension 24:1–7, 1994.

55. Ahn J, Varagic J, Slama M, et al: Cardiac structural and functional responses to salt loading in SHR. Am J Physiol Heart Circ Physiol 287:H767–H772, 2004.

56. Sander S, Rettig R, Ehrig B: Role of the native kidney in experimental post-transplantation hypertension. Pflugers Arch 431:971–976, 1996.

57. Grisk O, Frey BAJ, Uber A, Rettig R: Sympathetic activity in early renal posttransplantation hypertension in rats. Am J Physiol Regul Integr Comp Physiol 279:R1737–R1744, 2000.

58. Grisk O, Rose HJ, Lorenz G, Rettig R: Sympathetic-renal interaction in chronic arterial pressure control. Am J Physiol Regul Integr Comp Physiol 283:R441–R450, 2002.

59. Curtis JJ, Luke RG, Dustan HP, et al: Remission of essential hypertension after renal transplantation. N Engl J Med 309:1009–1015, 1983.

60. Guidi E, Menghetti D, Milani S, et al: Hypertension may be transplanted with the kidney in humans: A long-term historical prospective follow-up of recipients grafted with kidneys coming from donors with or without hypertension in their families. J Am Soc Nephrol 7:1131–1138, 1996.

61. Lund-Johansen P: Newer thinking on the hemodynamics of hypertension. Curr Opin Cardiol 9:505–511, 1994.

62. van Hooft IM, Grobbee DE, Waal-Manning HJ, Hofman A: Hemodynamic characteristics of the early phase of primary hypertension. The Dutch Hypertension and Offspring Study. Circulation 87:1100–1106, 1993.

63. Touyz RM: Impaired vasorelaxation in hypertension: Beyond the endothelium. J Hypertens 20:371–373, 2002.

64. Chitaley K, Weber D, Webb RC: RhoA/Rho-kinase, vascular changes, and hypertension. Curr Hypertens Rep 3:139–144, 2001.

65. Sowers JR: Insulin resistance and hypertension. Am J Physiol Heart Circ Physiol 286:H1597–H602, 2004.

66. Iwamoto T, Kita S, Zhang J, et al: Salt-sensitive hypertension is triggered by Ca^{2+} entry via Na$^+$Ca^{2+} exchanger type-1 in vascular smooth muscle. Nat Med 10:1193–1199, 2004.

67. Kim HS, Krege JH, Kluckman KD, et al: Genetic control of blood pressure and the angiotensinogen locus. Proc Natl Acad Sci U S A 92:2735–2739, 1995.

68. Tian B, Meng QC, Chen YF, et al: Blood pressures and cardiovascular homeostasis in mice having reduced or absent angiotensin-converting enzyme gene function. Hypertension 30:128–133, 1997.

69. Cole JM, Xiao H, Adams JW, et al: New approaches to genetic manipulation of mice: Tissue-specific expression of ACE. Am J Physiol Renal Physiol 284:F599–F607, 2003.

70. Ito M, Oliverio MI, Mannon PJ, et al: Regulation of blood pressure by the type 1A angiotensin II receptor gene. Proc Natl Acad Sci U S A 92:3521–3525, 1995.

71. Katovich MJ, Reaves PY, Francis SC, et al: Gene therapy attenuates the elevated blood pressure and glucose intolerance in an insulin-resistant model of hypertension. J Hypertens 19:1553–1558, 2001.

72. Stec DE, Keen HL, Sigmund CD: Lower blood pressure in floxed angiotensinogen mice after adenoviral delivery of Cre-recombinase. Hypertension 39:629–633, 2002.

73. Crowley SD, Gurley SB, Herrera MJ, et al: Angiotensin II causes hypertension and cardiac hypertrophy through its receptors in the kidney. Proc Natl Acad Sci U S A 103:17985–17990, 2006.

73a. Crowley SD, Gurley SB, Oliverio MI, et al: Distinct roles for the kidney and systemic tissues in blood pressure regulation by the renin-angiotensin system. J Clin Invest 115:1092–1099, 2005.

74. Wu JN, Berecek KH: Prevention of genetic hypertension by early treatment of spontaneously hypertensive rats with the angiotensin converting enzyme inhibitor captopril. Hypertension 22:139–146, 1993.

75. Smith PA, Meaney JF, Graham LN, et al: Relationship of neurovascular compression to central sympathetic discharge and essential hypertension. J Am Coll Cardiol 43:8453–8458, 2004.

76. Schlaich MP, Lambert E, Kaye DM, et al: Sympathetic augmentation in hypertension: Role of nerve firing, norepinephrine reuptake, and angiotensin neuromodulation. Hypertension 43:269–275, 2004.

77. Folkow B, Hallback M, Lundgren Y, Weiss L: The effects of immunosympathectomy on blood pressure and vascular reactivity in normal and spontaneously hypertensive rats. Acta Physiol Scand 84:512–523, 1975.

78. Aileru AA, Logan E, Callahan M, et al: Alterations in sympathetic ganglionic transmission in response to angiotensin II in (mRen2) 27 transgenic rats. Hypertension 43:270–275, 2004.

79. Lundin S, Ricksten SE, Thoren P: Interaction between mental stress and baroreceptor reflexes concerning effects on heart rate, mean arterial pressure and renal sympathetic nerve activity in conscious spontaneously hypertensive rats. Acta Physiol Scand 120:273–281, 1984.

80. Grisk O, Heukaufer M, Steinbach A, et al: Analysis of arterial pressure regulating systems in renal post-transplantation hypertension. J Hypertens 22:199–207, 2004.

81. Zeng C, Wang D, Asico LD, et al: Aberrant D1 and D3 dopamine receptor transregulation in hypertension. Hypertension 43:654–660, 2004.

82. Bughi S, Horton R, Antonipillai I, et al: Comparison of dopamine and fenoldopam effects on renal blood flow and prostacyclin excretion in normal and essential hypertensive subjects. J Clin Endocrinol Metab 69:1116–1121, 1989.

83. Chatziantoniou C, Ruan X, Arendshorst WJ: Defective G protein activation of the cAMP pathway in rat kidney during genetic hypertension. Proc Natl Acad Sci U S A 92:2924–2928, 1995.

84. de Vries PA, Navis G, de Jong PE, et al: Impaired renal vascular response to a D1-like receptor agonist but not to an ACE inhibitor in conscious spontaneously hypertensive rats. J Cardiovasc Pharmacol 34:191–198, 1999.

85. Fridovich I: Superoxide anion radical (O_2^-), superoxide dismutases, and related matters. J Biol Chem 272:18515–18517, 1997.

86. Swain SD, Rohn TT, Quinn MT: Neutrophil priming in host defense: Role of oxidants as priming agents. Antioxid Redox Signal 4:69–83, 2002.

87. Wolf G: Free radical production and angiotensin. Curr Hypertens Rep 2:167–173, 2000.

88. Griendling KK, Ushio-Fukai M: NADH/NADPH oxidase. Trends Cardiovasc Med 7:301–307, 1997.

89. Cai H, Griendling KK, Harrison DG: The vascular NAD(P)H oxidases as therapeutic targets in cardiovascular diseases. Trends Pharmacol Sci 24:471–478, 2003.

90. Alexander RW: Theodore Cooper Memorial Lecture. Hypertension and the pathogenesis of atherosclerosis. Oxidative stress and the mediation of arterial inflammatory response: A new perspective. Hypertension 25:155–161, 1995.

91. Kumar KV, Das UN: Are free radicals involved in the pathobiology of human essential hypertension? Free Radic Res Commun 19:59–66, 1993.

92. Kourie I: Interaction of reactive oxygen species with ion transport mechanisms. Am J Physiol 275:C1–C24, 1998.

93. Dalton TP, Shertzer HG, Puga A: Regulation of gene expression by reactive oxygen. Annu Rev Pharmacol Toxicol 39:67–101, 1999.

94. Lacy F, O'Connor DT, Schmid-Schonbein GW: Plasma hydrogen peroxide production in hypertensives and normotensive subjects at genetic risk of hypertension. J Hypertens 16:291–303, 1998.

95. Touyz RM, Schiffrin EL: Reactive oxygen species in vascular biology: Implications in hypertension. Histochem Cell Biol 122:339–352, 2004.

96. Zhang H, Schmeisser A, Garlichs CD, et al: Angiotensin II-induced superoxide anion generation in human vascular endothelial cells: Role of membrane-bound NADH-/NADPH-oxidases. Cardiovasc Res 44:215–222, 1999.

97. Cosentino F, Patton S, d'Uscio LV, et al: Tetrahydrobiopterin alters superoxide and nitric oxide release in prehypertensive rats. J Clin Invest 101:1530–1537, 1998.

98. Amico JA, Corder CN, McDonald RH Jr, Robinson AG: Levels of the oxytocin-associated and vasopressin-associated neurophysins in plasma and their responses in essential hypertension. Clin Endocrinol (Oxf) 20:289–297, 1984.

99. Krieger-Brauer HI, Kather H: The stimulus-sensitive H_2O_2-generating system present in human fat-cell plasma membranes is multireceptor-linked and under antagonistic control by hormones and cytokines. Biochem J 307:543–548, 1995.

100. Mukherjee SP, Mukherjee C: Stimulation of pyruvate dehydrogenase activity in adipocytes by oxytocin: Evidence for mediation of the insulin-like effect by endogenous hydrogen peroxide independent of glucose transport. Arch Biochem Biophys 214:211–222, 1982.

101. Cowley AW Jr: Control of the renal medullary circulation by vasopressin V1 and V2 receptors in the rat. Exp Physiol 85 (Spec No):223S–231S, 2000.

102. Bakris G, Bursztyn M, Gavras I, et al: Role of vasopressin in essential hypertension: Racial differences. J Hypertens 15:545–550, 1997.

103. Li L, Galligan JJ, Fink GD, Chen AF: Vasopressin induces vascular superoxide via endothelin-1 in mineralocorticoid hypertension. Hypertension 41:663–668, 2003.

104. Nickenig G, Strehlow K, Baumer AT, et al: Negative feedback regulation of reactive oxygen species on AT1 receptor gene expression. Br J Pharmacol 131:795–803, 2000.

105. Yang, Z, Asico LD, Yu P, et al: D5 dopamine receptor regulation of phospholipase D. Am J Physiol Heart Circ Physiol 288:H55–H61, 2005.

106. Yan Z, Asico LD, Yu P, et al: D5 dopamine receptor regulation of reactive oxygen species production, NADPH oxidase, and blood pressure. Am J Physiol Regul Integr Comp Physiol 290:R96–R104, 2006.
107. Yasunari K, Kohno M, Kano H, et al: Dopamine as a novel antioxidative agent for rat vascular smooth muscle cells through dopamine D1-like receptors. Circulation 101:2302–2308, 2000.
108. White BH, Sidhu A: Increased oxidative stress in renal proximal tubules of the spontaneously hypertensive rat: A mechanism for defective dopamine D1A receptor/G-protein coupling. J Hypertens 16:1659–1665, 1998.
109. Ishige K, Chen Q, Sagara Y, Schubert D: The activation of dopamine D4 receptors inhibits oxidative stress-induced nerve cell death. J Neurosci 21:6069–6076, 2001.
110. Carvey PM, McGuire SO, Ling ZD: Neuroprotective effects of D3 dopamine receptor agonists. Parkinsonism Relat Disord 7:213–223, 2001.
111. Nair VD, Sealfon SC: Agonist-specific transactivation of phosphoinositide 3-kinase signaling pathway mediated by the dopamine D2 receptor. J Biol Chem 278:47053–47061, 2003.
112. Gabbai FB, Blantz RC: Role of nitric oxide in renal hemodynamics. Semin Nephrol 19:242–250, 1999.
113. Wilcox CS: Redox regulation of the afferent arteriole and tubuloglomerular feedback. Acta Physiol Scand 179:217–223, 2003.
114. Kone BC: Nitric oxide synthesis in the kidney: Isoforms, biosynthesis, and functions in health. Semin Nephrol 24:299–315, 2004.
115. Komlosi P, Fintha A, Bell PD: Current mechanisms of macula densa cell signalling. Acta Physiol Scand 181:463–469, 2004.
116. Guzman NJ, Fang MZ, Tang SS, et al: Autocrine inhibition of Na$^+$K$^+$ ATPase by nitric oxide in mouse proximal tubule epithelial cells. J Clin Invest 95:2083–2088, 1995.
117. Liang M, Knox FG: Nitric oxide enhances paracellular permeability of opossum kidney cells. Kidney Int 55:2215–2223, 1999.
118. Varela M, Herrera M, Garvin JL: Inhibition of Na-K-ATPase in thick ascending limbs by NO depends on O$_2^-$ and is diminished by a high-salt diet. Am J Physiol Renal Physiol 287:F224–F230, 2004.
119. Wang T: Role of iNOS and eNOS in modulating proximal tubule transport and acid-base balance. Am J Physiol Renal Physiol 283:F658–F662, 2002.
120. Ortiz PA, Hong NJ, Garvin JL: NO decreases thick ascending limb chloride absorption by reducing Na$^+$K$^+$2Cl$^-$ cotransporter activity. Am J Physiol Renal Physiol 281:F819–F825, 2001.
121. Kawasaki T, Delea CS, Bartter FC, Smith H: The effect of high-sodium and low-sodium intakes on blood pressure and other related variables in human subjects with idiopathic hypertension. Am J Med 64:193–198, 1978.
122. Sullivan JM: Salt sensitivity. Definition, conception, methodology, and long-term issues. Hypertension 17:161–168, 1991.
123. Draaijer P, de Leeuw P, Maessen J, et al: Salt-sensitivity testing in patients with borderline hypertension: reproducibility and potential mechanisms. J Hum Hypertens 9:263–269, 1995.
124. Weinberger MH: Salt sensitivity and blood pressure in humans. Hypertension 27:481–490, 1996.
125. de la Sierra A, Giner V, Bragulat E, Coca A: Lack of correlation between two methods for the assessment of salt sensitivity in essential hypertension. J Hum Hypertens 16:255–260, 2002.
126. Kato N, Kanda T, Sagara M, et al: Proposition of a feasible protocol to evaluate salt sensitivity in a population-based setting. Hypertens Res 25:801–809, 2002.
127. Burt VL, Cutler JA, Higgins M, et al: Trends in the prevalence, awareness, treatment, and control of hypertension in the adult US population. Data from the health examination surveys, 1960 to 1991. Hypertension 26:60–69, 1995.
128. Weinberger MH, Fineberg NS, Fineberg SE, Weinberger M: Salt sensitivity, pulse pressure, and death in normal and hypertensive humans. Hypertension 37:429–432, 2001.
129. Bihorac A, Tezcan H, Ozener C, et al: Association between salt sensitivity and target organ damage in essential hypertension. Am J Hypertens 13:864–872, 2000.
130. de Wardener HE, MacGregor GA: Harmful effects of dietary salt in addition to hypertension. J Hum Hypertens 16:213–223, 2002.
131. Hu G, Qiao Q, Tuomilehto J: Nonhypertensive cardiac effects of a high salt diet. Curr Hypertens Rpt 4:13–17, 2002.
132. He J, Ogden LG, Vupputuri S, et al: Dietary sodium intake and subsequent risk of cardiovascular disease in overweight adults. JAMA 282:2027–2034, 1999.
133. Tuomilehto J, Jousilahti P, Rastenyte D, et al: Urinary sodium excretion and cardiovascular mortality in Finland: A prospective study. Lancet 357:848–851, 2001.
134. Kotchem TA, Kotchen JM: Dietary sodium and blood pressure: interactions with other nutrients. Am J Clin Nutr 65(Suppl):708S–711S, 1997.
135. Kurtz TW, Al-Bander HA, Morris RC Jr, et al: "Salt-sensitive essential hypertension in men: Is the sodium ion alone important? N Engl J Med 317:1043–1048, 1987.
136. Shore AC, Markandu ND, MacGregor GA: A randomized crossover study to compare the blood pressure response to sodium loading with and without chloride in patients with essential hypertension. J Hypertens 6:613–617, 1988.
137. Whitescarver SA, Ott CE, Jackson BA, et al: Salt-sensitive hypertension: Contribution of chloride. Science 223:1430–1432, 1984.
138. Luft FC, Steinberg H, Ganten U, et al: Effect of sodium chloride and sodium bicarbonate on blood pressure in stroke-prone spontaneously hypertensive rats. Clin Sci (Lond) 74:577–585, 1988.
139. Kurtz TW, Morris RC Jr: Dietary chloride as a determinant of "sodium-dependent" hypertension. Science 222:1139–1141, 1983.
140. Sato Y, Ogata E, Fujita T: Role of chloride in angiotensin II-induced salt-sensitive hypertension. Hypertension 18:622–629, 1991.
141. Brunner HR, Laragh JH, Baer L, et al: Essential hypertension: Renin and aldosterone, heart attack and stroke. N Engl J Med 286:441–449, 1972.
142. Laragh JH: Discordant nephron function. A pathogenic factor in hypertension and its vascular complications of stroke and heart attack. Am J Hypertens 4(1 Pt 2):2S–6S, 1991.
143. Tuck ML, Williams GH, Cain JP, et al: Relation of age, diastolic pressure and known duration of hypertension to presence of low renin essential hypertension. Am J Cardiol 32:637–642, 1973.
144. Grant FD, Romero JR, Jeunemaitre X, et al: Low-renin hypertension, altered sodium homeostasis, and an α-adducin polymorphism. Hypertension 39:191–196, 2002.
145. Sugimoto K, Hozawa A, Katsuya T, et al: α-adducin Gly460Trp polymorphism is associated with low renin hypertension in younger subjects in the Ohasama study. J Hypertens 20:1779–1784, 2002.
146. Hollenberg NK, Williams GH: Abnormal renal function, sodium-volume homeostasis and renin system behavior in normal renin-hypertension: The evolution of the nonmodulator concept. In Laragh JH, Brenner BM (eds): Hypertension: Pathophysiology, Diagnosis, and Management, 2nd ed. New York, Raven Press, 1995, pp 1837–1856.
147. Sanada H, Yatabe J, Midorikawa S, et al: Single-nucleotide polymorphisms for diagnosis of salt-sensitive hypertension. Clin Chem 52:352–360, 2006.
148. de la Sierra A, Lluch MM, Coca A, et al: Fluid, ionic and hormonal changes induced by high salt intake in salt-sensitive

and salt-resistant hypertensive patients. Clin Sci 91:155–161, 1996.

149. Sanchez R, Gimenez MI, Ramos F, et al: Non-modulating hypertension: Evidence for the involvement of kallikrein/kinin activity associated with overactivity of the renin-angiotensin system. Successful blood pressure control during long-term Na⁺ restriction. J Hypertens 14:1287–1291, 1996.

150. Burgess ED, Keane PM, Watanabe M: Norepinephrine and calcium responses to altered sodium intake in modulating and non-modulating high-renin hypertension. J Hypertens Suppl 6:S85–S87, 1988.

151. Gordon MS, Steunkel CA, Conlin PR, et al: The role of dopamine in nonmodulating hypertension. Clin Endocrinol Metab 69:426–432, 1989.

152. Lee MR: Dopamine and the kidney. Clin Sci (Lond) 62:439–448, 1982.

153. Gill JR Jr, Grossman E, Goldstein DS: High urinary dopa and low urinary dopamine-to-dopa ratio in salt-sensitive hypertension. Hypertension 18:614–621, 1991.

154. Kuchel O: Peripheral dopamine in hypertension and associated conditions. J Hum Hypertens 13:605–615, 1999.

155. Sowers JR, Zemel MB, Zemel P, et al: Salt sensitivity in blacks. Salt intake and natriuretic substances. Hypertension 12:485–490, 1988.

156. Cuspidi C, Meani S, Salerno M, et al: Cardiovascular target organ damage in essential hypertensives with or without reproducible nocturnal fall in blood pressure. J Hypertens 22:273–280, 2004.

157. Profant J, Dimsdale JE: Race and diurnal blood pressure patterns. A review and meta-analysis. Hypertension 33:1099–1104, 1999

158. Higashi Y, Nakagawa K, Kimura M, et al: Circadian variation of blood pressure and endothelial function in patients with essential hypertension: A comparison of dippers and non-dippers. J Am Coll Cardiol 40:2039–2043, 2002.

159. Jonas M, Garfinkel D, Zisapel N, et al: Impaired nocturnal melatonin secretion in non-dipper hypertensive patients. Blood Press 12:19–24, 2003.

160. Nakano Y, Oshima T, Ozono R, et al: Non-dipper phenomenon in essential hypertension is related to blunted nocturnal rise and fall of sympatho-vagal nervous activity and progress in retinopathy. Auton Neurosci 88:181–186, 2001.

161. Watanabe Y, Nishimura H, Sanaka S, et al: Does sodium sensitivity affect nocturnal blood pressure variation in outpatients with hypertension? Clin Exp Hypertens 24:99–107, 2002.

162. Polonia J, Diogo D, Caupers P, Damasceno A: Influence of two doses of irbesartan on non-dipper circadian blood pressure rhythm in salt-sensitive black hypertensives under high salt diet. J Cardiovasc Pharmacol 42:98–104, 2003.

163. Lapinski M, Lewandowski J, Januszewicz A, et al: Hormonal profile of dipper and non-dipper patients with essential hypertension. J Hypertens Suppl 11(Suppl 5):S294–S295, 1993.

164. Benetos A, Gardner JP, Zureik M, et al: Short telomeres are associated with increased carotid atherosclerosis in hypertensive subjects. Hypertension 43:182–185, 2004.

165. Aviv A: Chronology versus biology: Telomeres, essential hypertension, and vascular aging. Hypertension 40:229–232, 2002.

166. Serrano AL, Andres V: Telomeres and cardiovascular disease: Does size matter? Circ Res 94:575–584, 2004.

167. Glazier AM, Nadeau JH, Aitman TJ: Finding genes that underlie complex traits. Science 298:2345–2349, 2002.

168. Ranade K, Hinds D, Hsiung CA, et al: A genome scan for hypertension susceptibility loci in populations of Chinese and Japanese origins. Am J Hypertens 16:158–162, 2003.

169. Garcia EA, Newhouse S, Caulfield MJ, Munroe PB: Genes and hypertension. Curr Pharm Des 9:1679–1689, 2003.

170. Sharma P, Fatibene J, Ferraro F, et al: A genome-wide search for susceptibility loci to human essential hypertension. Hypertension 35:1291–1296, 2000.

171. von Wowern F, Bengtsson K, Lindgren CM, et al: A genome wide scan for early onset primary hypertension in Scandinavians. Hum Mol Genet 12:2077–2081, 2003.

172. Pharoah PD, Dunning AM, Ponder BA, Easton DF: Association studies for finding cancer-susceptibility genetic variants. Nat Rev Cancer 4:850–860, 2004.

173. Nagelkerke NJ, Hoebee B, Teunis P, Kimman TG: Combining the transmission disequilibrium test and case-control methodology using generalized logistic regression. Eur J Hum Genet 12:964–970, 2004.

174. Cardon LR, Palmer LJ: Population stratification and spurious allelic association. Lancet 361:598–604, 2003.

175. Ritchie MD, Hahn LW, Roodi N, et al: Multifactor-dimensionality reduction reveals high-order interactions among estrogen-metabolism genes in sporadic breast cancer. Am J Hum Genet 69:138–147, 2001.

176. Hahn LW, Ritchie MD, Moore JH: Multifactor dimensionality reduction software for detecting gene-gene and gene-environment interactions. Bioinformatics 19:376–382, 2003.

176a. Lou XY, Chen GB, Yan L, et al: A generalized combinatorial approach for detecting gene-by-gene and gene-by-environment interactions with application to nicotine dependence. Am J Hum Genet 80:1125–1137, 2007.

177. Felder RA, Sanada H, Xu J, et al: G protein–coupled receptor kinase 4 gene variants in human essential hypertension. Proc Natl Acad Sci U S A 99:3872–3877, 2002.

178. Zeng C, Sanada H, Watanabe H, et al: Functional genomics of the dopaminergic system in hypertension. Physiol Genomics 19:233–246, 2004.

179. O'Connell DP, Ragsdale NV, Boyd DG, et al: Differential human renal tubular responses to dopamine type 1 receptor stimulation are determined by blood pressure status. Hypertension 29:115–122, 1997.

180. Williams SM, Ritchie MD, Phillips JA, et al: Identification of multilocus genotypes that associate with high-risk and low-risk for hypertension. Hum Hered 57:28–38, 2004.

181. Williams SM, Addy JA, Phillips JA, et al: Combinations of variations in multiple genes are associated with hypertension. Hypertension 36:2–6, 2000.

182. Bengra C, Mifflin TE, Khripin Y, et al: Genotyping essential hypertension SNPs using a homogenous PCR method with universal energy transfer primers. Clin Chem 48:2131–2140, 2002.

183. Bianchi G, Tripodi G: Genetics of hypertension: The adducin paradigm. Ann NY Acad Sci 986:660–668, 2003.

184. Manunta P, Burnier M, D'Amico M, et al: Adducin polymorphism affects renal proximal tubule reabsorption in hypertension. Hypertension 33:694–697, 1999.

185. Beeks E, Kessels AG, Kroon AA, et al: Genetic predisposition to salt-sensitivity: A systematic review. J Hypertens 22:1243–1249, 2004.

186. Casari G, Barlassina C, Cusi D, et al: Association of the α-adducin locus with essential hypertension. Hypertension 25:320–326, 1995.

187. Allayee H, Dominguez KM, Aouizerat BE, et al: Genome scan for blood pressure in Dutch dyslipidemic families reveals linkage to a locus on chromosome 4p. Hypertension 38:773–778, 2001.

188. Pedrosa R, Jose PA, Soares-Da Silva P: Defective D1-like receptor-mediated inhibition of Cl⁻/HCO₃⁻ exchanger in immortalized SHR proximal tubular epithelial cells. Am J Physiol Renal Physiol 86:F1120–F1126, 2004.

188a. Blaustein MP, Zhang J, Chen L, Hamilton BP: How does salt retention raise blood pressure? Am J Physiol Regul Integr Comp Physiol 290: R514–523, 2006.

189. Zeng C, Wang D, Yang Z, et al: Dopamine D1 receptor augmentation of D3 receptor action in rat aortic or mesenteric vascular smooth muscles. Hypertension 43:673–679, 2004.

190. Lund-Johansen P, Omvik P: Hemodynamic patterns of untreated hypertensive disease. In Laragh JH, Brenner BM (eds): Hypertension: Pathophysiology, Diagnosis, and Management, 2nd ed. New York, Raven Press, 1995, pp 323–342.

191. Burnier M, Biollaz J, Magnin JL, et al: Renal sodium handling in patients with untreated hypertension and white coat hypertension. Hypertension 23:496–502, 1994.

192. Ducher M, Bertram D, Pozet N, et al: Stress-induced renal alterations in normotensives offspring of hypertensives and in hypertensives. Am J Hypertens 5:346–350, 2002.

193. Weder AB: Red-cell lithium-sodium countertransport and renal lithium clearance in hypertension. N Engl J Med 314:198–201, 1986.

194. Siani A, Russo P, Paolo Cappuccio F, et al: Combination of renin-angiotensin system polymorphisms is associated with altered renal sodium handling and hypertension. Hypertension 43:598–602, 2004.

195. Barlassina C, Schork NJ, Manunta P, et al: Synergistic effect of α-adducin and ACE genes causes blood pressure changes with body sodium and volume expansion. Kidney Int 57:1083–1090, 2000.

196. Sanada H, Yatabe J, Midorikawa S, et al: Single-nucleotide polymorphisms for diagnosis of salt-sensitive hypertension. Clin Chem 52:352–360, 2006.

197. Bianchi G, Tripodi G, Casari G, et al: Two point mutations within the adducin genes are involved in blood pressure variation. Proc Natl Acad Sci U S A 91:3999–4003, 1994.

198. Efendiev R, Krmar RT, Ogimoto G, et al: Hypertension-linked mutation in the adducin α-subunit leads to higher AP2-μ 2 phosphorylation and impaired Na^+,K^+-ATPase trafficking in response to GPCR signals and intracellular sodium. Circ Res 95:1100–1108, 2004.

199. Marro ML, Scremin OU, Jordan MC, et al: Hypertension in β-adducin–deficient mice. Hypertension 36:449–453, 2000.

200. Sanada H, Yatabe J, Midorikawa S, et al: Amelioration of genetic hypertension by suppression of renal G protein-coupled receptor kinase type 4 expression. Hypertension 47: 1131–1139, 2006.

SECTION 4

Acquired and Polygenic Renal Disease

Chapter 21

Molecular Mechanisms of Proteinuria

J. Ashley Jefferson and Stuart J Shankland

Proteinuria is one of the signature markers of kidney disease and a key determinant of progressive renal injury. The degree of proteinuria is the best predictor of end-stage renal disease in both diabetic[1] and nondiabetic glomerular disease.[2]

In this chapter we will review the physiologic processes limiting urine protein excretion and describe some of the cellular and molecular abnormalities that occur in proteinuric states.

NORMAL URINE PROTEIN EXCRETION

Although around 20% (180 L) of renal plasma flow is filtered at the glomerulus each day, only small amounts of protein are found in the urine (40–80 mg/day). The upper limit for normal is usually considered 150 mg/day, although children and adolescents may have slightly higher values (<250 mg/day). Of note, transient increases in protein excretion may occur with fever, marked exercise, or exacerbations of congestive heart failure or hypertension.

The composition of urine protein is mostly albumin (30%–40%) and Tamm Horsfall protein (50%) with smaller contributions from immunoglobulins (5%–10%) and light chains (5%). It is generally accepted that any protein that is filtered at the glomerulus is taken up and degraded in proximal tubular cells. However, recent evidence has suggested that there may be large amounts of peptide fragments present in human urine (2–3 g/day) that are not detected by standard protein assays.[3,4]

RENAL HANDLING OF ALBUMIN

Glomerular Filtration of Albumin

Albumin accounts for approximately 60% of all plasma proteins, and it is generally considered that only small amounts of albumin are filtered at the glomerulus.[5] Early electron microscopy studies suggested that albumin (molecular weight [MW] 69 kD) was mostly excluded from the glomerular capillary wall.[6] Although micropuncture studies are technically challenging, estimates of albumin concentration in glomerular filtrate are generally low (~22–32 mg/L), in keeping with a daily filtered albumin load of 4 to 5 g per day.[7–9]

An alternative view has suggested that large amounts of albumin may be filtered at the glomerulus each day with a glomerular sieving coefficient of approximately 7.5%.[10] Russo and colleagues estimate a daily filtered load of albumin of approximately 400 g per day and a high-efficiency albumin retrieval system returning tubular albumin to the renal vein. Criticism of this hypothesis has included (1) sheer amount, (2) studies employing toxins to impair tubular uptake may also cause glomerular injury, (3) cooling (8°C) to inhibit tubular protein reabsorption does not markedly increase urine protein excretion,[11] and (4) slit-diaphragm abnormalities lead to massive proteinuria.

Tubular Reabsorption of Albumin

Albumin that is filtered by the glomerulus is reabsorbed throughout the proximal tubule (predominantly S1 and S2 segments)[7] (Fig. 21-1). Albumin is not cleaved in the tubular lumen, but binds to a megalin-cubulin receptor complex in clathrin-coated pits and undergoes receptor-mediated endocytosis.[12] Inhibitors of 3-hydroxy-3 methylglutaryl-CoA reductase (statins) have recently been shown to inhibit this endocytosis.[13] Endocytic vesicles detach from the apical membrane and deliver the albumin-megalin-cubulin complex to a sorting endosomal compartment, where the albumin dissociates (due to the low pH) and megalin/cubulin are recycled to plasma membrane. Albumin subsequently reaches the lyzosomal compartment, where it is cleaved and the amino acids reabsorbed.

Interruption of this retrieval mechanism by antimegalin antibodies,[14] in megalin-knockout mice,[15] or in cubulin-deficient dogs[16] results in tubular proteinuria. Of note, cubulin is the intestinal vitamin B_{12} receptor, and humans with cubulin deficiency (Imerslund-Grasbeck disease) have hereditary megaloblastic anemia associated with tubular proteinuria.[17]

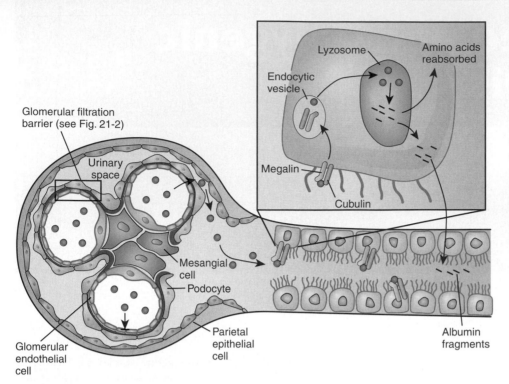

Figure 21-1 Renal handling of albumin. Small amounts of albumin are normally filtered at the glomerulus (4–5 g/day) and are reabsorbed in the proximal tubule by megalin-cubulin receptor-mediated endocytosis. Albumin is digested in lyzosomes, with amino acids being reabsorbed across the basolateral membrane. Small amounts of digested albumin fragments may return to the tubular lumen and be excreted in urine (depicted as black lines).

CLASSIFICATION OF PROTEINURIA

Proteinuria may be classified according to pathophysiologic mechanisms. The identification of the degree and type of proteinuria is vital in determining the underlying etiology. Thus, proteinuria is classified as follows:

1. *Glomerular proteinuria*—This typically causes the greatest degree of proteinuria, and when greater than 3.5 g/day is termed nephrotic range proteinuria. This consists mostly of albumin (70%) and other high-molecular-weight proteins (transferrin, immunoglobulin G) (30%).
2. *Tubular proteinuria*—This is usually more modest (<2 g/day) and consists of low-molecular-weight (LMW) proteins (α_1-microglobulin, retinol binding protein) with albumin accounting for smaller amounts (<30%). Importantly, there is some evidence that this LMW proteinuria may correlate better with degree of interstitial damage than urine total protein (see review[18]).
3. *Overflow proteinuria*—Increased filtration of LMW proteins may overload tubular reabsorptive mechanisms. Examples include light chains in multiple myeloma, myoglobinuria, hemoglobinuria, or lysozymuria in leukemia.
4. *Urinary tract proteinuria* (<500 mg)—This may occur with infections or neoplastic lesions in the urinary tract and resembles glomerular proteinuria but may be identified by the additional presence of α_2-macroglobulin.

Selective Proteinuria

This occurs when permeability to albumin is increased, but without a marked increase in the filtration of other higher-molecular-weight proteins (immunoglobulins, α_2-macroglobulin). This typically occurs in minimal change disease, and has been used to differentiate minimal change disease from focal segmental glomerulosclerosis (FSGS).

However, selective proteinuria may also be found at early stages of FSGS, membranous nephropathy (MN), and diabetic nephropathy (DN). Most believe that selective proteinuria is secondary to deficits in the glomerular charge barrier.

CLINICAL SIGNIFICANCE OF PROTEINURIA

Proteinuria is the best predictor of end-stage renal disease in both diabetic[1,19] and nondiabetic glomerular disease.[20,21] It has also been shown that therapies that reduce proteinuria slow the progression of diabetic[22-24] and nondiabetic glomerular disease.[2,25] It should also be recognized that proteinuria is a strong risk factor for cardiovascular disease.[26,27]

Proteinuria is clearly a predictor of renal progression, but is it only a marker of disease severity or is proteinuria harmful per se? The progression of renal disease correlates better with the degree of tubulo-interstitial injury than glomerular injury, and there is now convincing evidence that proteinuria may have pro-inflammatory, profibrogenic, and direct toxic effects on renal tubular cells (see review[28]).

Large amounts of filtered proteins may be taken up by proximal tubular cells and activate inflammatory pathways via nuclear factor-κB (NF-κB)[29,30] or complement-mediated pathways.[31] The lack of disease amelioration in Nagase analbuminemic rats with puromycin aminonucleoside nephritis or anti–glomerular basement membrane models of injury suggests that filtered albumin may not be the most critical portion of filtered protein.[32] Other pathogenic factors in proteinuric conditions may include the filtration of transferrin and iron-mediated oxidant injury,[33] filtration of toxic fatty acids bound to albumin,[34] filtration of cytokines and growth factors, luminal protein cast obstruction,[35] and increased proximal tubular cell apoptosis.[36]

Proximal tubular cells that are injured by filtered proteins may release chemokines such as RANTES and monocyte chemoattractant protein-1 (MCP-1), leading to influx of interstitial macrophages contributing to interstitial fibrosis.[37] Inhibition of chemokine receptors,[38] irradiation,[39] or immunosuppression with mycophenolate mofetil[40] have been shown to improve renal function in predominantly nonimmune forms of proteinuric renal disease.

GLOMERULAR FILTRATION BARRIER

The glomerular capillary wall is composed of three layers: a glomerular basement membrane (GBM), which is lined on the blood side by the fenestrated glomerular endothelium and on the urinary space side by a specialized epithelial cell, the podocyte (Table 21-1 and Fig. 21-2). These three layers compose the glomerular filtration barrier, but the relative contribution of each of the layers to the filtration barrier remains debated. The focus has recently moved to the podocyte slit-diaphragm as being predominant, but each layer may provide significant contributions as discussed below.

Functional Studies

Ultrafiltration occurs across the glomerulus at a high rate (~180 L/day) with a relatively low ultrafiltration pressure (estimated at <20 mmHg). Despite these large volumes of filtrate, the kidney is very efficient at ensuring that minimal protein is lost in the urine. Functional studies have used the concept of a glomerular sieving coefficient (GSC) to define the characteristics of the filtration barrier (see review[41]). The GSC is the ratio of the concentration of a substance in Bowman's space to its plasma concentration, and can be assessed measuring the fractional clearance of nonprotein polymers (dextrans, Ficoll, polyvinylpyrrolidone), which are neither secreted nor reabsorbed in the tubule. It should be recognized that estimating the GSC from urine collections may be challenging and that direct measurement by micropuncture techniques is also very difficult.

On the basis of early classical studies by Brenner and others, studying dextran sieving, a size, charge, and conformational barrier was postulated.[42–44] Technical concerns regarding the use of dextrans have led to some aspects of this model being questioned.[45]

Table 21-1 Disorders of the Glomerular Filtration Barrier

	Inherited Diseases	Acquired Diseases
Endothelial cell	Familial hemolytic-uremic syndrome (factor H)	Thrombotic microangiopathy Small vessel vasculitis Postinfectious glomerulonephritis Lupus nephritis
Glomerular basement membrane	Alport syndrome (type IV collagen) Thin basement membrane disease (type IV collagen) Nail patella syndrome (LMx1b)	Anti-GBM disease
Podocyte	Congenital nephrotic syndrome of the Finnish type (nephrin) Focal segmental glomerulosclerosis (podocin, CD2-AP, α-actinin-4)	Minimal change disease Focal segmental glomerulosclerosis Membranous nephropathy Diabetic nephropathy

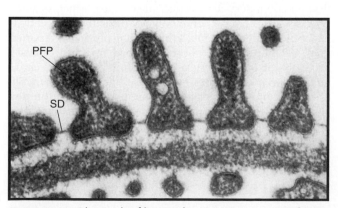

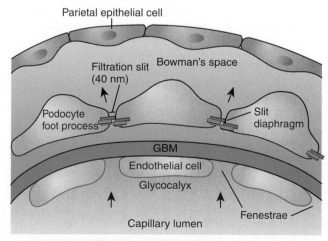

Figure 21-2 Glomerular filtration barrier: transmission electron micrograph (A) and illustration (B). The filtration barrier comprises the glomerular endothelial cell with fenestrations and an overlying negatively charged glycocalyx, glomerular basement membrane (GBM), and podocyte. The specialized cell junction between podocytes, the slit-diaphragm (SD), serves as the major size barrier to protein.

Size Barrier

There is little debate about the role of molecular size on glomerular permeability. Early sieving studies using charged and uncharged dextrans showed that as molecular size increases, barrier permeability decreases.[43] LMW proteins (MW <40 kD, radius <30 Å) are essentially freely filtered[7] (see review[18]), whereas high-molecular-weight proteins (MW >100 kD, radius >55 Å) are almost completely restricted.[18,46]

In microalbuminuria, no change in size selectivity (radius of pores, spread distribution of small pores, or magnitude of large pores) has been reported.[47,48] Early changes in diabetic nephropathy, by dextran sieving, show a small increase in large pores, but a marked increase in albumin passage through small selective pores.[47–49] An increase in large pores becomes more evident at higher degrees of proteinuria (3 g/g creatinine).[48]

Charge Barrier

The significance of a glomerular charge barrier is debated. It was first proposed on the basis of tracer studies showing that anionic ferritin was excluded from entering the GBM; however, cationic ferritin was able to reach the podocyte slit-diaphragm.[50] Additional studies comparing negatively charged dextrans (dextran sulfate) with either neutral dextran or positively charged dextrans showed increased permeability to cationic but restricted permeability to anionic dextrans.[42,43,51]

Technical issues with dextran sieving experiments include the binding of dextrans to plasma proteins,[51] the cellular uptake and intracellular desulfation of dextrans, and the binding of cationic dextrans to anionic sites on the capillary wall, damaging the filtration barrier.[45] This has led to the use of Ficolls, nonprotein polymers, for more recent glomerular sieving experiments. The results of these studies have been conflicting. Some have suggested a reduction in fractional clearances of anionic charged Ficolls compared with neutral,[11,52,53] but others have not noted a difference.[54,55] In nephrotic syndrome, some experiments have suggested a loss of charge barrier as the predominant functional abnormality accounting for the proteinuria.[46,51] Recently, clearance studies using albumin and uncharged Ficoll in the puromycin aminonucleoside model of nephrotic syndrome showed an increased clearance of Ficoll, and by estimating the ratio of albumin to Ficoll suggested only a small decrease in charge density.[56]

Steric Configuration

The use of uncharged polymers eliminates any charge barrier effect and has demonstrated that as molecular size increases the glomerular sieving coefficient decreases. In solution, dextrans uncoil, and this conformational change may reduce their effective molecular radius and overestimate the sieving coefficient. Recent data using Ficoll (which behaves as a nonconforming sphere) has demonstrated the importance of molecular shape on filtration.[46,57]

Hemodynamic Factors

Proteinuria may be increased by Starling type forces across the glomerulus due to increased renal plasma flow or increased glomerular capillary hydrostatic pressure (mediated by angiotensin II). This may account for the transient proteinuria associated with exercise, fever, uncontrolled hypertension, and congestive heart failure.

Theoretical Models of Pore Size

Using the sieving studies described above, several theoretical models of macromolecular transport across the glomerular filtration barrier have been proposed. A bimodal pore size model seems to most accurately fit the polymer sieving data.[46,58] According to this model, numerous restrictive pores exist (diameter 37–48 Å), as well as a small number of large pores (60–80 Å), which may act as a shunt pathway. Charge and size selectivity may be changed independently of each other, suggesting different sites or mechanisms. A gel membrane model has also recently been suggested.[9]

Structural Correlations

Studies have recently sought to explain these functional studies at a structural and molecular level. As described above, the glomerular filtration barrier consists of three elements in series within the glomerular capillary wall. Filtration initially occurs across the fenestrated glomerular endothelium, followed by the glomerular basement membrane and finally across the podocyte slit-diaphragms into the urinary space of Bowman's capsule (see Fig. 21-2). Early studies suggested that the GBM was the principal site of the filtration barrier, but more recently the critical role of the cellular elements has been recognized. We will discuss each of these in turn.

GLOMERULAR ENDOTHELIUM

The glomerular endothelium lines the capillary loops in the glomerulus and is in direct contact with the circulating blood. Unlike most other endothelial beds, the glomerular endothelium has characteristic fenestrations (60–100 nm in diameter), which facilitate ultrafiltration. Although caveolin-1 is expressed by the glomerular endothelial cell, these fenestrae are not dependent on caveolae for formation, as caveolin-1-deficient mice are able to form fenestrae.[59]

The glomerular endothelium is covered by a cell surface coat called the endothelial glycocalyx.[60] Due to standard tissue fixation techniques for electron microscopy, which degrade glycocalyx, this layer is commonly not recognized. Recently it has been reported to be much thicker than previously reported (300–400 nm).[61] It has been described in other capillary beds,[62] but in the glomerular endothelium it covers the entire luminal surface, including the fenestrae.[63] It consists primarily of sulfated proteoglycans and plasma proteins bound to the glycosaminoglycan side chains, which form an extracellular matrix. Glomerular endothelial cells express numerous proteoglycans, but only syndecan, perlecan, and versican are exported to the cell surface.[64]

Filtration Barrier

The heavily fenestrated endothelium has not previously been considered to have prominent restrictive properties.

Experiments using ferritin as a tracer molecule have suggested that the fenestrated endothelium is mostly porous to proteins that accumulate under the GBM.[65,66] However, if the glomerular endothelium does not play a prominent role in the filtration barrier, the issue of clogging of the filtration barrier and the question of how large amounts of albumin are returned to the circulation remain unanswered.

Recent data have suggested a more significant role for the endothelium and overlying endothelial glycocalyx (Fig. 21-3). In the puromycin aminonucleoside model of proteinuria, a decrease in both the number and size of endothelial fenestrations has been described.[67] Puromycin downregulates the expression of versican, which may inhibit the formation of the endothelial glycocalyx, and downregulates the transferases required for glycosaminoglycan (GAG) side chain biosynthesis, resulting in a decreased net negative charge.[64,68] Enzymatic cleavage of hyaluronic acid and chondroitin sulfate (hyaluronidase, heparanase) in mice decreases the negative charge barrier and increases the fractional clearance of albumin.[53] Importantly, electron microscopy shows no alteration in the glomerular cell structures or basement membrane, although an effect on the charge characteristics of these structures cannot be excluded.

Other supportive evidence for the endothelial glycocalyx as a site for the glomerular charge barrier includes the beneficial effect of serum orsomucoid[69]; alterations in glomerular charge density associated with changes in perfusate ionic strength[52,70]; and the presence of an exclusion zone for anionic molecules from the glomerular endothelium visible by electron microscopy.[71]

The exact role of the endothelial glycocalyx in the glomerular filtration barrier is still being determined. Endothelial fenestrae may permit high hydraulic permeability with the overlying glycocalyx, helping to restrict filtration of macromolecules[41,68] (see Fig. 21-3). Some of the conflicting views on the glomerular charge barrier may be partly due to the effects of different experimental protocols on the integrity of the endothelial cell glycocalyx.

Role of Vascular Endothelial Growth Factor in Proteinuria

Vascular endothelial growth factor (VEGF) is highly expressed in podocytes and acts as a growth and survival factor for vascular endothelium via VEGF receptors (VEGFR1 and VEGFR2). VEGF may also signal within the podocyte in an autocrine fashion (via VEGFR1).[72,73] VEGF exists as several splice variants, with $VEGF_{165}$ and $VEGF_{121}$ the main circulating forms in humans. VEGF is a critical growth factor during development, as deletion of even one allele results in embryonic lethality.[74] Selective $VEGF_{164}$/$VEGF_{188}$-knockout mice (i.e., only expressing $VEGF_{120}$) develop glomerulosclerosis with loss endothelial cells, but with normal podocytes.[75] Angiopoietin 1, another factor produced by the podocyte, acts on endothelial cells and may counterbalance the effects of VEGF.

VEGF may also play a role in maintaining glomerular endothelial fenestration. It induces fenestra in vitro[76,77] and has been linked to fusion of caveolin-1-containing vesicles.[78] However, this growth factor is not an absolute requirement, as fenestrations still develop in mice with inactivated VEGF.[79] This is reviewed in more detail in Chapter 25. Recent studies have shown that the inhibition of VEGF activity may lead to proteinuria. Anti-VEGF antibody or VEGF receptor antagonists used in cancer trials have been associated with proteinuria.[80,81] Soluble VEGFR1 (sFlt-1) receptor has been identified in patients with preeclampsia and proteinuria.[82]

Using recombinant technology with a Cre-loxP system, podocyte-specific, VEGF-deficient mice fail to form a glomerular barrier, resulting in embryonic lethality.[83] By contrast, loss of one VEGF-A allele leads to glomerular endothelial cell swelling (endotheliosis), nephrotic syndrome, and renal failure by 9 to 12 weeks.[83] The mechanism of proteinuria secondary to VEGF deficiency remains unclear. The absence of WT1, nephrin, and VEGF-A suggests a loss of podocytes in the majority of glomeruli at ESRD.[83] However, anti-VEGF antibodies or injection of soluble VEGF receptor

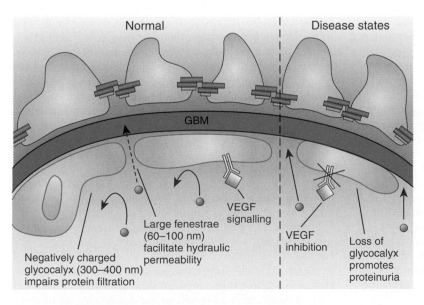

Figure 21-3 Glomerular endothelial cell and mechanisms of proteinuria. Normal glomerular endothelial cell integrity and function requires vascular endothelial growth factor (VEGF), which binds to its receptor. Under normal conditions, the anionic glycocalyx covering the endothelial cell prevents albumin from crossing the filtration barrier. In disease states, lack of VEGF and loss of glycocalyx promote proteinuria.

(sFlt-1) into rats or mice leads to proteinuria within a few hours of injection associated with endothelial cell hypertrophy and detachment, and downregulation of nephrin with the loss of occasional slit-diaphragms.[81]

It should be recognized that overexpression of VEGF may also produce proteinuria. Overexpression of VEGF-A in the podocyte may be injurious leading to a form of collapsing FSGS with proteinuria.[83]

GLOMERULAR BASEMENT MEMBRANE

Composition

The GBM is a 300- to 400-nm thick gel-like structure (90% water) that arises during development from the fusion of two distinct basement membranes (one derived from glomerular endothelium and one from the glomerular epithelium). It consists predominantly of type IV collagen, laminin-521 ($\alpha5\beta2\gamma1$), nidogen, and heparan sulfate proteoglycans.

Type IV collagen forms a highly cross-linked network, creating the basic structure of the GBM. Mammals express six different chains of type IV collagen ($\alpha1$–$\alpha6$ chains) encoded by separate genes, which associate into trimers, the predominant building blocks of the type IV collagen network. Embryonic kidney and young children have predominantly fetal type IV collagen consisting of $\alpha1$ and $\alpha2$ chains, which only later is replaced by adult type containing $\alpha3$, $\alpha4$, and $\alpha5$ chains. Persistence of the embryonic form of type IV collagen, due to mutations in the genes encoding $\alpha5$ (X-linked) or $\alpha3$ or $\alpha4$ (autosomal) chains, leads to hereditary nephritis (Alport syndrome) (see Chapter 10).

Laminins are extracellular matrix proteins, ubiquitous in basement membranes, which are formed by cruciform heterotrimers. Laminin $\alpha5\beta2\gamma1$ (LM-521) is the predominant laminin in the GBM, but analogous to type IV collagen, a fetal form, laminin $\alpha1\beta1\gamma1$ (LM-111), is initially laid down and replaced postnatally by laminin-11.[84] LM-521 interacts with other GBM components (nidogen, agrin, perlecan) and with cell surface receptors (integrins, α-dystroglycan). Mesangial cells maintain folded capillary loops by binding to LM-521 ($\alpha5$) via integrin $\alpha3\beta1$ and the Lutheran blood group glycoprotein.[85] Other functions include cell differentiation, adhesion, migration, and survival.

Heparan sulfate proteoglycan (HSPG) accounts for approximately 1% of the GBM dry weight.[86] Proteoglycans consist of a central core protein with GAG side chains. These GAG side chains contain multiple negative charges (sulfate and carboxyl groups). Agrin is the main HSPG core protein in the GBM (along with perlecan and collagen type XVIII, although these are more abundant in mesangial matrix).[87,88] HSPGs are synthesized both by podocytes[89] and endothelial cells.[68]

HSPGs have multiple roles within the GBM. They stabilize the GBM (by binding to laminin, type IV collagen, and nidogen); they act as adhesion contact points for podocytes and endothelial cells; and they can bind and sequester cytokines, anti-thrombin III, and growth factors (fibroblast growth factor-2 [FGF2], VEGF, FGF1), but critically, they are strongly negatively charged and may contribute to the charge-selective properties of the GBM.

Mechanisms of Proteinuria from GBM Injury

Early studies concluded that proteinuria was primarily due to a loss of charge and size selectivity of the GBM. This was based on early tracer studies showing that cationic ferritin readily passed through the glomerular endothelium, but became trapped by the GBM.[90,91] Electron microscopy using cationic probes demonstrated anionic sites on GBM, and anionic probes were mostly excluded by the GBM, implying that this was the site of glomerular charge selectivity.[50] The contribution of the GBM to the glomerular filtration barrier has recently been questioned.

Loss of Heparan Sulfate Proteoglycan Charge Barrier

HSPGs, with multiple sulfate and carboxyl groups on their glycosaminoglycan side chains, are strongly negatively charged. The loss of HSPG integrity may reduce the charge barrier imparted by the GBM and increase glomerular permselectivity (Fig. 21-4). Injury to HSPG may also impair podocyte and glomerular endothelial cell binding, and may release HSPG-bound growth factors (FGF, VEGF, heparin-binding epidermal growth factor–like growth factor).[92] Importantly, agents that injure HSPG in the GBM may also affect HSPG in the endothelial glycocalyx.

A reduction in GBM anionic sites or decreased heparan sulfate staining have been described in several animal models of glomerulonephritis.[93–98] It has also been described in human glomerular disease.[99,100] In some, the degree of heparan sulfate staining has been inversely correlated with albuminuria.[97,99–101] In diabetic nephropathy, functional studies have demonstrated an increase in pore size and decrease in charge barrier.[47,49,102] These functional changes have been correlated with a decrease in heparan sulfate staining, mostly without a reduction in HSPG core protein.[99,101] Both decreased synthesis of heparan sulfate (35S-sulfate incorporation)[103,104] and structural modification (undersulfation) have been described.[104]

Injury to the heparan sulfate components of the GBM may be caused by several mechanisms, including oxidative stress and enzymatic digestion (neutral serine proteases, heparanases). Reactive oxygen species (ROS) may be formed in the kidney from resident or infiltrating cells[105] and play a central pathogenic role in several models of proteinuria, including passive Heymann nephritis,[106] adriamycin nephropathy,[107,108] and puromycin aminonucleoside nephropathy.[109,110] Although ROS may directly cause podocyte injury, or can be derived from podocytes that are injured, there is also evidence that ROS may promote degradation of heparan sulfate. In vitro, heparan sulfate side chains of agrin may be depolymerized by ROS.[100] Peroxynitrite, derived from nitric oxide, can degrade hyaluronic acid and possibly other glycosaminoglycans.[111] In adriamycin nephropathy, albuminuria correlates with the decreased heparan sulfate staining, and both are ameliorated by the antioxidant dimethylthiourea.[100]

Enzymatic cleavage of HS side chains may also be an important factor in the development of proteinuria.[93,112] Neutral serine proteinases (elastase, cathepsin G) are released by activated polymorphonuclear cells. In vitro, cationic elastase binds to anionic heparan sulfate.[113] Renal infusion of these cationic enzymes results in the degradation of heparan

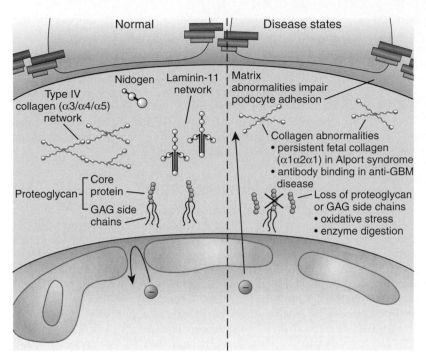

Figure 21-4 Glomerular basement membrane (GBM) and mechanisms of proteinuria. The normal GBM comprises several extracellular matrix proteins, including type IV collagen, nidogen, laminin-11, and heparan sulfate proteoglycans. In disease states, loss of heparan sulfate may diminish the net negative charge and impair the charge barrier to filtration. Other mechanisms of proteinuria due to GBM injury include structural abnormalities in type IV and impaired attachment of overlying podocytes.

sulfate and is associated with marked proteinuria, notably without foot process fusion seen on electron microscopy.[114] There was also no change in the other structural GBM components (type IV collagen, laminin, fibronectin).[115] In murine anti-GBM nephritis, proteinuria is ameliorated by elastase inhibitors[116] or abrogated in beige mice, which are deficient in elastase and cathepsin G.[117]

Heparanase, an endoglycosidase specific for heparan sulfate, is released from activated polymorphonuclear cells and platelets, and has been shown to degrade heparan sulfate in extracellular matrix.[118] Transgenic animals that overexpress heparanase develop spontaneous proteinuria associated with foot process effacement and renal impairment.[119] Heparanase expression in the podocyte (and glomerular endothelial cell) is upregulated in several models of proteinuria.[120,121] Blocking heparanase activity with an anti-heparanase antibody[121] or synthetic inhibitor PI-88[122] has been shown to ameliorate proteinuria in passive Heymann nephritis without changing the binding of antibody or C5b-9.

By contrast, although perlecan knockout mice die during embryonic development, mice with mutant perlecan leading to the loss of heparan sulfate side chains do not develop hematuria or proteinuria and do not have GBM structural abnormalities.[123] However, other proteoglycans such as agrin compensate for this loss. Agrin-deficient mice develop abnormalities at the neuromuscular junction, but GBM abnormalities have not been studied.[124]

Injury to GBM Structural Components

In the past few years, major insights into the significance of the GBM in the filtration barrier have been gained by studies of genetically engineered mice. Alport's syndrome is a hereditary nephritis due to mutations in genes encoding the α chains of type IV collagen, which result in abnormalities of GBM structure, proteinuria, and progressive renal impairment (see Chapter 10). *COL4A3*-knockout mice, an animal model of autosomal-recessive Alport syndrome, are unable to form the α3/α4/α5 protomers of type IV collagen and develop GBM abnormalities with alterations in GBM type IV collagen and laminin.[125] These mice do not develop immediate proteinuria; rather, this is delayed until the 5th postnatal week. It should be noted that during the first 4 weeks, the podocyte slit-diaphragms are ultrastructurally normal, with normal expression of podocyte and slit-diaphragm proteins. Associated with the onset of proteinuria, these mice develop morphologic abnormalities in the slit-diaphragm, foot process effacement, and altered nephrin expression,[126] implying that it is the slit-diaphragm proteins and not the GBM structural components that are the critical regulators of proteinuria. The mechanism of slit-diaphragm abnormalities in this condition is unclear but may relate to alterations in podocyte foot process attachment. The Alport GBM contains no LM-521, but retains the expression of fetal laminins (α2 and β1), which may provide abnormal signals or adhesion to podocyte foot processes.[127]

LMX1B-deficient mice, a model of nail-patella syndrome, develop similar GBM changes and die shortly after birth with massive proteinuria.[128] LMX1B is a transcription factor for the α3 and α4 chains of type IV collagen, explaining the GBM abnormalities. At birth these mice also have absent slit-diaphragms, with foot process effacement and decreased expression of nephrin, podocin, and CD2AP.[126] The promoter region of these genes also contains an Lmx1b binding site. Nidogen-deficient mice demonstrate only minor structural GBM abnormalities without proteinuria.[129,130]

By contrast, laminin β2 knockout mice, which have absent LM-521 and persistent fetal laminins (LM-111, LM-511), develop congenital nephrosis with profound neuromuscular disorders.[131] Remarkably, these mice develop severe proteinuria that precedes changes in the expression of slit-diaphragm proteins and prior to the development of foot process effacement.[115] This argues for a primary role for the GBM in the glomerular filtration barrier independent of podocyte abnormalities. LAMB2 mutations have been detected in human congenital nephrotic syndrome (Pierson syndrome).[132]

How Does the GBM Compare to the Cellular Elements as the Primary Filtration Barrier?

Studies looking at the isolated GBM (removing cellular components by digestion) have suggested that the charge barrier resides predominantly in cellular components of the filtration barrier. The isolated GBM shows size selectivity, but not charge selectivity in vitro[133]; however, preparation of the isolated GBM may alter its filtration properties. Glomerular sieving coefficients for albumin and large dextrans are much lower in the intact rat glomerulus in vivo than from the isolated GBM in vitro.[134] Treating the isolated GBM with heparatinase, adding protamine (to neutralize anionic polyanions), or reducing pH had little effect on sieving coefficient of albumin, whereas in the isolated intact glomerulus, albumin permselectivity increased, implying that the charge selectivity of glomerular barrier requires the presence of glomerular cells.[135]

As described above, inherited disorders of the GBM structural components such as Alport's syndrome are associated with proteinuria, but this is often relatively low grade (<3 g/day). By contrast, genetic disorders affecting the proteins of the podocyte slit-diaphragm such as congenital nephrotic syndrome of the Finnish type lead to massive proteinuria despite apparently normal GBM morphology.

GLOMERULAR VISCERAL EPITHELIAL CELL (PODOCYTE)

The podocyte is a highly specialized terminally differentiated cell lying on the outside (in the urinary space) of the

glomerular capillary, providing structural support to the capillary loop and forming the outermost layer of the glomerular filtration barrier. The podocyte consists of a primary cell body with secondary processes, which further branch to form interdigitating foot processes interacting with the glomerular basement membrane. Foot processes are connected by the slit-diaphragm, which may be the main size barrier to protein filtration. As will be discussed below, podocytes prevent proteinuria due to size (slit-diaphragm) and charge (podocalyxin) barriers.

Podocyte Slit-diaphragm

The slit-diaphragm is considered a type of gap junction. It is a thin membrane (40 nm) bridging the filtration pore close to the GBM[136,137] (Fig. 21-5). The structure was first described by transmission electron micrography as having a central pole with lateral rodlike structures producing a zipper-like appearance.[138] More recent imaging studies have supported and refined this configuration[139] (see Chapter 9).

Molecular studies have localized a number of specific proteins to the slit-diaphragm complex, including nephrin,[140] Neph1,[141] P-cadherin,[142] and FAT[143] (see review[144] and Fig. 21-5). Nephrin appears to be the major structural component of the slit-diaphragm. The extracellular domains of this transmembrane protein form dimers across the slit-diaphragm,[145,146] producing pores with a predicted diameter slightly smaller than the radius of albumin.[139] The slit-diaphragm also contains Neph1, a homolog of nephrin, and forms homo- and heterodimers with it.[146]

The slit-diaphragm proteins bind to the actin cytoskeleton of the podocyte via adaptor proteins (podocin, CD2AP, ZO-1, and catenins).[147] The intracellular domains of nephrin interact with CD2AP and podocin,[145,148,149] whereas Neph1 interacts with ZO-1 and podocin.[150]

It should also be recognized that the slit-diaphragm not only has structural functions, but more recently has been

Figure 21-5 Podocyte slit-diaphragm.

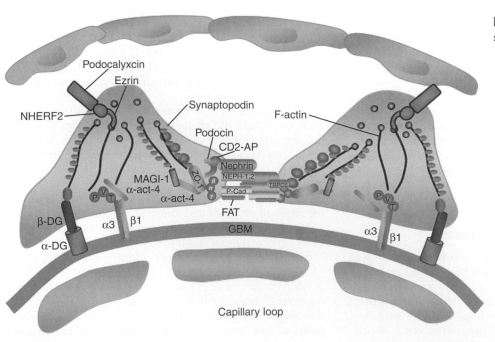

Capillary loop

recognized to perform signaling roles. The plasma membrane around the slit-diaphragm contains lipid raft microdomains,[151] and podocin and nephrin have been shown to localize here.[148,151] The slit-diaphragm complex, in association with TRPC6 (an epithelial calcium channel),[152,153] signals through a phosphoinositide 3-OH kinase–dependent AKT pathway to modulate cellular processes such as organization of the actin cytoskeleton, maintenance of cell polarity, and cell survival.[154]

MECHANISMS OF PROTEINURIA FOLLOWING PODOCYTE INJURY

Multiple factors may produce podocyte injury, including immune complexes, toxins, circulating factors, raised intraglomerular pressures, and mechanical stretch, hyperglycemia, and infections. The result of these insults often follows a common pathway leading to proteinuria and nephrotic syndrome. Over time, the inability of podocytes to proliferate and repair is pivotal in progressive glomerular scarring.[155] We will describe potential molecular mechanisms by which podocyte injury may lead to proteinuria (Fig. 21-6 and Table 21-2).

Loss of Podocyte Slit-diaphragm Integrity
Congenital and Hereditary Disorders

The slit-diaphragm is predicted to contain pores smaller than the radius of albumin (36 Å), inhibiting glomerular permeability to macromolecules.[139] Defects in slit-diaphragm proteins lead to massive proteinuria, suggesting that the slit-diaphragm is critical to maintaining the glomerular filtration barrier. Nephrin-deficient mice, a model of congenital

nephrotic syndrome of the Finnish type, display massive proteinuria at birth associated with the absence slit-diaphragms and foot process effacement. They have normal expression of GBM structural components, suggesting that the GBM is not the principal site of permselectivity.[126] Antibodies to nephrin lead to severe proteinuria within hours, with only focal foot process effacement.[156,157] Neph1 knockout mice also present with nephrotic syndrome at birth.[158]

The slit-diaphragm is anchored to the podocyte by adaptor proteins (CD2-AP, podocin, α-actinin-4). Recombinant mice deficient in CD2-AP,[159] podocin,[160] or α-actinin-4[161] all develop significant proteinuria, although typically less severe than in nephrin-deficient mice.

A number of inherited human proteinuric diseases have been described and attributed to defects in proteins of the slit-diaphragm complex, including congenital nephrotic syndrome of the Finnish type (nephrin,[162] WT1,[163] PLCe1[164]) and familial focal and segmental glomerulosclerosis (podocin,[165] TRPC6,[152,153] CD2-AP,[166] α-actinin-4[167]). These diseases are reviewed in Chapter 9.

Acquired Disorders

In acquired human proteinuric disease, a decreased density of slit-diaphragms has been described morphometrically in patients with nephrotic syndrome.[168] Studies have also sought to examine the expression of individual slit-diaphragm proteins in these conditions.[169,170] Abnormalities of nephrin expression have been described in minimal change disease,[171] diabetic nephropathy,[172] and membranous nephropathy.[173] Redistribution of nephrin and other slit-diaphragm components to intracellular locations has been described.[174–176] Interestingly, angiotensin II blockade prevents the decrease in nephrin in experimental glomerular disease.[177]

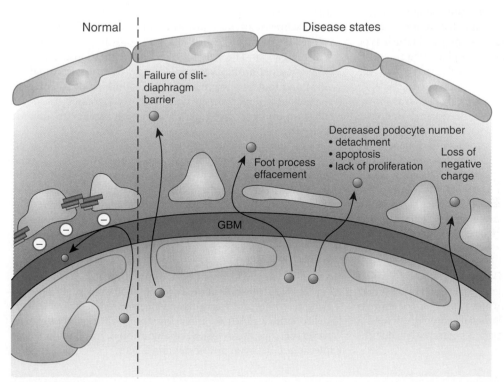

Figure 21-6 Podocyte injury and mechanisms of proteinuria. Injury to podocytes in disease states leads to proteinuria by several mechanisms, which are shown in this illustration.

Table 21-2 Mechanisms of Proteinuria Secondary to Podocyte Injury

Mechanism	Specific Podocyte Defect
Loss of slit-diaphragm integrity	Inherited (mutations in nephrin[162], podocin[165], CD2-AP[166], FAT-1, Neph-1) Acquired (altered expression or position of slit-diaphragm proteins[171–176])
Detachment of foot processes	Abnormalities in $\alpha3\beta1$ integrin[181,193–195] or α-β dystroglycan[183]
Reduced podocyte number[217]	Detachment Apoptosis Failure to proliferate
Podocyte effacement (?)	Changes in slit-diaphragm proteins[178] Abnormal podocyte-GBM interaction[131,181,182,184] Actin cytoskeleton reorganization (synaptopodin, α-actinin-4[167,180], CDK5[185]) Altered negative charge Disturbances in transcriptional regulation
Loss of podocyte negative charge	Decreased levels podocalyxin[228], GLEPP-1
Altered GBM permeability	Production of proteases or oxidants[106] leading to GBM injury or loss of heparan sulfate proteoglycan[231] GBM thickening due to matrix accumulation[232]
Altered glomerular endothelial cell function	Decreased VEGF production by podocyte[83]

GBM, glomerular basement membrane; GLEPP-1, glomerular epithelial protein-1; VEGF, vascular endothelial growth factor.

Foot Process Effacement

Effacement of podocyte foot processes is typically seen in proteinuric conditions, and, indeed, may be the only histologic abnormality (minimal change disease). Effacement is an active process resulting from retraction of the foot processes into the cell body, resulting in large areas of flattened epithelium covering the capillary loop. The exact molecular mechanisms resulting in effacement remain unclear. Podocytes have an abundant actin cytoskeleton, which is likely central to the abnormal shape changes that characterize effacement. Loss of slit-diaphragms may partly explain this abnormality,[178] although open slit pores with absent slit-diaphragms may be seen in congenital nephrotic syndrome of the Finnish type and minimal change disease without complete effacement.[179] Disruption of the podocyte actin cytoskeleton[167,180] or the podocyte-GBM interaction have also been proposed.[131,181–184] More recently, a role for cyclin-dependent kinase 5 was shown to be important in the maintenance of normal podocyte morphology.[185]

It is not clear, however, that foot process effacement alone can explain proteinuria, and indeed may be simply a consequence of podocyte injury. The podocyte flattening covers wide expanses of the GBM, and the total area for ultrafiltration is probably much decreased. Effacement may result in focal epithelial defects, allowing increased plasma flux across these denuded areas. There are also several experimental models where proteinuria occurs in the absence of foot process effacement, including anti-nephrin[156] or anti-neph1 antibodies[141]; aging male MWF rats[186]; and infusion of elastase[187] or H_2O_2[188] into rat renal arteries. Human data suggest a poor correlation between the degree of proteinuria and foot process effacement in glomerulonephritis,[189] and a familial form of nephrotic syndrome has been described without foot process effacement.[190]

Detachment of Foot Processes

Podocyte foot processes are connected to the GBM via several receptors, including $\alpha3\beta1$ integrin and α-β dystroglycan. $\alpha3\beta1$ binds to the type IV collagen $\alpha3$, $\alpha4$, and $\alpha5$ chains, as well as fibronectin, laminin-11, and nidogen, all constituents of the normal GBM.[191] However, the role of $\alpha3$ integrin in attachment has recently been questioned since, in vitro, $\alpha3$ knockout podocytes are less likely to detach.[192] By contrast, anti-$\beta1$ integrin antibody or blocking RGD peptides lead to foot process effacement, proteinuria, and podocyte detachment from the GBM.[193–195]

Detachment of foot processes may lead to focal gaps in epithelial covering of the capillary loop, leading to proteinuria (see review[184]). The $\alpha3$ integrin knockout mouse develops congenital nephrotic syndrome associated with an immature GBM and foot process fusion.[181] Cross-linking of $\beta1$ integrin receptors on podocytes in vitro leads to decreased podocyte adhesion and increased glomerular permeability to macromolecules.[196]

Detachment of foot processes from the GBM has been correlated with the onset of proteinuria in animal models,[197–199] and focal defects or tunnels have been described in human disease.[200,201] Live podocytes can also be recovered from the urine of patients with glomerular disease[202] and from animals with membranous[203] or diabetic nephropathy.[204]

By contrast, focal areas of detachment have been described in normal human kidneys.[201,205] In kidneys from patients with congenital nephrotic syndrome of the Finnish type and minimal change disease, denuded areas of GBM were rarely detected using scanning and transmission electron microscopy.[179] Also in proteinuric diseases, integrin expression is generally well preserved (despite cytoskeletal alterations), implying a stable interaction between podocytes and GBM.[206,207]

Decrease in Podocyte Number (Podocytopenia)

A decrease in podocyte number may result in denuded areas of GBM without epithelial covering. Experimental and human studies have shown a correlation between decreased podocyte number and the onset of proteinuria and glomerulosclerosis.[208–210] The mechanisms underlying podocytopenia include detachment (discussed above), apoptosis, and lack of proliferation.

Apoptosis

Increased apoptosis (programmed cell death) is a leading cause of reduced podocyte number. Apoptosis reflects a balance between signals/factors that favor survival versus death. Pro-apoptotic factors in the podocyte include transforming growth factor-β (TGF-β), angiotensin II, ROS, mechanical stretch, and detachment. TGF-β is increased in diabetic and nondiabetic proteinuric renal diseases, and podocyte apoptosis is increased in TGF-β transgenic mice, which correlates with glomerulosclerosis.[211] Angiotensin II can directly cause podocyte apoptosis, an effect mediated through the AT1 receptor.[212] Therapeutic angiotensin II blockade may therefore have additional glomeruloprotective effects independent of its hemodynamic actions.

Podocyte survival factors include nephrin, CD2-AP, VEGF collagen IV, and possibly insulin-like growth factor.[213] Thus, slit-diaphragm proteins not only provide a structural role, they also have a pro-survival function. Nephrin and CD2-AP facilitate the phosphorylation of Akt, a critical survival factor.[214] VEGF has been shown to protect podocytes from apoptosis induced by serum withdrawal by phosphorylating nephrin.[215] Dexamethasone protects podocytes from apoptosis by reducing levels of p53 and may partly explain why steroids can reduce proteinuria.[216]

Lack of Podocyte Proliferation

Podocytes are terminally differentiated cells and do not typically proliferate in response to injury. Indeed, the lack of adequate proliferation by these cells to replace those lost by detachment or apoptosis leads to reduced podocyte number. It should be noted that podocytes do proliferate in certain conditions, including human immunodeficiency virus (HIV)–associated nephropathy, cellular/collapsing FSGS, and crescentic glomerulonephritis. Altered levels of specific inhibitors of the cell cycle, called cyclin-dependent kinase inhibitors, have been shown to govern the inability of podocytes to proliferate. Levels of p21 and p27 increase in podocytes following experimental and human injury.[217] Proof of principle for their role derives from inducing experimental podocyte injury in p21- and p27-null mice, where the podocyte phenotype switches from a quiescent to a proliferative one that is associated with increased proteinuria.[218–220] More recent studies have shown that not only is DNA synthesis limited in podocytes due to increased cell cycle inhibitors, but there is also reduced mitosis, which may be due to the induction of DNA damage.[221]

Loss of Podocyte Charge

The podocyte slit-diaphragm and foot processes are covered with negatively charged glycocalyx consisting of sialoglycoproteins, including podocalyxin and podoendin.[222,223] Podocalyxin is synthesized by the podocyte and inserted into the apical membrane close to foot processes and filtration slits,[224] where it may act as an anti-adhesive molecule maintaining open filtration slits.[225,226] Podocalyxin-deficient mice have impaired glomerular development and fail to develop podocyte foot processes or slit-diaphragms.[227] Defective sialylation of podocalyxin has been described in the puromycin aminonucleoside model of nephrotic syndrome.[228] Thus, although the notion that podocalyxin and possibly podoendin reduce proteinuria based on negative charge, the verdict remains inconclusive.

Podocyte Endocytosis of Proteins

Could large amounts of protein pass through podocytes by active endocytosis? On electron microscopy, large amounts of pinocytic vesicles, phagosomes, and lyzosomes may be found in human proteinuric kidneys,[91,229,230] and defects in podocyte endocytosis have been proposed to cause glomerular injury.[166] Nevertheless, no difference in pinocytic invaginations in the cell membrane (apical or basal surfaces) was detected in minimal change disease between patients with proteinuria and those in remission.[179]

Podocyte Injury May Alter GBM Permeability or Glomerular Endothelial Cell Function

We should also recognize that podocyte injury may not only have local effects on the slit-diaphragm or podocyte structure, but may have secondary effects on the GBM or glomerular endothelial cell. The podocyte is partly responsible for the synthesis and turnover of the GBM, and podocyte-derived growth factors, particularly VEGF, are critical to the endothelial function. Despite this, the absence of obvious morphological features in the GBM and endothelial cell, and the very rapid onset of proteinuria following slit-diaphragm injury (e.g., anti-nephrin antibodies[156]) suggests that these factors may be less important.

CONCLUSION

The glomerular filtration barrier consists of the glomerular endothelial cell, the glomerular basement membrane, and the podocyte. Although there are data supporting a contribution from each of these layers to glomerular permselectivity, recent evidence suggests that the podocyte slit-diaphragm may be the major impediment to glomerular filtration of protein.

References

1. Keane WF, Brenner Bm, De Zeeuw D, et al: The risk of developing end-stage renal disease in patients with type 2 diabetes and nephropathy: The RENAAL study. Kidney Int 63:1499–1507, 2003.

2. Ruggenenti P, Perna A, Gherardi G, et al: Renal function and requirement for dialysis in chronic nephropathy patients on long-term ramipril: REIN follow-up trial. Gruppo Italiano di Studi Epidemiologici in Nefrologia (GISEN). Ramipril efficacy in nephropathy. Lancet 352:1252–1256, 1998.

3. Singh A, Gudehithlu KP, Le G, et al: Decreased urinary peptide excretion in patients with renal disease. Am J Kidney Dis 44:1031–1038, 2004.

4. Gudehithlu KP, Pegoraro AA, Dunea G, et al: Degradation of albumin by the renal proximal tubule cells and the subsequent fate of its fragments. Kidney Int 65:2113–2122, 2004.

5. Gekle M: Renal tubule albumin transport. Annu Rev Physiol 67:573–594, 2005.

6. Ryan GB, Hein SJ, Karnovsky MJ: Glomerular permeability to proteins. Effects of hemodynamic factors on the distribution of endogenous immunoglobulin G and exogenous catalase in the rat glomerulus. Lab Invest 34:415–427, 1976.

7. Tojo A, Endou H: Intrarenal handling of proteins in rats using fractional micropuncture technique. Am J Physiol 263:F601–F606, 1992.

8. Lund U, Rippe A, Venturoli D, et al: Glomerular filtration rate dependence of sieving of albumin and some neutral proteins in rat kidneys. Am J Physiol Renal Physiol 284:F1226–F1234, 2003.

9. Ohlson M, Sorensson J, Haraldsson B: A gel-membrane model of glomerular charge and size selectivity in series. Am J Physiol Renal Physiol 280:F396–F405, 2001.

10. Russo LM, Bakris GL, Comper WD: Renal handling of albumin: A critical review of basic concepts and perspective. Am J Kidney Dis 39:899–919, 2002.

11. Ohlson M, Sorensson J, Haraldsson B: Glomerular size and charge selectivity in the rat as revealed by FITC-ficoll and albumin. Am J Physiol Renal Physiol 279:F84–F91, 2000.

12. Christensen EI, Birn H: Megalin and cubilin: Synergistic endocytic receptors in renal proximal tubule. Am J Physiol Renal Physiol 280:F562–F573, 2001.

13. Sidaway JE, Davidson RG, Mctaggart F, et al: Inhibitors of 3-hydroxy-3-methylglutaryl-CoA reductase reduce receptor-mediated endocytosis in opossum kidney cells. J Am Soc Nephrol 15:2258–2265, 2004.

14. Zhai Xy, Nielsen R, Birn H, et al: Cubilin- and megalin-mediated uptake of albumin in cultured proximal tubule cells of opossum kidney. Kidney Int 58:1523–1533, 2000.

15. Christensen EI, Birn H: Megalin and cubilin: Multifunctional endocytic receptors. Nat Rev Mol Cell Biol 3:256–266, 2002.

16. Birn H, Fyfe JC, Jacobsen C, et al: Cubilin is an albumin binding protein important for renal tubular albumin reabsorption. J Clin Invest 105:1353–1361, 2000.

17. Aminoff M, Carter JE, Chadwick RB, et al: Mutations in CUBN, encoding the intrinsic factor-vitamin B12 receptor, cubilin, cause hereditary megaloblastic anaemia 1. Nat Genet 21:309–313, 1999.

18. D'amico G, Bazzi C: Pathophysiology of proteinuria. Kidney Int 63:809–825, 2003.

19. De Zeeuw D, Remuzzi G, Parving HH, et al: Proteinuria, a target for renoprotection in patients with type 2 diabetic nephropathy: Lessons from RENAAL. Kidney Int 65:2309–2320, 2004.

20. Hunsicker LG, Adler S, Caggiula A, et al: Predictors of the progression of renal disease in the Modification of Diet in Renal Disease Study. Kidney Int 51:1908–1919, 1997.

21. Ruggenenti P, Perna A, Remuzzi G: Retarding progression of chronic renal disease: The neglected issue of residual proteinuria. Kidney Int 63:2254–2261, 2003.

22. Lewis EJ, Hunsicker LG, Bain RP, Rohde RD: The effect of angiotensin-converting-enzyme inhibition on diabetic nephropathy. The Collaborative Study Group. N Engl J Med 329:1456–1462, 1993.

23. Brenner BM, Cooper ME, De Zeeuw D, et al: Effects of losartan on renal and cardiovascular outcomes in patients with type 2 diabetes and nephropathy. N Engl J Med 345:861–869, 2001.

24. Lewis EJ, Hunsicker LG, Clarke WR, et al: Renoprotective effect of the angiotensin-receptor antagonist irbesartan in patients with nephropathy due to type 2 diabetes. N Engl J Med 345:851–860, 2001.

25. Jafar TH, Stark PC, Schmid CH, et al: Proteinuria as a modifiable risk factor for the progression of non-diabetic renal disease. Kidney Int 60:1131–1140, 2001.

26. Yusuf S, Sleight P, Pogue J, et al: Effects of an angiotensin-converting-enzyme inhibitor, ramipril, on cardiovascular events in high-risk patients. The Heart Outcomes Prevention Evaluation Study Investigators. N Engl J Med 342:145–153, 2000.

27. De Zeeuw D, Remuzzi G, Parving HH, et al: Albuminuria, a therapeutic target for cardiovascular protection in type 2 diabetic patients with nephropathy. Circulation 110:921–927, 2004.

28. Zandi-Nejad K, Eddy AA, Glassock RJ, Brenner BM: Why is proteinuria an ominous biomarker of progressive kidney disease? Kidney Int Suppl 92:76–89, 2004.

29. Zoja C, Morigi M, Remuzzi G: Proteinuria and phenotypic change of proximal tubular cells. J Am Soc Nephrol 14(Suppl 1):36–41, 2003.

30. Hirschberg R, Wang S: Proteinuria and growth factors in the development of tubulointerstitial injury and scarring in kidney disease. Curr Opin Nephrol Hypertens 14:43–52, 2005.

31. Hsu SI, Couser WG: Chronic progression of tubulointerstitial damage in proteinuric renal disease is mediated by complement activation: A therapeutic role for complement inhibitors? J Am Soc Nephrol 14(Suppl):186–191, 2003.

32. Osicka TM, Strong KJ, Nikolic-Paterson DJ, et al: Renal processing of serum proteins in an albumin-deficient environment: An in vivo study of glomerulonephritis in the Nagase analbuminaemic rat. Nephrol Dial Transplant 19:320–328, 2004.

33. Harris DC, Tay YC, Chen J, et al: Mechanisms of iron-induced proximal tubule injury in rat remnant kidney. Am J Physiol 269:F218–F224, 1995.

34. Thomas ME, Harris KP, Walls J, et al: Fatty acids exacerbate tubulointerstitial injury in protein-overload proteinuria. Am J Physiol Renal Physiol 283:F640–F647, 2002.

35. Bertani T, Cutillo F, Zoja C, et al: Tubulo-interstitial lesions mediate renal damage in adriamycin glomerulopathy. Kidney Int 30:488–496, 1986.

36. Thomas ME, Brunskill NJ, Harris KP, et al: Proteinuria induces tubular cell turnover: A potential mechanism for tubular atrophy. Kidney Int 55:890–898, 1999.

37. Eddy A: Role of cellular infiltrates in response to proteinuria. Am J Kidney Dis 37(Suppl):25–29, 2001.

38. Anders HJ, Vielhauer V, Frink M, et al: A chemokine receptor CCR-1 antagonist reduces renal fibrosis after unilateral ureter ligation. J Clin Invest 109:251–259, 2002.

39. Diamond JR, Pesek-Diamond I: Sublethal X-irradiation during acute puromycin nephrosis prevents late renal injury: Role of macrophages. Am J Physiol 260:F779–F786, 1991.

40. Romero F, Rodriguez-Iturbe B, Parra G, et al: Mycophenolate mofetil prevents the progressive renal failure induced by 5/6 renal ablation in rats. Kidney Int 55:945–955, 1999.

41. Deen WM, Lazzara MJ, Myers BD: Structural determinants of glomerular permeability. Am J Physiol Renal Physiol 281:F579–F596, 2001.

42. Bohrer MP, Baylis C, Humes HD, et al: Permselectivity of the glomerular capillary wall. Facilitated filtration of circulating polycations. J Clin Invest 61:72–78, 1978.

43. Chang RL, Ueki IF, Troy JL, et al: Permselectivity of the glomerular capillary wall to macromolecules. II. Experimental

studies in rats using neutral dextran. Biophys J 15:887–906, 1975.

44. Deen WM, Bohrer MP, Robertson CR, Brenner BM: Determinants of the transglomerular passage of macromolecules. Fed Proc 36:2614–2618, 1977.

45. Comper WD, Glasgow EF: Charge selectivity in kidney ultrafiltration. Kidney Int 47:1242–1251, 1995.

46. Blouch K, Deen WM, Fauvel JP, et al: Molecular configuration and glomerular size selectivity in healthy and nephrotic humans. Am J Physiol 273:F430–F437, 1997.

47. Scandling JD, Myers BD: Glomerular size-selectivity and microalbuminuria in early diabetic glomerular disease. Kidney Int 41:840–846, 1992.

48. Lemley KV, Blouch K, Abdullah I, et al: Glomerular permselectivity at the onset of nephropathy in type 2 diabetes mellitus. J Am Soc Nephrol 11:2095–2105, 2000.

49. Deckert T, Kofoed-Enevoldsen A, Vidal P, et al: Size- and charge selectivity of glomerular filtration in type 1 (insulin-dependent) diabetic patients with and without albuminuria. Diabetologia 36:244–251, 1993.

50. Rennke HG, Cotran RS, Venkatachalam MA: Role of molecular charge in glomerular permeability. Tracer studies with cationized ferritins. J Cell Biol 67:638–646, 1975.

51. Guasch A, Deen WM, Myers BD: Charge selectivity of the glomerular filtration barrier in healthy and nephrotic humans. J Clin Invest 92:2274–2282, 1993.

52. Sorensson J, Ohlson M, Haraldsson B: A quantitative analysis of the glomerular charge barrier in the rat. Am J Physiol Renal Physiol 280:F646–F656, 2001.

53. Jeansson M, Haraldsson B: Glomerular size and charge selectivity in the mouse after exposure to glucosaminoglycan-degrading enzymes. J Am Soc Nephrol 14:1756–1765, 2003.

54. Guimaraes MA, Nikolovski J, Pratt LM, et al: Anomalous fractional clearance of negatively charged Ficoll relative to uncharged Ficoll. Am J Physiol Renal Physiol 285:F1118–F1124, 2003.

55. Schaeffer RC Jr, Gratrix ML, Mucha DR, Carbajal JM: The rat glomerular filtration barrier does not show negative charge selectivity. Microcirculation 9:329–342, 2002.

56. Hjalmarsson C, Ohlson M, Haraldsson B: Puromycin aminonucleoside damages the glomerular size barrier with minimal effects on charge density. Am J Physiol Renal Physiol 281:F503–F512, 2001.

57. Oliver JD 3rd, Anderson S, Troy JL, et al: Determination of glomerular size-selectivity in the normal rat with Ficoll. J Am Soc Nephrol 3:214–228, 1992

58. Myers BD, Guasch A: Mechanisms of proteinuria in nephrotic humans. Pediatr Nephrol 8:107–112, 1994.

59. Sorensson J, Fierlbeck W, Heider T, et al: Glomerular endothelial fenestrae in vivo are not formed from caveolae. J Am Soc Nephrol 13:2639–2647, 2002.

60. Avasthi PS, Koshy V: The anionic matrix at the rat glomerular endothelial surface. Anat Rec 220:258–266, 1988.

61. Rostgaard J, Qvortrup K: Electron microscopic demonstrations of filamentous molecular sieve plugs in capillary fenestrae. Microvasc Res 53:1–13, 1997.

62. Vink H, Duling BR: Identification of distinct luminal domains for macromolecules, erythrocytes, and leukocytes within mammalian capillaries. Circ Res 79:581–589, 1996.

63. Rostgaard J, Qvortrup K: Sieve plugs in fenestrae of glomerular capillaries—Site of the filtration barrier? Cells Tissues Organs 170:132–138, 2002.

64. Bjornson A, Moses J, Ingemansson A, et al: Primary human glomerular endothelial cells produce proteoglycans, and puromycin affects their posttranslational modification. Am J Physiol Renal Physiol 288:F748–F756, 2005.

65. Farquhar MG, Wissig SL, Palade GE: Glomerular permeability. I. Ferritin transfer across the normal glomerular capillary wall. J Exp Med 113:47–66, 1961.

66. Anderson WA: The use of exogenous myoglobin as an ultrastructural tracer. Reabsorption and translocation of protein by the renal tubule. J Histochem Cytochem 20:672–684, 1972.

67. Avasthi PS, Evan AP: Glomerular permeability in aminonucleoside-induced nephrosis in rats. A proposed role of endothelial cells. J Lab Clin Med 93:266–276, 1979.

68. Sorensson J, Bjornson A, Ohlson M, et al: Synthesis of sulfated proteoglycans by bovine glomerular endothelial cells in culture. Am J Physiol Renal Physiol 284:F373–F380, 2003.

69. Haraldsson BS, Johnsson EK, Rippe B: Glomerular permselectivity is dependent on adequate serum concentrations of orsomucoid. Kidney Int 41:310–316, 1992.

70. Sorensson J, Ohlson M, Lindstrom K, Haraldsson B: Glomerular charge selectivity for horseradish peroxidase and albumin at low and normal ionic strengths. Acta Physiol Scand 163:83–91, 1998.

71. Hjalmarsson C, Johansson BR, Haraldsson B: Electron microscopic evaluation of the endothelial surface layer of glomerular capillaries. Microvasc Res 67:9–17, 2004.

72. Chen S, Kasama Y, Lee JS, et al: Podocyte-derived vascular endothelial growth factor mediates the stimulation of alpha3(IV) collagen production by transforming growth factor-beta1 in mouse podocytes. Diabetes 53:2939–2949, 2004.

73. Foster RR, Hole R, Anderson K, et al: Functional evidence that vascular endothelial growth factor may act as an autocrine factor on human podocytes. Am J Physiol Renal Physiol 284:F1263–F1273, 2003.

74. Carmeliet P, Ferreira V, Breier G, et al: Abnormal blood vessel development and lethality in embryos lacking a single VEGF allele. Nature 380:435–439, 1996.

75. Mattot V, Moons L, Lupu F, et al: Loss of the VEGF(164) and VEGF(188) isoforms impairs postnatal glomerular angiogenesis and renal arteriogenesis in mice. J Am Soc Nephrol 13:1548–1560, 2002.

76. Roberts WG, Palade GE: Increased microvascular permeability and endothelial fenestration induced by vascular endothelial growth factor. J Cell Sci 108(Pt 6):2369–2379, 1995.

77. Esser S, Wolburg K, Wolburg H, et al: Vascular endothelial growth factor induces endothelial fenestrations in vitro. J Cell Biol 140:947–959, 1998.

78. Vasile E, Qu H, Dvorak HF, Dvorak AM: Caveolae and vesiculo-vacuolar organelles in bovine capillary endothelial cells cultured with VPF/VEGF on floating Matrigel-collagen gels. J Histochem Cytochem 47:159–167, 1999.

79. Gerber HP, Hillan KJ, Ryan AM, et al: VEGF is required for growth and survival in neonatal mice. Development 126:1149–1159, 1999.

80. Yang JC, Haworth L, Sherry RM, et al: A randomized trial of bevacizumab, an anti-vascular endothelial growth factor antibody, for metastatic renal cancer. N Engl J Med 349:427–434, 2003.

81. Sugimoto H, Hamano Y, Charytan D, et al: Neutralization of circulating vascular endothelial growth factor (VEGF) by anti-VEGF antibodies and soluble VEGF receptor 1 (sFlt-1) induces proteinuria. J Biol Chem 278:12605–12608, 2003.

82. Maynard SE, Min JY, Merchan J, et al: Excess placental soluble fms-like tyrosine kinase 1 (sFlt1) may contribute to endothelial dysfunction, hypertension, and proteinuria in preeclampsia. J Clin Invest 111:649–658, 2003.

83. Eremina V, Sood M, Haigh J, et al: Glomerular-specific alterations of VEGF-A expression lead to distinct congenital and acquired renal diseases. J Clin Invest 111:707–716, 2003.

84. Miner JH: Building the glomerulus: A matricentric view. J Am Soc Nephrol 16:857–861, 2005.

Chapter 22

Diabetic Nephropathy

Matthew Breyer and Raymond Harris

In the industrialized world, diabetes mellitus represents the leading cause of end-stage renal disease (ESRD). Both the incidence and prevalence of ESRD secondary to diabetes are on the rise. In the Unites States, over 30% of patients receiving either dialytic therapy or renal transplantation have ESRD as a result of diabetic nephropathy, and 40% of the new (incident) cases of ESRD are attributable to diabetes.

In the United States, Europe, and Japan, approximately 92% of diabetes represents type II rather than type I (insulinopenic). Correspondingly, over 80% of the ESRD secondary to diabetes is also seen in patients with type II diabetes. Although it was previously supposed that ESRD secondary to type II diabetes was less common than with type I diabetes, when cohorts of patients with type I and type II diabetes are followed for an extended period, the incidence of renal disease is similar. The demographics for ESRD due to type II diabetes mirror the prevalence of type II diabetes in the U.S. population, with a higher incidence in females and in African Americans, Hispanics, Native Americans, and Asian Americans, and with a peak incidence in the fifth to seventh decades of life.

PROPOSED MECHANISMS UNDERLYING DEVELOPMENT OF DIABETIC NEPHROPATHY

Hyperglycemia

Results from the Diabetes Control and Complications Trial (DCCT) and United Kingdom Prospective Diabetes Study (UKPDS) clinical trials in patients with type I and type II diabetes provide conclusive evidence that improved glucose control with lower hemoglobin A_{1C} (HbA_{1C}) is associated with reduced microvascular complications, including retinopathy, neuropathy, and the development of microalbuminuria.[1–5] Conversely, increased hyperglycemia results in several deleterious cellular events, including generation of reactive oxygen species (ROS), depletion of NAD(P)H, and production of advanced glycosylation end products.[6] These changes will be discussed in greater detail below. Nevertheless, it is humbling to acknowledge that while we can identify several pathogenic biochemical pathways, we still don't know which ones are most important and/or which of these disordered pathways distinguish the 40% of diabetics prone to developing nephropathy from the majority who fail to develop nephropathy despite comparable levels of glycemia.[7–9] The diversity of the biochemical pathways proposed to contribute to diabetic complications hints that diabetic nephropathy could be the result of lesions in any one of several distinct biochemical pathways, with some pathways being more important in one

individual than another, yet leading to a similar phenotype. Regardless of the importance of these unanswered questions, it is at least comforting to have firmly established the primacy of hyperglycemia as an initiating factor in the genesis of diabetic complications.

Hemodynamics

Patients with type I and, to a lesser extent, type II diabetes exhibit an increased glomerular filtration rate (GFR), the so-called "hyperfiltration" that has been suggested to be mediated by proportionately greater relaxation of the afferent arteriole than the efferent arteriole, leading to increased glomerular blood flow and elevated glomerular capillary pressure.[10] There is also glomerular hypertrophy, with increased glomerular capillary surface area. It has been suggested that these intraglomerular hemodynamic alterations may contribute to development and/or progression of diabetic renal injury. Since angiotensin-converting enzyme (ACE) inhibitors and decreased dietary protein reduce this increased intraglomerular capillary pressure in experimental animals, the hyperfiltration hypothesis provides one rationale for the success of these interventions in the progression of diabetic nephropathy.

Cellular Glucose Uptake

Increased cellular glucose has been implicated in the pathogenesis of diabetic nephropathy from studies of primary dysregulation of cellular glucose uptake[11,12] (Fig. 22-1). Primary increases in cellular glucose levels have been achieved in mesangial cells by overexpressing the facilitative glucose transporter 1 (GLUT1). This causes similar intracellular consequences as hyperglycemia, including increased aldose reductase, myo-inositol, lactate production, cell sorbitol content,[12] and increased net collagen accumulation.[13,14] Mesangial sclerosis is also observed in transgenic mice overexpressing GLUT1 driven by a modified human β-actin promoter, which is predominantly expressed in glomerular mesangial cells.[11] Another glucose transporter, the insulin-sensitive glucose transporter GLUT4, is most highly expressed in renal microvessels.[15] Dysregulation of glucose uptake in different tissues by these transporters is suggested by studies showing differential regulation of glucose uptake by vascular smooth muscle versus endothelial cells. Glucose transport activity in vascular smooth muscle cells is inversely and reversibly regulated by glucose, but glucose uptake in endothelial cells is not allosterically regulated by glucose levels.[16] The distinct regulation of glucose regulation in different tissues likely contributes to different susceptibility of nerve and endothelial cells to diabetic complications versus other tissues.

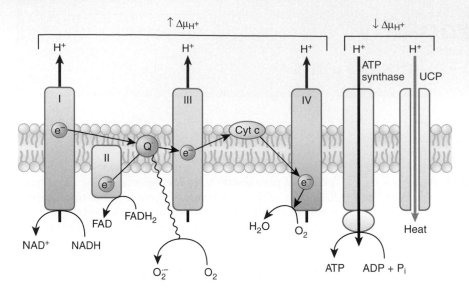

Figure 22-1 In response to hyperglycemia, the mitochondria is a major source of free radical production.

Generation of Reactive Oxygen Species from Intracellular Hyperglycemia

A major consequence of elevated cellular glucose is the inefficient utilization of this excess substrate, resulting in the formation of excess reactive free radicals. Hyperglycemia thus increases ROS production in cultured bovine aortic endothelial cells. A major mechanism by which intracellular hyperglycemia drives production of electron donors derives from their mitochondrial synthesis (see Fig. 22-1). This increase in reducing equivalents is a consequence of increased glucose flux through the tricarboxylic acid (TCA) cycle (NADH and $FADH_2$) generating a high mitochondrial membrane potential (μH^+), resulting from increased pumping of protons across the mitochondrial inner membrane. The high μH^+ impairs electron transport at complex III and increases the half-life of free-radical intermediates of coenzyme Q (ubiquinone), thus facilitating the reduction of O_2 to superoxide.[6,17] The possible contribution of increased oxidative stress to the complications of diabetes mellitus is supported by findings in diabetic humans of increased urinary isoprostanes, which are endogenous markers of oxidant formation.[18–21]

Other potential enzymatic sources of ROS include the arachidonic acid pathway enzymes lipoxygenase and cyclooxygenase, cytochrome p450s, xanthine oxidase, NADH/NADPH oxidases, NO synthase, peroxidases, and other hemoproteins.[22] The NADH/NADPH oxidases are a major contributor to renal vascular superoxide production in diabetes. This enzyme activity is mediated by the interaction of multiple protein subunits, including gp91phox/NOX, p22phox, rac, and p67phox[23] (Fig. 22-2). Together, gp91phox and p22phox form an integral membrane complex termed cytochrome b558, located in cytoplasmic vesicles and the plasma membrane. The catalytic subunit gp91phox binds three prosthetic groups, one FAD and two heme molecules.[24] Expression of these subunits is regulated by a variety of biologic factors, including growth factors and hormones.

NOX4 is one of several newly recognized gp91phox homologs.[25] NOX4 has been proposed to produce O_2^- preferentially using NADH, for its electron donor, as opposed to

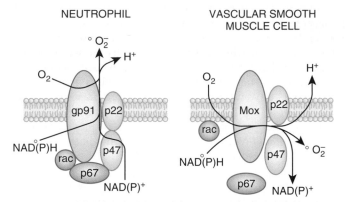

Figure 22-2 Subunit composition of the NADH/NADPH oxidases, a major contributor to renal vascular superoxide production in diabetes.

NADPH.[24] Aortas from old OLETF rats with hyperglycemia exhibit enhanced NADH oxidase activity in association with upregulated expression of p22phox and gp91phox.[26] Further studies of homogenates from endothelial and vascular smooth muscle cells indicate that the predominant substrate capable of driving O_2^- production is NADH and, to a lesser extent, NADPH,[23,27–29] so NOX4 may play a key role in this circumstance. Expression of the NAD(P)H oxidase subunits p22phox and NOX4 are increased in kidneys of diabetic rats, and immunostains show that expression of NOX4 and p22phox is increased in both distal tubular cells and glomeruli.[26] These findings are consistent with a contribution of increased renal NAD(P)H oxidase expression to the generation of ROS in the setting of diabetes.

Following their formation, ROS may be oxidized to inert species by diverse enzymatic systems, including catalase, glutathione peroxidase, Cu/Zn superoxide dismutase, and heme oxygenase-1 (HO-1), providing a defense system against oxidative injury. In diabetic glomeruli, heme oxygenase-1 is dramatically increased and could therefore play a major protective role.[30] Two weeks after the induction of diabetes in rats, expression of catalase, glutathione peroxidase, and Cu/Zn superoxide dismutase messenger RNAs (mRNAs) was not significantly different from that in control rats; however, it has been reported by others[30] that mRNA and protein expression of HO-1 was induced by 16-fold in glomeruli after the induction of,[31] and similar upregulation of, HO-1 in diabetic rat glomeruli.

Other antioxidant systems may also play roles in diabetes. In cultured mesangial cells exposed to high glucose, several thiol-reactive antioxidative genes (glutathione peroxidase 1, peroxiredoxin 6, and thioredoxin 2) were found to be increased by microarray and were confirmed to be upregulated by real-time polymerase chain reaction (PCR).[32] Impaired induction of catalase and glutathione peroxidase 1 has also been identified in fibroblasts harvested from patients with diabetic nephropathy.[33] In high-glucose conditions, Cu/Zn superoxide-dismutase mRNA and activity increased in fibroblasts from diabetics with or without nephropathy, while Mn superoxide dismutase did not change. In contrast, catalase mRNA and activity as well as glutathione-peroxidase mRNA and activity are increased in fibroblasts from type I diabetic patients without nephropathy, and in fibroblasts from nondiabetic nephropathic patients, but not in fibroblasts from type I diabetic patients with nephropathy,[33] implicating systemic impairment of these antioxidant pathways in patients with diabetic nephropathy.

Consequences of Increased Reactive Oxygen Species

Increased superoxide production can damage DNA, activate aldose reductase, induce diacylglycerol (DAG) production, activate protein kinase C (PKC), induce advanced glycation end product (AGE) formation, and activate the pleiotropic transcription factor nuclear factor-κB (NF-κB)[6,34] (Fig. 22-3). Increased ROS leads to single-strand DNA breaks,[35–37] providing an obligatory stimulus for the activation of the nuclear enzyme poly(ADP-ribose) polymerase (PARP). Poly(ADP-ribose) polymerase transfers ADP-ribose from NAD$^+$ to nuclear proteins through an energy-consuming process.[38,39] PARP activation in turn depletes the intracellular concentration of its substrate NAD$^+$, slowing the rate of glycolysis, electron transport, and adenosine triphosphate (ATP) formation, possibly as result of ADP-ribosylation of GAPDH.[40–42] The inhibition of GAPDH leads to increased glyceraldehyde-3 phosphate levels and its degradation products, yielding methylglyoxal-associated intracellular AGE production.[43,44]

PARP protein expression also appears to be involved in NF-κB-mediated activation of inflammatory gene transcription. Tissue obtained from PARP knockout mice does not exhibit NF-κB activation following endotoxin.[45] Other studies indicate that activation of NF-κB is dependent on the presence of PARP but is unaffected by inhibition of PARP activity,[46]

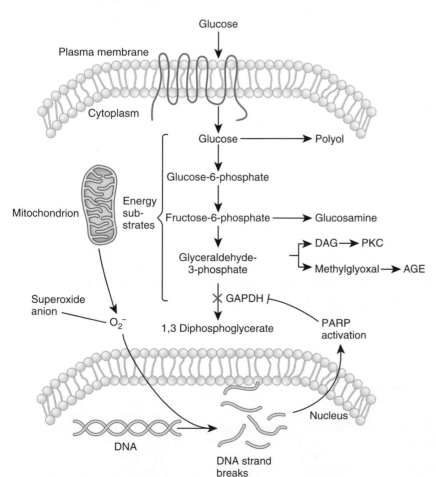

Figure 22-3 High glucose flux through constitutive glucose transporters present in endothelial cells overwhelms the mitochondrial electron transport system. Excess mitochondrial substrate flux results in the generation of reactive oxygen species that cause DNA strand breaks and activation of poly(ADP-ribose) polymerase (PARP). PARP ribosylates and inactivates GAPDH, thereby disrupting normal glucose metabolism. Inactivation of GAPDH effectively shunts glucose into the polyol pathway and leads to activation of protein kinase C (PKC) and accumulation of advanced glycosylation end products (AGEs) and glucosamine. DAG, diacylglycerol. (From Reusch, JEB: Diabetes, microvascular complications, and cardiovascular complications: What is it about glucose? J Clin Invest 112:986–988, 2003.)

suggesting that PARP protein but not its enzymatic activity is the relevant variable. PARP levels may also be upregulated in tissues during increased oxidative injury,[47] so it is conceivable that altered PARP expression might contribute to NF-κB activation in diabetic tissues.

ROS has been implicated in activating the mitogen-activated protein kinase (MAPK) signal transduction cascade.[48] Studies demonstrate that antioxidants, including *N*-acetyl-cysteine, vitamin E, and diphenyliodonium, blunt the activation of the MAPK pathway in cells chronically cultured in high glucose.[49–51] Similarly, studies show extracellular signal-regulated kinase 1 (ERK-1) and ERK-2 are activated by angiotensin and endothelin by a superoxide-dependent mechanism in vascular smooth muscle cells.[52,53] The molecular mechanisms whereby ROS activate these pathways remain uncertain.

Changes in the cellular redox state may also exert diverse effects on cell protein structure. A recent study shows that the cellular redox state can affect calcium flux via the type I inositol trisphosphate (IP3) receptor through its physical association with a thioredoxin protein (Erp44), and this association is dependent on the number of free cysteinyl sulfhydryl groups in IP3r1,[54] suggesting that reduction of protein S-S bonds plays an important role in intracellular calcium regulation. Whether this or some other mechanism plays a direct role in the activation of MAPKs by hyperglycemia remains undetermined.

Hexosamine Pathway

Under normal circumstances, 2% to 5% of glucose taken up into the cell is converted by the hexosamine pathway to UDP-GlcNAc.[55,56] Glutamine fructose-6-P amidotransferase (GFAT, also called transaminase or synthase) is the first and rate-limiting step in hexosamine biosynthesis, catalyzing an essentially irreversible reaction wherein L-glutamine donates an amino group to D-fructose-6-P, producing one molecule of glutamate and one molecule of aminated product, glucosamine-6-phosphate. Subsequent *N*-acetylation and reaction with UTP form UDP-*N*-acetylglucosamine (UDP-GlcNAc) (Fig. 22-4). The initial enzyme (glutamine fructose-6-P amidotransferase) is subject to feedback inhibition by the hexosamine UDP-*N*-acetylglucosamine and can be experimentally inhibited by glutamine analogs.

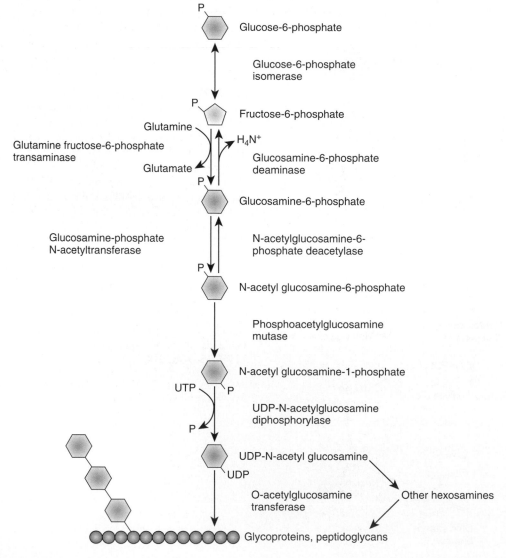

Figure 22-4 Hexosamine pathway. (From Bouché C, Serdy S, Kahn CR, Goldfine AB: The cellular fate of glucose and its relevance in type 2 diabetes. Endocr Rev 25:830, 2004.)

The final step in hexosamine biosynthesis is the formation of UDP-*N*-acetyl-glucosamine and other nucleotide hexosamines, which are major substrates for glycosylation of proteins. Many cytoplasmic and nuclear proteins are glycosylated on their serine and/or threonine residues by the addition of a single molecule of O-linked β-*N*-acetylglucosamine.[57,58] O-linked glycosylation can alter the activity and stability of several transcription factors, including Sp1, p53, and myc.[57,59] It has been suggested that these modifications may underlie gluco-toxicity,[43,60,61] glucose-induced changes in cell growth,[57] and glucose-induced insulin resistance.[55]

Alterations in the hexosamine pathway flux rate may induce defects involved in insulin secretion and action.[62] When rodents are infused with glucosamine, there is reduced glucose uptake as assessed by euglycemic-hyperinsulinemic clamping.[63] However, recent studies in patients with type II diabetes and Zucker diabetic fatty rats have not confirmed alteration in tissue UDP-GlcNAc levels,[64,65] so whether it is the flux through this pathway rather than the absolute levels of hexosamines that is relevant remains unclear. Glycosylation modifies activity of nuclear and cytoplasmic proteins,[61,66] including endothelial nitric oxide synthase,[60] and pathways involved in PKC and protein kinase A[67] or insulin signaling,[68] contributing to endothelial dysfunction.[43,60] In glomerular epithelial and mesangial cells from diabetic kidneys and in atherosclerotic plaques of diabetic patients, there is increased glycosylation and GFAT expression.[61,66] Activation of the hexosamine pathway may therefore contribute, in part, to the increased risk for vascular disease in diabetic patients.

Aldose Reductase

Increased intracellular glucose provides substrate for increased flux through the polyol pathway, metabolizing glucose to sorbitol via aldose reductase and then to fructose via sorbitol dehydrogenase (Fig. 22-5). The Km for glucose is relatively high and therefore dependent on intracellular glucose levels. Increased expression and activity of aldose reductase has been demonstrated in experimental diabetes and diabetic human tissues, including the diabetic kidney.[69] In the diabetic eye, increased sorbitol accumulation contributes to osmotic stress and cataract development[70]; however, osmotic stress does not appear to contribute to the development of neuropathy,[71] although an associated increase in oxidative stress may play a role.[72]

Conversion of glucose to sorbitol competes with GSSH for the availability of NADPH, blunting the formation of GSH

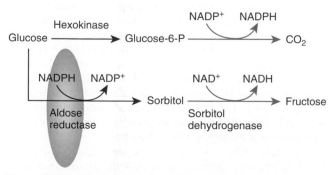

Figure 22-5 Aldose reductase and increased oxidant stress.

from GSSH and thereby the antioxidant capacity of the cell. Sorbitol is subsequently metabolized by sorbitol dehydrogenase to fructose accompanied by NAD^+ conversion to NADH. The consequent increased $NADH:NAD^+$ ratio resulting from the conversion of sorbitol to fructose can lead to de novo synthesis of PKC-activating DAGs[73,74] (see Protein Kinase C, following). Increased NADH also provides substrate for NADH oxidase (NOX),[75-77] enhancing ROS formation via NOX. Increased fructose also efficiently contributes to enhanced formation of AGEs,[78-81] which by activating RAGE (receptor for advanced glycosylation end products) increases ROS formation.[82,83] Through these multiple mechanisms, increased glucose flux via the polyol pathway contributes to increased oxidative injury in the diabetic milieu.

Advanced Glycosylation End Products

In the setting of diabetes mellitus and long-term hyper-glycemia, nonenzymatic modification of proteins (or lipids) by glucose, or its metabolic products, results in their stable modification and altered function. This process is thought to underlie a major pathogenic pathway leading to tissue injury in diabetes. A major pathway for AGE formation involves triose phosphate intermediaries derived from metabolism of glucose (Fig. 22-6). Triose phosphates build up as intracellular glucose increases and can nonenzymatically form the early glycosylation product methyglyoxal by spontaneous decomposition.[84,85] Amine-catalyzed sugar fragmentation reactions then modify protein lysine residues directly, forming *N*-(epsilon)-(carboxymethyl)lysine (CML), a major product of oxidative modification of glycated proteins.[85] Alternatively, reaction of terminal amino groups (e.g., on lysine) with glucose itself may form from early glycation products (i.e., Amadori products),[86,87] which rearrange to produce stable moieties that possess distinctive chemical cross-linking and biologic properties, designated AGEs.[88] Other glucose-derived Amadori products and fructose are thought to be potential precursors of 3-deoxyglucosone (3-DG) in vivo. Fructose generated by the aldose reductase pathway is converted into fructose-3-phosphate by the action of 3-phosphokinase (3-PK). This leads to the generation of 3-deoxyglucosone, a central precursor in the generation of an array of AGEs, in particular, CML-adducts and others.[89] 3-DG can further react with proteins to form pyrrolines or pentosidine.

AGEs have been suggested to represent a general marker of oxidative stress and long-term damage to proteins in aging, atherosclerosis, and diabetes.[84,85] Renal CML-AGE is increased in diabetes.[90,91] Immunolocalization of CML in skin, lung, heart, kidney, intestine, intervertebral discs, and particularly in arteries provide evidence for age-dependent increases in CML accumulation in distinct locations, and acceleration of this process in diabetes.[92] Immunostaining and immunoblots of diabetic human kidneys show increased CML in diabetic glomeruli, especially in the mesangial matrix and capillary walls.[1]

AGE Receptors

The consequences of increased tissue AGE expression includes activation of pro-inflammatory pathways, in large part due to receptor-mediated interaction of these products with specific cell surface receptors (Fig. 22-7). These receptors include

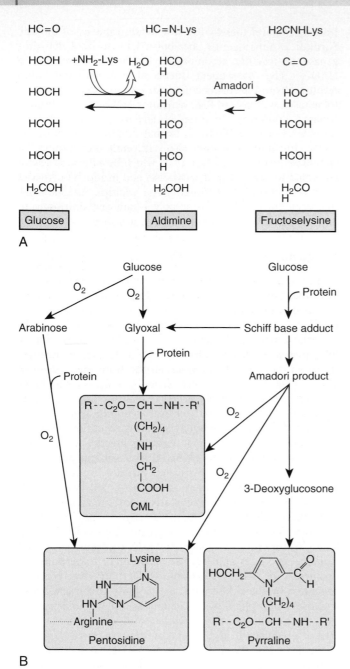

Figure 22-6 *A,* Amadori reaction. *B,* Maillard reaction pathway for formation of *N*-(epsilon)-(carboxymethyl)lysine (CML), pentosidine, and pyrroline. Fructoselysine is the Amadori compound, the first intermediate in the Maillard reaction occurring between glucose and protein. Pentosidine and CML are formed by sequential glycation and oxidation reactions. CML can form in two pathways: oxidative cleavage of fructoselysine, and reaction of protein with glyoxal, which is an autoxidation product of glucose or Schiff base adduct. Pentosidine is a cross-link between lysine and arginine residues resulting from glycoxidation of Amadori products or the reaction of arabinose, which is an autoxidative product of glucose. Pyrraline is formed by the reaction of protein with 3-deoxyglucosone. (*B* from Horie K, Miyata T, Maeda K, et al: Immunohistochemical colocalization of glycoxidation products and lipid peroxidation products in diabetic renal glomerular lesions. Implication for glycoxidative stress in the pathogenesis of diabetic nephropathy. J Clin Invest 100:2995–3004, 1997.)

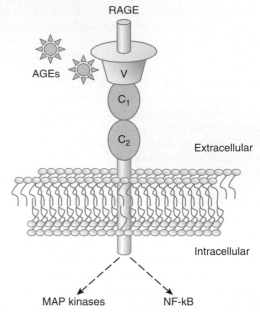

Figure 22-7 Advanced glycosylation end product (AGE) interaction with the receptor for AGE (RAGE) and subsequent activation of cell signaling.

CD36, macrophage scavenger receptor (MSR) type II, OST-48, 80K-H,[79,93,94] and a signal-transducing receptor designated RAGE.[91] RAGE activation appears to be a key to the development of diabetic complications, since blocking RAGE reduces diabetic atherosclerosis and nephropathy.[79,90,95] RAGE was first identified as a "receptor" for AGE using membranes from cultured mesangial cells and bovine lung extract and an iodine 125–radiolabeled probe of in vitro–prepared AGE albumin.[96,97] Molecular cloning analyses reveal that RAGE is a member of the immunoglobulin superfamily of cell surface molecules[98] and is composed of a large N-terminal extracellular portion of 332 amino acid residues consisting of a distal V-type immunoglobulin domain, followed by two C-type immunoglobulin domains (see Fig. 22-7). A series of studies of truncations of the extracellular region demonstrated that its ligands interacted with the V-domain of the receptor.[91,99,100] CML adducts as well as endogenous ligands including S100/calgranulin amyloid-β peptide and amphoterin proteins are major ligands for RAGE, binding the V domain.[101,102] Following ligation of the extracellular region, transmembrane signaling is thought to be transduced in part by a single hydrophobic transmembrane spanning domain followed by a short, highly charged cytosolic tail at the carboxyl-terminus. The intracellular portion of the molecule is essential for RAGE-triggered signaling and activates NF-κB-coupled signaling[101,102] as well as Cdc42-Rac-1-MAPK kinase 6-p38 MAPK pathways.[103,104] RAGE is upregulated in kidneys of diabetic animals, and nephropathy is ameliorated by blocking RAGE activation.[91] Binding of AGEs to RAGE activates cell-signaling mechanisms coupled to increased transforming growth factor-β (TGF-β) and vascular endothelial growth factor (VEGF) expression that are thought to contribute to the pathogenesis of diabetic complications.[90,91]

Conversely, other AGE receptors, designated AGE1 and AGE3 (galectin-3), appear to counteract the pro-inflammatory effects of RAGE and macrophage scavenger receptors.

Overexpression of AGE1 in mesangial cells markedly suppressed AGE-stimulated NF-κB activity and MAPK (p44/42) phosphorylation and activation.[105] Genetic disruption of galectin-3 exacerbates renal injury in diabetic mice.[106,107] These results support the possibility of utilizing selective AGE1 and AGE3 agonists to ameliorate diabetic complications.

Protein Kinase C

The PKC family is a group of structurally related serine and threonine kinases that are typically activated by certain lipids, particularly DAG, together with phosphatidylserine.[108] Activation of the cPKC subfamily (PKCα, β1, β2, and γ) also requires increased cell calcium, typically initiated by accompanying generation of IP3 as a result of phospholipase C (PLC)–mediated hydrolysis of phosphatidylinositol trisphosphate (PIP3) to IP3 and DAG.[109,110] The nPKCs (δ, ε, η, μ, αvδ, and θ) are also activated by DAG but do not require calcium as a co-factor.[111] Finally, atypical PKCs like PKCζ are activated by neither Ca^{2+} nor DAG, but by other atypical pathways. Agonist-induced production of DAG occurs through multiple mechanisms, including receptor tyrosine kinases and receptors linked to nonreceptor tyrosine kinases recruiting phosphatidylinositol-4,5-bisphosphate (PtdIns4,52)-specific PLC1/2 through their Src-homology-2 domains. Seven transmembrane receptors, such as AT1 and ET1 receptors, couple to the PIP3 active phospholipase Cβ family members through Gq-GTP and Gβ family member interactions.[108]

PKC isoforms exhibit differential tissue expression.[112,113] In the kidney there is segmental expression of several of the PKC isoforms along the nephron. Glomeruli predominantly express PKC-α, -βI (which, as discussed further below, has been particularly implicated in the pathogenesis of diabetic complications), and PKC-ε.[114] High glucose has been shown to activate several PKC isoforms in cultured mesangial cells, including PKC-α, -β, -δ, and -ε.[115,116] PKC-θ is primarily expressed in skeletal muscle, and its action has been implicated in the development of insulin resistance.[117] Altered adipocyte PKC-ε activity has been implicated in obesity.[118] This differential tissue distribution has important implications for therapies designed to inhibit PKC in target tissues of diabetic complications.

PKC activation has been implicated in the pathogenesis of microvascular diabetic complications in both the eye and kidney[2] (Fig. 22-8). Increased intracellular glucose contributes to PKC activation, in part via increased synthesis of DAG.[73,119,120] DAG can be formed de novo from the glycolytic intermediates dihydroxyacetone phosphate and glycerol 3-phosphate after stepwise acylation to lysophosphatidic acid and phosphatidic acid. Increased PKC activity has been detected in tissues from diabetic humans, dogs, and rats.[121,122] After elevating either in vivo or in vitro (medium) glucose

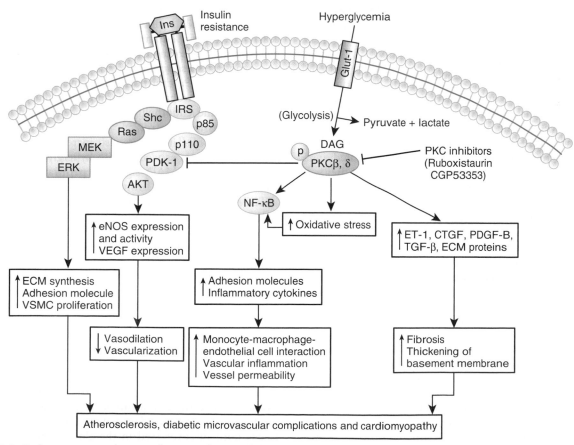

Figure 22-8 Pathogenic contribution of protein kinase C (PKC) activation to vascular complications of diabetes mellitus. (From He Z, King GL: Protein kinase Cbeta isoform inhibitors: A new treatment for diabetic cardiovascular diseases. Circulation 110:7–9, 2004.)

increased incidence with the D allele, which predisposes to increased levels of ACE. This polymorphism has been associated with development or severity of a variety of nondiabetic renal diseases,[259–269] although negative studies have also been reported.[270–274]

The angiotensinogen polymorphism M235T, associated with hypertension, has also been associated with diabetic nephropathy in some,[262,270,275–277] but not all,[267,272,273,276] studies. There have also been studies for[272,278,279] and against[263,270,273] association with the angiotensin AT1 receptor. There is also a report of a polymorphism in the prorenin gene that is associated with development of diabetic nephropathy.[280]

Other candidate genes have also been suggested based on their suggested role in pathogenesis of diabetic nephropathy and/or by linkage studies. Aldose reductase is the first and rate-limiting enzyme of the polyol pathway and converts glucose to sorbitol in an NADPH-dependent reaction. There is increased aldose reductase expression in patients with diabetic nephropathy and other microvascular complications,[69] and some, but not all, studies have indicated increased propensity for development of diabetic nephropathy in patients with polymorphisms of the aldose reductase gene that predispose to increased expression.[281,282]

Endothelial dysfunction is present in diabetes and is associated with impaired vascular NO synthesis. Linkage studies suggesting an association of polymorphisms in eNOS with nephropathy has been reported in Pima Indians with type II diabetes.[283] There have subsequently been some studies in other populations that have implicated eNOS polymorphisms that may lead to decreased expression and/or activity, although not all studies have been confirmatory.[284–289]

It has also been suggested that genetic abnormalities in lipid metabolism may underlie a predisposition to development of diabetic nephropathy. ApoE plays an important role in the metabolism of lipids and lipoproteins. It is found in chylomicrons, chylomicron remnants, very-low-density lipoproteins (VLDLs), VLDL remnants, and a subfraction of the high-density lipoproteins (HDLs). It acts as a ligand for their receptor-mediated catabolism through the low-density lipoprotein (LDL) receptor (ApoB100/E) and the ApoE receptor. Polymorphisms have been associated with altered plasma lipid values and have been associated with development of diabetic nephropathy in some patients as well as development and progression of atherosclerosis.[290,291]

A variety of other genes, including RAGE, Glut1, PAI-1, TGF-β, B2 bradykinin receptor, paroxonase, the homocyteine metabolism related enzyme methylenetetrahydrofolate reductase, atrial natriuretic peptide, RANTES, manganese SOD, lipoprotein lipase, decorin, VEGF, and PPARγ, have also been linked in some but not all studies. Suffice it to say, the identity of the predisposing genes continues to be the subject of intensive current research, and our understanding of the involved genetic interactions will very likely increase dramatically in the next few years.

Genome-wide scans have recently been employed in the study of the genetic basis of diabetic nephropathy. These scans allow a comprehensive survey of the entire genome for chromosome regions that are linked to diabetic nephropathy. Recent scans in Pima Indians and in African Americans have identified susceptibility loci on chromosome 3q, 7,18q, and 20p.[292–294] In addition, there is recent evidence for a susceptibility locus on chromosome 10 in both whites and African Americans for development of ESRD from diabetic nephropathy.[9]

CELLULAR SITES OF INJURY IN DIABETIC NEPHROPATHY

Endothelial Cells

Endothelial damage has been proposed as a common denominator of diabetic tissue injury in all target organs, including kidney, eye, nerve, and other micro- and macrovascular beds.[295,296] Endothelial cells may be particularly susceptible to the injurious effects of increased blood glucose because GLUT1, the major glucose transporter in endothelial cells,[297] provides a high-affinity uptake mechanism contributing to unregulated glucose uptake and intracellular hyperglycemia.[298] The precise mechanisms by which cellular hyperglycemia leads to endothelial damage are likely to involve increased mitochondrial ROS generation, by overwhelming the electron transport chain with substrate.[299,300]

Altered endothelial function contributes to enhanced atherosclerosis in large vessels. The factors contributing to accelerated atherosclerosis in diabetes mellitus undoubtedly include the associated dyslipidemia; however, other mechanisms also contribute to endothelial dysfunction. The endothelium is a major site of COX2 expression,[301] and normal endothelium primarily produces prostacyclin (PGI$_2$), an inhibitor of platelet aggregation. Although hyperglycemia increases cyclooxygenase-2 (COX2) though PKC-β activation, it shifts endothelial prostanoid production from PGI$_2$ to the prothombotic product thromboxane A$_2$.[302] Reduced PGI$_2$ receptor (IP) activation results in enhanced atherosclerosis in mice[303]; however, it remains to be determined whether reduced IP receptor activation contributes to atherosclerosis in the setting of diabetes.

Hyperglycemia and PKC-β activation also increase eNOS expression[302]; however, in the diabetic this is accompanied not by increased NO production, but rather ROS production.[304] The contribution of eNOS to atherosclerosis is complex, but appears to depend on the tissue levels of tetrahydrobiopterin (BH4).[304] It has been hypothesized that BH4 serves as an intermediary for electron donation to the eNOS heme-bound oxygen coupled to NO production.[305,306] In the absence of BH4, electrons associated with the eNOS flavin moiety preferentially react with uncoupled oxygen, thereby contributing to ROS formation, promoting atherosclerosis.[307] The complexities of eNOS expression level with respect to atherosclerosis may underlie the apparent conflicting results obtained regarding increased atheroma formation seen in double transgenic ApoE-null mice either overexpressing eNOS[308] or with genetic disruption of eNOS — independent of effects on blood pressure.[309] In the former studies, treatment of eNOS transgenic mice with BH4 reduced atherosclerotic plaque size,[308] consistent with a role for superoxide derived from eNOS. In pathologic circumstances, including diabetes, endothelial BH4 levels are reduced,[310] resulting in a switch of eNOS product from NO to the production of ROS, consistent with an increase in eNOS-derived oxidative injury in diabetes.

Dysfunctional endothelium in arterial resistance vessels also contributes to the development of hypertension.[311–315]

Impaired eNOS-dependent acetylcholine vasodilation has been demonstrated in patients with type II diabetes and is correlated with dyslipidemia and increased LDL levels.[314,315] Insulin resistance may contribute to endothelial dysfunction by downregulation of the phosphoinositide-3 kinase (PI3K)/ Akt pathway, reducing phosphorylation and impairing eNOS-dependent NO production.[316,317] Hyperglycemia occurring in either type I or type II diabetes mellitus may also impair eNOS activity via enhanced O-linked glycosylation of this enzyme.[68] Increased endothelial-derived ROS formation in diabetes[299] also appears to contribute to increased blood pressure.[52]

Altered capillary endothelial function also occurs in diabetics. Hyperglycemia impairs both endothelial proliferation and angiogenesis in the chick chorioallantoic membrane model.[318] Vasodilator NOS activity is suppressed in the renal glomerular capillary endothelial cells by both type I and type II diabetes.[319] Increased ambient glucose concentration decreases generation of NO production in freshly isolated glomeruli.[319] Conversely, in early diabetes induced by streptozotocin in rats, glomerular capillary eNOS immuno-reactivity is increased.[320] Taken together, these findings are consistent with the possibility that increased glomerular eNOS might serve as a source for superoxide production rather than NO.[304,321,322] Indeed, antioxidant treatment of afferent arterioles isolated from diabetic rabbits restores defective endothelium-dependent vasodilation.[323]

Mesangial Cells

Mesangial expansion and nodular sclerosis are major histopathologic features of diabetic nephropathy.[324,325] This observation has focused attention on the mesangial cell as a target of injury in diabetes mellitus. The major collagen produced in diabetic nephropathy is type IV.[326] Diverse mechanisms contribute to increased mesangial production of collagen in diabetes.

In mesangial cells, hyperglycemia exerts similar intracellular events as described in endothelial and other vascular cells. GLUT1 is the major facilitative glucose transporter present in mesangial cells,[31,327] and mesangial cells express only low levels of the insulin-sensitive glucose transporter GLUT4. Overexpression of GLUT1 in cultured mesangial cells increases collagen synthesis in normal glucose medium,[12] consistent with an important role of increased intracellular glucose entry in the genesis of mesangial sclerosis.

Increased cell glucose provides substrate for the enzymes of the polyol pathway, including aldose reductase and sorbitol dehydrogenase, both of which have been identified in mesangial cells.[328–330] Administration of the aldose reductase inhibitor epalrestat to streptozotocin-induced diabetic rats prevented the development of renal dysfunction and mesangial expansion without affecting levels of blood glucose.[74] Similarly, administration of tolrestat to streptozotocin-induced diabetic rats prevented glomerular hyperfiltration, mesangial cell hypocontractility, and reduced albuminuria.[331]

Advanced AGEs stimulate the production of collagen by mesangial cells by binding to their receptors, including RAGE and CD36. Mesangial cells exhibit specific binding of AGE-modified proteins, including albumin and collagen.[96] Binding of AGE to its mesangial receptors, including RAGE, stimulates cellular production of ROS[332] and STAT5-p21, which may lead to mesangial cell proliferation,[333] thereby contributing to

mesangial expansion in diabetic nephropathy. AGEs also activate pro-inflammatory pathways, including NF-κB and p42/44 MAPK in cultured mesangial cells[105] as well as podocytes.[91] Consequences of this include the induction of TGF-β and TGF-β type II receptor expression[179] with attendant increase in collagen synthesis by mesangial cells.[154,334,335] Treatment of cultured mesangial cells with AGE also induces the expression of ALK1, one of the type I receptor members for TGF-β family proteins.[336] Although ALK1 was originally described as an orphan receptor, recent reports show that ALK1 transduces TGF-β signals via Smad1.[337] Recent studies demonstrate Smad1 signaling activates transcription of the Col4a gene.[336] Importantly, induction of ALK1 is also demonstrated by immunostaining in glomeruli from diabetic kidneys.[336]

Diabetes is associated with increased expression and activity of mesangial extracellular response kinases, including ERK-5 (BMK1) and ERK-1/2, but not p38 in the glomeruli of OLETF rats at 52 weeks of age, which exhibit diabetic nephropathy.[338] In vitro, both glucose and raffinose caused rapid and significant activation of ERK-5 in cultured rat mesangial cells, suggesting that in tissue culture this may be a consequence of hypertonic stress rather than high glucose per se. The specific role of chronic hypertonicity imposed by hyperglycemia as a contributor to the cardiovascular complications of diabetes has not been rigorously explored.

Podocytes

The glomerular epithelial cell, or podocyte, is increasingly recognized as a primary target for glomerular injury, including diabetic nephropathy. The podocyte has a cell body with numerous foot processes that interdigitate with adjacent foot processes arising from different podocyte cell bodies. The surface of the podocyte, like the basement membrane, is covered in negatively charged molecules, including the transmembrane molecule podocalyxin, which is attached to the cytoskeleton via adaptor molecules. The slit-diaphragms between the podocyte foot processes contain nephrin, among other molecules, that form a zipper-like structure. In both experimental and human diabetes, podocytes are abnormal, with broadened and effaced foot processes and abnormalities in expression of many of the podocyte-specific proteins, including nephrin.[339–344]

Since the remaining podocytes have minimal ability to proliferate after podocyte loss, it is thought that podocyte protein abnormalities and progressive cell loss[345–348] may contribute to the development of proteinuria and ultimate glomerulosclerosis in both type I and type II diabetes. Podocytes are also a source of VEGF, which has been postulated to induce increased permeability and proteinuria.[91] In a study of 16 Pima Indians with type II diabetes for an average duration of 13.3 years, the subsequent progression of microalbuminuria or conversion to microalbuminuria in the next 4 years was strongly correlated with the number of podocytes.[345] Whether this represented destruction due to diabetes or was genetically determined could not be determined, although a previous cross-sectional analysis in the same population had demonstrated decreased podocyte number with overt nephropathy.[349] Although similar findings have recently been observed in cross-sectional studies of whites with type II diabetes,[348,346] proteinuria may correlate best with podocyte density, which may reflect some combination of decrease in podocyte number and glomerular hypertrophy.[346] Decreased numbers of podocytes have also been reported in cross-sectional studies of type I diabetes,[347,350] and a longitudinal study in normotensive type I diabetics also found a correlation between podocyte loss and increase in proteinuria[350]

There is evidence that nephrin expression decreases with increased proteinuria in diabetic nephropathy,[340] but this observation may be an effect rather than a cause of podocyte dysfunction, since decreased nephrin expression is also observed in other nondiabetic proteinuric conditions. In experimental animal models, ROS, angiotensin II, PKC, hypertension, and AGEs have all been proposed to mediate the podocyte injury and alterations in podocyte nephrin expression.[340]

Hypertrophy

In poorly controlled diabetes, there is increased renal mass, with both glomerular and tubular components increasing in size.[351] This growth is predominantly the result of hypertrophy, an increase in the size of existing cells, rather than hyperplasia, and an increase in cell number. Studies in cultured cells indicate that either high glucose or angiotensin II will induce hypertrophy of both glomerular and tubular cells, and TGF-β has been suggested to mediate both angiotensin II and hyperglycemia-induced hypertrophy.[170,178]

When cells proliferate, they must progress from a quiescent state (G_0) through the cell cycle (G_1, S, G_2, M). The cell cycle is regulated by cell cycle regulatory proteins (cyclins) that bind to and activate cyclin-dependent kinases (CDKs). Counter-regulation of this cell cycle activation is provided by CDK inhibitors. There are two families of CDK inhibitors, the p21(Cip1) (p21)/p27(Kip1) (p27) family and the p15(Ink4B)/16(Ink4A) family.[172,352] Cells undergoing hypertrophy demonstrate cell cycle arrest in late G_1 phase and fail to progress into the S phase. The G_1-phase cyclins D and E activate CDK4/6 and CDK2, respectively, which leads to phosphorylation of the retinoblastoma protein (Rb). Although p16 interacts only with CDK4/6, p21 and p27 families inhibit almost all cyclin-CDK complexes, and both p21 and p27 have been implicated in renal hypertrophy in diabetes.[353–357] Although still an area of uncertainty, there is some experimental and clinical evidence linking renal hypertrophy with the subsequent development of diabetic nephropathy.[358,359]

Tubulo-interstitial Injury

To the accumulated knowledge concerning mechanisms of glomerular injury must also be added the seminal insights of Risdon and colleagues[360] concerning the role of tubulo-interstitial injury in the ultimate outcome of chronic renal injury, which was subsequently confirmed by others.[361–365] It has long been recognized that in general glomerular injury with greater proteinuria progresses faster to end-stage disease. In the MDRD study, patients with proteinuria greater than 3 g/24 hr had a mean decrease in GFR of 10 mL/min/yr, while those with less than 1 g/24 hr had a decrease of 3 mL/min/yr, and reduction in proteinuria independent of blood pressure reduction decreased the rate of decline of GFR.[366] Although diabetic nephropathy was traditionally considered a primarily glomerular disease, it is now widely accepted that the rate of

deterioration of function correlates best with the degree of renal tubulo-interstitial fibrosis.[367,368] There is increasing interest in the role of tubule epithelial cells, especially the proximal tubule, and interstitial myofibroblasts, in the initiation of fibrosis and ultimate development of end-stage disease. An intriguing hypothesis to explain progressive tubulo-interstitial injury that accompanies glomerular damage is that the ensuing proteinuria is not only a marker of glomerular injury but is itself an active participant in the tubular destruction. This hypothesis has been stated most explicitly by Remuzzi and colleagues.[369,370] Studies utilizing proximal tubule cells in culture indicate that albumin activates tubular expression of chemokines, including MCP-1 and RANTES, through an NF-κB-dependent mechanism.[371–373] MCP-1 has been proposed to induce tubulo-interstitial fibrosis through recruitment and activation of macrophages, which then synthesize TGF-β. In this regard, studies have indicated that blocking MCP-1 attenuates interstitial nephritis.[374] Macrophages can also induce tubular apoptosis. It is also important to note that in addition to intrinsic renal cells, both tubular cells and glomerular mesangial cells, MCP-1 is also produced by macrophages, such that initiating tubulo-interstitial damage can lead to self-perpetuating propagation of the injury. In vivo studies with the puromycin model of proteinuria have also demonstrated increased tubular expression of osteopontin, which can also mediate macrophage recruitment.[375] In addition to increased chemokine expression, proteinuria has also been shown to increase tubule expression of ET-1.[202]

Recent studies have suggested that in the normal kidney there may be 1–2 g or more of albumin filtered by the glomerulus.[376] With the recent elucidation of the mechanisms of proximal tubule endocytosis, involving megalin and cubulin,[377,378] there is increasing awareness that the proximal tubule's capacity for protein reabsorption is so great that urinary protein levels may significantly underestimate the filtered protein load. Therefore, proteinuria may induce direct injury to intracellular lysomal pathways, and lysosomal rupture may produced direct tubule damage.[379] Normally albumin acts as an antioxidant, but it has been suggested that it may bring along tubule-activating substances such as LPS, as well as free fatty acids, prostaglandins, heavy metals, and steroid-based hormones.[380] It has also been suggested that oxidative injury may occur secondary to increased reabsorption of complexed iron and transferrin, with intracellular dissociation and activation-increased production of free radicals through the Fenton reaction.[381] Finally there may be increased presentation of lipid-bound chemotactic factors[382] and growth factors such as IGF-1, TGF-β, and hepatic growth factor (HGF).[383,384] Cell culture studies have usually utilized delipidated albumin to demonstrate proximal tubule cell injury and activation, although similar observations have been made with transferrin or IgG. However, the observation that conditions that induce relatively selective albuminuria, such as is seen with minimal change disease, rarely induce significant tubulo-interstitial injury and progressive decline in renal function, even in the face of significant proteinuria. Therefore, in vivo, it may be filtered proteins other than or in addition to albumin that induce the observed tubule dysfunction. One potential filtered protein is complement. In nonselective proteinuria, there is C3 and C5b-9 staining in the proximal tubule brush border membranes and intratubular complement activation, leading to sublytic attack and subsequent activation of proximal tubules.[369,375,385,386] It should also be noted that once tubule cells are activated, they can also activate the alternative pathway of complement activation.[387]

CLINICAL MANIFESTATIONS

Although a minority of patients presenting with diabetic nephropathy have type I diabetes, the natural history of the disease is best exemplified in this population; the onset of diabetes is more clearly definable in type I diabetes, and patients do not usually present initially with other co-morbid conditions commonly associated with type II diabetes (including essential hypertension, atherosclerotic cardiovascular disease, and obesity) that may independently produce chronic renal injury. Furthermore, the relatively advanced age of onset of type II diabetes and the increased cardiovascular mortality in this population may preclude development of all manifestations of diabetic nephropathy. In this regard, definitive descriptions of diabetic nephropathy in type II diabetes have been obtained in studies of Pima Indians, who exhibit a strong genetic predisposition to development of type II diabetes around the fourth decade of life, and who develop diabetic nephropathy that progresses in a similar pattern as is seen in type I diabetics.

In type I diabetes, it is possible to characterize the progression of diabetic nephropathy as occurring in four relatively distinct stages. In stage I, which commences soon after the overt manifestations of diabetes, the kidney undergoes hypertrophy compared to age- and weight-matched normal controls. Both the glomeruli and tubules are hypertrophied. In addition, there is up to 50% increase in renal blood flow and glomerular filtration rate in the initial phase of diabetic nephropathy. There is no detectable macroalbuminuria, but transient microalbuminuria (measurable by radioimmunoassay, enzyme-linked immunosorbent assay, or special dipsticks) is occasionally evident, especially induced by stress, physical exertion, intercurrent illness, or poor glycemic control. In type I diabetes, hypertension is usually absent in the early stages of the disease but is often present in type II diabetes at the time of presentation.

Approximately 30% of type I diabetic patients progress to stage II, characterized by fixed microalbuminuria of at least 30 mg/24 hr. The median duration of diabetes for progression to this clinically silent stage is 10 years. Although GFR either remains elevated or is within the normal range, abnormal renal histology is present, characterized by glomerular and tubular basement membrane thickening and inception of mesangial matrix expansion. The risk for developing microalbuminuria is greatly increased if other microvascular insults co-exist, and in particular, the presence of proliferative retinopathy increases the likelihood that detected microalbuminuria reflects the presence of diabetic nephropathy. In this regard, the predictive value of microalbuminuria for diabetic nephropathy is greater in type I than type II diabetics because of the high incidence in the latter population of hypertension, which may itself lead to microalbuminuria.

The great majority of patients who present with fixed microalbuminuria progress to overt nephropathy (stage III) within 5–7 years. In this stage, patients manifest overt proteinuria (>500 mg of total protein/24 hr) and macro-albuminuria (>200 mg/24 hr), which is detectable by a routine urinary protein dipstick. Blood pressure begins to rise in type I patients with stage III nephropathy, and in type II patients, who frequently have preexistent hypertension, blood pressure control becomes more problematic.

Diabetic nephropathy is characterized by progressive glomerular basement membrane thickening and mesangial matrix expansion, which progresses to glomerular sclerosis. Renal biopsy reveals diffuse or nodular (Kimmelsteil-Wilson) glomerulosclerosis. Although the Kimmelsteil-Wilson lesion is considered pathognomonic for advanced diabetic nephropathy, only approximately 25% of patients manifest this lesion. A nodular pattern of glomerulopathy mimicking Kimmelsteil-Wilson lesions may also be seen in light-chain nephropathy. Older descriptions of "diabetic nephropathy without overt hyperglycemia" that were based solely on light microscopic analysis may have actually represented light-chain disease. Nodular glomerular lesions can also be observed in amyloidosis and membranoproliferative glomerulonephritis type II. An additional pathognomonic finding of diabetic nephropathy is the co-existence of both afferent and efferent arteriolar hyalinosis, unlike the arteriolar lesion of essential hypertension, which is restricted to the afferent arteriole. In overt diabetic nephropathy, there is also progressive tubulo-interstitial fibrosis, which correlates most closely with the decline in renal function in a number of progressive renal diseases, including diabetic nephropathy. The GFR begins to decline from the normal range, but serum creatinine may remain in the normal range.

In stage IV, or advanced diabetic nephropathy, there is relentless decline in renal function to end-stage disease. The patients have nephrotic range proteinuria (>3.5 g/24 hr) and systemic hypertension, but no evidence of inflammatory glomerular (red blood cell casts) or tubulointerstitial (white blood cells [WBCs], WBC casts) lesions. The kidneys may be inappropriately large for the observed degree of renal insufficiency.

Although patients with type II diabetes also tend to have elevated GFR during their early presentation, the GFR increases are usually not as pronounced as are seen with insulin-dependent diabetes mellitus. In addition, there is a greater incidence of hypertension and microalbuminuria present at the time of detection of diabetes, with as many as 10% to 25% of patients presenting with these abnormalities. It is still unclear whether this difference in presentation represents a fundamental difference in the pathophysiology of the two conditions or, more likely, is due to the fact that type II patients may have unrecognized diabetes for many years because they are not ketosis prone and may have other associated conditions predisposing to renal abnormalities.

OTHER RENAL COMPLICATIONS

In addition to the clinical presentation of diabetic nephropathy described above, there are other kidney and genitourinary abnormalities that can ensue in the diabetic patient. Type IV (hyporeninemic, hypoaldosteronemic) metabolic acidosis with hyperkalemia is commonly encountered in patients with diabetes and mild to moderate renal insufficiency. These patients should be carefully monitored for development of severe hyperkalemia in response to volume depletion or after inception of drugs that interfere with the renin-angiotensin system, such as ACE inhibitors, AT1 receptor blockers, β-adrenergic blockers, nonsteroidal anti-inflammatory agents, heparin, or potassium-sparing diuretics.

Patients with diabetes have an increased incidence of bacterial and fungal infections of the genitourinary tract. In addition to lower urinary tract infections, there is an increased risk for pyelonephritis and intrarenal and perinephric abscess formation.

Unilateral or bilateral renal artery stenosis is more frequent in the type II diabetic population than in age-matched nondiabetic individuals and should be considered if a diabetic patient manifests intractable hypertension or a rapidly rising serum creatinine immediately after initiation of therapy with an ACE inhibitor or AT1 receptor blockers. Other causes of acute deterioration of renal function include papillary necrosis, with ureteral obstruction secondary to sloughing a papilla, obstructive uropathy due to bladder dysfunction resulting from autonomic neuropathy, and contrast media–induced acute tubular necrosis. In addition, diabetics may develop prerenal azotemia or acute tubular necrosis as a result of congestive heart failure or of volume depletion secondary to vomiting induced by gastroparesis or diarrhea due to autonomic neuropathy.

PREVENTION OF DIABETIC NEPHROPATHY

As mentioned above, studies have convincingly demonstrated that tight glycemic control significantly lessens but does not completely eliminate the incidence of diabetic nephropathy. Furthermore, in the DCCT, the incidence of clinically significant hypoglycemic episodes was increased threefold in the patients receiving intensive insulin therapy. Although the role of systemic hypertension as a pathogenic factor in development of diabetic nephropathy remains unresolved, it is well established to be the most important single risk factor in its progression, and blood pressure levels should be lowered to levels below what is considered to be the upper levels of normal pressure in the nondiabetic population. There is also evidence that smoking and elevated cholesterol may be predisposing factors in the development of diabetic nephropathy in type II diabetics.

TREATMENT OF LATENT (STAGE II) AND OVERT (STAGE III) DIABETIC NEPHROPATHY

Although the Stockholm Diabetes Intervention Study and the DCCT demonstrated that strict glycemic control was effective in preventing development of fixed microalbuminuria, subgroup analysis of the DCCT patients who initially presented with microalbuminuria, as well as a subsequent study by the Microalbuminuria Collaborative Study Group, has determined that tight control of type I patients may not prevent progression to macroalbuminuria, although it does prevent other microvascular complications, such as retinopathy and peripheral neuropathy. There is increasing evidence that better glycemic control will slow the progression of nephropathy in type II diabetics.

It is clear that optimal blood pressure control will retard progression of diabetic nephropathy. Studies have determined that interfering with the renin-angiotensin system by administration of either ACE inhibitors or AT1 receptor blockers has additional benefit beyond lowering systemic blood pressure to retard progression in both type I and type II patients. Conversely, there is evidence that dihydropyridine calcium channel blockers may be less effective or even detrimental in preventing progression of diabetic nephropathy. The underlying pathophysiologic explanation may relate to the ability of ACE inhibitors and AT1 receptor blockers to lower intraglomerular capillary pressure by decreasing efferent arteriolar pressure while dihydropyridine calcium channel blockers increase intraglomerular capillary pressure by inducing selective afferent arteriolar vasodilatation.

When administering ACE inhibitors or AT1 receptor blockers to patients with diabetic nephropathy, both serum potassium and creatinine should be monitored closely in the first week after initiation, given the associated co-morbid conditions of type IV RTA and renal artery stenosis. If blood pressure control is not achieved with these agents, addition of diuretics and other antihypertensive agents, including cardioselective β blockers, α blockers, and nonhydropyridine calcium channel blockers can be added. As mentioned previously, smoking cessation and antihyperlipidemic medication to patients with documented lipid abnormalities should be encouraged. Judicious restriction of dietary protein (to 0.8 g/kg of ideal body weight/day) is recommended by the American Diabetes Association. Although there are some data suggesting that further dietary protein restriction may retard progression of diabetic nephropathy, such an intervention must also take into account the individual nutritional carbohydrate and lipid requirements of the patient.

Efficacy of treatment can be determined by monitoring albuminuria and/or total proteinuria. For patients with deterioration of renal function, GFR determined by creatinine clearance and/or plots of 1/sCr are effective indicators of whether interventions are affecting the rate of progression of the nephropathy.

Renal Replacement Therapy

Currently, over 80% of the patients with end-stage diabetic nephropathy receive dialysis as their modality of renal replacement therapy, with 5.7 times as many of these patients receiving hemodialysis compared with peritoneal dialysis. Because of the associated macrovascular complications (cardiovascular, cerebrovascular, peripheral vascular) and the increased risk for infection, the survival of diabetic patients who receive either type of dialysis is lower than that of the nondiabetic dialysis population, with a mortality rate that is 1.5 to 2.0 times that of nondiabetic patients, and the 5-year survival rate of diabetic patients on maintenance dialysis is less than 20%. The survival rate of diabetic patients is slightly worse on peritoneal dialysis than on hemodialysis. It is not established whether this difference is a consequence of the therapy itself (dialytic adequacy may not be as easily obtained in larger patients, and systemic absorption of the high glucose solutions used in peritoneal dialysis may lead to poorer glycemic control and accelerate microvascular and/or macrovascular complications), or whether it is a reflection of the patients who may be more likely to be initiated on peritoneal dialysis (i.e., those patients whose associated vascular complications preclude hemodialysis). In general, the treatment of a diabetic patient nearing ESRD is similar to that of the nondiabetic patient. The patient should be under the care of a nephrologist and planning initiated for the modality of dialysis. Although dialysis is usually initiated when GFR declines to approximately 10 to 15 mL/min, in diabetic patients, early initiation of dialysis is sometimes necessary when either volume-dependent hypertension or hyperkalemia are not manageable by nondialytic therapy or when uremia, combined with gastroparesis, leads to anorexia and malnutrition and/or uncontrollable recurrent emesis.

Approximately 25% of the renal transplantations performed in the United States are in diabetic patients. The vast majority (>90%) are type I diabetics, due to their younger age and decreased associated macrovascular co-morbidity compared with type II patients. The long-term survival and quality of life after transplantation is generally superior to that seen with dialytic therapy. However, the other microvascular complications (retinopathy, neuropathy) are not improved by renal transplantation alone. The advent of pancreas and combined kidney-pancreas transplantation has been shown to improve significantly the quality of life of patients with diabetic nephropathy, by improving autonomic neuropathy, either retarding or possibly correcting retinopathy, and avoiding the potential complications of insulin administration. However, all transplantation options remain limited by organ availability.

Hopefully, through the identification of those molecular disturbances most relevant to the genesis of diabetic nephropathy, more specific targeted pharmaceutical interventions can forestall the progressive decline to ESRD in the future.

References

1. The Diabetes Control and Complications Trial / Epidemiology of Diabetes Interventions and Complications (DCCT/EDIC) Study Research Group: Intensive diabetes treatment and cardiovascular disease in patients with type 1 diabetes. N Eng J Med 353:2643–2653, 2005.
2. Retnakaran R, Cull CA, Thorne KI, et al: Risk factors for renal dysfunction in type 2 diabetes. UK Prospective Diabetes Study 74. Diabetes 55:1832–1839, 2006.
3. Reusch JE: Diabetes microvascular complications and cardiovascular complications: What is it about glucose? J Clin Invest 112:986–988, 2003.
4. Fukui M, Nakamura T, Ebihara I, et al: Gene expression for endothelins and their receptors in glomeruli of diabetic rats. J Lab Clin Med 122:149–156, 1993.
5. Stratton IM, Adler AI, Neil HA, et al: Association of glycaemia with macrovascular and microvascular complications of type 2 diabetes (UKPDS 35): Prospective observational study. BMJ 321:405–412, 2000.
6. Brownlee M: Biochemistry and molecular cell biology of diabetic complications. Nature 414:813–820, 2001.
7. Krolewski AS: Genetics of diabetic nephropathy: Evidence for major and minor gene effects [clinical conference]. Kidney Int 55:1582–1596, 1999.
8. Parving HH, Tarnow L, Rossing P: Genetics of diabetic nephropathy. J Am Soc Nephrol 7:2509–2517, 1996.
9. Iyengar SK, Fox KA, Schachere M, et al: Linkage analysis of candidate loci for end-stage renal disease due to diabetic nephropathy. J Am Soc Nephrol 14(Suppl):195–201, 2003.
10. Brenner BM, Lawler EV, Mackenzie HS: The hyperfiltration theory: A paradigm shift in nephrology. Kidney Int 49:1774–1777, 1996.
11. Heilig CW, Brosius FC, Cunningham C: Role for GLUT1 in diabetic glomerulosclerosis. Expert Rev Mol Med 8:1–18, 2006.
12. Heilig CW, Concepcion LA, Riser BL, et al: Overexpression of glucose transporters in rat mesangial cells cultured in a normal glucose milieu mimics the diabetic phenotype. J Clin Invest 96:1802–1814, 1995.
13. Heilig CW, Kreisberg JI, Freytag S, et al: Antisense GLUT-1 protects mesangial cells from glucose induction of GLUT-1 and fibronectin expression. Am J Physiol Renal Physiol 280:F657–F666, 2001.
14. Henry DN, Busik JV, Brosius FC 3rd, Heilig CW: Glucose transporters control gene expression of aldose reductase PKCalpha and GLUT1 in mesangial cells in vitro. Am J Physiol 277:F97–F104, 1999.
15. Brosius FC 3rd, Briggs JP, Marcus RG, et al: Insulin-responsive glucose transporter expression in renal microvessels and glomeruli. Kidney Int 42:1086–1092, 1992.
16. Kaiser N, Sasson S, Feener EP, et al: Differential regulation of glucose transport and transporters by glucose in vascular endothelial and smooth muscle cells. Diabetes 42:80–89, 1993.
17. Raha S, Robinson BH: Mitochondria oxygen free radicals disease and ageing. Trends Biochem Sci 25:502–508, 2000.
18. Davi G, Chiarelli F, Santilli F, et al: Enhanced lipid peroxidation and platelet activation in the early phase of type 1 diabetes mellitus: Role of interleukin-6 and disease duration. Circulation 107:3199–3203, 2003.
19. Morrow JD: Quantification of isoprostanes as indices of oxidant stress and the risk of atherosclerosis in humans. Arterioscler Thromb Vasc Biol 25:279–286, 2004.
20. Flores L, Rodela S, Abian J, et al: F2 isoprostane is already increased at the onset of type 1 diabetes mellitus: Effect of glycemic control. Metabolism 53:1118–1120, 2004.
21. Davi G, Ciabattoni G, Consoli A, et al: In vivo formation of 8-iso-prostaglandin f2alpha and platelet activation in diabetes mellitus: Effects of improved metabolic control and vitamin E supplementation. Circulation 99:224–229, 1999.
22. Cai H, Harrison DG: Endothelial dysfunction in cardiovascular diseases: The role of oxidant stress. Circ Res 87:840–844, 2000.
23. Griendling KK, Sorescu D, Ushio-Fukai M: NAD(P)H oxidase: Role in cardiovascular biology and disease. Circ Res 86:494–501, 2000.
24. Lassegue B, Clempus RE: Vascular NAD(P)H oxidases: Specific features expression and regulation. Am J Physiol Regul Integr Comp Physiol 285:R277–R297, 2003.
25. Lambeth JD, Cheng G, Arnold RS, Edens WA: Novel homologs of gp91phox. Trends Biochem Sci 25:459–461, 2000.
26. Etoh T, Inoguchi T, Kakimoto M, et al: Increased expression of NAD(P)H oxidase subunits NOX4 and p22phox in the kidney of streptozotocin-induced diabetic rats and its reversibility by interventive insulin treatment. Diabetologia 46:1428–1437, 2003.
27. Ushio-Fukai M, Zafari AM, Fukui T, et al: p22phox is a critical component of the superoxide-generating NADH/NADPH oxidase system and regulates angiotensin II-induced hypertrophy in vascular smooth muscle cells. J Biol Chem 271:23317–23321, 1996.
28. Zafari AM, Ushio-Fukai M, Akers M, et al: Role of NADH/NADPH oxidase-derived H_2O_2 in angiotensin II-induced vascular hypertrophy. Hypertension 32:488–495, 1998.
29. Ambasta RK, Kumar P, Griendling KK, et al: Direct interaction of the novel Nox proteins with p22phox is required for the formation of a functionally active NADPH oxidase. J Biol Chem 279:45935–45941, 2004.
30. Hayashi K, Haneda M, Koya D, et al: Enhancement of glomerular heme oxygenase-1 expression in diabetic rats. Diabetes Res Clin Pract 52:85–96, 2001.

106. Iacobini C, Amadio L, Oddi G, et al: Role of galectin-3 in diabetic nephropathy. J Am Soc Nephrol 14(Suppl):264–270, 2003.

107. Iacobini C, Menini S, Oddi G, et al: Galectin-3/AGE-receptor 3 knockout mice show accelerated AGE-induced glomerular injury: Evidence for a protective role of galectin-3 as an AGE receptor. FASEB J 18:1773–1775, 2004.

108. Parker PJ, Murray-Rust J: PKC at a glance. J Cell Sci 117:131–132, 2004.

109. Porte D Jr, Schwartz MW: Diabetes complications: Why is glucose potentially toxic? Science 272:699–700, 1996.

110. Nishizuka Y: Intracellular signaling by hydrolysis of phospholipids and activation of protein kinase C. Science 258:607–614, 1992.

111. Newton AC: Diacylglycerol's affair with protein kinase C turns 25. Trends Pharmacol Sci 25:175–177, 2004.

112. Idris I, Gray S, Donnelly R: Protein kinase C activation: Isozyme-specific effects on metabolism and cardiovascular complications in diabetes. Diabetologia 44:659–673, 2001.

113. Gutcher I, Webb PR, Anderson NG: The isoform-specific regulation of apoptosis by protein kinase C. Cell Mol Life Sci 60:1061–1070, 2003.

114. Redling S, Pfaff IL, Leitges M, Vallon V: Immunolocalization of protein kinase C isoenzymes alpha beta I beta II delta and epsilon in mouse kidney. Am J Physiol Renal Physiol 287:F289–F298, 2004.

115. Hua H, Munk S, Goldberg H, et al: High glucose-suppressed endothelin-1 Ca^{2+} signaling via NADPH oxidase and diacylglycerol-sensitive protein kinase C isozymes in mesangial cells. J Biol Chem 278:33951–33962, 2003.

116. Dlugosz JA, Munk S, Zhou X, Whiteside CI: Endothelin-1-induced mesangial cell contraction involves activation of protein kinase C-alpha, -delta and -epsilon. Am J Physiol 275:F423–F432, 1998.

117. Kim JK, Fillmore JJ, Sunshine MJ, et al: PKC-theta knockout mice are protected from fat-induced insulin resistance. J Clin Invest 114:823–827, 2004.

118. Frevert EU, Kahn BB: Protein kinase C isoforms epsilon, eta, delta and zeta in murine adipocytes: Expression subcellular localization and tissue-specific regulation in insulin-resistant states. Biochem J 316(Pt 3):865–871, 1996.

119. Lee TS, Saltsman KA, Ohashi H, King GL: Activation of protein kinase C by elevation of glucose concentration: Proposal for a mechanism in the development of diabetic vascular complications. Proc Natl Acad Sci U S A 86:5141–5145, 1989.

120. Kikkawa R, Haneda M, Uzu T, et al: Translocation of protein kinase C alpha and zeta in rat glomerular mesangial cells cultured under high glucose conditions. Diabetologia 37:838–841, 1994.

121. Xia P, Inoguchi T, Kern TS, et al: Characterization of the mechanism for the chronic activation of diacylglycerol-protein kinase C pathway in diabetes and hypergalactosemia. Diabetes 43:1122–1129, 1994.

122. Considine RV, Nyce MR, Allen LE, et al: Protein kinase C is increased in the liver of humans and rats with non-insulin-dependent diabetes mellitus: An alteration not due to hyperglycemia. J Clin Invest 95:2938–2944, 1995.

123. Kapor-Drezgic J, Zhou X, Babazono T, et al: Effect of high glucose on mesangial cell protein kinase C-delta and -epsilon is polyol pathway-dependent. J Am Soc Nephrol 10:1193–1203, 1999.

124. Ziyadeh FN, Fumo P, Rodenberger CH, et al: Role of protein kinase C and cyclic AMP/protein kinase A in high glucose-stimulated transcriptional activation of collagen alpha 1 (IV) in glomerular mesangial cells. J Diabetes Complications 9:255–261, 1995.

125. Taguchi A, Blood DC, del Toro G, et al: Blockade of RAGE-amphoterin signalling suppresses tumour growth and metastases. Nature 405:354–360, 2000.

126. Thornalley PJ: Cell activation by glycated proteins. AGE receptors receptor recognition factors and functional classification of AGEs. Cell Mol Biol (Noisy-le-grand) 44:1013–1023, 1998.

127. Heidland A, Sebekova K, Schinzel R: Advanced glycation end products and the progressive course of renal disease. Am J Kidney Dis 38(Suppl):100–106, 2001.

128. Leitges M, Plomann M, Standaert ML, et al: Knockout of PKC alpha enhances insulin signaling through PI3K. Mol Endocrinol 16:847–858, 2002.

129. Marumo T, Schini-Kerth VB, Fisslthaler B, Busse R: Platelet-derived growth factor-stimulated superoxide anion production modulates activation of transcription factor NF-kappaB and expression of monocyte chemoattractant protein 1 in human aortic smooth muscle cells. Circulation 96:2361–2367, 1997.

130. Seshiah PN, Weber DS, Rocic P, et al: Angiotensin II stimulation of NAD(P)H oxidase activity: Upstream mediators. Circ Res 91:406–413, 2002.

131. Sheetz MJ, King GL: Molecular understanding of hyperglycemia's adverse effects for diabetic complications. JAMA 288:2579–2588, 2002.

132. Koya D, Jirousek MR, Lin YW, et al: Characterization of protein kinase C beta isoform activation on the gene expression of transforming growth factor-beta extracellular matrix components and prostanoids in the glomeruli of diabetic rats. J Clin Invest 100:115–126, 1997.

133. Wakasaki H, Koya D, Schoen FJ, et al: Targeted overexpression of protein kinase C beta2 isoform in myocardium causes cardiomyopathy. Proc Natl Acad Sci U S A 94:9320–9325, 1997.

134. Cotter MA, Jack AM, Cameron NE: Effects of the protein kinase C beta inhibitor LY333531 on neural and vascular function in rats with streptozotocin-induced diabetes. Clin Sci (Lond) 103:311–321, 2002.

135. Kelly DJ, Zhang Y, Hepper C, et al: Protein kinase C beta inhibition attenuates the progression of experimental diabetic nephropathy in the presence of continued hypertension. Diabetes 52:512–518, 2003.

136. Koya D, Haneda M, Nakagawa H, et al: Amelioration of accelerated diabetic mesangial expansion by treatment with a PKC beta inhibitor in diabetic *db/db* mice a rodent model for type 2 diabetes. FASEB J 14:439–447, 2000.

137. Piek E, Heldin CH, Ten Dijke P: Specificity diversity and regulation in TGF-beta superfamily signaling. FASEB J 13:2105–2124, 1999.

138. Koli K, Saharinen J, Hyytiainen M, et al: Latency activation and binding proteins of TGF-beta. Microsc Res Tech 52:354–362, 2001.

139. Wrana JL, Attisano L, Wieser R, et al: Mechanism of activation of the TGF-beta receptor. Nature 370:341–347, 1994.

140. Hayashida T, Decaestecker M, Schnaper HW: Cross-talk between ERK MAP kinase and Smad signaling pathways enhances TGF-beta-dependent responses in human mesangial cells. FASEB J 17:1576–1578, 2003.

141. Gupta S, Clarkson MR, Duggan J, Brady HR: Connective tissue growth factor: Potential role in glomerulosclerosis and tubulointerstitial fibrosis. Kidney Int 58:1389–1399, 2000.

142. Shi Y: Structural insights on Smad function in TGFbeta signaling. Bioessays 23:223–232, 2001.

143. Yamamoto T, Noble NA, Cohen AH, et al: Expression of transforming growth factor-beta isoforms in human glomerular diseases. Kidney Int 49:461–469, 1996.

144. Hill C, Flyvbjerg A, Gronbaek H, et al: The renal expression of transforming growth factor-beta isoforms and their receptors in acute and chronic experimental diabetes in rats. Endocrinology 141:1196–1208, 2000.

145. Isono M, Cruz MC, Chen S, et al: Extracellular signal-regulated kinase mediates stimulation of TGF-beta1 and matrix by high

glucose in mesangial cells. J Am Soc Nephrol 11:2222–2230, 2000.

146. Rocco MV, Chen Y, Goldfarb S, Ziyadeh FN: Elevated glucose stimulates TGF-beta gene expression and bioactivity in proximal tubule. Kidney Int 41:107–114, 1992.

147. Yang CW, Vlassara H, Peten EP, et al: Advanced glycation end products up-regulate gene expression found in diabetic glomerular disease. Proc Natl Acad Sci U S A 91:9436–9440, 1994.

148. Ziyadeh FN, Han DC, Cohen JA, et al: Glycated albumin stimulates fibronectin gene expression in glomerular mesangial cells: Involvement of the transforming growth factor-beta system. Kidney Int 53:631–638, 1998.

149. Kolm-Litty V, Sauer U, Nerlich A, et al: High glucose-induced transforming growth factor beta1 production is mediated by the hexosamine pathway in porcine glomerular mesangial cells. J Clin Invest 101:160–169, 1998.

150. Riser BL, Cortes P, Heilig C, et al: Cyclic stretching force selectively up-regulates transforming growth factor-beta isoforms in cultured rat mesangial cells. Am J Pathol 148:1915–1923, 1996.

151. Yasuda T, Kondo S, Homma T, Harris RC: Regulation of extracellular matrix by mechanical stress in rat glomerular mesangial cells. J Clin Invest 98:1991–2000, 1996.

152. Wolf G, Ziyadeh FN: Renal tubular hypertrophy induced by angiotensin II. Semin Nephrol 17:448–454, 1997.

153. Dolan V, Hensey C, Brady HR: Diabetic nephropathy: Renal development gone awry? Pediatr Nephrol 18:75–84, 2003.

154. Isono M, Mogyorosi A, Han DC, et al: Stimulation of TGF-beta type II receptor by high glucose in mouse mesangial cells and in diabetic kidney. Am J Physiol Renal Physiol 278:F830–F838, 2000.

155. Isono M, Chen S, Hong SW, et al: Smad pathway is activated in the diabetic mouse kidney and Smad3 mediates TGF-beta-induced fibronectin in mesangial cells. Biochem Biophys Res Commun 296:1356–1365, 2002.

156. Ziyadeh FN: Mediators of diabetic renal disease: The case for TGF-beta as the major mediator. J Am Soc Nephrol 15(Suppl 1):55–57, 2004.

157. Kim SI, Han DC, Lee HB: Lovastatin inhibits transforming growth factor-beta1 expression in diabetic rat glomeruli and cultured rat mesangial cells. J Am Soc Nephrol 11:80–87, 2000.

158. Gilbert RE, Cox A, Wu LL, et al: Expression of transforming growth factor-beta1 and type IV collagen in the renal tubulointerstitium in experimental diabetes: Effects of ACE inhibition. Diabetes 47:414–422, 1998.

159. Pankewycz OG, Guan JX, Bolton WK, et al: Renal TGF-beta regulation in spontaneously diabetic NOD mice with correlations in mesangial cells. Kidney Int 46:748–758, 1994.

160. Cohen MP, Sharma K, Guo J, et al: The renal TGF-beta system in the db/db mouse model of diabetic nephropathy. Exp Nephrol 6:226–233, 1998.

161. Azar ST, Salti I, Zantout MS, Major S: Alterations in plasma transforming growth factor beta in normoalbuminuric type 1 and type 2 diabetic patients. J Clin Endocrinol Metab 85:4680–4682, 2000.

162. Sharma K, Ziyadeh FN, Alzahabi B, et al: Increased renal production of transforming growth factor-beta1 in patients with type II diabetes. Diabetes 46:854–859, 1997.

163. Sharma K, Eltayeb BO, McGowan TA, et al: Captopril-induced reduction of serum levels of transforming growth factor-beta1 correlates with long-term renoprotection in insulin-dependent diabetic patients. Am J Kidney Dis 34:818–823, 1999.

164. Sharma K, Ziyadeh FN: Biochemical events and cytokine interactions linking glucose metabolism to the development of diabetic nephropathy. Semin Nephrol 17:80–92, 1997.

165. Ziyadeh FN, Sharma K, Ericksen M, Wolf G: Stimulation of collagen gene expression and protein synthesis in murine

mesangial cells by high glucose is mediated by autocrine activation of transforming growth factor-beta. J Clin Invest 93:536–542, 1994.

166. Martin J, Steadman R, Knowlden J, et al: Differential regulation of matrix metalloproteinases and their inhibitors in human glomerular epithelial cells in vitro. J Am Soc Nephrol 9:1629–1637, 1998.

167. Shankland SJ, Ly H, Thai K, Scholey JW: Glomerular expression of tissue inhibitor of metalloproteinase (TIMP-1) in normal and diabetic rats. J Am Soc Nephrol 7:97–104, 1996.

168. Singh R, Song RH, Alavi N, et al: High glucose decreases matrix metalloproteinase-2 activity in rat mesangial cells via transforming growth factor-beta1. Exp Nephrol 9:249–257, 2001.

169. McLennan SV, Death AK, Fisher EJ, et al: The role of the mesangial cell and its matrix in the pathogenesis of diabetic nephropathy. Cell Mol Biol (Noisy-le-grand) 45:123–135, 1999.

170. Sharma K, Ziyadeh FN: Renal hypertrophy is associated with upregulation of TGF-beta 1 gene expression in diabetic BB rat and NOD mouse. Am J Physiol 267:F1094–F1001, 1994.

171. Ziyadeh FN, Sharma K: Role of transforming factor-beta in diabetic glomerulosclerosis and renal hypertrophy. Kidney Int Suppl 51:34–36, 1995.

172. Wolf G, Ziyadeh FN: Molecular mechanisms of diabetic renal hypertrophy. Kidney Int 56:393–405, 1999.

173. Kagami S, Border WA, Miller DE, Noble NA: Angiotensin II stimulates extracellular matrix protein synthesis through induction of transforming growth factor-beta expression in rat glomerular mesangial cells. J Clin Invest 93:2431–2437, 1994.

174. Hill C, Logan A, Smith C, et al: Angiotensin converting enzyme inhibitor suppresses glomerular transforming growth factor beta receptor expression in experimental diabetes in rats. Diabetologia 44:495–500, 2001.

175. Liao J, Kobayashi M, Kanamuru Y, et al: Effects of candesartan an angiotensin II type 1 receptor blocker on diabetic nephropathy in KK/Ta mice. J Nephrol 16:841–849, 2003.

176. King GL, Ishii H, Koya D: Diabetic vascular dysfunctions: A model of excessive activation of protein kinase C. Kidney Int Suppl 60:77–85, 1997.

177. Ishii H, Jirousek MR, Koya D, et al: Amelioration of vascular dysfunctions in diabetic rats by an oral PKC beta inhibitor. Science 272:728–731, 1996.

178. Sharma K, Jin Y, Guo J, Ziyadeh FN: Neutralization of TGF-beta by anti-TGF-beta antibody attenuates kidney hypertrophy and the enhanced extracellular matrix gene expression in STZ-induced diabetic mice. Diabetes 45:522–530, 1996.

179. Ziyadeh FN, Hoffman BB, Han DC, et al: Long-term prevention of renal insufficiency excess matrix gene expression and glomerular mesangial matrix expansion by treatment with monoclonal antitransforming growth factor-beta antibody in db/db diabetic mice. Proc Natl Acad Sci U S A 97:8015–8020, 2000.

180. Chen S, Iglesias-de la Cruz MC, Jim B, et al: Reversibility of established diabetic glomerulopathy by anti-TGF-beta antibodies in db/db mice. Biochem Biophys Res Commun 300:16–22, 2003.

181. Han DC, Hoffman BB, Hong SW, et al: Therapy with antisense TGF-beta1 oligodeoxynucleotides reduces kidney weight and matrix mRNAs in diabetic mice. Am J Physiol Renal Physiol 278:F628–F634, 2000.

182. Leask A, Abraham DJ: The role of connective tissue growth factor a multifunctional matricellular protein in fibroblast biology. Biochem Cell Biol 81:355–363, 2003.

183. Grotendorst GR, Okochi H, Hayashi N: A novel transforming growth factor beta response element controls the expression of the connective tissue growth factor gene. Cell Growth Differ 7:469–480, 1996.

184. Murphy M, Godson C, Cannon S, et al: Suppression subtractive hybridization identifies high glucose levels as a stimulus for expression of connective tissue growth factor and other genes in human mesangial cells. J Biol Chem 274:5830–5834, 1999.

185. Leask A, Abraham DJ: TGF-beta signaling and the fibrotic response. FASEB J 18:816–827, 2004.

186. McLennan SV, Wang XY, Moreno V, et al: Connective tissue growth factor mediates high glucose effects on matrix degradation through tissue inhibitor of matrix metalloproteinase type 1: Implications for diabetic nephropathy. Endocrinology 145:5646–5655, 2004.

187. Hogan BL: Bone morphogenetic proteins in development. Curr Opin Genet Dev 6:432–438, 1996.

188. Davies JA, Fisher CE: Genes and proteins in renal development. Exp Nephrol 10:102–113, 2002.

189. Klahr S: The bone morphogenetic proteins (BMPs). Their role in renal fibrosis and renal function. J Nephrol 16:179–185, 2003.

190. Zeisberg M, Kalluri R: The role of epithelial-to-mesenchymal transition in renal fibrosis. J Mol Med 82:175–181, 2004.

191. Murphy M, McMahon R, Lappin DW, Brady HR: Gremlins: Is this what renal fibrogenesis has come to? Exp Nephrol 10:241–244, 2002.

192. Wang SN, Lapage J, Hirschberg R: Loss of tubular bone morphogenetic protein-7 in diabetic nephropathy. J Am Soc Nephrol 12:2392–2399, 2001.

193. Woolf AS, Yuan HT: Angiopoietin growth factors and Tie receptor tyrosine kinases in renal vascular development. Pediatr Nephrol 16:177–184, 2001.

194. Kang DH, Johnson RJ: Vascular endothelial growth factor: A new player in the pathogenesis of renal fibrosis. Curr Opin Nephrol Hypertens 12:43–49, 2003.

195. Cooper ME, Vranes D, Youssef S, et al: Increased renal expression of vascular endothelial growth factor (VEGF) and its receptor VEGFR-2 in experimental diabetes. Diabetes 48:2229–2239, 1999.

196. Barleon B, Sozzani S, Zhou D, et al: Migration of human monocytes in response to vascular endothelial growth factor (VEGF) is mediated via the VEGF receptor flt-1. Blood 87:3336–3343, 1996.

197. Pertovaara L, Kaipainen A, Mustonen T, et al: Vascular endothelial growth factor is induced in response to transforming growth factor-beta in fibroblastic and epithelial cells. J Biol Chem 269:6271–6274, 1994.

198. Naicker S, Bhoola KD: Endothelins: Vasoactive modulators of renal function in health and disease. Pharmacol Ther 90:61–88, 2001.

199. Kohan DE: Production of endothelin-1 by rat mesangial cells: Regulation by tumor necrosis factor. J Lab Clin Med 119:477–484, 1992.

200. Marsden PA, Dorfman DM, Collins T, et al: Regulated expression of endothelin 1 in glomerular capillary endothelial cells. Am J Physiol 261:F117–F125, 1991.

201. Karet FE, Davenport AP: Localization of endothelin peptides in human kidney. Kidney Int 49:382–387, 1996.

202. Zoja C, Morigi M, Figliuzzi M, et al: Proximal tubular cell synthesis and secretion of endothelin-1 on challenge with albumin and other proteins. Am J Kidney Dis 26:934–941, 1995.

203. Hargrove GM, Dufresne J, Whiteside C, et al: Diabetes mellitus increases endothelin-1 gene transcription in rat kidney. Kidney Int 58:1534–1545, 2000.

204. Shin SJ, Lee YJ, Lin SR, et al: Decrease of renal endothelin 1 content and gene expression in diabetic rats with moderate hyperglycemia. Nephron 70:486–493, 1995.

205. Takahashi K, Suda K, Lam HC, et al: Endothelin-like immunoreactivity in rat models of diabetes mellitus. J Endocrinol 130:123–127, 1991.

206. Hocher B, Lun A, Priem F, et al: Renal endothelin system in diabetes: Comparison of angiotensin-converting enzyme inhibition and endothelin-A antagonism. J Cardiovasc Pharmacol 31(Suppl 1):492–495, 1998.

207. Hocher B, Schwarz A, Reinbacher D, et al: Effects of endothelin receptor antagonists on the progression of diabetic nephropathy. Nephron 87:161–169, 2001.

208. Cosenzi A, Bernobich E, Trevisan R, et al: Nephroprotective effect of bosentan in diabetic rats. J Cardiovasc Pharmacol 42:752–756, 2003.

209. Ding SS, Qiu C, Hess P, et al: Chronic endothelin receptor blockade prevents both early hyperfiltration and late overt diabetic nephropathy in the rat. J Cardiovasc Pharmacol 42:48–54, 2003.

210. Yao J, Morioka T, Li B, Oite T: Endothelin is a potent inhibitor of matrix metalloproteinase-2 secretion and activation in rat mesangial cells. Am J Physiol Renal Physiol 280:F628–F635, 2001.

211. Kone BC, Baylis C: Biosynthesis and homeostatic roles of nitric oxide in the normal kidney. Am J Physiol 272:F561–F578, 1997.

212. Komers R, Anderson S: Paradoxes of nitric oxide in the diabetic kidney. Am J Physiol Renal Physiol 284:F1121–F1137, 2003.

213. Noh H, Ha H, Yu MR, et al: High glucose increases inducible NO production in cultured rat mesangial cells. Possible role in fibronectin production. Nephron 90:78–85, 2002.

214. De Vriese AS, Stoenoiu MS, Elger M, et al: Diabetes-induced microvascular dysfunction in the hydronephrotic kidney: Role of nitric oxide. Kidney Int 60:202–210, 2001.

215. Schwartz D, Schwartz IF, Blantz RC: An analysis of renal nitric oxide contribution to hyperfiltration in diabetic rats. J Lab Clin Med 137:107–114, 2001.

216. Kiff RJ, Gardiner SM, Compton AM, Bennett T: The effects of endothelin-1 and NG-nitro-L-arginine methyl ester on regional haemodynamics in conscious rats with streptozotocin-induced diabetes mellitus. Br J Pharmacol 103:1321–1326, 1991.

217. Komers R, Lindsley JN, Oyama TT, et al: Role of neuronal nitric oxide synthase (NOS1) in the pathogenesis of renal hemodynamic changes in diabetes. Am J Physiol Renal Physiol 279:F573–F583, 2000.

218. Zatz R, Dunn BR, Meyer T, et al: Prevention of diabetic glomerulopathy by pharmacological amelioration of glomerular capillary hypertension. J Clin Invest 77:1925–1930, 1986.

219. Lewis EJ, Hunsicker LG, Bain RP, Rohde RD: The effect of angiotensin-converting-enzyme inhibition on diabetic nephropathy. The Collaborative Study Group. N Engl J Med 329:1456–1462, 1993.

220. Lewis EJ, Hunsicker LG, Clarke WR, et al: Renoprotective effect of the angiotensin-receptor antagonist irbesartan in patients with nephropathy due to type 2 diabetes. N Engl J Med 345:851–860, 2001.

221. Brenner BM, Cooper ME, de Zeeuw D, et al: Effects of losartan on renal and cardiovascular outcomes in patients with type 2 diabetes and nephropathy. N Engl J Med 345:861–869, 2001.

222. Parving HH, Lehnert H, Brochner-Mortensen J, et al: The effect of irbesartan on the development of diabetic nephropathy in patients with type 2 diabetes. N Engl J Med 345:870–878, 2001.

223. Vidotti DB, Casarini DE, Cristovam PC, et al: High glucose concentration stimulates intracellular renin activity and angiotensin II generation in rat mesangial cells. Am J Physiol Renal Physiol 286:F1039–F1045, 2004.

224. Hsieh TJ, Fustier P, Zhang SL, et al: High glucose stimulates angiotensinogen gene expression and cell hypertrophy via activation of the hexosamine biosynthesis pathway in rat kidney proximal tubular cells. Endocrinology 144:4338–4349, 2003.

225. Zimpelmann J, Kumar D, Levine DZ, et al: Early diabetes mellitus stimulates proximal tubule renin mRNA expression in the rat. Kidney Int 58:2320–2330, 2000.

226. Burns KD: Angiotensin II and its receptors in the diabetic kidney. Am J Kidney Dis 36:449–467, 2000.

227. Ballermann BJ, Skorecki KL, Brenner BM: Reduced glomerular angiotensin II receptor density in early untreated diabetes mellitus in the rat. Am J Physiol 247:F110–F116, 1984.

228. Cheng HF, Burns KD, Harris RC: Reduced proximal tubule angiotensin II receptor expression in streptozotocin-induced diabetes mellitus. Kidney Int 46:1603–1610, 1994.

229. Wehbi GJ, Zimpelmann J, Carey RM, et al: Early streptozotocin-diabetes mellitus downregulates rat kidney AT2 receptors. Am J Physiol Renal Physiol 280:F254–F265, 2001.

230. Anderson S, Meyer TW, Rennke HG, Brenner BM: Control of glomerular hypertension limits glomerular injury in rats with reduced renal mass. J Clin Invest 76:612–619, 1985.

231. Remuzzi A, Gagliardini E, Donadoni C, et al: Effect of angiotensin II antagonism on the regression of kidney disease in the rat. Kidney Int 62:885–894, 2002.

232. Noda M, Matsuo T, Nagano-Tsuge H, et al: Involvement of angiotensin II in progression of renal injury in rats with genetic non-insulin-dependent diabetes mellitus (Wistar fatty rats). Jpn J Pharmacol 85:416–422, 2001.

233. Nankervis A, Nicholls K, Kilmartin G, et al: Effects of perindopril on renal histomorphometry in diabetic subjects with microalbuminuria: A 3-year placebo-controlled biopsy study. Metabolism 47:12–15, 1998.

234. Chan JC, Ko GT, Leung DH, et al: Long-term effects of angiotensin-converting enzyme inhibition and metabolic control in hypertensive type 2 diabetic patients. Kidney Int 57:590–600, 2000.

235. Rodby RA, Rohde RD, Clarke WR, et al: The Irbesartan Type II Diabetic Nephropathy Trial: Study design and baseline patient characteristics. For the Collaborative Study Group. Nephrol Dial Transplant 15:487–497, 2000.

236. Mizuno M, Sada T, Kato M, Koike H: Renoprotective effects of blockade of angiotensin II AT1 receptors in an animal model of type 2 diabetes. Hypertens Res 25:271–278, 2002.

237. Carey RM: Update on the role of the AT2 receptor. Curr Opin Nephrol Hypertens 14:67–71, 2005.

238. Bortz JD, Rotwein P, DeVol D, et al: Focal expression of insulin-like growth factor I in rat kidney collecting duct. J Cell Biol 107:811–819, 1988.

239. Flyvbjerg A, Schrijvers BF, De Vriese AS, et al: Compensatory glomerular growth after unilateral nephrectomy is VEGF dependent. Am J Physiol Endocrinol Metab 283:E362–E366, 2002.

240. Schrijvers BF, Rasch R, Tilton RG, Flyvbjerg A: High protein-induced glomerular hypertrophy is vascular endothelial growth factor-dependent. Kidney Int 61:1600–1604, 2002.

241. Sayed-Ahmed N, Besbas N, Mundy J, et al: Upregulation of epidermal growth factor and its receptor in the kidneys of rats with streptozotocin-induced diabetes. Exp Nephrol 4:330–339, 1996.

242. Rall LB, Scott J, Bell GI, et al: Mouse prepro-epidermal growth factor synthesis by the kidney and other tissues. Nature 313:228–231, 1985.

243. Lee YJ, Shin SJ, Lin SR, et al: Increased expression of heparin binding epidermal growth-factor-like growth factor mRNA in the kidney of streptozotocin-induced diabetic rats. Biochem Biophys Res Commun 207:216–222, 1995.

244. Sakai M, Tsukada T, Harris RC: Oxidant stress activates AP-1 and heparin-binding epidermal growth factor-like growth factor transcription in renal epithelial cells. Exp Nephrol 9:28–39, 2001.

245. Fava S, Hattersley AT: The role of genetic susceptibility in diabetic nephropathy: Evidence from family studies. Nephrol Dial Transplant 17:1543–1546, 2002.

246. Seaquist ER, Goetz FC, Rich S, Barbosa J: Familial clustering of diabetic kidney disease. Evidence for genetic susceptibility to diabetic nephropathy. N Engl J Med 320:1161–1165, 1989.

247. Borch-Johnsen K, Norgaard K, Hommel E, et al: Is diabetic nephropathy an inherited complication? Kidney Int 41:719–722, 1992.

248. The Diabetes Control and Complications Trial Research Group. Clustering of long-term complications in families with diabetes in the diabetes control and complications trial. Diabetes 46:1829–1839, 1997.

249. Pettitt DJ, Saad MF, Bennett PH, et al: Familial predisposition to renal disease in two generations of Pima Indians with type 2 (non-insulin-dependent) diabetes mellitus. Diabetologia 33:438–443, 1990.

250. Fava S, Azzopardi J, Hattersley AT, Watkins PJ: Increased prevalence of proteinuria in diabetic sibs of proteinuric type 2 diabetic subjects. Am J Kidney Dis 35:708–712, 2000.

251. Faronato PP, Maioli M, Tonolo G, et al: Clustering of albumin excretion rate abnormalities in Caucasian patients with NIDDM. The Italian NIDDM Nephropathy Study Group. Diabetologia 40:816–823, 1997.

252. Canani LH, Gerchman F, Gross JL: Familial clustering of diabetic nephropathy in Brazilian type 2 diabetic patients. Diabetes 48:909–913, 1999.

253. Vijay V, Snehalatha C, Shina K, et al: Familial aggregation of diabetic kidney disease in type 2 diabetes in south India. Diabetes Res Clin Pract 43:167–171, 1999.

254. Roglic G, Colhoun HM, Stevens LK, et al: Parental history of hypertension and parental history of diabetes and microvascular complications in insulin-dependent diabetes mellitus: The EURODIAB IDDM Complications Study. Diabetes Med 15:418–426, 1998.

255. Canani LH, Gerchman F, Gross JL: Increased familial history of arterial hypertension coronary heart disease and renal disease in Brazilian type 2 diabetic patients with diabetic nephropathy. Diabetes Care 21:1545–1550, 1998.

256. Jacobsen P, Rossing P, Tarnow L, et al: Birth weight—A risk factor for progression in diabetic nephropathy? J Intern Med 253:343–350, 2003.

257. Keller G, Zimmer G, Mall G, et al: Nephron number in patients with primary hypertension. N Engl J Med 348:101–108, 2003.

258. Lei HH, Perneger TV, Klag MJ, et al: Familial aggregation of renal disease in a population-based case-control study. J Am Soc Nephrol 9:1270–1276, 1998.

259. Fava S, Azzopardi J, Ellard S, Hattersley AT: ACE gene polymorphism as a prognostic indicator in patients with type 2 diabetes and established renal disease. Diabetes Care 24:2115–2120, 2001.

260. Viswanathan V, Zhu Y, Bala K, et al: Association between ACE gene polymorphism and diabetic nephropathy in South Indian patients. JOP 2:83–87, 2001.

261. Solini A, Dalla Vestra M, Saller A, et al: The angiotensin-converting enzyme DD genotype is associated with glomerulopathy lesions in type 2 diabetes. Diabetes 51:251–255, 2002.

262. Lovati E, Richard A, Frey BM, et al: Genetic polymorphisms of the renin-angiotensin-aldosterone system in end-stage renal disease. Kidney Int 60:46–54, 2001.

263. Wu S, Xiang K, Zheng T, et al: Relationship between the renin-angiotensin system genes and diabetic nephropathy in the Chinese. Chin Med J (Engl) 113:437–441, 2000.

264. Hsieh MC, Lin SR, Hsieh TJ, et al: Increased frequency of angiotensin-converting enzyme DD genotype in patients with type 2 diabetes in Taiwan. Nephrol Dial Transplant 15:1008–1013, 2000.

265. Ha SK, Park HC, Park HS, et al: ACE gene polymorphism and progression of diabetic nephropathy in Korean type 2 diabetic patients: Effect of ACE gene DD on the progression of diabetic nephropathy. Am J Kidney Dis 41:943–949, 2003.

266. Gohda T, Makita Y, Shike T, et al: Association of the DD genotype and development of Japanese type 2 diabetic nephropathy. Clin Nephrol 56:475–480, 2001.

267. Hadjadj S, Belloum R, Bouhanick B, et al: Prognostic value of angiotensin-I converting enzyme I/D polymorphism for nephropathy in type 1 diabetes mellitus: A prospective study. J Am Soc Nephrol 12:541–549, 2001.

268. Jacobsen P, Tarnow L, Carstensen B, et al: Genetic variation in the renin-angiotensin system and progression of diabetic nephropathy. J Am Soc Nephrol 14:2843–2850, 2003.

269. Rudberg S, Rasmussen LM, Bangstad HJ, Osterby R: Influence of insertion/deletion polymorphism in the ACE-I gene on the progression of diabetic glomerulopathy in type 1 diabetic patients with microalbuminuria. Diabetes Care 23:544–548, 2000.

270. Chang HR, Cheng CH, Shu KH, et al: Study of the polymorphism of angiotensinogen angiotensin-converting enzyme and angiotensin receptor in type II diabetes with end-stage renal disease in Taiwan. J Chin Med Assoc 66:51–56, 2003.

271. Orchard TJ, Chang YF, Ferrell RE, et al: Nephropathy in type 1 diabetes: A manifestation of insulin resistance and multiple genetic susceptibilities? Further evidence from the Pittsburgh Epidemiology of Diabetes Complication Study. Kidney Int 62:963–970, 2002.

272. Fradin S, Goulet-Salmon B, Chantepie M, et al: Relationship between polymorphisms in the renin-angiotensin system and nephropathy in type 2 diabetic patients. Diabetes Metab 28:27–32, 2002.

273. Tarnow L, Kjeld T, Knudsen E, et al: Lack of synergism between long-term poor glycaemic control and three gene polymorphisms of the renin angiotensin system on risk of developing diabetic nephropathy in type I diabetic patients. Diabetologia 43:794–799, 2000.

274. Crook ED, Genous L, Oliver B: Angiotensin-converting enzyme genotype in blacks with diabetic nephropathy: Effects on risk of diabetes and its complications. J Invest Med 51:360–365, 2003.

275. Rogus JJ, Moczulski D, Freire MB, et al: Diabetic nephropathy is associated with AGT polymorphism T235: Results of a family-based study. Hypertension 31:627–631, 1998.

276. Wang J, Zhu X, Yang L, et al: Relationship between angiotensinogen gene M235T variant with diabetic nephropathy in Chinese NIDDM. Chin Med J (Engl) 112:797–800, 1999.

277. Oue T, Namba M, Nakajima H, et al: Risk factors for the progression of microalbuminuria in Japanese type 2 diabetic patients—A 10 year follow-up study. Diabetes Res Clin Pract 46:47–55, 1999.

278. Tomino Y, Makita Y, Shike T, et al: Relationship between polymorphism in the angiotensinogen angiotensin-converting enzyme or angiotensin II receptor and renal progression in Japanese NIDDM patients. Nephron 82:139–144, 1999.

279. Miller JA, Thai K, Scholey JW: Angiotensin II type 1 receptor gene polymorphism and the response to hyperglycemia in early type 1 diabetes. Diabetes 49:1585–1589, 2000.

280. Deinum J, Tarnow L, van Gool JM, et al: Plasma renin and prorenin and renin gene variation in patients with insulin-dependent diabetes mellitus and nephropathy. Nephrol Dial Transplant 14:1904–1911, 1999.

281. Moczulski DK, Scott L, Antonellis A, et al: Aldose reductase gene polymorphisms and susceptibility to diabetic nephropathy in type 1 diabetes mellitus. Diabet Med 17:111–118, 2000.

282. Park HK, Ahn CW, Lee GT, et al: (AC)(n) polymorphism of aldose reductase gene and diabetic microvascular complications in type 2 diabetes mellitus. Diabetes Res Clin Pract 55:151–157, 2002.

283. Zanchi A, Moczulski DK, Hanna LS, et al: Risk of advanced diabetic nephropathy in type 1 diabetes is associated with endothelial nitric oxide synthase gene polymorphism. Kidney Int 57:405–413, 2000.

284. Frost D, Chitu J, Meyer M, et al: Endothelial nitric oxide synthase (ecNOS) 4 a/b gene polymorphism and carotid artery intima-media thickness in type-1 diabetic patients. Exp Clin Endocrinol Diabetes 111:12–15, 2003.

285. Suzuki T, Okumura K, Sone T, et al: The Glu298Asp polymorphism in endothelial nitric oxide synthase gene is associated with coronary in-stent restenosis. Int J Cardiol 86:71–76, 2002.

286. Nagase S, Suzuki H, Wang Y, et al: Association of ecNOS gene polymorphisms with end stage renal diseases. Mol Cell Biochem 244:113–118, 2003.

287. Shin Shin Y, Baek SH, Chang KY, et al: Relations between eNOS Glu298Asp polymorphism and progression of diabetic nephropathy. Diabetes Res Clin Pract 65:257–265, 2004.

288. Neugebauer S, Baba T, Watanabe T: Association of the nitric oxide synthase gene polymorphism with an increased risk for progression to diabetic nephropathy in type 2 diabetes. Diabetes 49:500–503, 2000.

289. Shimizu T, Onuma T, Kawamori R, et al: Endothelial nitric oxide synthase gene and the development of diabetic nephropathy. Diabetes Res Clin Pract 58:179–185, 2002.

290. Araki S, Koya D, Makiishi T, et al: APOE polymorphism and the progression of diabetic nephropathy in Japanese subjects with type 2 diabetes: Results of a prospective observational follow-up study. Diabetes Care 26:2416–2420, 2003.

291. Eto M, Saito M, Okada M, et al: Apolipoprotein E genetic polymorphism remnant lipoproteins and nephropathy in type 2 diabetic patients. Am J Kidney Dis 40:243–251, 2002.

292. Imperatore G, Hanson RL, Pettitt DJ, et al: Sib-pair linkage analysis for susceptibility genes for microvascular complications among Pima Indians with type 2 diabetes. Pima Diabetes Genes Group. Diabetes 47:821–830, 1998.

293. Bowden DW, Colicigno CJ, Langefeld CD, et al: A genome scan for diabetic nephropathy in African Americans. Kidney Int 66:1517–1526, 2004.

294. Imperatore G, Knowler WC, Nelson RG, Hanson RL: Genetics of diabetic nephropathy in the Pima Indians. Curr Diabetes Rep 1:275–281, 2001.

295. Creager MA, Luscher TF, Cosentino F, Beckman JA: Diabetes and vascular disease: Pathophysiology clinical consequences and medical therapy: Part I. Circulation 108:1527–1532, 2003.

296. Singleton JR, Smith AG, Russell JW, Feldman EL: Microvascular complications of impaired glucose tolerance. Diabetes 52:2867–2873, 2003.

297. Mann GE, Yudilevich DL, Sobrevia L: Regulation of amino acid and glucose transporters in endothelial and smooth muscle cells. Physiol Rev 83:183–252, 2003.

298. Knott RM, Robertson M, Muckersie E, Forrester JV: Regulation of glucose transporters (GLUT-1 and GLUT-3) in human retinal endothelial cells. Biochem J 318(Pt 1):313–317, 1996.

299. Nishikawa T, Edelstein D, Brownlee M: The missing link: A single unifying mechanism for diabetic complications. Kidney Int Suppl 77:26–30, 2000.

300. Nishikawa T, Edelstein D, Du XL, et al: Normalizing mitochondrial superoxide production blocks three pathways of hyperglycaemic damage. Nature 404:787–790, 2000.

301. Topper JN, Cai J, Falb D, Gimbrone MA Jr: Identification of vascular endothelial genes differentially responsive to fluid mechanical stimuli: Cyclooxygenase-2 manganese superoxide dismutase and endothelial cell nitric oxide synthase are

selectively up-regulated by steady laminar shear stress. Proc Natl Acad Sci U S A 93:10417–10422, 1996.

302. Cosentino F, Eto M, De Paolis P, et al: High glucose causes upregulation of cyclooxygenase-2 and alters prostanoid profile in human endothelial cells: Role of protein kinase C and reactive oxygen species. Circulation 107:1017–1023, 2003.

303. Egan KM, Lawson JA, Fries S, et al: COX-2-derived prostacyclin confers atheroprotection on female mice. Science 306:1954–1957, 2004.

304. Kawashima S, Yokoyama M: Dysfunction of endothelial nitric oxide synthase and atherosclerosis. Arterioscler Thromb Vasc Biol 24:998–1005, 2004.

305. Vasquez-Vivar J, Martasek P, Whitsett J, et al: The ratio between tetrahydrobiopterin and oxidized tetrahydrobiopterin analogues controls superoxide release from endothelial nitric oxide synthase: An EPR spin trapping study. Biochem J 362:733–739, 2002.

306. Vasquez-Vivar J, Kalyanaraman B, Martasek P: The role of tetrahydrobiopterin in superoxide generation from eNOS: Enzymology and physiological implications. Free Radic Res 37:121–127, 2003.

307. Channon K: Tetrahydrobiopterin regulator of endothelial nitric oxide synthase in vascular disease. Trends Cardiovasc Med 14:323–327, 2004.

308. Ozaki M, Kawashima S, Yamashita T, et al: Overexpression of endothelial nitric oxide synthase accelerates atherosclerotic lesion formation in apoE-deficient mice. J Clin Invest 110:331–340, 2002.

309. Chen J, Kuhlencordt PJ, Astern J, et al: Hypertension does not account for the accelerated atherosclerosis and development of aneurysms in male apolipoprotein E/endothelial nitric oxide synthase double knockout mice. Circulation 104:2391–2394, 2001.

310. Meininger CJ, Marinos RS, Hatakeyama K, et al: Impaired nitric oxide production in coronary endothelial cells of the spontaneously diabetic BB rat is due to tetrahydrobiopterin deficiency. Biochem J 349:353–356, 2000.

311. Endemann DH, Schiffrin EL: Endothelial dysfunction. J Am Soc Nephrol 15:1983–1992, 2004.

312. De Vriese AS, Verbeuren TJ, Van de Voorde J, et al: Endothelial dysfunction in diabetes. Br J Pharmacol 130:963–974, 2000.

313. Beckman JA, Goldfine AB, Gordon MB, et al: Oral antioxidant therapy improves endothelial function in type 1 but not type 2 diabetes mellitus. Am J Physiol Heart Circ Physiol 285:H2392–H2398, 2003.

314. Malik RA, Schofield IJ, Izzard A, et al: Effects of angiotensin type-1 receptor antagonism on small artery function in patients with type 2 diabetes mellitus. Hypertension 45:264–269, 2005.

315. Schofield I, Malik R, Izzard A, et al: Vascular structural and functional changes in type 2 diabetes mellitus: Evidence for the roles of abnormal myogenic responsiveness and dyslipidemia. Circulation 106:3037–3043, 2002.

316. Cusi K, Maezono K, Osman A, et al: Insulin resistance differentially affects the PI 3-kinase- and MAP kinase-mediated signaling in human muscle. J Clin Invest 105:311–320, 2000.

317. Montagnani M, Ravichandran LV, Chen H, et al: Insulin receptor substrate-1 and phosphoinositide-dependent kinase-1 are required for insulin-stimulated production of nitric oxide in endothelial cells. Mol Endocrinol 16:1931–1942, 2002.

318. Larger E, Marre M, Corvol P, Gasc JM: Hyperglycemia-induced defects in angiogenesis in the chicken chorioallantoic membrane model. Diabetes 53:752–761, 2004.

319. Chu S, Bohlen HG: High concentration of glucose inhibits glomerular endothelial eNOS through a PKC mechanism. Am J Physiol Renal Physiol 287:F384–F392, 2004.

320. Veelken R, Hilgers KF, Hartner A, et al: Nitric oxide synthase isoforms and glomerular hyperfiltration in early diabetic nephropathy. J Am Soc Nephrol 11:71–79, 2000.

321. Schnackenberg CG: Oxygen radicals in cardiovascular-renal disease. Curr Opin Pharmacol 2:121–125, 2002.

322. Welch WJ, Blau J, Xie H, et al: Angiotensin-induced defects in renal oxygenation: Role of oxidative stress. Am J Physiol Heart Circ Physiol 288:H22–H28, 2005.

323. Schnackenberg CG, Wilcox CS: The SOD mimetic tempol restores vasodilation in afferent arterioles of experimental diabetes. Kidney Int 59:1859–1864, 2001.

324. Chavers BM, Bilous RW, Ellis EN, et al: Glomerular lesions and urinary albumin excretion in type I diabetes without overt proteinuria [see comments]. N Engl J Med 320:966–970, 1989.

325. Kimmelstiel P, Wilson C: Intercapillary lesions in the glomeruli of kidney. Am J Pathol 12:83–97, 1936.

326. Nerlich A, Schleicher E: Immunohistochemical localization of extracellular matrix components in human diabetic glomerular lesions. Am J Pathol 139:889–899, 1991.

327. Heilig CW, Liu Y, England RL, et al: D-glucose stimulates mesangial cell GLUT1 expression and basal and IGF-I-sensitive glucose uptake in rat mesangial cells: Implications for diabetic nephropathy. Diabetes 46:1030–1039, 1997.

328. Wada J, Makino H, Kanwar YS: Gene expression and identification of gene therapy targets in diabetic nephropathy. Kidney Int Suppl 61(Suppl 1):73–78, 2002.

329. Kikkawa R, Umemura K, Haneda M, et al: Evidence for existence of polyol pathway in cultured rat mesangial cells. Diabetes 36:240–243, 1987.

330. Kikkawa R, Umemura K, Haneda M, et al: Identification and characterization of aldose reductase in cultured rat mesangial cells. Diabetes 41:1165–1171, 1992.

331. Donnelly SM, Zhou XP, Huang JT, Whiteside CI: Prevention of early glomerulopathy with tolrestat in the streptozotocin-induced diabetic rat. Biochem Cell Biol 74:355–362, 1996.

332. Fukami K, Ueda S, Yamagishi S, et al: AGEs activate mesangial TGF-beta-Smad signaling via an angiotensin II type I receptor interaction. Kidney Int 66:2137–2147, 2004.

333. Brizzi MF, Dentelli P, Rosso A, et al: RAGE- and TGF-beta receptor-mediated signals converge on STAT5 and p21waf to control cell-cycle progression of mesangial cells: A possible role in the development and progression of diabetic nephropathy. FASEB J 18:1249–1251, 2004.

334. Kim HW, Kim BC, Song CY, et al: Heterozygous mice for TGF-betaIIR gene are resistant to the progression of streptozotocin-induced diabetic nephropathy. Kidney Int 66:1859–1865, 2004.

335. Park IS, Kiyomoto H, Abboud SL, Abboud HE: Expression of transforming growth factor-beta and type IV collagen in early streptozotocin-induced diabetes. Diabetes 46:473–480, 1997.

336. Abe H, Matsubara T, Iehara N, et al: Type IV collagen is transcriptionally regulated by Smad1 under advanced glycation end product (AGE) stimulation J Biol Chem 279:14201–14206, 2004.

337. Oh SP, Seki T, Goss KA, et al: Activin receptor-like kinase 1 modulates transforming growth factor-beta 1 signaling in the regulation of angiogenesis. Proc Natl Acad Sci U S A 97:2626–2631, 2000.

338. Suzaki Y, Yoshizumi M, Kagami S, et al: BMK1 is activated in glomeruli of diabetic rats and in mesangial cells by high glucose conditions. Kidney Int 65:1749–1760, 2004.

339. Yamamoto Y, Maeshima Y, Kitayama H, et al: Tumstatin peptide an inhibitor of angiogenesis prevents glomerular hypertrophy in the early stage of diabetic nephropathy. Diabetes 53:1831–1840, 2004.

340. Toyoda M, Suzuki D, Umezono T, et al: Expression of human nephrin mRNA in diabetic nephropathy. Nephrol Dial Transplant 19:380–385, 2004.

341. Aaltonen P, Luimula P, Astrom E, et al: Changes in the expression of nephrin gene and protein in experimental diabetic nephropathy. Lab Invest 81:1185–1190, 2001.

342. Bonnet F, Cooper ME, Kawachi H, et al: Irbesartan normalises the deficiency in glomerular nephrin expression in a model of diabetes and hypertension. Diabetologia 44:874–877, 2001.

343. Doublier S, Salvidio G, Lupia E, et al: Nephrin expression is reduced in human diabetic nephropathy: Evidence for a distinct role for glycated albumin and angiotensin II. Diabetes 52:1023–1030, 2003.

344. Forbes JM, Bonnet F, Russo LM, et al: Modulation of nephrin in the diabetic kidney: Association with systemic hypertension and increasing albuminuria. J Hypertens 20:985–992, 2002.

345. Meyer TW, Bennett PH, Nelson RG: Podocyte number predicts long-term urinary albumin excretion in Pima Indians with type II diabetes and microalbuminuria. Diabetologia 42:1341–1344, 1999.

346. Dalla Vestra M, Masiero A, Roiter AM, et al: Is podocyte injury relevant in diabetic nephropathy? Studies in patients with type 2 diabetes. Diabetes 52:1031–1035, 2003.

347. Steffes MW, Schmidt D, McCrery R, Basgen JM: Glomerular cell number in normal subjects and in type 1 diabetic patients. Kidney Int 59:2104–2113, 2001.

348. White KE, Bilous RW: Structural alterations to the podocyte are related to proteinuria in type 2 diabetic patients. Nephrol Dial Transplant 19:1437–1440, 2004.

349. Pagtalunan ME, Miller PL, Jumping-Eagle S, et al: Podocyte loss and progressive glomerular injury in type II diabetes. J Clin Invest 99:342–348, 1997.

350. White KE, Bilous RW, Marshall SM, et al: Podocyte number in normotensive type 1 diabetic patients with albuminuria. Diabetes 51:3083–3089, 2002.

351. Seyer-Hansen K: Renal hypertrophy in experimental diabetes mellitus. Kidney Int 23:643–646, 1983.

352. Preisig P: What makes cells grow larger and how do they do it? Renal hypertrophy revisited. Exp Nephrol 7:273–283, 1999.

353. Kuan CJ, al-Douahji M, Shankland SJ: The cyclin kinase inhibitor p21WAF1 CIP1 is increased in experimental diabetic nephropathy: potential role in glomerular hypertrophy. J Am Soc Nephrol 9:986–993, 1998.

354. Al-Douahji M, Brugarolas J, Brown PA, et al: The cyclin kinase inhibitor p21WAF1/CIP1 is required for glomerular hypertrophy in experimental diabetic nephropathy. Kidney Int 56:1691–1699, 1999.

355. Wolf G, Schroeder R, Thaiss F, et al: Glomerular expression of p27Kip1 in diabetic db/db mouse: Role of hyperglycemia. Kidney Int 53:869–879, 1998.

356. Wolf G, Reinking R, Zahner G, et al: Erk 12 phosphorylates p27(Kip1): Functional evidence for a role in high glucose-induced hypertrophy of mesangial cells. Diabetologia 46:1090–1099, 2003.

357. Huang HC, Preisig PA: G1 kinases and transforming growth factor-beta signaling are associated with a growth pattern switch in diabetes-induced renal growth. Kidney Int 58:162–172, 2000.

358. Hostetter TH: Hypertrophy and hyperfunction of the diabetic kidney. J Clin Invest 107:161–162, 2001.

359. Hostetter TH: Progression of renal disease and renal hypertrophy. Annu Rev Physiol 57:263–278, 1995.

360. Risdon RA, Sloper JC, De Wardener HE: Relationship between renal function and histological changes found in renal-biopsy specimens from patients with persistent glomerular nephritis. Lancet 2:363–366, 1968.

361. Striker GE, Schainuck LI, Cutler RE, Benditt EP: Structural-functional correlations in renal disease I A method for assaying and classifying histopathologic changes in renal disease. Human Pathol 1:615–630, 1970.

362. Mackensen-Haen S, Bader R, Grund KE, Bohle A: Correlations between renal cortical interstitial fibrosis atrophy of the proximal tubules and impairment of the glomerular filtration rate. Clin Nephrol 15:167–171, 1981.

363. Schainuck LI, Striker GE, Cutler RE, Benditt EP: Structural-functional correlations in renal disease II. The correlations. Human Pathol 1:631–641, 1970.

364. Nath KA: Tubulointerstitial changes as a major determinant in the progression of renal damage. Am J Kidney Dis 20:1–17, 1992.

365. Hruby Z, Smolska D, Filipowski H, et al: The importance of tubulointerstitial injury in the early phase of primary glomerular disease. J Intern Med 243:215–222, 1998.

366. Walls J: Relationship between proteinuria and progressive renal disease Am J Kidney Dis 37(Suppl):13–16, 2001.

367. Mauer SM, Steffes MW, Ellis EN, et al: Structural-functional relationships in diabetic nephropathy. J Clin Invest 74:1143–1155, 1984.

368. Bohle A, Wehrmann M, Bogenschutz O, et al: The pathogenesis of chronic renal failure in diabetic nephropathy. Investigation of 488 cases of diabetic glomerulosclerosis. Pathol Res Pract 187:251–259, 1991.

369. Abbate M, Zoja C, Rottoli D, et al: Antiproteinuric therapy while preventing the abnormal protein traffic in proximal tubule abrogates protein- and complement-dependent interstitial inflammation in experimental renal disease. J Am Soc Nephrol 10:804–813, 1999.

370. Abbate M, Zoja C, Rottoli D, et al: Proximal tubular cells promote fibrogenesis by TGF-beta1-mediated induction of peritubular myofibroblasts. Kidney Int 61:2066–2077, 2002.

371. Donadelli R, Abbate M, Zanchi C, et al: Protein traffic activates NF-κB gene signaling and promotes MCP-1-dependent interstitial inflammation. Am J Kidney Dis 36:1226–1241, 2000.

372. Morigi M, Macconi D, Zoja C, et al: Protein overload-induced NF-kappaB activation in proximal tubular cells requires $H^2(2)$ through a PKC-dependent pathway. J Am Soc Nephrol 13:1179–1189, 2002.

373. Zoja C, Donadelli R, Colleoni S, et al: Protein overload stimulates RANTES production by proximal tubular cells depending on NF-kappa B activation. Kidney Int 53:1608–1615, 1998.

374. Shimizu H, Maruyama S, Yuzawa Y, et al: Anti-monocyte chemoattractant protein-1 gene therapy attenuates renal injury induced by protein-overload proteinuria. J Am Soc Nephrol 14:1496–1505, 2003.

375. Nangaku M, Pippin J, Couser WG: Complement membrane attack complex (C5b-9) mediates interstitial disease in experimental nephrotic syndrome. J Am Soc Nephrol 10:2323–2331, 1999.

376. Eppel GA, Osicka TM, Pratt LM, et al: The return of glomerular filtered albumin to the rat renal vein—The albumin retrieval pathway. Renal Fail 23:347–363, 2001.

377. Brunskill NJ: Molecular interactions between albumin and proximal tubular cells. Exp Nephrol 6:491–495, 1998.

378. Brunskill NJ: Albumin and proximal tubular cells—Beyond endocytosis. Nephrol Dial Transplant 15:1732–1734, 2000.

379. Olbricht CJ, Cannon JK, Garg LC, Tisher CC: Activities of cathepsins B and L in isolated nephron segments from proteinuric and nonproteinuric rats. Am J Physiol 250:F1055–F1062, 1986.

380. Iglesias J, Levine JS: Albuminuria and renal injury—Beware of proteins bearing gifts. Nephrol Dial Transplant 16:215–218, 2001.

381. Alfrey AC: Toxicity of tubule fluid iron in the nephrotic syndrome. Am J Physiol 263:F637–F641, 1992.

382. Kees-Folts D, Sadow JL, Schreiner GF: Tubular catabolism of albumin is associated with the release of an inflammatory lipid. Kidney Int 45:1697–1709, 1994.

383. Wang SN, Lapage J, Hirschberg R: Glomerular ultrafiltration and apical tubular action of IGF-I TGF-beta and HGF in nephrotic syndrome. Kidney Int 56:1247–1251, 1999.

384. Hirschberg R, Wang S: Proteinuria and growth factors in the development of tubulointerstitial injury and scarring in kidney disease. Curr Opin Nephrol Hypertens 14:43–52, 2005.

385. Nath KA, Hostetter MK, Hostetter TH: Pathophysiology of chronic tubulo-interstitial disease in rats. Interactions of dietary acid load ammonia and complement component C3. J Clin Invest 76:667–675, 1985.

386. Nangaku M, Pippin J, Couser WG: C6 mediates chronic progression of tubulointerstitial damage in rats with remnant kidneys. J Am Soc Nephrol 13:928–936, 2002.

387. Baker PJ, Adler S, Yang Y, Couser WG: Complement activation by heat-killed human kidney cells: Formation activity and stabilization of cell-bound C3 convertases. J Immunol 133:877–881, 1984.

Chapter 23

Pathogenesis of HIV-Associated Nephropathy

Michael J. Ross and Paul E. Klotman

In 1984, 3 years after the first reported cases of acquired immunodeficiency syndrome (AIDS), clinicians reported the occurrence of a renal syndrome characterized by proteinuria and progressive renal failure. The most common pathologic abnormality in these patients was focal segmental glomerulosclerosis.[1] Since this original description of human immunodeficiency virus (HIV)–associated nephropathy (HIVAN), this disease has become recognized as the most common cause of chronic renal failure in HIV-1 seropositive patients and has become the third most common cause of end-stage renal disease (ESRD) in blacks aged 20 through 64. Despite advances in the treatment of patients with HIV/AIDS,[2] the incidence of HIVAN has not decreased even with the advent of highly active antiretroviral treatment (HAART).[3] However, major advances have been made in our understanding of the pathogenesis of HIVAN.

HISTOPATHOLOGIC ABNORMALITIES IN HIVAN

Because nearly 40% of HIV-seropositive patients suspected to have HIVAN by clinical criteria will have other renal diseases found at biopsy, renal biopsy remains necessary to establish the diagnosis of HIVAN. Histopathologic abnormalities in HIVAN affect nearly every region of the kidney, involving glomeruli, tubules, and interstitium. Typical glomerular histopathologic findings in HIVAN include collapsing focal glomerulosclerosis, which may be segmental (FSGS) or global in distribution. Most commonly, the glomerulosclerosis is the collapsing variant, with retraction of the glomerular basement membrane resulting in occlusion of capillary tufts. The podocytes overlying the collapsing glomerulus are usually proliferative and may form a "pseudocrescent" surrounding the glomerulus that may fill the Bowman space (Fig. 23-1A).[4–6] Within glomeruli, endothelial tubuloreticular inclusions (TRIs) had previously been reported to be present in more than 90% of glomeruli. However, since the advent of HAART, the proportion of HIVAN biopsy specimens containing TRIs has decreased. Because the presence of TRIs is thought to be induced by high systemic levels of interferon, it is likely that the decreased prevalence of TRIs in HIVAN reflects lower levels of interferon when HIV-1 replication is suppressed by HAART.[7] Immunofluorescence microscopy in HIVAN is generally nonspecific, with varying degrees of positivity for IgG, IgM, and IgA as well as complement in glomeruli.[5]

Severe tubulointerstitial disease is also present in HIVAN, and the severity is often out of proportion to the degree of glomerulosclerosis. Tubules develop microcystic dilatation, as well as simplification and atrophy of the tubular epithelial cells (Fig. 23-1B). Microcysts are tubules that are dilated at least threefold as compared with normal tubules[5] and may form in any segment of the nephron in HIVAN.[8] Microcyst formation is probably responsible for the marked echogenicity and the increase in renal size that is often noted during ultrasonographic evaluation of patients with HIVAN. Tubular

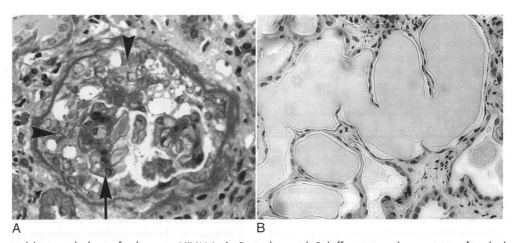

Figure 23-1 Typical histopathologic findings in HIVAN. **A,** Periodic acid–Schiff staining demonstrates focal glomerulosclerosis with collapse of the glomerular tuft (*arrow*) and overlying proliferative podocytes (*arrowheads*). **B,** Hematoxylin and eosin staining reveals tubular microcystic disease, interstitial leukocytic infiltration, and interstitial fibrosis.

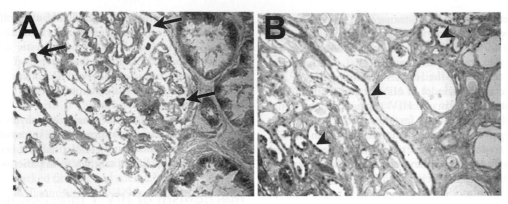

Figure 23-5 Detection of HIV-1 proviral DNA in renal biopsies by in situ DNA PCR in podocytes (**A,** *arrows*) and tubular epithelial cells (**B,** *arrowheads*). (Adapted from Marras D, Bruggeman LA, Gao F, et al: Replication and compartmentalization of HIV-1 in kidney epithelium of patients with HIV-associated nephropathy. Nat Med 8:522, 2002.)

primary RTECs in vitro. They also reported that infection was not inhibited by an anti-CD4 antibody, indicating that viral entry was not CD4 dependent, and they found no evidence that infection was a result of fusion of macrophages with renal epithelial cells.[34]

The distribution of HIV-1 infection in RTECs is striking, with focal tubular involvement. Within infected tubules, however, nearly every cell harbors virus (see Fig. 23-5). Thus, the initial viral infection of a cell within a tubule is a rare event, whereas subsequent spread of the viral infection to other epithelial cells in that tubule is very efficient. It is unclear whether propagation of the virus along the nephron occurs via direct cell-to-cell passage or by release of infectious virus from epithelial cells with subsequent receptor-mediated infection of neighboring cells.

Although HIV-1 can generally be detected in renal epithelial cells in patients with HIVAN, the prevalence of HIV-1 infection in the renal epithelium of seropositive patients without HIVAN has not been well studied.

THE KIDNEY IS A RESERVOIR FOR HIV-1

HIV-1 infection of renal epithelial cells has ramifications beyond the role of the virus in promoting the development of HIVAN. Renal epithelial cells are a reservoir wherein HIV-1 may persist in patients who have no detectable HIV-1 in plasma. In the series reported by Bruggeman et al,[28] 4 of the 21 HIV-1 seropositive patients with renal disease who underwent diagnostic renal biopsy had undetectable HIV-1 in plasma. In each of these patients, HIV-1 RNA was detected in renal epithelial cells. Winston et al reported a patient who developed HIVAN in the setting of acute seroconversion.[35] After treatment with HAART, the patient had clinical and histologic resolution of his renal disease. Despite the dramatic response of the clinical and histopathologic abnormalities of the patient's HIVAN to HAART (Fig. 23-6), HIV-1 RNA expression in the kidney remained unchanged (Fig. 23-7). To further explore this epithelial compartment, Marras et al used laser-capture microdissection followed by PCR to clone HIV-1 gp120 sequences from infected RTECs taken from HIVAN biopsy samples.[29] These gp120 clones were sequenced, along

with those derived from peripheral blood mononuclear cells (PBMCs) from the same patients. These studies resulted in two major findings. First, there was divergence in the gp120 sequences cloned from the renal epithelial cells. Because such sequence divergence occurs as a result of mutations in the viral genome introduced by reverse transcriptase during viral replication, these data indicate that renal epithelial cells are able to support full viral replication in vivo (which had not been shown previously). Second, phylogenetic analysis revealed that the gp120 sequences from kidney clustered separately within the radiation of gp120 sequences from the same patients' PBMCs (Fig. 23-8). These data suggest that the renal epithelium is a reservoir for HIV-1 that is not in equilibrium with the blood compartment and supports the evolution of divergent viral quasispecies.

Thus, the renal epithelium is a reservoir where HIV-1 persists despite "optimal" treatment with HAART and a lack of detectable virus in the plasma. Whether virus from the renal epithelium contributes to rebound of plasma viral loads in patients who had previously been well controlled is unknown. There is also very little known about the ability of antiretroviral medications to achieve therapeutic levels in renal epithelial cells and whether the effects of these medications on the HIV-1 life cycle in renal epithelial cells is similar to that in leukocytes. Future therapeutic strategies that aim to completely eradicate HIV-1 virus from patients will therefore need to address the renal epithelial compartment.

HIV-1 INFECTION INDUCES DISEASE IN THE RENAL EPITHELIUM

Many of the characteristic epithelial phenotypic changes found in HIVAN in vivo are recapitulated by expression of HIV-1 proteins in epithelial cells in vitro. Podocytes from HIV-1 transgenic mice demonstrate increased levels of proliferation and anchorage-independent growth as compared with podocytes from normal mice (Fig. 23-9A). Moreover, the proliferative phenotype is recapitulated by infection of wild-type podocytes with the same HIV-1 construct used to generate the HIV-1 transgenic HIVAN model (Fig. 23-9B).[36] Podocytes that express HIV-1 also become dedifferentiated and have

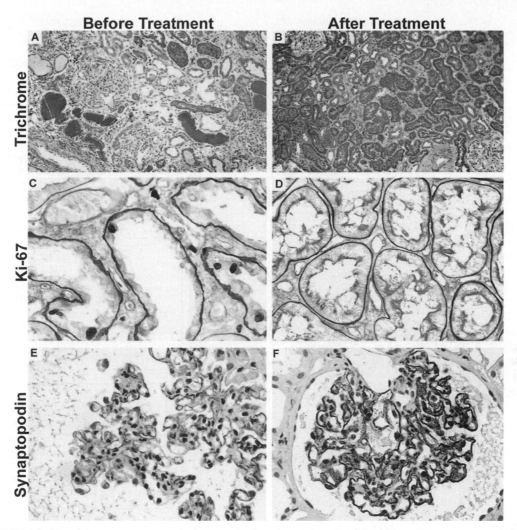

Figure 23-6 HIVAN kidney biopsy specimens before and after the initiation of highly active antiretroviral therapy. Biopsy specimen before treatment (**A**) shows one of three glomeruli with collapsing sclerosis and marked hyperplasia of podocytes. The tubules are separated by edema, mild fibrosis, and patchy interstitial inflammatory infiltrates. Many proximal tubules show degenerative changes, and there are focal tubular microcysts containing large casts. Biopsy specimen after HAART treatment (**B**) shows normal glomeruli and mild focal interstitial fibrosis, with restoration of normal tubular architecture. No tubular microcysts or interstitial inflammation is apparent. In the pretreatment biopsy specimen (**C**) many nuclei in the renal tubular epithelial cells stain for Ki-67, whereas in the biopsy specimen obtained after the initiation of antiretroviral therapy (**D**), a representative field shows no staining for Ki-67. Immunostaining for synaptopodin in the pretreatment biopsy specimen shows weak staining or no staining in the podocytes of a collapsed glomerulus (**E**). There is strong, global positivity for synaptopodin in the podocytes of a representative glomerulus from the biopsy specimen obtained after 3 months of highly active antiretroviral therapy (**F**). (Adapted from Winston JA, Bruggeman LA, Ross MD, et al: Nephropathy and establishment of a renal reservoir of HIV type 1 during primary infection. N Engl J Med 344:1979, 2001.)

reduced expression of the podocyte markers synaptopodin, CALLA, and WT-1.[37] Remarkably, in some patients with HIVAN, viral inhibition by treatment with HAART is able to reverse many of these phenotypic changes (see Fig. 23-6).[35]

RTECs isolated from HIV-1 transgenic mice also demonstrate increased proliferation compared to wild-type RTECs.[38] In contrast to podocytes, in which HIV-1 infection leads to a primarily proliferative response, the RTEC response to HIV-1 expression is more complex. HIV infection of RTECs induces not only the expression of proliferative markers (see Fig. 23-6C) but apoptosis as well (Fig. 23-10).[14,15,34]

WHICH HIV-1 GENES CONTRIBUTE TO HIVAN PATHOGENESIS?

The HIV-1 Viral Genome

The HIV-1 genome encodes 9 genes (Fig. 23-11). Proteolytic processing of polypeptides encoded by these genes results in the generation of 15 proteins during the viral life cycle. Two of the major structural genes, *gag* (encodes matrix, capsid, nucleocapsid, and p6 proteins) and *pol* (encodes reverse transcriptase, protease, RNase H, and integrase) encode 8 of the 15 HIV-1 proteins.[39]

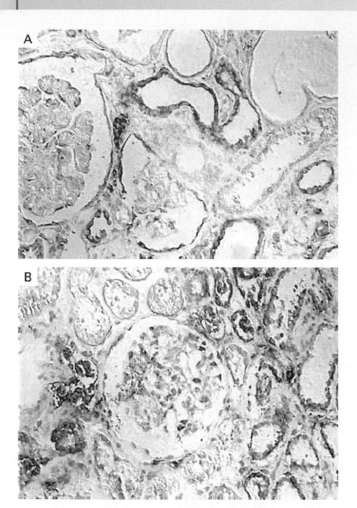

Figure 23-7 HIV-1 RNA in situ hybridization of kidney biopsy specimens obtained before and after the initiation of HAART. The use of an antisense probe generated from the *gag* region demonstrates the presence of HIV-1 RNA in tubular cells and podocytes as well as in interstitial inflammatory cells before (**A**) and after (**B**) the initiation of HAART. (Adapted from Winston JA, Bruggeman LA, Ross MD, et al: Nephropathy and establishment of a renal reservoir of HIV type 1 during primary infection. N Engl J Med 344:1979, 2001.)

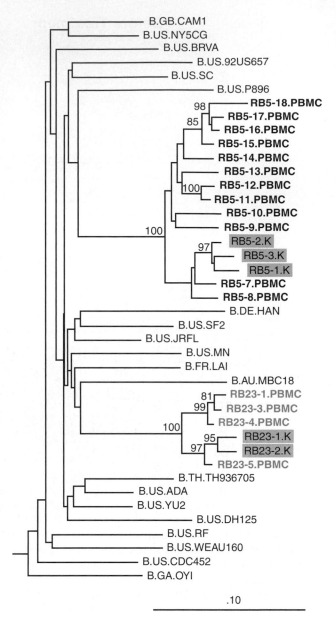

Figure 23-8 HIV-1 quasispecies complexity of kidney and PBMC-derived gp120 from two patients with HIVAN. gp120 sequence tree constructed from deduced amino acid sequences. Newly derived kidney (*highlighted*) and PBMC sequences from two patients, RB5 and RB23, are shown, along with 20 subtype B reference sequences from the Los Alamos Sequence Database. (Adapted from Marras D, Bruggeman LA, Gao F, et al: Replication and compartmentalization of HIV-1 in kidney epithelium of patients with HIV-associated nephropathy. Nat Med 8:522, 2002.)

The HIV-1 transgenic mouse[21] and rat[23] models of HIVAN express a *gag/pol*-deleted HIV-1 transgene under control of the native viral LTR promoter. Thus, in these rodent models of HIVAN, the *gag* and *pol* gene products are not required for development of the HIVAN phenotype. The major viral determinants of HIVAN pathogenesis are therefore likely to be mediated via the remaining viral genes. These genes are the envelope gene (*env*), the regulatory genes *tat*, *rev*, and *nef*, or the accessory genes, *vif*, *vpr*, and *vpu*. Animal models and in vitro studies have been used to map the HIV-1 genes that are important for HIVAN pathogenesis.

Nef

Nef is a 206–amino acid N-terminally myristoylated protein that has pleiotropic effects on the HIV-1 life cycle and host cell function. Functions ascribed to *nef* include immune evasion via reduction in cell surface expression of CD4 and major

histocompatibility complex class I molecules, increased viral production and infectivity, and prevention of apoptosis.[40]

Several studies have implicated a role for *nef* in HIVAN pathogenesis. To determine the HIV-1 genes necessary for the development of an AIDS-like phenotype, Hanna et al created 18 transgenic mouse lines expressing five different HIV-1 mutant constructs, each under control of the human CD4 regulatory sequences.[41] Each of these constructs contained different combinations of HIV-1 genes. In these transgenic

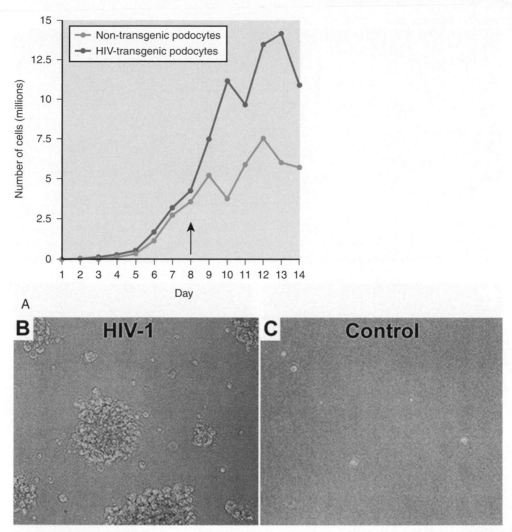

Figure 23-9 HIV-1 gene expression induces proliferation and loss of contact inhibition in podocytes. (A) Total number of nontransgenic (O) and HIV-1 transgenic (λ) cells after 14 days' culture. The *arrow* marks the time point at which cells became confluent (day 8). Murine podocytes infected with vesicular stomatitis virus G–pseudotyped HIV-1 transgenic construct proliferate in soft agar (B), whereas podocytes infected with control virus do not (C). (Adapted from Schwartz EJ, Cara A, Snoeck H, et al: Human immunodeficiency virus-1 induces loss of contact inhibition in podocytes. J Am Soc Nephrol 12:1677, 2001.)

mice, expression of HIV-1 *nef* was both necessary and sufficient to induce an AIDS-like phenotype and renal disease. The transgene was expressed under control of the CD4 promoter so that *nef* was primarily expressed in leukocytes. Because RTECs have been shown to express CD4 in vitro,[15] however, minimal expression in RTECs was possible. The relevance of this study to HIVAN pathogenesis is limited in that the renal phenotype was primarily interstitial nephritis, with little or no focal glomerulosclerosis or tubular microcystic disease. Since the $P_{72}XXP_{75}$ SH3-binding domain of Nef is important for mediating adhesion of important effector proteins including the Src-family tyrosine kinases Hck, Lck, and Fyn, the same group of investigators generated transgenic mice that express a *nef* transgene with a mutated SH3 binding domain, under control of the human CD4 promoter. These transgenic mice did not develop the AIDS phenotype or renal disease, suggesting that the ability of Nef to bind cellular proteins via the SH3 binding domain is necessary for pathogenesis.[42] To investigate the role of Hck as an effector of Nef-

mediated renal pathogenesis, the same group bred wild-type *nef*-transgenic mice with *hck*-mutant mice. The progeny had a delay in development of disease but there was otherwise no difference in renal pathology. Therefore, Hck is not crucial for Nef activity in the CD4-*nef* disease model.

These studies by Hanna et al did not recreate the most definitive phenotype of HIVAN, glomerular podocyte proliferation. To determine the HIV-1 gene(s) that are responsible for inducing the proliferative phenotype of podocytes in HIVAN, Husain et al transduced murine podocytes with scanning mutant constructs in which stop codon mutations were introduced sequentially into each of the HIV-1 open reading frames. In addition, individual HIV-1 gene expression constructs were generated and introduced into podocytes using HIV-1 retroviral vectors.[43] The multigenic vectors contained the same parental backbone pNL4-3 that was used in the generation of the HIV-1 transgenic model of HIVAN. Using this approach, they found that expression of *nef* alone, without other HIV-1 genes, resulted in increased proliferation and

Unstained frozen section

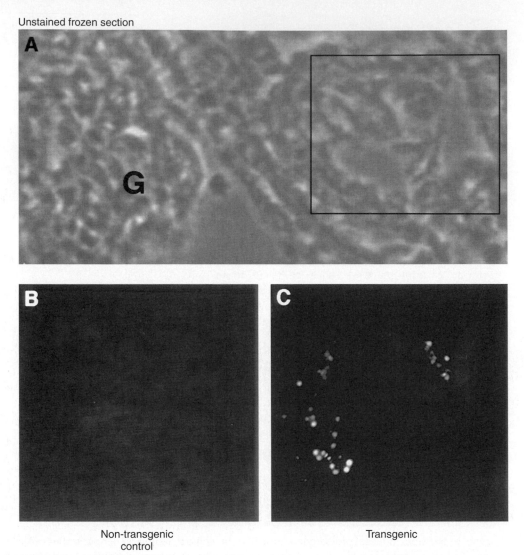

Figure 23-10 Identification of apoptotic cells in HIV-transgenic mouse kidneys by terminal transferase dUTP nick end labeling (TUNEL) assay. TUNEL assay was performed on adult, diseased transgenic, and nontransgenic mice. (**A**) Unstained frozen section. G, glomerulus. (**B**) TUNEL fluorescence of a nontransgenic control in region of tubules. (**C**) TUNEL fluorescence in transgenic kidney corresponding to the boxed region of **A** exhibiting tubular dilatation. (Adapted from Bruggeman LA, Dikman S, Meng C, et al: Nephropathy in human immunodeficiency virus-1 transgenic mice is due to renal transgene expression. J Clin Invest 100:84, 1997.)

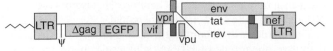

Figure 23-11 Schematic representation of HIV-1 genome.

anchorage-independent growth in the podocytes and that expression of the other HIV-1 genes in the absence of *nef* did not induce the proliferative phenotype. In a subsequent study, Nef expression was shown to induce loss of expression of markers of differentiation in podocytes in vitro, including synaptopodin and CALLA.[37] Thus, Nef expression in podocytes in vitro is capable of recapitulating the altered podocyte phenotype found in HIVAN in vivo.

He et al have elucidated the molecular mechanisms by which Nef induces proliferation and dedifferentiation of podocytes.[44] Nef expression in murine podocytes strongly induces Src kinase activity, the signal transducer and activator of transcription 3 (Stat3) phosphorylation, and activates the Ras-c-Raf-MAPK1,2 pathway (Fig. 23-12A). These pathways were also activated in podocytes in vivo in the HIV-transgenic model of HIVAN and in kidneys from patients with HIVAN. Mutation of the SH3 domain that mediates the interaction of Nef with Src family kinases completely prevented activation of Src signaling and also prevented podocyte proliferation and dedifferentiation. Moreover, Nef-induced proliferation and dedifferentiation is completely abrogated in vitro by expression of dominant-negative Src and partially prevented by inhibition of either Stat3 or MAPK1,2 individually (Fig. 23-12B and C). Thus, the ability of Nef to induce proliferation and

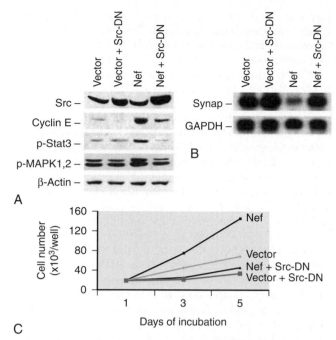

A

B

C

Figure 23-12 Role of Src activation in Nef-induced MAPK1,2 and Stat3 phosphorylation and phenotypic changes in podocytes. Control vector-infected (Vector) or Nef-infected (Nef) podocytes were transfected with dominant negative Src (Src-DN) and then selected with hygromycin B. Inhibition of Src by Src-DN inhibited Nef-induced activation of Cyclin E, Stat3, and MAPK1,2 (**A**), as well as Nef-induced decrease in expression of synaptopodin (**B**) and Nef-induced podocyte proliferation (**C**). (Adapted from He JC, Husain M, Sunamoto M, et al: Nef stimulates proliferation of glomerular podocytes through activation of Src-dependent Stat3 and MAPK1,2 pathways. J Clin Invest 114:643, 2004.)

dedifferentiation of podocytes is mediated via SH3-dependent interaction with Src family kinase(s).

Tat

The HIV-1 Tat protein is a 101–amino acid protein that is released from HIV-infected cells and is detectable in serum from infected patients. Extracellular Tat is capable of entering cells via endocytosis, resulting in multiple effects on viral and cellular gene expression. Tat has been shown to promote and/or inhibit apoptosis depending upon the cell type and dosage used. Studying the effects of Tat in isolation is difficult, because it is a potent transactivator of the HIV-1 LTR promoter and increases expression of the integrated HIV-1 provirus.[45] HIV-1 constructs and transgenes using the endogenous LTR viral promoter have much lower expression in the absence of Tat.

In studies using immortalized human podocytes derived from whites, investigators reported that exogenous Tat protein is capable of inducing podocyte proliferation and dedifferentiation.[46] A problem limiting the relevance of this study to HIVAN, however, is that it used podocytes derived from whites, an ethnic group in whom the development of HIVAN is exceedingly rare. Also, other groups have found that in animal models of HIVAN and in vitro podocyte assays, expression of

tat-encoding constructs does not induce significant renal disease, podocyte proliferation, or expression of differentiation markers.[41,43] It is possible, however, that free extracellular Tat may have different biologic effects than Tat expressed within cells. Also, the effects of Tat differ significantly according to the dosage used. In summary, a direct role for *tat* in HIVAN pathogenesis is possible but awaits corroboration.

Vpr

Vpr is a 96–amino acid protein that has several important functions in the HIV-1 life cycle.[47] Vpr contains a noncanonical nuclear localization sequence that is important for nuclear import of the HIV-1 preintegration complex in nondividing cells such as macrophages. It is possible that this function of Vpr is also important in HIV-1 infection of renal epithelial cells. Vpr expression can induce apoptosis in several cell types and also results in cell cycle arrest at the G2-M phase. This cell cycle arrest is likely to be important for viral production, because transcription of the viral LTR promoter is enhanced during G2. Similar to Tat, Vpr is detectable in serum of HIV-infected patients and extracellular Vpr is taken up by cells and becomes localized to the nucleus.

Dickie et al recently reported that mutation of *vpr* in mice expressing the same proviral HIV-1 *gag/pol* deletion construct used in the HIV-1 transgenic model of HIVAN resulted in abrogation of the renal phenotype.[48] The same group found that expression of a *tat/vpr* transgene under control of the viral LTR promoter in a single transgenic line was able to induce significant proteinuria in homozygous offspring. The most characteristic feature of HIVAN, the proliferation of podocytes, was not induced by Vpr, however. Crossing the *tat/vpr* transgenic mice with the *vpr*-mutant mice resulted in offspring with significantly increased proteinuria. Interestingly, expression of *vpr* as a transgene expressed in mice under control of the macrophage-specific promoter resulted in proteinuria and focal glomerulosclerosis. Although these studies support a role for *vpr* in HIVAN pathogenesis, it is not clear whether the macrophage-specific expression may have caused disease via systemic release of Vpr with subsequent uptake into renal cells or whether dysregulated macrophages had a direct role in causing the renal phenotype.

gp120

The HIV-1 *env* gene encodes the gp160 glycoprotein, which is subsequently cleaved into the envelope proteins gp120 and gp41. gp120 is the viral surface protein that mediates attachment of the virus to target cells via binding to the CD4 receptor and a co-receptor, most commonly the chemokine receptors CCR5 or CXCR4. gp41 is a transmembrane protein that mediates fusion of the viral and cellular lipid membranes once gp120 has bound its cognate receptor and co-receptor.

Singhal and colleagues have reported that exposure of mesangial cells and tubular epithelial cells to gp120 in vitro causes several abnormalities. They have reported that gp120 induces aberrant proliferation and apoptosis of human mesangial cells[49] and apoptosis of human tubular epithelial cells[50] in vitro. The same group also determined that induction of apoptosis in tubular epithelial cells was CD4 and p38 MAPK dependent. The relevance of these studies to HIVAN pathogenesis in vivo is limited in that although several groups have demonstrated subsets of tubular epithelial cells expression of CD4 and/or the common HIV-1 co-receptors in vitro, these findings have not been reproduced using human kidney specimens.[19,31]

THE ROLE OF HOST GENES IN THE PATHOGENESIS OF HIVAN

Studies of the Genetic Predisposition to HIVAN

Soon after the first descriptions of HIVAN as a clinical entity, it became clear that most affected patients were of African descent. In cities such as San Francisco, where most of the HIV-infected patients were white, HIVAN was rarely diagnosed, whereas urban centers with large numbers of HIV-seropositive blacks saw an ever-increasing number of patients with HIVAN. Recently, the predisposition of blacks to developing HIVAN has been studied more rigorously.

Although blacks have been found to be more susceptible than most other racial groups to the development of several renal diseases, the predisposition of blacks for HIVAN is stronger than virtually any other form of renal disease. In a study analyzing data from the U.S. Renal Data System, HIVAN was found to be 12.2 times more common in blacks than in other racial groups, and the only cause of ESRD that was more closely associated with black race was sickle cell disease.[51] In our experience at Mount Sinai Medical Center in New York City, every patient who has been diagnosed with HIVAN in the past 10 years has been black or Hispanic. Many of the Hispanic patients with HIVAN are from Caribbean or Latin American regions with a high admixture of individuals of African descent.

The predisposition of blacks to developing HIVAN has also been reported in series from Europe. In two case series, 7/7 patients from London[52] and 97/102 patients in France[53] who were diagnosed with HIVAN were black. In an autopsy series from Switzerland that examined 239 patients who had died with HIV/AIDS between 1981 and 1989, only one case of HIVAN was detected. The individual with HIVAN was one of the only six black patients in the study.[54]

Among blacks, the risk of developing HIVAN is heterogeneous. Freedman et al found that HIVAN tends to occur in blacks with a family history of renal diseases.[55] In this series, investigators compared the prevalence of non-HIVAN ESRD in first- and second-degree family members of patients with HIVAN to the prevalence of affected family members in HIV-infected blacks without renal disease. They found that 24% of patients with HIVAN had at least one family member with ESRD as compared with only 6% of controls. After controlling for multiple factors, the authors reported that patients with ESRD due to HIVAN were 5.4 times more likely to have family members with ESRD than controls.

Despite clear evidence that genetic factors are important for HIVAN pathogenesis, the genes that modulate HIVAN susceptibility remain unknown. Genetic linkage studies have been difficult to perform because of a paucity of available multiplex families with HIVAN. One study reported that the Duffy antigen/receptor for chemokines (DARC), a chemokine receptor, is upregulated in the kidneys of HIV-seropositive children with renal disease.[56] Because polymorphisms in the promoter for DARC are common in blacks, Woolley et al studied whether there is an association between DARC polymorphisms and the development of HIVAN. However, no such association was detected.[57]

WT-1 is a transcription factor that is constitutively expressed in normal differentiated podocytes and is necessary for normal renal and genital development.[58] In HIVAN, podocytes demonstrate markedly decreased expression of WT-1. No studies evaluating whether the loss of WT-1 expression has a direct pathogenic role in HIVAN have been published. A recent study by Orloff et al, however, found an association between single nucleotide polymorphisms (SNPs) in the WT-1 gene and the development of FSGS.[59] Their study groups consisted entirely of black participants, and the groups were stratified by HIV-1 status. The investigators found that one SNP in the sixth intron of WT-1 was associated with an odds ratio of 0.23 for developing HIVAN. Interestingly, this SNP was not associated with the development of FSGS in HIV-negative subjects. Another SNP, in the WT-1 promoter, approached statistical significance for association with a decreased risk for FSGS in HIV-positive subjects. This same SNP, however, was associated with an increased risk of FSGS in the HIV-negative population. Further analysis indicated that certain haplotypes of SNPs were associated with significantly different odds ratios for the development of FSGS in HIV-positive patients. More studies are required to confirm whether SNPs in WT-1 alter susceptibility to HIVAN and to determine the molecular mechanisms by which they may exert such an effect.

The Genetics of HIVAN in HIV-1 Transgenic Mice

Similar to humans, mice with different genetic backgrounds display marked differences in susceptibility to developing the HIVAN phenotype. For instance, when the *gag/pol*-deleted HIV-1 transgene is bred onto the FVB/N background, the penetrance of the renal phenotype approaches 100%. However, when the FVB/N transgenic mice (TgFVB) are bred with CAST mice, the HIVAN phenotype is completely abolished in the F1 offspring. Breeding of the transgene onto other strains of mice results in intermediate renal phenotypes. The HIVAN phenotype in these mice is independent of the level of renal expression of the HIV-1 transgene. To ascertain loci that are linked to the HIVAN phenotype, Gharavi et al backcrossed F1 animals from the TgFVB × CAST cross with TgFVB animals and used the progeny to perform genome-wide linkage analysis. Using this approach, they found several loci that were linked to the development of renal disease. The locus with the strongest linkage (Lod score 4.9) was subsequently named *HIVAN1* (Fig. 23-13).[60]

Interestingly, the *HIVAN1* locus is syntenic to human chromosome 3q25–27. This region of the human genome has previously been linked to the development of diabetic nephropathy in Pima Indians with type 2 diabetes,[61] whites with type 1 diabetes,[62] and creatinine clearance in blacks.[63] The 95% confidence interval for the *HIVAN1* locus encompasses 30 centimorgans (cM) and a large number of genes, limiting the ability of the investigators to speculate on particular candidate genes until they are able to significantly reduce the size of the interval. Thus, this study demonstrated that the genetic background of the host strongly influences whether expression of HIV-1 will lead to the development of HIVAN.

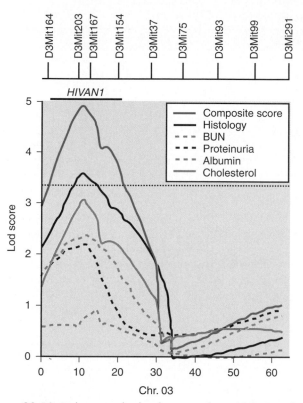

Figure 23-13 Linkage in the backcross cohort. Multipoint lod score plot for phenotypes on chromosomes 3 for the six primary phenotypes are shown. Map distance is presented in centimorgans. The positions of informative markers genotyped are shown above each plot. The dashed horizontal bar indicates the threshold for genome-wide significance for a backcross. The solid bar above the chromosome 3 lod plot indicates the 95% confidence interval for *HIVAN1* computed by bootstrap resampling (composite score). (Adapted from Gharavi AG, Ahmad T, Wong RD, et al: Mapping a locus for susceptibility to HIV-1-associated nephropathy to mouse chromosome 3. Proc Natl Acad Sci U S A 101:2488, 2004.)

Host Factors for HIVAN Pathogenesis

Although genetic linkage studies have yet to reveal polymorphisms in specific genes that confer increased risk for developing HIVAN, several studies have shed light upon host factors that mediate HIVAN pathogenesis. Most of these factors are known to influence cellular processes that are perturbed in HIVAN, including proliferation, apoptosis, inflammation, and fibrogenesis. Recent studies have also identified novel genes that are upregulated in HIVAN, but whose function and role in the disease are just beginning to be elucidated. Table 23-1 summarizes the host genes that have putative roles in the pathobiology of HIVAN.

Proliferation

In "classic" idiopathic FSGS and most other progressive glomerular diseases, podocyte number decreases. In the collapsing form of FSGS that is observed in HIVAN, however, there is vigorous proliferation of podocytes, leading to "pseudo-crescent" formation (see Figs. 23-1A and 23-2B).[4] As

discussed previously in the chapter, the HIV-1 *nef* gene has been shown to be an important mediator of this proliferative phenotype, probably via activation of Src family kinases with subsequent phosphorylation and activation of MAPK1,2 and Stat3.[41,44]

The dysregulation of podocyte proliferation present in HIVAN is also manifested by alterations in the expression of cyclins and cyclin-dependent kinases. Cyclin E is upregulated in podocytes in response to HIV-1 infection. This effect is mediated by Nef.[37] There are also reports by some investigators of increased expression of cyclin D1 in HIVAN,[64] whereas others reported decreased glomerular cyclin D1.[65] Shankland et al reported that the CDK inhibitors p27 and p57 were downregulated in podocytes in HIVAN biopsy specimens, whereas p21 was upregulated. These findings contrast with glomerular diseases without podocyte proliferation and normal podocytes, where there is stable constitutive expression of p27 and p57 and no expression of p21.[66]

Basic fibroblast growth factor is upregulated in HIVAN and has been shown previously to increase proliferation of renal epithelial cells in vitro.[38,67,68] The combined actions of growth factors and cell cycle–regulatory proteins probably contribute to the increased epithelial proliferation observed in HIVAN.

Apoptosis and Fibrogenesis

Apoptotic cells are also increased in the renal epithelium in HIV-1 transgenic mice and of patients with HIVAN.[16] HIV-1 infection of RTECs may lead to receptor-mediated apoptosis in renal tubular epithelial cells (Fig. 23-14). Conaldi et al found that HIV-1 infection of human proximal tubular cells led to apoptosis of infected cells. They also found that infection of tubular epithelial cells induced increased expression of Fas and that infected cells are susceptible to Fas-mediated apoptosis. Apoptosis in these experiments was inhibited by adding a caspase inhibitor to the cells before Fas stimulation.[15]

Transforming growth factor-β (TGF-β), another proapoptotic molecule, is upregulated in HIVAN.[69–71] TGF-β has been implicated in the pathogenesis of several renal diseases and is an important mediator of apoptosis and fibrosis in the kidney.[72] TGF-β expression has been detected in glomeruli and tubular epithelial cells in HIVAN specimens. It is possible that some of the glomerular expression of TGF-β may be induced by HIV-1 Tat protein. One group reported that exposure of mesangial cells to Tat results in increased production of TGF-β and increased production of matrix proteins.[71] Another group reported that HIV-1–expressing mesangial cells demonstrate increased apoptosis and proliferation.[73] There is no clear evidence that mesangial cells are infected by HIV-1 in HIVAN. However, because extracellular Tat is capable of transducing cells, extracellular Tat may have been responsible for inducing TGF-β production.

HIV-1 envelope protein may also stimulate TGF-β. Kapasi et al reported that gp120 induced expression of TGF-β in RTECs and that TGF-β could then aid in the recruitment of monocytes into the renal interstitium.[74] The stress response MAPK, p38 MAPK, was suggested to mediate the apoptotic response of tubular epithelial cells to the CD4 gp120 interaction in vitro.[50] Because tubular epithelial cells are not known to express either CD4 or the major co-receptors for HIV-1, the in vivo significance of these experiments remains unclear. Smad proteins, the downstream effectors of TGF-β signaling,

Table 23-1 Epithelial Factors with Putative Roles in HIVAN Pathogenesis

Epithelial Factors	References
Proliferation/Growth Factors	
Src family kinases	41, 44
Mitogen activated protein kinase (MAPK) 1, 2	41, 44
Cyclin D	64, 65, 91
Cyclin E	37
Cyclin-dependent kinase inhibitors p27, p57, p21	65, 66
Basic fibroblast growth factor	38
Vascular endothelial growth factor (VEGF)	90
Apoptosis	
Transforming growth factor-β (TGF-β)	69–71
p38 MAPK	50
Fas/ FasL	15, 49
Transcription Factors	
Nuclear factor-κB (NF-κB)	75
SP-1	75
WT-1	11, 12, 37, 46
Pro-fibrogenic Factors	
TGF-β	69–71
Proinflammatory Mediators	
NF-κB	75
Monocyte chemoattractant protein-1 (MCP-1)	74, 83
MHC Class II	83
Interleukin-8 (IL-8)	83
RANTES	83
Interferon-α (IFN-α)	83
IFN-γ receptor	83
Cell-Cell/Cell-Matrix Interactions	
Synaptopodin	11, 12, 37, 46, 65, 76
Podocalyxin	12, 37, 76
Podocan	86

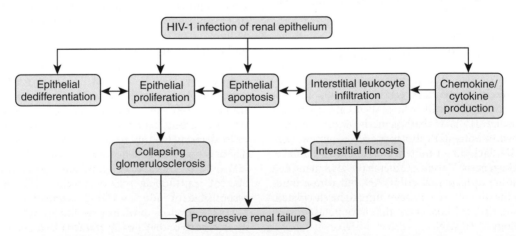

Figure 23-14 Schema of cellular processes that are perturbed in response to expression of HIV-1 genes in renal epithelial cells leading to progressive renal failure.

have not been studied in the context of HIVAN, and the relative contributions of the different Smads to HIVAN pathogenesis have yet to be defined.

Transcription Factors

Regulation of HIV-1 transcription in podocytes seems to occur via mechanisms similar to those in lymphocytes. The activity of the viral LTR promoter in murine podocytes requires binding of inducible nuclear factor-κB (NF-κB) and Sp1 to the viral LTR.[75] These same factors are important regulators of HIV-1 transcription in human lymphocytes. Inhibition of HIV-1 transcription in murine podocytes using an inhibitor of cyclin-dependent kinase-9 (CDK-9) resulted in decreased proliferation and re-expression of podocyte differentiation markers in vitro.[64,76] CDK-9 binds RNA polymerase II and is a component of multiprotein complex including cyclin T and Tat that potentiates transcriptional activation of the LTR promoter.[77] Systemic administration of these CDK-9 inhibitors to HIV-1 transgenic mice resulted in amelioration of the HIVAN phenotype.[78] Both of these studies used mice or murine cell lines. Given the markedly decreased efficiency of HIV-1 transcription in murine cells due to the lack of cyclin T,[77] however, it is unclear whether CDK-9 inhibition would have similar therapeutic effects in podocytes from humans with HIVAN. It is also unclear whether the therapeutic effect of the CDK-9 inhibitors was mediated predominantly via inhibition of viral transcription or via inhibition of cell cycle progression through interference with the function of CDKs.

Inflammatory Mediators

Interstitial infiltration by leukocytes is a prominent pathologic finding in HIVAN,[4] and these infiltrating cells may have an important role in HIVAN pathogenesis. Several small case series have suggested that treatment with steroids has beneficial effects upon renal outcome in HIVAN.[53,79–81] The most prominent pathologic change in one patient who had received a renal biopsy after treatment with steroids for HIVAN was a decrease in the interstitial inflammatory infiltrate.[82]

Several inflammatory mediators have been reported to be upregulated in kidneys from patients with HIVAN or HIV-transgenic mice. Kimmel et al reported that RANTES, interleukin-8 (IL-8), and monocyte chemoattractant protein-1 (MCP-1) are present in higher levels in kidneys from HIV-infected patients than in kidneys from controls; however, there was no difference in levels of these proteins in patients with HIVAN as compared with HIV-positive patients without renal disease. They did find, however, that nonpolymorphic major histocompatibility complex class II protein, interferon-α (IFN-α), and the γ-interferon receptor were all present in higher levels in HIVAN biopsy specimens than in HIV-positive patients without renal disease.[83] Although these studies implicate potential roles for the latter three proteins in HIVAN pathogenesis, it is also possible that RANTES, IL-8, and/or MCP-1 also contribute to the recruitment of inflammatory cells into the infected kidney.

NF-κB is expressed in podocytes in HIV-transgenic mice.[75] Expression of this protein, however, has not been well studied in human kidney specimens. NF-κB is known to be capable of inducing expression of a wide variety of chemokines, cytokines, and other mediators of inflammation.[84] It is likely that this protein may have important roles not only in facilitating viral transcription but also in increasing production of pro-inflammatory molecules by infected epithelial cells, thereby contributing to the influx of leukocytes into the renal interstitium.

Production of inflammatory mediators by renal epithelial cells may have important effects upon viral expression in immune cells. O'Donnell et al reported that co-culture of human tubular epithelial cells with HIV-1–infected monocytes induced increased viral production by the monocytes. Most of this effect was mediated by the production of IL-6 and tumor necrosis factor-α by the epithelial cells.[85]

Mediators of Cell-Matrix and Cell-Cell Interactions

Ross et al recently reported a novel gene, podocan, that is upregulated in podocytes from HIV-1 transgenic mice.[86] Podocan was identified using complementary DNA representational difference analysis to ascertain differentially expressed genes in podocytes from HIV-1 transgenic and normal mice. Podocan is a novel small leucine-rich repeat protein that represents a new family of small leucine-rich repeat proteins. Podocan is developmentally regulated in the kidney during embryogenesis and is expressed at low levels in normal adult podocytes. However, podocan protein markedly accumulates in sclerotic glomerular lesions in HIV-1 transgenic mice. The role of podocan in the pathogenesis of HIVAN and other diseases is currently under study.

Another gene that was found to be upregulated in podocytes from HIV-1 transgenic mice is sidekick-1 (sdk-1).[87] Sdk-1 is a transmembrane protein of the immunoglobulin superfamily. Sdk-1 and its ortholog, sidekick-2 (sdk-2), were recently shown to guide axonal terminals to specific synapses in developing neurons.[88] Sdk-1, like podocan, is developmentally regulated in the kidney during embryogenesis and is expressed at low levels in podocytes in normal adult kidneys. In HIVAN biopsy specimens, glomerular expression of Sdk-1 protein is greatly increased. Because podocyte processes share many similarities with neuronal axons, it is possible that dysregulation of Sdk-1 may contribute to the podocyte abnormalities that are characteristic of HIVAN, with subsequent disruption of the slit diaphragm and glomerulosclerosis.

Synaptopodin and podocalyxin are both expressed in quiescent, differentiated podocytes.[13] In HIVAN, however, expression of both of these proteins decreases markedly.[11,12] Although these proteins are increasingly recognized as being important for normal podocyte structure and function, their roles in the pathogenesis of HIVAN have not been studied.

Vascular endothelial growth factor (VEGF) is normally expressed in podocytes and tubular epithelial cells. Although the roles of VEGF in normal kidney function and homeostasis are poorly defined, glomerular expression of VEGF is elevated in some renal diseases, including diabetic nephropathy.[89] Podocyte-specific dysregulation of VEGF using a transgenic murine model has recently been shown to be capable of inducing a variety of renal phenotypes. Decreased expression of VEGF in podocytes led to endotheliosis, similar to the lesions of preeclampsia, whereas podocyte-specific overexpression of VEGF led to collapsing glomerulosclerosis, closely resembling the glomerular phenotype found in HIVAN.[90] The role of VEGF in the pathobiology of the collapsing glomerular lesion found in HIVAN warrants further study.

CONCLUSIONS

HIVAN is the most common cause of chronic renal failure in HIV-seropositive patients. Characteristic pathologic findings in HIVAN include collapsing focal glomerulosclerosis with podocyte proliferation, microcystic dilatation of the tubules, leukocytic infiltration of the interstitium, and interstitial fibrosis. HIV-1 infects the renal epithelium, and epithelial expression of HIV-1 genes is a critical component of pathogenesis. The renal epithelium is a reservoir of HIV-1 infection that is capable of harboring transcriptionally active virus even in patients on HAART with undetectable plasma viral loads.

Several HIV-1 genes have been studied for their roles in HIVAN pathogenesis. Although HIV-1 *nef* seems to be an important mediator of podocyte proliferation in HIVAN, it is likely that other HIV-1 genes also contribute to the development of renal disease. Although there are clearly genetic factors that contribute to HIVAN susceptibility in humans and animal models, these factors remain largely undefined. Several cellular genes, including mediators of proliferation, apoptosis, inflammation, cell-cell and cell-matrix interactions, have been reported to have putative roles in HIVAN pathogenesis. Much has been learned regarding the factors that contribute to progressive renal disease in HIVAN in the two decades since it was first described. However, the recent dramatic improvements in mortality of patients with HIV/AIDS have not translated into decreased incidence of ESRD due to HIVAN. Further research is therefore desperately needed to rationally design new strategies for prevention and treatment of this disease.

References

1. Rao TK, Filippone EJ, Nicastri AD, et al: Associated focal and segmental glomerulosclerosis in the acquired immunodeficiency syndrome. N Engl J Med 310:669, 1984.
2. Centers for Disease Control and Prevention: HIV/AIDS Surveillance Report 13 (No. 2), 2001.
3. U.S. Renal Data System: USRDS 2003 Annual Data Report: Atlas of End-Stage Renal Disease in the United States. Bethesda, MD, National Institutes of Health, National Institute of Diabetes and Digestive and Kidney Diseases, 2003.
4. D'Agati V, Suh JI, Carbone L, et al: Pathology of HIV-associated nephropathy: A detailed morphologic and comparative study. Kidney Int 35:1358, 1989.
5. D'Agati V, Appel GB: Renal pathology of human immunodeficiency virus infection. Semin Nephrol 18:406, 1998.
6. D'Agati V, Appel GB: HIV infection and the kidney. J Am Soc Nephrol 8:138, 1997.
7. Stylianou E, Aukrust P, Bendtzen K, et al: Interferons and interferon (IFN)-inducible protein 10 during highly active anti-retroviral therapy (HAART)—Possible immunosuppressive role of IFN-α in HIV infection. Clin Exp Immunol 119:479, 2000.
8. Ross MJ, Bruggeman LA, Wilson PD, Klotman PE: Microcyst formation and HIV-1 gene expression occur in multiple nephron segments in HIV-associated nephropathy. J Am Soc Nephrol 12:2645, 2001.
9. Rey L, Viciana A, Ruiz P: Immunopathological characteristics of in situ T-cell subpopulations in human immunodeficiency virus–associated nephropathy. Hum Pathol 26:408, 1995.
10. Bodi I, Abraham AA, Kimmel PL: Macrophages in human immunodeficiency virus–associated kidney diseases. Am J Kidney Dis 24:762, 1994.
11. Barisoni L, Bruggeman LA, Mundel P, et al: HIV-1 induces renal epithelial dedifferentiation in a transgenic model of HIV-associated nephropathy. Kidney Int 58:173, 2000.
12. Barisoni L, Kriz W, Mundel P, D'Agati V: The dysregulated podocyte phenotype: A novel concept in the pathogenesis of collapsing idiopathic focal segmental glomerulosclerosis and HIV-associated nephropathy. J Am Soc Nephrol 10:51, 1999.
13. Mundel P, Shankland SJ: Podocyte biology and response to injury. J Am Soc Nephrol 13:3005, 2002.
14. Bruggeman LA, Dikman S, Meng C, et al: Nephropathy in human immunodeficiency virus-1 transgenic mice is due to renal transgene expression. J Clin Invest 100:84, 1997.
15. Conaldi PG, Biancone L, Bottelli A, et al: HIV-1 kills renal tubular epithelial cells in vitro by triggering an apoptotic pathway involving caspase activation and Fas upregulation. J Clin Invest 102:2041, 1998.
16. Bodi I, Abraham AA, Kimmel PL: Apoptosis in human immunodeficiency virus–associated nephropathy. Am J Kidney Dis 26:286, 1995.
17. Cohen AH, Sun NC, Shapshak P, Imagawa DT: Demonstration of human immunodeficiency virus in renal epithelium in HIV-associated nephropathy. Mod Pathol 2:125, 1989.
18. Kimmel PL, Ferreira-Centeno A, Farkas-Szallasi T, et al: Viral DNA in microdissected renal biopsy tissue from HIV infected patients with nephrotic syndrome. Kidney Int 43:1347, 1993.
19. Eitner F, Cui Y, Hudkins KL, et al: Chemokine receptor (CCR5) expression in human kidneys and in the HIV infected macaque [see Comments]. Kidney Int 54:1945, 1998.
20. Barbiano di Belgiojoso G, Genderini A, Vago L, et al: Absence of HIV antigens in renal tissue from patients with HIV-associated nephropathy. Nephrol Dial Transplant 5:489, 1990.
21. Dickie P, Felser J, Eckhaus M, et al: HIV-associated nephropathy in transgenic mice expressing HIV-1 genes. Virology 185:109, 1991.
22. Kopp JB, Klotman ME, Adler SH, et al: Progressive glomerulosclerosis and enhanced renal accumulation of basement membrane components in mice transgenic for human immunodeficiency virus type 1 genes. Proc Natl Acad Sci U S A 89:1577, 1992.
23. Reid W, Sadowska M, Denaro F, et al: An HIV-1 transgenic rat that develops HIV-related pathology and immunologic dysfunction. Proc Natl Acad Sci U S A 98:9271, 2001.
24. Gattone VH, 2nd, Tian C, Zhuge W, et al: SIV-associated nephropathy in rhesus macaques infected with lymphocyte-tropic SIVmac239. AIDS Res Hum Retroviruses 14:1163, 1998.
25. Liu ZQ, Muhkerjee S, Sahni M, et al: Derivation and biological characterization of a molecular clone of SHIV(KU-2) that causes AIDS, neurological disease, and renal disease in rhesus macaques. Virology 260:295, 1999.
26. Stephens EB, Tian C, Li Z, et al: Rhesus macaques infected with macrophage-tropic simian immunodeficiency virus (SIVmacR71/17E) exhibit extensive focal segmental and global glomerulosclerosis. J Virol 72:8820, 1998.
27. Stephens EB, Tian C, Dalton SB, Gattone VH, 2nd: Simian-human immunodeficiency virus–associated nephropathy in macaques. AIDS Res Hum Retroviruses 16:1295, 2000.
28. Bruggeman LA, Ross MD, Tanji N, et al: Renal epithelium is a previously unrecognized site of HIV-1 infection. J Am Soc Nephrol 11:2079, 2000.
29. Marras D, Bruggeman LA, Gao F, et al: Replication and compartmentalization of HIV-1 in kidney epithelium of patients with HIV-associated nephropathy. Nat Med 8:522, 2002.
30. Tokizawa S, Shimizu N, Hui-Yu L, et al: Infection of mesangial cells with HIV and SIV: Identification of GPR1 as a coreceptor. Kidney Int 58:607, 2000.
31. Eitner F, Cui Y, Hudkins KL, et al: Chemokine receptor CCR5 and CXCR4 expression in HIV-associated kidney disease. J Am Soc Nephrol 11:856, 2000.

32. Bhattacharya J, Peters PJ, Clapham PR: CD4-independent infection of HIV and SIV: Implications for envelope conformation and cell tropism in vivo. AIDS 17(Suppl 4):S35, 2003.

33. van der Meer P, Ulrich AM, Gonzalez-Scarano F, Lavi E: Immunohistochemical analysis of CCR2, CCR3, CCR5, and CXCR4 in the human brain: Potential mechanisms for HIV dementia. Exp Mol Pathol 69:192, 2000.

34. Ray PE, Liu XH, Henry D, et al: Infection of human primary renal epithelial cells with HIV-1 from children with HIV-associated nephropathy. Kidney Int 53:1217, 1998.

35. Winston JA, Bruggeman LA, Ross MD, et al: Nephropathy and establishment of a renal reservoir of HIV type 1 during primary infection. N Engl J Med 344:1979, 2001.

36. Schwartz EJ, Cara A, Snoeck H, et al: Human immunodeficiency virus-1 induces loss of contact inhibition in podocytes. J Am Soc Nephrol 12:1677, 2001.

37. Sunamoto M, Husain M, He JC, et al: Critical role for Nef in HIV-1-induced podocyte dedifferentiation. Kidney Int 64:1695, 2003.

38. Ray PE, Bruggeman LA, Weeks BS, et al: bFGF and its low affinity receptors in the pathogenesis of HIV-associated nephropathy in transgenic mice. Kidney Int 46:759, 1994.

39. Frankel AD, Young JA: HIV-1: Fifteen proteins and an RNA. Annu Rev Biochem 67:1, 1998.

40. Fackler OT, Baur AS: Live and let die: Nef functions beyond HIV replication. Immunity 16:493, 2002.

41. Hanna Z, Kay DG, Rebai N, et al: Nef harbors a major determinant of pathogenicity for an AIDS-like disease induced by HIV-1 in transgenic mice. Cell 95:163, 1998.

42. Hanna Z, Weng X, Kay DG, et al: The pathogenicity of human immunodeficiency virus (HIV) type 1 Nef in CD4C/HIV transgenic mice is abolished by mutation of its SH3-binding domain, and disease development is delayed in the absence of Hck. J Virol 75:9378, 2001.

43. Husain M, Gusella GL, Klotman ME, et al: HIV-1 Nef induces proliferation and anchorage-independent growth in podocytes. J Am Soc Nephrol 13:1806, 2002.

44. He JC, Husain M, Sunamoto M, et al: Nef stimulates proliferation of glomerular podocytes through activation of Src-dependent Stat3 and MAPK1,2 pathways. J Clin Invest 114:643, 2004.

45. Pugliese A, Vidotto V, Beltramo T, et al: A review of HIV-1 Tat protein biological effects. Cell Biochem Funct 23:223, 2004.

46. Conaldi PG, Bottelli A, Baj A, et al: Human immunodeficiency virus-1 Tat induces hyperproliferation and dysregulation of renal glomerular epithelial cells. Am J Pathol 161:53, 2002.

47. Sherman MP, De Noronha CM, Williams SA, Greene WC: Insights into the biology of HIV-1 viral protein R. DNA Cell Biol 21:679, 2002.

48. Dickie P, Roberts A, Uwiera R, et al: Focal glomerulosclerosis in proviral and c-fms transgenic mice links Vpr expression to HIV-associated nephropathy. Virology 322:69, 2004.

49. Kapasi AA, Fan S, Singhal PC: Role of 14-3-3ε, c-Myc/Max, and Akt phosphorylation in HIV-1 gp 120-induced mesangial cell proliferation. Am J Physiol Renal Physiol 280:F333, 2001.

50. Kapasi AA, Patel G, Franki N, Singhal PC: HIV-1 gp120-induced tubular epithelial cell apoptosis is mediated through p38-MAPK phosphorylation. Mol Med 8:676, 2002.

51. Abbott KC, Hypolite I, Welch PG, Agodoa LY: Human immunodeficiency virus/acquired immunodeficiency syndrome–associated nephropathy at end-stage renal disease in the United States: Patient characteristics and survival in the pre highly active antiretroviral therapy era. J Nephrol 14:377, 2001.

52. Williams DI, Williams DJ, Williams IG, et al: Presentation, pathology, and outcome of HIV-associated renal disease in a specialist centre for HIV/AIDS. Sex Transm Infect 74:179, 1998.

53. Laradi A, Mallet A, Beaufils H, et al: HIV-associated nephropathy: Outcome and prognosis factors. Groupe d' Etudes Nephrologiques d'Ile de France. J Am Soc Nephrol 9:2327, 1998.

54. Hailemariam S, Walder M, Burger HR, et al: Renal pathology and premortem clinical presentation of Caucasian patients with AIDS: An autopsy study from the era prior to antiretroviral therapy. Swiss Med Wkly 131:412, 2001.

55. Freedman BI, Soucie JM, Stone SM, Pegram S: Familial clustering of end-stage renal disease in blacks with HIV-associated nephropathy. Am J Kidney Dis 34:254, 1999.

56. Liu XH, Hadley TJ, Xu L, et al: Up-regulation of Duffy antigen receptor expression in children with renal disease. Kidney Int 55:1491, 1999.

57. Woolley IJ, Kalayjian R, Valdez H, et al: HIV nephropathy and the Duffy antigen/receptor for chemokines in African Americans. J Nephrol 14:384, 2001.

58. Pritchard-Jones K, Fleming S, Davidson D, et al: The candidate Wilms' tumour gene is involved in genitourinary development. Nature 346:194, 1990.

59. Orloff MS, Iyengar SK, Winkler CA, et al: Variants in the Wilms tumor gene are associated with focal segmental glomerulosclerosis in the African American population. Physiol Genomics 21:212, 2005.

60. Gharavi AG, Ahmad T, Wong RD, et al: Mapping a locus for susceptibility to HIV-1-associated nephropathy to mouse chromosome 3. Proc Natl Acad Sci U S A 101:2488, 2004.

61. Imperatore G, Hanson RL, Pettitt DJ, et al: Sib-pair linkage analysis for susceptibility genes for microvascular complications among Pima Indians with type 2 diabetes. Pima Diabetes Genes Group. Diabetes 47:821, 1998.

62. Moczulski DK, Rogus JJ, Antonellis A, et al: Major susceptibility locus for nephropathy in type 1 diabetes on chromosome 3q: Results of novel discordant sib-pair analysis. Diabetes 47:1164, 1998.

63. DeWan AT, Arnett DK, Miller MB, et al: Refined mapping of suggestive linkage to renal function in African Americans: The HyperGEN study. Am J Hum Genet 71:204, 2002.

64. Nelson PJ, Sunamoto M, Husain M, Gelman IH: HIV-1 expression induces cyclin D1 expression and pRb phosphorylation in infected podocytes: Cell-cycle mechanisms contributing to the proliferative phenotype in HIV-associated nephropathy. BMC Microbiol 2:26, 2002.

65. Barisoni L, Mokrzycki M, Sablay L, et al: Podocyte cell cycle regulation and proliferation in collapsing glomerulopathies. Kidney Int 58:137, 2000.

66. Shankland SJ, Eitner F, Hudkins KL, et al: Differential expression of cyclin-dependent kinase inhibitors in human glomerular disease: Role in podocyte proliferation and maturation. Kidney Int 58:674, 2000.

67. Ray PE, Liu XH, Robinson LR, et al: A novel HIV-1 transgenic rat model of childhood HIV-1-associated nephropathy. Kidney Int 63:2242, 2003.

68. Liu XH, Aigner A, Wellstein A, Ray PE: Up-regulation of a fibroblast growth factor binding protein in children with renal diseases. Kidney Int 59:1717, 2001.

69. Yamamoto T, Noble NA, Miller DE, et al: Increased levels of transforming growth factor-β in HIV-associated nephropathy. Kidney Int 55:579, 1999.

70. Shukla RR, Kumar A, Kimmel PL: Transforming growth factor β increases the expression of HIV-1 gene in transfected human mesangial cells. Kidney Int 44:1022, 1993.

71. Bodi I, Kimmel PL, Abraham AA, et al: Renal TGF-β in HIV-associated kidney diseases. Kidney Int 51:1568, 1997.

72. Bottinger EP, Bitzer M: TGF-β signaling in renal disease. J Am Soc Nephrol 13:2600, 2002.

73. Singhal PC, Sharma P, Loona R, et al: Enhanced proliferation, apoptosis, and matrix accumulation by mesangial cells derived from HIV-1 transgenic mice. J Investig Med 46:297, 1998.

74. Kapasi A, Bhat P, Singhal PC: Tubular cell and HIV-1 gp120 interaction products promote migration of monocytes. Inflammation 22:137, 1998.

75. Bruggeman LA, Adler SH, Klotman PE: Nuclear factor-kappa B binding to the HIV-1 LTR in kidney: Implications for HIV-associated nephropathy. Kidney Int 59:2174, 2001.

76. Nelson PJ, Gelman IH, Klotman PE: Suppression of HIV-1 expression by inhibitors of cyclin-dependent kinases promotes differentiation of infected podocytes. J Am Soc Nephrol 12:2827, 2001.

77. Wei P, Garber ME, Fang SM, et al: A novel CDK9-associated C-type cyclin interacts directly with HIV-1 Tat and mediates its high-affinity, loop-specific binding to TAR RNA. Cell 92:451, 1998.

78. Nelson PJ, D'Agati VD, Gries JM, et al: Amelioration of nephropathy in mice expressing HIV-1 genes by the cyclin-dependent kinase inhibitor flavopiridol. J Antimicrob Chemother 51:921, 2003.

79. Smith MC, Austen JL, Carey JT, et al: Prednisone improves renal function and proteinuria in human immunodeficiency virus–associated nephropathy. Am J Med 101:41, 1996.

80. Eustace JA, Nuermberger E, Choi M, et al: Cohort study of the treatment of severe HIV-associated nephropathy with corticosteroids. Kidney Int 58:1253, 2000.

81. Szczech LA, Edwards LJ, Sanders LL, et al: Protease inhibitors are associated with a slowed progression of HIV-related renal diseases. Clin Nephrol 57:336, 2002.

82. Briggs WA, Tanawattanacharoen S, Choi MJ, et al: Clinicopathologic correlates of prednisone treatment of human immunodeficiency virus–associated nephropathy. Am J Kidney Dis 28:618, 1996.

83. Kimmel PL, Cohen DJ, Abraham AA, et al: Upregulation of MHC class II, interferon-α and interferon-γ receptor protein expression in HIV-associated nephropathy. Nephrol Dial Transplant 18:285, 2003.

84. Richmond A: NF-κB, chemokine gene transcription and tumour growth. Nat Rev Immunol 2:664, 2002.

85. O'Donnell MP, Chao CC, Gekker G, et al: Renal cell cytokine production stimulates HIV-1 expression in chronically HIV-1-infected monocytes. Kidney Int 53:593, 1998.

86. Ross MD, Bruggeman LA, Hanss B, et al: Podocan, a novel small leucine-rich repeat protein expressed in the sclerotic glomerular lesion of experimental HIV-associated nephropathy. J Biol Chem 278:33248, 2003.

87. Kaufman L, Hayashi K, Ross MJ, et al: Sidekick-1 is upregulated in glomeruli in HIV-associated nephropathy. J Am Soc Nephrol 15:1721, 2004.

88. Yamagata M, Weiner JA, Sanes JR: Sidekicks: Synaptic adhesion molecules that promote lamina-specific connectivity in the retina. Cell 110:649, 2002.

89. Schrijvers BF, Flyvbjerg A, De Vriese AS: The role of vascular endothelial growth factor (VEGF) in renal pathophysiology. Kidney Int 65:2003, 2004.

90. Eremina V, Sood M, Haigh J, et al: Glomerular-specific alterations of VEGF-A expression lead to distinct congenital and acquired renal diseases. J Clin Invest 111:707, 2003.

Pathogenesis of Paraproteinemic Renal Disease

Paul W. Sanders

Paraproteinemic renal diseases represent a large class of renal lesions that are associated with deposition of intact immunoglobulins or immunoglobulin fragments that include heavy chains and light chains (Table 24-1). The list of associated diseases includes AL-amyloidosis (composed of light chains), AH-amyloidosis (composed of heavy chains), monoclonal light-chain and light- and heavy-chain deposition disease (collectively termed *ML(H)CDD* in this review), monoclonal heavy-chain deposition disease, Waldenström's macroglobulinemia, immunotactoid glomerulopathy,[1] glomerulonephritis associated with monoclonal immunoglobulin deposition,[2] glomerulonephritis associated with type I cryoglobulin deposition, cast nephropathy (also known as "myeloma kidney"), epithelial cell injury related to light-chain deposition in proximal tubule,[3–5] and tubulointerstitial nephritis.[4] This review focuses primarily on two glomerular lesions, AL-amyloid and ML(H)CDD, and two tubulointerstitial lesions (proximal tubular injury and cast nephropathy).

IMMUNOGLOBULIN METABOLISM AND STRUCTURE

Because of the central role of the immunoglobulin light chain and, to a lesser extent, heavy chain and intact immunoglobulin in the molecular pathogenesis of paraproteinemic renal diseases, developing an understanding of these processes initially requires comprehension of the synthesis and metabolism of the immunoglobulin molecule and immunoglobulin fragments. Immunoglobulin G (IgG) is a heteromeric protein composed of two different gene products that are known as heavy and light chains. Before secretion, these immunoglobulin precursor proteins undergo post-translational modifications that produce intermolecular disulfide bridges between two heavy chains and two light chains to form the intact immunoglobulin molecule.[6] The presence of a slight excess of light chains, as compared with heavy chains, seems to facilitate the assembly and secretion of an intact immunoglobulin.[7] Thus, immunoglobulin light chains can also be secreted, and small amounts of polyclonal light chains can normally be found in the circulation. Circulating free heavy chains indicate a pathologic state. When a clone of plasma cells is present, significant concentrations of monoclonal light chain may be observed in the serum. Unlike the intact immunoglobulin, free light chains, with a molecular weight of about 22 kDa (one-third that of albumin), are filtered at the glomerulus.[8] Glomerular filtration is the primary route of removal of light chains from the circulation.[9] Light chains, particularly the lambda isotype, can undergo dimerization before secretion, and the dimers are also removed by glomerular filtration, albeit at a more restricted rate. Light chains in the glomerular ultrafiltrate may either bind to megalin or to cubilin, which compose the endocytic heteromeric complex that is present on the apical surface of proximal tubule epithelial cells,[10–12] or escape reabsorption in the proximal tubule to appear in the lumen of the distal nephron and ultimately the urine. Following endocytosis, these low-molecular-weight proteins are hydrolyzed and the constituent amino acids are returned to the circulation across the basolateral membrane of the proximal tubule.

The immunoglobulin light chain is composed of a variable (V_L) and a constant (C_L) peptide domain (Fig. 24-1).[13] Within

Table 24-1 Paraproteinemic Renal Diseases

Diseases with Predominant Glomerular Involvement
Amyloidosis with amyloid composed of light chains
Amyloidosis with amyloid composed of heavy chains
Monoclonal light-chain and light- and heavy-chain deposition disease
Monoclonal heavy-chain deposition disease
Waldenström's macroglobulinemia
Immunotactoid glomerulopathy
Glomerulonephritis associated with monoclonal immunoglobulin deposition
Glomerulonephritis associated with type I cryoglobulin deposition
Diseases with Predominant Tubulointerstitial Involvement
Cast nephropathy, or "myeloma kidney"
Proximal tubulopathy including Fanconi syndrome
Tubulointerstitial nephritis

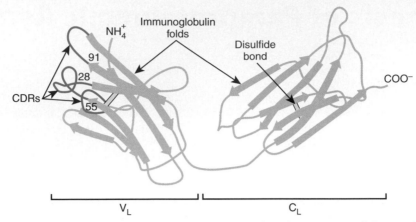

Figure 24-1 Structural model of the immunoglobulin light-chain molecule. The structure of the V_L domain is created by the framework regions, which form the classical immunoglobulin folds that permit exposure of the complementarity-determining regions (CDRs). Intramolecular disulfide bridges stabilize the layers. The CDRs are the sites of sequence diversity and are largely responsible for the uniqueness of the light chain. The numbers represent the approximate locations of the amino acid residues.

the globular V_L domain are framework regions (FR1, FR2, FR3, and FR4), which form β-sheet structures that permit development of a hydrophobic core.[14–19] Between the framework regions are complementarity-determining regions (CDR1, CDR2, and CDR3), which form part of the antigen-binding site of the immunoglobulin molecule; these regions generally provide the sequence variability among light chains.[14–16] Diversity among the CDRs occurs because the V_L domain is synthesized from multiple gene segments, termed V and J segments. The number of human V_κ and V_λ gene segments are estimated to be 30 to 50 and 20 to 30, respectively, whereas there are probably 5 J_κ and 20 to 30 J_λ gene segments.[20] The V_L domain is a product of one V and J region, so a large number of combinatorial possibilities exists. Thus, although light chains have a similar structure, each light chain is unique. A similar process also produces the structural diversity observed with heavy chains.

The course that light chains take in the kidney permits them to interact potentially with any segment of the nephron. Unique, but not yet completely defined, peptide domains of light chains confer a tropism for certain parts of the nephron. As described in the following paragraphs, it is this tropism that produces the wide spectrum of pathology associated with light chains.

PARAPROTEINEMIC RENAL DISEASES WITH PREDOMINANT GLOMERULAR INVOLVEMENT

Although light chains are the underlying cause of most of these renal lesions, the larger molecular weight proteins that include immunoglobulin heavy chains and intact immunoglobulins can participate directly in the pathogenesis of certain renal lesions. Diseases associated with isolated deposition of monoclonal heavy chains are particularly rare and include AH-amyloidosis[21] and monoclonal heavy-chain deposition disease.[22] Deposition of intact monoclonal immunoglobulin can also produce renal dysfunction. The usual causes of renal insufficiency associated with accumulation of monoclonal

immunoglobulin M (IgM) in Waldenström's macroglobulinemia are hyperviscosity syndrome and type I cryoglobulinemia with IgM deposition within the glomerular capillary lumen. In immunotactoid glomerulopathy, deposition of monoclonal IgG in the mesangium and along the glomerular basement membrane produces fibrillar deposits reminiscent of amyloid but are larger and do not stain with Congo red.[1] A recent report presented 10 patients who had proliferative glomerulonephritis associated with monoclonal immunoglobulin deposition apparently unassociated with type I cryoglobulinemia.[2]

The two major glomerular lesions associated with light chains are AL-amyloidosis[23–28] and ML(H)CDD.[4,18,29–38] Some light chains interact directly with mesangial cells to alter their function.[27,37–39] It now appears that light chains that promote glomerular injury bind to receptors on the surface of the mesangial cell and undergo endocytosis via a clathrin-mediated process.[40] Endocytosis of light chains also seems to promote phenotypic transformation of the mesangial cell, with amyloidogenic light chains promoting a macrophage-like phenotype and light chains associated with ML(H)CDD promoting a myofibroblastic phenotype.[41] Thus, although monoclonal light-chain deposition is the basic cause for both diseases, the pathogenetic processes are very different.

When primary cultures of rat mesangial cells were exposed to two different light chains isolated from patients who had ML(H)CDD, cell proliferation was inhibited and production of matrix proteins (type IV collagen, laminin, and fibronectin) increased. By immunocytochemistry and bioassay, transforming growth factor-β (TGF-β) production and activity increased when mesangial cells were exposed specifically to these monoclonal light-chain proteins. Furthermore, anti-TGF-β antibody abolished the inhibition of cell proliferation and matrix production caused by the two light chains. None of these findings was observed in mesangial cells exposed to human albumin and two other light chains previously characterized to have tubular, but not glomerular, cell toxicity.[37] These observations were expanded by determining if these light chains directly altered mesangial cell calcium homeostasis.[38] Intracellular Ca^{+2} signaling was determined in suspensions of rat mesangial cells using the fluorescent dye Fura-2AM with a calcium removal-addback protocol. Pretreatment of cultured rat mesangial cells with a κ light chain from a patient with ML(H)CDD produced reversible dose- and time-dependent attenuation of adenosine triphosphate (ATP)- and thrombin-evoked Ca^{+2} transients and capacitative calcium influx. Mesangial cells treated with this κ light chain and supplemented with *myo*-inositol (450 μM) did not demonstrate the attenuation of the ATP-evoked Ca^{+2} transient and capacitative calcium influx. The light chain also decreased mean Ca^{+2} transient and capacitative calcium influx in response to thapsigargin, a Ca^{+2} ATPase inhibitor. This inhibition was not reversed by exogenous *myo*-inositol. Another κ light chain (10 μg/mL), obtained from a patient who did not have ML(H)CDD, did not affect mesangial cell calcium signaling.

Thus, light chains that cause ML(H)CDD interact directly with the mesangial cell to promote functional changes that include increased production of TGF-β, which perhaps facilitated the myofibroblastic transformation of the mesangial cells and increased matrix protein production. Together with clinical studies that demonstrated increased production of TGF-β and extracellular matrix proteins in affected glomeruli of patients with ML(H)CDD,[34,42] light chain–mediated stimulation of mesangial cells to produce TGF-β seems to be a key pathogenetic mechanism of this disease.[37] The final result is development of glomerular sclerosis.

Internalization and processing of amyloidogenic light chains by mesangial cells facilitates the formation of amyloid in vitro.[27,39,43] Although production of TGF-β was integrally involved in development of ML(H)CDD, active TGF-β inhibited amyloid formation in vitro.[39] Unlike ML(H)CDD, the mechanism of glomerular injury in amyloidosis is largely related to replacement of the glomerular architecture with the amyloid protein.

The biochemical property(ies) of the light chain that confers nephrotoxicity remains under investigation, although advances have been made. Generally, sequence abnormalities in the V_L domain seem to be responsible for both processes. AL-amyloid is composed of the V_L of κ or λ light chains as well as intact light chains.[25,44,47] Comenzo et al[48] showed a preferential use of immunoglobulin V_L germ-line gene segments in AL-amyloidosis, including several genes that make minimal contributions to the normal repertoire. In addition, the tropism of organ involvement in AL-amyloidosis is significantly influenced by the V_L germline gene use and clonal plasma cell burden; patients with λVI clonal disease were more likely to have dominant renal involvement.[48] Several studies have shown that sequence variations in the V_L domain confer amyloidogenicity,[23,28,49] although the ambient composition of solutes such as urea may facilitate fibril formation by partially denaturing the light chain.[50] Variations in the amino acid sequence of the V_L domain have also been identified in light chains responsible for ML(H)CDD.[18,31,32,35]

PARAPROTEINEMIC RENAL DISEASES WITH PREDOMINANT TUBULOINTERSTITIAL INVOLVEMENT

Tubulointerstitial involvement related to monoclonal intact immunoglobulins or heavy chains does not occur, perhaps

because of significant restriction from the glomerular ultrafiltrate. In contrast, interaction of segments of the nephron with immunoglobulin light chains can result in a variety of tubulointerstitial lesions. Reabsorption of light chains by the proximal tubule can produce functional and morphologic alterations that seem to be related to distention of the endolysosomal system because of an inability to rapidly hydrolyze the light chains.[51–53] Clinical manifestations of this altered process can include renal failure from proximal tubular cell necrosis, or in less severe cases, acquired Fanconi syndrome. Sequence variations have been identified in the V_L domain of several κ light chains that cause Fanconi syndrome. These variations promote resistance to proteolysis.[54,55] There has also been recent interest in understanding the effect of reabsorption of filtered proteins on function of the proximal tubule in proteinuric conditions. Sengul et al demonstrated that endocytosis of light chains promoted the production of inflammatory cytokines by cells in culture through activation of NF-κB[56]; this process may promote tubulointerstitial inflammation and damage.

A mechanism of light chain–mediated tubule injury that is independent of proximal tubule toxicity is intratubular obstruction from precipitation of light chains in the distal nephron (Fig. 24-2).[52] Intraluminal protein precipitation was also shown to be the more common cause of tubular injury than isolated proximal tubule damage.[52] The mechanism of cast formation by light chains has been clarified and involves the co-precipitation of light chain with Tamm-Horsfall protein (THP) (Fig. 24-3).[52,53,57–60]

Only cells of the thick ascending limb of the loop of Henle synthesize and secrete THP, the major protein constituent of normal urine.[61,62] This fibrillar glycoprotein is composed of 616 amino acids and has a carbohydrate component that

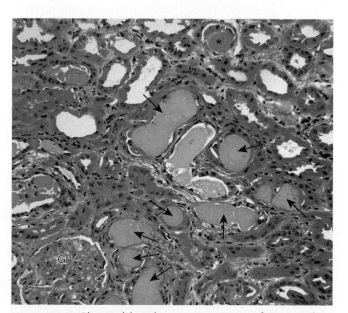

Figure 24-2 Classical histologic appearance of cast nephropathy. Numerous casts (*arrows*) are present within the tubular lumen. The surrounding epithelial cells of the nephron are compressed and distorted by the cast. Multinucleated giant cells surround one cast (*asterisk*). The glomeruli (G) are typically spared.

approaches 30% of the apparent molecular weight and consists of N-linked sugars (see Fig. 24-3).[63] Sialic acid residues confer an isoelectric point of 3.2; thus, the protein has a net negative charge at physiologic pH. In dilute salt solutions, THP forms filamentous strands that may exceed 7×10^6 Da[61]; a zona pellucida domain near the C terminus (see Fig. 24-3) promotes the homotypic aggregation into filaments.[64] THP belongs to the class of phosphatidylinositol-linked proteins,[65] permitting anchoring into the lipid bilayer of the apical surface of the cell and extension into the tubular lumen of the distal nephron. Cleavage from the glycophospholipid anchor produces a soluble form that appears in the urine. Viscosity of THP-containing solutions markedly increases when the NaCl concentration is greater than 60 mM. Increasing the concentrations of THP, H^+, and Ca^{+2} also increases viscosity of THP-containing solutions.[61] Although constitutively expressed, increased dietary salt intake increases expression of THP in rats.[66]

Intravenous infusions of nephrotoxic human light chains in rats acutely elevates proximal tubule pressure and simultaneously decreases single-nephron glomerular filtration rate; intraluminal protein casts were identified in these kidneys.[67] Isolated in vivo microperfusion experiments demonstrated that the casts form exclusively in the distal portion of the nephron, beginning with the thick ascending limb of Henle's loop. Removal of THP by pretreatment of rats with colchicine prevented cast formation in vivo.[57] Casts are seen primarily in the distal portion of the nephron in humans, although on occasion casts may also be found in proximal tubular segments and even in glomeruli in renal biopsy specimens. When examined, however, these casts generally contain THP, suggesting reflux of co-precipitated THP and light chain into the proximal nephron.[68,69]

Human light chains that precipitate in the rat nephron in vivo co-aggregate in vitro with human THP.[53] Light chains bind THP with differing affinities in a competitive fashion.[58,60,70] Enzymatic removal of the carbohydrate moiety of THP did not alter binding to light chains.[58] A single nine–amino acid binding domain for light chain has been mapped on THP (see Fig. 24-3).[60] By use of the yeast two-hybrid assay originally designed by Fields and Song,[71] the CDR3 region of both κ and λ light chains was identified as the site involved in binding THP.[70] A synthetic peptide that was identical to the CDR3 region of a light chain, which showed moderate

binding affinity to THP, effectively competed for binding to THP with six different light chains obtained from patients with myeloma and cast nephropathy.

In addition to intrinsic binding affinity, the environment in which THP interacts with light chains also modulates this binding and subsequent cast formation. Volume depletion slows tubular fluid flow rates, which promotes cast formation. Light chains that have a low affinity for THP and are ordinarily nontoxic can form casts in vivo under these conditions.[57] Increasing the concentrations of sodium, hydrogen, calcium, light chain, and THP facilitates co-precipitation in vitro.[53] Addition of furosemide promotes cast formation in a dose-dependent fashion.[57] Both low urinary pH and the presence of contrast agents also facilitate renal failure from light chains.[72] These laboratory findings suggest that altering the environment in which light chains interact with THP can regulate cast formation and further suggest a useful clinical approach to prevent cast formation in patients who have light-chain proteinuria. In addition to efforts to eradicate the clone of plasma cells responsible for production of the offending monoclonal light chain, it seems prudent to ensure high tubule fluid flow rates through the use of water consumption and avoidance of nonsteroidal anti-inflammatory agents. Because a diet high in salt content facilitates THP production,[66] dietary intake of salt should be restricted. Furosemide, and presumably all loop diuretics, should be avoided. Hypercalcemia should be corrected promptly with bisphosphonates. Although the interaction between some light chains and THP diminishes as pH increases,[59] it is difficult to administer bicarbonate without increasing sodium intake and should therefore not be considered.

SUMMARY

Scientific discoveries in the past decade have provided a clearer understanding of the pathogenesis of the multiple and varied clinical and pathologic presentations of paraproteinemic renal diseases. A central feature of many of these pathogenetic processes is the immunoglobulin light chain. As research into the molecular basis of paraproteinemic renal diseases continues, new therapeutic approaches will be designed to limit the morbidity and mortality associated with these intricate disease processes.

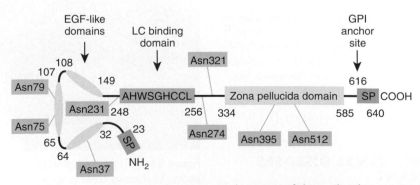

Figure 24-3 Human Tamm-Horsfall protein domains. The N-terminal portion of the molecule contains three epidermal growth factor (EGF)-like motifs, the functional significance of which is unknown. A zona pellucida domain near the C terminus is required for homotypic aggregation. Between these domains is the light-chain (LC) binding site. N-linked glycosylation sites are shown (Asn), as well as the glycosylphosphatidylinisotol (GPI)-anchor recognition site

Acknowledgments

This work was supported by the Office of Research and Development, Medical Research Service, Department of Veterans Affairs, by a grant from the Multiple Myeloma Research Foundation, and by generous donations from friends and family of Nila and Larry Minor. The author thanks Drs. Daniel F. Balkovetz and Anupam Agarwal and Mr. Ryan Corrick for critical evaluation of this review.

References

1. Rosenstock JL, Markowitz GS, Valeri AM, et al: Fibrillary and immunotactoid glomerulonephritis: Distinct entities with different clinical and pathologic features. Kidney Int 63:450, 2003.

2. Nasr SH, Markowitz GS, Stokes MB, et al: Proliferative glomerulonephritis with monoclonal IgG deposits: A distinct entity mimicking immune-complex glomerulonephritis. Kidney Int 65:5, 2004.

3. Martinez-Maldonado M, Yium J, Suki WN, Eknoyan G: Renal complications in multiple myeloma: Pathophysiology and some aspects of clinical management. J Chron Dis 24:221, 1971.

4. Sanders PW, Herrera GA, Kirk KA, et al: Spectrum of glomerular and tubulointerstitial renal lesions associated with monotypical immunoglobulin light chain deposition. Lab Invest 64:527, 1991.

5. Decourt C, Bridoux F, Touchard G, Cogne M: A monoclonal V κI light chain responsible for incomplete proximal tubulopathy. Am J Kidney Dis 41:97, 2003.

6. Bergman LW, Kuehl WM: Formation of intermolecular disulfide bonds on nascent immunoglobulin polypeptides. J Biol Chem 254:5690, 1979.

7. Morrison SL, Scharff MD: A mouse myeloma variant with a defect in light chain synthesis. Eur J Immunol 9:461, 1979.

8. Baylis C, Falconer-Smith J, Ross B: Glomerular and tubular handling of differently charged human immunoglobulin light chains by the rat kidney. Clin Sci (Lond) 74:639, 1988.

9. Wochner RD, Strober W, Waldmann TA: The role of the kidney in the catabolism of Bence Jones proteins and immunoglobulin fragments. J Exp Med 126:207, 1967.

10. Batuman V, Dreisbach AW, Cyran J: Light-chain binding sites on renal brush-border membranes. Am J Physiol 258(5 Pt 2):F1259, 1990.

11. Batuman V, Verroust PJ, Navar GL, et al: Myeloma light chains are ligands for cubilin (gp280). Am J Physiol 275(2 Pt 2):F246, 1998.

12. Klassen RB, Allen PL, Batuman V, et al: Light chains are a ligand for megalin. J Appl Physiol 98:257, 2005.

13. Day ED: The light chairs of immunoglobins. In Day ED (ed): Advanced Immunochemistry. New York, Wiley-Liss, 1990, pp 3–51.

14. Bruccoleri RE, Haber E, Novotny J: Structure of antibody hypervariable loops reproduced by a conformational search algorithm. Nature (Lond) 335:564, 1988.

15. Chothia C, Lesk AM: Canonical structures for the hypervariable regions of immunoglobulins. J Mol Biol 196:901, 1987.

16. Chothia C, Lesk AM, Tramontano A, et al: Conformations of immunoglobulin hypervariable regions. Nature (Lond) 342:877, 1989.

17. Glockshuber R, Steipe B, Huber R, Plückthun A: Crystallization and preliminary x-ray studies of the V_L domain of the antibody McPC603 produced in *Escherichia coli*. J Mol Biol 213:613, 1990.

18. Rocca A, Khamlichi AA, Aucouturier P, et al: Primary structure of a variable region of the $V_{κI}$ subgroup (ISE) in light chain deposition disease. Clin Exp Immunol 91:506, 1993.

19. Poljak RJ, Amzel LM, Chen BL, et al: The three-dimensional structure of the Fab′ fragment of a human myeloma immunoglobulin at 2.0-Å resolution. Proc Natl Acad Sci U S A 71:3440, 1974.

20. Solomon A: Light chains of immunoglobulins: Structural-genetic correlates. Blood 68:603, 1986.

21. Eulitz M, Weiss DT, Solomon A: Immunoglobulin heavy-chain-associated amyloidosis. Proc Natl Acad Sci U S A 87:6542, 1990.

22. Katz A, Zent R, Bargman JM: IgG heavy-chain deposition disease. Mod Pathol 7:74, 1994.

23. Schormann N, Murrell JR, Liepnieks JJ, Benson MD: Tertiary structure of an amyloid immunoglobulin light chain protein: A proposed model for amyloid fibril formation. Proc Natl Acad Sci U S A 92:9490, 1995.

24. Kyle RA, Greipp PR: Amyloidosis (AL): Clinical and laboratory features in 229 cases. Mayo Clin Proc 58:665, 1983.

25. Klafki H-W, Kratzin HD, Pick AI, et al: Complete amino acid sequence determinations demonstrate identity of the urinary Bence Jones protein (BJP-DIA) and the amyloid fibril protein (AL-DIA) in a case of AL-amyloidosis. Biochemistry 31:3265, 1992.

26. Klafki H-W, Pick AI, Pardowitz I, et al: Reduction of disulfide bonds in an amyloidogenic Bence Jones protein leads to formation of "amyloid-like" fibrils in vitro. Biol Chem Hoppe Seyler 374:1117, 1993.

27. Tagouri YM, Sanders PW, Picken MM, et al: In vitro AL-amyloid formation by rat and human mesangial cells. Lab Invest 74:290, 1996.

28. Wall JS, Gupta V, Wilkerson M, et al: Structural basis of light chain amyloidogenicity: Comparison of the thermodynamic properties, fibrillogenic potential and tertiary structural features of four V_l6 proteins. J Mol Recognit 17:23, 2004.

29. Randall RE, Williamson WC, Mullinax F, et al: Manifestations of systemic light chain deposition. Am J Med 60:293, 1976.

30. Alpers CE, Tu W-H, Hopper J, Biava CG: Single light chain subclass (κ-chain) immunoglobulin deposition in glomerulonephritis. Human Pathol 16:294, 1985.

31. Bellotti V, Stoppini M, Merlini G, et al: Amino acid sequence of k Sci, the Bence Jones protein isolated from a patient with light chain deposition disease. Biochim Biophys Acta 1097:177, 1991.

32. Cogné M, Preud'homme J-L, Bauwens M, et al: Structure of a monoclonal κ-chain of the Vκ$_{IV}$ subgroup in the kidney and plasma cells in light chain deposition disease. J Clin Invest 87:2186, 1991.

33. Ganeval D, Noël L-H, Preud'homme J-L, et al: Light-chain deposition disease: Its relation with AL-type amyloidosis. Kidney Int 26:1, 1984.

34. Herrera GA, Shultz JJ, Soong S-j, Sanders PW: Growth factors in monoclonal light chain–related renal diseases. Hum Pathol 25:883, 1994.

35. Khamlichi AA, Rocca A, Touchard G, et al: Role of light chain variable region in myeloma with light chain deposition disease: Evidence from an experimental model. Blood 86:655, 1995.

36. Preud'homme J-L, Aucouturier P, Touchard G, et al: Monoclonal immunoglobulin deposition disease (Randall type). Relationship with structural abnormalities of immunoglobulin chains. Kidney Int 46:965, 1994.

37. Zhu L, Herrera GA, Murphy-Ullrich JE, et al: Pathogenesis of glomerulosclerosis in light chain deposition disease: Role for transforming growth factor-β. Am J Pathol 147:375, 1995.

38. Zhu L, Herrera GA, White CR, Sanders PW: Immunoglobulin light chain alters mesangial cell calcium homeostasis. Am J Physiol 272(3 Pt 2):F319, 1997.

39. Isaac J, Kerby JD, Russell WJ, et al: In vitro modulation of AL-amyloid formation by human mesangial cells exposed to amyloidogenic light chains. Amyloid 5:238, 1998.

40. Teng J, Russell WJ, Gu X, et al: Different types of glomerulopathic light chains interact with mesangial cells using a common receptor but exhibit different intracellular trafficking patterns. Lab Invest 84:40, 2004.

41. Keeling J, Teng J, Herrera GA: AL-amyloidosis and light-chain deposition disease light chains induce divergent phenotypic transformations of human mesangial cells. Lab Invest 84:322, 2004.

42. Turbat-Herrera EA, Isaac J, Sanders PW, et al: Integrated expression of glomerular extracellular matrix proteins and β1 integrins in monoclonal light chain–related renal diseases. Mod Pathol 10:85, 1997.

43. Herrera GA, Russell WJ, Isaac J, et al: Glomerulopathic light chain–mesangial cell interactions modulate in vitro extracellular matrix remodeling and reproduce mesangiopathic findings documented in vivo. Ultrastruct Pathol 23:107, 1999.

44. Glenner GG, Ein D, Eanes ED, et al: Creation of "amyloid" fibrils from Bence Jones proteins in vitro. Science 174:712, 1971.

45. Glenner GG, Terry W, Harada M, et al: Amyloid fibril proteins: Proof of homology with immunoglobulin light chains by sequence analysis. Science 172:1150, 1971.

46. Epstein WV, Tan M, Wood IS: Formation of "amyloid" fibrils in vitro by action of human kidney lysosomal enzymes on Bence Jones proteins. J Lab Clin Med 84:107, 1974.

47. Hurle MR, Helms LR, Li L, et al: A role for destabilizing amino acid replacements in light-chain amyloidosis. Proc Natl Acad Sci U S A 91:5446, 1994.

48. Comenzo RL, Zhang Y, Martinez C, et al: The tropism of organ involvement in primary systemic amyloidosis: Contributions of Ig V(L) germ line gene use and clonal plasma cell burden. Blood 98:14, 2001.

49. Solomon A, Frangione B, Franklin EC: Bence Jones proteins and light chains of immunoglobulins: Preferential association of the V$_{IVI}$ subgroup of human light chains with amyloidosis AL(l). J Clin Invest 70:453, 1982.

50. Kim YS, Cape SP, Chi E, et al: Counteracting effects of renal solutes on amyloid fibril formation by immunoglobulin light chains. J Biol Chem 276:626, 2001.

51. Sanders PW, Herrera GA, Galla JH: Human Bence Jones protein toxicity in rat proximal tubule epithelium in vivo. Kidney Int 32:851, 1987.

52. Sanders PW, Herrera GA, Chen A, et al: Differential nephrotoxicity of low molecular weight proteins including Bence Jones proteins in the perfused rat nephron in vivo. J Clin Invest 82:2086, 1988.

53. Sanders PW, Booker BB, Bishop JB, Cheung HC: Mechanisms of intranephronal proteinaceous cast formation by low molecular weight proteins. J Clin Invest 85:570, 1990.

54. Messiaen T, Deret S, Mougenot B, et al: Adult Fanconi syndrome secondary to light chain gammopathy. Clinicopathologic heterogeneity and unusual features in 11 patients. Medicine (Baltimore) 79:35, 2000.

55. Deret S, Denoroy L, Lamarine M, et al: Kappa light chain–associated Fanconi's syndrome: Molecular analysis of monoclonal immunoglobulin light chains from patients with and without intracellular crystals. Protein Eng 12:63, 1999.

56. Sengul S, Zwizinski C, Simon EE, et al: Endocytosis of light chains induces cytokines through activation of NF-κB in human proximal tubule cells. Kidney Int 62:977, 2002.

57. Sanders PW, Booker BB: Pathobiology of cast nephropathy from human Bence Jones proteins. J Clin Invest 89:630, 1992.

58. Huang Z-Q, Kirk KA, Connelly KG, Sanders PW: Bence Jones proteins bind to a common peptide segment of Tamm-Horsfall glycoprotein to promote heterotypic aggregation. J Clin Invest 92:2975, 1993.

59. Huang Z-Q, Sanders PW: Biochemical interaction of Tamm-Horsfall glycoprotein with Ig light chains. Lab Invest 73:810, 1995.

60. Huang Z-Q, Sanders PW: Localization of a single binding site for immunoglobulin light chains on human Tamm-Horsfall glycoprotein. J Clin Invest 99:732, 1997.

61. Hoyer JR, Seiler MW: Pathophysiology of Tamm-Horsfall protein. Kidney Int 16:279, 1979.

62. Kumar S, Muchmore A: Tamm-Horsfall protein-uromodulin. 1950–1990. Kidney Int 37:1395, 1990.

63. Williams J, Marshall RD, van Halbeek H, Vliegenthart JFG: Structural analysis of the carbohydrate moieties of human Tamm-Horsfall glycoprotein. Carbohydr Res 134:141, 1984.

64. Jovine L, Qi H, Williams Z, et al: The ZP domain is a conserved module for polymerization of extracellular proteins. Nat Cell Biol 4:57, 2002.

65. Rindler MJ, Naik SS, Li N, et al: Uromodulin (Tamm-Horsfall glycoprotein/uromucoid) is a phosphatidylinositol-linked membrane protein. J Biol Chem 265:20784, 1990.

66. Ying W-Z, Sanders PW: Expression of Tamm-Horsfall glycoprotein is regulated by dietary salt in rats. Kidney Int 54:1150, 1998.

67. Weiss JH, Williams RH, Galla JH, et al: Pathophysiology of acute Bence-Jones protein nephrotoxicity in the rat. Kidney Int 20:198, 1981.

68. Start DA, Silva FG, Davis LD, et al: Myeloma cast nephropathy: Immunohistochemical and lectin studies. Modern Pathol 1:336, 1988.

69. Winearls CG: Acute myeloma kidney. Kidney Int 48:1347, 1995.

70. Ying W-Z, Sanders PW: Mapping the binding domain of immunoglobulin light chains for Tamm-Horsfall protein. Am J Pathol 158:1859, 2001.

71. Fields S, Song O: A novel genetic system to detect protein-protein interactions. Nature 340:245, 1989.

72. Holland MD, Galla JH, Sanders PW, Luke RG: Effect of urinary pH and diatrizoate on Bence Jones protein nephrotoxicity in the rat. Kidney Int 27:46, 1985.

Preeclampsia

Sharon E. Maynard and S. Ananth Karumanchi

CLINICAL FEATURES AND EPIDEMIOLOGY

Preeclampsia affects about 5% of all pregnancies,[1,2] and is classically defined as the new onset of hypertension and proteinuria after the 20th week of gestation. The onset of preeclampsia is often insidious and asymptomatic, but may include headache, visual disturbances, epigastric pain, weight gain, and edema of the hands and face. These early signs and symptoms are important to recognize clinically, since they may herald progression to more severe, often life-threatening, disease. Severe complications of preeclampsia can include acute renal failure, cerebral edema, cerebral hemorrhage, seizures (eclampsia), pulmonary edema, thrombocytopenia, hemolytic anemia, coagulopathy, and liver injury—including the syndrome of hemolysis, elevated liver enzymes, and low platelets (HELLP). Although antihypertensive medications help to lower blood pressure and magnesium sulfate is effective in seizure prophylaxis,[3] delivery remains the only definitive treatment. When preeclampsia threatens to lead to severe maternal complications, urgent delivery of the fetus and placenta are often undertaken to preserve maternal health.

In the developed world, where safe emergent cesarean delivery is available, the burden of morbidity and mortality due to preeclampsia is on the neonate. Preeclampsia is associated with placental hypoperfusion, which can lead to intrauterine growth restriction and oligohydramnios. But neonatal morbidity is most often due to the sequelae of prematurity and low birth weight, including prolonged neonatal intensive care unit stays, respiratory distress, necrotizing enterocolitis, intraventricular hemorrhage, sepsis, and death.[4,5] The HELLP syndrome has been associated with a 15% to 20% incidence of perinatal mortality, attributable to premature delivery.[6]

The epidemiology of preeclampsia provides hints about pathophysiology, which are still being deciphered. Although most preeclampsia occurs in healthy nulliparous women, several risk factors are reminiscent of cardiovascular risk factors, including chronic hypertension,[7,8] renal disease,[9,10] diabetes mellitus,[11,12] morbid obesity,[7,13,14] and family history of cardiovascular disease.[15] Congenital or acquired thrombophilia has been associated with preeclampsia in some[16,17] but not all[18,19] studies. Rheumatologic disorders such as systemic lupus and antiphospholipid antibody syndrome also increase risk.[20] The importance of cardiovascular risk factors has strengthened the hypothesis that preexisting maternal vascular dysfunction or susceptibility has a pathologic role in at least some cases of preeclampsia.

THE ROLE OF THE PLACENTA

Observational evidence suggests the placenta has a central role in preeclampsia. Preeclampsia only occurs in the presence of a placenta—though not necessarily a fetus, as in the case of hyatidiform mole—and almost always remits after its delivery. In a case of preeclampsia with extrauterine pregnancy, removal of the fetus alone was not sufficient; symptoms persisted until the placenta was delivered.[21] A recent report suggests that in cases of preeclampsia with discordant twins, selective fetocide reverses preeclampsia, with the attenuation of symptoms occurring in a time frame consistent with placental involution.[22]

Long-standing and severe preeclampsia is associated with pathologic evidence of placental hypoperfusion and ischemia. Findings include acute atherosis, a lesion of diffuse vascular obstruction first described in 1945,[23] which includes fibrin deposition, intimal thickening, necrosis, atherosclerosis, and endothelial damage. Infarcts, likely resulting directly from occlusion of maternal spiral arteries,[24] are also common. Although these findings are not universal, they appear to be correlated with severity of clinical disease.[25]

Abnormal uterine artery Doppler ultrasound results, suggesting increased uteroplacental resistance to blood flow, are observed before the clinical onset of preeclampsia,[26] although this finding is nonspecific, limiting its use as a screening test.[27] The incidence of preeclampsia is increased two- to fourfold in women residing at high altitude, implying hypoxia may be a contributing factor.[28] Hypertension and proteinuria can be induced by constriction of uterine blood flow in pregnant primates[29,30] and other mammals. These observations suggest placental ischemia may be an early event.

However, evidence for a causative role for placental ischemia remains circumstantial, and several observations call the hypothesis into question. For example, the animal models based on uterine hypoperfusion universally fail to induce several of the multiorgan features of preeclampsia, including seizures and glomerular endotheliosis, the hallmark renal pathologic finding. In most cases of preeclampsia, there is no evidence of growth restriction or fetal intolerance of labor, which would be an expected consequence of placental ischemia. It may be that the pathologic evidence of placental ischemic damage that accompanies late-stage preeclampsia may be a secondary event: no studies have examined placental changes prior to the onset of clinical signs of preeclampsia. Nevertheless, recent evidence suggests that early abnormalities in placental vascular remodeling may be present in preeclampsia.

PLACENTAL VASCULAR REMODELING

Early in normal placental development, extravillous cytotrophoblasts invade the uterine spiral arteries of the decidua and myometrium. These invasive fetal cells replace the endothelial layer of the uterine vessels, transforming them from small resistance vessels to flaccid, high-caliber capacitance vessels.[31,32] This vascular transformation allows the increase in uterine blood flow needed to sustain the fetus through the pregnancy (Fig. 25-1).

In preeclampsia, this transformation is incomplete (see Fig. 25-1).[33,34] Cytotrophoblast invasion of the arteries is limited to the superficial decidua, and the myometrial segments remain narrow and undilated.[35,36] Fisher and colleagues

have shown that in normal placental development, invasive cytotrophoblasts downregulate the expression of adhesion molecules characteristic of their epithelial cell origin and adopt an endothelial cell surface adhesion phenotype, a process referred to as pseudovasculogenesis.[37,38] In preeclampsia, cytotrophoblasts do not undergo this switching of cell surface

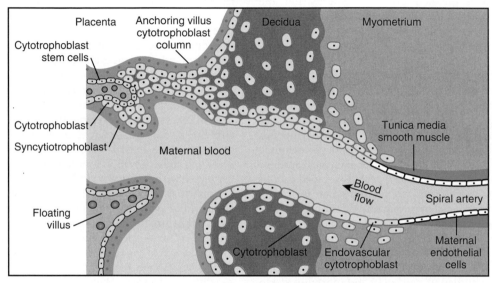

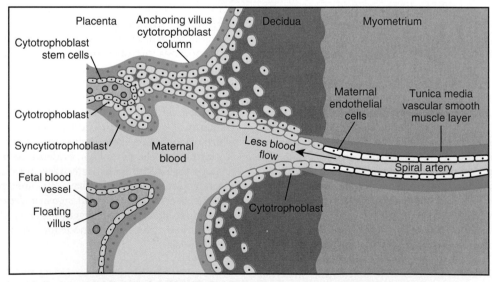

Figure 25-1 Abnormal placentation in preeclampsia. Exchange of oxygen, nutrients, and waste products between the fetus and the mother depends on adequate placental perfusion by maternal vessels. In normal placental development, invasive cytotrophoblasts of fetal origin invade the maternal spiral arteries, transforming them from small-caliber resistance vessels to high-caliber capacitance vessels capable of providing placental perfusion adequate to sustain the growing fetus. During the process of vascular invasion, the cytotrophoblasts differentiate from an epithelial phenotype to an endothelial phenotype, a process referred to as "pseudovasculogenesis" *(top).* In preeclampsia, cytotrophoblasts fail to adopt an invasive endothelial phenotype. Instead, invasion of the spiral arteries is shallow and they remain small-caliber resistance vessels *(bottom).* This may result in the placental ischemia. (From Karumanchi SA, Maynard SE, Stillman IE, et al: Preeclampsia: A renal perspective. Kidney Int 67:2101–2113, 2005.)

integrins and adhesion molecules[39] and fail to adequately invade the myometrial spiral arteries. The factors that regulate this process are just beginning to be elucidated. Invasive cytotrophoblasts express several angiogenic factors and receptors, including vascular endothelial growth factor (VEGF), placental growth factor (PlGF), and VEGFR-1 (Flt1); expression of these proteins by immunolocalization is altered in preeclampsia.[40] Liu and colleagues found that expression of CD146, an endothelial adhesion molecule normally expressed by invasive/migratory cytotrophoblasts, was absent in preeclampsia.[41] More work is needed to uncover the molecular signals governing cytotrophoblast invasion early in placentation. These mechanisms are sure to hold key insights into the pathogenesis of preeclampsia.

MATERNAL ENDOTHELIAL DYSFUNCTION

The clinical manifestations of preeclampsia reflect widespread endothelial dysfunction, often resulting in vasoconstriction and end-organ ischemia.[42,43] Several serum markers of endothelial activation are altered in women with preeclampsia, including von Willebrand antigen,[44] cellular fibronectin,[45] soluble tissue factor, soluble E-selectin, platelet-derived growth factor, and endothelin.[46] C-reactive protein[47] and leptin[48] levels are increased early in gestation. There is evidence for oxidative stress,[49] increased lipid peroxidation,[50] and platelet activation.[51] Decreased production of prostaglandin I_2, an endothelial-derived prostaglandin, occurs well before the onset of clinical symptoms.[52] Inflammation is often present; for example, there is neutrophil infiltration in the vascular smooth muscle of subcutaneous fat, with increased vascular smooth muscle expression of interleukin-8 and intracellular adhesion molecule-1.[53] Several of these aberrations occur well before the onset of symptoms, suggesting that they are primary, rather than secondary, effects.

In the kidney, endothelial damage results in proteinuria and produces glomerular endotheliosis This pathologic lesion is characterized by generalized swelling and vacuolization of the endothelial cells, obliteration of the endothelial fenestrae, and loss of the capillary space.[54,55] There are deposits of fibrinogen and fibrin within and under the endothelial cells.[56] The injury is specific to endothelial cells: the podocyte foot processes are almost completely normal in appearance early in disease, a finding atypical of other nephrotic diseases. Changes in the afferent arteriole, including atrophy of the macula densa and hyperplasia of the juxtaglomerular apparatus, have also been described.[57] Although once considered pathognomonic for preeclampsia, recent studies have shown that mild glomerular endotheliosis also can occur in pregnancy without preeclampsia, especially in pregnancy-induced hypertension.[58] This suggests the endothelial dysfunction of preeclampsia may in fact be an exaggeration of a process present near term in many pregnancies.

Long-term outcomes among women with a history of preeclampsia suggest the endothelial damage is not limited to pregnancy. Impaired endothelium-dependent vasodilatation, a marker for endothelial dysfunction, persists for years postpartum.[59,60] Cardiovascular morbidity and mortality are increased among women with a history of preeclampsia, including stroke,[61] ischemic heart disease,[62,63] and chronic hypertension.[64] An increased incidence of the metabolic syndrome after preeclampsia has been described.[65] Whether these observations result from endothelial damage accompanying preeclampsia, or simply reflect the consequences of risk factors common between preeclampsia and cardiovascular disease, remains speculative.

MECHANISMS OF PREECLAMPSIA

Genetic Factors

Although most preeclampsia occurs in women with no family history, the presence of preeclampsia in a first-degree relative increases a woman's risk for severe preeclampsia two- to fourfold,[66–68] suggesting a genetic contribution to the disease.

Early genetic studies have focused on maternal genes, but evidence is now strong that paternal genes, expressed in the fetus, are also important. There is a striking lack of concordance in the incidence of preeclampsia between mothers who are monozygous twins,[69] suggesting that the maternal genetic contribution is only part of the story. Men who were products of pregnancies complicated by preeclampsia were twice as likely to father a child who was the product of a pregnancy complicated by preeclampsia compared to control men with no such history.[68] If a woman becomes pregnant by a man who has already fathered a preeclamptic pregnancy in a different woman, her risk for developing preeclampsia is nearly doubled.[70] While a woman who has completed a normotensive pregnancy increases her preeclampsia risk by changing partners in the second pregnancy, a woman with prior preeclampsia will decrease her subsequent preeclampsia risk by changing partners.[71]

These studies, implicating a strong paternal (thus fetal) component to the genetic predisposition, might be consistent with a single-gene inheritance model, which requires homozygosity for the same recessive gene in both mother and fetus.[72] Others have hypothesized a role for genomic imprinting, a type of gene control in which the allele from one parent is expressed and the allele from the other parent is silenced. According to this model, preeclampsia may arise from a mutation in a paternally imprinted, maternally active gene, which must be expressed by the fetus in order to establish a normal placenta in the first pregnancy.[73] Perhaps the most popular model, however, is that preeclampsia is polygenetic with many susceptibility genes contributing to the disease.

Many case-control studies have looked at polymorphisms and mutations in specific maternal susceptibility genes. The list of genes for which associations have been described is large and has recently been reviewed in detail.[74] Several of these have been disappointing, with early studies suggesting an association that was not borne out in later, larger studies. For example, early work suggested an association between the factor V Leiden mutation and pregnancy-induced hypertension, but subsequent work did not bear out a strong association.[75]

Elevated homocysteine levels, associated with vascular disease in other populations, have been noted in preeclampsia.[76] Although nutritional factors such as folate deficiency may contribute, especially in developing countries,[77] some reports suggest that mutations in the 5,10-methylenetetrahydrofolate reductase (MTHFR) gene may be at play. Several early reports suggested that the common missense mutation of MTHFR

(677T polymorphism) is more prevalent among nulliparous preeclamptic women compared with controls.[78,79] However, the majority of studies in a variety of ethnic populations have not confirmed an association.[77,80–85]

Other candidate genes that have been studied, with mixed epidemiologic results, include mutations in genes coding for prothrombin, lipoprotein lipase, superoxide dismutase, nitric oxide synthetase, and apolipoprotein E.[74] The possible contributions of these mutations and polymorphisms remain to be determined. As with the candidate gene approach, several large genome-wide scans seeking a specific linkage to preeclampsia have been fairly discordant and disappointing. Of published studies, only one Icelandic analysis produced a significant logarithm of the odds (LOD) score (>3.6) for the 2p13 locus.[86] Even in this study, however, most of the support came from two large families yielding 17 affected patients. Other studies have produced suggestive LOD scores, each for different loci. This discordance suggests that a single genetic inheritance model is unlikely. Susceptibility may in fact be due to complex interactions between two or more maternal and fetal genes and environmental factors. It is interesting to note that all these genome-wide studies and candidate gene studies have focused on maternal genetic factors only. More recently, a small Dutch genetic study suggested that polymorphism in STOX1 (a member of the winged helix gene family), a gene that is paternally imprinted, may be linked to the occurrence of preeclampsia.[87] The Genetics of Preeclampsia Collaborative (GOPEC) study now in progress has collected genomic information from 1,000 women with preeclampsia throughout Great Britain, along with the proband's parents, child, and partner. This study will explore both maternal and fetal contributions to risk, and its results are eagerly anticipated.

Changes in the Renin-Angiotensin-Aldosterone System

Preeclampsia is a state of sympathetic overactivity. Maternal vascular reactivity to the vasopressors angiotensin II and norepinephrine is increased.[88] Endothelium-dependent vasorelaxation is impaired, both in the myometrial vessels in vitro[88] and in forearm blood flow in vivo.[60] In normal pregnancy, the renin-angiotensin-aldosterone system is activated; in preeclampsia, plasma renin levels are low compared with normal pregnancy,[89] likely suppression resulting from hypertension.

Wallukat and colleagues identified circulating angiotensin I (AT1) receptor autoantibodies in women with preeclampsia.[90] They found that these autoantibodies activated the AT1 receptor, and hypothesized that they might account for the increased angiotensin II sensitivity of preeclampsia. The same investigators later showed that these AT1 autoantibodies, like angiotensin II itself, stimulate endothelial cells to produce tissue factor, an early marker of endothelial dysfunction. Xia and colleagues found that AT1 autoantibodies decreased invasiveness of immortalized human trophoblasts in an in vitro Matrigel invasion assay.[91] These autoantibodies are not limited to pregnancy; they also appear to be increased in malignant renovascular hypertension in nonpregnancy.[92]

The angiotensinogen T235 polymorphism, a common molecular variant associated with essential hypertension and microvascular disease, was associated with preeclampsia in a U.S. and Japanese cohort.[93,94] Functional aspects of this mutation are unclear, however, and the association was not confirmed in a British population.[95] Work by AbdAlla and colleagues has suggested that heterodimerization of AT1 receptors with bradykinin-2 receptors may also contribute to angiotensin II hypersensitivity in preeclampsia.[96]

Oxidative Stress and Inflammation

Oxidative stress, the presence of active oxygen species in excess of available antioxidant buffering capacity, is a prominent feature of preeclampsia. Oxidative stress is known to damage proteins, cell membranes, and DNA and is a potential mediator of endothelial dysfunction. It has been hypothesized that in preeclampsia, placental oxidative stress is transferred to the systemic circulation, resulting in oxidative damage to the vascular endothelial cells throughout the body. According to proponents of this theory, oxidative stress itself may be the link between placenta and end-organ disease.[97]

Many studies in both mother and placenta document markers of oxidative stress in preeclampsia. In preeclamptic placentas, there is decreased expression of enzymatic antioxidants.[98–100] Abnormally high superoxide generation by placental tissue from women with preeclampsia has been noted.[101,102] Several studies have documented higher placental levels of lipid peroxidation, and increased production and secretion of isoprostanes.[103] Maternal serum markers for oxidative stress in preeclampsia include peroxynitrite,[104] protein carbonyls,[105] and others. Volatile organic compounds in alveolar breath (marker for oxidative stress) are increased in women with preeclampsia.[106]

Increased circulating fetal DNA in women with preeclampsia has been attributed to placental oxidative stress. Several studies have shown that fetal DNA in the maternal circulation rises prior to preeclampsia onset,[107,108] as early as 16 to 20 weeks of gestation.[109,110] Redman and others have suggested that reactive oxygen species (ROS) may result in deportation of syncytiotrophoblast fragments.[111,112] This material may contribute to endothelial activation in the mother.

Several theories exist regarding the source of free radical generation in placenta. Burton and colleagues theorized that the trigger for increased placental free radical generation is hypoxia-reperfusion,[111] presumably a consequence of placental vascular insufficiency outlined earlier in this chapter. Others have posited defects in the usual cellular defenses against oxidative stress. For example, glutathione S-transferases (GSTs) are an important enzyme system that provides protection against oxidative stress. Polymorphism in GST P1 is associated with preeclampsia, both in the maternal[113] and in the paternal[114] genome. There is some evidence that uric acid, consistently elevated in preeclampsia, may contribute to oxidative stress by decreasing nitric oxide production by human umbilical vein endothelial cells.[115]

NAD(P)H oxidases are a major source of oxygen free radical production in several cell types. Human placenta contains a functional NAD(P)H oxidase that is highly active, which could be an important source of superoxide during pregnancy and preeclampsia.[116] Raijmakers and colleagues showed that early-onset preeclampsia, but not late-onset preeclampsia, was associated with increased NAD(P)H-derived placental superoxide production.[117] AT1 receptor autoantibodies, described in the previous section, increase ROS production by activation of NADPH oxidase,[118] suggesting a mechanism by which these antibodies may contribute to the oxidative stress seen in preeclampsia.

Animal models and human trials also suggest a role for oxidative stress. One of the major animal models of preeclampsia is produced by infusion of L-NAME (L-nitro-arginine methylester), an inhibitor of NO synthesis, into pregnant rats. This produces a preeclampsia-like syndrome with hypertension, proteinuria, and thrombocytopenia.[119] A U.K. study showed that deficiency of selenium, a trace element with antioxidant properties, was associated with an increased risk for preeclampsia[120] But the most clinically relevant insights come from human trials: if oxidative stress is a key element in preeclampsia, antioxidant treatment might be expected to be beneficial. A randomized controlled trial by Chappell and colleagues showed that supplementation with vitamin C and E decreased preeclampsia in high-risk pregnant women (odds ratio 0.4). PAI-1 and PAI-2, markers of endothelial activation, were also decreased in the treatment group.[121] Similarly, treatment with the antioxidant lycopene was found to decrease the risk for preeclampsia by almost 50% in a small randomized trial.[122] These studies suggest that oxidative stress plays a central role in the propagation of the preeclampsia syndrome, and larger studies are ongoing.

Imbalance in Circulating Angiogenic Factors

If placental secretion of a soluble factor into the maternal bloodstream contributes to preeclampsia, it may be detectable using gene expression profiling. Using messenger RNA microarray analysis of placenta, our group found sFlt1 (soluble fms-like tyrosine kinase, also referred to as sVEGFR1), a truncated form of the VEGF receptor, was upregulated in the placenta of women with preeclampsia.[123] The in vitro effects of sFlt1 included vasoconstriction and endothelial dysfunction, mimicking the effects of plasma from women with preeclampsia. Exogenous sFlt1 administered to pregnant rats produced a syndrome resembling preeclampsia, including hypertension, proteinuria, and glomerular endotheliosis.[123] Proteinuria and glomerular endothelial damage has also been reported by exogenous sFlt1 therapy in nonpregnant mice.[124] This work has generated considerable enthusiasm for sFlt1 as an important mediator in preeclampsia.

sFlt1 is an anti-angiogenic molecule that antagonizes VEGF and PlGF (Fig. 25-2). VEGF is important in both angiogenesis (the growth of new blood vessels) and in the maintenance of endothelial cell health in the basal state. Although the function of PlGF is still ill defined, it appears to act synergistically with VEGF, and may be necessary for wound healing and angiogenesis in ischemic tissues.[125,126] VEGF has a family of receptors, the most important of which are Flt1 (VEGFR1) and Flk1 (VEGFR2).[127] sFlt1 is a truncated form of the Flt1 receptor. It includes the extracellular ligand-binding domain, but not the transmembrane and intracellular domains; it is secreted (hence "soluble") and antagonizes VEGF and PlGF in the circulation by binding and preventing their interaction with their endothelial receptors (see Fig. 25-2).[128] Although sFlt1 is made in small amounts by other tissues (endothelial cells and monocytes), the placenta seems to be the major source of circulating sFlt1 during pregnancy, as evidenced by the dramatic fall in circulating concentrations of sFlt1 after the delivery of the placenta.[123]

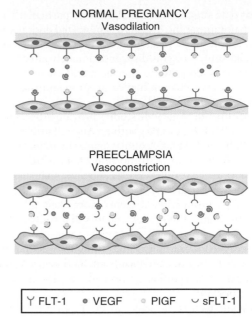

Figure 25-2 A schematic of the mechanism of action of sFlt1 in the vasculature of normal and preeclamptic pregnancy. Excess circulating sFlt1 binds VEGF and PlGF in the circulation, preventing these ligands from binding with their endogenous endothelial receptors. (From Bdolah Y, Sukhatme VP, Karumanchi SA: Angiogenic imbalance in the pathophysiology of preeclampsia: Newer insights. Semin Nephrol 24:548–556, 2004.)

sFlt1 levels are increased, and free (unbound) PlGF and free VEGF levels are suppressed, in the serum of women with preeclampsia.[123] The increase in sFlt1 precedes the onset of clinical disease by at least 5 weeks[129,130] and appears to more pronounced in severe and early-onset preeclampsia.[131,132] In several studies, decreased free PlGF levels were observed before 20 weeks of gestation in women who developed preeclampsia later in pregnancy,[131,133,134] though not all investigators have confirmed this finding.[135] Although reduction in free PlGF may be predominantly explained by increased sFlt1 production, some data suggest that the fall in PlGF may actually precede the rise in sFlt1, implicating other mechanisms such as decreased PlGF production. Since free PlGF is readily filtered through an intact glomerulus, urinary PlGF measurements can also be used for the prediction of preeclampsia.[136]

Derangements in other angiogenic molecules have also been observed. Levels of endostatin, an anti-angiogenic factor, are also elevated in preeclampsia.[137] A naturally occurring soluble form of Flk (VEGFR-2), the other major VEGF receptor, has recently been identified as being produced by the placenta.[138] Its role, if any, in placental vasculogenesis or preeclampsia remains unknown.

There is significant supportive evidence suggesting that VEGF and PlGF antagonism by sFlt1 could produce the endothelial dysfunction in preeclampsia. VEGF is highly expressed by glomerular podocytes, and VEGF receptors are present on glomerular endothelial cells.[139,140] In experimental glomerulonephritis, VEGF is necessary for glomerular capillary repair.[141,142] In anti-angiogenesis cancer trials, VEGF antagonists produce proteinuria and hypertension in human subjects.[143,144]

Recent data suggest that VEGF may be particularly important in maintaining the health of fenestrated endothelium,[145] which is found in the renal glomerulus, choroids plexus, and hepatic sinusoids—organs disproportionately affected in preeclampsia. It is tempting to speculate that cigarette smoking may exert its protective influence on preeclampsia risk[146] by its pro-angiogenic effects.[147]

On the other hand, genetic studies provide little support for a role for sFlt1. For example, both an Australian/New Zealand cohort[148] and an Icelandic cohort[86] have suggested a maternal susceptibility locus on chromosome 2, bearing no known relationship to sFlt1. Although it is possible that such loci are associated with transcription factors or splicing factors affecting sFlt1 production, it seems more likely that there are other as yet unidentified genetic factors that contribute to this multifactorial disease. The Flt1/sFlt1 gene is located on chromosome 13q12, and it is interesting to note that trisomy 13 has long been associated with an increased incidence of preeclampsia,[149] suggesting that a gene on this chromosome may be important.

Angiogenic factors are likely to be important in placental vasculogenesis. Generally speaking, VEGF is involved in all aspects of vascular development, including proliferation, migration, survival, and regulation of vascular permeability.[40] VEGF ligands and receptors are highly expressed by placental tissue in the first trimester.[150] In vitro, sFlt1 decreases invasiveness in primary cytotrophoblast culture.[40] Circulating sFlt1 levels are relatively low early in pregnancy, and begin to rise in the third trimester. This may reflect a physiologic antiangiogenic shift in the placental milieu toward the end of pregnancy, corresponding to completion of the vasculogenic phase of placental growth. It is intuitive to hypothesize that placental vascular development might be regulated by a local balance between pro- and anti-angiogenic factors, and that excess anti-angiogenic sFlt1 in early gestation could contribute to inadequate cytotrophoblast invasion in preeclampsia. By the third trimester, excess placental sFlt1 is detectable in the maternal circulation, producing end-organ effects. In this case, placental ischemia may not be causative, but rather the earliest organ affected by this derangement angiogenic balance. It is also interesting to note that women with preeclampsia appeared to have a decreased risk for malignancy in several studies,[61,151–153] suggesting an anti-angiogenic milieu that may extend beyond the pregnancy itself.

Immune Mechanisms

The possibility of immune maladaption remains one of the most enigmatic theories of preeclampsia. Normal placentation requires the development of immune tolerance between the fetus and the mother. The fact that preeclampsia occurs more often in first pregnancies or after a change in partners suggests that abnormal maternal immune response to paternally derived fetal antigens may play a role. This could result in failure of fetal-derived cells to successfully invade the maternal vessels in placental vascular development. These factors are reviewed in detail elsewhere.[154]

Observational studies suggest that preeclampsia risk increased in cases with exposure to novel paternal antigens: not only first pregnancies, but especially first pregnancies with a new partner[155] and long interpregnancy interval.[156] Women impregnated by intracytoplasmic sperm injection (ICSI), in which sperm were surgically obtained (i.e., the woman was never exposed to her partner's sperm in intercourse), had a threefold increased risk for preeclampsia compared with ICSI cases where sperm were obtained by ejaculation.[157] Conversely, prior exposure to paternal antigens appears to be protective. The duration of sexual relationship is inversely related to incidence of preeclampsia,[158] and oral tolerization to paternal antigens by oral sex and swallowing is associated with decreased risk.

An intact immune system seems necessary for the development of preeclampsia: women with human immunodeficiency virus (HIV) infection on no retroviral medication have a very low incidence of preeclampsia, but the incidence returns to normal in HIV-positive women who are taking highly active antiretroviral therapy (HAART).[159] Other immunologic phenomena have been observed in women with preeclampsia, providing circumstantial evidence for an immunologic role, such as increased circulating immune complexes, complement activation, complement and immune complex deposits in spiral arteries, placenta, liver, kidney, skin, and increased pro-inflammatory cytokines.[154] None of these clinical and biochemical observations have provided insights into immunologic triggers, however.

On a molecular level, human leukocyte antigen-G (HLA-G) expression appears to be abnormal in preeclampsia. HLA-G is a major histocompatibility tissue-specific antigen expressed in extravillous trophoblast (tissue of fetal origin), which may play a role in inducing immune tolerance at the maternal-fetal interface. Soluble HLA-G1 isoform downregulates both CD8+ and CD4+ T-cell reactivity. HLA-G also modulates innate immunity by binding to several natural killer (NK) and/or decidual receptors. In normal pregnancy, HLA-G is highly expressed by the most invasive cytotrophoblasts. Goldman-Wohl and colleagues have shown that in preeclampsia, HLA-G expression by cytotrophoblasts is either absent or reduced.[160] HLA-G protein concentrations are reduced in both maternal serum and in placental tissue in preeclampsia.[161] These investigators have hypothesized that this may affect the ability of trophoblasts to invade effectively, and could contribute to the ineffective trophoblasts invasion seen in preeclampsia. The molecular mechanisms that govern HLA-G expression, and how they might be deranged in preeclampsia, are still being elucidated.

It has been recently suggested that the NK cells in the maternal-fetal interface may play a role in maternal vascular remodeling and thus may be involved in the pathogenesis of preeclampsia. Genetic studies looking at polymorphisms in the killer immunoglobulin receptors (KIRs) on maternal NK cells and the fetal HLA-C haplotype suggest that patients with KIR-AA genotype and fetal HLA-C2 genotype were at greatly increased risk for preeclampsia.[162]

The possibility that infectious agents may play an etiologic or precipitory role in at least some cases of preeclampsia has continued to have sporadic support. Both anti-cytomegalovirus and anti-chlamydia antibody (immunoglobulin G) titers were increased in women with early-onset preeclampsia compared with late-onset preeclampsia and normal controls.[163] Another group confirmed increased titers against *Chlamydia pneumoniae* in patients with preeclampsia.[164] The association with *Chlamydia* is particularly interesting given its known association with coronary and other vascular disease, which shares many common risk factors with preeclampsia. Case reports have described preeclampsia with parvovirus B19 infection.[165] Other viral infections, such as herpes simplex virus-2 and

Epstein-Barr virus, have been associated with a lower incidence of preeclampsia.[166] Overall, it is safe to conclude that known infectious agents do not have a primary role in the majority of cases of preeclampsia.

DIAGNOSIS AND THERAPY: FUTURE DIRECTIONS

Currently, there is no useful and practical screening test for preeclampsia. Management is supportive and nonspecific, centering on bed rest, antihypertensive agents, magnesium, and early delivery. As our understanding of the pathophysiology of preeclampsia becomes more complete, specific and sensitive diagnostic tools and targeted therapies may be developed. It is difficult to predict which of the many leads described in this chapter will lead to changes in preeclampsia management. Indeed, given the polygenic and multifactorial nature of preeclampsia, diagnosis and treatment seem likely to have multiple arms. For example, the combination of low PlGF and low sex hormone binding globulin (SHBG), a marker of insulin resistance, was found to be more predictive of preeclampsia than either test alone.[167] Other groups are examining the utility of combining abnormalities in uterine artery Doppler waveform, a promising but nonspecific marker of preeclampsia risk, with serum markers.[168–170] Recent retrospective studies demonstrating the feasibility of urine screening test (PlGF) followed by a confirmatory blood test for circulating angiogenic proteins (sFlt1 and PlGF) for the prediction of preeclampsia are promising.[136] A prospective longitudinal study examining both urine and serum serially throughout gestation for alterations in angiogenic factors is needed to determine the relevance of these markers for the early identification of preeclampsia and the prediction of its severity.

Of course, a screening or diagnostic test will become truly useful only when an effective treatment or preventative intervention becomes available. A large multicenter trial of antioxidants for primary prevention of preeclampsia is currently underway with results expected in late 2006. Pharmacologic approaches to counteract the effects of sFlt1 might prove to be an effective treatment for established preeclampsia. It is clear that in cases of early, severe preeclampsia, a treatment that would allow clinicians to safely postpone delivery even a few weeks would result in a significant impact on neonatal morbidity. Therefore, there is a great opportunity to make a substantial clinical impact if effective treatments are developed.

Clearly, a multifactorial approach is required as we continue to deepen our understanding of the preeclampsia syndrome. As our understanding continues to advance based on molecular and genetic techniques, we are hopeful that new interventions may improve our management of this important syndrome in the near future.

References

1. World Health Organization: The Hypertensive Disorders of Pregnancy. WHO Technical Report Series 758. Geneva, World Health Organization, 1987.
2. Walker JJ: Pre-eclampsia. Lancet 356:1260–1265, 2000.
3. Lucas MJ, Leveno KJ, Cunningham FG: A comparison of magnesium sulfate with phenytoin for the prevention of eclampsia. N Engl J Med 333:201–206, 1995.
4. Sibai BM, et al: Maternal and perinatal outcome of conservative management of severe preeclampsia in midtrimester. Am J Obstet Gynecol 152:32–37, 1985.
5. Friedman SA, et al: Neonatal outcome after preterm delivery for preeclampsia. Am J Obstet Gynecol 172:1785–1788, 1995.
6. Roelofsen AC, van Pampus MG, Aarnoudse JG: The HELLP-syndrome; maternal-fetal outcome and follow up of infants. J Perinatal Med 31:201–208, 2003.
7. Sibai BM, et al: Risk factors associated with preeclampsia in healthy nulliparous women. The Calcium for Preeclampsia Prevention (CPEP) Study Group. Am J Obstet Gynecol 177:1003–1010, 1997.
8. Caritis S, et al: Predictors of pre-eclampsia in women at high risk. National Institute of Child Health and Human Development Network of Maternal-Fetal Medicine Units. Am J Obstet Gynecol 179:946–951, 1998.
9. Mostello D, et al: Preeclampsia in the parous woman: Who is at risk? Am J Obstet Gynecol 187:425–429, 2002.
10. Cunningham FG, et al: Chronic renal disease and pregnancy outcome. Am J Obstet Gynecol 163:453–459, 1990.
11. Sibai BM: Risk factors pregnancy complications and prevention of hypertensive disorders in women with pregravid diabetes mellitus. J Maternal Fetal Med 9:62–65, 2000.
12. Garner PR, et al: Preeclampsia in diabetic pregnancies. Am J Obstet Gynecol 163:505–508, 1990.
13. Weiss JL, et al: Obesity obstetric complications and cesarean delivery rate—A population-based screening study. Am J Obstet Gynecol 190:1091–1097, 2004.
14. Thadhani R, et al: High body mass index and hypercholesterolemia: Risk of hypertensive disorders of pregnancy. Obstet Gynecol 94:543–550, 1999.
15. Ness RB, et al: Family history of hypertension heart disease and stroke among women who develop hypertension in pregnancy. Obstet Gynecol 102:1366–1371, 2003.
16. Roque H, et al: Maternal thrombophilias are not associated with early pregnancy loss. Thrombos Haemost 91:290–295, 2004.
17. Rasmussen A, Ravn P: High frequency of congenital thrombophilia in women with pathological pregnancies? Acta Obstet Gynecol Scand 83:808–817, 2004.
18. Branch DW, et al: Antiphospholipid antibodies in women at risk for preeclampsia. Am J Obstet Gynecol 184:825–832, 2001.
19. Kujovich JL: Thrombophilia and pregnancy complications. Am J Obstet Gynecol 191:412–424, 2004.
20. Wolfberg AJ, et al: Association of rheumatologic disease with preeclampsia. Obstet Gynecol 103:1190–1193, 2004.
21. Shembrey MA, Noble AD: An instructive case of abdominal pregnancy. Aust N Z J Obstet Gynaecol 35:220–221, 1995.
22. Heyborne KD, Porreco R: Selective fetocide reverses preeclampsia in discordant twins. Am J Obstet Gynecol 191:477–480, 2004.
23. Hertig AT: Vascular pathology in the hypertensive albuminuric toxemias of pregnancy. Clinics 4:602–614, 1945.
24. Zeek PM, Assali NS: Vascular changes with eclamptogenic toxemia of pregnancy. Am J Clin Pathol 20:1099–1109, 1950.
25. Salafia CM, et al: Clinical correlations of patterns of placental pathology in preterm pre-eclampsia. Placenta 19:67–72, 1998.
26. Bower SK, Schuchter, Campbell S: Doppler ultrasound screening as part of routine antenatal scanning: Prediction of pre-eclampsia and intrauterine growth retardation. Br J Obstet Gynaecol 100:989–994, 1993.
27. North RA, et al: Uterine artery Doppler flow velocity waveforms in the second trimester for the prediction of preeclampsia and fetal growth retardation. Obstet Gynecol 83:378–386, 1994.
28. Palmer SK, et al: Altered blood pressure course during normal pregnancy and increased preeclampsia at high altitude (3100 meters) in Colorado. Am J Obstet Gynecol 180:1161–1168, 1999.

29. Cavanagh D, et al: Pregnancy-induced hypertension: Development of a model in the pregnant primate (Papio anubis). Am J Obstet Gynecol 151:987–999, 1985.

30. Combs CA, et al: Experimental preeclampsia produced by chronic constriction of the lower aorta: Validation with longitudinal blood pressure measurements in conscious rhesus monkeys. Am J Obstet Gynecol 169:215–223, 1993.

31. De Wolf F, et al.: The human placental bed: Electron microscopic study of trophoblastic invasion of spiral arteries. Am J Obstet Gynecol 137:58–70, 1980.

32. Brosens IA, Robertson WB, Dixon HG: The role of the spiral arteries in the pathogenesis of preeclampsia. Obstet Gynecol Annu 1:177–191, 1972.

33. Kumar D: Chronic placental ischemia in relation to toxemias of pregnancy. A preliminary report. Am J Obstet Gynecol 84:1323–1329, 1962.

34. Robertson WB, Brosens I, Dixon HG: The pathological response of the vessels of the placental bed to hypertensive pregnancy. J Pathol Bacteriol 93:581–592, 1967.

35. Meekins JW, et al: A study of placental bed spiral arteries and trophoblast invasion in normal and severe pre-eclamptic pregnancies. Br J Obstet Gynaecol 101:669–674, 1994.

36. Pijnenborg R, et al: Placental bed spiral arteries in the hypertensive disorders of pregnancy. Br J Obstet Gynaecol 98:648–55, 1991.

37. Zhou Y, et al: Preeclampsia is associated with abnormal expression of adhesion molecules by invasive cytotrophoblasts. J Clin Invest 91:950–960, 1993.

38. Zhou Y, et al: Human cytotrophoblasts adopt a vascular phenotype as they differentiate. A strategy for successful endovascular invasion? J Clin Invest 99:2139–2151, 1997.

39. Zhou Y, Damsky CH, Fisher SJ: Preeclampsia is associated with failure of human cytotrophoblasts to mimic a vascular adhesion phenotype. One cause of defective endovascular invasion in this syndrome? J Clin Invest 99:2152–2164, 1997.

40. Zhou Y, et al: Vascular endothelial growth factor ligands and receptors that regulate human cytotrophoblast survival are dysregulated in severe preeclampsia and hemolysis elevated liver enzymes and low platelets syndrome. Am J Pathol 160:1405–1423, 2002.

41. Liu Q, et al: Pre-eclampsia is associated with the failure of melanoma cell adhesion molecule (MCAM/CD146) expression by intermediate trophoblast. Lab Invest 84:221–228, 2004.

42. Ferris TF: Pregnancy preeclampsia and the endothelial cell. N Engl J Med 325:1439–1440, 1991.

43. Roberts JM, et al: Preeclampsia: An endothelial cell disorder. Am J Obstet Gynecol 161:1200–1204, 1989.

44. Calvin S, et al: Factor VIII: von Willebrand factor patterns in the plasma of patients with pre-eclampsia. Am J Perinatol 5:29–32, 1988.

45. Lockwood CJ, Peters JH: Increased plasma levels of ED1+ cellular fibronectin precede the clinical signs of preeclampsia. Am J Obstet Gynecol 162:358–362, 1990.

46. Nova A, et al: Maternal plasma level of endothelin is increased in preeclampsia. Am J Obstet Gynecol 165:724–727, 1991.

47. Qiu C, et al: A prospective study of maternal serum C-reactive protein concentrations and risk of preeclampsia. Am J Hypertens 17:154–160, 2004.

48. Chappell LC, et al: A longitudinal study of biochemical variables in women at risk of preeclampsia. Am J Obstet Gynecol 187:127–136, 2002.

49. Davidge ST: Oxidative stress and altered endothelial cell function in preeclampsia. Semin Reprod Endocrinol 16:65–73, 1998.

50. Hubel CA, et al: Fasting serum triglycerides free fatty acids and malondialdehyde are increased in preeclampsia are positively correlated and decrease within 48 hours post partum. Am J Obstet Gynecol 174:975–982, 1996.

51. Kolben M et al: Measuring the concentration of various plasma and placenta extract proteolytic and vascular factors in pregnant patients with HELLP syndrome preeclampsia and highly pathologic Doppler flow values. Gynakol Geburtshilfliche Rundsch 35(Suppl 1):126–131, 1995.

52. Mills JL, et al: Prostacyclin and thromboxane changes predating clinical onset of preeclampsia: A multicenter prospective study. JAMA 282:356–362, 1999.

53. Leik CE, Walsh SW: Neutrophils infiltrate resistance-sized vessels of subcutaneous fat in women with preeclampsia. Hypertension 44:72–77, 2004.

54. Spargo BH, McCartney C, Winemiller R: Glomerular capillary endotheliosis in toxemia of pregnancy. Arch Pathol 13:593–599, 1959.

55. Fisher KA, et al: Hypertension in pregnancy: Clinical-pathological correlations and remote prognosis. Medicine (Baltimore) 60:267–276, 1981.

56. Pirani CL, et al: The renal glomerular lesions of pre-eclampsia: Electron microscopic studies. Am J Obstet Gynecol 87:1047–1070, 1963.

57. Govan AD: Renal changes in eclampsia. J Pathol Bacteriol 67:311–322, 1954.

58. Strevens H, et al: Glomerular endotheliosis in normal pregnancy and pre-eclampsia. Br J Obstet Gynaecol 110:831–836, 2003.

59. Agatisa PK, et al: Impairment of endothelial function in women with a history of preeclampsia: An indicator of cardiovascular risk. Am J Physiol Heart Circ Physiol 286:1389–1393, 2004.

60. Chambers JC, et al: Association of maternal endothelial dysfunction with preeclampsia. JAMA 285:1607–1612, 2001.

61. Irgens HU, et al: Long term mortality of mothers and fathers after pre-eclampsia: Population based cohort study. BMJ 323:1213–1217, 2001.

62. Haukkamaa L, et al: Risk for subsequent coronary artery disease after preeclampsia. Am J Cardio 93:805–808, 2004.

63. Smith GC, Pell J, Walsh D: Pregnancy complications and maternal risk of ischaemic heart disease: A retrospective cohort study of 129290 births [see comment]. Lancet 357:2002–2006, 2001.

64. Epstein FH: Late vascular effects of toxemia of pregnancy. N Engl J Med 271:391–395, 1964.

65. Pouta A, et al: Manifestations of metabolic syndrome after hypertensive pregnancy. Hypertension 43:825–831, 2004.

66. Cincotta RB, Brennecke S: Family history of pre-eclampsia as a predictor for pre-eclampsia in primigravidas. Int J Gynecol Obstet 60:23–27, 1998.

67. Mogren I, et al: Familial occurrence of preeclampsia. Epidemiology 10:518–522, 1999.

68. Esplin MS, et al: Paternal and maternal components of the predisposition to preeclampsia [see comment]. N Engl J Med 344:867–872, 2001.

69. Thornton JG, Onwude JL: Pre-eclampsia: Discordance among identical twins. BMJ (Clinical Research Ed) 303:1241–1242, 1991.

70. Lie RT, et al: Fetal and maternal contributions to risk of pre-eclampsia: Population based study. BMJ 316:1343–1347, 1998.

71. Li DK, Wi S: Changing paternity and the risk of preeclampsia/eclampsia in the subsequent pregnancy. Am J Epidemiol 151:57–62, 2000.

72. Liston WA, Kilpatrick DC: Is genetic susceptibility to pre-eclampsia conferred by homozygosity for the same single recessive gene in mother and fetus? Br J Obstet Gynaecol 98:1079–1086, 1991.

73. Graves JA: Genomic imprinting development and disease—Is pre-eclampsia caused by a maternally imprinted gene? Reprod Fertil Dev 10:23–29, 1998.

74. Wilson ML, et al: Molecular epidemiology of preeclampsia. Obstet Gynecol Surv 58:39–66, 2003.

75. Kosmas IA, Tatsioni, Ioannidis J: Association of Leiden mutation in factor V gene with hypertension in pregnancy and pre-eclampsia: A meta-analysis. J Hypertens 21:1221–1228, 2003.

76. Dekker GA, et al: Underlying disorders associated with severe early-onset preeclampsia. Am J Obstet Gynecol 173:1042–1048, 1995.

77. Rajkovic A, et al: Methylenetetrahydrofolate reductase 677 C → T polymorphism plasma folate vitamin B12 concentrations and risk of preeclampsia among black African women from Zimbabwe. Mol Genet Metab 69:33–39, 2000.

78. Sohda S, et al: Methylenetetrahydrofolate reductase polymorphism and pre-eclampsia. J Med Genet 34:525–526, 1997.

79. Grandone E, et al: Factor V Leiden C → T MTHFR polymorphism and genetic susceptibility to preeclampsia. Thromb Haemost 77:1052–1054, 1997.

80. Chikosi AB, et al: 510 methylenetetrahydrofolate reductase polymorphism in black South African women with pre-eclampsia. Br J Obstet Gynaecol 106:1219–1220, 1999.

81. Kaiser T, Brennecke S, Moses EK: Methylenetetrahydrofolate reductase polymorphisms are not a risk factor for pre-eclampsia/eclampsia in Australian women. Gynecol Obstet Invest 50:100–102, 2000.

82. Laivuori H, et al: 677 C→T polymorphism of the methylenetetrahydrofolate reductase gene and preeclampsia. Obstet Gynecol 96:277–280, 2000.

83. Powers RW, et al: Methylenetetrahydrofolate reductase polymorphism folate and susceptibility to preeclampsia. J Soc Gynecol Invest 6:74–79, 1999.

84. Lachmeijer AMA, et al: Mutations in the gene for methylenetetrahydrofolate reductase homocysteine levels and vitamin status in women with a history of preeclampsia. Am J Obstet Gynecol 184:394–402, 2001.

85. Kobashi G, et al: Absence of association between a common mutation in the methylenetetrahydrofolate reductase gene and preeclampsia in Japanese women American. J Med Genet 93:122–125, 2000.

86. Arngrimsson R, et al: A genome-wide scan reveals a maternal susceptibility locus for pre-eclampsia on chromosome 2p13. Hum Mol Genet 8:1799–1805, 1999.

87. van Dijk M, et al: Maternal segregation of the Dutch preeclampsia locus at 10q22 with a new member of the winged helix gene family. Nat Genet 37:514–519, 2005.

88. Ashworth JR, et al: Loss of endothelium-dependent relaxation in myometrial resistance arteries in pre-eclampsia. Br J Obstet Gynaecol 104:1152–1158, 1997.

89. Brown MA, Wang J, Whitworth JA: The renin-angiotensin-aldosterone system in pre-eclampsia. Clin Exp Hypertens (New York) 19:713–726, 1997.

90. Wallukat G, et al: Patients with preeclampsia develop agonistic autoantibodies against the angiotensin AT1 receptor. J Clin Invest 103:945–52, 1999.

91. Xia Y, et al: Maternal autoantibodies from preeclamptic patients activate angiotensin receptors on human trophoblast cells. J Soc Gynecol Invest 10:82–93, 2003.

92. Fu ML, et al: Autoantibodies against the angiotensin receptor (AT1) in patients with hypertension. J Hypertens 18:945–953, 2000.

93. Ward K, et al: A molecular variant of angiotensinogen associated with preeclampsia. Nat Genet 4:59–61, 1993.

94. Kobashi G, et al: Multivariate analysis of genetic and acquired factors; T235 variant of the angiotensinogen gene is a potent independent risk factor for preeclampsia. Semin Thromb Hemost 27:143–147, 2001.

95. Morgan L, et al: Maternal and fetal angiotensinogen gene allele sharing in pre-eclampsia. Br J Obstet Gynaecol 106:244–251, 1999.

96. AbdAlla S, et al: Increased AT[1] receptor heterodimers in preeclampsia mediate enhanced angiotensin II responsiveness. Nat Med 7:1003–1009, 2001.

97. Roberts JM, Hubel CA: Is oxidative stress the link in the two-stage model of pre-eclampsia? [comment]. Lancet 354:788–789, 1999.

98. Walsh SW: Maternal-placental interactions of oxidative stress and antioxidants in preeclampsia. Semin Reprod Endocrinol 16:93–104, 1998.

99. Wang Y, Walsh SW: Antioxidant activities and mRNA expression of superoxide dismutase catalase and glutathione peroxidase in normal and preeclamptic placentas. J Soc Gynecol Invest 3:179–184, 1996.

100. Zusterzeel PL, et al: Glutathione S-transferase isoenzymes in decidua and placenta of preeclamptic pregnancies. Obstet Gynecol 94:1033–1038, 1999.

101. Wang Y, Walsh SW: Increased superoxide generation is associated with decreased superoxide dismutase activity and mRNA expression in placental trophoblast cells in pre-eclampsia. Placenta 22:206–212, 2001.

102. Sikkema JM et al: Placental superoxide is increased in pre-eclampsia. Placenta 22:304–308, 2001.

103. Walsh SW, et al: Placental isoprostane is significantly increased in preeclampsia. FASEB J 14:1289–1296, 2000.

104. Roggensack AM, Zhang Y, Davidge ST: Evidence for peroxynitrite formation in the vasculature of women with preeclampsia. Hypertension 33:83–89, 1999.

105. Zusterzeel PL, et al: Protein carbonyls in decidua and placenta of pre-eclamptic women as markers for oxidative stress. Placenta 22:213–219, 2001.

106. Moretti M, et al: Increased breath markers of oxidative stress in normal pregnancy and in preeclampsia. Am J Obstet Gynecol 190:1184–1190, 2004.

107. Leung TN, et al: Increased maternal plasma fetal DNA concentrations in women who eventually develop preeclampsia. Clin Chem 47:137–139, 2001.

108. Zhong XY, Holzgreve W, Hahn S: The levels of circulatory cell free fetal DNA in maternal plasma are elevated prior to the onset of preeclampsia. Hypertens Pregnancy 21:77–83, 2002.

109. Cotter AM, et al: Increased fetal DNA in the maternal circulation in early pregnancy is associated with an increased risk of preeclampsia. Am J Obstet Gynecol 191:515–520, 2004.

110. Levine RJ, et al: Two-stage elevation of cell-free fetal DNA in maternal sera before onset of preeclampsia. Am J Obstet Gynecol 190:707–713, 2004.

111. Hung TH, et al: Hypoxia-reoxygenation: A potent inducer of apoptotic changes in the human placenta and possible etiological factor in preeclampsia. Circ Res 90:1274–1281, 2002.

112. Redman CW, Sargent IL: Pre-eclampsia the placenta and the maternal systemic inflammatory response—A review. Placenta 24(Suppl A):21–27, 2003.

113. Zusterzeel PL, et al: Polymorphism in the glutathione S-transferase P1 gene and risk for preeclampsia. Obstet Gynecol 96:50–54, 2000.

114. Zusterzeel PL, et al: Paternal contribution to the risk for pre-eclampsia. J Med Genet 39:44–45, 2002.

115. Kang DH, et al: Uric acid endothelial dysfunction and pre-eclampsia: Searching for a pathogenetic link [see comment]. J Hypertens 22:229–235, 2004.

116. Poston L, Raijmakers MT: Trophoblast oxidative stress antioxidants and pregnancy outcome—A review. Placenta 25(Suppl A):72–78, 2004.

117. Raijmakers MT, et al: NAD(P)H oxidase associated superoxide production in human placenta from normotensive and pre-eclamptic women. Placenta 25(Suppl A):85–89, 2004.
118. Dechend R, et al: AT1 receptor agonistic antibodies from preeclamptic patients stimulate NADPH oxidase. Circulation 107:1632–1639, 2003.
119. Yallampalli C, Garfield RE: Inhibition of nitric oxide synthesis in rats during pregnancy produces signs similar to those of preeclampsia. Am J Obstet Gynecol 169:1316–1320, 1993.
120. Rayman M, Bode P, Redman CWG: Low selenium status is associated with the occurrence of the pregnancy disease preeclampsia in women from the United Kingdom. Am J Obstet Gynecol 189:1343–1349, 2003.
121. Chappell LC, et al: Effect of antioxidants on the occurrence of pre-eclampsia in women at increased risk: A randomised trial. Lancet 354:810–816, 1999.
122. Sharma JB, et al: Effect of lycopene on pre-eclampsia and intra-uterine growth retardation in primigravidas. Int J Gynaecol Obstet 81:257–262, 2003.
123. Maynard SE, et al: Excess placental soluble fms-like tyrosine kinase 1 (sFlt1) may contribute to endothelial dysfunction hypertension and proteinuria in preeclampsia. J Clin Invest 111:649–658, 2003.
124. Sugimoto H, et al: Neutralization of circulating vascular endothelial growth factor (VEGF) by anti-VEGF antibodies and soluble VEGF receptor 1 (sFlt-1) induces proteinuria. J Biol Chem 278:12605–12608, 2003.
125. Luttun A, et al: Revascularization of ischemic tissues by PlGF treatment and inhibition of tumor angiogenesis arthritis and atherosclerosis by anti-Flt1. Nat Med 8:831–840, 2002.
126. Carmeliet P, et al: Synergism between vascular endothelial growth factor and placental growth factor contributes to angiogenesis and plasma extravasation in pathological conditions. Nat Med 7:575–583, 2001.
127. Dvorak HF: Vascular permeability factor/vascular endothelial growth factor: A critical cytokine in tumor angiogenesis and a potential target for diagnosis and therapy. J Clin Oncol 20:4368–4380, 2002.
128. Kendall RL, Thomas KA: Inhibition of vascular endothelial cell growth factor activity by an endogenously encoded soluble receptor. Proc Natl Acad Sci U S A 90:10705–10709, 1993.
129. McKeeman GC, et al: Soluble vascular endothelial growth factor receptor-1 (sFlt-1) is increased throughout gestation in patients who have preeclampsia develop. Am J Obstet Gynecol 191:1240–1246, 2004.
130. Hertig A, et al: Maternal serum sFlt1 concentration is an early and reliable predictive marker of preeclampsia. Clin Chem 50:1702–1703, 2004.
131. Levine RJ, et al: Circulating angiogenic factors and the risk of preeclampsia [see comment]. N Engl J Med 350:672–683, 2004.
132. Chaiworapongsa T, et al: Evidence supporting a role for blockade of the vascular endothelial growth factor system in the pathophysiology of preeclampsia. Young Investigator Award. Am J Obstet Gynecol 190:1541–1550, 2004.
133. Thadhani R, et al: First trimester placental growth factor and soluble fms-like tyrosine kinase 1 and risk for preeclampsia. J Clin Endocrinol Metab 89:770–775, 2004.
134. Taylor RN, et al: Longitudinal serum concentrations of placental growth factor: Evidence for abnormal placental angiogenesis in pathologic pregnancies. Am J Obstet Gynecol 188:177–182, 2003.
135. Livingston JC, et al: Placenta growth factor is not an early marker for the development of severe preeclampsia. Am J Obstet Gynecol 184:1218–1220, 2001.
136. Levine RJ, et al: Urinary placental growth factor and risk of preeclampsia. JAMA 293:77–85, 2005.
137. Hirtenlehner K, et al: Elevated serum concentrations of the angiogenesis inhibitor endostatin in preeclamptic women. J Soc Gynecol Invest 10:412–417, 2003.
138. Ebos JML, et al: A naturally occurring soluble form of vascular endothelial growth factor receptor 2 detected in mouse and human plasma. Mol Cancer Res 2:315–326, 2004.
139. Simon M, et al: Expression of vascular endothelial growth factor and its receptors in human renal ontogenesis and in adult kidney. Am J Physiol 268:F240–F250, 1995.
140. Simon M, et al: Receptors of vascular endothelial growth factor/vascular permeability factor (VEGF/VPF) in fetal and adult human kidney: Localization and (125I)VEGF binding sites. J Am Soc Nephrol 9:1032–1044, 1998.
141. Masuda Y, et al: Vascular endothelial growth factor enhances glomerular capillary repair and accelerates resolution of experimentally induced glomerulonephritis. Am J Pathol 159:599–608, 2001.
142. Ostendorf T, et al: VEGF(165) mediates glomerular endothelial repair. J Clin Invest 104:913–923, 1999.
143. Kabbinavar F, et al: Phase II randomized trial comparing bevacizumab plus fluorouracil (FU)/leucovorin (LV) with FU/LV alone in patients with metastatic colorectal cancer. J Clin Oncol 21:60–65, 2003.
144. Yang JC, et al: A randomized trial of bevacizumab an anti-vascular endothelial growth factor antibody for metastatic renal cancer. N Engl J Med 349:427–434, 2003.
145. Esser S, et al: Vascular endothelial growth factor induces endothelial fenestrations in vitro. J Cell Biol 140:947–959, 1998.
146. Lain KY, et al: Smoking during pregnancy is associated with alterations in markers of endothelial function. Am J Obstet Gynecol 189:1196–1201, 2003.
147. Heeschen C, et al: Nicotine stimulates angiogenesis and promotes tumor growth and atherosclerosis. Nat Med 7:833–839, 2001.
148. Moses EK, et al: A genome scan in families from Australia and New Zealand confirms the presence of a maternal susceptibility locus for pre-eclampsia on chromosome 2. Am J Hum Genet 67:1581–1585, 2000.
149. Tuohy JF, James DK: Pre-eclampsia and trisomy 13. Br J Obstet Gynaecol 99:891–894, 1992.
150. Yancopoulos GD, et al: Vascular-specific growth factors and blood vessel formation. Nature 407:242–248, 2000.
151. Polednak A, Janerich DT: Characteristics of first pregnancy in relation to early breast cancer. A case-control study. J Reprod Med 28:314–318, 1983.
152. Vatten LJ, et al: Pre-eclampsia in pregnancy and subsequent risk for breast cancer. Br J Cancer 87:971–973, 2002.
153. Innes KE, Byers TE: First pregnancy characteristics and subsequent breast cancer risk among young women. Int J Cancer 112:306–311, 2004.
154. Dekker GA, Sibai BM: Etiology and pathogenesis of preeclampsia: Current concepts. Am J Obstet Gynecol 179:1359–1375, 1998.
155. Tubbergen P, et al: Change in paternity: A risk factor for preeclampsia in multiparous women? J Reprod Immunol 45:81–88, 1999.
156. Skjaerven R, Wilcox AJ, Lie RT: The interval between pregnancies and the risk of preeclampsia. N Engl J Med 346:33–38, 2002.
157. Wang JX, et al: Surgically obtained sperm and risk of gestational hypertension and pre-eclampsia. Lancet 359:673–674, 2002.
158. Robillard P-Y, et al: Association of pregnancy-induced hypertension with duration of sexual cohabitation before conception. Lancet 344:973–975, 1994.
159. Wimalasundera RC, et al: Pre-eclampsia antiretroviral therapy and immune reconstitution. Lancet 360:1152–1154, 2002.

160. Goldman-Wohl DS, et al: Lack of human leukocyte antigen-G expression in extravillous trophoblasts is associated with pre-eclampsia. Mol Hum Reprod 6:88–95, 2000.

161. Yie SM, et al: HLA-G protein concentrations in maternal serum and placental tissue are decreased in preeclampsia. Am J Obstet Gynecol 191:525–529, 2004.

162. Hiby SE, et al: Combinations of maternal KIR and fetal HLA-C genes influence the risk of preeclampsia and reproductive success. J Exp Med 200:957–965, 2004.

163. von Dadelszen P, et al: Levels of antibodies against cytomegalovirus and Chlamydophila pneumoniae are increased in early onset pre-eclampsia. Br J Obstet Gynaecol 110:725–730, 2003.

164. Heine RRB, Ness RB, Roberts JM: Seroprevalence of antibodies to Chlamydia pneumoniae in women with preeclampsia [see comment]. Obstet Gynecol 101:221–226, 2003.

165. Yeh S, et al: Evidence of parvovirus B19 infection in patients of pre-eclampsia and eclampsia with dyserythropoietic anaemia. Br J Haematol 126:428–433, 2004.

166. Trogstad LI, et al: Is preeclampsia an infectious disease? Acta Obstet Gynecol Scand 80:1036–1038, 2001.

167. Thadhani R, et al: Insulin resistance and alterations in angiogenesis: Additive insults that may lead to preeclampsia. Hypertension 43:988–992, 2004.

168. Savvidou MD, et al: Endothelial dysfunction and raised plasma concentrations of asymmetric dimethylarginine in pregnant women who subsequently develop pre-eclampsia. Lancet 361:1511–1517, 2003.

169. Florio P, et al: The addition of activin A and inhibin A measurement to uterine artery Doppler velocimetry to improve the early prediction of pre-eclampsia. Ultrasound Obstet Gynecol 21:165–169, 2003.

170. Aquilina J, et al: Improved early prediction of pre-eclampsia by combining second-trimester maternal serum inhibin—A and uterine artery. Doppler Ultrasound Obstet Gynecol 17:477–484, 2001.

Chapter 26

Molecular Insights into the Thrombotic Microangiopathies

Charles C. Matouk and Philip A. Marsden

INTRODUCTION TO THE THROMBOTIC MICROANGIOPATHIES

The thrombotic microangiopathies are a heterogeneous group of serious disorders characterized by thrombocytopenia, microangiopathic hemolytic anemia, and varying degrees of renal dysfunction.[1] Prominent neurologic symptoms and signs often accompany this clinical syndrome and constitute a major cause of morbidity and mortality. Histopathologically, lesions are defined by intravascular platelet aggregates that result in microvascular occlusion and secondary ischemic tissue injury.[2] It is generally accepted that a dysfunctional, activated endothelium is the primary cellular target that precipitates this pathologic state.[2–4]

Three distinct clinical syndromes comprise the thrombotic microangiopathies, differing in the severity of renal dysfunction and neurologic involvement. First described by Gasser and colleagues in 1955,[5] the hemolytic uremic syndrome (HUS) is the most common of the thrombotic microangiopathies and is characterized by severe renal impairment. The vast majority of patients are children who suffer a prodromal, bloody diarrheal illness typically 1 week before the onset of HUS.[6,7] With the institution of appropriate supportive therapies, most children have an excellent prognosis and are not prone to relapses.[7] This form of the disease is referred to as diarrhea-associated HUS (D+HUS). A minority of patients with HUS do not present with prodromal hemorrhagic colitis, are prone to relapses, and progress to end-stage renal disease (ESRD) despite institution of aggressive therapeutic measures.[8,9] These patients are said to have diarrhea-negative HUS (D–HUS), or atypical HUS. Finally, patients with prominent extrarenal manifestations, particularly neurologic involvement, and milder renal impairment constitute a syndrome first described by Moschcowitz in 1924, thrombotic thrombocytopenic purpura (TTP).[10,11] Without institution of prompt, daily plasma exchange, the disease is almost universally fatal. With appropriate therapy, however, over 90% of patients improve in dramatic fashion.[12] Because these clinical definitions are somewhat vague, clinician dependent, and overlapping, significant controversy exists in the differentiation of these clinical syndromes that may cause delays in the institution of appropriate therapies, or even institution of ineffective ones.[13]

In the past 20 years, significant progress has been made in our understanding of the molecular mechanisms that contribute to disease pathogenesis in the thrombotic microangiopathies.[1] Three major breakthroughs served as catalysts to ignite an explosion of detailed molecular and genetic investigations into these disorders. In 1982, Moake and colleagues were the first to report "unusually large" von Willebrand factor (vWF) multimers in the plasma of patients with chronic, relapsing TTP, and hypothesized that a deficiency in a plasma-borne processing activity may be causally associated with the disease.[14] Soon thereafter, an epidemiologic association was established between infection with Shiga toxin–producing Escherichia coli O157:H7, hemorrhagic colitis, and HUS.[15] Most recently, in 1998, Warwicker and colleagues provided the first molecular evidence th.at patients with atypical HUS have defects in the ability of host cells, particularly renal glomerular endothelial cells, to protect themselves against activation of the alternative pathway of complement.[16] Today, these novel molecular insights have brought us to the cusp of a revolution in the diagnosis and targeted therapy of these disorders. They are individually discussed below.

DIARRHEA-ASSOCIATED HEMOLYTIC UREMIC SYNDROME ESCHERICIA— INFECTION WITH ESCHERICIA COLI O157:H7

D+HUS is the most common of the thrombotic microangiopathies, and a major cause of acute renal failure in children. As its name implies, and distinct from other thrombotic microangiopathies, a bloody diarrheal illness with low-grade or absent fever generally precedes the onset of HUS by 2 to 14 days (median 6 days).[6,15] The pathology reveals hemorrhagic colitis, which can be severe. Patients display the characteristic features of microangiopathic nonimmune hemolytic anemia, thrombocytopenia, and acute renal failure. Extrarenal manifestations may also occur and involve numerous tissues, including the pancreas, skeletal muscle, and myocardium.[17] Central nervous system (CNS) complications occur in 20% of children with D+HUS during the acute phase of the illness.[7] Seizure, stroke, and coma are responsible for the majority of deaths, especially in young children and the elderly.[7,17,18] Histopathologically, renal glomeruli demonstrate fibrin-rich thrombi, swelling, and detachment of endothelial cells from the basement membrane, capillary wall thickening, and concomitant narrowing of the capillary lumen.[2,19] Evidence of vasculitis or perivascular infiltration is conspicuously absent. Accompanying cortical necrosis is often a prominent feature. Fibrin deposition and thrombosis in larger preglomerular arterioles and medium-sized vessels have also been documented.[18,19] The venous circulation is typically spared. Similar histopathologic lesions with accompanying parenchymal ischemic changes are also characteristic of other affected organ systems, particularly the human gastrointestinal tract[20] and brain.[21–23] These pathologic stigmata belie the central role of endothelial injury in the pathogenesis of D+HUS.[4]

The Major Breakthrough—Epidemiologic Association of *E. coli* O157:H7, Hemorrhagic Colitis, and HUS

The major breakthrough in our understanding of this disease was the epidemiologic association of infection with a novel human pathogen, *E. coli* O157:H7, hemorrhagic colitis ,and HUS.[24–26] In particular, Karmali and colleagues proposed that a virulence factor produced by this enterohemorrhagic pathotype of *E. coli*, Shiga-like toxin (or verotoxin), was likely the causative agent.[15,27,28] Since these initial descriptions, *E. coli* O157:H7 has effectively made the transition from a medical curiosity to a major public health concern.[7] With an incidence of approximately eight infections per 100,000 persons per year in North America,[29,30] infection with *E. coli* O157:H7 has been linked to both sporadic cases and numerous disease outbreaks worldwide.[7,31,32] The vast majority of infections are caused by food or water contamination with cattle excrement, the principal reservoir for human infection with *E. coli* O157:H7.[1,7] Major outbreaks have been reported from the consumption of contaminated, undercooked hamburger meat,[31] commercial salami[33] and even alfalfa[34,35] and radish sprouts,[36] as was the case in a massive epidemic affecting elementary school children in Sakai City, Japan, in 1996. Drinking or swimming in contaminated water have also been linked to several large *E. coli* O157:H7 outbreaks.[37] In May 2000, the municipal water supply of the small town of Walkerton, Ontario, Canada, was contaminated by surface water draining into their wells. Of the nearly 5,000 residents of Walkerton, 2,300 persons developed gastroenteritis, 65 persons required hospitalization and 27 persons developed D+HUS. Of this latter group, seven persons died from their illness,[38,39] making D+HUS the most serious and dreaded complication of infection with *E. coli* O157:H7.[1,7] In most reported series, the risk for progression to D+HUS ranges from 1% to 8%,[39–41] but rates higher than 20% have been reported in several outbreaks.[42,43] Risk factors for progression to D+HUS include bloody diarrhea, elevated serum leukocyte count, extremes of age, and, though arguable, treatment with antibiotics.[7,37,44] During the acute phase of the disease, nearly 50% of patients require dialysis.[7] Although the vast majority of patients recover from an episode of D+HUS, and recurrence is very unlikely, 3% to 5% develop chronic renal failure and a similar percentage die of the disease.[7,45] Perhaps most alarming are the lack of specific therapies and apparent rise in disease incidence worldwide.[46,47]

E. coli O157:H7, Shiga-Like Toxins (Verotoxins), and the Classical Paradigm of D+HUS Pathogenesis

Commensal *E. coli* organisms colonize the colonic mucosa of human infants shortly after birth and quickly emerge as the most abundant facultative anaerobe in the human intestine. Here, they enjoy a symbiotic relationship with their host for many decades.[48] In contrast, other *E. coli* organisms have acquired specific virulence attributes and are important agents of human disease, in particular, gastroenteritis, urinary tract infections, and sepsis/meningitis.[48] Depending on the specific combination of acquired virulence factors, these pathogenic *E. coli* are categorized into various pathotypes comprising different clonal groups (serotypes) characterized by shared O (lipopolysaccharide) and H (flagellar) antigens.[48,49] Among

enterohemorrhagic *E. coli* (EHEC) organisms, the O157:H7 serotype is responsible for the majority of cases of hemorrhagic colitis and D+HUS in North America, the United Kingdom, and Japan.[6,48] Because EHEC organisms are noninvasive and remain in the gut after ingestion of contaminated food or water, the pathogenic properties of *E. coli* O157:H7, especially in relation to the pathogenesis of D+HUS, are in large part ascribed to its key secreted virulence factors, the Shiga-like toxins.[50] Although intensive research efforts have focused on the roles of Shiga-like toxins in D+HUS, host-pathogen relationships are complex and it is likely that other determinants (both human and bacterial) contribute to disease pathogenesis. For example, it is now well appreciated that over 200 serotypes of *E. coli* produce Shiga-like toxins, but only a few (most prominently the O157 and O111 serogroups) are associated with human disease.[6,48] It is of interest that these pathogenic strains also harbor a chromosomal pathogenicity island termed the locus for enterocyte effacement (LEE), whose gene products are required for the development of characteristic attaching and effacing (A/E) lesions in the human intestine.[48,51] If, and how, these additional virulence factors specifically contribute to the pathogenesis of D+HUS remains to be elucidated.[52] Other lines of evidence that underscore the importance of non-Shiga-like toxin bacterial determinants of D+HUS include the identification of novel chromosomal pathogenicity islands discovered during the complete sequencing of the *E. coli* O157:H7 genome,[53] the recent characterization of a subtilase cytotoxin from EHEC that induces microvascular thrombosis in target organs after intraperitoneal injection in mice,[54] and the observation that some strains of *E. coli* O157:H7 associated with D+HUS do not produce Shiga-like toxins.[55] Notwithstanding, research on Shiga-like toxins forms the basis for our current understanding of the molecular mechanisms underlying D+HUS.[1]

The Shiga Family of Toxins—Potent Inhibitors of Protein Synthesis

The Shiga family of toxins belong to a larger family of clinically relevant bacterial and plant AB toxins.[50] These include the bacterial cholera, diphtheria, and pertussis toxins, among others, as well as the plant toxin ricin.[56] The latter is derived from the seeds of the castor plant (*Ricinus communis*) used in the production of castor oil.[57] The AB toxins are so named because they share a common structural organization that is characteristic of nearly all intracellularly acting protein toxins. One or more B subunits mediate binding of the holotoxin to glycolipid receptors on the surface of target cells. This ligand-receptor interaction initiates internalization of the holotoxin and transport of the enzymatically active A subunit to the cytosol.[56] The Shiga family of toxins are AB_5 hexamers consisting of identical B subunits (7.7 kD each) noncovalently bonded to a helix at the carboxyl-terminus of the single A subunit (32 kD) in a doughnut-shaped pentameric ring.[58,59] The A subunit is composed of two fragments linked by disulfide bonding: the enzymatically active A1 fragment (27 kD) and the smaller (4 kD) A2 fragment required for holotoxin assembly[18,60] (Fig. 26-1, upper right corner). Kiyoshi Shiga described the first member of this family, Shiga toxin, from *Shigella dysenteriae*, and it is in his honor that the family of toxins is named.[61,62] EHEC organisms are known to produce at least two genetically and antigenically distinct Shiga-like

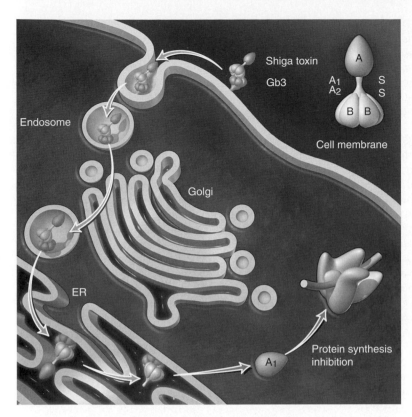

Figure 26-1 Classical paradigm of verotoxin-induced cellular toxicity in diarrhea-associated hemolytic-uremic syndrome. Verotoxins (VTs) are AB_5 exotoxins produced by pathogenic strains of enterohemorrhagic *Escherichia coli*, most prominently *E. coli* O157:H7. They are composed of five identical B subunits noncovalently bonded to a single A subunit in a donut-shaped pentameric ring. The A subunit consists of the enzymatically active A1 fragment and smaller A2 fragment. VT binds to susceptible cell surfaces, particularly endothelial cells, via a Gb_3 glycolipid receptor. This initial binding is followed by receptor-mediated endocytosis, retrograde transport of the toxin through the *trans*-Golgi apparatus and endoplasmic reticulum (ER). During its retrograde transport through the cell's acidic, intracellular compartments, VT is cleaved by furin to release the enzymatically active A1 fragment into the cytosol, where it potently inhibits protein synthesis by a direct and specific activity on ribosomes. **(See Color Plate 1.)**

toxins: Shiga toxin 1 (Stx1) and Shiga toxin 2 (Stx2).[63] These toxins are also known as verotoxin-1 (VT1) and verotoxin-2 (VT2), respectively, in reference to their initial characterization as cytotoxic activities against an African green monkey kidney cell line (Vero).[24] VT1 is nearly identical to Shiga toxin, differing by a single amino acid substitution from serine to threonine at position 45 in the toxin's A subunit.[64,65] The A subunits of VT1 and VT2 share only 56% amino acid sequence identity.[66] Unlike VT1, the VT2 subfamily of toxins is composed of a number of variants, including VT2c and VT2e. *E. coli* O157:H7 commonly produces VT1 and VT2, VT2 alone, or VT2 and VT2c; all combinations have been associated with D+HUS.[66,67] Intriguingly, *E. coli* O157:H7 strains that produce only VT2 family members, in particular, VT2c,[68] are most closely linked with progression to D+HUS in epidemiologic studies[69–72] and several animal models.[73–75] The molecular explanation for this observation is unclear; however, slower association and dissociation rates than VT1 with their cognate receptor,[76] increased cytotoxicity against human renal microvascular endothelial cells,[77] and associated virulence factors may be contributory.[63] VT2e causes the systemic edema disease of weaning piglets.[78]

The A subunits of the various AB toxins possess different catalytic activities. For example, diphtheria, cholera, and pertussis toxins catalyze the transfer of the adenosine diphosphate (ADP)-ribose moiety of nicotinamide adenine dinucleotide (NAD) to the cytosolic protein targets elongation factor-2 (EF-2, a component of the eukaryotic protein synthesis machinery)[79] and the α subunits of G_s[80] and $G_{i/o}$[81] adenylate cyclase regulatory proteins, respectively. Alternatively, the A subunits of the Shiga family of toxins and ricin possess intrinsic RNA *N*-glycosidase activity and catalyze the depurination of a specific adenosine at position 4,324 from the 5′

terminus of the eukaryotic 28S ribosomal RNA (rRNA) of the 60S ribosomal subunit.[82–84] Although the mechanism by which this occurs has not been fully elucidated, it likely involves "base-flipping" after targeting of the toxin to the evolutionarily conserved sarcin/ricin loop (SRL) of 28S rRNA, a structural element known to be important for elongation factor binding.[85,86] This *N*-glycosidase-mediated depurination of 28S rRNA prevents amino-acyl-tRNA from engaging the 60S ribosomal subunit and antagonizes the binding and coordinated function of elongation factor-1 and -2. The result is potent and irreversible inhibition of protein synthesis and cell death.[50,82–84] Verotoxins, like other AB toxins, are enzymes; even minute quantities of toxin can have pronounced effects on target cells.[87–89]

Verotoxin Receptors and the Classical Paradigm of D+HUS Pathogenesis

For the catalytic A subunit to reach its cytosolic target, the holotoxin must first bind to a susceptible cell surface and become internalized. This specificity is achieved by binding of the B subunits to cell surface glycolipid receptors in a classical receptor-ligand interaction.[18] Each of the five B subunit monomers is composed of a single α helix and adjacent antiparallel β strands (or barrels) among which are housed three carbohydrate-binding sites.[90,91] Two sites per monomer (10 per pentamer) mediate high-avidity binding to receptor surfaces, while a third site in the monomer (5 per pentamer) seems to facilitate binding of the high-avidity sites to receptor groupings.[92] The third site appears to be absent from members of the VT2 family.[66] Two prominent membrane glycolipid receptors are characterized by the core carbohydrate sequence, galactose $\alpha(1\rightarrow4)$-galactose $\beta(1\rightarrow4)$-glucose ceramide; namely, globotriaosyl ceramide (Gb$_3$, CD77) and globotetraosyl ceramide (Gb$_4$).[93–96] Gb$_3$ and Gb$_4$ glycolipid receptors are also known as the Pk and P antigens, respectively, of the P blood group system expressed on the surface of red blood cells.[97,98] The B subunits of VT1, VT2, and VT2c, which are the variants most important in the pathogenesis of D+HUS, bind Gb$_3$, while VT2e, important in the pig edema disease, preferentially binds Gb$_4$.

Cell surface expression of the glycolipid receptor Gb$_3$ is the major determinant of host cell sensitivity to verotoxin.[97] This is substantiated by the tissue distribution of Gb$_3$ in humans and animal models coincident with the pattern of affected host tissues in D+HUS.[99–102] In particular, endothelial and epithelial cells (e.g., renal proximal tubule and cortical epithelial cells) demonstrate high surface levels of Gb$_3$.[97] Endothelial cell expression of Gb$_3$ varies with the vascular bed of origin.[2] For example, microvascular endothelial cells express high levels of Gb$_3$ and are exquisitely sensitive to verotoxin, whereas endothelial cell cultures derived from glomeruli and medium-sized vessels such as human umbilical vein endothelial cells (HUVECs) have a much lower cell surface expression of Gb$_3$ and are more resistant to the toxin.[88,103,104] These studies are in keeping with the histopathology of D+HUS characterized by preferential involvement of the microcirculation.[2,19] Nevertheless, it is probable that other factors contribute to a susceptible phenotype in a host cell's response to verotoxin. For example, decreasing levels of renal Gb$_3$ expression from infancy to adulthood have been postulated to explain the preferential involvement of children in D+HUS epidemics.[105] This dogma has recently been called into question with the demonstration that prominent renal Gb$_3$ staining may persist into adulthood, suggesting that other factors help determine disease predilection for infants and young children.[106] It is also now recognized that Gb$_3$-independent mechanisms exist for verotoxin internalization by host cells. Their physiologic relevance and contribution to the pathogenesis of D+HUS remain to be elucidated.[107–109]

After binding to a susceptible host cell surface, verotoxin is rapidly internalized by endocytosis from clathrin-coated pits into the endosomal compartment.[89] Although clathrin-independent uptake has been described, it is much slower and of uncertain in vivo relevance. Verotoxin is then transported in a retrograde fashion to the Golgi apparatus. Although the molecular details of this transport are currently unclear, it is in this manner that verotoxin escapes targeting to lysosomes for subsequent degradation. Within the *trans*-Golgi network (TGN), or possibly within endosomes themselves, the enzyme furin cleaves the verotoxin A subunit to generate two proteolytic fragments: the enzymatically active A1 fragment (27 kD), and a smaller, residual A2 fragment (4 kD) that remains covalently linked to the B subunit. This enzymatic reaction is potentiated by the acidic environment of these intracellular compartments, and is essential for cellular intoxication. Verotoxin is then transported in a retrograde fashion from the TGN to the endoplasmic reticulum (ER), and finally, to the cytosol where it is now available to exert its protein synthesis inhibitory activity.[89,109] This pathway constitutes the classical paradigm for the central role of verotoxin in the pathogenesis of D+HUS (see Fig. 26-1). Intriguingly, aberrant proteins in the ER are normally targeted to the 26S proteasome in the cytosol for ubiquitin-dependent proteasomal degradation. In the vast majority of cases, proteins destined for degradation in

this fashion are "tagged" on lysine residues with ubiquitin chains of variable length.[110] That verotoxin has evolved in such a way that it possesses lysine residue at a reduced frequency compared to a majority of mammalian proteins is an extremely elegant system for evading eukaryotic host defenses.[110,111]

Newer Concepts in the Pathogenesis of D+HUS

In recent years, exciting newer concepts have evolved regarding the roles of verotoxin in the pathogenesis of D+HUS. The classical paradigm, although providing important mechanistic insights, cannot explain many of the disease subtleties.[112] For example, how does a potent protein synthesis inhibitor induce a marked inflammatory response characterized by cytokines in patients' blood and serum?[113–115] How does circulating verotoxin promote endothelial cell activation and a prothrombotic luminal surface in susceptible vascular beds of the microcirculation?[116–118] The newer concepts address these fundamental questions and add substantively to the classical paradigm by shifting the focus away from protein synthesis inhibition to other novel and equally important pathogenic properties of the toxin.

The Ribotoxic Stress Response and Subinhibitory Concentrations of Verotoxin

It is now well appreciated that a pronounced inflammatory response accompanies D+HUS.[112] This has been repeatedly documented in patients[113–115] and various animal models.[74,119,120] Indeed, an exuberant inflammatory response likely plays a major role in disease pathogenesis by activating susceptible endothelial cells, aggravating vascular injury, and promoting microvascular thombosis.[116] These observations, however, create a paradox in which the inflammatory response, an active process that requires *de novo* protein synthesis, is induced by a potent translational inhibitor. The same paradox confounds recent observations of apoptosis,[121] the active process of programmed cell death, in various in vitro cell culture models,[104,122–124] animal models,[125–127] as well as renal biopsies of patients with D+HUS.[123,128] How is the observation of these cellular phenomena that are dependent on *de novo* protein synthesis reconciled with the well-characterized mechanism of action of verotoxin?

The ribotoxic stress response (RSR) is an evolutionarily conserved cellular reaction to toxins and other stimuli that target the 3' end of 28S rRNA.[129] Central to this molecular paradigm is the activation of intracellular signaling cascades, most prominently, mitogen-activated kinases (MAPKs), which leads to the induction of specific gene expression profiles involved in the cellular response to stress.[129,130] This includes genes important in differentiation, cell survival, apoptosis, and cellular activation, among others.[129,131] Importantly, induction of the RSR is not a general feature of protein synthesis inhibitors, but appears to be a highly specific phenomenon restricted to those stimuli that interfere with the functioning of the SRL or damage the SRL in the 3' end of 28S rRNA; for example, ricin and α-sarcin.[130] In contrast, other AB$_5$ toxins that act as potent protein synthesis inhibitors by different mechanisms (for example, diphtheria toxin and *Pseudomonas aeruginosa* exotoxin A catalyze the specific ADP-ribosylation of EF-2) fail to induce the RSR.[129,130,132] Recently,

Kojima and colleagues demonstrated that VT1, but not mutant VT1 lacking N-glycosidase activity, specifically activates MAPKs and the RSR in a human epithelial cell culture model.[133]

Greater credence was given to induction of the RSR in the pathobiology of verotoxin-associated D+HUS when it was discovered that even subinhibitory concentrations of verotoxin, that is, toxin concentrations that demonstrate no or minimal effects on nascent protein synthesis, could have dramatic effects of cellular gene expression profiles. First documented by Bitzan and colleagues for endothelin-1 (ET-1), a prominent physiologic vasoconstrictor,[87] it is now appreciated that subinhibitory concentrations of verotoxin can act as potent activators of the endothelial phenotype characterized by genes known to be important in the inflammatory response, and apoptosis.[104,134,135] In this fashion, lesioning of 28S rRNA may serve as an intracellular sensor for stress by initiating specific signaling cascades that result in the induction of specific gene expression programs. Although the molecular transducers and in vivo relevance of this newer molecular paradigm remain to be definitively established, verotoxin-induced RSR (independent of protein synthesis inhibition) represents a major conceptual advance in our understanding of verotoxin-associated D+HUS.

Nuclear DNA is an Alternative Substrate for Verotoxin

Both protein synthesis inhibition and induction of the RSR require depurination of a specific adenosine in the 3′ end of 28S rRNA. Recently, however, it has been appreciated that nuclear DNA can also serve as an important enzymatic substrate for verotoxin.[136,137] This reaction involves the specific removal of adenines from multiple sites within the DNA template, and appears to be common to toxins that possess N-glycosidase activity (e.g., ricin) rather than a consequence of generalized protein synthesis inhibition.[137–139] Unlike DNA glycosylases involved in DNA repair, single-strand breaks are thought to result from a weakening of the DNA sugar-phosphate backbone rather than specific apurinic/apyrimidinic lyase activity, consistent with the known mechanism of action of these enzymes.[140,141] Importantly, Brigotti and colleagues demonstrated that VT1 depurinates DNA in HUVECs after the onset of potent protein synthesis inhibition but prior to the onset of apoptosis.[142] These researchers speculate that this novel action of the toxin may be important in the induction of apoptosis, and may promote more insidious perturbations in gene expression by targeting critical regulatory regions of the genome. The relevance of this novel action of verotoxin in the pathogenesis of D+HUS remains to be determined.

Implications for Therapy and the Way Ahead

Prior to the ready availability of dialysis therapy for patients with D+HUS in acute renal failure, mortality rates as high as 25% were reported.[63] Today, early disease recognition and rapid institution of dialysis have significantly improved disease outcomes. Nevertheless, 3% to 5% of patients still progress to chronic renal failure and a similar percentage die from the disease.[7,45] Indeed, D+HUS remains the most dreaded complication of infection with EHEC and a major cause of acute renal failure among children.[6,15]

The most effective therapeutic strategy to date remains prevention of infection with disease-causing strains of E. coli through public education and improved food and water safety.[143] No specific therapies currently exist for the treatment of D+HUS.[63,144] Therapy remains entirely supportive. For example, the role of antibiotics in the treatment of D+HUS is currently uncertain and extremely controversial.[145] While some groups proport major beneficial effects on prevention and improvement in the clinical course of D+HUS,[146] others report no benefit[147,148] or even significant harm associated with their prescription early on in the disease.[37,44] Similarly, antiplatelet agents[149] and plasmapheresis[150] are used at the discretion of the treating clinician with unclear supporting evidence. Anticoagulants,[151–153] fibrinolytics,[154] intravenous gammaglobulin (IVIG),[155] plasma infusion,[156] and steroids[157] are likely of no clinical benefit. It is hoped that recent molecular insights highlighting the central role of verotoxins in the pathogenesis of D+HUS will lead to novel therapeutic strategies.

In this regard, two general strategies have been pursued by the research community: first, the development of a vaccine to protect at-risk populations[158]; and second, agents to prevent the binding of verotoxin to its cognate receptor, Gb$_3$, on susceptible host cell surfaces.[63,143,144] Vaccines may be employed to protect cattle from colonization with E. coli O157:H7[159] or humans against infection after consuming contaminated beef. These measures have proven to be effective in several animal models,[160,161] but their safety and efficacy remain to be tested in humans.[158] In recent years, however, it is the potential of verotoxin binders used early in the diarrheal phase of illness to prevent D+HUS that has received the most attention and research dollars. Verotoxin binders can be categorized as synthetic toxin binders, probiotic therapy, or monoclonal antibodies.[144] Synsorb-Pk is a synthetic toxin binder composed of the trisaccharide moiety of Gb$_3$ bound to a silicon-based carrier.[162] Despite its ability to protect Vero cells in culture from the cytotoxic activity of verotoxins, it failed to improve outcomes in patients with D+HUS in a double-blind, randomized, placebo-controlled trial.[162] Currently, synthetic binders and monoclonal antibody cocktails with greater affinity for verotoxins that may be administered intravenously are currently under development and remain to be tested in clinical trials.[63,144,163,164] It is likely that these agents will need to be administered early in the diarrheal phase of illness and not subsequent to the development of D+HUS if they are to be maximally effective.

ATYPICAL HEMOLYTIC UREMIC SYNDROME—DEFECTIVE HOST PROTECTION AGAINST ACTIVATION OF THE ALTERNATIVE PATHWAY OF COMPLEMENT

A subgroup of patients do not present with a prodromal diarrheal illness and infection with Shiga toxin–producing bacteria and are therefore categorized as having diarrhea-negative HUS (D-HUS).[1] These "atypical" patients constitute a heterogeneous population.[9] In most, a clear inciting factor precedes the development of HUS; for example, drugs, non-diarrheal infection, solid organ and hematologic transplantation, other systemic diseases, and pregnancy.[1] Patients are most often older and portend a worse prognosis.[1,165] These patients will be discussed separately in the final section. In others, atypical HUS develops in the absence of easily recognizable, exogenous triggers.[1,9] In stark contrast to patients with D+HUS, mortality rates higher than 50% have been reported, with approximately half of survivors suffering relapses and as many as 81% progressing to ESRD.[1,8,9] Histopathologically, lesions are very similar to those seen in D+HUS, characterized by the accumulation of platelet- and fibrin-rich thrombi in affected renal glomeruli and, to a lesser extent, small vessels of the CNS. Renal arteriolar lesions are especially prominent.[166–168] Notably, evidence of vasculitis and immune complex deposition is lacking. Familial clustering of atypical HUS has been documented in 10% to 15% of all cases.[1] Both autosomal-dominant and -recessive modes of inheritance have been described.[8,16,169,170] The incomplete penetrance and variable phenotypes most characteristic of these pedigrees likely reflect a complex disease with important genetic and environmental contributions. It is the molecular and genetic analyses of these rare families that have provided the greatest insights into disease pathogenesis and have helped establish atypical HUS as the prototypical disease of inefficient protection against activation of the alternative pathway of complement on susceptible cell surfaces—notably, of renal glomerular and arteriolar endothelial cells.[16,171,172]

Atypical HUS, the Human Complement System, and Regulator of Complement Activation Gene Cluster

Dysregulation of the human complement system has long since been implicated in the pathogenesis of renal disease.[173,174] Initial reports on the role of complement in HUS, appearing as a series of letters in *Lancet*, provided two important insights. First, low plasma levels of C3 and high levels of complement degradation products suggested overactivity of the human complement system as a possible etiologic factor; and second, only a small percentage (10%–15%) of patients with HUS manifested these plasma-derived laboratory abnormalities.[175–178] It is only in the past 10 years that careful investigations have helped to resolve this paradox and firmly establish abnormalities in the regulation of complement activation on host cell surfaces as predisposing to the condition.[172,179]

The Alternative Pathway of the Human Complement System

The human complement system is a versatile and powerful effector of innate immunity. Its functional complexity is belied by its more than 30 protein constituents in the plasma and on cell surfaces. The complement system not only provides a robust first-line defense against pyogenic bacterial infection, but also bridges innate and adaptive immunity and rids the body of immune complexes and damaged (apoptotic) host cells.[180] Three distinct pathways lead to activation of the complement system: the classical, mannose-binding lectin, and alternative pathways. Although they differ in their modes of activation, each pathway results in the generation of C3 convertase enzymes responsible for cleaving C3 into proteolytic fragments, C3a and C3b. C3b then contributes to the creation of the C5 convertase enzymes with subsequent formation of the membrane attack complex (MAC), a porelike, lipophilic protein complex consisting of complement components C5b to C9 that inserts into cellular membranes and results in cell lysis.[181] In addition, other complement components serve as opsonins and anaphylatoxins. Inherent to the complement system's ability to subserve host defense is the capacity to discriminate between self and nonself. It is therefore not surprising that many of the complement components are dedicated regulators of the complement system, focusing complement activities on microbial cell surfaces while at the same time protecting normal host cells from bystander injury. When these regulators are compromised by inherited or acquired defects, they can result in pathologic states that manifest as human disease.[180–182] It is indeed an inability of host cells, particularly glomerular endothelial cells, to adequately protect themselves against activation of the alternative pathway of complement that predisposes to atypical HUS.[172,179,183]

The alternative pathway of complement, unlike the classical pathway, does not require an antibody–cell surface interaction for activation. Low levels of C3 are spontaneously activated in vivo through the "C3 tick-over" pathway.[181,184] This intramolecular reaction involves the nucleophilic attack (or water hydrolysis) of an internal thioester bond in native C3 to generate a metastable, functionally "C3b-like" C3 capable of binding to exposed hydroxyls or amines on biologic surfaces. This in turn leads to an amplification step with the generation of the alternative pathway C3 convertase enzyme, C3bBb. C3bBb cleaves more plasma-borne C3, which is deposited as active C3b on permissive cell surfaces, and is thereby available (in a feedback loop) for the generation of more C3 convertase enzyme.[180,184]

Atypical HUS, Inefficient Protection Against Activation of the Alternative Pathway of Complement and the RCA Gene Cluster

Combining a constitutively active pathway with the inherent nonspecificity of its downstream effectors, it is intuitive that regulation of the alternative pathway C3 convertase is paramount to mounting an efficient antimicrobial attack without damaging normal host cells. This is accomplished by complement proteins collectively referred to as the "regulators of complement activation." Most prominent among these is factor I, a serine esterase that is uniquely capable of cleaving membrane-bound C3b so that it is not available to participate in the generation of C3bBb. Factor I, however, cannot accomplish this task alone, and relies on the participation of co-factors, including factor H, membrane co-factor protein (MCP, CD46), decay-accelerating factor (DAF, CD55) and complement receptor type 1 (CR1, CD35). In large part, it is these co-factors that discriminate self from nonself and help to focus the activities of the alternative pathway on appropriate biologic targets.[180]

All known regulators of the alternative pathway C3 convertase, with the exception of factor I (located on human chromosome 4), are encoded by closely linked genes on the long arm of human chromosome 1 (1q32), a chromosomal region known as the regulator of complement activation (RCA) gene cluster.[185–189] This genetic locus contains more than 60 genes, at least 16 of which constitute components of the complement system.[186,190] These complement-related genes are clustered together in tandem (head-to-tail) within two distinct gene groups: a centromeric group (approximately

650 kb of genomic DNA) containing the factor H gene (*HF1*) and factor H–related genes 1 to 5 (*FHR1-5*), and a telomeric group (approximately 900 kb long) housing *DAF*, *CR1*, and *MCP* genes, among others. In keeping with their close physical proximity in the human genome and singular biologic purpose, it is generally accepted that these complement regulatory genes share a common ancestor from which they arose by multiple events of gene duplication.[185,186,191]

Several earlier reports suggested a possible association between the regulators of complement activation, particularly factor H, and atypical HUS.[192–195] Molecular evidence, however, was lacking. The breakthrough study was reported by Warwicker and colleagues in 1998.[16] These investigators undertook a linkage analysis using a candidate gene approach in three families with multiple affected members. They successfully mapped the disease phenotype to the RCA gene cluster. In one of these families, and in a 36-year-old man with nonfamilial, sporadic/relapsing HUS, they found two disease mutations in the coding region of the factor H gene. This disease association has subsequently been corroborated by independent laboratories in diverse populations from around the world.[8,9,196] More recently, the same group sequenced the coding region of another complement regulatory protein located within the RCA gene cluster, the *MCP* gene, in 30 families with atypical HUS, and identified probable disease mutations in three families, including one of the original families initially screened for *HF1* mutations.[197] Again, this disease association was corroborated by an independent laboratory.[198] These findings provide the molecular underpinnings of an emerging paradigm for atypical HUS as a disease of inefficient regulation in the activation of the alternative pathway of complement on host cell surfaces.

Complement Factor H and Atypical HUS

Human factor H, first identified as β1H globulin, is the major fluid-phase regulator of the alternative pathway of complement.[189,199] Synthesized and secreted constitutively by the liver,[200] factor H consists of a single polypeptide chain glycoprotein (150 kD) normally present at plasma concentrations of approximately 110 to 615 µg/mL.[201] Extrahepatic synthesis of factor H has also been documented in various cell types in vitro, including endothelial cells.[202] Although the contribution of non–liver–derived factor H in vivo in the regulation of the alternative pathway of complement is currently unknown, it is interesting to speculate that it affords enhanced local protection against complement-mediated tissue injury at sites of infection, inflammation, or otherwise damaged endothelium.[189]

Factor H is composed of 20 homologous units of approximately 60 amino acids termed short consensus repeats (SCRs) or complement control protein (CCP) modules, much like "beads on a string"[203] (Fig. 26-2). This organizational strategy of contiguous, globular protein domains is shared with other complement proteins,[204] and is reflected in the genomic structure of its single gene, *HF1*. Located in the centromeric group of complement-related genes in the RCA gene cluster, *HF1* spans over 94 kb of genomic DNA and consists of 23 exons.[189,205] Each SCR is encoded by a single exon, with the exception of SCR2, which is encoded by exons 3 and 4. Its single, TATA-less promoter is responsible for the generation of at least two prominent protein-coding transcripts in the liver: full-length factor H and the alternatively spliced transcript, factor H-like 1 (FHL-1).[206,207] This latter transcript is translated into a 43-kD protein comprising the identical N-terminal seven SCRs of factor H, in addition to a unique four–amino acid C-terminus.[208,209] It is normally present in human plasma at much lower concentrations than factor H (10–50 µg/mL).[201] Several reports have documented cell-type and stimulus-dependent differential regulation of both proteins and demonstrated factor H-like complement regulatory activity for FHL-1.[189,202,208–211] To date, most research has focused on factor H itself. The role of FHL-1 in the pathogenesis of atypical HUS, if any, remains to be determined.

Plasma-Borne Factor H Protects Endothelial Cell Surfaces Against Activation of the Alternative Pathway of Complement

Targeting the alternative pathway C3 convertase is the primary function of factor H in the regulation of complement.[180,189] In fluid phase, factor H rapidly binds to and inactivates C3b. On cell surfaces, this molecular interaction is modulated by the specific chemical composition of the local environment. In particular, the presence of sialic acids, polyanionic molecules (e.g., glycosaminoglycans), or sulphated polysaccharides (e.g., heparin) potentiates factor H binding to surface-bound C3b.[212–216] Inactivation of the C3 convertase is then achieved by one (or a combination of) three mechanisms: (1) diminishing engagement of factor B with C3b, thereby preventing the generation of C3 convertase and arresting its amplification loop; (2) promoting dissociation of the C3bBb complex (also

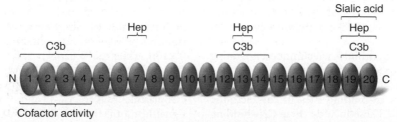

Figure 26-2 Modular organization and critical binding sites of human factor H. Factor H is a plasma-borne regulator of complement activation composed of 20 homologous subunits of approximately 60 amino acids termed short consensus repeats (SCRs) or complement control protein (CCP) modules. C3b, heparin (Hep), and sialic acid binding sites are depicted, as is the functional importance of SCR1-4 in conferring "co-factor activity" to the functional molecule. SCR19-20 represents a mutational "hot spot" in patients with atypical hemolytic-uremic syndrome, comprising over 70% of all disease mutations. **(See Color Plate 1.)**

known as "decay-accelerating activity"); and (3) acting as a co-factor for factor I in the cleavage of membrane-bound C3b (also known as "co-factor activity").[217–220] This permissive environment is characteristic of normal host surfaces, including the fenestrated endothelial lining of glomeruli, but not of invading microorganisms. It is therefore a fundamental determinant of self-nonself discrimination.

Deficiency of Factor H Predisposes to Atypical HUS

Deficiency or homozygous deletion of factor H in two animal models (pig and mouse, respectively) leads to overactivity of the alternative pathway of complement, an associated consumptive hypocomplementemia and spontaneous progression to renal failure.[183,221–223] This clinicopathologic syndrome is akin to human type II membranoproliferative glomerulonephritis (MPGNII). In both humans and animals, renal histopathology is characterized by glomerular capillary wall thickening, mesangial cell proliferation, intramembranous electron-dense deposits along the glomerular basement membrane, and the notable absence of immune complex deposition. In the Norwegian Yorkshire piglet model, plasma factor H was severely reduced by aberrant secretion of a mutant protein secondary to its intracellular retention.[224] In a very elegant experiment using sophisticated murine transgenic techniques, it was demonstrated that the spontaneous development of renal pathology in factor H–deficient mice [Cfh(-/-)] was abrogated in double-knockouts unable to efficiently activate the alternative pathway because of concomitant homozygous deletion of factor B [Bf(-/-)].[222] Taken together, these experiments suggest that (1) the glomerular endothelium is particularly sensitive to depletion of factor H and (2) overactivity of the alternative pathway of complement is responsible for the development of animal MPGNII. Human cases of MPGNII have rarely been described with constitutional deficiency of plasma factor H.[225] However, biochemical analyses of patients' sera almost always demonstrate a profound hypocomplementemia and circulating levels of C3 nephritic factor, a predominantly IgG autoantibody that binds to and stabilizes the alternative pathway C3bBb convertase, at least in part, by antagonizing factor H–mediated degradation.[226–228] Indeed, a unique monoclonal immunoglobulin lambda light (L) chain dimer (lambda L) has also been isolated from the sera of MPGNII patients that directly targets factor H and interferes with its complement regulatory functions.[229,230] In contradistinction, 10% to 15% of patients with atypical HUS carry heterozygous mutations in HF1, but do not share all the pathologic hallmarks of MPGNII and may not demonstrate low levels of plasma C3. This apparent paradox has been partially reconciled by careful structure-function analyses of normal factor H and mutants observed in patients with atypical HUS.[171,189]

Using a battery of molecular biology techniques, including inhibitory monoclonal antibodies, enzymatic digestion, and site-directed mutagenesis, a number of investigators have characterized distinct protein-binding sites in the factor H molecule[189] (see Fig. 26-2). These include three C3b-binding sites (SCR1-4, SCR12-14, and SCR19-20), three heparin- and sialic acid–binding sites (SCR7, SCR13, and SCR19-20),[179,189,231] and distinct binding sites for C-reactive protein (CRP)[232,233] and adrenomedullin.[234–236] Although functional

characterization of these domains is incomplete, the N-terminal SCR1-4 protein module appears to confer co-factor activity.[189,237] Based on these analyses, one might predict that factor H mutations in atypical HUS would preferentially target the N-terminus; however, the C-terminal SCR19-20 protein domains are the "hot-spot" for genetic mutation in atypical HUS, accounting for over 70% of all HF1 disease mutations to date.[8,189] Subsequent in vitro analyses of these factor H mutants have convincingly documented preserved co-factor activity and efficient regulation of the alternative pathway of complement in fluid phase. In contrast, the control of complement activation on cell surfaces was severely diminished.[189,231,238–242] These findings are consistent with the normocomplementemia often observed in the plasma of patients with atypical HUS.[8,175–178] Taken together, these studies support an emerging paradigm for atypical HUS as a disease of inefficient regulation in the activation of the alternative pathway of complement on host cell surfaces (Fig. 26-3). This situation is likely distinct from the massive overactivity of the alternative pathway of complement and secondary consumptive hypocomplementemia in patients with MPGNII.[189]

Membrane Co-factor Protein (CD46) and Atypical HUS

Human MCP, a type I transmembrane glycoprotein (gp), was first identified as a C3b-binding protein expressed on the surface of human peripheral blood leukocytes.[243] Initially named gp45-70 to reflect its broad eletrophoretic mobility pattern on sodium dodecyl sulphate polyacrylamide gel electrophoresis (SDS-PAGE), it was subsequently renamed when it was discovered that it possessed co-factor activity in the factor I–dependent cleavage of membrane-bound C3b.[244] MCP is now known to be ubiquitously expressed on the surface of nearly all human cell types (with the exception of erythrocytes), including endothelial cells of the renal glomerulus, where expression is thought to be particularly prominent.[245–250]

Located in the telomeric group of complement-related genes in the RCA gene cluster, MCP spans over 43 kb of genomic DNA and contains 14 exons.[251–253] Its single, TATA-less promoter[254] drives the expression of multiple protein-coding, alternatively spliced transcripts.[253,255–258] All isoforms of MCP possess four extracellular, N-terminal SCR (or CCP) domains encoded by exons 2 to 6 (Fig. 26-4). These SCRs are followed by a domain rich in serine, threonine, and proline (STP region), a 12–amino acid juxtamembranous region of unknown sequence homology, a transmembrane domain, a cytoplasmic anchor, and a cytoplasmic tail.[257] The STP region is encoded by three separate exons (7 to 9, more commonly referred to as A, B and C, respectively) and represents an important site of alternative splicing.[257] The four major isoforms of MCP do not contain the A exon and all utilize the C exon, while the B exon is alternatively spliced to generate BC- and C-containing STP regions.[257,259] These two isoform types are further distinguished by attachment to one of two cytoplasmic tails (CYT-1 and CYT-2) possessing distinct signaling motifs that also arise by alternative splicing in MCP's C-terminal end.[172,257,259,260] Multiple isoforms may be co-expressed by a single cell type and, together with differential, isoform-specific O-glycosylation of the STP region, are major determinants of MCP's characteristic broad electrophoretic

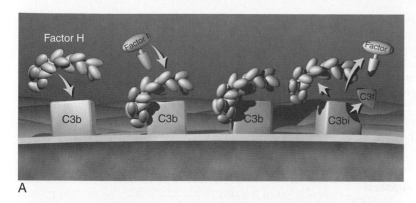

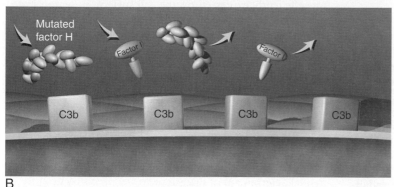

A

B

Figure 26-3 Mechanism of action of plasma-borne factor H in protection of endothelial cell surfaces against activation of the alternative pathway of complement in diarrhea-negative hemolytic-uremic syndrome (D-HUS). In the normal individual **(A)**, plasma-borne factor H binds C3b deposited on a damaged (or activated) endothelial cell surface. This interaction is critical in regulating the formation of C3bBb, the alternative pathway C3 convertase, and mitigating complement-mediated host cellular injury. Factor H accomplishes this important task by (1) diminishing factor B binding to C3b, thereby preventing the formation of C3bBb; (2) promoting the dissociation of C3bBb (so-called "decay-accelerating activity"); and (3) acting as a co-factor for factor I in the cleavage of membrane-bound C3b (so-called "co-factor activity"). In a patient with atypical HUS **(B)**, factor H is functionally deficient and cannot efficiently regulate the formation of C3bBb deposited on endothelial surfaces. Membrane-bound C3b is now left unchecked to generate C3bBb in an amplification loop that results in endothelial injury and pathologic thrombosis. **(See Color Plate 2.)**

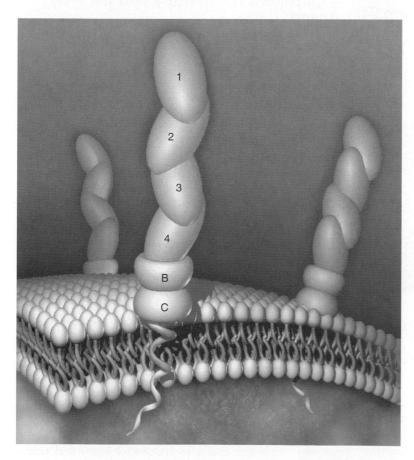

Figure 26-4 Structure of human membrane co-factor protein (MCP, CD46). MCP is a membrane-bound regulator of complement activation that may exist as multiple isoforms in a single cell type. All isoforms share four extracellular, N-terminal SCR domains, akin to those of factor H and other regulators of complement activation. These SCRs are followed by a domain rich in serine, threonine, and proline (STP region), a 12–amino acid juxtamembranous region of unknown sequence homology, transmembrane domain, cytoplasmic anchor, and cytoplasmic tail. The four major isoforms of MCP do not contain the A exon, and all utilize the C exon, while the B exon is alternatively spliced to generate BC- and C-containing STP regions. To date, all disease mutations in atypical hemolytic-uremic syndrome target the shared SCR4 domain. **(See Color Plate 2.)**

mobility pattern on SDS-PAGE analysis.[259,261] Tissue-specific expression patterns of the various MCP isoforms have previously been described; for example, the less O-glycosylated CYT-2 isoform predominates in the brain and germ cells, while the kidneys preferentially express the more heavily O-glycosylated CYT-2 isoform.[247,257] The functional relevance of this considerable diversity in the expression of MCP and its differential posttranslational modifications is of unclear physiologic significance. Its contribution to the pathogenesis of atypical HUS, if any, remains to be elucidated.[172,259]

Cell Surface MCP Protects Endothelial Cells Against Activation of the Alternative Pathway of Complement

Like factor H, MCP regulates activation of the alternative pathway of complement on susceptible host cell surfaces by targeting the alternative pathway C3 convertase. In particular, it acts as a co-factor for the factor I–mediated cleavage of surface-bound C3b.[262,263] Unlike factor H, it does not possess decay-accelerating activity, nor does it interfere with the engagement of factor B and C3b in the assembly of the alternative pathway C3 convertase.[172] Structure-function analyses of human MCP using deletion constructs, site-directed mutagenesis, and inhibitory antibodies have identified SCR3-4 domains as responsible for C3b-binding, while the partially overlapping SCR2-4 domains are required for optimal co-factor activity.[264-266] MCP also binds to and displays co-factor activity against C4b, a constituent of the classical pathway C3 convertase. However, the ability of MCP to protect cells against classical pathway-mediated complement cytolysis is currently uncertain. Regulation of the alternative pathway of

complement on cell surfaces is likely its primary physiologic role.[263,267]

Deficiency of MCP Predisposes to Atypical HUS

To date, a total of four families have been described by two independent research groups with atypical HUS and putative disease mutations in the *MCP* gene.[197,198] One family harbored a six–base pair deletion in *MCP*, resulting in the loss of two amino acids and intracellular retention of the mutant protein.[197] Two other families reported by the same research group demonstrated a T822C transition resulting in the substitution of a serine to proline. While this mutant protein was efficiently expressed on the cell surface, it demonstrated markedly reduced C3b binding activity.[197] A fourth family had a heterozygous two–base pair deletion, resulting in the insertion of a premature stop codon and loss of the MCP protein's C-terminus (including the transmembrane domain).[198] These genetic defects all target the SCR4 domain, a region common to all major isoforms of MCP and known to be critical in the regulation of the alternative pathway of complement (Fig. 26-5). Taken together, these studies substantiate the role of factor H in the pathogenesis of atypical HUS, and highlight inefficient regulation in the activation of the alternative pathway of complement on cell surfaces as a fundamental determinant of disease.

Implications for Therapy and the Way Ahead

Currently, the care of patients with atypical HUS is largely supportive, and includes removal of clear inciting factors and

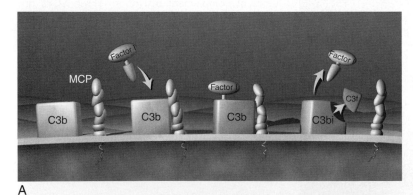

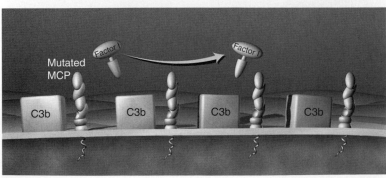

Figure 26-5 Mechanism of action of cell surface human membrane co-factor protein (MCP) in protection of endothelial cells against activation of the alternative pathway of complement in diarrhea-negative hemolytic-uremic syndrome (D-HUS). In the normal individual **(A)**, cell surface MCP binds C3b deposited on a damaged (or activated) endothelial cell surface. This interaction is critical in regulating the formation of C3bBb, the alternative pathway C3 convertase, and mitigating complement-mediated host cellular injury. MCP accomplishes this important task by acting as a co-factor for factor I in the cleavage of membrane-bound C3b, so-called "co-factor activity." In a patient with atypical HUS **(B)**, MCP is functionally deficient and cannot efficiently regulate the formation of C3bBb deposited on endothelial surfaces. All known mutations of the *MCP* gene target the SCR4 domain. As illustrated, the mutant MCP protein is most representative of a T822C transition previously described in two families (see text). Membrane-bound C3b is now left unchecked to generate C3bBb in an amplification loop that results in endothelial injury and pathologic thrombosis. **(See Color Plate 3.)**

appropriate support of renal function. Attempts at plasma infusion or exchange during acute episodes, at best, provide only transient relief, and are notoriously ineffective at halting or slowing progression to ESRD.[1] It is this newer, molecular paradigm of atypical HUS that offers novel targets for therapeutic intervention and renewed hope for patients. First, it is now appreciated that overactivity of the alternative pathway of complement on susceptible host cell surfaces is a fundamental mechanistic determinant of disease. It is conceivable that inhibitors of complement activation, already in clinical development for many years, may diminish renal endothelial injury, prevent relapses, and protect against progression to ESRD.[268–270] Some investigators have recently called for the initiation of clinical trials in patients with atypical HUS.[197] Second, therapeutic replacement of factor H and MCP, respectively, in patients with corresponding disease mutations is a very elegant treatment approach. This could be accomplished by replacement with a recombinant, soluble form of the factor or gene therapy protocols. Indeed, replacement therapy with a recombinant, soluble form of MCP has already demonstrated efficacy in reducing complement-mediated injury in a mouse-to-rat xenograft model, and represents an important proof-of-principle experiment.[271,272] Although infusion of normal fresh-frozen plasma (which contains normal factor H) in patients harboring *HF1* mutations does not prevent relapses or slow progression to ESRD,[16,195,273,274] it remains to be determined whether more potent, recombinant factor H or gene replacement strategies have greater clinical efficacy.[1] Third, outcomes of patients with atypical HUS undergoing renal transplantation have been disappointing, with recurrence of HUS in transplanted kidneys of approximately 50%.[1,8] Patients carrying *HF1* mutations fare especially poorly, with recurrence rates reported to be as high as 80%.[8,275–277] This situation differs markedly with outcomes of renal transplantation in patients with D+HUS, where recurrence is decidedly uncommon.[7,276] It is of great clinical interest that cadaveric renal transplantation in three relatives with *MCP* mutations was not complicated by disease recurrence.[197,278] Although it is still too early to comment on the generalizability of these preliminary observations, these favorable results are consistent with the current molecular paradigm. Unlike factor H, which is a soluble factor produced predominantly by the liver, MCP is ubiquitously expressed on the cell surfaces of a myriad of host cells, including glomerular and renal arteriolar endothelial cells of the transplanted kidney. It is therefore plausible that wild-type MCP on the engrafted kidney is protective against recurrence in patients harboring *MCP* mutations. Alternatively, any wild-type factor H produced by cells of the renal transplant is likely insufficient to protect against disease recurrence in patients with *HF1* mutations. Combined hepatorenal transplantation may be a more rationale therapeutic strategy to ameliorate graft survival in this subset of patients.[279] Knowledge of the molecular mechanisms underlying disease pathogenesis may help to facilitate genetic counseling, selection of appropriate candidates (and donors) for renal transplantation, and decision making with regard to the type of transplantation that should be performed in patients with atypical HUS.[172,278]

Much, however, remains to be learned. Atypical HUS is a heterogeneous condition with probable multilocus, genetic contributions and important environmental influences. These important facets of a complex, nonmendelian disease are reflected in the partial penetrance characteristic of affected pedigrees and highly variable disease phenotypes, even among family members with identical mutations.[172,197,278] Implicit to the original work of Warwicker and colleagues, who linked the RCA gene cluster to familial atypical HUS,[16] it is probable that disease mutations in other regulators of complement activation will be identified.[172,278] In this regard, probable disease mutations in factor I, the critical serine esterase responsible for cleavage of C3b and degradation of the alternative pathway C3 convertase, have recently been identified in three patients with atypical HUS.[280] Why renal endothelial cells are preferentially targeted by mutations in complement regulatory genes and whether these disease mutations are implicated in the pathogenesis of the more common D+HUS remain to be elucidated.

Thrombotic Thrombocytopenic Purpura— Defective Processing of vWF Multimer Size

Thrombotic thrombocytopenic purpura (TTP), referred to as the "systemic clumping plague" by Joel Moake, is the most deadly of the thrombotic microangiopathies and universally fatal if left untreated.[12] With daily plasma exchange, however, over 90% of patients respond in dramatic fashion.[281,282] This contrasts markedly with the often disappointing treatment results in atypical HUS. Patients with TTP present with the clinical triad of severe thrombocytopenia (with platelet counts often less than 20,000 per cubic millimeter during acute episodes), microangiopathic hemolytic anemia, and neurologic dysfunction.[1,12] Fever and renal failure are less frequently observed, and complete the classical pentad ascribed to the condition by Moschcowitz.[283] As implied by its moniker, nearly all other organ systems may be affected. The gastrointestinal tract, pancreas, heart, lungs, and retina, for unknown reasons, are particularly vulnerable.[12] It is sometimes difficult to distinguish between atypical HUS and TTP on clinical grounds alone. Most clinicians agree that prominent extrarenal manifestations, especially neurologic involvement, is most consistent with a diagnosis of TTP, whereas severe renal involvement is most characteristic of HUS.[1,12] These clinical distinctions are, however, at best subjective and at worst ambiguous and misleading. For example, CNS complications are observed in as many as 20% of children with D+HUS,[7] but few clinicians would label their clinical condition as TTP. Later in this section, we will discuss how newer molecular insights may more clearly differentiate between these overlapping clinical entities, and guide clinicians to the most appropriate therapeutic strategy.

Clinically, two major subgroups of TTP are distinguished. Acute idiopathic TTP is the most common variant and typically occurs in adults (20–60 years old), preferentially affects women, and is characterized by a single acute episode.[12] A minority of patients (10%–30%) may suffer recurrences at irregular intervals.[12,281,282,284] An even smaller percentage of patients have identifiable triggers, for example, drugs (classically, the adenosine diphosphate inhibitors, ticlopidine, and clopidogrel),[285] pregnancy,[286] and infection (particularly late-stage human immunodeficiency virus [HIV] disease).[12,287] This latter subgroup will be discussed separately in the last section. Alternatively, patients may present with a chronic relapsing form of the disease that is typically first diagnosed in early infancy.[12,288] This rare disease variant is likely indistinguishable from the Upshaw-Schulman syndrome,[289,290] a congenital disorder characterized by chronic thrombocytopenia, microangiopathic hemolytic anemia, and a dramatic (albeit transient) response to transfusion with normal fresh-frozen plasma.[283,291–293] Insights from both patients with the common, idiopathic, and rare chronic relapsing forms of the disease have been important for defining a shared, underlying mechanism of disease.

The Critical Observation—Unusually Large Circulating vWF Multimers in TTP

Three early lines of evidence implicated vWF biology in the pathogenesis of TTP.[294] First, thrombus formation in TTP, like atypical HUS, has a predilection for small arterioles.[1] These small-caliber, high-flow vessels demonstrate the highest fluid shear rates in the human circulatory system, and are dependent on the presence of plasma and subendothelial matrix-bound vWF multimers for efficient hemostasis. Second, the thrombi in patients with TTP are enriched in platelets and vWF protein, a pathologic entity distinct from the fibrin-rich lesions most characteristic of HUS and disseminated intravascular coagulation (DIC).[1,295] Like patients with HUS, characteristic secondary ischemic tissue injury and lack of perivascular inflammation complete the classical histopathologic picture and may obscure definitive diagnosis. Finally, the most compelling early evidence was the critical observation by Moake and colleagues in 1982 that patients with the chronic relapsing form of the disease demonstrated unusually large circulating vWF multimers.[14] They later reported dramatic resolution of symptoms in these patients and, importantly, concomitant disappearance of ultralarge vWF multimers after transfusion with normal fresh-frozen plasma.[296] These researchers hypothesized that patients with this form of the disease were susceptible to periodic relapses as a result of defective processing of these unusually large thrombogenic multimers because of an activity that was lacking in their plasma.[10,14,296] The nature of this activity, however, would remain elusive for many years.

vWF Biology, Multimer Size, and TTP

vWF is a critical determinant of vascular hemostasis.[297] An intrinsic component of the subendothelial matrix,[298,299] it mediates attachment of circulating platelets to exposed collagen and other substrates (e.g., proteoglycans and sulfatides)[300,301] at sites of vessel wall injury.[302,303] This interaction between circulating platelets and vWF is mediated by at least two prominent platelet receptors: platelet membrane gp1bα and platelet integrin $\alpha_{IIb}\beta_3$.[304] The former constitutively active receptor engages the vWF protein via its A1 domain and serves to tether circulating platelets to immobilized vWF in exposed subendothelial matrix. Characterized by fast association and dissociation rates, this molecular interaction results in the slow translocation of circulating platelets along the vessel wall, and thus permits the subsequent activation and binding of platelet integrin $\alpha_{IIb}\beta_3$ by an RGDS sequence in the vWF protein carboxy-terminal C1 domain.[305] It is this second ligand-receptor interaction that is responsible for firm platelet adhesion at sites of vascular injury. Acting in synergy, these vWF-bound platelet receptors promote the recruitment of other platelets, at least partially by vWF homotypic self-association, and constitute the nidus of an evolving platelet thrombus.[297,306] Indirectly, vWF contributes to vascular hemostasis by binding procoagulant factor VIII, thereby preventing its rapid clearance from plasma and ensuring its availability for the generation of thrombin.[304,307]

vWF Multimer Size is a Major Determinant in Platelet-Dependent Vascular Hemostasis Under Conditions of High Fluid Shear Stress

The potential of vWF to act as a biologic adhesive in platelet-dependent vascular hemostasis is directly proportional to the extent of polymerization of secreted vWF. Encoded by a single large gene (178 kb of genomic DNA) on the short arm of human chromosome 12 (12p13), vWF synthesis is restricted to endothelial cells and megakaryocytes. It is initially translated as a 2,813 amino acid pre-pro-peptide consisting of a 22–amino acid signal peptide, 741 amino acid pro-peptide, and 2,050 residue mature subunit sequence.[308,309] Extensive post-translational modification includes tail-to-tail dimerization of individual pro-vWF molecules within the ER by disulfide-bonding of their C-terminal ends,[310] and subsequent multimerization within the acidic environment of the *trans*-Golgi network in a head-to-head configuration by additional disulfide bonding at their N-terminal ends.[311] These large vWF multimers are stored within specialized endothelial and megakaryocyte intracellular storage compartments, Weibel-Palade bodies, and platelet α granules, respectively. Secretion of vWF multimers occurs constitutively in endothelial cells after proteolysis of the pro-peptide sequence and release of this fragment (von Willebrand antigen II) along with mature vWF multimers (as a polymer of the mature 220-kD polypeptide) into the circulation and onto the subendothelial matrix.[294] Typically, the vWF released constitutively by endothelial cells is composed of dimers and small multimers; and consequently, constitute the majority of vWF in normal plasma. In contrast, vWF multimers released by endothelial cells upon stimulation by secretagogues (e.g., vasopressin [or the V_1 receptor agonist, dDAVP], thrombin, fibrin, complement components C5–9, and histamine) are almost exclusively of high molecular weight.[297,304] Indeed, they may be composed of more than 40 individual subunits with a molecular mass in excess of 20,000 kD.[297,304,312] These large and unusually large multimers,[14] typically absent in normal plasma, are functionally multivalent and therefore capable of binding to the subendothelial matrix and activated platelets with many more sites and with much greater affinity (approximately 100-fold) than vWF dimers.[313–315] Their importance in efficient vascular hemostasis is underscored by their selective deficiency in the bleeding diathesis, type IIA von Willebrand disease.[297] Of particular relevance to the vascular pathology observed in TTP, the role of these large and unusually large multimers as biological adhesives is perhaps most relevant in situations of high fluid shear, a situation most characteristic of the flow dynamics in the small arterioles of the human circulatory tree. In the presence of high shear stress, the normally globular vWF multimers "uncoil" and appear to stretch out as extraordinarily long, thin filaments (potentially as long as several millimeters).[297,304,316,317] Under these high shear stress conditions, the critical initial binding of platelet gp1bα receptors to outstretched, unusually large vWF multimers is potentiated.[315,318] In this fashion, the unusually large vWF multimers serve to efficiently tether circulating platelets to sites of vascular injury. In contrast, vWF is not required for initial platelet binding to exposed subendothelial matrix in a low shear stress environment, for example, as is observed in the venous circulation.[14,303,319,320] The arteriolar thrombosis prominent in TTP is in keeping with the pathologic association of large and unusually large vWF multimers in patients' plasma.[14]

ADAMTS13, The vWF-Cleaving Ptotease, and TTP

Proteolytic cleavage of vWF multimers was first suggested by the presence of characteristic vWF degradation products in the plasma of normal individuals.[321–326] Specifically, secreted vWF multimers were known to be cleaved into a series of smaller multimers that also produced, as a byproduct, stereotypic 140- and 176-kD disulfide-linked homodimers.[294] Although several proteases demonstrated vWF-cleaving activity in vitro, none produced these conserved proteolytic fragments normally observed in vivo.[322,327–334] In 1996, Miha Furlan and Han-Mou Tsai independently reported the presence of vWF-specific protease activity in the plasma of normal individuals capable of generating proteolytic fragments of the appropriate size.[314,335] Soon thereafter, a constitutive deficiency of this activity was documented in four patients with chronic relapsing TTP, and an inhibitory autoantibody against the vWF-cleaving protease was observed in a single patient with the more common, acquired form of the disease.[288,336] These preliminary reports were substantiated by the same two research groups in 1998 in two independent, large series of patients.[337,338] These researchers concluded that patients with the chronic relapsing form of the disease had a constitutional deficiency of the vWF-cleaving protease consistent with the persistence of ultralarge vWF multimers in their plasma even during periods of remission. In contrast, patients with acute episodes of TTP were more likely to have a plasma-borne inhibitor of the vWF-cleaving protease detectable only during acute episodes, with normalization of plasma vWF multimer profiles and vWF-cleaving protease activity accompanying clinical improvement. The nature of this inhibitor was an IgG autoantibody in all cases.[10] These critical observations provided the first important insights into the pathogenesis of TTP, even before full characterization of the vWF-cleaving protease itself.

Identification of ADAMTS13 as the vWF-Cleaving Protease

Three different approaches were successfully pursued by independent laboratories to identify the vWF-cleaving protease. Gerritsen and colleagues utilized sequential chromatographic methodologies, including immunoadsorption on autoantibodies from a patient with acquired TTP, to isolate sufficient quantities of purified protein from the plasma of normal individuals for sequencing of the first 15 amino acids of its N-terminal end.[339] In a simultaneous report, Fujikawa and colleagues used a commercial preparation of factor VIII/vWF concentrate as starting material to successfully purify and sequence the first 20 amino acids of the vWF-cleaving protease N-terminus.[340] These two reports produced nearly identical sequences. In addition, by performing a sequence search of the human genome and expressed sequence tags (EST)

databases, the latter group was able to predict that the vWF-cleaving protease was encoded by a novel gene on human chromosome 9q34 that shared significant homology with members of a recently described family of metalloproteinases, namely, the ADAMTS (a disintegrin-like and metalloprotease with thombospondin type I motifs) family. These findings were corroborated by Levy and colleagues using a fundamentally different, and very elegant, approach.[341] These investigators undertook a genome-wide linkage scan of four pedigrees with familial, chronic-relapsing TTP. None of the affected members carried plasma-borne inhibitors to vWF-cleaving protease, and all demonstrated ultralarge vWF multimers in their plasma. Instead of using inherently nebulous clinical criteria as the basis for their phenotypic trait, they demonstrated that vWF-cleaving protease activity reliably distinguished between affected individuals (2%–7% of normal), carriers (51%–68% of normal), and noncarrier family members. With this simple observation, they significantly increased the genetic power of their linkage analysis and potential to map the corresponding locus. These investigators successfully mapped the disease phenotype to human chromosome 9q34, and subsequently found disease mutations in the ADAMTS13 gene in all four pedigrees (and three additional patients with chronic, relapsing TTP). Unlike the mutations found in the HF1 gene linked to atypical HUS, these 12 disease mutations were distributed throughout the length of the coding sequence. To date, no overt mutational "hot-spot" has been identified. In keeping with low-level vWF-cleaving protease activity in affected individuals, no obvious null alleles were detected, implying that homozygous deficiency of ADAMTS13 may be lethal.[341,342] Taken together, these studies strongly suggest that ADAMTS13 is the elusive vWF-cleaving protease and its constitutional deficiency causally responsible for most (if not all) cases of familial, chronic-relapsing TTP.

Structure and Function of the ADAMTS13 Gene

The ADAMTS13 gene is the most divergent member of the recently described ADAMTS protease family consisting of 19 known members in the human genome. All are secreted metalloproteases of the reprolysin-type with conserved ancillary domains that contain at least one thrombospondin type I repeat (TSR).[343,344] ADAMTS13 is comprised of 29 exons and spans 37 kb of genomic DNA.[341,345] Full-length ADAMTS13 mRNA is synthesized primarily in the liver; however, expression in many other tissues and cell types has been reported.[346] Alternatively spliced transcripts have been detected in several tissues (including the liver), and may encode for smaller ADAMTS13 protein species lacking various C-terminal protein motifs.[341,345,347,348] The biologic relevance of these mRNA variants is currently unclear. The primary translation product is 1,427 amino acids in length and is detected in the plasma of normal individuals at a concentration of approximately 1 μg/mL.[339] It is composed of a series of protein motifs including (from the N-terminus): a signal peptide, propeptide, reprolysin-like metalloprotease domain, disintegrin-like domain, TSR, cysteine-rich domain, ADAMTS spacer domain, seven additional TSRs, and two CUB (complement components C1r/C1s, urinary epidermal growth factor and bone morphogenic protein-1) domains[341–343,345] (Fig. 26-6). This multidomain structure is highly conserved between human, mouse, rat, fish, and bird, suggesting that critical "selectable properties" of the constituent protein motifs contribute to the normal in vivo function of the ADAMTS13 protein.[342,349]

To date, vWF is the only known biological substrate of ADAMTS13, and vWF-cleaving activity its only biologic function. This activity is mediated by its reprolysin-like metalloprotease domain and can be inhibited, like other metalloproteases, by chelation of Ca^{2+} or Zn^{2+} divalent ions. In vitro, it cleaves a specific Tyr1605Met1606 bond in the A2 domain of the vWF subunit, thereby reducing vWF multimer size, generating the characteristic in vivo proteolytic fragments and inhibiting platelet adhesion.[342] Preliminary studies using deletion-mutation constructs and epitope mapping with IgG autoantibodies from three patients with acquired TTP suggested the critical importance of the cysteine-rich and spacer domains for vWF-cleaving activity.[349,350] These results were further substantiated when an independent group reported that 25 of 25 patients with acquired TTP demonstrated inhibitory autoantibodies specific for these regions.[351] Although these researchers postulate a role for the cysteine-rich and spacer domains in substrate recognition, their specific contribution to vWF-cleaving protease activity in vivo is not proven. Recent studies have also focused on the TSR2-8 and CUB domains in the ADAMTS13 C-terminus. TSR domains are a defining feature of the ADAMTS protease family and may serve as ligands for cellular receptors and points of attachment to components of the extracellular matrix.[352] Their physiologic relevance, however, is uncertain. CUB domains are not shared by other members of the ADAMTS family. They are generally thought to participate in protein-protein and protein-carbohydrate interactions.[353] With respect to ADAMTS13 vWF-cleaving protease activity, seemingly contradictory reports have emerged. It was previously demonstrated that deletion-mutation constructs lacking the two CUB (and TSR2-8) domains were not required for vWF cleavage in vitro.[349,350] Further credence was given to these findings when it was recently reported that the *Adamts13* gene in some inbred mouse strains (BALB/c, C3H/He, C57BL/6, and DBA/2) contained an intracisternal A particle (IAP) retrotransposon that included a premature stop codon. This results in the homozygous production of a truncated ADAMTS13 enzyme lacking its C-terminal TSR7-8 and CUB domains.[354] Others have suggested that the ADAMTS13 C-terminal protein motifs are critical for in vivo function, and that they serve as important points of attachment to endothelial cell surfaces, surface-bound, ultralarge vWF multimers, and/or components of the extracellular matrix. This view is substantiated by the discovery of inhibitory IgG autoantibodies[351] and disease mutations[293,355–358] involving these C-terminal domains in patients with acquired and chronic-relapsing TTP, respec-

tively. The physiologic relevance of these protein motifs, and others, in the normal functioning of the ADAMTS13 protein remains to be elucidated.

Most recently, elegant cell biology experiments have provided unique insights into the mechanism by which ADAMTS13 may cleave vWF multimers in vivo, and contribute to pathologic thrombosis in TTP. The impetus for these studies was the observation that classical in vitro vWF activity assays require strong denaturation of the substrate and long incubation periods (up to 24 hours) under nonphysiologic conditions.[335,359] This long time course is not in keeping with the postulated role of the enzyme in vivo, or the rapid clinical improvement after plasma infusion/exchange in TTP patients.[296] It was therefore speculated that conditions present in vivo, but absent in the in vitro assays, enhanced vWF multimer cleavage. In support of this hypothesis, Dong and colleagues demonstrated extremely rapid cleavage (within seconds) of ultralarge vWF multimers anchored to endothelial cell surfaces under conditions of fluid shear stress by normal plasma or partially purified ADAMTS13, but not plasma from patients with TTP.[317] This interaction is likely mediated by a conformational change induced in ultralarge vWF multimers under conditions of fluid shear stress that enhance the availability of vWF binding sites to circulating ADAMTS13.[360] This same research group subsequently showed that inflammatory cytokines can dramatically impede cleavage of ultralarge vWF multimers in vitro, thereby providing important mechanistic evidence for a putative link between inflammation and pathologic thrombosis.[361] In particular, interleukin-8 and tumor necrosis factor-α stimulated the release of ultralarge vWF multimers by endothelial cells. It is conceivable that this increased production could overwhelm plasma ADAMTS13 activity. These in vitro findings are consistent with the increased levels of cytokines detected in the plasma of patients with TTP during acute episodes.[362] It is also of significant interest that P-selectin, an adhesion molecule expressed on the surface of activated endothelial cells (and platelets),[363] may anchor newly secreted ultralarge vWF multimers to the endothelial cell surface at multiple sites.[317,364] Under normal conditions of high fluid shear stress, these cellular attachments might induce a structural conformation in surface-bound ultralarge vWF multimers amenable to cleavage by ADAMTS13. In the absence of plasma-borne ADAMTS13 activity and high fluid shear stress, however, these same interactions might subserve adherence of circulating platelets via platelet gp1bα receptors and promote pathologic thrombosis.[364] Taken together, these studies support an emerging paradigm for the role of ADAMTS13 in the control of vWF multimer size on endothelial cell surfaces under conditions of high fluid shear stress, and how its deficiency leads to pathologic thombosis

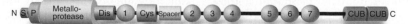

Figure 26-6 Structure of ADAMTS13 (a disintegrin-like and metalloprotease with thombospondin type I motifs). ADAMTS13 is the plasma-borne von Willebrand factor-protease. It is composed of a series of protein motifs including (from the N-terminus) a signal peptide, propeptide, reprolysin-like metalloprotease domain, disintegrin-like domain, thrombospondin repeat (TSR), cysteine-rich domain, ADAMTS spacer domain, seven additional TSRs, and two CUB (complement components C1r/C1s, urinary epidermal growth factor and bone morphogenic protein-1) domains. Acquired or inherited deficiencies of ADAMTS13 activity are causally linked with thrombotic thrombocytopenic purpura. **(See Color Plate 3.)**

(Fig. 26-7). They also highlight repeated bouts of inflammation as a possible etiologic trigger in pathologic thrombosis. Whether binding of ADAMTS13 to the endothelial cell surface is required for cleavage of vWF multimers in vivo is currently not known. This finding could have important clinical implications, as it might explain why some patients with TTP and unusually large circulating vWF multimers demonstrate normal ADAMTS13 activity in in vitro assays.[357,365] Of course, other determinants of vWF multimer size may also contribute to the pathologic thrombosis observed in patients with TTP, and are briefly discussed below.

Other Genetic Modifiers of vWF Multimer Size—Thrombospondin-1 and the ABO Blood Group Locus

To date, most research has focused on proteolytic cleavage by ADAMTS13 as the primary mechanism for regulation of vWF multimer size in plasma. More recently, additional mechanisms have been implicated in the control of plasma vWF levels, particularly thrombospondin-1 (TSP-1) and the ABO blood group. TSP-1 is a homotrimeric glycoprotein whose individual subunits are linked by disulfide bonding. It is predominantly synthesized in megakaryocytes and endothelial cells. Part of a family of five known thrombospondin extracellular glycoproteins, TSP-1 generated significant interest in the cancer community as an endogenous inhibitor of angiogenesis; however, other roles in cell-cell and cell-matrix adhesion have also been described.[297] Philip Hogg's laboratory has postulated an important function for TSP-1 in the control of vWF multimer size. In this model, an unpaired cysteine at position 974 in the molecule's C-terminal end acts as a free thiol capable of mounting a nucleophilic attack on the vWF intersubunit disulfide bonds. It thereby disrupts the "glue" holding the large vWF multimers together, and leads to their disassembly.[297,366–368] A recent report from the same laboratory using *Tsp-1* null-mice failed to recapitulate these findings.[369] Paradoxically, average plasma vWF multimer size was reduced in *Tsp-1* null-mice with more efficient processing of endothelial cell-derived large vWF multimers. These in vivo results suggest an inhibitory role for Tsp-1 in the control of vWF multimer size, at least in the murine model.[369] Regardless of its specific role, it is of particular interest that patients with acquired, sporadic TTP harbor autoantibodies against CD36, the cellular receptor for TSP-1 in microvascular endothelial cells.[1,370] Whether these autoantibodies affect TSP-1 binding, inhibit ADAMTS13 binding via its TSR domains, or play some other disparate role remains to be elucidated.

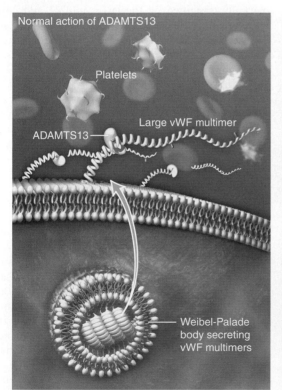 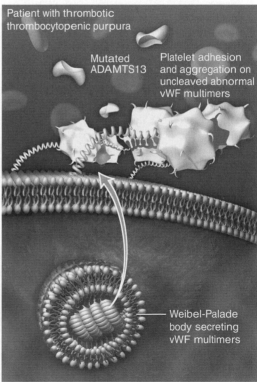

Figure 26-7 Mechanism of action of ADAMTS13 in normal individuals and patients with thrombotic thrombocytopenic purpura (TTP). Secretagogues stimulate endothelial cells to secrete "unusually large" von Willebrand factor (vWF) multimers from their intracellular storage sites, the Weibel-Palade bodies. Attached to the cell surface (and any exposed subendothelial matrix), these vWF multimers uncoil under the influence of high fluid shear stress, exposing sites for attachment of circulating platelets (via an interaction with platelet gp1bα receptors) and cleavage by ADAMTS13. In the normal individual **(A)**, ADAMTS13 successfully competes for target sites on uncoiled, surface-bound vWF multimers and cleaves them to produce characteristic vWF degradation products. In a patient with TTP **(B)**, ADAMTS13 activity is severely deficient and cannot effectively compete with circulating platelets for exposed binding sites. This results in platelet aggregation and pathologic thrombosis. **(See Color Plate 4.)**

The ABO blood group and plasma vWF levels have long since been implicated in human diseases characterized by pathologic thrombosis, such as, coronary heart disease, atherosclerosis, and venous thromboembolism.[371] In these studies, a non-O blood type and increased plasma vWF were associated with increased thrombogenicity. These earlier claims were substantiated by Souto and colleagues, who recently reported the results of a genome-wide linkage analysis that identified the ABO locus as the major determinant of vWF plasma levels in the Spanish population.[372] These researchers, and others, postulated that different ABO blood groups might cause different vWF posttranslational glycosylation patterns that influence steady-state vWF plasma levels. In support of this hypothesis, it was recently shown by multimeric analysis that ADAMTS13 cleaved vWF associated with blood group O more efficiently than vWF associated with other blood groups.[373] These results need to be interpreted with caution. First, this effect was modest, and of uncertain physiologic significance. And second, it is perhaps not coincidental that the ABO locus identified in the above linkage analysis is on chromosome 9q34, just 140,000 nucleotides centromeric to *ADAMTS13*.[374] At the present time, the biologic relevance of TSP-1 and the ABO blood group in the regulation of plasma vWF multimer size is unclear, as are their contributions to the pathologic thrombosis observed in patients with TTP.

Is Deficiency of ADAMTS13 Activity Specific for TTP?

The appropriate classification of patients with thrombotic microangiopathies into its two major subgroups, HUS and TTP, remains a point of strong contention in the field. To date, no objective clinical or laboratory findings reliably categorize patients into one group or the other.[1,13] Both groups share the hallmarks of thrombotic microangiopathies: thrombocytopenia and microangiopathic hemolytic anemia. If renal impairment is prominent and severe, a diagnosis of HUS is made. On the other hand, if renal impairment is mild and CNS manifestations dominate the clinical picture, the patient is considered to have TTP. Clearly, the clinical and laboratory findings overlap and cannot readily distinguish between these two subgroups of patients. For example, it is not unusual for patients with D+HUS to demonstrate prominent CNS involvement; indeed, it is perhaps the most important cause of mortality in D+HUS.[7,17] Other patients only manifest thrombocytopenia and microangiopathic anemia without prominent renal or extrarenal manifestations, especially early on in the course of the disease.[375] On the ward, it is common experience, even among experienced clinicians, to change a patient's diagnostic label depending on the emergence of severe renal impairment, new neurologic symptoms and signs, and disease recurrence. This diagnostic quandary is exacerbated by the inherent phenotypic heterogeneity characteristic of all thrombotic microangiopathies, even among affected family members with inherited forms of the disease. This issue is not semantics. The different thrombotic microangiopathies portend different natural histories and warrant specific therapeutic strategies. Greater clarity in the assignment of clinical diagnoses would substantively move the field forward and improve patient care. The discovery that vWF biology, and particularly severe plasma ADAMTS13 activity deficiency, causes TTP is primed to resolve this controversy. Important questions, then, are, "Is

deficiency of ADAMTS13 activity specific for TTP? And if so, can this knowledge be used in the clinic to facilitate diagnosis, improve prognostication, and guide therapy?" These questions have elicited spirited and scholarly debates.[375,376]

It is now undeniable that decreased ADAMTS13 activity is causally related to TTP as the result of an inherited enzyme mutation or, more commonly, acquired plasma-borne inhibitor.[10,337,338,341] When clinical suspicion of TTP is high, that is, adult patients presenting with mild renal dysfunction, no antecedent diarrheal episode, and the absence of easily identifiable triggers, severe ADAMTS13 deficiency ($\leq$ 0.1 U/mL) during an exacerbation is nearly universal and diagnostic for TTP.[338,375] Tsai and colleagues tested the specificity of this association by measuring plasma ADAMTS13 activity in randomly selected hospital patients with or without other thrombotic disorders, as well as a group of children with classical D+HUS. By and large, ADAMTS13 activity was demonstrated to be normal or mildly decreased with none demonstrating severe ADAMTS13 deficiencies akin to those observed in the TTP group.[338,375,377] Disenters point to numerous sporadic case reports and small case series of patients with a myriad of systemic conditions, including idiopathic thrombocytopenic purpura, systemic lupus erythematosus,[378] metastatic carcinoma,[379] and decompensated liver cirrhosis,[380] with documented severe ADAMTS13 deficiency.[376] While these results seemingly implicate severe ADAMTS13 deficiency in various disorders not related to TTP, they are likely to be at least partially explained by the large number and complexity of different assays used in the assessment of plasma ADAMTS13 activity, thereby frustrating meaningful comparisons of measurements obtained by different laboratories.[375,381,382] In addition, normal ranges for plasma ADAMTS13 activity for any single assay are typically very wide and established arbitrarily. For example, in the study examining ADAMTS13 activity levels in patients with decompensated liver cirrhosis, only the two patients tested with chronic, relapsing TTP had undetectable ADAMTS13 plasma activity levels.[380] Caution must be exercised in the interpretation of these studies.

Whether severe ADAMTS13 deficiency is specific for TTP will only be definitively answered when sensitive and specific tests are developed that are more easily translated to clinical practice and with the adoption of reference standards by the research community.[283,294,375] Currently, determinations of ADAMTS13 plasma activity levels are confined to a few expert research laboratories worldwide. The original methodologies developed by Furlan and colleagues[337] and Tsai and colleagues[338] are Western blotting protocols designed to demonstrate the disappearance of large vWF multimers or appearance of characteristic 176- and 140-kD degradation products, respectively, as markers for the presence of functional, plasma-derived ADAMTS13. Unfortunately, these assays are technically challenging and require the cooperation of skilled biochemists. They are also labor intensive, costly, and time consuming (>24 hours). Another major limitation is that these assays are performed under nonphysiologic (static, denaturing) conditions and may not detect all physiologically relevant mutations. In the last few years, several methodologies have emerged that differ in the substrate for cleavage, extent of protein denaturation, and technique for measurement of cleaved vWF.[383–389] Unfortunately, they suffer from many of the same limitations. Other methodologies have sought to more closely recapitulate the in vivo situation by adopting flow conditions and/or performing the in vitro activity assays on an endothelial monolayer.[317,390] The utility of these newer methodologies in the assessment of severe ADAMTS13 deficiency is currently uncertain, but their complexity almost certainly precludes their widespread usage in clinical practice. The field eagerly awaits the validation and adoption of appropriate standards for enzyme-linked immunosorbent assay (ELISA)-based methodologies that are simple, more economical, less labor intensive, and highly sensitive and specific for the determination of severe plasma ADAMTS13 deficiency.[391]

Implications for Therapy and the Way Ahead

Left untreated, TTP is almost universally fatal.[12] With the institution of therapeutic plasma exchange or plasma infusion as soon as TTP is suspected, over 90% of patients respond in dramatic fashion.[283,284] Nevertheless, these highly efficacious therapeutic modalities are not without limitations and complications.[375,392] Plasma infusion is limited by the volume of infused plasma that can be tolerated by a patient. This is especially problematic in patients with compromised renal function. Repeated infusions expose the patient to plasma derived from a large number of donors, increasing the risk for transmission of blood-borne viruses and alloimmune reactions.[392] Plasma exchange necessitates placement of a central venous catheter, often in patients with severe thrombocytopenia and increased risk for hemorrhage.[392–394] In some adults and older children with acquired acute idiopathic TTP, daily plasma exchange may be required for prolonged periods of time, in some cases longer than 30 days.[282,392] These prolonged treatment periods increase the likelihood of catheter-related and systemic infections. Disease recurrence is commonplace (30%–60%) and requires the reinstitution of plasma exchange and long hospitalizations.[392,395,396] Other complications of plasma exchange include citrate-related paresthesias and muscle cramps, cardiorespiratory compromise, and chills and rigors.[392–394] It is clear that a more rationale approach to treatment would greatly improve the care of these patients.

The discovery that a severe, inherited deficiency of plasma ADAMTS13 activity causes familial TTP offers the realistic hope of specific replacement therapy in the treatment of this condition.[1,375] This could be accomplished by infusion of purified or recombinant ADAMTS13 protein or gene therapy protocols. Because as little as 5% enzyme activity is required to prevent or alleviate thrombotic episodes, optimism in the success of these novel therapeutic strategies is not misgiven.[1,397,398] Perhaps even more exciting is the possibility of testing for ADAMTS13 deficiency in at-risk children and siblings prior to the development of thrombotic complications, so that preventive replacement therapy can be instituted.[375] Efforts are ongoing to bring this new molecular understanding of inherited TTP to clinical fruition.

The identification of inhibitory autoantibodies against ADAMTS13 during acute episodes of acquired idiopathic TTP suggests an underlying autoimmune etiology. It is therefore conceivable that interfering with autoantibody production may be beneficial during acute episodes, especially in patients who fail to respond to plasma exchange or develop severe, treatment-associated complications.[1,375] These efforts have included treatment with various immunosuppressive agents (glucocorticoids, vincristine, cyclophosphamide, intravenous immunoglobulins) and splenectomy.[1,284,392,399,400] This is also the therapeutic rationale for clinical trials of rituximab, a chimeric monoclonal anti-CD20 antibody that targets B cells, in patients with refractory, chronic relapsing TTP.[401,402] Although it is still too early to judge its efficacy, preliminary results are very encouraging.[402] As our understanding of the role of ADAMTS13 and vWF biology in thrombotic microangiopathies matures, more focused therapeutic strategies will emerge that target the molecular underpinnings of this frustrating disease.

ASSOCIATED THROMBOTIC MICROANGIOPATHIES

It is increasingly recognized that thrombotic microangiopathies may complicate other systemic conditions and their therapies (Table 26-1).[375] These inciting triggers likely damage or activate the endothelial lining of the microcirculation in susceptible vascular beds to trigger pathologic thrombosis, hemolytic anemia, and a consumptive thrombocytopenia. Organ damage may be mild or severe, with prominent renal or extrarenal manifestations, depending on the specific trigger and individual. As such, it is often difficult (and misleading) to classify these associated thrombotic microangiopathies as either HUS or TTP. Prominent among these are drug-,[403] transplantation-,[404–407] cancer-,[408,409] HIV-,[410,411] and pregnancy-associated thrombotic microangiopathies.[412] Together, they comprise a significant proportion of all thrombotic microangiopathies, especially in adulthood. To date, the roles of factor H, MCP, and ADAMTS13 in the pathogenesis of these associated thrombotic microangiopathies is unclear,[413–417] but will undoubtedly lead to more rationale therapeutic strategies for a significant number of these patients.

CONCLUSION

The past 5 years have seen exciting advances in our understanding of the molecular mechanisms responsible for endothelial dysfunction in the thrombotic microangiopathies. These include novel mechanisms of action for verotoxin in the pathogenesis of D+HUS, the unexpected role of inefficient protection of host cell surfaces against activation of the alternative pathway of complement in D-HUS, and deficiency of the plasma-borne vWF-cleaving protease, ADAMTS13, in TTP. In addition to providing exciting potential therapeutic targets for disease intervention, these newer molecular insights offer hope for an improved molecular classification of thrombotic microangiopathies. This would substantively improve clinicians' current abilities to prognosticate and prescribe rationale and targeted therapeutic strategies for their patients.

Acknowledgments

P.A.M. is a recipient of a Career Investigator Award from the Heart and Stroke Foundation of Canada and is supported by a grant from the Kidney Foundation of Canada. C.C.M. is a recipient of a Canadian Institutes of Health Research (CIHR) Postdoctoral Fellowship.

Table 26-1 Associated Thrombotic Microangiopathies

Categories	Examples
Drugs	Chemotherapeutics (mitomycin C, tamoxifen, cisplatin, bleomycin) Posttransplantation/antirejection drugs (cyclosporin, tacrolimus) Antiplatelet agents (clopidogrel, ticlopidine) Others (interferon, quinine)
Viruses	Human immunodeficiency virus (HIV) Cytomegalovirus (CMV) Human herpesvirus-6 (HHV-6) Hepatitis C virus (HCV)
Transplantation	Bone marrow transplantation Solid organ transplantation
Cancer	Hematologic malignancies Solid malignancies (especially widely disseminated cancers)
Rheumatologic disorders	Systemic lupus erythematosis (SLE) Rheumatoid arthritis Scleroderma (limited and diffuse)
Pregnancy	Pre-eclampsia, eclampsia HELLP syndrome
Other	Prosthetic heart valves Coronary artery bypass grafts Postvascular surgery

HELLP, hemolysis, elevated liver enzymes and low platelet count.

References

1. Moake JL: Thrombotic microangiopathies. N Engl J Med 347:589–600, 2002.
2. Ruggenenti P, Noris M, Remuzzi G: Thrombotic microangiopathy, hemolytic uremic syndrome, and thrombotic thrombocytopenic purpura. Kidney Int 60:831–846, 2001.
3. Nangaku M, Shankland SJ, Couser WG, et al: A new model of renal microvascular injury. Curr Opin Nephrol Hypertens 7:457–462, 1998.
4. Zoja C, Morigi M, Remuzzi G: The role of the endothelium in hemolytic uremic syndrome. J Nephrol 14(Suppl 4):58–62, 2001.
5. Gasser C, Gautier E, Steck A, et al: [Hemolytic-uremic syndrome: bilateral necrosis of the renal cortex in acute acquired hemolytic anemia]. Schweiz Med Wochenschr 85:905–909, 1955.
6. Boyce TG, Swerdlow DL, Griffin PM: Escherichia coli O157:H7 and the hemolytic-uremic syndrome. N Engl J Med 333:364–368, 1995.
7. Mead PS, Griffin PM: Escherichia coli O157:H7. Lancet 352:1207–1212, 1998.
8. Neumann HP, Salzmann M, Bohnert-Iwan B, et al: Haemolytic uraemic syndrome and mutations of the factor H gene: A registry-based study of German speaking countries. J Med Genet 40:676–681, 2003.
9. Noris M, Ruggenenti P, Perna A, et al: Hypocomplementemia discloses genetic predisposition to hemolytic uremic syndrome and thrombotic thrombocytopenic purpura: Role of factor H abnormalities. Italian Registry of Familial and Recurrent Hemolytic Uremic Syndrome/Thrombotic Thrombocytopenic Purpura. J Am Soc Nephrol 10:281–293, 1999.
10. Moake JL: Moschcowitz, multimers, and metalloprotease. N Engl J Med 339:1629–1631, 1998.
11. Moschcowitz E: Hyaline thrombosis of the terminal arterioles and capillaries: A hitherto undescribed disease. Proc NY Pathol Soc 24:21–24, 1924.
12. Moake JL: Thrombotic thrombocytopenic purpura: the systemic clumping "plague." Annu Rev Med 53:75–88, 2002.
13. Shah NT, Rand JH: Controversies in differentiating thrombotic thrombocytopenic purpura and hemolytic uremic syndrome. Mt Sinai J Med 70:344–351, 2003.
14. Moake JL, Rudy CK, Troll JH, et al: Unusually large plasma factor VIII:von Willebrand factor multimers in chronic relapsing thrombotic thrombocytopenic purpura. N Engl J Med 307:1432–1435, 1982.
15. Karmali MA, Petric M, Lim C, et al: The association between idiopathic hemolytic uremic syndrome and infection by verotoxin-producing Escherichia coli. J Infect Dis 151:775–782, 1985.
16. Warwicker P, Goodship TH, Donne RL, et al: Genetic studies into inherited and sporadic hemolytic uremic syndrome. Kidney Int 53:836–844, 1998.
17. Siegler RL: Spectrum of extrarenal involvement in postdiarrheal hemolytic-uremic syndrome. J Pediatr 125:511–518, 1994.
18. O'Loughlin EV, Robins-Browne RM: Effect of Shiga toxin and Shiga-like toxins on eukaryotic cells. Microbes Infect 3:493–507, 2001.
19. Richardson SE, Karmali MA, Becker LE, et al: The histopathology of the hemolytic uremic syndrome associated with verocytotoxin-producing Escherichia coli infections. Hum Pathol 19:1102–1108, 1988.
20. Griffin PM, Olmstead LC, Petras RE: Escherichia coli O157:H7-associated colitis. A clinical and histological study of 11 cases. Gastroenterology 99:142–149, 1990.
21. Rooney JC, Anderson RM, Hopkins IJ: Clinical and pathologic aspects of central nervous system involvement in the

haemolytic uraemic syndrome. Proc Aust Assoc Neurol 8:67–75, 1971.

22. Sheth KJ, Swick HM, Haworth N: Neurological involvement in hemolytic-uremic syndrome. Ann Neurol 19:90–93, 1986.

23. Upadhyaya K, Barwick K, Fishaut M, et al: The importance of nonrenal involvement in hemolytic-uremic syndrome. Pediatrics 65:115–120, 1980.

24. Konowalchuk J, Speirs JI, Stavric S: Vero response to a cytotoxin of Escherichia coli. Infect Immun 18:775–779, 1977.

25. Koster F, Levin J, Walker L, et al: Hemolytic-uremic syndrome after shigellosis. Relation to endotoxemia and circulating immune complexes. N Engl J Med 298:927–933, 1978.

26. Riley LW, Remis RS, Helgerson SD, et al: Hemorrhagic colitis associated with a rare Escherichia coli serotype. N Engl J Med 308:681–685, 1983.

27. Karmali MA, Petric M, Lim C, et al: Escherichia coli cytotoxin, haemolytic-uraemic syndrome, and haemorrhagic colitis. Lancet 2:1299–1300, 1983.

28. Karmali MA, Steele BT, Petric M, et al: Sporadic cases of haemolytic-uraemic syndrome associated with faecal cytotoxin and cytotoxin-producing Escherichia coli in stools. Lancet 1:619–620, 1983.

29. MacDonald KL, O'Leary MJ, Cohen ML, et al: Escherichia coli O157:H7, an emerging gastrointestinal pathogen. Results of a one-year, prospective, population-based study. JAMA 259:3567–3570, 1988.

30. Waters JR, Sharp JC, Dev VJ: Infection caused by Escherichia coli O157:H7 in Alberta, Canada, and in Scotland: A five-year review, 1987–1991. Clin Infect Dis 19:834–843, 1994.

31. Bell BP, Goldoft M, Griffin PM, et al: A multistate outbreak of Escherichia coli O157:H7-associated bloody diarrhea and hemolytic uremic syndrome from hamburgers. The Washington experience. JAMA 272:1349–1353, 1994.

32. Fukushima H, Hashizume T, Morita Y, et al: Clinical experiences in Sakai City Hospital during the massive outbreak of enterohemorrhagic Escherichia coli O157 infections in Sakai City, 1996. Pediatr Int 41:213–217, 1999.

33. Tilden J Jr, Young W, McNamara AM, et al: A new route of transmission for Escherichia coli: Infection from dry fermented salami. Am J Public Health 86:1142–1145, 1996.

34. From the Centers for Disease Control and Prevention. Outbreaks of Escherichia coli O157:H7 infection associated with eating alfalfa sprouts—Michigan and Virginia, June–July 1997. JAMA 278:809–810, 1997.

35. Breuer T, Benkel DH, Shapiro RL, et al: A multistate outbreak of Escherichia coli O157:H7 infections linked to alfalfa sprouts grown from contaminated seeds. Emerg Infect Dis 7:977–982, 2001.

36. Michino H, Araki K, Minami S, et al: Massive outbreak of Escherichia coli O157:H7 infection in schoolchildren in Sakai City, Japan, associated with consumption of white radish sprouts. Am J Epidemiol 150:787–796, 1999.

37. Slutsker L, Ries AA, Maloney K, et al: A nationwide case-control study of Escherichia coli O157:H7 infection in the United States. J Infect Dis 177:962–966, 1998.

38. Leadership and fecal coliforms: Walkerton 2000. CMAJ 163:1417–1419, 2000.

39. Waterborne outbreak of gastroenteritis associated with a contaminated municipal water supply, Walkerton, Ontario, May–June 2000. Can Commun Dis Rep 26:170–173, 2000.

40. Le Saux N, Spika JS, Friesen B, et al: Ground beef consumption in noncommercial settings is a risk factor for sporadic Escherichia coli O157:H7 infection in Canada. J Infect Dis 167:500–502, 1993.

41. Slutsker L, Ries AA, Greene KD, et al: Escherichia coli O157:H7 diarrhea in the United States: Clinical and epidemiologic features. Ann Intern Med 126:505–513, 1997.

42. Carter AO, Borczyk AA, Carlson JA, et al: A severe outbreak of Escherichia coli O157:H7-associated hemorrhagic colitis in a nursing home. N Engl J Med 317:1496–1500, 1987.

43. Wall PG, McDonnell RJ, Adak GK, et al: General outbreaks of vero cytotoxin producing Escherichia coli O157 in England and Wales from 1992 to 1994. Commun Dis Rep CDR Rev 6:R26–R33, 1996.

44. Wong CS, Jelacic S, Habeeb RL, et al: The risk of the hemolytic-uremic syndrome after antibiotic treatment of Escherichia coli O157:H7 infections. N Engl J Med 342:1930–1936, 2000.

45. Siegler RL: The hemolytic uremic syndrome. Pediatr Clin North Am 42:1505–1529, 1995.

46. Griffin PM, Tauxe RV: The epidemiology of infections caused by Escherichia coli O157:H7, other enterohemorrhagic E. coli, and the associated hemolytic uremic syndrome. Epidemiol Rev 13:60–98, 1991.

47. Tarr PI, Neill MA, Allen J, et al: The increasing incidence of the hemolytic-uremic syndrome in King County, Washington: Lack of evidence for ascertainment bias. Am J Epidemiol 129:582–586, 1989.

48. Kaper JB, Nataro JP, Mobley HL: Pathogenic Escherichia coli. Nat Rev Microbiol 2:123–140, 2004.

49. Nataro JP, Kaper JB: Diarrheagenic Escherichia coli. Clin Microbiol Rev 11:142–201, 1998.

50. Sandvig K: Shiga toxins. Toxicon 39:1629–1635, 2001.

51. Paton AW, Manning PA, Woodrow MC, et al: Translocated intimin receptors (Tir) of Shiga-toxigenic Escherichia coli isolates belonging to serogroups O26, O111, and O157 react with sera from patients with hemolytic-uremic syndrome and exhibit marked sequence heterogeneity. Infect Immun 66:5580–5586, 1998.

52. Karmali MA: Infection by Shiga toxin-producing Escherichia coli: An overview. Mol Biotechnol 26:117–122, 2004.

53. Perna NT, Plunkett G 3rd, Burland V, et al: Genome sequence of enterohemorrhagic Escherichia coli O157:H7. Nature 409:529–533, 2001.

54. Paton AW, Srimanote P, Talbot UM, et al: A new family of potent AB5 cytotoxins produced by Shiga toxigenic Escherichia coli. J Exp Med 200:35–46, 2004.

55. Schmidt H, Scheef J, Huppertz HI, et al: Escherichia coli O157:H7 and O157:H⁻ strains that do not produce Shiga toxin: Phenotypic and genetic characterization of isolates associated with diarrhea and hemolytic-uremic syndrome. J Clin Microbiol 37:3491–3496, 1999.

56. Falnes PO, Sandvig K: Penetration of protein toxins into cells. Curr Opin Cell Biol 12:407–413, 2000.

57. Olsnes S, Kozlov JV: Ricin. Toxicon 39:1723–1728, 2001.

58. Fraser ME, Chernaia MM, Kozlov YV, et al: Crystal structure of the holotoxin from Shigella dysenteriae at 2.5 A resolution. Nat Struct Biol 1:59–64, 1994.

59. Sixma TK, Pronk SE, Kalk KH, et al: Crystal structure of a cholera toxin-related heat-labile enterotoxin from E. coli. Nature 351:371–377, 1991.

60. Austin PR, Jablonski PE, Bohach GA, et al: Evidence that the A2 fragment of Shiga-like toxin type I is required for holotoxin integrity. Infect Immun 62:1768–1775, 1994.

61. Felsenfeld O: K. Shiga, bacteriologist. Science 126:113, 1957.

62. Trofa AF, Ueno-Olsen H, Oiwa R, et al: Dr. Kiyoshi Shiga: Discoverer of the dysentery bacillus. Clin Infect Dis 29:1303–1306, 1999.

63. Tzipori S, Sheoran A, Akiyoshi D, et al: Antibody therapy in the management of Shiga toxin-induced hemolytic uremic syndrome. Clin Microbiol Rev 17:926–941, 2004.

64. Calderwood SB, Auclair F, Donohue-Rolfe A, et al: Nucleotide sequence of the Shiga-like toxin genes of Escherichia coli. Proc Natl Acad Sci U S A 84:4364–4368, 1987.

65. De Grandis S, Ginsberg J, Toone M, et al: Nucleotide sequence and promoter mapping of the Escherichia coli Shiga-like toxin operon of bacteriophage H-19B. J Bacteriol 169:4313–4319, 1987.

66. Fraser ME, Fujinaga M, Cherney MM, et al: Structure of Shiga toxin type 2 (Stx2) from Escherichia coli O157:H7. J Biol Chem 279:27511–27517, 2004.

67. Russmann H, Schmidt H, Heesemann J, et al: Variants of Shiga-like toxin II constitute a major toxin component in Escherichia coli O157 strains from patients with haemolytic uraemic syndrome. J Med Microbiol 40:338–343, 1994.

68. Friedrich AW, Bielaszewska M, Zhang WL, et al: Escherichia coli harboring Shiga toxin 2 gene variants: Frequency and association with clinical symptoms. J Infect Dis 185:74–84, 2002.

69. Kleanthous H, Smith HR, Scotland SM, et al: Haemolytic uraemic syndromes in the British Isles, 1985-8: Association with verocytotoxin producing Escherichia coli. Part 2: Microbiological aspects. Arch Dis Child 65:722–727, 1990.

70. Milford DV, Taylor CM, Guttridge B, et al: Haemolytic uraemic syndromes in the British Isles 1985–8: Association with verocytotoxin producing Escherichia coli. Part 1: Clinical and epidemiological aspects. Arch Dis Child 65:716–721, 1990.

71. Ostroff SM, Tarr PI, Neill MA, et al: Toxin genotypes and plasmid profiles as determinants of systemic sequelae in Escherichia coli O157:H7 infections. J Infect Dis 160:994–998, 1989.

72. Scotland SM, Willshaw GA, Smith HR, et al: Properties of strains of Escherichia coli belonging to serogroup O157 with special reference to production of Vero cytotoxins VT1 and VT2. Epidemiol Infect 99:613–624, 1987.

73. Donohue-Rolfe A, Kondova I, Oswald S, et al: Escherichia coli O157:H7 strains that express Shiga toxin (Stx) 2 alone are more neurotropic for gnotobiotic piglets than are isotypes producing only Stx1 or both Stx1 and Stx2. J Infect Dis 181:1825–1829, 2000.

74. Siegler RL, Obrig TG, Pysher TJ, et al: Response to Shiga toxin 1 and 2 in a baboon model of hemolytic uremic syndrome. Pediatr Nephrol 18:92–96, 2003.

75. Tesh VL, Burris JA, Owens JW, et al: Comparison of the relative toxicities of Shiga-like toxins type I and type II for mice. Infect Immun 61:3392–3402, 1993.

76. Nakajima H, Kiyokawa N, Katagiri YU, et al: Kinetic analysis of binding between Shiga toxin and receptor glycolipid Gb3Cer by surface plasmon resonance. J Biol Chem 276:42915–42922, 2001.

77. Louise CB, Obrig TG: Specific interaction of Escherichia coli O157:H7-derived Shiga-like toxin II with human renal endothelial cells. J Infect Dis 172:1397–1401, 1995.

78. Linggood MA, Thompson JM: Verotoxin production among porcine strains of Escherichia coli and its association with oedema disease. J Med Microbiol 24:359–362, 1987.

79. Collier RJ: Understanding the mode of action of diphtheria toxin: A perspective on progress during the 20th century. Toxicon 39:1793–1803, 2001.

80. De Haan L, Hirst TR: Cholera toxin: A paradigm for multi-functional engagement of cellular mechanisms (Review). Mol Membr Biol 21:77–92, 2004.

81. Bokoch GM, Katada T, Northup JK, et al: Identification of the predominant substrate for ADP-ribosylation by islet activating protein. J Biol Chem 258:2072–2075, 1983.

82. Furutani M, Kashiwagi K, Ito K, et al: Comparison of the modes of action of a Vero toxin (a Shiga-like toxin) from Escherichia coli, of ricin, and of alpha-sarcin. Arch Biochem Biophys 293:140–146, 1992.

83. O'Brien AD, Tesh VL, Donohue-Rolfe A, et al: Shiga toxin: Biochemistry, genetics, mode of action, and role in pathogenesis. Curr Top Microbiol Immunol 180:65–94, 1992.

84. Wool IG, Gluck A, Endo Y: Ribotoxin recognition of ribosomal RNA and a proposal for the mechanism of translocation. Trends Biochem Sci 17:266–269, 1992.

85. Correll CC, Yang X, Gerczei T, et al: RNA recognition and base flipping by the toxin sarcin. J Synchrotron Radiat 11:93–96, 2004.

86. Yang X, Gerczei T, Glover LT, et al: Crystal structures of restrictocin-inhibitor complexes with implications for RNA recognition and base flipping. Nat Struct Biol 8:968–973, 2001.

87. Bitzan MM, Wang Y, Lin J, et al: Verotoxin and ricin have novel effects on preproendothelin-1 expression but fail to modify nitric oxide synthase (ecNOS) expression and NO production in vascular endothelium. J Clin Invest 101:372–382, 1998.

88. Ohmi K, Kiyokawa N, Takeda T, et al: Human microvascular endothelial cells are strongly sensitive to Shiga toxins. Biochem Biophys Res Commun 251:137–141, 1998.

89. Sandvig K, Spilsberg B, Lauvrak SU, et al: Pathways followed by protein toxins into cells. Int J Med Microbiol 293:483–490, 2004.

90. Ling H, Boodhoo A, Hazes B, et al: Structure of the Shiga-like toxin I B-pentamer complexed with an analogue of its receptor Gb3. Biochemistry 37:1777–1788, 1998.

91. Bast DJ, Banerjee L, Clark C, et al: The identification of three biologically relevant globotriaosyl ceramide receptor binding sites on the Verotoxin 1 B subunit. Mol Microbiol 32:953–960, 1999.

92. Soltyk AM, MacKenzie CR, Wolski VM, et al: A mutational analysis of the globotriaosylceramide-binding sites of verotoxin VT1. J Biol Chem 277:5351–5359, 2002.

93. Jacewicz M, Clausen H, Nudelman E, et al: Pathogenesis of shigella diarrhea. XI. Isolation of a shigella toxin-binding glycolipid from rabbit jejunum and HeLa cells and its identification as globotriaosylceramide. J Exp Med 163:1391–1404, 1986.

94. Keusch GT, Jacewicz M, Donohue-Rolfe A: Pathogenesis of shigella diarrhea: Evidence for an N-linked glycoprotein shigella toxin receptor and receptor modulation by beta-galactosidase. J Infect Dis 153:238–248, 1986.

95. Lindberg AA, Brown JE, Stromberg N, et al: Identification of the carbohydrate receptor for Shiga toxin produced by Shigella dysenteriae type 1. J Biol Chem 262:1779–1785, 1987.

96. Lingwood CA, Law H, Richardson S, et al: Glycolipid binding of purified and recombinant Escherichia coli produced verotoxin in vitro. J Biol Chem 262:8834–8839, 1987.

97. Lingwood CA: Role of verotoxin receptors in pathogenesis. Trends Microbiol 4:147–153, 1996.

98. Marcus DM, Kundu SK, Suzuki A: The P blood group system: Recent progress in immunochemistry and genetics. Semin Hematol 18:63–71, 1981.

99. Boyd B, Tyrrell G, Maloney M, et al: Alteration of the glycolipid binding specificity of the pig edema toxin from globotetraosyl to globotriaosyl ceramide alters in vivo tissue targeting and results in a verotoxin 1-like disease in pigs. J Exp Med 177:1745–1753, 1993.

100. Mobassaleh M, Donohue-Rolfe A, Jacewicz M, et al: Pathogenesis of shigella diarrhea: Evidence for a developmentally regulated glycolipid receptor for shigella toxin involved in the fluid secretory response of rabbit small intestine. J Infect Dis 157:1023–1031, 1988.

101. Tyrrell GJ, Ramotar K, Toye B, et al: Alteration of the carbohydrate binding specificity of verotoxins from Gal alpha 1-4Gal to GalNAc beta 1-3Gal alpha 1-4Gal and vice versa by site-directed mutagenesis of the binding subunit. Proc Natl Acad Sci U S A 89:524–528, 1992.

102. Zoja C, Corna D, Farina C, et al: Verotoxin glycolipid receptors determine the localization of microangiopathic process in rabbits given verotoxin-1. J Lab Clin Med 120:229–238, 1992.

103. Obrig TG, Louise CB, Lingwood CA, et al: Endothelial heterogeneity in Shiga toxin receptors and responses. J Biol Chem 268:15484–15488, 1993.

104. Pijpers AH, van Setten PA, van den Heuvel LP, et al: Verocytotoxin-induced apoptosis of human microvascular endothelial cells. J Am Soc Nephrol 12:767–778, 2001.

105. Lingwood CA: Verotoxin-binding in human renal sections. Nephron 66:21-8, 1994.

106. Ergonul Z, Clayton F, Fogo AB, et al: Shigatoxin-1 binding and receptor expression in human kidneys do not change with age. Pediatr Nephrol 18:246–253, 2003.

107. Devenish J, Gyles C, LaMarre J: Binding of Escherichia coli verotoxins to cell surface protein on wild-type and globotriaosylceramide-deficient Vero cells. Can J Microbiol 44:28–34, 1998.

108. Philpott DJ, Ackerley CA, Kiliaan AJ, et al: Translocation of verotoxin-1 across T84 monolayers: Mechanism of bacterial toxin penetration of epithelium. Am J Physiol 273:G1349–G1358, 1997.

109. Sandvig K, Ryd M, Garred O, et al: Retrograde transport from the Golgi complex to the ER of both Shiga toxin and the nontoxic Shiga B-fragment is regulated by butyric acid and cAMP. J Cell Biol 126:53–64, 1994.

110. Roos-Mattjus P, Sistonen L: The ubiquitin-proteasome pathway. Ann Med 36:285–295, 2004.

111. Lord JM, Deeks E, Marsden CJ, et al: Retrograde transport of toxins across the endoplasmic reticulum membrane. Biochem Soc Trans 31:1260–1262, 2003.

112. Heyderman RS, Soriani M, Hirst TR: Is immune cell activation the missing link in the pathogenesis of post-diarrhoeal HUS? Trends Microbiol 9:262–266, 2001.

113. Fitzpatrick MM, Shah V, Trompeter RS, et al: Interleukin-8 and polymorphoneutrophil leucocyte activation in hemolytic uremic syndrome of childhood. Kidney Int 42:951–956, 1992.

114. Litalien C, Proulx F, Mariscalco MM, et al: Circulating inflammatory cytokine levels in hemolytic uremic syndrome. Pediatr Nephrol 13:840–845, 1999.

115. van Setten PA, van Hinsbergh VW, van den Heuvel LP, et al: Monocyte chemoattractant protein-1 and interleukin-8 levels in urine and serum of patents with hemolytic uremic syndrome. Pediatr Res 43:759–767, 1998.

116. Ballermann BJ: Endothelial cell activation. Kidney Int 53:1810–1826, 1998.

117. Mawji IA, Marsden PA: Perturbations in paracrine control of the circulation: Role of the endothelial-derived vasomediators, endothelin-1 and nitric oxide. Microsc Res Tech 60:46–58, 2003.

118. Morigi M, Galbusera M, Binda E, et al: Verotoxin-1-induced up-regulation of adhesive molecules renders microvascular endothelial cells thrombogenic at high shear stress. Blood 98:1828–1835, 2001.

119. Singer M, Sansonetti PJ: IL-8 is a key chemokine regulating neutrophil recruitment in a new mouse model of Shigella-induced colitis. J Immunol 173:4197–4206, 2004.

120. Taylor FB Jr, Tesh VL, DeBault L, et al: Characterization of the baboon responses to Shiga-like toxin: Descriptive study of a new primate model of toxic responses to Stx-1. Am J Pathol 154:1285–1299, 1999.

121. Cherla RP, Lee SY, Tesh VL: Shiga toxins and apoptosis. FEMS Microbiol Lett 228:159-166, 2003.

122. Erwert RD, Eiting KT, Tupper JC, et al: Shiga toxin induces decreased expression of the anti-apoptotic protein Mcl-1 concomitant with the onset of endothelial apoptosis. Microb Pathog 35:87–93, 2003.

123. Karpman D, Hakansson A, Perez MT, et al: Apoptosis of renal cortical cells in the hemolytic-uremic syndrome: In vivo and in vitro studies. Infect Immun 66:636–644, 1998.

124. Kodama T, Nagayama K, Yamada K, et al: Induction of apoptosis in human renal proximal tubular epithelial cells by Escherichia coli verocytotoxin 1 in vitro. Med Microbiol Immunol (Berl) 188:73–78, 1999.

125. Keenan KP, Sharpnack DD, Collins H, et al: Morphologic evaluation of the effects of Shiga toxin and E coli Shiga-like toxin on the rabbit intestine. Am J Pathol 125:69–80, 1986.

126. Pai CH, Kelly JK, Meyers GL: Experimental infection of infant rabbits with verotoxin-producing Escherichia coli. Infect Immun 51:16–23, 1986.

127. Wolski VM, Soltyk AM, Brunton JL: Tumour necrosis factor alpha is not an essential component of verotoxin 1-induced toxicity in mice. Microb Pathog 32:263–271, 2002.

128. Kaneko K, Kiyokawa N, Ohtomo Y, et al: Apoptosis of renal tubular cells in Shiga-toxin-mediated hemolytic uremic syndrome. Nephron 87:182–185, 2001.

129. Laskin JD, Heck DE, Laskin DL: The ribotoxic stress response as a potential mechanism for MAP kinase activation in xenobiotic toxicity. Toxicol Sci 69:289–291, 2002.

130. Iordanov MS, Pribnow D, Magun JL, et al: Ribotoxic stress response: Activation of the stress-activated protein kinase JNK1 by inhibitors of the peptidyl transferase reaction and by sequence-specific RNA damage to the alpha-sarcin/ricin loop in the 28S rRNA. Mol Cell Biol 17:3373–3381, 1997.

131. Rolli-Derkinderen M, Gaestel M: p38/SAPK2-dependent gene expression in Jurkat T cells. Biol Chem 381:193–198, 2000.

132. Yamasaki C, Nishikawa K, Zeng XT, et al: Induction of cytokines by toxins that have an identical RNA N-glycosidase activity: Shiga toxin, ricin, and modeccin. Biochim Biophys Acta 1671:44–50, 2004.

133. Kojima S, Yanagihara I, Kono G, et al: mkp-1 encoding mitogen-activated protein kinase phosphatase 1, a verotoxin 1 responsive gene, detected by differential display reverse transcription-PCR in Caco-2 cells. Infect Immun 68:2791–2796, 2000.

134. Matussek A, Lauber J, Bergau A, et al: Molecular and functional analysis of Shiga toxin-induced response patterns in human vascular endothelial cells. Blood 102:1323–1332, 2003.

135. Yamasaki C, Natori Y, Zeng XT, et al: Induction of cytokines in a human colon epithelial cell line by Shiga toxin 1 (Stx1) and Stx2 but not by non-toxic mutant Stx1 which lacks N-glycosidase activity. FEBS Lett 442:231–234, 1999.

136. Barbieri L, Valbonesi P, Brigotti M, et al: Shiga-like toxin I is a polynucleotide:adenosine glycosidase. Mol Microbiol 29:661–662, 1998.

137. Barbieri L, Valbonesi P, Bonora E, et al: Polynucleotide:adenosine glycosidase activity of ribosome-inactivating proteins: Effect on DNA, RNA and poly(A). Nucleic Acids Res 25:518–522, 1997.

138. Barbieri L, Gorini P, Valbonesi P, et al: Unexpected activity of saporins. Nature 372:624, 1994.

139. Brigotti M, Barbieri L, Valbonesi P, et al: A rapid and sensitive method to measure the enzymatic activity of ribosome-inactivating proteins. Nucleic Acids Res 26:4306–4307, 1998.

140. Barbieri L, Valbonesi P, Righi F, et al: Polynucleotide:adenosine glycosidase is the sole activity of ribosome-inactivating proteins on DNA. J Biochem (Tokyo) 128:883–889, 2000.

141. Brigotti M, Accorsi P, Carnicelli D, et al: Shiga toxin 1: Damage to DNA in vitro. Toxicon 39:341–348, 2001.

142. Brigotti M, Alfieri R, Sestili P, et al: Damage to nuclear DNA induced by Shiga toxin 1 and ricin in human endothelial cells. Faseb J 16:365–372, 2002.

143. Andreoli SP, Trachtman H, Acheson DW, et al: Hemolytic uremic syndrome: Epidemiology, pathophysiology, and therapy. Pediatr Nephrol 17:293–298, 2002.

229. Meri S, Koistinen V, Miettinen A, et al: Activation of the alternative pathway of complement by monoclonal lambda light chains in membranoproliferative glomerulonephritis. J Exp Med 175:939–950, 1992.

230. Jokiranta TS, Solomon A, Pangburn MK, et al: Nephritogenic lambda light chain dimer: A unique human miniautoantibody against complement factor H. J Immunol 163:4590–4596, 1999.

231. Zipfel PF, Skerka C, Hellwage J, et al: Factor H family proteins: On complement, microbes and human diseases. Biochem Soc Trans 30:971–978, 2002.

232. Giannakis E, Jokiranta TS, Male DA, et al: A common site within factor H SCR 7 responsible for binding heparin, C-reactive protein and streptococcal M protein. Eur J Immunol 33:962–969, 2003.

233. Jarva H, Jokiranta TS, Hellwage J, et al: Regulation of complement activation by C-reactive protein: Targeting the complement inhibitory activity of factor H by an interaction with short consensus repeat domains 7 and 8-11. J Immunol 163:3957–3962, 1999.

234. Martinez A, Pio R, Zipfel PF, et al: Mapping of the adrenomedullin-binding domains in human complement factor H. Hypertens Res 26(Suppl):55–59, 2003.

235. Pio R, Elsasser TH, Martinez A, et al: Identification, characterization, and physiological actions of factor H as an adrenomedullin binding protein present in human plasma. Microsc Res Tech 57:23–27, 2002.

236. Pio R, Martinez A, Unsworth EJ, et al: Complement factor H is a serum-binding protein for adrenomedullin, and the resulting complex modulates the bioactivities of both partners. J Biol Chem 276:12292–12300, 2001.

237. Sharma AK, Pangburn MK: Identification of three physically and functionally distinct binding sites for C3b in human complement factor H by deletion mutagenesis. Proc Natl Acad Sci U S A 93:10996–11001, 1996.

238. Manuelian T, Hellwage J, Meri S, et al: Mutations in factor H reduce binding affinity to C3b and heparin and surface attachment to endothelial cells in hemolytic uremic syndrome. J Clin Invest 111:1181–1190, 2003.

239. Pangburn MK: Cutting edge: Localization of the host recognition functions of complement factor H at the carboxyl-terminal: Implications for hemolytic uremic syndrome. J Immunol 169:4702–4706, 2002.

240. Sanchez-Corral P, Gonzalez-Rubio C, Rodriguez de Cordoba S, et al: Functional analysis in serum from atypical hemolytic uremic syndrome patients reveals impaired protection of host cells associated with mutations in factor H. Mol Immunol 41:81–84, 2004.

241. Sanchez-Corral P, Perez-Caballero D, Huarte O, et al: Structural and functional characterization of factor H mutations associated with atypical hemolytic uremic syndrome. Am J Hum Genet 71:1285–1295, 2002.

242. Schreiber RD, Pangburn MK, Lesavre PH, et al: Initiation of the alternative pathway of complement: recognition of activators by bound C3b and assembly of the entire pathway from six isolated proteins. Proc Natl Acad Sci U S A 75:3948–3952, 1978.

243. Cole JL, Housley GA, Jr., Dykman TR, et al: Identification of an additional class of C3-binding membrane proteins of human peripheral blood leukocytes and cell lines. Proc Natl Acad Sci U S A 82:859–863, 1985.

244. Seya T, Turner JR, Atkinson JP: Purification and characterization of a membrane protein (gp45-70) that is a cofactor for cleavage of C3b and C4b. J Exp Med 163:837–855, 1986.

245. Endoh M, Yamashina M, Ohi H, et al: Immunohistochemical demonstration of membrane cofactor protein (MCP) of complement in normal and diseased kidney tissues. Clin Exp Immunol 94:182–188, 1993.

246. Ichida S, Yuzawa Y, Okada H, et al: Localization of the complement regulatory proteins in the normal human kidney. Kidney Int 46:89–96, 1994.

247. Johnstone RW, Loveland BE, McKenzie IF: Identification and quantification of complement regulator CD46 on normal human tissues. Immunology 79:341–347, 1993.

248. McNearney T, Ballard L, Seya T, et al: Membrane cofactor protein of complement is present on human fibroblast, epithelial, and endothelial cells. J Clin Invest 84:538–545, 1989.

249. Nakanishi I, Moutabarrik A, Hara T, et al: Identification and characterization of membrane cofactor protein (CD46) in the human kidneys. Eur J Immunol 24:1529–1535, 1994.

250. Liszewski MK, Farries TC, Lublin DM, et al: Control of the complement system. Adv Immunol 61:201–283, 1996.

251. Bora NS, Lublin DM, Kumar BV, et al: Structural gene for human membrane cofactor protein (MCP) of complement maps to within 100 kb of the 3' end of the C3b/C4b receptor gene. J Exp Med 169:597–602, 1989.

252. Lublin DM, Liszewski MK, Post TW, et al: Molecular cloning and chromosomal localization of human membrane cofactor protein (MCP). Evidence for inclusion in the multigene family of complement-regulatory proteins. J Exp Med 168:181–194, 1988.

253. Post TW, Liszewski MK, Adams EM, et al: Membrane cofactor protein of the complement system: alternative splicing of serine/threonine/proline-rich exons and cytoplasmic tails produces multiple isoforms that correlate with protein phenotype. J Exp Med 174:93–102, 1991.

254. Cui W, Hourcade D, Post T, et al: Characterization of the promoter region of the membrane cofactor protein (CD46) gene of the human complement system and comparison to a membrane cofactor protein-like genetic element. J Immunol 151:4137–4146, 1993.

255. Purcell DF, Jonstone RW, McKenzie IF: Identification of four different CD46 (MCP) molecules with anti-peptide antibodies. Biochem Biophys Res Commun 180:1091–1097, 1991.

256. Purcell DF, Russell SM, Deacon NJ, et al: Alternatively spliced RNAs encode several isoforms of CD46 (MCP), a regulator of complement activation. Immunogenetics 33:335–344, 1991.

257. Seya T, Hirano A, Matsumoto M, et al: Human membrane cofactor protein (MCP, CD46): Multiple isoforms and functions. Int J Biochem Cell Biol 31:1255–1260, 1999.

258. Pollard AJ, Flanagan BF, Newton DJ, et al: A novel isoform of human membrane cofactor protein (CD46) mRNA generated by intron retention. Gene 212:39–47, 1998.

259. Riley-Vargas RC, Gill DB, Kemper C, et al: CD46: Expanding beyond complement regulation. Trends Immunol 25:496–503, 2004.

260. Wang G, Liszewski MK, Chan AC, et al: Membrane cofactor protein (MCP; CD46): Isoform-specific tyrosine phosphorylation. J Immunol 164:1839–1846, 2000.

261. Seya T, Atkinson JP: Functional properties of membrane cofactor protein of complement. Biochem J 264:581–588, 1989.

262. Barilla-LaBarca ML, Liszewski MK, Lambris JD, et al: Role of membrane cofactor protein (CD46) in regulation of C4b and C3b deposited on cells. J Immunol 168:6298–6304, 2002.

263. Devaux P, Christiansen D, Fontaine M, et al: Control of C3b and C5b deposition by CD46 (membrane cofactor protein) after alternative but not classical complement activation. Eur J Immunol 29:815–822, 1999.

264. Adams EM, Brown MC, Nunge M, et al: Contribution of the repeating domains of membrane cofactor protein (CD46) of the complement system to ligand binding and cofactor activity. J Immunol 147:3005–3011, 1991.

265. Liszewski MK, Leung M, Cui W, et al: Dissecting sites important for complement regulatory activity in membrane cofactor protein (MCP; CD46). J Biol Chem 275:37692–37701, 2000.

266. Iwata K, Seya T, Yanagi Y, et al: Diversity of sites for measles virus binding and for inactivation of complement C3b and C4b on membrane cofactor protein CD46. J Biol Chem 270:15148–15152, 1995.

267. Kojima A, Iwata K, Seya T, et al: Membrane cofactor protein (CD46) protects cells predominantly from alternative complement pathway-mediated C3-fragment deposition and cytolysis. J Immunol 151:1519–1527, 1993.

268. Couser WG: Complement inhibitors and glomerulonephritis: Are we there yet? J Am Soc Nephrol 14:815–818, 2003.

269. Inal JM, Pascual M, Lesavre P, et al: Complement inhibition in renal diseases. Nephrol Dial Transplant 18:237–240, 2003.

270. Morgan BP, Harris CL: Complement therapeutics; history and current progress. Mol Immunol 40:159–170, 2003.

271. Christiansen D, Milland J, Thorley BR, et al: A functional analysis of recombinant soluble CD46 in vivo and a comparison with recombinant soluble forms of CD55 and CD35 in vitro. Eur J Immunol 26:578–585, 1996.

272. Christiansen D, Milland J, Thorley BR, et al: Engineering of recombinant soluble CD46: An inhibitor of complement activation. Immunology 87:348–354, 1996.

273. Rougier N, Kazatchkine MD, Rougier JP, et al: Human complement factor H deficiency associated with hemolytic uremic syndrome. J Am Soc Nephrol 9:2318–2326, 1998.

274. Warwicker P, Donne RL, Goodship JA, et al: Familial relapsing haemolytic uraemic syndrome and complement factor H deficiency. Nephrol Dial Transplant 14:1229–1233, 1999.

275. Donne RL, Abbs I, Barany P, et al: Recurrence of hemolytic uremic syndrome after live related renal transplantation associated with subsequent de novo disease in the donor. Am J Kidney Dis 40:E22, 2002.

276. Loirat C, Niaudet P: The risk of recurrence of hemolytic uremic syndrome after renal transplantation in children. Pediatr Nephrol 18:1095–1101, 2003.

277. Ruggenenti P: Post-transplant hemolytic-uremic syndrome. Kidney Int 62:1093–1104, 2002.

278. Bonnardeaux A, Pichette V: Complement dysregulation in haemolytic uraemic syndrome. Lancet 362:1514–1515, 2003.

279. Cheong HI, Lee BS, Kang HG, et al: Attempted treatment of factor H deficiency by liver transplantation. Pediatr Nephrol 19:454–458, 2004.

280. Fremeaux-Bacchi V, Dragon-Durey MA, Blouin J, et al: Complement factor I: A susceptibility gene for atypical haemolytic uraemic syndrome. J Med Genet 41:e84, 2004.

281. Bell WR, Braine HG, Ness PM, et al: Improved survival in thrombotic thrombocytopenic purpura-hemolytic uremic syndrome. Clinical experience in 108 patients. N Engl J Med 325:398–403, 1991.

282. Rock GA, Shumak KH, Buskard NA, et al: Comparison of plasma exchange with plasma infusion in the treatment of thrombotic thrombocytopenic purpura. Canadian Apheresis Study Group. N Engl J Med 325:393–397, 1991.

283. Amorosi EL, Ultmann JE: Thrombotic thrombocytopenic purpura: Report of 16 cases and review of the literature. Medicine (Baltimore) 45:139–159, 1966.

284. Byrnes JJ, Moake JL: Thrombotic thrombocytopenic purpura and the haemolytic-uraemic syndrome: Evolving concepts of pathogenesis and therapy. Clin Haematol 15:413–442, 1986.

285. Medina PJ, Sipols JM, George JN: Drug-associated thrombotic thrombocytopenic purpura-hemolytic uremic syndrome. Curr Opin Hematol 8:286–293, 2001.

286. George JN: The association of pregnancy with thrombotic thrombocytopenic purpura-hemolytic uremic syndrome. Curr Opin Hematol 10:339–344, 2003.

287. Sutor GC, Schmidt RE, Albrecht H: Thrombotic microangiopathies and HIV infection: Report of two typical cases, features of HUS and TTP, and review of the literature. Infection 27:12–15, 1999.

288. Furlan M, Robles R, Solenthaler M, et al: Deficient activity of von Willebrand factor-cleaving protease in chronic relapsing thrombotic thrombocytopenic purpura. Blood 89:3097–3103, 1997.

289. Schulman I, Pierce M, Lukens A, et al: Studies on thrombopoiesis. I. A factor in normal human plasma required for platelet production; chronic thrombocytopenia due to its deficiency. Blood 16:943–957, 1960.

290. Upshaw JD Jr: Congenital deficiency of a factor in normal plasma that reverses microangiopathic hemolysis and thrombocytopenia. N Engl J Med 298:1350–1352, 1978.

291. Fujimura Y: Is Upshaw-Schulman syndrome congenital thrombotic thrombocytopenic purpura or hemolytic-uremic syndrome? Yes to both. J Thromb Haemost 1:2457–2458, 2003.

292. Fujimura Y, Matsumoto M, Yagi H, et al: Von Willebrand factor-cleaving protease and Upshaw-Schulman syndrome. Int J Hematol 75:25–34, 2002.

293. Veyradier A, Lavergne JM, Ribba AS, et al: Ten candidate ADAMTS13 mutations in six French families with congenital thrombotic thrombocytopenic purpura (Upshaw-Schulman syndrome). J Thromb Haemost 2:424–429, 2004.

294. Tsai HM: Advances in the pathogenesis, diagnosis, and treatment of thrombotic thrombocytopenic purpura. J Am Soc Nephrol 14:1072–1081, 2003.

295. Asada Y, Sumiyoshi A, Hayashi T, et al: Immunohistochemistry of vascular lesion in thrombotic thrombocytopenic purpura, with special reference to factor VIII related antigen. Thromb Res 38:469–479, 1985.

296. Moake JL, Byrnes JJ, Troll JH, et al: Effects of fresh-frozen plasma and its cryosupernatant fraction on von Willebrand factor multimeric forms in chronic relapsing thrombotic thrombocytopenic purpura. Blood 65:1232–1236, 1985.

297. Pimanda J, Hogg P: Control of von Willebrand factor multimer size and implications for disease. Blood Rev 16:185–192, 2002.

298. Stel HV, Sakariassen KS, de Groot PG, et al: Von Willebrand factor in the vessel wall mediates platelet adherence. Blood 65:85–90, 1985.

299. Wagner DD: Cell biology of von Willebrand factor. Annu Rev Cell Biol 6:217–246, 1990.

300. Christophe O, Obert B, Meyer D, et al: The binding domain of von Willebrand factor to sulfatides is distinct from those interacting with glycoprotein Ib, heparin, and collagen and resides between amino acid residues Leu 512 and Lys 673. Blood 78:2310–2317, 1991.

301. Fujimura Y, Titani K, Holland LZ, et al: A heparin-binding domain of human von Willebrand factor. Characterization and localization to a tryptic fragment extending from amino acid residue Val-449 to Lys-728. J Biol Chem 262:1734–1739, 1987.

302. de Groot PG, Ottenhof-Rovers M, van Mourik JA, et al: Evidence that the primary binding site of von Willebrand factor that mediates platelet adhesion on subendothelium is not collagen. J Clin Invest 82:65–73, 1988.

303. Savage B, Almus-Jacobs F, Ruggeri ZM: Specific synergy of multiple substrate-receptor interactions in platelet thrombus formation under flow. Cell 94:657–666, 1998.

304. Ruggeri ZM: Von Willebrand factor, platelets and endothelial cell interactions. J Thromb Haemost 1:1335–1342, 2003.

305. Ruggeri ZM: von Willebrand factor. J Clin Invest 99:559–564, 1997.

306. Savage B, Sixma JJ, Ruggeri ZM: Functional self-association of von Willebrand factor during platelet adhesion under flow. Proc Natl Acad Sci U S A 99:425–430, 2002.

307. Nogami K, Shima M, Nishiya K, et al: A novel mechanism of factor VIII protection by von Willebrand factor from activated protein C-catalyzed inactivation. Blood 99:3993–3998, 2002.

308. Bonthron D, Orr EC, Mitsock LM, et al: Nucleotide sequence of pre-pro-von Willebrand factor cDNA. Nucleic Acids Res 14:7125–7127, 1986.

387. He S, Cao H, Magnusson CG, et al: Are increased levels of von Willebrand factor in chronic coronary heart disease caused by decrease in von Willebrand factor cleaving protease activity? A study by an immunoassay with antibody against intact bond 842Tyr-843Met of the von Willebrand factor protein. Thromb Res 103:241–248, 2001.

388. Obert B, Tout H, Veyradier A, et al: Estimation of the von Willebrand factor-cleaving protease in plasma using monoclonal antibodies to vWF. Thromb Haemost 82:1382–1385, 1999.

389. Knovich MA, Craver K, Matulis MD, et al: Simplified assay for VWF cleaving protease (ADAMTS13) activity and inhibitor in plasma. Am J Hematol 76:286–290, 2004.

390. Shenkman B, Inbal A, Tamarin I, et al: Diagnosis of thrombotic thrombocytopenic purpura based on modulation by patient plasma of normal platelet adhesion under flow condition. Br J Haematol 120:597–604, 2003.

391. Whitelock JL, Nolasco L, Bernardo A, et al: ADAMTS-13 activity in plasma is rapidly measured by a new ELISA method that uses recombinant VWF-A2 domain as substrate. J Thromb Haemost 2:485–491, 2004.

392. Barz D, Budde U, Hellstern P: Therapeutic plasma exchange and plasma infusion in thrombotic microvascular syndromes. Thromb Res 107(Suppl 1):23–27, 2002.

393. McLeod BC, Sniecinski I, Ciavarella D, et al: Frequency of immediate adverse effects associated with therapeutic apheresis. Transfusion 39:282–288, 1999.

394. Rizvi MA, Vesely SK, George JN, et al: Complications of plasma exchange in 71 consecutive patients treated for clinically suspected thrombotic thrombocytopenic purpura-hemolytic-uremic syndrome. Transfusion 40:896–901, 2000.

395. Bandarenko N, Brecher ME: United States Thrombotic Thrombocytopenic Purpura Apheresis Study Group (US TTP ASG): Multicenter survey and retrospective analysis of current efficacy of therapeutic plasma exchange. J Clin Apheresis 13:133–141, 1998.

396. Rock G, Shumak KH, Sutton DM, et al: Cryosupernatant as replacement fluid for plasma exchange in thrombotic thrombocytopenic purpura. Members of the Canadian Apheresis Group. Br J Haematol 94:383–386, 1996.

397. Allford SL, Harrison P, Lawrie AS, et al: Von Willebrand factor-cleaving protease activity in congenital thrombotic thrombocytopenic purpura. Br J Haematol 111:1215–1222, 2000.

398. Barbot J, Costa E, Guerra M, et al: Ten years of prophylactic treatment with fresh-frozen plasma in a child with chronic relapsing thrombotic thrombocytopenic purpura as a result of a congenital deficiency of von Willebrand factor-cleaving protease. Br J Haematol 113:649–651, 2001.

399. Winslow GA, Nelson EW: Thrombotic thrombocytopenic purpura: indications for and results of splenectomy. Am J Surg 170:558–563, 1995.

400. Rock GA: Management of thrombotic thrombocytopenic purpura. Br J Haematol 109:496–507, 2000.

401. Chemnitz J, Draube A, Scheid C, et al: Successful treatment of severe thrombotic thrombocytopenic purpura with the monoclonal antibody rituximab. Am J Hematol 71:105–108, 2002.

402. Reddy PS, Deauna-Limayo D, Cook JD, et al: Rituximab in the treatment of relapsed thrombotic thrombocytopenic purpura. Ann Hematol 84:232–235, 2005.

403. Pisoni R, Ruggenenti P, Remuzzi G: Drug-induced thrombotic microangiopathy: Incidence, prevention and management. Drug Saf 24:491–501, 2001.

404. Karthikeyan V, Parasuraman R, Shah V, et al: Outcome of plasma exchange therapy in thrombotic microangiopathy after renal transplantation. Am J Transplant 3:1289–1294, 2003.

405. Reynolds JC, Agodoa LY, Yuan CM, et al: Thrombotic microangiopathy after renal transplantation in the United States. Am J Kidney Dis 42:1058–1068, 2003.

406. Woywodt A, Haubitz M, Buchholz S, et al: Counting the cost: Markers of endothelial damage in hematopoietic stem cell transplantation. Bone Marrow Transplant 34:1015–1023, 2004.

407. Daly AS, Xenocostas A, Lipton JH: Transplantation-associated thrombotic microangiopathy: Twenty-two years later. Bone Marrow Transplant 30:709–715, 2002.

408. Chang JC, Naqvi T: Thrombotic thrombocytopenic purpura associated with bone marrow metastasis and secondary myelofibrosis in cancer. Oncologist 8:375–380, 2003.

409. Murgo AJ: Thrombotic microangiopathy in the cancer patient including those induced by chemotherapeutic agents. Semin Hematol 24:161–177, 1987.

410. Gervasoni C, Ridolfo AL, Vaccarezza M, et al: Thrombotic microangiopathy in patients with acquired immunodeficiency syndrome before and during the era of introduction of highly active antiretroviral therapy. Clin Infect Dis 35:1534–1540, 2002.

411. Becker S, Fusco G, Fusco J, et al: HIV-associated thrombotic microangiopathy in the era of highly active antiretroviral therapy: An observational study. Clin Infect Dis 39(Suppl 5):267–275, 2004.

412. McCrae KR, Cines DB: Thrombotic microangiopathy during pregnancy. Semin Hematol 34:148–158, 1997.

413. Blot E, Decaudin D, Veyradier A, et al: Cancer-related thrombotic microangiopathy secondary to Von Willebrand factor-cleaving protease deficiency. Thromb Res 106:127–130, 2002.

414. Forman RB, Benkel SA, Novik Y, et al: Presence of ADAMTS13 activity in a patient with metastatic cancer and thrombotic microangiopathy. Acta Haematol 109:150–152, 2003.

415. Lattuada A, Rossi E, Calzarossa C, et al: Mild to moderate reduction of a von Willebrand factor cleaving protease (ADAMTS-13) in pregnant women with HELLP microangiopathic syndrome. Haematologica 88:1029–1034, 2003.

416. Orimo S, Ozawa E, Yagi H, et al: Simple plasma exchange reduced autoantibody to von Willebrand factor-cleaving protease in a Japanese man with ticlopidine-associated thrombotic thrombocytopenic purpura. J Intern Med 251:280–281, 2002.

417. Sahud MA, Claster S, Liu L, et al: von Willebrand factor-cleaving protease inhibitor in a patient with human immunodeficiency syndrome-associated thrombotic thrombocytopenic purpura. Br J Haematol 116:909–911, 2002.

The Molecular Basis of IgA Nephropathy

Stephen I-Hong Hsu and John Feehally

The initiating event in the pathogenesis of immunoglobulin A nephropathy (IgAN) is the mesangial deposition of IgA, which is predominantly polymeric IgA of the IgA1 subclass (pIgA1). With or without the additional deposition of IgG and C3 complement, this may be associated with glomerular inflammation and injury with the potential for that injury either to resolve or heal with sclerosis. Co-deposits of IgG and complement components are not mandatory for disease activity or progression, and their presence at diagnosis does not correlate with clinical outcome. Tubular atrophy and interstitial fibrosis may follow, leading to progressive renal failure (Fig. 27-1). While the deposition of IgA and the mechanisms by which IgA provokes glomerular inflammation are specific to IgAN, subsequent "downstream" inflammatory events and their consequences are generic, and appear to differ little from common mechanisms in progression of chronic renal disease.

A number of clinical observations in patients with IgAN are relevant to any description of its pathogenesis. These include:

- Mesangial IgA deposition may occur in apparently healthy individuals who have little or no clinical evidence of renal disease.
- The extent and intensity of the glomerular injury in response to mesangial IgA deposition are very variable. There may be low-grade glomerular inflammation that resolves completely; others develop slowly progressive renal insufficiency. A minority has a more fulminant necrotizing inflammation with crescent formation.
- Recurrent mesangial IgA deposition is very common after renal transplantation, increasing with duration of transplantation, occurring eventually in approximately 50% of all patients.[1] In addition, occasional unwitting "experiments" in which cadaveric kidneys with mesangial IgA deposits were transplanted into recipients with primary renal disease other than IgAN have usually resulted in resolution of the IgA deposits within weeks.[2,3] These findings strongly suggest that IgAN is a consequence of altered host susceptibility, including abnormalities of the IgA immune system, rather than an intrinsic kidney abnormality.
- Elevated serum IgA per se is not sufficient to cause IgAN. For example, in IgA myeloma there may be a large circulating load of pIgA1, but cast nephropathy rather than IgAN is the characteristic renal lesion. In human immunodeficiency virus (HIV) and acquired immunodeficiency syndrome (AIDS), even though there may be very high quantities of circulating polyclonal pIgA, IgAN is only one of a number of patterns of glomerular disease that are seen.[4]
- Some patients with IgAN also develop Henoch-Schönlein purpura (HSP), a systemic vasculitis in which skin, joint,

and gut involvement coincide with a renal lesion that may be indistinguishable from IgAN. The relationship between IgAN and HSP has been reviewed[5] and is not further discussed here.

OVERVIEW OF THE IMMUNOPATHOGENESIS OF IgA NEPHROPATHY

There are three elements that may contribute to the development of IgAN, and the extent to which each is operational decides the severity, tempo, and eventual outcome of IgAN in any individual. These elements are:

1. Synthesis and release into the circulation of pIgA1 with characteristics that favor mesangial deposition.
2. The "responsiveness" of the glomerular mesangium as judged by susceptibility to mesangial IgA deposition, the mesangial inflammatory response to IgA deposition, and the ability to follow this by resolution of inflammation rather than ongoing sclerosis.

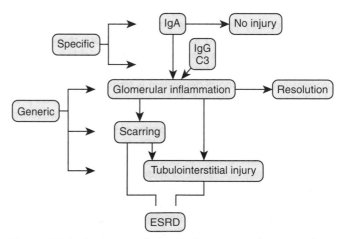

Figure 27-1 Overview of the pathogenesis of IgA nephropathy (IgAN). IgA deposition with or without associated IgG and complement leads to mesangial inflammation and injury, which may resolve or lead to progressive renal scarring and eventually end-stage renal disease (ESRD). While the deposition of IgA and the initiation of mesangial injury are specific to IgAN, subsequent "downstream" events are likely to be generic, differing little from those in other progressive renal disease. (Redrawn from Barratt J, Feehally J, Smith AC: Pathogenesis of IgA nephropathy. Semin Nephrol 24:197–217, 2004.)

Control of Human IgA Production

Systemic production of IgA appears to be under similar T-cell control mechanisms to IgG production: antigen exposure resulting in serum IgA antibody production showing broadly similar patterns of primary and secondary immune responses and affinity maturation as seen with IgG.[10] Type 2 T-cell cytokines (IL-4, -5, and -6) promote B-cell class switching to IgA, and subsequent proliferation and differentiation of IgA-producing cells.[11] IgA production is also specifically promoted by the cytokines IL-10 and TGF-β,[12] which have suppressive effects on IgG production. The control of mucosal IgA production is less well understood, although Th2 T cells are undoubtedly involved.[13,14] A variety of cell types probably contribute to the maintenance of a mucosal microenvironment strongly favoring pIgA production. The factors that influence co-expression of J chain by mucosal but not systemic IgA plasma cells are unknown, but may be of great relevance to our understanding of the immunopathogenesis of IgAN.[15]

The mucosal and systemic immune systems produce IgA with differing features and functions. The homing of subpopulations of activated T and B cells to the correct effector sites is mediated by highly specific receptor-ligand interactions; lymphocyte cell surface homing and chemokine receptors interact with location-specific vascular endothelial cell ligands.[16] Mucosally and systemically activated cells migrating through the circulation express distinct receptors and are recruited back to their priming tissue by recognition of the relevant vascular ligands in order to effect an immune response in the appropriate location. However, there appears to be a "mucosa–bone marrow axis," in which there is continual trafficking of antigen specific lymphocytes and antigen-presenting cells between mucosal sites and primary lymphoid tissues such as the tonsils, spleen, and bone marrow.[17–19] This is illustrated by the phenomenon of oral tolerance, by which systemic immune responses to mucosally encountered antigens—such as frequently encountered non-pathogenic antigens, including those derived from food or commensal bacteria—are actively suppressed.[20] Oral tolerance occurs in humans, but most of the evidence on its control comes from experimental animals. Oral tolerance is mediated by antigen-specific T cells that arise in the mucosa but migrate to the systemic compartment. T-cell subsets implicated in oral tolerance include Th2 cells, Tr (T-regulatory) cells, and Th3 cells, which produce the immunosuppressive cytokines IL-10 and TGF-β,[21] and γδ T cells.[22] γδ T cells are a minority T-cell population in most compartments of the immune system, but they have particular importance in mucosal immunity and play a pivotal role in mucosal IgA production.[23] The polymorphic V regions of the γ and δ T-cell receptor genes are grouped in families, and characteristic Vγ and δ families predominate in the γδ T cell populations found in different immune system compartments. Furthermore, γδ T-cell subsets expressing different V region families also differ in their homing receptor and cytokine expression,[24] suggesting that V region usage may define functional γδ T-cell subsets.

All cell types implicated in the control of oral tolerance are associated with promotion of IgA production. TGF-β is a key cytokine in the control of IgA production, not only promoting IgA production, and suppressing other isotype responses, but also inducing expression of the mucosal retention receptor αEβ7 by mucosal lymphocytes.[25] Functional analysis of these

T-cell subtypes has not yet made clear the extent of overlap between Th3 cells, Tr cells, and γδ T cells.

Clearance of Human IgA

IgA and IgA-immune complexes IgA-IC are cleared from the circulation at least partly via the liver. The hepatic asialoglycoprotein receptor (ASGPR) and the Fcα receptor CD89 are IgA-binding receptors expressed in the liver, although in the human their relative contributions to IgA catabolism have yet to be fully elucidated.[26–28] IgA is also catabolized by monocytes/macrophages and neutrophils via their expression of CD89; this is another potentially important route of clearance.[29]

ABNORMALITIES OF IgA AND ITS PRODUCTION IN IgA NEPHROPATHY

Numerous aspects of IgA and IgA production are abnormal in patients with IgAN (Table 27-1). Patients are heterogeneous with respect to many of these abnormalities, supporting the notion that more than one pathogenic mechanism may result in the production of pathogenic circulating IgA.

Deposited mesangial IgA must come from the blood. High plasma IgA alone is not sufficient to produce mesangial IgA deposits; therefore, patients with IgAN must produce a pool of circulating IgA molecules with special characteristics that particularly promote mesangial deposition. For these molecules to accumulate in the kidney, the rate of their deposition must exceed that of clearance.

Characteristics of Circulating IgA in IgA Nephropathy

Physicochemical Properties of Circulating IgA in IgA Nephropathy

Serum IgA levels are modestly increased in IgAN. The increase in serum IgA is accounted for by pIgA1, with mIgA and IgA2 levels generally being normal.[30] The serum IgA of patients is anionic,[31,32] λ light chains are over-represented,[33] and the IgA1 O-glycosylation profile is altered in comparison to controls (see Table 27-1).[34]

There is increasing evidence that abnormal O-glycosylation of IgA1 has a role in the pathogenesis of IgAN. Early studies evaluated binding of O-glycan-specific lectins to serum IgA1 from patients with IgAN.[35] Although lectins are convenient tools for indicating abnormal glycosylation patterns, they cannot provide precise structural information about O-glycan chains because their specificities are not absolute, and their binding may be affected by factors other than the individual O-glycan moieties present.[35] Nevertheless such studies have clearly and consistently demonstrated that serum IgA1 in IgAN is abnormally O-glycosylated, and strongly suggested that the abnormality takes the form of reduced galactosylation of the O-glycans, leading to increased frequency of truncated glycan chains consisting of GalNAc alone and possibly to increased exposure of the hinge region peptide itself.[36] More precise analysis of IgA1 O-glycosylation using carbohydrate electrophoresis,[37] chromatography,[36,38] and mass spectroscopy[39,40] all support a lack of O-linked galactosyl chains in IgA1 from patients with IgAN. Altered sialylation of the

Table 27-1 Properties of IgA in Normal Subjects and in IgA Nephropathy (IgAN): The Common Features of Serum and Mesangial IgA in IgAN

Properties of IgA	Controls		IgAN	
	Serum IgA	Mucosal IgA	Serum IgA	Mesangial IgA
Size	Mostly mIgA	Mostly pIgA	Increased pIgA	pIgA
Subclass	Mostly IgA1	IgA1 & IgA2	Increased IgA	IgA1
Proportion of l light chain compared with normal serum IgA	—	Not known	Increased	Increased
Charge compared with normal serum IgA	—	Not known	Anionic	Anionic
O-glycosylation	Heavily galactosylated and sialylated	Unknown galactosylation Decreased sialylation	Reduced galactosylation Increased or decreased sialylation	Reduced galactosylated and sialylation

Reproduced from Barratt J, Feehally J: IgA nephropathy. J Am Soc Nephrol 16:2088–2097, 2005.

O-glycans in IgA1 is more debatable as the specificity of sialic acid-binding lectins is unsatisfactory. Both increased[41] and decreased[40] O-sialylation have been suggested. Further confirmation will required improved analytical techniques.

There is no evidence that IgAN results from a clonal abnormality of IgA-producing plasma cells. The changes in IgA1 O-glycosylation do not result in a tightly restricted pattern with IgA1 molecules all showing a specific abnormality; rather, there is a shift that slightly favors the appearance of IgA1 molecules with glycoforms less likely to contain galactose (and perhaps sialic acid).

Any functional effects of altered IgA1 hinge region O-glycosylation are as yet unproven, but may be expected given the pivotal position of the hinge region in the IgA1 molecule. The hinge region is a short sequence consisting of only 18 amino acids, but it typically carries 10 to 12 O-glycan chains, which contribute about half of the molecular weight of the region, depending on the completeness of O-glycosylation. As the glycans extend from the peptide core, they shield it from external exposure and will influence the physical shape and electrical charge of the IgA1 molecule, thus potentially affecting interactions with proteins and receptors.[42,43] They may also determine the antigenicity of IgA1, as discussed below. IgA1 glycosylation also appears to influence matrix interactions; molecules lacking terminal sialic acid and galactose units have been shown in vitro to exhibit increased affinity for the extracellular matrix components fibronectin and type IV collagen.[44] There have been some reports that serum IgA1 glycosylation pattern is associated with variations in the extent and pattern of histopathologic glomerular injury.[45]

Antigen Specificity of IgA in IgA Nephropathy

In IgAN there is no convincing evidence of circulating IgA autoantibodies against a mesangial antigen,[46] but there are reports of increased levels of circulating IgA-IC. This may arise from increased antigen load and persistent IgA antibody production, or from failure of IgA-IC clearance from the circulation. Increases in circulating IgA antibodies against a variety of antigens have been described, although no single pathogenic antigen has been established. As is the case for total serum IgA, the increase in IgA antibody titers seems to be restricted to IgA1,[47,48] and pIgA may be over-represented.[49] Since the majority of pIgA is mucosal in origin, particular attention has been focused on mucosally encountered antigens as potential triggers for the development of IgAN, and there is convincing evidence for an increase in circulating pIgA1 antibodies against a variety of mucosal antigens, both microbial and environmental. However, the same can also be seen for systemically encountered antigens,[47,48,50] suggesting that there is a general tendency to overproduce pIgA1 antibodies in IgAN.

Large immune complexes that persist in the circulation are most susceptible to mesangial trapping. IgA-IC composed of pIgA will be likely to meet these criteria: they will be large by virtue of the polymeric nature of the IgA, and the low efficiency of IgA complement fixation may favor both large size and persistence in the circulation, as complement interrupts IC lattice formation and is involved in immune complex internalization by phagocytes. Furthermore, in a study of antibody responses to systemic immunization with tetanus toxoid in IgAN, the pIgA1 antibody response was not only increased and prolonged,[49] but the IgA was also of low affinity, although IgG affinity was normal.[10] This suggests that some IgA antibodies may be functionally abnormal in IgAN, leading to failure of antigen clearance and consequent persistence of IgA production and circulating IgA-IC. Another intriguing explanation for the presence of circulating IgA-IC in IgAN is provided by the demonstration in patients' serum of IgG and IgA antibodies against agalactosyl IgA1 O-glycans and the "naked" IgA1 hinge region peptide.[51,52] This raises the possibility that in some IgA-IC, abnormally O-glycosylated IgA1 is actually the antigen rather than the antibody, and therefore continued production of abnormally O-glycosylated IgA1 will ensure the persistence of circulating IgA-IC.

It remains unclear which physicochemical characteristics of pathogenic IgA dictate mesangial deposition, and may therefore be found in individuals with mesangial IgA but no GN, and which features are responsible for the initiation of a pro-inflammatory glomerular response in susceptible individuals. In animal models of GN, macromolecular Ig-containing complexes are particularly prone to mesangial deposition, and therefore it seems likely that the increased levels of serum IgA macromolecules in IgAN will promote mesangial deposition through nonspecific, size-dependent mesangial trapping. The exaggerated O-glycosylation defect detected in mesangial IgA1 may promote this phenomenon: it has been shown that aberrantly glycosylated IgA1 molecules have an increased tendency both to self-aggregate[44] and form antigen-antibody complexes with IgG antibodies directed against IgA1 hinge epitopes.[52] Furthermore, altered IgA1 O-glycosylation is a feature also seen in other conditions associated with glomerular IgA deposition.[39,95] There is also evidence from transgenic mice that soluble CD89-IgA complexes generated after binding of IgA to membrane bound CD89 are associated with massive mesangial IgA deposition.[96] It is possible that circulating FcαRI-IgA complexes may form part of the circulating pool of macromolecular "pathogenic" IgA in human IgAN, although more recent data suggest that CD89-IgA complexes may not be specific to IgAN.[97]

In addition to nonspecific, size-dependent mesangial trapping, there is also evidence that IgA deposition may be influenced by interactions between IgA and specific mesangial matrix components. Studies in renal biopsy material show rebinding of IgA eluates to autologous glomeruli and to some other IgAN samples but not to normal glomeruli, suggesting that specific IgA-matrix interactions may be present.[98] IgA1 glycosylation again appears to influence matrix interactions; molecules lacking terminal sialic acid and galactose units in vitro have increased affinity for the extracellular matrix components fibronectin and type IV collagen.[44] The anionic pI of mesangial IgA may also promote interactions with such mesangial proteins.

Although immunoglobulins using λ light chains do seem to predominate in glomerular deposits in various renal diseases,[94,99] it is unlikely that λ light chain usage per se is the driving force behind deposition in IgAN, since significant amounts of IgA1λ are found in the circulation of all individuals.

Mesangial Cell IgA Receptors and IgA Clearance

For there to be mesangial IgA accumulation, the rate of mesangial IgA deposition must exceed that of mesangial clearance. The principal candidate pathway for IgA clearance is through mesangial cell (MC) receptor-mediated endocytosis and catabolism of IgA deposits. Unfortunately, the published data on the expression of IgA receptors by MC are inconsistent (Table 27-2). Although preliminary evidence has been reported that MCs express known IgA receptors, including CD89 (FcαRI), polymeric Ig receptor, and hepatic ASGPR,[100,101] none of these reports have been definitely confirmed. It has been reported that human MCs express the transferrin receptor (CD71), which can act as an IgA receptor, and that this may be overexpressed in the mesangium in IgAN.[102,103] There is some in vitro evidence that CD71 may

also enhance MC proliferation through a positive feedback loop with pIgA1.[104] Understanding of the range and significance of MC IgA receptor(s) is still incomplete; for example, there is also preliminary evidence that human MCs may in addition express a novel FcαR.[105]

Independent of the receptor involved, there is in vitro evidence that MCs are capable of receptor-mediated endocytosis and catabolism of IgA, supporting the role of the MC as a major contributor to mesangial IgA clearance.[102,106] It is not yet known whether there are abnormalities of MC IgA binding in IgAN; however, it is possible that impaired binding could lead to defective mesangial IgA clearance and thereby contribute to IgA accumulation and the development of GN.

Mechanisms of Initiation and Progression of Glomerular Inflammation in IgA Nephropathy

Although IgG and complement components are often co-deposited, IgA alone appears sufficient to provoke glomerular injury in the susceptible individual. In animal models it has been shown that passive transfer of either "pathogenic" IgA or T–cell-depleted allogeneic bone marrow cells from IgAN-prone mice can trigger the development of IgAN in previously normal animals.[107,108] Furthermore, bone marrow transplanted from normal donors lowers total serum IgA, including the macromolecular IgA fraction, while simultaneously attenuating the glomerular lesions seen in these IgAN-prone mice.[109] Separately it has been shown that deposition of pIgA, but not mIgA, initiates GN, suggesting that those IgA macromolecules prone to mesangial trapping are also capable of initiating inflammation.[110] The development of GN following IgA deposition is believed to result from both IgA-induced activation of MC and local complement activation.

Mesangial Cell Activation

There is strong in vitro evidence that cross-linking of MC IgA receptors with macromolecular IgA elicits pro-inflammatory and pro-fibrotic transformation in MC. Consistent with the mesangial hypercellularity seen in renal biopsy specimens, MCs proliferate in response to IgA.[111,112] Furthermore, exposure to IgA upregulates secretion of both extracellular matrix components and the pro-fibrotic growth factor TGF-β.[113] IgA is also capable of altering MC-matrix interactions by modulating integrin expression, and this may have an important role in remodeling of the mesangium following glomerular injury.[114] Exposure of MC to IgA is also capable of initiating a pro-inflammatory cascade involving MC secretion of platelet activating factor (PAF), IL-1β, IL-6, tumor necrosis factor-α (TNF-α), and migration inhibitory factor (MIF); the release of the chemokines monocyte chemotactic protein-1 (MCP-1), IL-8, IL-10; and development of an amplifying pro-inflammatory loop involving IL-6- and TNF-α-induced upregulation of MC IgA receptors.[115] There is also evidence that activation of MCs by co-deposited IgG may synergistically contribute to the development of a pro-inflammatory MC phenotype and thereby influence the degree of glomerular injury.[116]

pIgA1 from patients with IgAN enhances mesangial activation compared with the response to normal human pIgA1.[117,118] It is not yet certain which specific physicochemical properties of mesangial IgA affect MC activation; however, there is some

Table 27-2 Review of Evidence on Identification of the Mesangial Cell (MC) IgA Receptor(s)

Receptor	Demonstration of Receptor mRNA Using Human MC or Renal Biopsies	Demonstration of Receptor Protein Using Human MC or Renal Biopsies	Functional Effects of MC Receptor Cross-linking
pIgR	No	No	N/A
Hepatic ASGPR	No	No	N/A
FcαRI (CD89)	Yes	No	N/A
Transferrin receptor (CD71)	Yes	Yes	Not known
Novel FcαR	N/A	Yes	MC proliferation Cytokine & ECM synthesis Activation of 2nd messenger pathways and upregulation of transcription factors*
Fcα/μR	Yes	No	No
Novel ASGPR	N/A	Yes	Catabolism of desIgA

Only studies using human MC or human renal biopsy data have been included (reviewed by Monteiro[109]).
*These functional effects of receptor cross-linking have been observed with whole IgA molecules and most have been shown to be Fcα dependent. This does not therefore exclude the possibility that the observed effects could have been due to cross-linking of CD71 or Fcα/μR.
pIgR, polymeric immunoglobulin receptor; ASGPR, asioaloglycoprotein receptor; FcαR, receptor binding the Fc region of IgA; Fcα/μR, receptor binding both IgA and IgM; ECM, extracellular matrix components; desIgA, desialylated IgA.
Reproduced from Barrat J, Feehally J, Smith AC: Pathogenesis of IgA nephropathy. Semin Nephrol 24:197–217, 2004.

in vitro evidence that undergalactosylated IgA glycoforms from patients with IgAN reduce proliferation, increase nitric oxide synthesis and the rate of apoptosis, and enhance integrin synthesis in cultured MCs.[117,119,120] IgA1-immune complexes that contain galactose-deficient IgA1 enhance MC proliferation in vitro.[121]

Complement

Although involvement of the complement cascade is not essential for the development of IgAN, there is evidence that local complement activation can influence the extent of glomerular injury. In rats, dIgA and pIgA, but not mIgA, can activate complement to induce glomerular damage.[113] Mesangial IgA activation of C3 probably occurs through the mannan-binding lectin (MBL) pathway, leading to the generation of C5b-9, sublytic concentrations of which can activate MCs to produce inflammatory mediators as well as matrix proteins.[122,123] C3 and MBL are not only deposited in the kidney in IgA,[56,112,124] but can also be synthesized locally by MCs, and in the case of C3, by podocytes as well.[125] It is likely, therefore, that once MCs have bound IgA, they are capable of activating complement, independent of any systemic complement activity, by utilizing endogenously generated C3 and MBL.[115,125] MCs also synthesize complement regulatory proteins,[126] which may explain why C5b-9 generation in IgAN does not usually result in mesangiolysis. By contrast, the downregulation of CR1 by podocytes in IgAN may render podocytes highly sensitive to complement attack.[127]

Cellular Effector Mechanisms

IgAN is not generally associated with a marked glomerular cellular infiltrate, suggesting that most of the glomerular injury is mediated by an expansion in resident glomerular cells. However, as glomerular lesions become more severe, the number of mononuclear cells increases both in the mesangium and Bowman's space.[128,129] In crescentic IgAN, not only macrophages but also activated T cells can be detected in glomeruli.[130]

Progression or Resolution of Mesangial Injury

While mesangial IgA deposition and the initiation by IgA of glomerular inflammation are specific to IgAN, mechanisms of the subsequent mesangial injury followed either by resolution or progressive sclerosis are likely to be generic, not differing substantially from those seen in other forms of chronic mesangial proliferative GN unrelated to IgA. These processes have been extensively studied in vitro and in animal models of mesangial proliferative GN (particularly the anti-Thy1.1 model). MCs have a tremendous capacity to reconstitute normal mesangial morphology even after pronounced mesangial proliferative injury. This occurs through MC apoptosis and the production of anti-mitogenic factors, the removal of excess matrix through the action of mesangial proteases and antifibrotic factors, and the production of factors that will counteract various pro-inflammatory products.[131]

ANIMAL MODELS OF IgA NEPHROPATHY

Several animal models that mimic the disease phenotype of human IgA nephropathy to varying degrees have been extensively characterized.[132] These include the outbred ddY mouse model of spontaneous IgAN associated with relatively high serum IgA levels with wide individual variation but in the

problem").[132,145,152] This has raised the question of validity and the need to reappraise the methodologic framework that has been the foundation of hundreds of such studies in IgAN genetics research that were conducted in the 1990s and that continue to the present day.

Repeated Nonreplication of Results—The Case of the *ACE* I/D Polymorphism

A widely studied example of the dilemma of repeated non-replication of results is represented by genetic case-control association studies of the angiotensin I–converting enzyme (*ACE*) gene insertion/deletion (I/D) polymorphism in the development and/or progression of IgA nephropathy, as well as a whole host of common human diseases and conditions, including cardiovascular disease; complications of diabetes such as retinopathy and nephropathy; glomerular, tubulo-interstitial, and renal cystic renal diseases; and even renal allograft survival.[132,152,168] The interest in studying the *ACE* I/D polymorphism is based on evidence for "biologic plausibility." Rigat and colleagues reported in 1990 that the *ACE* I/D polymorphism in intron 16 of the human *ACE* gene accounts for half of the variation in serum ACE levels in a white study cohort.[169] This is due to the presence of a transcriptional repressor element in the I allele.[170]

There have been numerous population-based studies that either support or refute an association between the D allele and progression of renal disease in these conditions.[132,152] Recent meta-analyses have concluded that the D allele is not associated with renal disease progression in patients with IgA nephropathy or diabetic nephropathy[168,171] Despite more than a dozen generally small genetic case-control studies of the *ACE* I/D polymorphism in both white and Asian IgAN cohorts, no conclusions can be confidently drawn from these studies regarding the association between the D allele or DD genotype and development and/or progression of IgAN. Population-based genetic association studies of other genes encoding proteins in the renin-angiotensin-aldosterone system (RAAS) such as angiotensinogen (AGT) and the angiotensin II type 1 receptor (ATR1), as well as renin (*REN*) and aldosterone synthase (CYP11β2), have also generated conflicting results, as have similar studies of the "expanded" RAAS that includes 11β-hydroxysteroid dehydrogenase type 2 (11βHSD2) and the mineralocorticoid receptor (MLR).[172] In general, the approach has been to genotype by polymerase chain reaction/restriction fragment length polymorphism (PCR-RFLP) a single common polymorphism in each gene. It is remarkable that to date, the role of the RAAS, whose components ACE and ATR1 are the targets of the important ACE inhibitor and ARB classes of drugs, respectively, has not been convincingly demonstrated by any genetic association study.

The Haplotype Block Structure of the Human Genome and Implications for Conducting Genetic Association Studies

In the post-genomic era, there has been a renewed interest in conducting genetic association studies, especially SNP-based, whole-genome association studies, to identify genetic variations associated with the development and/or progression of a number of common human diseases. This renewed interest reflects the important finding that linkage disequilibrium (LD), the phenomenon that particular alleles at nearby sites can co-occur on the same haplotype more often than expected by chance,[173,174] is highly structured into discrete blocks separated by hotspots for recombination.

The haplotype block model for LD has important implications for the way in which genetic association studies should now be conducted, and may explain at least in part the problem of repeated nonreplication of results that has plagued such studies in the past. Why might genotyping solely for the *ACE* I/D polymorphism in IgAN result in repeated nonreplication of results? Based on the haplotype block model of LD, the *ACE* I/D polymorphism is but a single marker variant in the *ACE* gene. Researchers have assumed that the D allele defines a single population of subjects at risk for disease. This assumption may prove incorrect since within the common SNP haplotype block that contains the *ACE* I/D polymorphism, more than one haplotype pattern may share the D allele, only one of which is associated with risk for disease. The lumping of such subgroups defined by haplotypes that share the D allele may explain at least in part the basis for discrepant reports of genetic association with disease.

Criteria for a Valid Genetic Case-Control Study

The *Journal of the American Society of Nephrology* has recently defined a set of minimum criteria for association studies using polymorphic genetic markers, in which it is acknowledged that the common SNP haplotype block model should ideally be taken into account in order for a manuscript to be considered seriously for peer review.[175] Based on these guidelines, only genetic association studies that employ one or more methodologically valid approaches and satisfy the minimum rigorous conditions for a reliable genetic association study (e.g., biologic plausibility, haplotype relative risk analysis to identify statistically significant "at-risk haplotype[s]" associated with small *P* values, use of family-based methodologies, such as the transmission equilibrium test [TDT/sib-TDT] or the family-based association test [FBAT] to directly study trios/sib-trios and extended families or to verify the absence of significant population stratification bias [admixture] inherent in population-based case-control association studies, and the study of moderately large [i.e., adequately powered] cohorts) will be reviewed in the following section. Since the existence of admixture has not been ruled out in any published population-based association study of IgAN, only family-based studies will be reviewed.

Post–Genomic Era Family-Based Association Studies to Identify "At-Risk Haplotypes" in Candidate Genes

Only five studies examining three candidate genes have employed the family-based TDT study methodology and/or analysis of "at-risk" haplotypes, the majority published in 2006, reflecting the emergence of the first studies to attempt to satisfy minimum criteria for a valid association study. Three SNP polymorphisms in two contiguous genes at the *selectin* gene cluster at chromosome 1q24-25 (712C>T[P238S] in the coding region and -642A>G in the promoter region of the *L-selectin* gene; 1402C>T[H468Y] in the coding region of the *E-selectin gene*) were previously reported to be in tight LD and to occur in two haplotypes (IgAN-associated TGT and wild-type [Wt] CAC).[176] The researchers have recently shown that overexpression of an adenoviral construct expressing the disease-associated P238S substitution of the *L-selectin* gene is associated with significantly less rolling adhesion of stably transfected Chinese hamster ovary (CHO) cells perfused over IL-1β-activated human umbilical vein endothelial cells, as compared with Wt and control adenovirus expressing CHO cells.[177] The disease-associated -642A>G promoter variant was also shown to be associated with significantly less transcriptional activity. In contrast, the H468Y substitution in the *E-selectin* gene did not exhibit a functional difference in rolling adhesion. These findings suggest that in Japanese subjects, the disease-associated TGT haplotype in the *selectin* gene cluster can influence the quality and quantity of *L-selectin* gene products, and may play a potential role in inflammatory processes such as leukocyte-endothelial interactions that may be important in the pathogenesis of IgAN. Notably, the *L-selectin* gene has been previously suggested as a candidate susceptibility gene based on the previously reported genome-wide scan of the ddY mouse model[164] and because of its well-known function as a T-cell homing receptor.

A family- and haplotype-based association study employing the TDT methodology has shown that 2093C and 2180T SNP variants in the 3′-untranslated region of the *Megsin* gene were significantly more frequently transmitted from heterozygous parents to patients than expected in the extended TDT analysis (increased co-transmission in 232 Chinese families, $P < 0.001$), while haplotype relative risk (HRR) analyses showed that these same SNP alleles were more often transmitted to patients (HRR = 1.568, $P < 0.014$ for the 2093C allele; HRR = 2.114, $P < 0.001$ for the 2180T allele).[178] The same group using a similar approach recently reported that the *Megsin* 23167G SNP variant is associated with both susceptibility and progression of IgAN in 435 Chinese patients and their family members using TDT and HRR analysis.[179] The GG genotype was found to be associated with severe histologic lesions and disease progression. Megsin is a member of the serpin (serine proteinase inhibitor) superfamily that is upregulated in the context of mesangial proliferation and extracellular matrix expansion in IgAN, and therefore represents a strong candidate gene for susceptibility to IgAN.

A haplotype of the interferon-γ (*IFNγ*) gene consisting of the 12-CA repeat allele in tight LD with the +874A SNP variant has recently demonstrated an association with susceptibility to IgAN without influencing survival in an FBAT analysis of 53 Italian patients, 45 complete trios, 4 incomplete trios, and 36 discordant siblings from the collection of the European IgAN Consortium.[180] The +874T/A SNP lies within a putative nuclear factor-κB (NF-κB) transcription factor binding site. Notably, the +874A variant is associated with transcriptional downregulation of *INFγ* gene promoter activity, consistent with the known role of NF-κB in the transcriptional regulation of the *INFγ* gene.

References

1. Floege J, Burg M, Kliem V: Recurrent IgA nephropathy after renal transplantation. Semin Nephrol 24:287–291, 2004.
2. Cuevas X, Lloveras J, Mir M, et al: Disappearance of mesangial IgA deposits from the kidneys of two donors after transplantation. Transplant Proc 19:2208–2209, 1987.
3. Sanfilippo F, Croker BP, Bollinger RR: Fate of four cadaveric donor renal allografts with mesangial IgA deposits. Transplantation 33:370–376, 1982.
4. Viertel A, Weidmann E, Rickerts V, et al: Renal involvement in HIV-infection. Results from the Frankfurt AIDS Cohort Study (FACS) and a review of the literature. Eur J Med Res 5:185–198, 2000.
5. Davin JC, Ten Berge IJ, Weening JJ: What is the difference between IgA nephropathy and Henoch-Schonlein purpura nephritis? Kidney Int 59:823–834, 2001.
6. Kerr MA: The structure and function of human IgA. Biochem J 271:285–296, 1990.
7. Johansen FE, Braathen R, Brandtzaeg P: Role of J chain in secretory immunoglobulin formation. Scand J Immunol 52:240–248, 2000.
8. Russell MW, Kilian M, Lamm ME: Biological activities of IgA. In Mestecky J, Bienenstock J, McGhee J, et al. (eds): Mucosal Immunology, 2nd ed. San Diego, CA, Academic Press, 1999, pp 225–240.
9. Mestecky J, Russell MW, Elson CO: Intestinal IgA: Novel views on its function in the defence of the largest mucosal surface. Gut 44:2–5, 1999.
10. Layward L, Allen AC, Hattersley JM, et al: Low antibody affinity restricted to the IgA isotype in IgA nephropathy. Clin Exp Immunol 95:35–41, 1994.
11. Lycke N: T cell and cytokine regulation of the IgA response. Chem Immunol 71:209–234, 1998.
12. Defrance T, Vanbervliet B, Briere F, et al: Interleukin 10 and transforming growth factor beta cooperate to induce anti-CD40-activated naive human B cells to secrete immunoglobulin A. J Exp Med 175:671–682, 1992.
13. Fujihashi K, Kweon MN, Kiyono H, et al: A T cell/B cell/epithelial cell internet for mucosal inflammation and immunity. Springer Semin Immunopathol 18:477–494, 1997.
14. Abreu-Martin MT, Targan SR: Regulation of immune responses of the intestinal mucosa. Crit Rev Immunol 16:277–309, 1996.
15. Brandtzaeg P, Farstad IN, Johansen FE, et al: The B-cell system of human mucosae and exocrine glands. Immunol Rev 171:45–87, 1999.
16. Wiedle G, Dunon D, Imhof BA: Current concepts in lymphocyte homing and recirculation. Crit Rev Clin Lab Sci 38:1–31, 2001.
17. Pabst R, Binns RM: In vivo labelling of the spleen and mesenteric lymph nodes with fluorescein isothiocyanate for lymphocyte migration studies. Immunology 44:321–329, 1981.
18. Pabst R, Reynolds JD: Peyer's patches export lymphocytes throughout the lymphoid system in sheep. J Immunol 139:3981–3985, 1987.
19. Alley CD, Kiyono H, McGhee JR: Murine bone marrow IgA responses to orally administered sheep erythrocytes. J Immunol 136:4414–4419, 1986.
20. Simecka JW: Mucosal immunity of the gastrointestinal tract and oral tolerance. Adv Drug Deliv Rev 34:235–259, 1998.
21. Roncarolo MG, Bacchetta R, Bordignon C, et al: Type 1 T regulatory cells. Immunol Rev 182:68–79, 2001.
22. Ke Y, Pearce K, Lake JP, et al: Gamma delta T lymphocytes regulate the induction and maintenance of oral tolerance. J Immunol 158:3610–3618, 1997.
23. Fujihashi K, McGhee JR, Kweon MN, et al: Gamma/delta T cell-deficient mice have impaired mucosal immunoglobulin A responses. J Exp Med 183:1929–1935, 1996.
24. Chao CC, Sandor M, Dailey MO: Expression and regulation of adhesion molecules by gamma delta T cells from lymphoid tissues and intestinal epithelium. Eur J Immunol 24:3180–3187, 1994.
25. Lim SP, Leung E, Krissansen GW: The beta7 integrin gene (Itgb-7) promoter is responsive to TGF-beta1: Defining control regions. Immunogenetics 48:184–195, 1998.

26. van Egmond M, van Garderen E, van Spriel AB, et al: FcalphaRI-positive liver Kupffer cells: Reappraisal of the function of immunoglobulin A in immunity. Nat Med 6:680–685, 2000.

27. Rifai A, Schena FP, Montinaro V, et al: Clearance kinetics and fate of macromolecular IgA in patients with IgA nephropathy. Lab Invest 61:381–388, 1989.

28. Rifai A, Fadden K, Morrison SL, et al: The N-glycans determine the differential blood clearance and hepatic uptake of human immunoglobulin (Ig)A1 and IgA2 isotypes. J Exp Med 191:2171–2182, 2000.

29. Grossetete B, Launay P, Lehuen A, et al: Down-regulation of Fc alpha receptors on blood cells of IgA nephropathy patients: Evidence for a negative regulatory role of serum IgA. Kidney Int 53:1321–1335, 1998.

30. Feehally J: Immune mechanisms in glomerular IgA deposition. Nephrol Dial Transplant 3:361–378, 1988.

31. Harada T, Hobby P, Courteau M, et al: Charge distribution of plasma IgA in IgA nephropathy. Clin Exp Immunol 77:211–214, 1989.

32. Monteiro RC, Chevailler A, Noel LH, et al: Serum IgA preferentially binds to cationic polypeptides in IgA nephropathy. Clin Exp Immunol 73:300–306, 1988.

33. Lam CW, Chui SH, Leung NW, et al: Light chain ratios of serum immunoglobulins in disease. Clin Biochem 24:283–287, 1991.

34. Allen A, Feehally J: IgA glycosylation in IgA nephropathy. Adv Exp Med Biol 435:175–183, 1998.

35. Allen AC: Methodological approaches to the analysis of IgA1 O-glycosylation in IgA nephropathy. J Nephrol 12:76–84, 1999.

36. Mestecky J, Tomana M, Crowley-Nowick PA, et al: Defective galactosylation and clearance of IgA1 molecules as a possible etiopathogenic factor in IgA nephropathy. Contrib Nephrol 104:172–182, 1993.

37. Allen AC, Bailey EM, Barratt J, et al: Analysis of IgA1 O-glycans in IgA nephropathy by fluorophore-assisted carbohydrate electrophoresis. J Am Soc Nephrol 10:1763–1771, 1999.

38. Hiki Y, Iwase H, Kokubo T, et al: Association of asialo-galactosyl beta 1-3N-acetylgalactosamine on the hinge with a conformational instability of Jacalin-reactive immunoglobulin A1 in immunoglobulin A nephropathy. J Am Soc Nephrol 7:955–960, 1996.

39. Hiki Y, Tanaka A, Kokubo T, et al: Analyses of IgA1 hinge glycopeptides in IgA nephropathy by matrix-assisted laser desorption/ionization time-of-flight mass spectrometry. J Am Soc Nephrol 9:577–582, 1998.

40. Hiki Y, Odani H, Takahashi M, et al: Mass spectrometry proves under-O-glycosylation of glomerular IgA1 in IgA nephropathy. Kidney Int 59:1077–1085, 2001.

41. Leung JC, Tang SC, Chan DT, et al: Increased sialylation of polymeric lambda-IgA1 in patients with IgA nephropathy. J Clin Lab Anal 16:11–19, 2002.

42. Boehm MK, Woof JM, Kerr MA, et al: The Fab and Fc fragments of IgA1 exhibit a different arrangement from that in IgG: A study by X-ray and neutron solution scattering and homology modelling. J Mol Biol 286:1421–1447, 1999.

43. Moura IC, Arcos-Fajardo M, Leroy V, et al: Glycosylation and size of IgA1 are essential for interaction with mesangial transferring receptor in IgA nephropathy. J Am Soc Nephrol 15:622–634, 2004.

44. Kokubo T, Hiki Y, Iwase H, et al: Protective role of IgA1 glycans against IgA1 self-aggregation and adhesion to extracellular matrix proteins. J Am Soc Nephrol 9:2048–2054, 1998.

45. Xu LH, Zhao MH: Aberrantly glycosylated serum IgA1 are closely associated with pathologic phenotypes of IgA nephropathy. Kidney Int 68:167–172, 2005.

46. O'Donoghue DJ, Feehally J: Autoantibodies in IgA nephropathy. Contrib Nephrol 111:93–103, 1995.

47. Layward L, Allen AC, Hattersley JM, et al: Elevation of IgA in IgA nephropathy is localized in the serum and not saliva and is restricted to the IgA1 subclass. Nephrol Dial Transplant 8:25–28, 1993.

48. van den Wall Bake AW, Beyer WE, Evers-Schouten JH, et al: Humoral immune response to influenza vaccination in patients with primary immunoglobulin A nephropathy. An analysis of isotype distribution and size of the influenza-specific antibodies. J Clin Invest 84:1070–1075, 1989.

49. Layward L, Allen AC, Harper SJ, et al: Increased and prolonged production of specific polymeric IgA after systemic immunization with tetanus toxoid in IgA nephropathy. Clin Exp Immunol 88:394–398, 1992.

50. Fortune F, Courteau M, Williams DG, et al: T and B cell responses following immunization with tetanus toxoid in IgA nephropathy. Clin Exp Immunol 88:62–67, 1992.

51. Kokubo T, Hashizume K, Iwase H, et al: Humoral immunity against the proline-rich peptide epitope of the IgA1 hinge region in IgA nephropathy. Nephrol Dial Transplant 15:28–33, 2000.

52. Tomana M, Novak J, Julian BA, et al: Circulating immune complexes in IgA nephropathy consist of IgA1 with galactose-deficient hinge region and antiglycan antibodies. J Clin Invest 104:73–81, 1999.

53. Roccatello D, Picciotto G, Coppo R, et al: The fate of aggregated immunoglobulin A injected in IgA nephropathy patients and healthy controls. Am J Kidney Dis 18:20–25, 1991.

54. Leung JC, Tsang AW, Chan LY, et al: Size-dependent binding of IgA to HepG2, U937, and human mesangial cells. J Lab Clin Med 140:398–406, 2002.

55. van Zandbergen G, van Kooten C, Mohamad NK, et al: Reduced binding of immunoglobulin A (IgA) from patients with primary IgA nephropathy to the myeloid IgA Fc-receptor, CD89. Nephrol Dial Transplant 13:3058–3064, 1998.

56. Hisano S, Matsushita M, Fujita T, et al: Mesangial IgA2 deposits and lectin pathway-mediated complement activation in IgA glomerulonephritis. Am J Kidney Dis 38:1082–1088, 2001.

57. Oortwijn BD, van der Boorg PJ, Roos A, et al: A pathogenic role for secretory IgA in IgA nephropathy. Kidney Int. 69:1131–1138, 2006.

58. Feehally J, Allen AC: Pathogenesis of IgA nephropathy. Ann Med Interne (Paris) 150:91–98, 1999.

59. Allen AC, Bailey EM, Brenchley PE, et al: Mesangial IgA1 in IgA nephropathy exhibits aberrant O-glycosylation: Observations in three patients. Kidney Int 60:969–973, 2001.

60. Leinikki PO, Mustonen J, Pasternack A: Immune response to oral polio vaccine in patients with IgA glomerulonephritis. Clin Exp Immunol 68:33–38, 1987.

61. Barratt J, Bailey EM, Buck KS, et al: Exaggerated systemic antibody response to mucosal Helicobacter pylori infection in IgA nephropathy. Am J Kidney Dis 33:1049–1057, 1999.

62. Ots M, Uibo O, Metskula K, et al: IgA-antigliadin antibodies in patients with IgA nephropathy: The secondary phenomenon? Am J Nephrol 19:453–458, 1999.

63. Westberg NG, Baklien K, Schmekel B, et al: Quantitation of immunoglobulin-producing cells in small intestinal mucosa of patients with IgA nephropathy. Clin Immunol Immunopathol 26:442–445, 1983.

64. Harper SJ, Pringle JH, Wicks AC, et al: Expression of J chain mRNA in duodenal IgA plasma cells in IgA nephropathy. Kidney Int 45:836–844, 1994.

65. de Fijter JW, Eijgenraam JW, Braam CA, et al: Deficient IgA1 immune response to nasal cholera toxin subunit B in primary IgA nephropathy. Kidney Int 50:952–961, 1996.

66. van den Wall Bake AW, Daha MR, Evers-Schouten J, et al: Serum IgA and the production of IgA by peripheral blood and bone marrow lymphocytes in patients with primary IgA nephropathy: Evidence for the bone marrow as the source of mesangial IgA. Am J Kidney Dis 12:410–414, 1988.

67. Harper SJ, Allen AC, Pringle JH, et al: Increased dimeric IgA producing B cells in the bone marrow in IgA nephropathy determined by in situ hybridisation for J chain mRNA. J Clin Pathol 49:38–42, 1996.
68. Layward L, Finnemore AM, Allen AC, et al: Systemic and mucosal IgA responses to systemic antigen challenge in IgA nephropathy. Clin Immunol Immunopathol 69:306–313, 1993.
69. Ichinose H, Miyazaki M, Koji T, et al: Detection of cytokine mRNA-expressing cells in peripheral blood of patients with IgA nephropathy using non-radioactive in situ hybridization. Clin Exp Immunol 103:125–132, 1996.
70. Lai KN, Ho RT, Lai CK, et al: Increase of both circulating Th1 and Th2 T lymphocyte subsets in IgA nephropathy. Clin Exp Immunol 96:116–121, 1994.
71. Ebihara I, Hirayama K, Yamamoto S, et al: Th2 predominance at the single-cell level in patients with IgA nephropathy. Nephrol Dial Transplant 16:1783–1789, 2001.
72. Lai KN, Ho RT, Leung JC, et al: Increased mRNA encoding for transforming factor-beta in CD4$^+$ cells from patients with IgA nephropathy. Kidney Int 46: 862–868, 1994.
73. de Caestecker MP, Bottomley M, Telfer BA, et al: Detection of abnormal peripheral blood mononuclear cell cytokine networks in human IgA nephropathy. Kidney Int 44:1298–1308, 1993.
74. de Fijter JW, Daha MR, Schroeijers WE, et al: Increased IL-10 production by stimulated whole blood cultures in primary IgA nephropathy. Clin Exp Immunol 111:429–434, 1998.
75. Allen AC, Harper SJ, Feehally J: Galactosylation of N- and O-linked carbohydrate moieties of IgA1 and IgG in IgA nephropathy. Clin Exp Immunol 100:470–474, 1995.
76. Greer MR, Barratt J, Harper SJ, et al: The nucleotide sequence of the IgA1 hinge region in IgA nephropathy. Nephrol Dial Transplant 13:1980–1983, 1998.
77. Allen AC, Topham PS, Harper SJ, et al: Leucocyte beta 1,3 galactosyltransferase activity in IgA nephropathy. Nephrol Dial Transplant 12:701–706, 1997.
78. Ju T, Cummings RD: A unique molecular chaperone Cosmc required for activity of the mammalian core 1 beta 3-galactosyltransferase. Proc Natl Acad Sci U S A 99:16613–16618, 2002.
79. Oin W, Zhou O, Ynag LC et al: Peripheral B lymphocyte beta1,3-galactosyltransferase and chaperone expression in immunoglobulin A nephropathy. J Intern Med 258:467–477, 2005.
80. Smith AC, de Woolff JF, Molyneux K, et al: O-glycosylation of serum IgD in IgA nephropathy. J Am Soc Nephrol 17:1192–1199, 2006.
81. Pierce-Cretel A, Pamblanco M, Strecker G, et al: Heterogeneity of the glycans O-glycosidically linked to the hinge region of secretory immunoglobulins from human milk. Eur J Biochem 114:169–178, 1981.
82. Smith AC, Molyneux K, Feehally J, Barratt J: O-glycosylation of serum IgA antibodies against mucosal and systemic antigens in IgA nephropathy. J Am Soc Nephrol 17:3520–3528, 2006.
83. Feehally J, Beattie TJ, Brenchley PE, et al: Response of circulating immune complexes to food challenge in relapsing IgA nephropathy. Pediatr Nephrol 1:581–586, 1987.
84. Nagy J, Scott H, Brandtzaeg P: Antibodies to dietary antigens in IgA nephropathy. Clin Nephrol 29:275–279, 1988.
85. Rostoker G, Petit-Phar M, Delprato S, et al: Mucosal immunity in primary glomerulonephritis: II. Study of the serum IgA subclass repertoire to food and airborne antigens. Nephron 59:561–566, 1991.
86. Kennel A, Bene MC, Hurault de Ligny B, et al: Serum anti-dextran antibodies in IgA nephropathy. Clin Nephrol 43:216–220, 1995.
87. Rantala I, Collin P, Holm K, et al: Small bowel T cells, HLA class II antigen DR, and GroEL stress protein in IgA nephropathy. Kidney Int 55:2274–2280, 1999.
88. Rostoker G, Delchier JC, Chaumette MT: Increased intestinal intra-epithelial T lymphocytes in primary glomerulonephritis: A role of oral tolerance breakdown in the pathophysiology of human primary glomerulonephritides? Nephrol Dial Transplant 16:513–517, 2001.
89. Olive C, Allen AC, Harper SJ, et al: Expression of the mucosal gamma delta T cell receptor V region repertoire in patients with IgA nephropathy. Kidney Int 52:1047–1053, 1997.
90. Buck KS, Foster EM, Watson D, et al: Expression of T cell receptor variable region families by bone marrow gamma delta T cells in patients with IgA nephropathy. Clin Exp Immunol 127:527–532, 2002.
91. Toyabe S, Harada W, Uchiyama M: Oligoclonally expanding gammadelta T lymphocytes induce IgA switching in IgA nephropathy. Clin Exp Immunol 124:110–117, 2001.
92. Batra A, Foster EM, Barratt J, et al: Increased systemic homing T cell numbers in IgA nephropathy. J Am Soc Nephrol 13:350A, 2002.
93. Waldherr R, Rambausek M, Duncker WD, et al: Frequency of mesangial IgA deposits in a non-selected autopsy series. Nephrol Dial Transplant 4:943–946, 1989.
94. Hotta O, Furuta T, Chiba S, et al: Regression of IgA nephropathy: A repeat biopsy study. Am J Kidney Dis 39:493–502, 2002.
95. Zickerman AM, Allen AC, Talwar V, et al: IgA myeloma presenting as Henoch-Schonlein purpura with nephritis. Am J Kidney Dis 36:E19, 2000.
96. Launay P, Grossetete B, Arcos-Fajardo M, et al: Fc alpha receptor (CD89) mediates the development of immunoglobulin A (IgA) nephropathy (Berger's disease): Evidence for pathogenic soluble receptor-Iga complexes in patients and CD89 transgenic mice. J Exp Med 191:1999–2009, 2000.
97. Van Der Boog PJ, De Fijter JW, Van Kooten C, et al: Complexes of IgA with Fc alphaRI/CD89 are not specific for primary IgA nephropathy. Kidney Int 63:514–521, 2003.
98. Tomino Y, Endoh M, Nomoto Y, et al: Specificity of eluted antibody from renal tissues of patients with IgA nephropathy. Am J Kidney Dis 1:276–280, 1982.
99. Orfila C, Rakotoarivony J, Manuel Y, et al: Immunofluorescence characterization of light chains in human nephropathies. Virchows Arch A Pathol Anat Histopathol 412:591–594, 1988.
100. Gomez-Guerrero C, Duque N, Egido J: Mesangial cells possess an asialoglycoprotein receptor with affinity for human immunoglobulin A. J Am Soc Nephrol 9:568–576, 1998.
101. McDonald KJ, Cameron AJ, Allen JM, et al: Expression of Fc-alpha/mu receptor by human mesangial cells: A candidate receptor for immune complex deposition in IgA nephropathy. Biochem Biophys Res Commun 290:438–442, 2002.
102. Moura IC, Centelles MN, Arcos-Fajardo M, et al: Identification of the transferrin receptor as a novel immunoglobulin (Ig)A1 receptor and its enhanced expression on mesangial cells in IgA nephropathy. J Exp Med 194:417–425, 2001.
103. Haddad E, Moura IC, Arcos-Fajardo M, et al: Enhanced expression of the CD71 mesangial IgA1 receptor in Berger disease and Henoch-Schonlein nephritis: Association between CD71 expression and IgA deposits. J Am Soc Nephrol 14:327–337, 2003.
104. Moura IC, Arcos-Fajardo M, Gdoura A et al: Engagement of transferrin receptor by polymeric IgA1: Evidence for a positive feedback loop involving increased receptor expression and mesangial cell proliferation in IgA nephropathy. J Am Soc Nephrol 16:2667–2676, 2005.

105. Barratt J, Greer MR, Pawluczyk IZ, et al: Identification of a novel Fcalpha receptor expressed by human mesangial cells. Kidney Int 57:1936–1948, 2000.

106. Gomez-Guerrero C, Lopez-Armada MJ, Gonzalez E, et al: Soluble IgA and IgG aggregates are catabolized by cultured rat mesangial cells and induce production of TNF-alpha and IL-6, and proliferation. J Immunol 153:5247–5255, 1994.

107. Yan D, Rumbeiha WK, Pestka JJ: Experimental murine IgA nephropathy following passive administration of vomitoxin-induced IgA monoclonal antibodies. Food Chem Toxicol 36:1095–1106, 1998.

108. Imasawa T, Utsunomiya Y, Kawamura T, et al: Evidence suggesting the involvement of hematopoietic stem cells in the pathogenesis of IgA nephropathy. Biochem Biophys Res Commun 249:605–611, 1998.

109. Imasawa T, Nagasawa R, Utsunomiya Y, et al: Bone marrow transplantation attenuates murine IgA nephropathy: Role of a stem cell disorder [see comments]. Kidney Int 56:1809–1817, 1999.

110. Stad RK, Bruijn JA, van Gijlswijk-Janssen DJ, et al: An acute model for IgA-mediated glomerular inflammation in rats induced by monoclonal polymeric rat IgA antibodies. Clin Exp Immunol 92:514–521, 1993.

111. Fujii K, Muller KD, Clarkson AR, et al: The effect of IgA immune complexes on the proliferation of cultured human mesangial cells. Am J Kidney Dis 16:207–210, 1990.

112. Chen A, Chen WP, Sheu LF, et al: Pathogenesis of IgA nephropathy: In vitro activation of human mesangial cells by IgA immune complex leads to cytokine secretion. J Pathol 173:119–126, 1994.

113. Lopez-Armada MJ, Gomez-Guerrero C, Egido J: Receptors for immune complexes activate gene expression and synthesis of matrix proteins in cultured rat and human mesangial cells: Role of TGF-beta. J Immunol 157:2136–2142, 1996.

114. Peruzzi L, Amore A, Cirina P, et al: Integrin expression and IgA nephropathy: In vitro modulation by IgA with altered glycosylation and macromolecular IgA. Kidney Int 58:2331–2340, 2000.

115. Monteiro RC, Moura IC, Launay P, et al: Pathogenic significance of IgA receptor interactions in IgA nephropathy. Trends Mol Med 8:464–468, 2002.

116. Van Dixhoorn MG, Sato T, Muizert Y, et al: Combined glomerular deposition of polymeric rat IgA and IgG aggravates renal inflammation [In Process Citation]. Kidney Int 58:90–99, 2000.

117. Lai KN, Tang SC, Guh JY et al: Polymeric IgA1 from patients with IgA nephropathy upregulates transforming growth factor-β synthesis and signal transduction in human mesangial cells via the renin-angiotensin system. J Am Soc Nephrol 14:3127–3137, 2003.

118. Wang Y, Zhao MH, Li XM, Wan HY: Binding capacity and pathophysiological effects of IgA1 from patients with IgA nephropathy on human glomerular mesangial cells. Clin Exp Immunol 136:168–175, 2004.

119. Amore A, Cirina P, Conti G, et al: Glycosylation of circulating IgA in patients with IgA nephropathy modulates proliferation and apoptosis of mesangial cells. J Am Soc Nephrol 12:1862–1871, 2001.

120. Coppo R, Amore A: Aberrant glycosylation in IgA nephropathy. Kidney Int 65:1544–1547, 2004.

121. Novak J, Tomana M, Matousovic K et al: IgA1-containing immune complexes in IgA nephropathy differentially affect proliferation of mesangial cells. Kidney Int 67:504–513, 2005.

122. Matsuda M, Shikata K, Wada J, et al: Deposition of mannan binding protein and mannan binding protein-mediated complement activation in the glomeruli of patients with IgA nephropathy. Nephron 80:408–413, 1998.

123. Hansch GM: The role of complement in mesangial cell damage [Editorial]. Nephrol Dial Transplant 8:4–5, 1993.

124. Endo M, Ohi H, Ohsawa I, et al: Glomerular deposition of mannose-binding lectin (MBL) indicates a novel mechanism of complement activation in IgA nephropathy. Nephrol Dial Transplant 13:1984–1990, 1998.

125. Abe K, Miyazaki M, Koji T, et al: Intraglomerular synthesis of complement C3 and its activation products in IgA nephropathy. Nephron 87:231–239, 2001.

126. Abe K, Miyazaki M, Koji T, et al: Expression of decay accelerating factor mRNA and complement C3 mRNA in human diseased kidney. Kidney Int 54:120–130, 1998.

127. Moll S, Miot S, Sadallah S, et al: No complement receptor 1 stumps on podocytes in human glomerulopathies. Kidney Int 59:160–168, 2001.

128. Yoshioka K, Takemura T, Aya N, et al: Monocyte infiltration and cross-linked fibrin deposition in IgA nephritis and Henoch-Schonlein purpura nephritis. Clin Nephrol 32:107–112, 1989.

129. Arima S, Nakayama M, Naito M, et al: Significance of mononuclear phagocytes in IgA nephropathy. Kidney Int 39:684–692, 1991.

130. Li HL, Hancock WW, Dowling JP, et al: Activated (IL-2R+) intraglomerular mononuclear cells in crescentic glomerulonephritis. Kidney Int 39:793–798, 1991.

131. Johnson RJ: The glomerular response to injury: Progression or resolution? Kidney Int 45:1769–1782, 1994.

132. Hsu SI, Ramirez SB, Winn MP, et al: Evidence for genetic factors in the development and progression of IgA nephropathy. Kidney Int 57:1818–1835, 2000.

133. Imai H, Nakamoto Y, Asakura K, et al: Spontaneous glomerular IgA deposition in ddY mice: An animal model of IgA nephritis. Kidney Int 27:756–761, 1985.

134. Miyawaki S, Muso E, Takeuchi E, et al: Selective breeding for high serum IgA levels from noninbred ddY mice: Isolation of a strain with an early onset of glomerular IgA deposition. Nephron 76:201–207, 1997.

135. Zhang Z, Kundu GC, Yuan CJ, et al: Severe fibronectin-deposit renal glomerular disease in mice lacking uteroglobin. Science 276:1408–1412, 1997.

136. Zheng F, Kundu GC, Zhang Z, et al: Uteroglobin is essential in preventing immunoglobulin A nephropathy in mice. Nat Med 5:1018–1025, 1999.

137. Yong D, Qing WQ, Hua L, et al: Association of uteroglobin G38A polymorphism with IgA nephropathy: A meta-analysis. Am J Kidney Dis 48:1–7, 2006.

138. Launay P, Grossetete B, Arcos-Fajardo M, et al: Fc alpha receptor (CD89) mediates the development of immunoglobulin A (IgA) nephropathy (Berger's disease). Evidence for pathogenic soluble receptor-IgA complexes in patients and CD89 transgenic mice. J Exp Med 191:1999–2009, 2000.

139. van der Boog PJ, van Kooten C, van Zandbergen G, et al: Injection of recombinant Fc alpha RI/CD89 in mice does not induce mesangial IgA deposition. Nephrol Dial Transplant 19:2729–2736, 2004.

140. Portis JL, Coe JE, et al: Deposition of IgA in renal glomeruli of mink affected with Aleutian disease. Am J Pathol 96:227–236, 1979.

141. Jessen RH, Emancipator SN, Jacobs GH, et al: Experimental IgA-IgG nephropathy induced by a viral respiratory pathogen. Dependence on antigen form and immune status. Lab Invest 67:379–386, 1992.

142. Schroeder C, Osman AA, Roggenbuck D, et al: IgA-gliadin antibodies, IgA-containing circulating immune complexes, and IgA glomerular deposits in wasting marmoset syndrome. Nephrol Dial Transplant 14: 1875–1880, 1999.

143. Marquina R, Diez MA, Lopez-Hoyos M, et al: Inhibition of B cell death causes the development of an IgA nephropathy in (New Zealand white x C57BL/6)(F1bcl)-2 transgenic mice. J Immunol 172:7177–7185, 2004.

144. Kennel-De March A, Prin-Mathieu C, Kohler CH, et al: Back-pack mice as a model of renal mesangial IgA dimers deposition. Int J Immunopathol Pharmacol 18:701–708, 2005.

145. Frimat L, Kessler M: Controversies concerning the importance of genetic polymorphism in IgA nephropathy. Nephrol Dial Transplant 2002;17: 42–45.

146. Johnstone DB, Holzman LB: Clinical impact of research on the podocyte slit diaphragm. Nat Clin Pract Nephrol 2:271–282, 2006.

147. Helms C, Cao L, Krueger JG, et al: A putative RUNX1 binding site variant between SLC9A3R1 and NAT9 is associated with susceptibility to psoriasis. Nat Genet 35:349–356, 2003.

148. Prokunina L, Castillejo-Lopez C, Oberg F, et al: A regulatory polymorphism in PDCD1 is associated with susceptibility to systemic lupus erythematosus in humans. Nat Genet 32:666–669, 2002.

149. Tokuhiro S, Yamada R, Chang X, et al: An intronic SNP in a RUNX1 binding site of SLC22A4, encoding an organic cation transporter, is associated with rheumatoid arthritis. Nat Genet 35:341–348, 2003.

150. Hoogendoorn B, Coleman SL, Guy CA, et al: Functional analysis of human promoter polymorphisms. Hum Mol Genet 12:2249–2254, 2003.

151. Lo HS, Wang Z, Hu Y, et al: Allelic variation in gene expression is common in the human genome. Genome Res 13:1855–1862, 2003.

152. Hsu SI: The molecular pathogenesis and experimental therapy of IgA nephropathy: Recent advances and future directions. Curr Mol Med 1:183–196, 2001.

153. Izzi C, Sanna-Cherchi S, Prati E, et al: Familial aggregation of primary glomerulonephritis in an Italian population isolate: Valtrompia study. Kidney Int 69:1033–1040, 2006.

154. Julian BA, Quiggins PA, Thompson JS, et al: Familial IgA nephropathy. Evidence of an inherited mechanism of disease. N Engl J Med 312:202–208, 1985.

155. Scolari F: Inherited forms of IgA nephropathy. J Nephrol 16:317–320, 2003.

156. Schena FP, Cerullo G, Rossini M, et al: Increased risk of end-stage renal disease in familial IgA nephropathy. J Am Soc Nephrol 13:453–460, 2002.

157. Izzi C, Ravani P, Torres D, et al: IgA nephropathy: The presence of familial disease does not confer an increased risk for progression. Am J Kidney Dis 47:761–769, 2006.

158. Li LS, Liu ZH: Epidemiologic data of renal diseases from a single unit in China: Analysis based on 13,519 renal biopsies. Kidney Int 66:920–923, 2004.

159. Mittal BV, Singh AK, Rennke HG: Spectrum of glomerular disease: Results of the Brigham database of glomerulonephritis. J Am Soc Nephrol 15:553A, 2004.

160. Hall YN, Fuentes EF, Chertow GM, et al: Race/ethnicity and disease severity in IgA nephropathy. BMC Nephrol 5:10, 2004.

161. Gharavi AG, Yan Y, Scolari F, et al: IgA nephropathy, the most common cause of glomerulonephritis, is linked to 6q22–23. Nat Genet 26:354–357, 2000.

162. Tsukaguchi H: A genetic mapping for a familial IgA nephropathy: Nephrology (Carlton) 9(Suppl 2):A65, 2004.

163. Schena FP, Cerullo G, Torres DD, et al: The IgA nephropathy Biobank. An important starting point for the genetic dissection of a complex trait. BMC Nephrol 6:14, 2005.

164. Suzuki H, Suzuki Y, Yamanaka T, et al: Genome-wide scan in a novel IgA nephropathy model identifies a susceptibility locus on murine chromosome 10, in a region syntenic to human IGAN1 on chromosome 6q22-23. J Am Soc Nephrol 16:1289–1299, 2005.

165. Oida E, Nogaki F, Kobayashi I, et al: Quantitative trait loci (QTL) analysis reveals a close linkage between the hinge region and trimeric IgA dominancy in a high IgA strain (HIGA) of ddY mice. Eur J Immunol 34:2200–2208, 2004.

166. Nogaki F, Oida E, Kamata T, et al: Chromosomal mapping of hyperserum IgA and glomerular IgA deposition in a high IgA (HIGA) strain of ddY mice. Kidney Int 68:2517–2525, 2005.

167. Schneider B, Hanke P, Jagla W, et al: Synergistic interaction of two independent genetic loci causes extreme elevation of serum IgA in mice. Genes Immun 5:375–380, 2004.

168. Schena FP, D'Altri C, Cerullo G, et al: ACE gene polymorphism and IgA nephropathy: An ethnically homogeneous study and a meta-analysis. Kidney Int 60:732–740, 2001.

169. Rigat B, Hubert C, Alhenc-Gelas F, et al: An insertion/deletion polymorphism in the angiotensin I-converting enzyme gene accounting for half the variance of serum enzyme levels. J Clin Invest 86:1343–1346, 1990.

170. Hunley TE, Julian BA, Phillips JA 3rd, et al: Angiotensin converting enzyme gene polymorphism: Potential silencer motif and impact on progression in IgA nephropathy. Kidney Int 49:571–577, 1996.

171. Kunz R, Bork JP, Fritsche L, et al: Association between the angiotensin-converting enzyme-insertion/deletion polymorphism and diabetic nephropathy: A methodologic appraisal and systematic review. J Am Soc Nephrol 9:1653–1663, 1998.

172. Poch E, Gonzalez D, Giner V, et al: Molecular basis of salt sensitivity in human hypertension. Evaluation of renin-angiotensin-aldosterone system gene polymorphisms. Hypertension 38:1204–1209, 2001.

173. Goldstein DB: Islands of linkage disequilibrium. Nat Genet 29:109–111, 2001.

174. Wahl JD, Pritchard JK: Haplotype blocks and linkage disequilibrium in the human genome. Nat Rev Genet 4:587–597, 2003.

175. Couser WG: Revisions to instructions to JASN authors regarding articles reporting studies using DNA arrays, DNA polymorphisms and randomized controlled clinical trials. J Am Soc Nephrol 14:2686–2687, 2003.

176. Takei T, Iida A, Nitta K, et al: Association between single-nucleotide polymorphisms in selectin genes and immunoglobulin A nephropathy. Am J Hum Genet 70:781–786, 2002.

177. Takei T, Hiraoka M, Nitta K, et al: Functional impact of IgA nephropathy-associated selectin gene haplotype on leukocyte-endothelial interaction. Immunogenetics 58:355–361, 2006.

178. Li YJ, Du Y, Li CX, et al: Family-based association study showing that immunoglobulin A nephropathy is associated with the polymorphisms 2093C and 2180T in the 3' untranslated region of the Megsin gene. J Am Soc Nephrol 15:1739–1743, 2004.

179. Xia YF, Huang S, Li X, et al: A family-based association study of megsin A23167G polymorphism with susceptibility and progression of IgA nephropathy in a Chinese population. Clin Nephrol 65:153–159, 2006.

180. Schena FP, Cerullo G, Torres DD, et al: Role of interferon-gamma gene polymorphisms in susceptibility to IgA nephropathy: A family-based association study. Eur J Hum Genet 14:488–496, 2006.

Chapter 28

Glomerulonephritis Caused by Anti-neutrophil Cytoplasmic Autoantibodies

Gloria A. Preston and Ronald J. Falk

Anti-neutrophil cytoplasmic autoantibodies (ANCAs) are directed against cytoplasmic constituents of granulocytes and monocytes and cause vasculitic lesions predominantly in small vessels of vulnerable organs, particularly the lungs and kidneys. ANCAs were first described by Davies in 1982, and then in 1985 an association of ANCA and Wegener's granulomatosis was reported.[1,2] Three years later, our own investigations of patients with pauci-immune necrotizing glomerulonephritis identified perinuclear ANCAs that were specific for myeloperoxidase (MPO-ANCAs).[3] Over the ensuing years, the ever-expanding ANCA community focused on understanding the role of MPO-ANCAs, and soon thereafter proteinase 3 (PR3) emerged as a target antigen for ANCAs (PR3-ANCAs) with a characteristic cytoplasmic staining pattern.[4–8]

ANCA effects are predominantly seen in vessels smaller than arteries, in particular glomerular capillaries and alveolar capillaries.[9] Histologically, the glomerular lesions in ANCA disease include segmental fibrinoid necrosis and crescent formation, with remarkably few if any immune deposits. Hematuria, proteinuria, and renal insufficiency caused by glomerulonephritis are frequent clinical features of these patients.

The lack of ANCA and ANCA antigen deposits along the vascular wall has made it particularly challenging to demonstrate a causal role for these autoantibodies in renal disease. Recently, an animal model developed by our group convincingly demonstrates that anti-MPO antibodies alone can cause necrotizing and crescentic glomerulonephritis. The model uses MPO knockout mice as the host to generate anti-MPO antibodies. The splenocytes from MPO$^{-/-}$ mice immunized with murine MPO are transferred into Rag2$^{-/-}$ mice, which lack the ability to initiate V(D)J rearrangement and thus lack T and B lymphocytes. These mice develop circulating anti-MPO antibodies and necrotizing and crescentic glomerulonephritis and small-vessel vasculitis in the lung, lymph node, and spleen.[10,11] Furthermore, intravenous infusion of purified anti-MPO immunoglobulin G (IgG) from immunized MPO$^{-/-}$ mice into Rag2$^{-/-}$ and wild-type B6 mice caused the development of necrosis and crescents in glomeruli in 100% of the animals, in contrast to the control anti–bovine serum albumin (anti-BSA) IgG, where 0% developed glomerular lesions. Equally important, immunofluorescence microscopy demonstrated a paucity of immunoglobulin or complement in the glomeruli of mice with anti-MPO antibody-induced glomerulonephritis, thus modeling the pauci-immune characteristic of human ANCA glomerulonephritis. There is a rat model of ANCA glomerulonephritis, and in this model immunization of the animal with human

MPO is done in combination with a second insult in order to induce crescentic glomerulonephritis and vasculitis.[12,13]

The strongest data supportive of the pathogenicity of ANCA come from the numerous in vitro studies over the last 14 years. Early in vitro studies documented that ANCA could activate neutrophils and monocytes. The ANCA pathogenic process, as depicted in Fig. 28-1, begins when ANCAs interact with neutrophils and monocytes. This interaction involves both the binding of the F(ab')$_2$ to ANCA antigens expressed on the cell surface and by the binding of the Fc region to its receptors.[6,14–20] This interaction results in leukocyte activation with induction of respiratory burst, degranulation, and release of neutrophil and monocyte products into the microenvironment. These activated leukocytes and their noxious products interact with the endothelium and other vessel wall structures, resulting in inflammatory damage. Observations that support this mechanism are (1) the presence of ANCAs in patients with

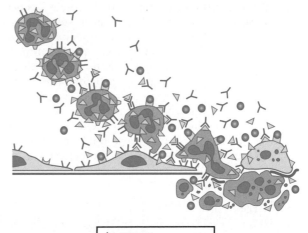

人	ANCA
△	ANCA antigen
●	Cytokine
⋈	Cytokine receptor
Ц	Fc receptor
▽	Adhesion molecule
Ⅴ	Adhesion molecule receptor

Figure 28-1 Schematic of ANCAs and their interaction with neutrophils causing neutrophil degranulation and tissue injury. (From Jennette JC, Falk RJ: Pathogenesis of the vascular and glomerular damage in ANCA-positive vasculitis. Nephrol Dial Transplant 13[Suppl 1]:19, 1998.) **(See Color Plate 5.)**

a distinctive pattern of pauci-immune glomerulonephritis that is shared by microscopic polyangiitis (MPA), Wegener's granulomatosis, and Churg-Strauss syndrome,[21,22] (2) the correlation of an ANCA-positive titer with disease activity,[23] and (3) the observation that some patients with drug-induced (e.g., by thiouracils) ANCAs develop vasculitis and glomerulonephritis, which resolves after discontinuation of the drug.[24]

In the following sections we will discuss recent advances in our understanding of the many components of ANCA disease, including what may be acting as an inciting immunogen, how the autoantibodies, once produced, affect neutrophils, and how the proteins released from activated neutrophils cause vascular injury.

WHAT INCITES AN AUTOIMMUNE RESPONSE?

A New Theory

A pressing quesiton in autoimmunity is "what causes or what allows autoantibodies to develop?" There have been a number of theories describing the origin of autoimmunity, including examples of molecular mimicry,[25–29] antigen drift, and aberrant T-cell regulation.[30,31] None of these have provided answers to the cause of this human autoimmune disease. A recent discovery in the field of ANCA glomerulonephritis opens new avenues of research that could lead to an understanding of how autoimmune disease develops in general.[32] The seminal observation was made while attempting to map epitopes on the PR3 molecule recognized by autoantibodies from PR3-ANCA patients. We were screening a bacterial library expressing small fragments of the human PR3 protein. Sequence analysis of positive colonies revealed that in some cases the patients' sera were reactive with a protein produced from DNA that had inserted into the vector in the wrong orientation, that is, the protein was translated from antisense RNA of the PR3 gene (*PRTN3*), thus producing a protein complementary to the PR3 protein (for definition of terms see Fig. 28-2). This finding, which we felt might have broad implications to the understanding of autoimmunity, set off a series of experiments to elucidate the basis for this observation. It took 4 years of research to be satisfied that what was observed was both

repeatable and had a valid explanation. These studies provide the foundation for a refined theory for the development of autoimmunity, the Theory of Autoantigen Complementarity. The theory proposes that the initiator of an autoimmune response is not necessarily the autoantigen, but instead may be a peptide that is "antisense" or *complementary* to the autoantigen. As depicted in Fig. 28-3, the first immune response is the production of an antibody specific for a complementary protein. Secondarily, an anti-antibody response produces an immunoglobulin that now reacts with the corresponding "sense" or self-protein (e.g., PR3), which is the autoantibody (e.g., PR3-ANCA). It appears that proteins, complementary in amino acid sequence to the known autoantigen, incite the initial immune response in PR3-ANCA glomerulonephritis. An invited commentary on this work states, "The work of Pendergraft et al. brings together what has, until now, been a set of peculiar and seemingly unrelated observations. What we must do now is hone, test and prod this new paradigm. We might just find that the idea of an antisense-initiated idiotypic network has something to offer for treating a wide range of autoimmune disorders."[33]

The theoretical framework for the Theory of Autoantigen Complementarity draws on concepts proposed in the late 1960s by Mekler[34,35] and also by Blalock and colleagues, who built on the concepts of Mekler and put forth the Molecular Recognition Theory.[36,37] Mekler founded the concept that a sense protein has a natural affinity for its complementary protein counterpart due to inverted hydropathy. For example, the complementary amino acid for the hydrophilic amino acid arginine (R) (codon CGG) is the hydrophobic amino acid proline (P) (coded by the antisense codon CCG). A review by Heal and colleagues cites numerous studies proving that sense proteins and their complementary counterparts have a natural affinity, and that increasing affinity correlates with increasing

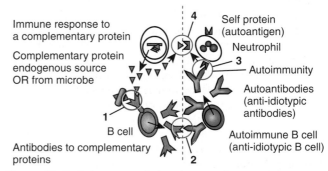

Figure 28-3 Schematic of the theory of autoantigen complementarity. The theory proposes that the immunogen that begins the sequence of events leading to the production of autoantibodies is not the autoantigen or its mimic, but rather its complementary peptide or its mimic. Step 1: The complementary proteins may be introduced by invading microbes or they may be produced by the individual through translation of antisense RNA. An antibody is produced in response to the complementary protein. Step 2: A second antibody is elicited against the first antibody, referred to as an anti-idiotypic response. Step 3: The resultant anti-idiotypic antibodies react with the autoantigen, whose amino acid sequence is complementary to the sequence of the initiating antigen. Step 4: Complementary proteins have a natural affinity because the hydropathy of one is the opposite of the other. **(See Color Plate 5.)**

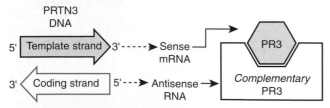

Figure 28-2 Definition of terms. *Antisense RNA* is a general term used to describe a sequence of RNA that is complementary to messenger RNA (mRNA). The sequence of the antisense RNA is the same as the DNA template strand or antisense strand. A *complementary protein* is one that is translated from antisense RNA. The hydropathy of the complementary protein is exactly opposite to that of the mRNA-coded protein from that same gene. Thus, the individual folding patterns result in contour structures that can interact in a lock and key manner.

peptide length.[38] Computational studies illustrate that ligands and their receptors share regions of complementarity, and this was demonstrated in a study showing interleukin-2 (IL-2) binding to its receptor is blocked by a complementary peptide of IL-2.[39–41] Specificity of this inhibitory peptide was confirmed using a scrambled version of the same amino acid.

A receptor binding its ligand is analogous to an antibody binding its antigen. Indeed, it was shown that an antigen is complementary to its antibody in the epitope-binding site.[42] To take this one step further, if one antibody is directed against a sense protein and a second antibody is directed against the complementary protein counterpart, these two antibodies are now complementary to each other.[42] In theory, these two antibodies would be considered to be an idiotypic pair. Is complementarity the molecular basis for Niels Kaj Jerne's idiotypic network theory? He hypothesized that the antigen-binding site of an antibody (idiotype) can act as an antigen and elicit anti-antibodies (anti-idiotypes).[43,44] In turn, anti-idiotypes elicit anti-anti-idiotypes directed against their complementarity-determining regions and so on. Under normal conditions the network is balanced, but when an antigen is introduced, the equilibrium is disturbed. The immune system attempts to restore balance, which leads to an immune response against the antibody. Jerne and colleagues demonstrated such a phenomenon in multiple scientific reports, including one in which they were able to precipitate anti-idiotypic antibodies from rabbits immunized with immunoglobulin.[45]

The principles of molecular recognition and idiotypy have been discussed in the context of autoimmunity by researchers for some time. Erlanger and colleagues reported that they could inhibit the binding of an antibody to thyroid-stimulating hormone by adding a second antibody specific for the hormone's receptor, that is, the antibodies bound each other in an idiotypic fashion, thus competing out one's binding to the hormone.[46–48] Shoenfeld and coworkers demonstrated in multiple animal models of autoimmunity that anti-idiotypes raised against autoantibodies induced the production of anti-anti-idiotypes that possessed characteristics of the initial autoantibodies and caused disease after immunization.[49] They hypothesized that antibodies regulate each other by suppressing or augmenting the immune reaction.[33] Specifically, anti–double-stranded DNA (anti-dsDNA) antibody-positive mice treated with anti-dsDNA anti-id antibodies, purified from commercial intravenous immunoglobulin, showed a decline in their anti-dsDNA antibody level, and had decreased proteinuria, reduced renal disease, and an increase in life span.[50,51]

Complementary Proteinase 3 Protein or its Mimic Incites the ANCA Immune Response

The Theory of Autoantigen Complementarity postulates that human ANCAs develop through a pathway that starts with exposure to a complementary PR3 protein. This was demonstrated in mice after immunization with complementary PR3 protein. The animals launched an immune response producing antibodies against the immunogen, and as predicted the animals secondarily produced antibodies against the immunogen's sense counterpart, PR3.[52] It follows that the question now is how and from where do PR3-ANCA patients get exposed to a complementary PR3 protein or its mimic. It is highly likely that microbes carry proteins that are molecular mimics of complementary PR3.[52,53] Many investigators have focused on potential associations between infection and vascular inflammation (see review[54]). Interestingly, the onset of ANCA disease is commonly associated with a flulike illness.[55] A database sequence analysis of complementary PR3 identified a variety of pathogenic organisms with homologous proteins, including Ross River virus, *Staphylococcus aureus*, and *Entamoeba histolytica*,[52] all shown earlier to be linked with ANCA disease.[1,56,57] Moreover, systemic administration of lipopolysaccharide (LPS) in conjunction with anti-MPO IgG in the murine ANCA model confirmed that ANCAs and proinflammatory stimuli act synergistically to induce vasculitis.[58]

Recent reports suggest that other autoimmune diseases might arise and/or progress, at least in part, through a process in line with the Theory of Autoantigen Complementarity.[59] A group led by Tzioufas showed that roughly half of anti-La-positive sera from patients with Sjögren's syndrome or systemic lupus erythematosus reacted with peptides complementary to the La/SSB and Ro/SSA autoantigens. This same group recapitulated their findings in a mouse model by immunizing mice with sense or complementary peptides corresponding to an epitope within La/SSB.[60,61]

Theoretically, a basic local alignment search tool (BLAST) database search of complementary proteins corresponding to other known autoantigens would identify potential microbial sources. We tested this idea, and the results were very intriguing.[62] Bullous pemphigoid (BP), a chronic, blistering, and subepidermal autoimmune skin disease occurring primarily in the elderly, is caused by pathogenic autoantibodies directed against the BP180 ectodomain of hemidesmosomes.[63] When the complementary protein sequence of BP180 (FYSIHAVPIGQYAP) was entered into the database, one microbe identified was the bacterium *Clostridium tetani*, and interestingly, there is historical documentation of an association between vaccination for tetanus and the onset of bullous pemphigoid.[64–67] As another example, patients with myasthenia gravis have autoantibodies that target the acetylcholine receptor, causing muscle weakness and fatigue due to impaired neuromuscular transmission. The main immunogenic region appears to be a continuous 10– to 15–amino acid fragment of the α subunit.[68] When we performed the complementary protein search (FHTAIVIWIPFZVVIH), two of the microbes that were identified were *Clostridium diphtheriae* and *C. tetani*; again, vaccinations for tetanus and diphtheria have been linked with onset of myasthenia gravis in children.[69,70] Identification of potential microbial mimics for other known autoantigens is straightforward, especially if the epitope is defined. The complementary protein sequence can be derived by an in-frame translation of the hypothetical antisense RNA strand of the autoantigen gene. This sequence can be entered into the basic local alignment search tool (http://www.ncbi.nlm.nih.gov/BLAST/) to generate a list of proteins with regions of homology.

A second source of complementary proteins that must be considered is the possibility that individuals transcribe and translate antisense RNA from their own genes, thus producing these proteins themselves. Evidently, 2% of the normal human transcriptome consists of natural antisense transcripts (NATs).[71] Indeed, approximately 50% of the PR3-ANCA patients tested synthesize antisense PR3 RNA.[52] Interestingly, this antisense PR3 transcript was not in the NAT database;

thus, it was termed pathologic antisense transcripts (PATs), since these transcripts appear to be strictly associated with ANCA disease.[52] ANCA disease may not be the only condition where antisense transcripts are associated with disease. Increased amounts of antisense RNAs were reported to be associated with tumor progression.[72] Whether these antisense transcripts are translated into protein product is in question, but it seems plausible, since others have identified proteins coded from sense messenger RNA (mRNA) and from antisense RNA of the same gene.[73] Interestingly an unprecedented report by Van den Eynde and colleagues described their discovery of a protein in humans that is translated from antisense RNA.[74] Transcription of the antisense RNA is initiated within its first intron extending into the promoter of the gene encoding the sense RNA. Examination of the protein sequences indicates that these two proteins (RU2S and RU2AS) are translated in the same reading frame, thus conforming to the definition of a "complementary protein pair." The sense RU2S transcript appears to encode a housekeeping mRNA, and is expressed in all tissues examined. The antisense RNA RU2AS mRNA is restricted to expression in the kidney, bladder, liver, and testis. These results are striking in that they clearly demonstrate that the antisense RNA of a gene can be transcribed and encode a protein product.

Heal and colleagues propose that one reason there are fewer genes in humans than expected is that proteins arise from translation of both sense RNA and antisense RNA.[38]

IS THE PRESENCE OF CIRCULATING PR3-ANCA OR MPO-ANCA SUFFICIENT TO CAUSE DISEASE IN HUMANS?

Aberrant Gene Expression in Circulating Leukocytes of ANCA Patients

Recent data point to a pathologic component in ANCA disease that might be equally as important as the presence of anti-MPO or anti-PR3 autoantibodies. It was discovered that mature leukocytes and monocytes from the majority of ANCA patients with active disease have high levels of PR3 and MPO mRNA.[75,76] This is astonishing in light of the dogma that these genes are silenced before the cells leave the bone marrow (Fig. 28-4). Increased transcripts correlated with disease activity and absolute neutrophil values, but not with "left shift," drug regimen, cytokine levels, hematuria, proteinuria, ANCA titer, serum creatinine, sex, or age.[75] This anomaly appears to be ANCA disease specific, since upregulation of these genes was not observed in patients with end-stage renal disease, rheumatoid arthritis, or lupus, or in healthy volunteers. To our knowledge, this is the first report of this phenomenon in non-neoplastic cells. This finding, which we feel has broad implications for understanding ANCA disease, raises the question of whether increased transcription of PR3 and MPO causes increased protein on the cell surface, thus placing these individuals at risk for the development of ANCA disease. Indeed, there are reports indicating a correlation between higher concentrations of surface PR3 and development of disease. One report introduced the concept that subsets of neutrophils express PR3 molecules on their surface and that the proportion of neutrophils presenting PR3 is genetically controlled and highly stable.[77] The researchers found that the

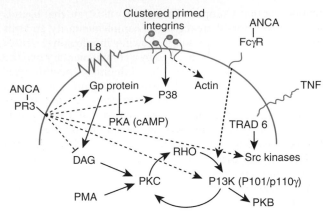

Figure 28-4 Schematic of signal transduction pathways associated with anti-neutrophil cytoplasmic autoantibodies.

phenotype of increased PR3 surface expression was significantly over-represented in patients with ANCA-associated vasculitis. These data raise the hypothesis that in addition to the presence of anti-MPO or anti-PR3 autoantibodies, a second critical component in the etiology of this disease is the reactivation of once-silenced genes leading to increased antigen availability.

An added note, the utility of leukocyte transcriptional profiles is underscored by the discovery of increased PR3 and MPO gene expression in patients. It is highly feasible that expression profiling will be an informative and noninvasive approach to following ANCA disease activity in the near future. This approach to predict disease activity in IgA nephropathy was successful in generating a unique profile using iterative bioinformatics.[78]

HOW DO ANCA AFFECT NEUTROPHILS AND MONOCYTES?

ANCA-mediated effects on neutrophils and monocytes are conferred by both the $F(ab')_2$ region binding to its antigen and the engagement of the Fc region with the Fc receptor.[15,20,79–84] The extent to which the $F(ab')_2$ region contributes has been debated for some years; however, now it is clear that antibody-antigen interactions are fundamental for the neutrophilic perturbations required for vascular injury.[16–18,83,85] Cross-linking of ANCA target antigens with the $F(ab')_2$ region triggers superoxide (O_2^-) release, which was reduced by only 33% after blocking FcγIIa receptors.[17] ANCAs uniquely affect gene expression through the $F(ab')_2$ portion of the antibody. In vitro treatment of leukocytes from healthy donors with ANCA IgG or $F(ab')_2$ results in activation of a number of differentially expressed genes, as compared with genes activated by normal IgG or $F(ab')_2$, such as differentiation-dependent gene 2 (DIF-2), IL-8, and cyclo-oxygenase-2 (COX-2). Activation of transcription by ANCA infers changes in cellular signaling pathways. How is signaling induced by binding of the $F(ab')_2$ to antigen? Feasibly, the $F(ab')_2$ serves as a tethering molecule. Perhaps cross-linking of surface antigens by ANCAs results in clusters of associated molecules, thereby forming lipid raft-like structures, particularly if the antigens are binding other proteins on the cell surface, such as Mac-1 (CD11b/CD18)[86] or a β_2-integrin.[87] Reportedly, ANCA F(ab')^2 fragments and the whole IgG molecule differentially activate K-ras through cooperative activation of Src kinase and phosphatidylinositol-3-kinase (PI3K).[88,89] A schematic of potential signal transduction pathways responsive to ANCAs is shown in Fig. 28-5. ANCAs antagonize IP3/DAG generation; thus, they could modulate the protein kinase (PKC)/PI3K pathways.[18] ANCA-induced signals are synergistic with tumor necrosis factor-α effects,[17,82] probably through the Src kinase pathways.[88,89] ANCAs activate transcription of the IL-1β gene,[90] indicating that ANCAs activate p38 map kinase (MAPK).[91] ANCAs affect integrin-mediated events, providing another link with p38 MAPK. The intertwined complexity of the signal transduction network makes it difficult to pinpoint the pathways crucial to ANCA pathogenesis with the currently available information. Research in this area is certainly needed for development of therapeutic interventions at the neutrophil level.

HOW DO AUTOANTIBODIES THAT TARGET NEUTROPHILS AND MONOCYTES CAUSE GLOMERULAR LESIONS?

The paradigm of ANCA pathogenesis must include several events that occur simultaneously or sequentially, including the generation of ANCAs, leukocyte activation, and injured endothelium. Indications are that renal tissue in patients has increased IL-18 deposition, resulting in increased neutrophil recruitment and priming on the endothelium.[92] The endothelium was originally considered a direct target of ANCA-mediated effects because of the histologic pattern of

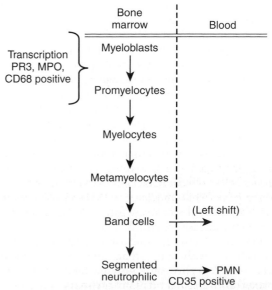

Figure 28-5 Transcription of primary granule constituents is terminally silenced once a granulocyte matures and leaves the bone marrow.[4] Myeloperoxidase (MPO) and proteinase 3 (PR3) mRNA transcripts are found almost exclusively at the early promyelocyte stage. Neutrophil maturation-linked gene silencing results in morphologic changes in nuclear DNA three or four lobes structures joined by thin DNA-containing filaments.[6,7]

necrotizing vascular injury, a pathologic hallmark of the ANCAs. A mechanism whereby ANCAs would physically interact with endothelial cells is not obvious, since the expression of ANCA antigens (PR3 and MPO) is restricted to myeloid lineage cells.[93,94] Nonetheless, there arose a controversy in the 1990s of whether or not cytokines could influence PR3 and MPO expression on the endothelial cell surface[95–97] rendering the endothelium a direct target for ANCA-induced injury.[98–100] Conflicting reports on PR3 expression in endothelial cells spurred another search for mRNA of PR3 and MPO using TaqMan polymerase chain reaction. These data confirmed the findings of King and coworkers that endothelial cells do not express ANCA antigens.[101] In light of this information, it is highly unlikely that PR3 or MPO production by an endothelial cell is a common feature or that such rare and undetected production would be responsible for the major pathogenic events in ANCA-associated systemic vasculitis. Current knowledge continues to support the view that ANCA pathogenesis is a direct result of the autoantibodies' effects on neutrophils and monocyte causing activation inappropriately, consequently leading to endothelial and vascular injury.

How do these inappropriately released granule constituents cause endothelial injury? Several years ago, it was discovered that PR3 can traverse the endothelial plasma membrane, and, once internalized, induce apoptosis.[102] It appears that this apoptotic function specifically affects endothelial cells because this effect was not observed in epithelial cells. Endothelial cells also internalize MPO.[102] Unlike PR3, MPO does not cause apoptosis, but does cause an increase in intracellular oxidant radicals. Currently, what is known about PR3-mediated endothelial cell apoptosis is that both the catalytically inactive and active forms of PR3 induce apoptosis; however, the kinetics of death are quite different. To study the mechanism(s) of inactive PR3-induced apoptosis, the PR3 molecule was subcloned and expressed as three fragments: N-terminal (PR3n), middle (PR3m), and C-terminal (PR3c). Each fragment contains only one member of the catalytic triad, rendering the fragments enzymatically inactive. We found that the 100–amino acid C-terminal region of the PR3 molecule carries the apoptotic function, and this fragment alone induced apoptosis in a time frame (12–24 hours) similar to that of the full-length inactive molecule (Fig. 28-6).[102] These findings support the hypothesis that the mechanism of PR3-induced apoptosis does not necessarily require its proteolytic function.

Proteolytically active PR3 can induce apoptosis in endothelial cells in 4 to 6 hours compared with the 24 hours required for inactive PR3.[102,103] This difference can be explained, in part, by data that show that PR3 is a caspase-like protease that can cleave proteins normally cleaved by caspases during the apoptotic program.[104,105] Thus, the speculation is that PR3 sidesteps caspase requirements and accelerates the apoptotic process. For example, nuclear factor-κB (NF-κB) is a substrate for PR3 and for caspases (Fig. 28-7). Sequence analysis showed that the PR3 cleavage site is unique with respect to the reported caspase cleavage site. Another caspase-3 substrate that is also cleaved by PR3 is p21 (Waf1/Cip1/Sdi1) (see Fig. 28-7),[52,106,107] a protein known as a major determinant of cell fate.[108] For example, cleavage of p21 is required for endothelial cell death.[105] Reportedly, PR3 mimics caspase-2 and -3 by cleaving the Sp1 transcription factor,[109] and mimics caspase-1 in its ability to process IL-1β.[110] It appears that PR3 performs similar functions in tissues at sites of neutrophil and monocyte recruitment based on findings that the p21 fragment was identified in inflamed bowel tissue, coincident with detectable PR3.[52] Moreover, PR3 has the capacity to specifically process biologically important proteins, such as angiotensinogen,[111] transforming growth factor-β1,[112] TNF-α[110,113] and IL-32.[114] The caspase-like function of PR3 provides a unique mechanism of cross talk between leukocytes and endothelial cells at sites of inflammation impacting both cytokine networks and cell viability.

PR3 can regulate signaling pathways.[115] PR3 causes sustained activation of c-Jun N-terminal kinase 1 (JNK 1), a primary apoptosis-signaling pathway.[103] PR3 can induce IL-8 production in endothelial cells, and furthermore, addition of α1-antitrypsin inhibitor does not significantly influence this effect, indicating that proteolytic activity is not required.[116] In addition, the pro-form of PR3 can compete with granulocyte colony-stimulating factor for binding to its receptor,[117] thus setting a precedent for the involvement of PR3 in receptor-mediated events.

MPO is internalized into endothelial cells by an energy-dependent process,[102,118] which is inhibitable by heparin or endoglycosidase, suggesting involvement of cell surface glycosaminoglycans.[49,119] In fact, MPO was shown to transcytose intact endothelium and co-localize with the extracellular matrix protein fibronectin. Exposure to MPO results in cellular damage by activation of the MPO-H_2O_2-halide system, which in the presence of chloride leads to the formation of potent oxidants. Chloramide intermediates are formed that lead to the fragmentation of extracellular matrix protein, a process that continues even after the consumption of HOCl has ceased.[120] In the presence of the substrates H_2O_2 and NO_2^-,

MPO catalyzes nitration of tyrosine residues on extracellular matrix proteins, especially fibronectin.[118,121] The radicals generated by MPO cause consumption of nitric oxide and alter nitric oxide's signaling and vasodilatory effects during inflammation.[122]

Identification of an endothelial receptor(s) for MPO and/or PR3 could reveal functional roles not yet associated with these proteins, and offer an explanation for the focal nature of vascular injury seen in ANCA vasculitis. It is possible that only those vascular beds expressing the receptor(s) are susceptible to injury. Of equal importance, unraveling the complex potentials of these proteins at the cellular level could impact approaches of therapeutic intervention in inflammatory diseases.

CONCLUSION

Studies of the molecular biology of ANCA glomerulonephritis have added much to our understanding, but much remains to be elucidated in terms of what causes and modifies this dreadful disease. A recent breakthrough was the identification of complementary proteins as a potential *cause* of ANCA glomerulonephritis offering an explanation of *how* it develops, as delineated in the Theory of Autoantigen Complementarity. The novelty and the tremendous potential of this research make it very exciting as we continue to ascertain the mechanistic processes surrounding complementary proteins in ANCA glomerulonephritis.

Neutrophils and monocytes, which contain abundant amounts of ANCA target antigens, are the critical cells in the pathogenesis of ANCA glomerulonephritis. Leukocytoclasia is a hallmark of this disease process, and recent observations in our animal model of anti-MPO antibody-induced glomerulonephritis demonstrated that the complete removal of neutrophils ameliorates disease activity.[123] Establishment of this credible mouse model of ANCA glomerulonephritis was a major accomplishment that will enable us to advance the understanding of the pathogenic processes that cause glomerular injury and the immunogenic events that give rise to the ANCA autoimmune response.

A second critical component in the etiology of ANCA glomerulonephritis is the reactivation of once-silenced genes in mature neutrophils and monocytes, leading to increased antigen availability. These observations raise a number of questions and open the intriguing possibility that a new therapeutic approach could be considered in these patients. If we could learn what regulates MPO and PR3 messages, conceivably we could selectively turn off antigen production and ameliorate disease activity.

We now have microarray data on leukocytes from over 30 ANCA patients with more than 200 controls, including patients with IgA nephropathy, systemic lupus erythematosus, rheumatoid arthritis, and inflammatory bowel diseases. Using

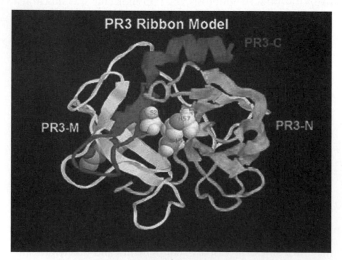

Figure 28-6 Ribbon model of proteinase 3 molecule. The 100–amino acid apoptosis domain appears as the darkest strand. **(See Color Plate 5.)**

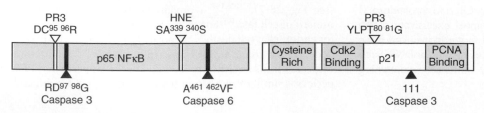

Figure 28-7 Proteinase 3 (PR3), human neutrophil elastase (HNE), and p21 cleavage sites compared with caspase cleavage sites.

an iterative bioinformatics approach, we have identified genes that correlate with ANCA glomerulonephritis disease activity and are still uncovering others. Now, we are ready to embark on an approach that uses candidate genes as markers of clinical disease activity. The clinical exigency is great, for there is no existing clinical marker of disease activity, including ANCA titers, that reliably answers the critical clinical conundrum of disease status for patients and their doctors with ANCA glomerulonephritis, or for any autoimmune disease.

References

1. Davies DJ, Moran JE, Niall JF, Ryan GB: Segmental necrotising glomerulonephritis with antineutrophil antibody: Possible arbovirus aetiology? BMJ 285:606–610, 1982.
2. van der Woude FJ, Rasmussen N, Lobatto S, et al: Autoantibodies against neutrophils and monocytes. Lancet 1:425–429, 1985.
3. Falk RJ, Jennette JC: Anti-neutrophil cytoplasmic autoantibodies with specificity for myeloperoxidase in patients with systemic vasculitis and idiopathic necrotizing and crescentic glomerulonephritis. N Engl J Med 318:1651–1657, 1988.
4. Jennette JC, Wilkman AS, Falk RJ: Anti-neutrophil cytoplasmic autoantibody-associated glomerulonephritis and vasculitis. Am J Pathol 135:921–930, 1989.
5. Ludemann J, Utecht B, Gross WL: Anti-neutrophil cytoplasm antibodies in Wegener's granulomatosis recognize an elastinolytic enzyme. J Exp Med 171:357–362, 1990.
6. Mulder AH, Heeringa P, Brouwer E, et al: Activation of granulocytes by anti-neutrophil cytoplasmic antibodies (ANCA): A Fc gamma RII-dependent process. Clin Exp Immunol 98:270–278, 1994.
7. Hagen EC, Ballieux BE, van Es LA, et al: Antineutrophil cytoplasmic autoantibodies: A review of the antigens involved, the assays, and the clinical and possible pathogenetic consequences. Blood 81:1996–2002, 1993.
8. Niles JL, Pan GL, Collins AB, et al: Antigen-specific radioimmunoassays for anti-neutrophil cytoplasmic antibodies in the diagnosis of rapidly progressive glomerulonephritis. J Am Soc Nephrol 2:27–36, 1991.
9. Jennette JC, Falk RJ: Disease associations and pathogenic role of antineutrophil cytoplasmic autoantibodies in vasculitis. Curr Opin Rheumatol 4:9–15, 1992.
10. Xiao H, Heeringa P, Hu P, et al: Antineutrophil cytoplasmic autoantibodies specific for myeloperoxidase cause glomerulonephritis and vasculitis in mice. J Clin Invest 110:955–963, 2002.
11. Falk RJ, Jennette JC: ANCA are pathogenic—Oh yes they are! J Am Soc Nephrol 13:1977–1979, 2002.
12. Brouwer E, Huitema MG, Klok PA, et al: Antimyeloperoxidase-associated proliferative glomerulonephritis: an animal model. J Exp Med 177:905–914, 1993.
13. Heeringa P, Brouwer E, Klok PA, et al: Autoantibodies to myeloperoxidase aggravate mild anti-glomerular-basement-membrane-mediated glomerular injury in the rat. Am J Pathol 149:1695–1706, 1996.
14. Falk RJ, Terrell RS, Charles LA, Jennette JC: Anti-neutrophil cytoplasmic autoantibodies induce neutrophils to degranulate and produce oxygen radicals in vitro. Proc Natl Acad Sci U S A 87:4115–4119, 1990.
15. Johnson PA, Alexander HD, McMillan SA, Maxwell AP: Up-regulation of the granulocyte adhesion molecule Mac-1 by autoantibodies in autoimmune vasculitis. Clin Exp Immunol 107:513–519, 1997.
16. Keogan MT, Esnault VL, Green AJ, et al: Activation of normal neutrophils by anti-neutrophil cytoplasm antibodies. Clin Exp Immunol 90:228–234, 1992.
17. Kettritz R, Jennette JC, Falk RJ: Crosslinking of ANCA-antigens stimulates superoxide release by human neutrophils. J Am Soc Nephrol 8:386–394, 1997.
18. Lai KN, Lockwood CM: The effect of anti-neutrophil cytoplasm autoantibodies on the signal transduction in human neutrophils. Clin Exp Immunol 85:396–401, 1991.
19. Savage CO, Pottinger BE, Gaskin G, et al: Autoantibodies developing to myeloperoxidase and proteinase 3 in systemic vasculitis stimulate neutrophil cytotoxicity toward cultured endothelial cells. Am J Pathol 141:335–342, 1992.
20. Porges AJ, Redecha PB, Kimberly WT, et al: Anti-neutrophil cytoplasmic antibodies engage and activate human neutrophils via Fc gamma RIIa. J Immunol 153:1271–1280, 1994.
21. Falk RJ, Jennette JC: Immune complex induced glomerular lesions in C5 sufficient and deficient mice. Kidney Int 30:678–686, 1986.
22. Gross WL, Schmitt WH, Csernok E: ANCA and associated diseases: Immunodiagnostic and pathogenetic aspects. Clin Exp Immunol 91:1–12, 1993.
23. De'Oliviera J, Gaskin G, Dash A, et al: Relationship between disease activity and anti-neutrophil cytoplasmic antibody concentration in long-term management of systemic vasculitis. Am J Kidney Dis 25:380–389, 1995.
24. Dolman KM, Gans RO, Vervaat TJ, et al: Vasculitis and antineutrophil cytoplasmic autoantibodies associated with propylthiouracil therapy. Lancet 342:651–652, 1993.
25. Benoist C, Mathis D: Autoimmunity. The pathogen connection [news]. Nature 394:227–228, 1998.
26. Kirvan CA, Swedo SE, Heuser JS, Cunningham MW: Mimicry and autoantibody-mediated neuronal cell signaling in Sydenham chorea. Nat Med 9:914–920, 2003.
27. Levin MC, Lee SM, Kalume F, et al: Autoimmunity due to molecular mimicry as a cause of neurological disease. Nat Med 8:509–513, 2002.
28. Oldstone MB: Molecular mimicry and autoimmune disease. Cell 50:819–820, 1987.
29. Weathington NM, Blalock JE: Rational design of peptide vaccines for autoimmune disease: Harnessing molecular recognition to fix a broken network. Expert Rev Vaccines 2:61–73, 2003.
30. Singh H: Genetic analysis of transcription factors implicated in B lymphocyte development. Immunol Res 13:280–290, 1994.
31. Griffith ME, Coulthart A, Pusey CD: T cell responses to myeloperoxidase (MPO) and proteinase 3 (PR3) in patients with systemic vasculitis. Clin Exp Immunol 103:253–258, 1996.
32. McGuire KL, Holmes DS: Role of complementary proteins in autoimmunity: An old idea re-emerges with new twists. Trends Immunol 26:367–372, 2005.
33. Shoenfeld Y: The idiotypic network in autoimmunity: Antibodies that bind antibodies that bind antibodies. Nat Med 10:17–18, 2004.
34. Mekler LB: Specific selective interaction between amino acid groups of polypeptide chains. Biofizika 14:581–584, 1969.
35. Mekler LB: On the specific mutual interaction of amino acid residues of polypeptide chains and amino acid residues with codons. Oncology 27:286–288, 1973.
36. Blalock JE, Smith EM: Hydropathic anti-complementarity of amino acids based on the genetic code. Biochem Biophys Res Commun 121:203–207, 1984.
37. Blalock JE: Complementarity of peptides specified by "sense" and "antisense" strands of DNA. Trends Biotechnol 8:140–144, 1990.
38. Heal JR, Roberts GW, Raynes JG, et al: Specific interactions between sense and complementary peptides: The basis for the proteomic code. Chembiochem 3:136–151, 2002.
39. Fassina G, Melli M: Identification of interactive sites of proteins and protein receptors by computer-assisted searches for

complementary peptide sequences. Immunomethods 5:114–120, 1994.

40. Fassina G: Complementary peptides as recognition molecules. Agents Actions Suppl 46:109–120, 1995.

41. Bost KL, Blalock JE: Preparation and use of complementary peptides. Methods Enzymol 168:16–28, 1989.

42. Bost KL, Blalock JE: Production of anti-idiotypic antibodies by immunization with a pair of complementary peptides. J Mol Recognit 1:179–183, 1989.

43. Smith LR, Bost KL, Blalock JE: Generation of idiotypic and anti-idiotypic antibodies by immunization with peptides encoded by complementary RNA: a possible molecular basis for the network theory. J Immunol 138:7–9, 1987.

44. Jerne NK: Towards a network theory of the immune system. Ann Immunol (Paris) 125C:373–389, 1974.

45. Jerne NK, Roland J, Cazenave PA: Recurrent idiotopes and internal images. EMBO J 1:243–247, 1982.

46. Erlanger BF: Auto-anti-idiotypy, autoimmunity and some thoughts on the structure of internal images. Int Rev Immunol 5:131–137, 1989.

47. Erlanger BF, Cleveland WL, Wassermann NH, et al: Auto-anti-idiotype: A basis for autoimmunity and a strategy for anti-receptor antibodies. Immunol Rev 94:23–37, 1986.

48. Hill BL, Erlanger BF: Monoclonal antibodies to the thyrotropin receptor raised by an autoantiidiotypic protocol and their relationship to monoclonal autoantibodies from Graves' patients. Endocrinology 122:2840–2850, 1988.

49. Shoenfeld Y: Idiotypic induction of autoimmunity: A new aspect of the idiotypic network. FASEB J 8:1296–1301, 1994.

50. Shoenfeld Y, Rauova L, Gilburd B, et al: Efficacy of IVIG affinity-purified anti-double-stranded DNA anti-idiotypic antibodies in the treatment of an experimental murine model of systemic lupus erythematosus. Int Immunol 14:1303–1311, 2002.

51. Shoenfeld Y: Anti-DNA idiotypes: From induction of disease to novel therapeutic approaches. Immunol Lett 100:73–77, 2005.

52. Pendergraft WF 3rd, Preston GA, Shah RR, et al: Autoimmunity is triggered by cPR-3(105–201) a protein complementary to human autoantigen proteinase-3. Nat Med 10:72–79, 2004.

53. Preston GA, Pendergraft WF 3rd, Falk RJ: New insights that link microbes with the generation of antineutrophil cytoplasmic autoantibodies: The theory of autoantigen complementarity. Curr Opin Nephrol Hypertens 14:217–222, 2005.

54. Rodriguez-Pla A, Stone JH: Vasculitis and systemic infections. Curr Opin Rheumatol 18:39–47, 2006.

55. Falk RJ, Hogan S, Carey TS, Jennette JC: Clinical course of anti-neutrophil cytoplasmic autoantibody-associated glomerulonephritis and systemic vasculitis. The Glomerular Disease Collaborative Network [see comments]. Ann Intern Med 113:656–663, 1990.

56. Stegeman CA, Tervaert JW, Sluiter WJ, et al: Association of chronic nasal carriage of Staphylococcus aureus and higher relapse rates in Wegener granulomatosis. Ann Intern Med 120:12–17, 1994.

57. Pudifin DJ, Duursma J, Gathiram V, Jackson TF: Invasive amoebiasis is associated with the development of anti-neutrophil cytoplasmic antibody. Clin Exp Immunol 97:48–51, 1994.

58. Huugen D, Xiao H, van Esch A, et al: Aggravation of anti-myeloperoxidase antibody-induced glomerulonephritis by bacterial lipopolysaccharide: role of tumor necrosis factor-alpha. Am J Pathol 167:47–58, 2005.

59. Routsias JG, Touloupi E, Dotsika E, et al: Unmasking the anti-La/SSB response in sera from patients with Sjogren's syndrome by specific blocking of anti-idiotypic antibodies to La/SSB antigenic determinants. Mol Med 8:293–305, 2002.

60. Routsias JG, Dotsika E, Touloupi E, et al: Idiotype-anti-idiotype circuit in non-autoimmune mice after immunization with the epitope and complementary epitope 289–308aa of La/SSB: implications for the maintenance and perpetuation of the anti-La/SSB response. J Autoimmun 21:17–26, 2003.

61. Papamattheou MG, Routsias JG, Karagouni EE, et al: T cell help is required to induce idiotypic-anti-idiotypic autoantibody network after immunization with complementary epitope 289-308aa of La/SSB autoantigen in non-autoimmune mice. Clin Exp Immunol 135:416–426, 2004.

62. Pendergraft WF 3rd, Pressler BM, Jennette JC, et al: Autoantigen complementarity: A new theory implicating complementary proteins as initiators of autoimmune disease. J Mol Med 83:12–25, 2005.

63. Mutasim DF: Autoimmune bullous dermatoses in the elderly: Diagnosis and management. Drugs Aging 20:663–681, 2003.

64. Lohrisch I, Haustein UF, Baumert A, Szeskus H: Immune response to tetanus toxoid in bullous pemphigoid. Dermatol Monatsschr 171:153–157, 1985.

65. Fournier B, Descamps V, Bouscarat F, et al: Bullous pemphigoid induced by vaccination. Br J Dermatol 135:153–154, 1996.

66. Baykal C, Okan G, Sarica R: Childhood bullous pemphigoid developed after the first vaccination. J Am Acad Dermatol 44:348–350, 2001.

67. Erbagci Z: Childhood bullous pemphigoid following hepatitis B immunization. J Dermatol 29:781–785, 2002.

68. Tzartos SJ, Kokla A, Walgrave SL, Conti-Tronconi BM: Localization of the main immunogenic region of human muscle acetylcholine receptor to residues 67-76 of the alpha subunit. Proc Natl Acad Sci U S A 85:2899–2903, 1988.

69. Ionescu-Drinea M, Serbanescu G, Nicolau C, Voiculescu V: Association of myasthenic and neuritic symptoms following administration of antitetanic serum. Rev Roum Neurol 10:239–243, 1973.

70. Giovanardi Rossi P, Nanni AG, Gambi D, Borromei A: [Juvenile myasthenia gravis of possible post-vaccinal inoculation: study of 2 cases]. Riv Neurol 46:265–296, 1976.

71. Lehner B, Williams G, Campbell RD, Sanderson CM: Antisense transcripts in the human genome. Trends Genet 18:63–65, 2002.

72. Lavorgna G, Dahary D, Lehner B, et al: In search of antisense. Trends Biochem Sci 29:88–94, 2004.

73. Labrador M, Mongelard F, Plata-Rengifo P, et al: Protein encoding by both DNA strands. Nature 409:1000, 2001.

74. Van Den Eynde BJ, Gaugler B, Probst-Kepper M, et al: A new antigen recognized by cytolytic T lymphocytes on a human kidney tumor results from reverse strand transcription. J Exp Med 190:1793–1800, 1999.

75. Yang JJ, Pendergraft WF, Alcorta DA, et al: Circumvention of normal constraints on granule protein gene expression in peripheral blood neutrophils and monocytes of patients with antineutrophil cytoplasmic autoantibody-associated glomerulonephritis. J Am Soc Nephrol 15:2103–2114, 2004.

76. Ohlsson S, Hellmark T, Pieters K, et al: Increased monocyte transcription of the proteinase 3 gene in small vessel vasculitis. Clin Exp Immunol 141:174–182, 2005.

77. Halbwachs-Mecarelli L, Bessou G, Lesavre P, et al: Bimodal distribution of proteinase 3 (PR3) surface expression reflects a constitutive heterogeneity in the polymorphonuclear neutrophil pool. FEBS Lett 374:29–33, 1995.

78. Preston GA, Waga I, Alcorta DA, et al: Gene expression profiles of circulating leukocytes correlate with renal disease activity in IgA nephropathy. Kidney Int 65:420–430, 2004.

79. Kobold AC, Kallenberg CG, Tervaert JW: Monocyte activation in patients with Wegener's granulomatosis. Ann Rheum Dis 58:237–245, 1999.

80. Kocher M, Edberg JC, Fleit HB, Kimberly RP: Antineutrophil cytoplasmic antibodies preferentially engage Fc gammaRIIIb on human neutrophils. J Immunol 161:6909–6914, 1998.

81. Locke IC, Leaker B, Cambridge G: A comparison of the characteristics of circulating anti-myeloperoxidase autoantibodies in vasculitis with those in non-vasculitic conditions. Clin Exp Immunol 115:369–376, 1999.

82. Reumaux D, Vossebeld PJ, Roos D, Verhoeven AJ: Effect of tumor necrosis factor-induced integrin activation on Fc gamma receptor II-mediated signal transduction: Relevance for activation of neutrophils by anti-proteinase 3 or anti-myeloperoxidase antibodies. Blood 86:3189–3195, 1995.

83. Yang JJ, Preston GA, Alcorta DA, et al: Expression profile of leukocyte genes activated by anti-neutrophil cytoplasmic autoantibodies (ANCA). Kidney Int 62:1638–1649, 2002.

84. Mulder AH, Stegeman CA, Kallenberg CG: Activation of granulocytes by anti-neutrophil cytoplasmic antibodies (ANCA) in Wegener's granulomatosis: A predominant role for the IgG3 subclass of ANCA. Clin Exp Immunol 101:227–232, 1995.

85. Alcorta D, Preston G, Munger W, et al: Microarray studies of gene expression in circulating leukocytes in kidney diseases. Exp Nephrol 10:139–149, 2002.

86. Kurosawa S, Esmon CT, Stearns-Kurosawa DJ: The soluble endothelial protein C receptor binds to activated neutrophils: Involvement of proteinase-3 and CD11b/CD18. J Immunol 165:4697–4703, 2000.

87. Calderwood JW, Williams JM, Morgan MD, et al: ANCA induces beta2 integrin and CXC chemokine-dependent neutrophil-endothelial cell interactions that mimic those of highly cytokine-activated endothelium. J Leukoc Biol 77:33–43, 2005.

88. Williams JM, Savage CO: Characterization of the regulation and functional consequences of p21ras activation in neutrophils by antineutrophil cytoplasm antibodies. J Am Soc Nephrol 16:90–96, 2005.

89. Williams JM, Ben-Smith A, Hewins P, et al: Activation of the G(i) heterotrimeric G protein by ANCA IgG F(ab')2 fragments is necessary but not sufficient to stimulate the recruitment of those downstream mediators used by intact ANCA IgG. J Am Soc Nephrol 14:661–669, 2003.

90. Brooks CJ, King WJ, Radford DJ, et al: IL-1 beta production by human polymorphonuclear leucocytes stimulated by anti-neutrophil cytoplasmic autoantibodies: Relevance to systemic vasculitis. Clin Exp Immunol 106:273–279, 1996.

91. Hashimoto S, Matsumoto K, Gon Y, et al: p38 Mitogen-activated protein kinase regulates IL-8 expression in human pulmonary vascular endothelial cells. Eur Respir J 13:1357–1364, 1999.

92. Hewins P, Morgan MD, Holden N, et al: IL-18 is upregulated in the kidney and primes neutrophil responsiveness in ANCA-associated vasculitis. Kidney Int 69:605–615, 2006.

93. Sturrock A, Franklin KF, Hoidal JR: Human proteinase-3 expression is regulated by PU.1 in conjunction with a cytidine-rich element. J Biol Chem 271:32392–32402, 1996.

94. Chen HM, Zhang P, Voso MT, et al: Neutrophils and monocytes express high levels of PU-1 (Spi-1) but not Spi-B. Blood 85:2918–2928, 1995.

95. Mayet WJ, Csernok E, Szymkowiak C, et al: Human endothelial cells express proteinase-3, the target antigen of anticytoplasmic antibodies in Wegener's granulomatosis. Blood 82:1221–1229, 1993.

96. Mayet WJ, Hermann EM, Csernok E, et al: In vitro interactions of c-ANCA (antibodies to proteinase 3) with human endothelial cells. Adv Exp Med Biol 336:109–113, 1993.

97. King WJ, Adu D, Daha MR, et al: Endothelial cells and renal epithelial cells do not express the Wegener's autoantigen, proteinase 3. Clin Exp Immunol 102:98–105, 1995.

98. Sibelius U, Hattar K, Schenkel A, et al: Wegener's granulomatosis: Anti-proteinase 3 antibodies are potent inductors of human endothelial cell signaling and leakage response. J Exp Med 187:497–503, 1998.

99. Mayet WJ, Schwarting A, Orth T, et al: Signal transduction pathways of membrane expression of proteinase 3 (PR-3) in human endothelial cells. Eur J Clin Invest 27:893–899, 1997.

100. Johnson PA, Alexander HD, McMillan SA, Maxwell AP: Up-regulation of the endothelial cell adhesion molecule intercellular adhesion molecule-1 (ICAM-1) by autoantibodies in autoimmune vasculitis. Clin Exp Immunol 108:234–242, 1997.

101. Pendergraft WF, Alcorta DA, Segelmark M, et al: ANCA antigens, proteinase 3 and myeloperoxidase, are not expressed in endothelial cells. Kidney Int 57:1981–1990, 2000.

102. Yang JJ, Preston GA, Pendergraft WF, et al: Internalization of proteinase 3 is concomitant with endothelial cell apoptosis and internalization of myeloperoxidase with generation of intracellular oxidants. Am J Pathol 158:581–592, 2001.

103. Preston GA, Zarella CS, Pendergraft WF 3rd, et al: Novel effects of neutrophil-derived proteinase 3 and elastase on the vascular endothelium involve in vivo cleavage of NF-kappaB and proapoptotic changes in JNK, ERK, and p38 MAPK signaling pathways. J Am Soc Nephrol 13:2840–2849, 2002.

104. Kang KH, Lee KH, Kim MY, Choi KH: Caspase-3-mediated cleavage of the NF-κB subunit p65 at the NH2-terminus potentiates naphtoquinone analog-induced apoptosis. J Biol Chem 24:24, 2001.

105. Levkau B, Koyama H, Raines EW, et al: Cleavage of p21Cip1/Waf1 and p27Kip1 mediates apoptosis in endothelial cells through activation of Cdk2: Role of a caspase cascade. Mol Cell 1:553–563, 1998.

106. Witko-Sarsat V, Canteloup S, Durant S, et al: Cleavage of P21/Waf1 by proteinase 3, a myeloid specific serine protease, potentiates cell proliferation. J Biol Chem 26:26, 2002.

107. Jiang H, Lin J, Su ZZ, Collart FR, et al: Induction of differentiation in human promyelocytic HL-60 leukemia cells activates p21, WAF1/CIP1, expression in the absence of p53. Oncogene 9:3397–3406, 1994.

108. Javelaud D, Besancon F: Inactivation of p21WAF1 sensitizes cells to apoptosis via an increase of both p14ARF and p53 levels and an alteration of the Bax/Bcl-2 ratio. J Biol Chem 277:37949–37954, 2002.

109. Piedrafita FJ, Pfahl M: Retinoid-induced apoptosis and Sp1 cleavage occur independently of transcription and require caspase activation. Mol Cell Biol 17:6348–6358, 1997.

110. Coeshott C, Ohnemus C, Pilyavskaya A, et al: Converting enzyme-independent release of tumor necrosis factor alpha and IL-1beta from a stimulated human monocytic cell line in the presence of activated neutrophils or purified proteinase 3. Proc Natl Acad Sci U S A 96:6261–6266, 1999.

111. Ramaha A, Patston PA: Release and degradation of angiotensin I and angiotensin II from angiotensinogen by neutrophil serine proteinases. Arch Biochem Biophys 397:77–83, 2002.

112. Csernok E, Szymkowiak CH, Mistry N, et al: Transforming growth factor-beta (TGF-beta) expression and interaction with proteinase 3 (PR3) in anti-neutrophil cytoplasmic antibody (ANCA)- associated vasculitis. Clin Exp Immunol 105:104–111, 1996.

113. Bank U, Ansorge S: More than destructive: Neutrophil-derived serine proteases in cytokine bioactivity control. J Leukoc Biol 69:197–206, 2001.

114. Novick D, Rubinstein M, Azam T, et al: Proteinase 3 is an IL-32 binding protein. Proc Natl Acad Sci U S A 103:3316–3321, 2006.

115. Sugawara S: Immune functions of proteinase 3. Crit Rev Immunol 25:343–360, 2005.

116. Berger SP, Seelen MA, Hiemstra PS, et al: Proteinase 3, the major autoantigen of Wegener's granulomatosis, enhances IL-8 production by endothelial cells in vitro. J Am Soc Nephrol 7:694–701, 1996.

117. Skold S, Rosberg B, Gullberg U, Olofsson T: A secreted proform of neutrophil proteinase 3 regulates the proliferation of granulopoietic progenitor cells. Blood 93:849–856, 1999.

118. Baldus S, Eiserich JP, Mani A, et al: Endothelial transcytosis of myeloperoxidase confers specificity to vascular ECM proteins as targets of tyrosine nitration. J Clin Invest 108:1759–1770, 2001.

119. Baldus S, Heitzer T, Eiserich JP, et al: Myeloperoxidase enhances nitric oxide catabolism during myocardial ischemia and reperfusion. Free Radic Biol Med 37:902–911, 2004.

120. Woods AA, Linton SM, Davies MJ: Detection of HOCl-mediated protein oxidation products in the extracellular matrix of human atherosclerotic plaques. Biochem J 370:729–735, 2003.

121. Brennan ML, Wu W, Fu X, et al: A tale of two controversies: Defining both the role of peroxidases in nitrotyrosine formation in vivo using eosinophil peroxidase and myeloperoxidase-deficient mice, and the nature of peroxidase-generated reactive nitrogen species. J Biol Chem 277:17415–17427, 2002.

122. Eiserich JP, Baldus S, Brennan ML, et al: Myeloperoxidase, a leukocyte-derived vascular NO oxidase. Science 296:2391–2394, 2002.

123. Xiao H, Heeringa P, Liu Z, et al: The role of neutrophils in the induction of glomerulonephritis by anti-myeloperoxidase antibodies. Am J Pathol 167:39–45, 2005.

Chapter 29

Systemic Lupus Erythematosus and the Kidney

Vicki Rubin Kelley, Laurence Morel, and Mary H. Foster

Systemic lupus erythematosus (SLE, lupus) is one of the most mysterious human diseases. This autoimmune illness afflicts more than 1 million persons in the United States and has a bewildering constellation of forms. Lupus is a heterogeneous disease; the clinical manifestations wax and wane, and range from mild to lethal. Lupus is triggered by the complex interactions of genetic and environmental susceptibility factors. The resulting immune dysregulation of B- and T-cell autoreactivity leads to diverse clinical manifestations, including nephritis, arthritis, serositis, skin lesions, hematopoietic cytopenias, cerebritis, and arteritis. Kidney disease occurs in a large proportion of patients with lupus (30%–50%).[1] Even with optimal therapy, up to one fourth of these patients progress to end-stage renal disease (ESRD). The survival rate in lupus patients at 10 years is 80% to 90%, but drops an additional 20% in patients with nephritis.[2] Thus, kidney disease is a major cause of morbidity and mortality in lupus.

Lupus nephritis (LN) is characterized by mononuclear cell infiltration, antibody deposits in the kidney, and aberrant cytokine expression. These features of inflammation result in renal damage. This chapter reviews the advances in the genetics and pathogenesis of lupus. In the first section, the genetics of human and animal models is reviewed. This is followed by a section on pathogenesis, encompassing the immune abnormalities (B and T cell) leading to the loss of tolerance and initiation of disease, humoral components such as nephritogenic autoantibodies, complement and Fcγ receptors that mediate disease, and downstream events that are responsible for inflammation, most notably the role of macrophage and T cells in LN. This overview highlights the need for continuing intensive and comprehensive studies on genetic susceptibility and critical pathogenetic factors to facilitate predicting and treating patients with LN.

GENETICS

SLE is a Multifactorial Disease

Susceptibility to develop SLE is a multifactorial process in which both genetic and environmental components play a role. The strength of the genetic contribution and familial aggregation to a multifactorial disease is measured with a parameter called λ_s, which compares the relative risk for disease in siblings of patients to that of the population at large. The λ_s value of 15 to 20 for SLE indicates a strong genetic basis.[3] Other major autoimmune diseases, such as type I diabetes and multiple sclerosis, have a λ_s similar to SLE.[4] The inheritance of this type of multigenic diseases has been coined "threshold liability."

Contrary to mendelian inheritance, in which there is an obligate relationship between the inheritance of an allele and a specific phenotype, a threshold liability disease develops when an individual cumulates a number of genetic and environmental factors that is greater than the disease threshold.[3] The involvement of nongenetic factors in SLE susceptibility is clearly illustrated by a concordance rate between monozygotic twins of 34% to 50%[4]; if SLE susceptibility were purely genetic, the concordance rate would be 100%. Although the existence of environmental/nongenetic factors is widely accepted, the nature of these factors is still hotly debated.

The existence of specific inbred strains of mice that spontaneously develop a lupus-like disease also strongly argues in favor of a genetic basis for SLE susceptibility.[5] As will be detailed below, parallel genetic studies have been conducted in murine models and human populations. Genetic analyses of the murine models have been very useful to understand the threshold liability mode of inheritance and the intricate level of interactions that exist between susceptibility genes.[6] It is not known yet if the same genes mediate lupus in mice and in humans, but it is strongly believed that many of these genes belong to the same functional pathways, as illustrated by the results of multiple gene-targeting experiments (Table 29-1).

The exact number of genes involved in SLE susceptibility is currently unknown. This value may actually be difficult to define, and may not be informative per se, because, as will be illustrated by the data discussed below, SLE susceptibility results from various combinations of different genes. With a few exceptions, the identity of these genes is also unknown. Rapid progress is being made, however, toward their identification, largely benefiting from the completion of the human and mouse genome sequencing projects and the development of high throughput genotyping techniques.[7] Two strategies have been employed in parallel to identify lupus susceptibility genes.

One approach evaluates candidate genes that have been selected based on their function in the immune system (e.g., FcγRIIIa) or their aberrant expression in lupus patients (e.g., IL-8). Statistical associations have then been evaluated on sequence variations within these genes (most often single nucleotide polymorphisms, or SNPs) between patients and controls (Table 29-2). This approach presents inherent limitations; the most obvious is the bias toward genes with an expected contribution to the disease, thus confining the search to the realm of known pathogenic pathways. In addition, a number of statistical issues can hinder result interpretation, which may explain why independent studies have reached opposite conclusions on the association of specific polymorphisms with SLE or LN (see Table 29-2).

Table 29-1 Mouse Genes, Deletion, Overexpression, or Mutation Resulting in Lupus Nephritis

Gene	Protein	Mm chr	Putative QTL*	Type	LN†	Reference
Apoptosis						
Cflar	FLIP	1	Bsxb1 SLEN2	Retroviral expression in lymphocytes	++	84
Bcl2	BCL-2	1		Tg with Eμ enhancer	++	85
Tnfsf6	FasL	1		Gld mutation	+	86
Bcl2l11	Bim	2		KO	+	87
Pik3r1	p85PI3K	3		Constitutive mutant Tg with Lck promoter	++	88
Gadd45a	GADD45α	3		KO	++	89
E2f2	E2F-2	4	Nbal	KO	++	90
Ier-3	IEX1	17		KO	++	91
Tnfrsf6	FAS	19		Lpr mutation	+++	92
Pten	PTEN	19		Hemizygosity	+	93
Lymphocyte activation						
Pdcd1	PD-1	1		KO	++	46
Ptprc	CD45	1		E613E mutation	++	94
Fcgr2b	FcγRIIB	1		KO	++	52
Lyn	LYN	4		KO, gain of function mutation	++	95,96
Tnfsf13b	BLyS	8		Tg	++	97
Csnk2a2	CK2α	8	16p12	Tg in MRL/lpr	+	98
Fli1	Fli-1	9		Tg H-2K^k promoter	++	99
Ifng	IFNγ	10		Tg involucrin promoter Plasmid encoded	++ +	100 101
Tnfrsf13b	TAC1	11		KO	++	102
Pecam1	CD31	11		KO	+	103
Gpr132	G2A	12		KO	+	104
Prkcd	PKCδ	14	SLEN1	KO	++	105
Ifnar1	IFNαR1	16		KO in MRL	++	106
Emk	Par-1	19		KO	++	107
Tnfsf5	CD40L	X		Tg K14 promoter Tg V_H promoter	+ +	108 109
Clearance						
Ssa2	SS-A/Ro	1		KO	++	110
Crp, Sap	CRP, SAP	1		hTg, KO	++	111,112
Tgm2	Tgase 2	2	Wbw1	KO	+	113
Mertk	MER	2	Wbw1	KO	+	114
C1qa	C1qα	4	Nba1	KO	+	115
Mfge8	MFG-E8	7	Nba	KO	+	116
Igh-6	secretory IgM	12		KO	+	117
Dnase1	DNase1	16		KO	++	118
C4	C4	17		KO	+	119

continued

Table 29-1 Mouse Genes, Which Deletion, Overexpression, or Mutation Resulted in Lupus Nephritis—cont'd

Gene	Protein	Mm chr	Putative QTL*	Type	LN†	Reference
Miscellaneous						
Mgat5	N-acetyl-glucosaminyl-transferase V	1		KO	+	120
Nrf2	NRF2	2		KO	++	121
Spp1	Osteopontin	5		Tg	|	56
Esr1	ERα	10		KO	++	122
Il4	IL-4	11		Tg class I promoter	++	123,124
Zfpn1a3	AIOLOS	11		KO	++	125
Man2a1	αMannosidase II	17		KO	+	126

*See Figure 29-1.
†Relative severity, age of onset, or penetrance of renal pathology in each model.
Mm chr, Mus musculas chromosome; QTL, quantitative trait loci; LN, lupus nephritis; KO, knockout.

This approach corresponds conceptually to the analysis of genetically engineered mice in which a gene of interest is either overexpressed as a transgene, or "knocked out," resulting in a null allele (see Table 29-1). This approach is obviously drastic, and does not correspond to the more subtle functional variants that are likely to occur in spontaneous mouse models or in SLE patients. Nonetheless, these studies have been very informative, and have shown that most of the genes whose aberrant expression result in SLE fall into three categories: apoptosis regulation, lymphocyte activation, and apoptotic products/immune complex clearance.[3] Overexpression or deficiency in a large number of genes has been found to result in a lupus-like syndrome in mice.[8,9] An obvious interpretation of this result is that there are many ways leading to SLE and that prevention of systemic autoimmunity has to be tightly controlled. However, these results have to be interpreted with caution, since the mixed genetic background in which many of the gene-targeting effects are evaluated (C57BL/6 X 129) results by itself in the development of autoantibodies.[10,11]

The other approach relies on genome-wide scans of families of SLE patients or specific crosses between susceptible and resistant mouse strains using anonymous DNA markers. Subsequent statistical analyses have mapped the location of genomic regions named quantitative trait loci (QTLs) linked to SLE or LN susceptibility (Tables 29-3 and 29-4). In contrast to the candidate gene approach, genome scans have the potential to identify susceptibility genes with either unknown function, or with functions not previously associated with SLE. However, the identification process for each of these genes is a long and complicated journey. The functional significance of a QTL is a probability that one or several susceptibility alleles are contained within this region. Validation of these statistical results in human studies is achieved through independent replications with other family sets. Several scans have been performed with various sets of SLE families that met the four American College of Rheumatology (ACR) criteria, and so far, eight QTLs have been validated[12] (Fig. 29-1). In the mouse,

standard validation requires the production of congenic strains, which can be accomplished in two ways. The QTL in the susceptible strain can be replaced with the corresponding interval from the resistant strain, and validation is obtained through a loss of phenotype, i.e., a decrease in SLE penetrance, severity, or time of onset. Alternatively, the susceptible interval is bred on the resistant strain, and validation is achieved with a gain of phenotype, i.e., the presentation of an SLE-related phenotype.[7] In addition to their validation value, the "gain-of-phenotype" congenic strains are also a powerful tool to perform functional studies to unravel the mechanisms by which the susceptibility alleles may contribute to the disease process. Congenic strains are also the necessary step toward the production of a high-resolution genetic map, and the eventual identification of the susceptibility alleles.

Genetic Determinants of Lupus Nephritis

SLE is a very heterogeneous disease, affecting various target organs, including the kidneys. It is still a matter of debate within the research community whether end organ targeting has a genetic basis. A number of studies, however, favor a genetic basis for renal involvement in SLE. The risk for developing ESRD is 2.6- to 5.6-fold greater in African Americans than in European Americans,[13] and a number of studies have shown a genetic component to ESRD, either in general[14] or associated with diabetic nephropathy[15] or LN.[16] In the mouse, susceptibility to experimental immune-mediated nephritis varies greatly among strains, which implies a genetic basis.[17] Interestingly, the NZW genome, which contributes to SLE pathogenesis when combined with other genomes such as NZB and BXSB, is associated with a high susceptibility to nephrotoxic autoantibodies.[18]

Nephritis is one of the most serious outcomes associated with a high mortality and morbidity in SLE. Consequently, renal involvement may represent a marker of disease severity rather than a distinct genetic etiology. LN is also strongly

Table 29-2 Genes and Polymorphisms Significantly Associated with Lupus Nephritis (LN), or Increased LN Severity, in SLE Patients

Gene	Protein	Position	Allele	LN*	Comments†	LN neg‡	Comments§
FcγRIIa	FcγRIIA	1q23	R/H131	20	Meta-analysis	22	Meta-analysis
FcγRIIIa	FcγRIIIA	1q23	V/F158	23	Meta-analysis		
IL-10	IL-10	1q31-q32	$(CA)_n$ in promoter	37	Mexican Americans		
			A-597C and	39	Taiwanese		
			T-824C	38	Chinese	60	mixed
PDCD1	PD-1	2q37	PD1.3A	61	Swedes and CA	62	RA
CCR5	CCR5	3p21	D32	63	Spaniards		
IL-8	IL-8	4q13-q21	C-845C	64	Mixed ethnicity U.S.		
SPP1	Osteopontin	4q21-q25	C707T	55	CA		
DRB1	DRβ1	6p21.3	DRB1*1501	34	Italians	66	CA**
						67	Koreans**
			DRB1*0301	34	Italians		
			DRB1*13	65	Mixed ethnicity U.S.		
DQA	DQα	6p21.3	DQA*0101	34	Italians		
DQB	DQβ	6p21.3	DQB*0201	34	Italians		
				65	Mixed ethnicity U.S.		
ER	Estrogen receptor	6q25.1	PpXx	68	Chinese		
eNOS	eNOS	7q36	Intron 4 repeat	69	Koreans		
PAI-I	Plasminogen activator inhibitor	7q21.3-q22	-675 4G4G INDE	70	Chinese		
MBL2	Mannose-binding lectin	10q11.2-q21	Gly 54 Asp	71	Spaniards		
UG	Uteroglobin	11q12.3-q13.1	A38G	72	Italians		
VDR	Vit D receptor	12q12-q14	bb Bsml RFLP allele	73	Japanese	74,75	Taiwanese
IFNγ	IFNγ	12q14	allele 114	76	Japanese		
IG VH3	Ig VH3	16p11.2	Hv3005	77	Koreans		
MCP-1	MCP-1	17q11.2-q21.1	A-2518G	40,41	Koreans	63	Spaniards
					Mixed ethnicity U.S.	78	Japanese
ACE	ACE	17q23	Alu I/D	79	Japanese	81	Koreans
				80	Mixed ethnicity U.S.	82	Israeli
EPCR	Endothelial protein C receptor	20q11.2	A6936G	83	Mixed ethnicity U.S.		

* Reference of the study reporting a significant association with LN.
† Ethnic groups analyzed in the study reporting significant association with LN.
‡ Reference of the study reporting a lack of association with LN.
§ Ethnic groups analyzed reporting a lack of association with LN.
** Association with SLE, but not LN.
CA, Caucasians; AA, African Americans.

Table 29-3 Quantitative Trait Loci (QTL) Linked to Human Lupus Nephritis (LN)

QTL	Position	Ethnicity	Reference	SLE QTL*	Candidate Gene†	Mouse QTL‡
SLEN2	2q34-35	CA	43,44	SLE2B	PCDC1	Bxsb1
SLEN	3q23	AA	43	3q21-23		
SLEN	4q13.1	CA	43		IL-18	
SLEN1	10q22.3	CA	43,44			
SLEN	11p13	AA	43			
SLEN3	11p15.6	AA	43			

*Overlap with a QTL identified in systemic lupus erythematosus (SLE) patients ascertained with 4 ACR criteria (see Fig. 29–1).
†Genes with polymorphisms significantly associated with LN co-localizing with the SLEN loci (see Table 29-2).
‡Overlap with a mouse locus that has been linked to GN (see Table 29-4 and Fig. 29.1).
CA, Caucasians; AA, African Americans.

associated with a number of other disease markers, most notably with the production of anti-double-stranded DNA (anti-dsDNA) immunoglobulin G (IgG) antibodies. It is therefore possible that some of the LN susceptibility genes are in fact genes that predispose to the production of these antibodies. One should keep in mind these considerations when interpreting the results compiled below associating a specific gene or linking a chromosomal region to LN susceptibility.

Genetics of Human Lupus Nephritis

Association Studies

Polymorphisms in about 20 genes have now been significantly associated with an increased LN frequency (see Table 29-2). Most of these studies were conducted with relatively small data sets, and were most likely underpowered. It is therefore not surprising that for nearly half of these genes, independent studies on unrelated data sets have reported an absence of association. The discrepancy in some results can also be the consequence of ethnic-specific associations. The frequency of the susceptibility alleles and interacting alleles may vary significantly among populations, making the ethnic stratification of the case and control population a critical parameter and a common source of statistical error in association studies.

Polymorphisms in only two genes, FcγRIIa and FcγRIIIa, have been the subject of enough independent studies to carry out meta-analyses of their association with LN. A large number of functional and genetic studies have implicated the Fcγ receptors in the development of systemic autoimmunity in both humans and animal models. The FcγRIIa and FcγRIIIa genes encode low-affinity IgG receptors, CD32 and CD16, respectively. Their primary role is to mediate immune complex clearance, with CD32 functioning as an inhibitory receptor and CD16 as an activating receptor, with far-reaching effects in the regulation of the immune response, including lymphocyte activation and B-cell tolerance.[19]

Two meta-analyses have been conducted on the association between the R/H 131 polymorphism in the FcγRIIa gene (which impacts CD32's avidity to bind IgG2) and LN. Although the first analysis concluded to a significant association,[20] the validity of the statistical methodology was questioned.[21] A subsequent meta-analysis conducted on the same data set[22]

concluded that the R/R genotype of FcγRIIa was significantly more frequent in SLE patients than in controls (odds ratio [OR] = 1.30, 95% confidence interval [CI] = 1.10–1.52), but a significant correlation was found with the absence of nephritis (OR = 1.27, 95% CI = 1.04–1.55).

A meta-analysis of 11 association studies of the V/F158 polymorphism in FcγRIIIa[23] showed that the F158 allele, which binds IgG1 and IgG3 with a lower affinity, was significantly associated with LN (OR = 1.2, 95% CI = 1.06–1.36). When comparing FF versus VV homozygotes, the risk was higher (OR = 1.47, 95% CI = 1.11–1.93). This analysis, however, did not find a significant association between V/F158 and SLE. This supports the hypothesis that FcγRIIIA plays an essential role in immune complex clearance, preventing the deposition of pathogenic autoantibodies in the kidney, in the absence of a direct role in immune dysregulation. Congruent with this hypothesis was the finding that autoimmune mice rendered deficient in the FcR γ chain, which forms part of the FcγRIII and FcγRI receptors, were protected from kidney disease, although the production of pathogenic autoantibodies was unchanged.[24] These later data and others[25] suggest that glomerular binding of pathogenic autoantibodies is FcγRIII dependent.

IgG2 and IgG3 are the most common isotypes forming the immune complexes that are deposited in the kidneys of LN patients. Consequently, the FcγRIIa-H/R131 and FcγRIIIa-V/F158 polymorphisms might not be independent risk factors, and it has been suggested that they are in linkage disequilibrium.[26] Polymorphisms in these two genes may therefore interact with other susceptibility alleles of genes affecting immune complex clearance to enhance SLE risk.[27] One should note that the relative risk associated with each individual FcγR allele is typically low, in spite of the associations being highly significant. It has been suggested that genotyping errors due to the high degree of sequence homology between the FcγR genes might contribute to underestimated OR values.[12] Nonetheless, the OR values for these alleles fall within the range reported for other individual susceptibility alleles in autoimmune diseases, such as CTLA-4 for type I diabetes and autoimmune thyroid disease.[28] Epistatic interactions, in which the co-expression of two susceptibility alleles results in a phenotype with a greater amplitude than would be expected from the simple sum of the two individual phenotypes, have been demonstrated with

Table 29-4 Quantitative Trait Loci (QTLs) Linked to Lupus Nephritis (LN) in Crosses Between Lupus-susceptible Strains and Various Resistant Strains, and Their Validation in Congenic Strains When Applicable

QTL	Position (chr, cM)	Susceptible Strain	Resistant Strain	Congenic Nephritis	References
Bxs1	**1 (32.8)**	**BXSB.Yaa**	**B10**	**Y**	**47,49**
Bxs2	1 (63.1)	BXSB.Yaa	B10	N	47,49
Sle1	1 (87.9)	NZM2410 (NZW)	B6	N	127–129
Hmr1	1 (92.3)	SJL	DBA/2*	NA†	130
Nba2	1 (92)	NZB	B6.H-2^z	N	131,132
Cgnz1	**1 (92.3)**	**NZM2328**	**C57/L**	**Y‡**	**133,134**
Sle1d	**1(95)**	**NZM2410 (NZW)**	**B6**	**Y§**	**57**
Bxs3	**1 (100)**	**BXSB.Yaa**	**B10**	**Y‖**	**47,49**
Agnz1	1 (106.3)	NZM2328	C57/L	Y‡	133,134
Wbw1	2 (85)	NZW	PL/J	NA	135
Bxs5¶	3 (63.1)	B10	BXSB.Yaa	NA	47
Nbwa2	4 (31)	NZB	BALB/c	NA	136
Sle2	4 (41)	NZM2410 (NZW/NZB)	B6	N	127,128,137
Lbw2	4 (53)	NZB	NZW	NA	138
Nba1	4 (60)	NZB	NZW	NA	139
Imh1/Mott	4 (69)	NZB	NZW	NA	140
Sle6	5 (20)	NZW	B6.Sle1	NA	141
Lxw2	6 (23)	NZW	BXSB	NA	142
Lrdm1	7 (2.7)	MRL.1pr	CAST/Ei	NA	143
Sle3	**7 (27.8)**	**NZM2410 (NZW)**	**B6**	**Y**	**127,128,144**
Nba3	7 (31)	NZB	SWR	NA	145
Nba**	7 (45)	NZB/W	SM	NA	146
Lmb4	10 (35)	MRL.1pr	B6.1pr	NA	147
Sle**	10 (69)	NZM2410 (NZW)	B6	N††	141
Nbal**	11 (9)	NZB	BALB/c.H-2^z	NA	148
Sle**	11 (20)	NZM2410 (NZW)	B6	N††	141
Nbaw1	12 (3.5)	NZB	BALB/c	NA	136
Lrdm2	12 (22.3)	MRL.1pr	CAST/Ei	NA	143
Bxs6	13 (24)	BXSB.Yaa	B10	NA	149
Nba**	13 (59)	NZB	B10.A^z	NA	150
Nba**	13 (72)	NZB/W	SM	NA	146
Swrl2	14 (35)	SWR	NZB	NA	151
Nba**	14 (40)	NZB	BALB/c.H-2^z	NA	148
Lprm3¶	14 (45)	C3H.1pr	MRL.1pr	NA	152
Nwa1	16 (38)	NZW	NZB	NA	148
Lbw1	17 (19.2)	NZW	NZB	NA	138
Sle4‡‡	17 (19.6)	NZM2410 (NZW)	B6	N	153–155
H-2	17 (19.8)	BXSB	NZW	NA	142
Wbw2	17 (24)	NZW	PL/J	NA	135
Agnz2	17 (48.5)	NZM2328	C57/L	NA	133
Lbw6	18 (49)	NZB	NZW	NA	138

Bold characters highlight LN susceptibility loci that have been confirmed through congenic analysis.
* $HgCl_2$-induced autoimmunity.
† NA: No congenic strain carrying this locus has been reported.
‡ Resistance of C57/L locus on NZM2328 background.
§ Not detected by linkage analysis, but only with B6.Sle1 subcongenic strains.
‖ QTL linked to anti-dsDNA Abs.
¶ Transgressive locus.
** Unnamed locus in the NZB or NZB/W strain.
†† Morel, unpublished.
‡‡ Protective locus.

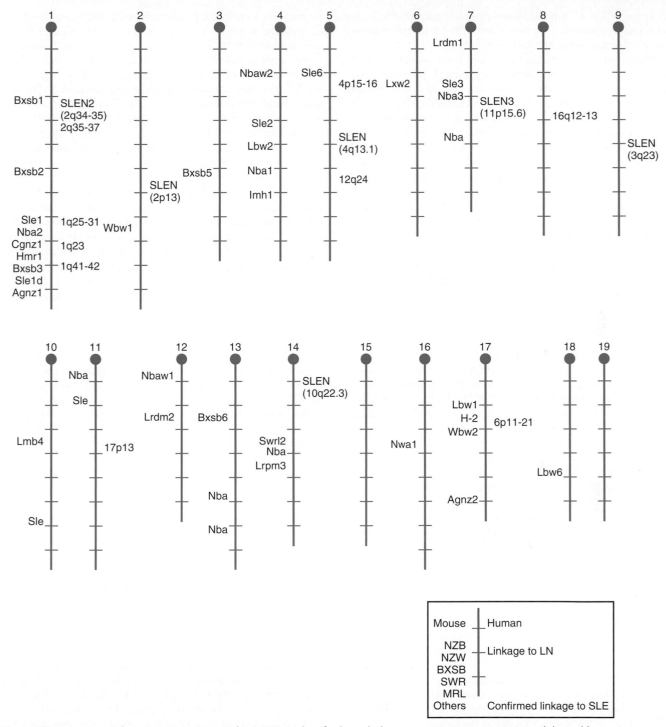

Figure 29-1 Lupus nephritis quantitative trait loci (QTLs) identified in whole genome scans in murine models and human systemic lupus erythematosus (SLE) patients. The 19 murine autosomes are represented by vertical lines with their centromere at the top and tick lines every 10 cM. On the left side are shown QTLs significantly linked to glomerulonephritis (GN), at the approximate position of the peak marker published for each locus. The colors correspond to the lupus strain in which the locus has been identified (see inset). Details on each locus are presented in Table 29-4. On the right are indicated in black the name and location of human QTLs linked to lupus nephritis (see Table 29-3). In addition, the location of confirmed QTLs linked to SLE[12] are indicated in gray. Alignments of the human loci of the mouse chromosomes were performed using http://www.informatics.jax.org/reports/homologymap/mouse_human.shtml.

congenic mice.[29,30] Similar interactions are suspected to occur in humans, although they have been difficult to demonstrate, largely due to genetic heterogeneity.

Most autoimmune diseases have been associated with specific major histocompatibility complex (MHC) alleles. For SLE, significant association has been reported with human leukocyte antigen (HLA) class II (DRB1 and DQA) or class III (C4 and TNF-α) genes.[31,32] In addition, a recent genome-wide analysis has provided a strong evidence of linkage (log of odds [LOD] = 4.19) between the MHC locus and SLE.[33] The association between these genes and LN has been more tenuous; this might be explained, at least in part, by the small number of LN patients considered. Significant associations have been reported, however, between DRβ1, DQα, and DQβ and LN (see Table 29-2). In the most extensive study reported so far, conducted on 244 Italian white LN patients,[34] a very high risk factor was found for the combination of the DRB1*1501 and DQA1*0101 alleles (OR = 65.96, 95% CI = 9.35–1326.25), illustrating how epistatic interactions between alleles can drastically alter disease susceptibility. However, association studies within the MHC locus have to be interpreted with great caution. This locus thus encompasses approximately 4.5 Mb of DNA in which more than 180 genes are expressed, 40% of which have known function in immune regulation. Moreover, many of these genes are in tight linkage disequilibrium (LD), which means that combinations of alleles of these genes are inherited in blocks, the size of which depends on the population structure. Consequently, association studies cannot discriminate which one among genes in LD contributes to the disease. To begin to address this question, the HLA locus in 334 SLE families was genotyped with 158 markers.[35] Three DRβ1/DQβ haplotypes were identified to be significantly associated with SLE, and two of these haplotypes were narrowed down to an approximately 500-kb region. The same type of analysis is still lacking for LN, but there is a strong likelihood that DRβ1 and DQβ, or genes in close proximity, correspond to SLE and LN susceptibility alleles. The definitive identification of these genes and alleles will require the upcoming completion of the haplotype map of the human genome (HapMap), and more specifically, the MHC HapMap.[36]

Besides the Fcγ receptors and the MHC class II genes, cytokines and chemokines are the most common class of genes that have been associated with LN (see Table 29-2). Noticeably, associations between *IL-10*[37–39] and *MCP-1*[40,41] polymorphisms and LN have been independently found in unrelated data sets, indicating that these genes are likely to play a role in the development of LN by regulating the level of inflammation, either systemically or locally in the kidney.

Linkage Analyses

A phenotype stratification strategy has been applied to genome scan results in order to address the genetic basis of various specific clinical manifestations.[42] Using this approach, six SLEN QTLs have been linked to LN, three of them in African Americans and three in white Americans[43] (see Fig. 29-1 and Table 29-3). Among them, SLEN2 (2q34-35) and SLEN1 (10q22.3) have subsequently been validated in an independent data set.[44] Interestingly, only one of the SLEN loci, SLEN2, overlaps with a validated SLE QTL, SLE2B at 2q35-37. *PDCD1*, a strong candidate gene for SLE2B,[45] produces an inhibitory

receptor on T cells, and its deletion in C57BL/6 mice results in a lupus-like disease.[46] The overlap between SLEN2 and SLE2B does not entail that the same gene accounts for both linkages, as the genomic intervals are not precisely defined and contain a large number of genes; finer mapping will be required to resolve this issue. Another potential overlap is at 3q21-23, a region in which nominal evidence of linkage has been obtained in two family collections ascertained with the four ACR criteria[3] and in one family collection stratified by LN.[43]

Interestingly, SLEN2 also overlaps with the mouse QTL *Bxsb1* (see Table 29-4 and Fig. 29-1). This locus was initially identified in a male progeny from a cross between lupus susceptible strain BXSB and resistant strain C57BL/10.[47] The BXSB strain is unique among the lupus models in that disease is greatly accelerated by the expression of *Yaa* (Y-linked autoimmune accelerating locus), which corresponds to an as yet unidentified gene.[48] Development of glomerulonephritis (GN) in a congenic line co-expressing *Bxsb1* and *Yaa* on a C57BL/10 background subsequently confirmed the presence of a GN susceptibility gene (or group of genes) in this locus.[49] *Bxsb1* linkage to GN in females (without *Yaa* expression) has not yet been evaluated. SLEN2 was identified in a data set in which the female:male ratio was likely to reflect the typical 9:1 ratio observed in SLE patients. If SLEN2 and *Bxsb1* correspond to the same gene, it would imply that other genes in the human genome could functionally replace *Yaa* and synergize with SLEN2.

It is noticeable that the 6p11-23 HLA locus was not found linked to LN, in spite of its significant linkage to SLE and the strong association between HLA class II genes and LN. LN linkage analysis was performed only by one group, although on two independent data sets. It is therefore not clear whether this discrepancy between linkage and association studies reflects population heterogeneity and/or statistical distortion resulting from the stratification scheme, or if it indicates that HLA genes contribute essentially to SLE susceptibility, but not as much to nephritis.

Genetic of Lupus Nephritis in Animal Models

Single Gene Studies

As noted above, a large number of gene knockout experiments or transgenic overexpression have resulted in the presentation of a lupus-like syndrome.[8,9] The majority of these mice show some form of immune complex–related renal pathology and could therefore be considered as models of LN (see Table 29-1). As for SLE in general, most of the single genes that affect LN are involved either in apoptosis regulation, lymphocyte activation, or apoptotic products/immune complex clearance (see Table 29-1), although some of these genes clearly overlap between these categories. Decreased apoptosis results in the accumulation of autoreactive lymphocytes, which are normally eliminated at peripheral tolerance checkpoints. Increased activation may allow autoreactive lymphocytes to respond to subthreshold signals, or bypass the necessity of appropriate secondary signals. Finally, impaired clearance of immune complexes and/or apoptotic materials may expose antigen-presenting cells (APCs) and lymphocytes to stimulatory signals for extended periods of time, or in an inappropriate form. More directly relevant for renal pathology, uncleared immune complexes can accumulate in the kidney and accelerate the inflammatory process.

With the exception of the Fcrγ gene[24] discussed earlier, the primary defect in each of these models is likely to be systemic autoimmunity, with GN developing as a consequence. It is interesting, however, that some of these mutations, such as Cbl-b[-/-],[50] result in the production of anti-dsDNA antibodies, without GN being reported. It is not clear whether this absence of renal outcome is due to quantitative or qualitative differences in the type and fine specificity of the autoantibodies being produced. The importance of the latter and the role played by the genetic background have been clearly illustrated by Pdcd1 (PD-1) deficiency. On a C57BL/6 genetic background, PD-1 deficiency results in the production of anti-dsDNA antibodies and GN,[46] whereas on a BALB/c background, the same mutation induces the production of antibodies against cardiac troponin I, and ensuing autoimmune cardiomyopathy.[51] Similarly, deficiency in Fcgr2 encoding FcγRIIb, an Fcγ receptor expressed on B cells that acts as a B-cell receptor signaling inhibitor, is strongly associated with GN when expressed on the appropriate background, such as C57BL/6,[52] FAS deficiency,[53] the Sle1 or Yaa loci,[54] but not on other backgrounds such as BALB/c (see Table 29-1). This shows that epistatic interactions are crucial in determining Fcgr2 contribution to SLE in general and LN in particular.

Interestingly, only a few genes that have a polymorphism associated with LN have resulted in nephritis in the mouse when either knocked out (Pdcd1 [PD-1], Esr1 [ERα]), or overexpressed as a transgene (Ifng [IFNγ]). On the other hand, an osteopontin polymorphism was significantly associated with increased susceptibility to LN,[55] but overexpression of the murine gene induced systemic autoimmunity but not nephritis.[56] A number of reasons probably contribute to this reduced overlap, chiefly the requirement for the appropriate genetic background and the absence of testing functional genetic variants associated with human LN in the mouse.

Finally, some of these single genes affecting GN are located within the support interval of human or mouse QTLs linked to this phenotype, and may therefore be considered as candidate genes (see Table 29-1). In all cases, however, the resolution of the genetic map is not sufficient to provide a significant weight to these co-localizations.

Murine Linkage Analyses

The large number of QTLs that have been reported for SLE susceptibility[8,9] result from multiple factors. First, there are several models of murine SLE, most frequently spontaneous models such as the (NZB X NZW)F$_1$, MRL-Fas(lpr), and BXSB-Yaa strains, but also induced, such as the mercury-induced model.[5] Second, each susceptible strain contains multiple loci associated with SLE. Third, complex genetic interactions between the susceptible and resistant genomes take place in a cross, and changes in the resistant strain reveal different loci. Finally, multiple SLE-related phenotypes have been ascertained in QTL analyses, and QTLs have been found linked to subsets of these phenotypes.

Among these SLE-related phenotypes, 40 QTLs show linkage to GN (see Table 29-4). Only 12 of these have been evaluated individually in a congenic strain. Six of these loci did not impact on the renal phenotype of congenic strains. It is probably safe to speculate that at least 50% of the remaining

28 loci would also fail to show a GN phenotype when individually evaluated by congenic analysis. This emphasizes again the power of genetic interactions, which allow for a QTL to be linked to phenotypes to which it contributes only in combination with other undetermined loci. QTL analyses rarely assess genetic interactions adequately. This is largely due to the insufficient statistical power provided by the sample size of the crosses typically produced for genome-wide scans. Four susceptible loci (Bxs1, Sle1d, Bxs3, and Sle3) resulted in renal pathology on a resistant background, and two resistance loci (Cgnz1 and Agnz1) resulted in an absence of nephritis when bred on the susceptible strain. Interestingly, all these loci but Sle3 are located on mouse chromosome 1, which is syntenic with regions linked or associated with human LN (Fig. 29-1). Bxs1 and Bxs3 were identified in BXSB-Yaa, while Sle1d, Sle3, Cgnz1, and Agnz1 correspond to NZW alleles in the NZM2410 strain for the Sle loci, and NZM2328 for the gnz loci. The Sle1d locus was not by itself identified via a genome scan, but through the generation of Sle1 congenic recombinants and their breeding to NZW to produce a disease phenotype.[57] By itself, Sle1d does not have a phenotype and may represent a true nephropathic locus, contrary to the other loci that are also associated with autoantibody production.

The true value of these loci will only be achieved when the underlying susceptibility gene is identified. This is not a simple task, and only a small number of susceptibility genes involved in autoimmune diseases have been identified.[7] The initial QTL identified through linkage analysis corresponds to a large genomic interval, typically 20 to 30 cM long, which contains hundreds of genes. The first task is to narrow down this interval by generating congenic recombinants and screening them for the presentation of the phenotype of interest, in this case GN. This task has been complicated by the fact that most strong QTLs correspond to clusters of weaker loci, such as for Sle1,[57] and that the phenotype of each of these individual subloci may have a very low penetrance, requiring interactions with other loci to reach a detectable level of disease. Once a locus is mapped down to a small "critical interval," usually less than 1 Mb, the list of genes contained in that region can be accessed thanks to the completion of the Mouse Genome Sequencing Project (http://www.ensembl.org/Mus_musculus/), and candidate genes can be selected based on their known function in the disease process. These candidate genes can then be evaluated for functional polymorphisms that could account for the phenotype associated with this locus. We have just recently completed this process for Sle1c[58] and Sle1b,[59] and proposed Cr2 and genes from the SLAM/CD2 family as candidate genes for these respective loci. Although polymorphisms in these genes do not by themselves contribute to GN, these studies pave the way to a true understanding of the genetics of LN.

PATHOGENESIS

Loss of Tolerance and Initiation of Systemic Lupus Erythematosus

SLE arises when environmental insults superimposed on genetic susceptibility disrupt normal immune regulation and tolerance. It has been estimated that in healthy individuals 55% to 75% of newly generated B-cell receptors and a similar percentage of positively selected thymocytes are autoreactive and subject to central regulation.[156–158] Autoreactive cells that escape deletion, receptor editing or anergy in the bone marrow or thymus, as well as autoreactive B cells generated in germinal centers by somatic hypermutation, are subsequently exposed to a peripheral network of mechanisms that prevent activation of mature lymphocytes. Insights into the mechanisms that control reactivity to prototypic lupus autoantigens and that fail in autoimmune-prone individuals have been revealed through study of T- and B-cell receptor transgenic models. Autoimmune-prone MRL-Fas(lpr) and NZBW/F1 strains bearing Ig transgenes reactive with prototypic lupus autoantigens produce transgenic autoantibodies, revealing defects in B-cell tolerance (reviewed in 159), and T-cell receptor (TCR)-transgenic T cells from lupus-prone MRL/++ mice transferred into mice bearing target self-antigen are resistant to anergy induction.[160] Altered tolerance may result from abnormalities in any of a large number of signaling and biologic pathways. Numerous intrinsic functional defects and abnormal signaling are reported in lymphocytes in both murine and human lupus (see review[161,162]). Moreover, transgenic overexpression or targeted disruption of diverse molecules involved in B- and T-cell signaling, activation, and survival can lead to a spontaneous lupus-like phenotype, with variable expression of nephritis (see review[163]). Certain exogenous agents that induce lupus-like syndromes similarly function by modulation of tolerance thresholds.[164,165]

Autoimmunity is also precipitated by disruption of B- and T-cell interactions that co-regulate their respective activation and proliferation. Autoreactive B cells can either tolerize or activate autoreactive T cells,[166,167] and regulatory T cells or T-cell tolerance can prevent activation of autoreactive B cells.[168,169] Conversely, inappropriate T-cell help can block tolerance induction or reactivate silenced B cells.[170–173] Autoreactive and deregulated T cells are a prominent feature of systemic lupus and are implicated in autoantibody production in murine and human disease.[174,175] Recent studies have provided important new insights into the mechanisms by which autoreactive cells are activated: nucleosomes provide peptide Ag to recruit T-cell help for anti-DNA B cells[176]; target nuclear antigen is exposed on the surface of apoptotic cells, such that defective clearance of apoptotic cells promotes lupus-like autoimmunity[177]; and, chromatin-containing immune complexes activate B cells through co-signaling via toll-like receptors.[178] Elucidation of these pathways has led to potential new therapies to re-establish tolerance in human lupus.[179]

Humoral Immunity in Lupus Nephritis

B Cells in Lupus Nephritis

The fundamental importance of antibodies and B cells in LN is clearly illustrated by abolition of autoimmune disease and early mortality in MRL-Fas(lpr) mice rendered deficient in B cells.[180] Parallels in human SLE are suggested by early reports of efficacy of therapeutic B-cell depletion using anti-CD20 monoclonal antibody. Efficacy is attributed in part to depletion of nuclear antigen–reactive autoantibodies, a cornerstone of diagnosis and a hallmark of lupus GN. The B-cell contribution to pathogenicity, however, is clearly not due solely to autoantibody production, in that MRL-Fas(lpr) mice bearing B cells incapable of secreting antibody also develop nephritis and early death.[181] These observations indicate a complex role for B cells in lupus pathogenesis.[182] Antibody-independent B-cell

functions include modulation of T-cell repertoire and memory, promotion of autoreactive T-cell activation and expansion, production of cytokines and co-signals that regulate dendritic cells and T-cell subsets, and formation of lymphoid organs.[167,183–186] There is evidence that these pathways are involved in lupus pathogenesis. B–cell-deficient MRL-Fas(lpr) mice fail to develop populations of activated T cells found in B–cell-sufficient mice.[187] B cells are highly efficient APCs, capable of capturing antigen via cell surface Ig receptors for subsequent internalization, processing, and presentation via class I or II MHC molecules. B-cell presentation of autoantigen peptides can directly activate T cells.[167] B-cell dependence of CD8 and CD4 T-cell activation in MRL-Fas(lpr) mice is thought to occur primarily via B cell–CD4 T-cell interactions, because enhanced CD8 T-cell activation remains intact in lupus mice lacking MHC class I antigen on B cells.[188] B cells were recently recognized to play a key role in early lymphogenesis, and may initiate organization of pathogenic lymphoid aggregates in lupus. B-cell chemoattractant is ectopically expressed in BWF1 mice, promoting abnormal thymic, kidney, and lung trafficking of B-1 B cells,[189,190] and antibody-secreting B cells are prominent in diseased BWF1 kidneys.[191] Infiltrating B cells isolated from diseased MRL-Fas(lpr) mouse kidneys secrete autoantibodies cross-reactive with glomerular antigens and DNA, suggesting an effector role in disease pathogenicity.[192] Conversely, a protective role for autoreactive IgM in nonautoimmune individuals was recently postulated, based on the observed worsening of lupus-like disease in C57Bl/6 and mixed 129/B6/MRL-Fas(lpr) mice lacking secreted IgM.[117,193]

Nephritogenic Autoantibodies and Mechanisms of Antibody-Mediated Injury

Glomerular antibody deposition is a hallmark of lupus GN. The properties that confer nephritogenicity to Ig have been inferred from study of spontaneous serum autoantibodies and monoclonal Ig derived through B-cell fusion and viral immortalization, and by elution of pathogenic Ig from diseased kidneys. These approaches revealed that nephritogenic autoantibodies comprise a diverse population with regard to antigen specificity, isotype, avidity, and charge, and suggest that pathogenic antibodies localize to the kidney by a variety of mechanisms (see reviews[194–196]). Specificity for DNA is important for pathogenesis for a subset of lupus Ig. Anti-DNA IgG is present in nephritic kidneys in both murine and human lupus, and a subset of monoclonal anti-dsDNA and anti-nucleosome IgG induce renal histopathologic lesions in naive animals.[197,198] Nonetheless, antinuclear, antihistone, or anti-dsDNA antibodies are neither necessary nor sufficient for development of LN. Serum anti-dsDNA titers and affinity can be dissociated from the presence and severity of renal disease in both rodent models and patients,[134] and a majority of Ig eluted from lupus kidneys do not bind DNA.[199]

Multiple mechanisms appear to contribute to renal antibody deposition in lupus. In situ formation of immune complexes, either via direct autoantibody binding to intrinsic renal components or via binding to self-antigen previously planted in the kidney, may be a dominant mechanism of Ig deposition (see reviews[194,196,200]). Cross-reactivity of anti-DNA autoantibodies with non-DNA glomerular antigens is well described,[201] and may account for renal deposition by anti-DNA Ig. Anti-DNA eluted from nephritic kidneys as well as serum and monoclonal anti-DNA Ig cross-react with polynucleotides, phospholipids, cytoskeletal proteins, and non-nuclear glomerular antigens.[199] Alpha-actinin and alpha-enolase are additional renal targets recently implicated in lupus pathogenesis.[202,203] Subsets of SLE Ig bind in vitro to isolated glomeruli, crude renal and glomerular extracts, cultured endothelial and mesangial cells, and purified glomerular antigens. Perfusion of kidneys ex vivo and administration of polyclonal human SLE IgG and both human and murine monoclonal lupus Ig to naive recipients results in glomerular Ig deposition. Small DNA fragments and soluble proteins targeted by lupus antibodies have an intrinsic affinity for glomerular cell or basement membrane structures. Collagen, laminin, and fibronectin possess binding sites for DNA, and some cells express DNA-binding receptors. Nuclear histones, nucleosomes (DNA-histone), and cationic immune complexes can bind polyanions in the glomerular basement membrane or negatively charged glycosaminoglycans in cell membranes and serve as planted antigen for subsequent binding by anionic DNA, antihistone, or anti-nucleosome Ig. Similar mechanisms may account for selective glomerular binding by preformed circulating DNA–anti-DNA immune complexes. These autoantibodies and corresponding antigens have been recovered from human and murine lupus renal lesions. Rheumatoid factors, antibodies to the collagen-like region of complement component C1q, and certain antibody idiotypes are defined by unique antigenic determinants in the antibody variable region; these are reported in high frequency in lupus serum and kidney deposits, suggesting that some antibodies bind to previously deposited Ig or C1q. Nephritogenicity of IgG3 in MRL-*Fas(lpr)* lupus is attributed in part to physicochemical properties independent of antigen specificity. Murine IgG3 can self-aggregate through Fc-Fc interactions, leading to decreased solubility and cryoglobulin formation. These different mechanisms may account for the distinct histopathologic patterns of injury and clinical phenotypes observed in LN.

Lupus autoantibodies may induce renal injury by mechanisms other than immune complex deposition. Antiphospholipid antibodies interfere with in vitro phospholipid-dependent coagulation, paradoxically causing a prothrombotic state in vivo; intrarenal thromboses consistent with antiphospholipid syndrome nephropathy may co-exist with lupus GN. A similar role has been proposed for antiheparan sulfate antibodies due to cross-reactivity with anionic phospholipids or binding to endothelial cell surface heparan sulfate, a physiologic ligand for antithrombin III. Select anti-dsDNA antibodies trigger complement-mediated cytotoxicity upon binding cultured kidney cells.[204] Direct renal cell injury, resulting in proteinuria and hypercellularity, due to autoantibody penetration of living cells with resultant disruption of cell functions, is described for select human and murine lupus antibodies.[205] Cell entry is triggered by antibody binding to membrane targets, such as myosin, with subsequent subcellular localization dependent on antibody specificity or expression of nuclear localization sequences within the antibody variable region (see review[206]).

Fc Receptors

The pathogenic potential of autoantibodies in LN is attributed largely to effector functions determined by constant region domains of IgG that contain the binding sites for Fcγ receptors and complement. Ig within renal immune deposits can engage activating FcγRs on macrophages, neutrophils, or renal parenchymal cells to promote leukocyte adhesion and trigger synthesis of multiple inflammatory mediators. Deposited Ig can also bind complement component C1q to trigger activation of the classical complement cascade to recruit anaphylatoxins and terminal complement components. However, unexpected outcomes in gene targeted experiments in rodent models of inflammation and recognition of the wide distribution and diverse functions of networks of FcRs, complement components, and their respective receptors and regulatory proteins have revealed additional and complex contributions to disease. The relevance of FcRs to the genetics of LN has been discussed in the genetics section of this chapter, and we will now briefly review the role of these molecules in the pathogenesis of this illness.

FcγRs comprise a complex family of constitutive and inducible cell surface proteins that vary in cell distribution, Ig affinity, signaling, and function. The relative balance of inhibitory (FcγRIIB) and activating (FcγRI, FcγRIIA, and FcγRIII) receptors expressed on lymphocytes, macrophages, neutrophils, and renal parenchymal cells determines the nature of the immune and inflammatory response. Engagement of activating FcγRs generally promotes, whereas inhibitory receptors dampen, immunity and inflammation. Therapeutic efficacy of intravenous immune globulin in human lupus is attributed in part to inhibition of effector responses through blockade of macrophage activatory receptors and/or engagement of inhibitory FcγRIIB receptors. In murine lupus models, activatory FcγR dependence of nephritis appears to be strain dependent. Activating FcγRs in mice share a common Fcγ chain that contains an immunoreceptor tyrosine-based activation motif (ITAM). Targeted deletion of the FcR γ chain gene (FcRγ-KO) dramatically attenuates nephritis in lupus-prone (NZBxNZW)F1 mice, despite persistence of autoantibodies and prominent glomerular IgG and C3 deposition.[24] Alleviation of renal inflammation in MRL-*Fas(lpr)* mice subjected to high-dose granulocyte-colony stimulating factor (G-CSF) infusions is attributed to G-CSF-induced downmodulation of glomerular activating FcγRIII.[207] Conversely, FcγR deficiency has no affect on autoimmunity, nephritis, and vasculitis in MRL-*Fas(lpr)* mice.[208] In nonlupus experimental systems, targeted deletion of FcγR dramatically increases immune complex deposition, suggesting an important role in normal immune complex clearance. FcγRIII also mediates uptake of immune complexes to promote antigen presentation by dendritic cells,[209] and is implicated with TLR9 in dendritic cell activation by chromatin-containing immune complexes.[210]

Deficiency of the inhibitory IgG Fc receptor FcγRIIB promotes development of spontaneous anti-dsDNA and antichromatin autoantibodies, fatal GN, and early mortality in susceptible B6, but not in resistant Balb/c, mice.[52] Bone marrow transfer experiments determined that disease is due to deficiency of FcγRIIB on B cells, and not due to modulation of myeloid cell effector functions. Engagement of FcγRIIB suppresses activation of B cells, and upon self-ligation, induces B-cell apoptosis, potentially contributing to maintenance of B-cell tolerance. FcγRIIB deficiency also accelerates nephritis in B6.Yaa mice, whereas contradictory outcomes are reported in B6.Fas/lpr mice.[53,211] These experiments must be interpreted with caution, however, because the FcγRIIB gene-targeted

Complement

deletion was originally constructed on a 129Sv/B6 hybrid background, and it was recently reported that strain 129–derived sequences near the FcγRIIB locus on mouse chromosome 1 are independently linked to autoimmunity.[11]

Complement

Complement components have diverse functions and play a complex role in the pathogenesis of lupus. Complement proteins, their receptors, and a network of cell-bound and soluble complement regulatory proteins are expressed by renal parenchymal cells as well as by myeloid and lymphoid cells. There are more than 30 known complement proteins, the functions, ligands, receptors, and regulation of which are only partially understood. Complement modulates B- and T-cell activation and maintains tolerance, promotes solubility and clearance of immune complexes and apoptotic cells, governs immune complex deposition, and mediates inflammation through production of anaphylatoxins C3a and C5a and terminal complement components. Blockade or targeted deletion of components of the complement system has been particularly useful in dissecting their relative importance in renal immune physiology and disease. A key role for complement in lupus pathogenesis is suggested by depression of C3 and C4 levels in lupus mouse and patient sera and by deposition of C1q and C3 in inflamed glomeruli and tubules. The presence in renal lesions of early complement component C1q suggests activation of the classical pathway. Notably, however, multiple observations suggest that proteins of the early classical complement pathway play primarily a protective, not a pathogenic, role in the development of SLE (see review[212]). Gene-targeted deletion of early components, C1qa or C4, leads to spontaneous autoantibody production and GN in genetically susceptible 129 and C57BL/6 mice, and accelerates disease in autoimmune MRL/++ and B6.Fas(lpr) mice.[115,119,213–216] Independent confirmation of C1q effects may be required, because like FcγRIIB, the targeted C1q locus sits on mouse chromosome 1 in a region independently linked to autoimmunity.[11] A protective role for C1q in human lupus is suggested by the paradoxical association of homozygous deficiency in early components of the classical pathway (C1q, C4) with development of SLE. The mechanism of protection is unclear, but C1q deficiency is linked to impaired opsonization and clearance of apoptotic cells, which in turn is linked to loss of self-tolerance. The protection provided by C1q is independent of glomerular C3 activation.[217] Protection also may be related to a crucial role for complement in maintaining B-cell tolerance. Anergy induction is prevented in autoreactive B cells deficient in complement protein C4 or complement receptors CD21 (CR2) and CD35 (CR1) (alternative splice products of the Cr2 locus).[119]

In contrast, the role of early components of the alternative complement pathway may be primarily proinflammatory. Genetic absence of alternative pathway proteins factor B or factor D protects against proliferative GN in the MRL-Fas(lpr) model.[218,219] Activation of the alternative pathway presumably occurs via C3b, a product of classical pathway activation. Alternative pathway deficiency may abrogate disease by limiting amplification of the complement inflammatory cascade, or by poorly understood effects on B-cell tolerance or activation.

C3 plays a complex role in LN, presumably related to the site and level of expression and biologic functions of complement components, metabolites, receptors, and regulatory proteins. C3 activation leads to release of C3a and C5a that recruit neutrophils, act as anaphylatoxins, induce vasodilation, and interact with myeloid, lymphoid, and parenchymal cell C3aR and C5aR, the functions of which remain poorly understood. Additionally, release of C5b initiates formation of the terminal membrane attack complex. Fragment C3b amplifies alternative pathway activation, fragments C3b/C4b bind CD35, and fragment C3d binds CD21 on B cells and phagocytic cells to paradoxically both amplify T-dependent humoral immune responses[220] and promote B-cell tolerance.[119] A dominant proinflammatory role for C3 in LN is suggested by the ability of soluble Crry-Ig fusion protein to protect MRL-Fas(lpr) mice from GN and vasculitis.[221] Crry, complement receptor 1-related gene/protein, is a potent membrane complement regulator in rodents that inhibits C3 activation. However, genetic C3 deficiency does not ameliorate nephritis in MRL-Fas(lpr) mice and is associated with increased glomerular IgG deposition in this background.[222] C3 deficiency similarly has little effect on autoantibody production and immune complex GN in mixed 129/B6.Fas(lpr) mice.[119,214] The reason for lack of protection by C3 deficiency is not known, but is consistent with the absence of an association between C3 deficiency and development of SLE in humans. The role of downstream complement components is less clear. Terminal complement components are reported in renal biopsy specimens of patients with LN and in serum of a subset of patients with active disease. A pathogenic role is suggested by amelioration of renal disease and prolonged survival in NZB/WF1 mice chronically administered anti-C5 monoclonal antibody that blocks C5 cleavage.[223]

How other aspects of complement biology contribute to lupus pathogenesis is not yet well explored. Cell protection from complement-induced injury is dependent in part on circulating, soluble, and renal cell membrane-associated complement regulatory proteins that limit complement consumption and bystander damage. Deletion of decay-accelerating factor (DAF, CD55), a membrane protein that restricts complement activation on autologous cells, does not alter MRL-Fas(lpr) LN,[224] a finding that may be explained by the very low level expression of DAF in MRL-Fas(lpr) kidney or DAF's dual role as a ligand for lymphocyte CD97. It was recently reported that human and mouse T-cell subsets express complement regulatory proteins that modulate T-cell responses (see review[212]); the relevance to lupus is currently unknown.

Cellular Immunity in Lupus Nephritis

Macrophages and T cells collaborate and mediate LN. The MRL-Fas(lpr) strain has proven particularly valuable for probing mononuclear cell contributions to lupus pathogenesis and testing therapeutic strategies. Disease in this strain is predictable and consistent, and the tempo is slow enough to tease apart the mechanisms, yet sufficiently rapid to be efficient and economical. Autoimmune disease in this strain shares features with the human illness. The phenotypic hallmarks include a massive lymphadenopathy, splenomegaly, circulating autoantibodies, and the infiltration of leukocytes into multiple tissues. Kidney disease is the major cause of fatality (50% = 5–6 months of age).[92] While the mutation in Fas(lpr) is not sufficient to cause lupus, the interaction of the MRL background genes and the Fas(lpr) mutation accelerates the tempo of nephritis. It is not clear whether this aggressive disease is attributable to the intrarenal infiltrating leukocytes, and/or autoantibodies. It is also not known whether these elements conspire to cause renal injury. Whereas the preceding section focused on features such as the breaking of tolerance that initiates LN, and the importance of B cells and autoantibodies in the pathogenesis, this section will provide an overview of macrophages and their growth factors, T cells, and their co-stimulatory pathways that are instrumental in inflammation in the kidney.

Macrophages and Macrophage Growth Factors in Lupus Nephritis

The macrophage is central to the pathogenesis of kidney diseases. Macrophages mediate the renal resident cell apoptosis. We have determined that activated macrophages release molecules that induce apoptosis of tubular epithelial cells,[225] while others have shown that macrophages induce apoptosis of mesangial cells, but require cell contact.[226] Macrophages are especially abundant in the kidney of MRL-Fas(lpr) mice, rendering this strain particularly valuable for identifying molecules responsible for macrophage recruitment into the kidney, and for determining the mechanisms that arm these cells to destroy. It is important to appreciate that macrophages within the kidney during disease are not end-stage cells. These cells are dividing, and their influx, survival, and proliferation and activation in the kidney is dependent on the principal macrophage growth factor (colony-stimulating factor-1, CSF-1).[227] Thus, it is logical that CSF-1 in the serum and kidney is a harbinger of autoimmune-mediated kidney disease.[228] In support of this concept, CSF-1 is increased in the circulation of neonatal MRL-Fas(lpr) mice, well in advance of clinically detectable kidney disease (3 mo), and increases even further in proportion to the severity of renal injury. Similarly, CSF-1 has been identified in the MRL-Fas(lpr) kidney at 1 month of age in the glomeruli and 2 months of age in vessels and tubules using in situ hybridization.[229] Intrarenal CSF-1 rises as kidney damage advances. By comparison, CSF-1 is not detectable in the circulation, or in the kidney in normal mouse strains. Moreover, the kidney is the major source of circulating CSF-1 in MRL-Fas(lpr) mice; transplanting a single CSF-1-expressing MRL-Fas(lpr) macrophage-rich nephritic kidney into a congenic MRL-++ strain after removal of normal kidneys results in an increase of CSF-1 in the serum to approximately one half the amount detected in MRL-Fas(lpr) mice with both kidneys.[230] Furthermore, rapidly (2 weeks) following transplantation, CSF-1 and macrophage-rich nephritis disappear within the donor kidney. Conversely, transplanting an MRL-++ kidney into MRL-Fas(lpr) recipients after bilateral removal of the nephritic kidneys rapidly induces (2 weeks) CSF-1 and macrophage-rich nephritis in the donor kidneys.[231] Taken together, this suggests that CSF-1 is a proximal stimulus in triggering cytopathic kidney autoimmune injury, and intrarenal expression of CSF-1 requires continual stimulation from a circulating factor(s).

To test the concept that CSF-1 incites autoimmune renal injury, a gene transfer strategy was constructed to deliver CSF-1 into the kidney. Renal tubular epithelial cells (TECs) were genetically modified using a recombinant retrovirus vector to express CSF-1.[232] These TECs are efficiently converted into "carrier cells" that secrete stable, sustained levels of CSF-1. Implanting these carrier cells under the renal capsule persistently delivers CSF-1 into the kidney and circulation. Using this gene transfer strategy, intrarenal CSF-1 elicited an influx

of macrophage and T cells, resulting in interstitial nephritis in strains with Fas(lpr), but not in normal strains. Since Fas is instrumental in deleting autoreactive T cells, we suspect that CSF-1 draws macrophages into the kidney, but requires autoreactive T cells to incite local inflammation.

Macrophage growth factors are increased in glomeruli of patients with lupus. Upregulation of CSF-1 and another macrophage growth factor (granulocyte-macrophage growth factor, GM-CSF), have been identified in glomeruli in patients with LN.[233] CSF-1 is increased earlier and more abundantly in the kidney than GM-CSF in MRL-Fas(lpr)mice. Clearly, a more comprehensive evaluation of human renal injury is required to determine the importance of macrophage growth factors in the expansion of macrophages within the kidney and the extent of kidney disease. Nevertheless, we would predict strategies that prevent the intrarenal expression of CSF-1, and perhaps GM-CSF, will protect the kidney from injury in individuals genetically susceptible to autoimmune illnesses.

CSF-1 is instrumental in nephritis. The genetic deletion of CSF-1 suppresses postobstructive nephritis and autoimmune nephritis in mice.[227,234] CSF-1-deficient MRL-Fas(lpr) mice are protected from nephritis and injury to other tissues as compared with the wild-type strain.[234] Kidney protection in CSF-1-deficient MRL-Fas(lpr) mice is attributed, at least in part, to a decrease in intrarenal leukocytes and a reduction in activated macrophages in the kidney. It follows that without activated macrophages, the kidney is spared from macrophage-induced renal resident cell apoptosis. On the other hand, CSF-1-deficient MRL-Fas(lpr) mice have a reduction in multiple autoantibody and Ig isotypes in the circulation, and a decrease in IgG and complement in glomeruli. This reduction of Ig's and autoantibodies may be related to an enhanced B-cell apoptosis in the bone marrow of these mice. Thus, CSF-1 regulates multiple cell and antibody functions that may be instrumental in the pathogenesis of LN.

While CSF-1 attracts macrophages into the kidney, the fate of these cells is regulated by the CSF-1 receptor, termed c-fms. Macrophages within the MRL background accumulate more rapidly in the kidney than other normal strains, and have a heightened response to CSF-1.[235] There is a defect in the downregulation of c-fms in the MRL strains, which is probably responsible for the notable presence of macrophages in the kidney of MRL-Fas(lpr) mice. Since the failure to downregulate the CSF-1 receptor may be linked to a modifying gene in the MRL background, it is intriguing to speculate that identification of these genes in mice may provide clues to identifying the counterpart in human lupus patients. Taken together, determining the expression and regulation of receptors for molecules that are integral in the pathogenesis of LN, such as CSF-1, may be prognostic indicators of the tempo of disease.

Macrophages in the MRL-Fas(lpr) strain have other abnormal functions. These include a decrease in cytokine production,[236–238] increased antibody-dependent cellular cytotoxicity and hydrogen peroxide production,[239] and decreased Fc-mediated binding and impaired phagocytosis.[240] In many of these studies it is not clear whether the impaired macrophage function is a consequence of the disease, or is genetically linked to either the Fas(lpr) mutation or MRL background. As in the mouse, defective macrophage functions are a feature of human SLE.[241] It is critical to determine whether these defects are identifiable in healthy individuals prior to the loss of renal function, or are a consequence of the disease. Nevertheless, a systematic exploration of the regulation of intrarenal macrophage functions and their impact on kidney disease will undoubtedly lead to the design of novel therapeutics.

T-Cell Effectors in Lupus Nephritis

T cells regulate a wide range of as diverse functions that are pivotal in tissue destruction and protection. T cells are notable within the kidneys in human and mouse forms of lupus. Therefore, it is important to elucidate their role in LN. The T cells in *Fas*-deficient *Fas(lpr)* strains that escape apoptosis are distinctive. The massive enlargement of lymph nodes and spleens in this strain is due to infiltration by unique double-negative cell (DN) T cells [TCRα/β, CD4⁻, CD8⁻, B220 epitope of CD45⁺], the origin, proliferation, and migration of which remain controversial.[242–247] The abundant expression of two activation determinants, B220 and FasL, and the spontaneous cytotoxic activity suggests that DN T cells were previously activated.[248] Notably, DN T-cell clones propagated from the kidney of MRL-*Fas(lpr)* mice exclusively proliferate to renal parenchymal TEC and mesangial cells and not to other tissues.[249] In addition, infiltrating DN cells are evident in the kidney, lymph nodes, and spleens simultaneously. Based on these findings, we suggest that DN T cells expand in the kidney. DN T cells are class I MHC selected, and are reduced in the MRL-*Fas(lpr)* strain deficient in β_2-microglobulin (i.e., class I).[250] Class I–deficient MRL-*Fas(lpr)* mice are spared from an infiltration of DN and CD8 T cells into the kidney and have drastically reduced CD4 T cells. These mice are protected from renal injury.[251,252] Thus, class I–selected T cells are necessary for autoimmune kidney injury in the MRL-*Fas(lpr)* strain.

The CD4 T cells in the MRL-*Fas(lpr)* strain are distinctive.[174,253,254] CD4⁺ and DN T cells account for the majority of T cells in nephritic MRL-*Fas(lpr)* kidneys. Elimination of CD4 T cells in MRL-*Fas(lpr)* mice protects the kidney from glomerular, tubular, and vascular pathology, an outcome similar to that achieved by eliminating TCR α/β cells. Thus, autoimmune kidney disease in this strain requires both multiple T-cell populations.[252]

Regulating T Cells: Co-stimulatory Pathways

Immune cell interactions and T-cell costimulatory pathways are instrumental in autoimmune disease induction and provide key targets for therapeutic intervention. Antigen recognition alone is not sufficient for full T-cell activation. T cells require two distinct signals to become fully activated.[255,256] The first signal is provided by the engagement of the TCR with the MHC and peptide complex on APCs. The second "co-stimulatory" signal is provided by engagement of one or more T-cell surface receptors with their specific ligands on APCs.[257–259] Signaling through the TCR alone in the absence of a co-stimulatory signal leads to prolonged T-cell unresponsiveness, or anergy.[256]

The CD28 Family

The engagement of CD28 on T cells with either B7-1 or B7-2 on APCs is the best characterized co-stimulatory pathway.[260] The CD28/CTLA4-B7-1/B7-2 T-cell co-stimulatory pathway is a unique and complex pathway that regulates T-cell activation.[261] Interaction of CD28, constitutively expressed on T cells, with B7-1 and B7-2, expressed on APCs, provides a second "positive" signal that results in T-cell activation. During T-cell activation cytokines are generated, the clones expand, and T-cell anergy is prevented. Furthermore, T-cell survival, clonal expansion, and differentiation are defective in CD28-/- mice (see review[262]). Thus, the CD28-B7 interaction is critical for T-cell survival.

The CD28 family is versatile; it provides "negative" signals to terminate T-cell responses. After activation, T cells express another CD28 family member, CTLA4 (CD152), with a higher affinity for B7-1 and B7-2. CTLA4 provides a "turn off" signal to terminate T-cell responses.[263,264] For example, CTLA4-deficient mice succumb to a fatal lymphoproliferative disorder with lymphocyte-mediated multi-organ tissue destruction, which shares some features with the MRL-*Fas(lpr)* phenotype.[265,266] Furthermore, CTLA4 is a plausible "master switch" for peripheral T-cell tolerance.[267]

The CD28 family molecules are promising therapeutic targets for LN. Eliminating the B7 pathway (genetic deletion of B7-1 and B7-2) in MRL-*Fas(lpr)* mice protects this strain from renal and other tissue injury.[268] Furthermore, prophylactic treatment of MRL-*Fas(lpr)* mice with CTLA4Ig (a fusion protein that binds to B7 and blocks this pathway) diminished kidney disease, but not lung disease in this strain.[269] This emphasizes the differential impact of the CD28/CTLA4 pathway on target tissues in the MRL-*Fas(lpr)* strain. Similarly, CD28-/-MRL-*Fas(lpr)* mice developed less severe GN, but greater splenomegaly than WT mice.[270] Treating mild renal disease in another form of LN, the NZB x NZW F1 hybrid females (BW) delayed the onset of proteinuria. However, delaying treatment until the BW mice have advanced nephritis requires CTLA4Ig in combination with cyclophosphamide to retard the onset of proteinuria.[271] Nevertheless, BW mice survived longer whether treatment with CTLA4Ig was initiated in mice with mild or advanced nephritis as compared with controls. We anticipate that these studies will seed clinical trials using CTLA4Ig for patients with LN.

New CD28 Homologs

The number of co-stimulatory pathways is rapidly expanding. There are several new members of the CD28 family, including the ICOS and PD-1 pathways. The functions of these pathways are complex and have not been defined in autoimmune kidney disease, including LN. These pathways are summarized below.

The ICOS-ICOS-L Pathway: Amplifying and Dampening Immune Responses

The more recently identified CD28 homolog, ICOS, is a T-cell costimulatory molecule first reported on activated human T cells.[272,273] Human ICOS shares 24% identity (and 39% similarity) with human CD28 and 17% identity (and 39% similarity) with human CTLA4.[274] B7-1 and B7-2 are ligands for CD28, but not ICOS. Similarly, the ligand for ICOS, ICOS-L (also termed B7h, LICOS, B7RP-1, B7H-2, GL-50), does not bind to CD28 or CTLA4.[275–277]

ICOS shares features that are similar to CD28. These include enhancing T-cell proliferation, cytokine production, upregulating CD154, and providing help for Ig production by B cells.[272] However, ICOS has properties that are distinct from

CD28 that are intriguing. Whereas CD28 is constitutively expressed on T cells, ICOS is induced upon TCR engagement. The inducible expression of ICOS shortly after T-cell activation suggests that ICOS may be critical for providing costimulatory signals to activate T cells.[278] ICOS is expressed on activated T cells and resting memory T cells.[273] ICOS expression is enhanced by CD28 costimulation, and ICOS upregulation is markedly reduced in the absence of B7-1 and B7-2, suggesting that some of the functions ascribed to CD28 are due in part to ICOS signaling.[279]

ICOS-L shares 20% sequence identity with the B7 molecules CD80 and CD86.[280] But unlike CD80 and CD86, ICOS-L does not bind to CD28 or CTLA4.[273] ICOS-L displayed on the cell surface has been detected on bone marrow–derived cells (B cells, dendritic cells, macrophages) and some T cells such as DN T cells.[280,281] ICOS-L messenger RNA expression has been detected in multiple tissues, spleen, lymph node, kidney, heart, and brain, and on parenchymal cells (TEC, endothelial).[275,281] And constitutive cell surface ICOS-L is upregulated by cytokines on endothelial cells.[281] Thus, ICOS-ICOS-L interactions between leukocytes and/or parencyhmal cells may regulate immune events.

The ICOS pathway in vivo may be as complex as the B7 pathway, imparting signals that promote and inhibit T-cell activation. In another autoimmune disease, experimental allergic encephalomyelitis (EAE), ICOS-deficient mice developed more severe disease as compared with the wild-type strain.[282] Similarly, ICOS blockade during antigen priming exacerbated EAE.[283] In contrast, ICOS blockade during the efferent immune response in EAE abrogated disease. These findings suggest that the function of the ICOS pathway is dictated by the nature of the immune reaction during stages of autoimmune disease.

The concept that parenchymal cells expressing ICOS-L are negative regulators of T cells in the kidney is supported by recent findings. Blocking ICOS-L expression on TECs (Ia+) enhances interleukin-2 production by T-cell hybridomas, suggesting that TECs may inactivate T cells.[284] We have recently established that renal disease in ICOS-deficient MRL-Fas(lpr) mice is more severe as compared with the wild-type strain (manuscript in preparation).[284a] The increase in disease appears to be related to local T-cell interactions within the kidney, since intrarenal nephritogenic T-cell cytokines, and not systemic cytokines, are increased in the ICOS-deficient MRL-Fas(lpr) strain. These studies suggest that ICOS-L on renal resident cells, such as TEC, may provide a negative regulatory signal to dampen T-cell activation, and thus are poised to protect the kidney.

The PD-1 Pathway: A Negative Regulator of Immune Responses

A new member of the CD28 superfamily is the PD-1 pathway. PD-1, like CD28, ICOS, and CTLA4, is a transmembrane protein and belongs to the Ig superfamily. As is the case for CTLA4, PD-1 possesses only a single V-like domain, and an immunoreceptor tyrosine-based inhibitory motif (ITIM) within its cytoplasmic tail. PD-1 is homologous (23%) with CTLA4, but lacks the MYPPPY motif required for B7-1 and B7-2 binding. The PD-1 receptor is expressed on activated T cells, B cells, and myeloid cells, including macrophages. It binds two known ligands, PD-L1 and PD-L2. These ligands

are expressed on professional APCs such as dendritic cells and monocytes, and are constitutively expressed on some T and B cells, and parenchymal cells within the kidneys, heart, and lungs.[285,286] PD-1 is functionally similar to CTLA4: (1) Each provides negative regulation, including inhibiting downstream cell signaling events, diminishing cell proliferation, and reducing cytokine production; and (2) deleting either gene results in autoimmune disease. PD-1-/- mice (normal strains) develop an autoimmune phenotype that is dictated by the strain's background genes and includes splenomegaly, B-cell expansion with increased serum Ig's, arthritis, and cardiomyopathy.[46] On the other hand, PD-1-/- on the B6 background resulted in a low incidence (3 of 10 mice) and mild GN, even in the second year of life. By comparison, PD-1-/- on the B6-Fas(lpr) background had a greater incidence (8 of 9 mice) and severity of GN, although based on the limited data, it remains modest.[46] Since T cells do not infiltrate the kidney in the B6-Fas(lpr) strain, we speculate that deleting PD-1 converts the kidney into a susceptible target for invading leukocytes, no longer providing a protective barrier to combat leukocytes. This may be related to T-cell interactions with leukocytes outside, or within, the kidney.

Weakly activated T cells are most readily downregulated by PD-L engagement. PD-1 signaling inhibits suboptimal levels of CD28-mediated co-stimulation.[285] Therefore, the threshold for T-cell activation may be a balance between activating signals, such as those delivered by CD28 and B7-1 and B7-2 interactions, and inhibitory signals mediated engagement of PD-1 and its ligands, although deleting PD-1 alters central selection in the thymus.[287] PD-L1 expressed on parenchymal cells in peripheral tissues may be the most formidable barrier preserving tolerance. The net effect of signaling through these different pathways on T cells present in inflamed tissues will therefore be complex, and the balance may dictate the final outcome of the immune response.

Renal Parenchymal Cells Regulate T-Cell Activation/Anergy

Hematopoietic cells, macrophages, dendritic cells, and B cells are well-recognized "professional" APCs. Since TECs comprise 80% of the renal cortex, TECs are well positioned to "turn on" or "turn off" T-cell activation. Thus, it seems logical to suggest that T-cell activation and anergy are regulated by TECs and other renal epithelial parenchymal cell (podocyte) surface determinants. Over a decade ago, we determined that TECs in MRL-Fas(lpr) mice expressed MHC Ia.[288] This prompted us to determine whether Ia+TEC, and other renal parenchymal cells, process and present antigen to T cells. We established that TECs, stimulated with IFN-γ, expressed Ia determinants and functioned as APCs capable of activating T-cell hybridomas.[289] However, this is not a sufficiently stringent test; T-cell hybridomas are easily activated. In contrast, antigen pulsed TEC (Ia+) did not stimulate a T helper cell (Th1) clone to proliferate, but rather rendered the Th1 clone unresponsive. The interaction of the CD28 displayed on T cells with its ligand B7 expressed on APCs (Ia+) is a potent costimulatory signal that induces T-cell proliferation. This suggested that the lack of B7 on TECs was responsible for anergy in these Th1 clones.[290] We transfected the B7-1 gene into a SV40-transformed TEC line. Th1 clones were not induced by TECs (B7+, Ia+) to proliferate; however, they were not anergic since they did proliferate to antigen-pulsed spleen cells (immunologic ignorance).[291] Cocultivating TECs (B7,[+] Ia,[+] antigen pulsed) with Th1 clones stimulated through the TCR via anti-CD3 antibody (Ab) caused these Th1 clones to proliferate; anti-B7 and anti-CD28 Abs blocked this response. Thus, parenchymal cells and "professional" APCs are governed by different rules. The parenchymal cells are poised to "turn off" T-cell activation. The CD28/CTLA4/B7 pathway, to date, is restricted to T cell– and bone marrow–derived APC interactions. By comparison, the ICOS and PD-1 pathways on bone marrow-derived and parenchymal cells regulate T cells. It is intriguing to speculate that converting parenchymal cells into APCs initiates autoimmune disease. Since regulation of Th1 clones and T cells is not necessarily similar, and naïve and memory T cells require different activation signals, it is critical to thoroughly determine how CD28 member co-stimulatory pathways (ICOS and PD-1) on TECs, and other kidney parenchymal cells, regulate T cells.

Kidneys in the vast majority of people remain normal. To protect the kidney following random T-cell contact with parenchymal cells, T cells must be more readily inactivated than activated. In addition, we have reported that TECs (IFN-γ stimulated) downregulate proliferation in autoreactive T-cell clones derived from MRL-*Fas(lpr)* kidneys.[292] These data suggest that TECs deliver signals that limit the expansion of autoreactive T cells within the kidney. It is conceivable that the initiation and maintenance of T-cell activation is a regulated process, and that an imbalance in activating and anergic signals results in autoimmune LN.

CONCLUSION

Systemic lupus is an autoimmune syndrome characterized by multiple-organ immune injury, including severe nephritis. We have presented an overview of the genetics of mouse and human lupus and selected immune features that are integral in LN. Although we are just beginning to appreciate the complex nature of genetic and immune interactions, we are encouraged by the identification of several promising therapeutic targets for human LN.

References

1. Klippel JH: Systemic lupus erythematosus: Demographics, prognosis, and outcome. J Rheumatol Suppl 48:67–71 1997.
2. Petri M: Long-term outcomes in lupus. Am J Manag Care 7(Suppl):480–485, 2001.
3. Wakeland EK, Liu K, Graham RR, Behrens TW: Delineating the genetic basis of systemic lupus erythematosus. Immunity 15:397–408, 2001.
4. Wandstrat AE, Wakeland EK: The genetics of complex autoimmune diseases: Non-MHC susceptibility genes. Nat Immunol 2:802–809, 2001.
5. Theofilopoulos AN, Dixon FJ: Murine models of systemic lupus erythematosus. Adv Immunol 37:269–390, 1985.
6. Wakeland E, Morel L, Mohan C, Yui M: Genetic dissection of lupus nephritis in murine models of SLE. J Clin Immunol 17:272–281, 1997.
7. Morahan G, Morel L: Genetics of autoimmune diseases in humans and in animal models. Curr Opin Immunol 14:803–811, 2002.
8. Raman K, Mohan C: Genetics underpinnings of autoimmunity—Lessons from studies in arthritis, diabetes, lupus and multiple sclerosis. Curr Opin Immunol 15:651–659, 2003.
9. Kono DH, Baccala R, Theofilopoulos AN: In Lahita RG (ed): Systemic Lupus Erythematosus. Oxford, UK, Elsevier Academic, 2004, pp 225–263.
10. Santiago-Raber ML, et al: Role of cyclin kinase inhibitor p21 in systemic autoimmunity. J Immunol 167:4067–4074, 2001.
11. Bygrave AE, et al: Spontaneous autoimmunity in 129 and C57BL/6 mice—Implications for autoimmunity described in gene-targeted mice. PLoS Biol 2:E243, 2004.
12. Tsao BP: Update on human systemic lupus erythematosus genetics. Curr Opin Rheumatol 16:513–521, 2004.
13. U.S. Renal Data System. USRDS 2003 annual report: Atlas of end-stage renal disease in the United States. NIH NDDK. Bethesda, Md., 2003.
14. Bowden DW: Genetics of kidney disease. Kidney Int 63:8–12, 2003.
15. Bowden DW, et al: A genome scan for diabetic nephropathy in African Americans. Kidney Int 66:1517–1526, 2004.
16. Freedman BI, et al: Familial clustering of end-stage renal disease in blacks with lupus nephritis. 29:729–732, 1997.
17. Xie C, Sharma R, Wang H, et al: Strain distribution pattern of susceptibility to immune-mediated nephritis. J Immunol 172:5047–5055, 2004.
18. Xie C, Zhou XJ, Liu XB, Mohan C: Enhanced susceptibility to end-organ disease in the lupus-facilitating NZW mouse strain. Arthritis Rheum 48:1080–1092, 2003.
19. Bolland S, Ravetch JV: IgG Fc Receptors. Annu Rev Immunol 19:275–290, 2001.
20. Lehrnbecher T, et al: Variant genotypes of the low-affinity Fcgamma receptors in two control populations and a review of low-affinity Fcgamma receptor polymorphisms in control and disease populations. Blood 94:4220–4232, 1999.
21. Trikalinos TA, Karassa FB, Ioannidis JPA: Meta-analysis of the association between low-affinity Fcγ receptor gene polymorphisms and hematologic and autoimmune diseases. Blood 98:1634–1635, 2001.
22. Karassa FB, Trikalinos TA, Ioannidis JPA: Role of the Fc gamma receptor IIa polymorphism in susceptibility to systemic lupus erythematosus and lupus nephritis—A meta-analysis. Arthritis Rheum 46:1563–1571, 2002.
23. Karassa FB, Trikalinos TA, Ioannidis JPA: The Fcγ RIIIA-F158 allele is a risk factor for the development of lupus nephritis: A meta-analysis. Kidney Int 63:1475–1482, 2003.
24. Clynes R, Dumitru C Jr: Uncoupling of immune complex formation and kidney damage in autoimmune glomerulonephritis. Science 279:1052–1054, 1998.
25. Ravetch JV: Fc receptors. Curr Opin Immunol 9:121–125, 1997.
26. Magnusson V, et al: Both risk alleles for Fc gamma RIIA and Fc gamma RIIIA are susceptibility factors for SLE: A unifying hypothesis. Genes Immunity 5:130–137, 2004.
27. Sullivan KE, et al: Analysis of polymorphisms affecting immune complex handling in systemic lupus erythematosus. Rheumatology 42:446–452, 2003.
28. Ueda H, et al: Association of the T-cell regulatory gene CTLA4 with susceptibility to autoimmune disease. Nature 423:506–511, 2003.
29. Cornall RJ, et al: Polygenic autoimmune traits: Lyn, CD22, and SHP-1 are limiting elements of a biochemical pathway regulating BCR signaling and selection. Immunity 8:497–508, 1998.
30. Croker BP, Gilkeson G, Morel L: Genetic interactions between susceptibility loci reveal epistatic pathogenic networks in murine lupus. Genes Immunity 4:575–585, 2003.
31. Fronek Z, et al: Major histocompatibility complex associations with systemic lupus erythematosus. Am J Med 85:42–44, 1988.
32. Moulds JM, Krych M, Holers VM, et al: Genetics of the complement system and rheumatic diseases. Rheum Dis Clin North Am 18:893–914, 1992.

33. Gaffney PM, et al: Genome screening in human systemic lupus erythematosus: Results from a second Minnesota cohort and combined analyses of 187 sib-pair families. Am J Hum Genet 66:547–556, 2000.
34. Marchini M, et al: HLA class II antigens associated with lupus nephritis in Italian SLE patients. Hum Immunol 64:462–468, 2003.
35. Graham RR, et al: Visualizing human leukocyte antigen class II risk haplotypes in human systemic lupus erythematosus. Am J Hum Genet 71:543–553, 2002.
36. Stewart CA, et al: Complete MHC haplotype sequencing for common disease gene mapping. Genome Res 14:1176–1187, 2004.
37. Mehrian R, et al: Synergistic effect between IL-10 and bcl-2 genotypes in determining susceptibility to systemic lupus erythematosus. Arthritis Rheum 41:596–602, 1998.
38. Mok CC, Lanchbury JS, Chan DW, Lau CS: Interleukin-10 promoter polymorphisms in Southern Chinese patients with systemic lupus erythematosus. Arthritis Rheum 41:1090–1095, 1998.
39. Ou TT, et al: Genetic analysis of interleukin-10 promoter region in patients with systemic lupus erythematosus in Taiwan. Kaohsiung J Med Sci 14:599–606, 1998.
40. Kim HL, et al: The polymorphism of monocyte chemoattractant protein-1 is associated with the renal disease of SLE. Arthritis Rheumatism 40:1146–1152, 2002.
41. Tucci M, et al: Strong association of a functional polymorphism in the monocyte chemoattractant protein 1 promoter gene with lupus nephritis. Arthritis Rheum 50:1842–1849, 2004.
42. Nath SW, Kelly JA, Harley JB, Scofield RH: In Perl A (ed): Autoimmunity Methods and Protocols. Totowa, NJ, Humana Press, 2004, pp 11–30.
43. Quintero-del-Rio AI, Kelly JA, Kilpatrick J, et al: The genetics of systemic lupus erythematosus stratified by renal disease: Linkage at 10q22.3 SLEN1, 2q34-35 SLEN2, and 11p 15.6 SLEN3. Genes Immunity 3(Suppl):57–62, 2002.
44. Quintero-del-Rio AI, et al: SLEN2 2q34-35 and SLEN1 10q22.3 replication in systemic lupus erythematosus stratified by nephritis. Am J Hum Genet 75:346–348, 2004.
45. Prokunina L, et al: A regulatory polymorphism in PDCD1 is associated with susceptibility to systemic lupus erythematosus in humans. Nat Genet 32:666–669, 2002.
46. Nishimura H, Nose M, Hiai H, et al: Development of lupus-like autoimmune diseases by disruption of the PD-1 gene encoding an ITIM motif-carrying immunoreceptor. Immunity 11:141–151, 1999.
47. Hogarth MB, et al: Multiple lupus susceptibility loci map to chromosome 1 in BXSB mice. J Immunol 161:2753–2761, 1998.
48. Murphy ED, Roths JB: A Y chromosome associated factor in strain BXSB producing accelerated autoimmunity and lymphoproliferation. Arthritis Rheum 22:1188–1194, 1979.
49. Haywood MEK, et al: Dissection of BXSB lupus phenotype using mice congenic for chromosome 1 demonstrates that separate intervals direct different aspects of disease. J Immunol 173:4277–4285, 2004.
50. Bachmaier K, et al: Negative regulation of lymphocyte activation and autoimmunity by the molecular adaptor Cbl-b. Nature 403:211–216, 2000.
51. Okazaki T, et al: Autoantibodies against cardiac troponin I are responsible for dilated cardiomyopathy in PD-1-deficient mice. Nat Med 9:1477–1483, 2003.
52. Bolland S, Ravetch J: Spontaneous autoimmune disease in FcgammaRIIB-deficient mice: Results from strain-specific epistasis. Immunity 13:277–285, 2000.
53. Yajima K, Nakamura A, Sugahara A, Takai T: FcgammaRIIB deficiency with Fas mutation is sufficient for the development of systemic autoimmune disease. Eur J Immunol 33:1020–1029, 2003.
54. Bolland S, Yim YS, Tus K, et al: Genetic modifiers of systemic lupus erythematosus in Fc gamma RIIB-/- mice. J Exp Med 195:1167–1174, 2002.
55. Forton AC, Petri MA, Goldman D, Sullivan KE: An osteopontin SPP1 polymorphism associated with systemic lupus erythematosus. Hum Mutat 19:459–463, 2002.
56. Iizuka J, et al: Introduction of an osteopontin gene confers the increase in B1 cell population and the production of anti-DNA autoantibodies. Lab Invest 78:1523–1533, 1998.
57. Morel L, Blenman KR, Croker BP, Wakeland EK: The major murine systemic lupus erythematosus susceptibility locus, Sle1, is a cluster of functionally related genes. Proc Natl Acad Sci U S A 98:1787–1792, 2001.
58. Boackle SA, et al: Cr2, a candidate gene in the murine Sle1c lupus susceptibility locus, encodes a dysfunctional protein. Immunity 15:775–785, 2001.
59. Wandstrat AE, et al: Association of extensive polymorphisms in the SLAM/CD2 gene cluster with murine lupus. Immunity 21:769–780, 2004.
60. Crawley E, Woo P, Isenberg DA: Single nucleotide polymorphic haplotypes of the interleukin-10 5' flanking region are not associated with renal disease or serology in Caucasian patients with systemic lupus erythematosus. Arthritis Rheum 42:2017–2018, 1999.
61. Prokunina L, et al: The systemic lupus erythematosus-associated PDCD1 polymorphism PD1.3A in lupus nephritis. Arthritis Rheum 50:327–328, 2004.
62. Prokunina L, et al: Association of the PD-1.3A allele of the PDCD1 gene in patients with rheumatoid arthritis negative for rheumatoid factor and the shared epitope. Arthritis Rheum 50:1770–1773, 2004.
63. Aguilar F, Gonzalez-Escribano MF, Sanchez-Roman J, Nunez-Roldan A: MCP-1 promoter polymorphism in Spanish patients with systemic lupus erythematosus. Tissue Antigens 58:335–338, 2001.
64. Rovin BH, Lu L, Zhang XL: A novel interleukin-8 polymorphism is associated with severe systemic lupus erythematosus nephritis—Rapid communication. Kidney Int 62:261–265, 2002.
65. Bastian HM, et al: Systemic lupus erythematosus in three ethnic groups. XII. Risk factors for lupus nephritis after diagnosis. Lupus 11:152–160, 2002.
66. Tsuchiya N, et al: Analysis of the association of HLA-DRB1, TNF alpha promoter and TNFR2 TNFRSF1B polymorphisms with SLE using transmission disequilibrium test. Genes Immunity 2:317–322, 2001.
67. Lee HS, et al: Independent association of HLA-DR and FCγ receptor polymorphisms in Korean patients with systemic lupus erythematosus. Rheumatology 42:1501–1507, 2003.
68. Liu ZH, et al: Sex differences in estrogen receptor gene polymorphism and its association with lupus nephritis in Chinese. Nephron 90:174–180, 2002.
69. Lee YH, et al: Intron 4 polymorphism of the endothelial nitric oxide synthase gene is associated with the development of lupus nephritis. Lupus 13:188–191, 2004.
70. Wang AYM, et al: Plasminogen activator inhibitor-1 gene polymorphism 4G/4G genotype and lupus nephritis in Chinese patients. Kidney Int 59:1520–1528, 2001.
71. Villarreal J, et al: Mannose binding lectin and FcγRIIa CD32 polymorphism in Spanish systemic lupus erythematosus patients. Rheumatology 40:1009–1012, 2001.
72. Menegatti E, et al: Polymorphism of the uteroglobin gene in systemic lupus erythematosus and IgA nephropathy. Lab Invest 82:543–546, 2002.
73. Ozaki Y, et al: Vitamin-D receptor genotype and renal disorder in Japanese patients with systemic lupus erythematosus. Nephron 85:86–91, 2000.

74. Huang CM, Wu MC, Wu JY, Tsai FJ: Association of vitamin D receptor gene BsmI polymorphisms in Chinese patients with systemic lupus erythematosus. Lupus 11:31–34, 2002.

75. Huang CM, Wu MC, Wu JY, Tsai FJ: No association of vitamin D receptor gene start codon Fok I polymorphisms in Chinese patients with systemic lupus erythematosus. J Rheumatol 29:1211–1213, 2002.

76. Miyake K, et al: Genetically determined interferon-gamma production influences the histological phenotype of lupus nephritis. Rheumatology 41:518–524, 2002.

77. Cho ML, et al: Association of homozygous deletion of the Humhv3005 and the VH3-30.3 genes with renal involvement in systemic lupus erythematosus. Lupus 12:400–405, 2003.

78. Nakashima H, et al: Absence of association between the MCP-1 gene polymorphism and histological phenotype of lupus nephritis. Lupus 13:165–167, 2004.

79. Akai Y, et al: Association of an insertion polymorphism of angiotensin-converting enzyme gene with the activity of lupus nephritis. Clin Nephrol 51:141–146, 1999.

80. Parsa A, et al: Association of angiotensin-converting enzyme polymorphisms with systemic lupus erythematosus and nephritis: analysis of 644 SLE families. Genes Immunity 3(Suppl):42–46, 2002.

81. Uhm WS, et al: Angiotensin-converting enzyme gene polymorphism and vascular manifestations in Korean patients with SLE. Lupus 11:227–233, 2002.

82. Molad Y, et al: Renal outcome and vascular morbidity in systemic lupus erythematosus SLE: Lack of association with the angiotensin-converting enzyme gene polymorphism. Semin Arthritis Rheum 30:132–137, 2000.

83. Sesin C, Yin X, Buyon JP, Clancy R: In vivo and in vitro evidence that shedding of endothelial protein C receptors (EPCR) contributes to the pathogenesis of SLE. Arthritis Rheum 50(Suppl):647, 2004.

84. Van Parijs L, et al: Uncoupling IL-2 signals that regulate T cell proliferation, survival, and Fas-mediated activation-induced cell death. Immunity 11:281–288, 1999.

85. Strasser A, et al: Enforced BCL2 expression in B-lymphoid cells prolongs antibody responses and elicits autoimmune disease. Proc Natl Acad Sci U S A 88:8661–8665, 1991.

86. Roths JB, Murphy ED, Eicher EM: A new mutation, gld, that produces lymphoproliferation and autoimmunity in C3H/HeJ mice. J Exp Med 159:1–20, 1984.

87. Bouillet P, et al: Proapoptotic Bcl-2 relative Bim required for certain apoptotic responses, leukocyte homeostasis, and to preclude autoimmunity. Science 286:1735–1738, 1999.

88. Borlado L, et al: Increased phosphoinositide 3-kinase activity induces a lymphoproliferative disorder and contributes to tumor generation in vivo. FASEB J 14:895–903, 2000.

89. Salvador JM, et al: Mice lacking the p53-effector gene Gadd45a develop a lupus-like syndrome. Immunity 16:499–508, 2002.

90. Murga M, et al: Mutation of E2F2 in mice causes enhanced T lymphocyte proliferation, leading to the development of autoimmunity. Immunity 15:959–970, 2001.

91. Zhang Y, et al: Impaired apoptosis, extended duration of immune responses, and a lupus-like autoimmune disease in IEX-1-transgenic mice. Proc Natl Acad Sci U S A 99:878–883, 2002.

92. Andrews BS, et al: Spontaneous murine lupus-like syndromes. Clinical and immunopathological manifestations in several strains. J Exp Med 148:1198–1215, 1978.

93. Di Cristofano A, et al: Impaired Fas response and autoimmunity in Pten+/ mice. Science 285:2122–2125, 1999.

94. Majeti R, et al: An inactivating point mutation in the inhibitory wedge of CD45 causes lymphoproliferation and autoimmunity. Cell 103:1059–1070, 2000.

95. Hibbs ML, et al: Multiple defects in the immune system of lyn-deficient mice, culminating in autoimmune disease. Cell 83:301–311, 1995.

96. Hibbs ML, et al: Sustained activation of Lyn tyrosine kinase in vivo leads to autoimmunity. J Exp Med 196:1593–1604, 2002.

97. Mackay F, et al: Mice transgenic for BAFF develop lymphocytic disorders along with autoimmune manifestations. J Exp Med 190:1697–1710, 1999.

98. Rifkin IR, et al: Acceleration of lpr lymphoproliferative and autoimmune disease by transgenic protein kinase CK2α. J Immunol 161:5164–5170, 1998.

99. Zhang L, et al: An immunological renal disease in transgenic mice that overexpress Fli-1, a member of the ets family of transcription factor genes. Mol Cell Biol 15:6961–6970, 1995.

100. Seery JP, Carroll JM, Cattell V, Watt FM: Antinuclear autoantibodies and lupus nephritis in transgenic mice expressing interferon gamma in the epidermis. J Exp Med 186:1451–1459, 1997.

101. Hasegawa K, Hayashi T, Maeda K: Promotion of lupus in NZB x NZWF1 mice by plasmids encoding interferon IFN-γ but not by those encoding interleukin IL-4. J Comp Path 127:1–6, 2002.

102. Seshasayee D, et al: Loss of TACI causes fatal lymphoproliferation and autoimmunity, establishing TACI as an inhibitory BLyS receptor. Immunity 18:279–288, 2003.

103. Wilkinson R, et al: Platelet endothelial cell adhesion molecule-1 PECAM-1/CD31 acts as a regulator of B-cell development, B-cell antigen receptor BCR-mediated activation, and autoimmune disease. Blood 100:184–193, 2002.

104. Le LQ, et al: Mice lacking the orphan G protein-coupled receptor G2A develop a late-onset autoimmune syndrome. Immunity 14:561–571, 2001.

105. Miyamoto A, et al: Increased proliferation of B cells and auto-immunity in mice lacking protein kinase C delta. Nature 416:865–869, 2002.

106. Hron JD, Peng SL: Type I IFN protects against murine lupus. J Immunol 173:2134–2142, 2004.

107. Hurov JB, et al: Immune system dysfunction and autoimmune disease in mice lacking Emk Par-1 protein kinase. Mol Cell Biol 21:3206–3219, 2001.

108. Mehling A, et al: Overexpression of CD40 ligand in murine epidermis results in chronic skin inflammation and systemic autoimmunity. J Exp Med 194:615–628, 2001.

109. Higuchi T, et al: Cutting edge: Ectopic expression of CD40 ligand on B cells induces lupus-like autoimmune disease. J Immunol 168:9–12, 2002.

110. Xue D, et al: A lupus-like syndrome develops in mice lacking the Ro 60-kDa protein, a major lupus autoantigen. Proc Natl Acad Sci U S A 100:7503–7508, 2003.

111. Bickerstaff MCM, et al: Serum amyloid P component controls chromatin degradation and prevents antinuclear autoimmunity. Nat Med 5:694–697, 1999.

112. Szalai AJ, et al: Delayed lupus onset in NZB x NZWF-1 mice expressing a human C-reactive protein transgene. Arthritis Rheum 48:1602–1611, 2003.

113. Szondy Z, et al: Transglutaminase 2-/- mice reveal a phagocytosis-associated crosstalk between macrophages and apoptotic cells. Proc Natl Acad Sci U S A 100:7812–7817, 2003.

114. Cohen PL, et al: Delayed apoptotic cell clearance and lupus-like autoimmunity in mice lacking the c-mer membrane tyrosine kinase. J Exp Med 196:135–140, 2002.

115. Botto M, et al: Homozygous C1q deficiency causes glomerulonephritis associated with multiple apoptotic bodies. Nat Genet 19:56–59, 1998.

116. Hanayama R, et al: Autoimmune disease and impaired uptake of apoptotic cells in MFG-E8-deficient mice. Science 304:1147–1150, 2004.

117. Boes M, et al: Accelerated development of IgG autoantibodies and autoimmune disease in the absence of secreted IgM. Proc Natl Acad Sci U S A 97:1184–1189, 2000.

118. Napirei M, et al: Features of systemic lupus erythematosus in Dnase1-deficient mice. Nat Genet 25:177–181, 2000.

119. Prodeus AP, et al: A critical role for complement in maintenance of self-tolerance. Immunity 9:721–731, 1998.

120. Demetriou M, Granovsky M, Quaggin S, Dennis JW: Negative regulation of T-cell activation and autoimmunity by Mgat5 N-glycosylation. Nature 409:733–739, 2001.

121. Yoh K, et al: Nrf2-deficient female mice develop lupus-like autoimmune nephritis. Kidney Int 60:1343–1353, 2001.

122. Shim GJ, Kis LL, Warner M, Gustafsson JA: Autoimmune glomerulonephritis with spontaneous formation of splenic germinal centers in mice lacking the estrogen receptor alpha gene. Proc Natl Acad Sci U S A 101:1720–1724, 2004.

123. Erb KJ, et al: Constitutive expression of interleukin IL-4 in vivo causes autoimmune-type disorders in mice. J Exp Med 185:329–339, 1997.

124. Ruger BM, et al: Interleukin-4 transgenic mice develop glomerulosclerosis independent of immunoglobulin deposition. Eur J Immunol 30:2698–2703, 2000.

125. Sun J, Matthias G, Mihatsch MJ, et al: Lack of the transcriptional coactivator OBF-1 prevents the development of systemic lupus erythematosus-like phenotypes in Aiolos mutant mice. J Immun 170:1699–1706, 2003.

126. Chui D, et al: Genetic remodeling of protein glycosylation in vivo induces autoimmune disease. Proc Natl Acad Sci U S A 98:1142–1147, 2001.

127. Morel L, et al: Functional dissection of systemic lupus erythematosus using congenic mouse strains. J Immunol 158:6019–6028, 1997.

128. Morel L, Rudofsky U, Longmate J, et al: Polygenic control of susceptibility to murine systemic lupus erythematosus. Immunity 1:219–229, 1994.

129. Mohan C, Alas E, Morel L, et al: Genetic dissection of SLE pathogenesis: Sle1 on murine chromosome 1 leads to a selective loss of tolerance to H2A/H2B/DNA subnucleosomes. J Clin Invest 101:1362–1372, 1998.

130. Kono DH, et al: Resistance to xenobiotic-induced autoimmunity maps to chromosome 1. J Immunol 167:2396–2403, 2001.

131. Vyse T, Rozzo S, Drake C, et al: Control of multiple autoantibodies linked with a lupus nephritis susceptibility locus in New Zealand Black Mice. J Immunol 158:5566–5574, 1997.

132. Rozzo SJ, et al: Evidence for an interferon-inducible gene Ifi202 in the susceptibility to systemic lupus. Immunity 15:435–443, 2001.

133. Waters ST, et al: NZM2328: A new mouse model of systemic lupus erythematosus with unique genetic susceptibility loci. Clin Immunol 100:372–383, 2001.

134. Waters ST, et al: Breaking tolerance to double stranded DNA nucleosome and other nuclear antigens is not required for the pathogenesis of lupus glomerulonephritis. J Exp Med 199:255–264, 2004.

135. Rahman ZS, et al: A novel susceptibility locus on chromosome 2 in the New Zealand Black x New Zealand WhiteF1 hybrid mouse model of systemic lupus erythematosus. J Immunol 168:3042–3049, 2002.

136. Rigby RJ, et al: New loci from New Zealand Black and New Zealand White on chromosomes 4 and 12 contribute to lupus-like disease in the context of BALB/c. J Immunol 172:4609–4617, 2004.

137. Mohan C, Morel L, Yang P, Wakeland EK: Genetic dissection of systemic lupus erythematosus pathogenesis—Sle2 on murine chromosome 4 leads to B cell hyperactivity. J Immunol 159:454–465, 1997.

138. Kono DH, et al: Lupus susceptibility loci in New Zealand mice. Proc Natl Acad Sci U S A 91:10168–10172, 1994.

139. Drake CG, Babcock SK, Palmer E, Kotzin BL: Genetic analysis of the NZB contribution to lupus-like autoimmune disease in NZB x NZWF1 mice. Proc Natl Acad Sci U S A 91:4062–4066, 1994.

140. Hirose S, Tsurui H, Nishimura H, et al: Mapping of a gene for hypergammaglobulinemia to the distal region of chromosome 4 in NZB mice and its contribution to systemic lupus erythematosus in NZB X NZWF1 mice. Int Immunol 6:1857–1864, 1994.

141. Morel L, Tian XH, Croker BP, Wakeland EK: Epistatic modifiers of autoimmunity in a murine model of lupus nephritis. Immunity 11:131–139, 1999.

142. Kono DH, Park MS, Theofilopoulos AN: Genetic complementation in female BXSB x NZWF-2 mice. J Immunol 171:6442–6447, 2003.

143. Watson ML, et al: Genetic analysis of MRL-lpr mice: Relationship of the Fas apoptosis gene to disease manifestations and renal disease-modifying loci. J Exp Med 176:1645–1656, 1992.

144. Mohan C, Yu Y, Morel L, et al: Genetic dissection of Sle pathogenesis: Sle3 on murine chromosome 7 impacts T cell activation differentiation and cell death. J Immunol 162:6492–6502, 1999.

145. Xie S, et al: Dominant NZB contributions to lupus in the SWR x NZBF1 model. Genes Immunity 3(Suppl):13–20, 2002.

146. Drake CG, et al: Analysis of the New Zealand Black contribution to lupus-like renal disease. Multiple genes that operate in a threshold manner. J Immunol 154:2441–2447, 1995.

147. Vidal S, Kono DH, Theofilopoulos AN: Loci predisposing to autoimmunity in MRL-Fas lpr and C57BL/6-Faslpr mice. J Clin Invest 101:696–702, 1998.

148. Rozzo SJ, Vyse TJ, Drake CG, Kotzin BL: Effect of genetic background on the contribution of New Zealand black loci to autoimmune lupus nephritis. Proc Nat Acad Sci U S A 93:15164–15168, 1996.

149. Haywood MEK, et al: Autoantigen glycoprotein 70 expression is regulated by a single locus which acts as a checkpoint for pathogenic anti-glycoprotein 70 autoantibody production and hence for the corresponding development of severe nephritis in lupus-prone BXSB mice. J Immunol 167:1728–1733, 2001.

150. Rozzo SJ, Vyse TJ, Menze K, et al: Enhanced susceptibility to lupus contributed from the nonautoimmune C57BL/10 but not C57BL/6 genome. J Immunol 164:5515–5521, 2000.

151. Xie SK, et al: Genetic contributions of nonautoimmune SWR mice toward lupus nephritis. J Immunol 167:7141–7149, 2001.

152. Wang Y, Nose M, Kamoto T, et al: Host modifier genes affect mouse autoimmunity induced by the lpr gene. Am J Pathol 151:1791–1798, 1997.

153. Morel G: Internalization and nuclear localization of peptide hormones. Biochem Pharmacol 47:63–76, 1994.

154. Morel L, Yykrbra C, Ek W: Production of congenic mouse strains carrying genomic intervals containing SLE-susceptibility genes derived from the SLE-prone NZM2410 strain. Mammal Genome 7:335–339, 1996.

155. Morel L, et al: Multiplex inheritance of component phenotypes in a murine model of lupus. Mammal Genome 10:176–181, 1999.

156. Nemazee D: Antigen receptor "capacity" and the sensitivity of self-tolerance. Immunol Today 17:25–29, 1996.

157. Mathis D, Benoist C: Back to central tolerance. Immunity 20:509–516, 2004.

158. Wardemann H, et al: Predominant autoantibody production by early human B cell precursors. Science 301:1374–1377, 2003.

159. Fields ML, Erikson J: The regulation of lupus-associated autoantibodies: Immunoglobulin transgenic models. Curr Opin Immunol 15:709–717, 2003.

160. Bouzahzah F, Jung S, Craft J: CD4$^+$ T cells from lupus-prone mice avoid antigen-specific tolerance induction in vivo. J Immunol 170:741–748, 2003.

161. Tsokos G, Wong H, Enyedy E, Nambiar M: Immune cell signaling in lupus. Curr Opin Rheumatol 12:355–363, 2000.

162. Kong PL, et al: Intrinsic T cell defects in systemic autoimmunity. Ann NY Acad Sci 987:60–67, 2003.

163. Yu CC, Mamchak AA, DeFranco AL: Signaling mutations and autoimmunity. Curr Dir Autoimmun 6:61–88, 2003.

164. Kretz-Rommel A, Rubin R: Disruption of positive selection of thymocytes causes autoimmunity. Nat Med 6:298–305, 2000.

165. Rao T: Richardson B. Environmentally induced autoimmune diseases: Potential mechanisms. Environ Health Perspect 107(Suppl 5):737–742, 1999.

166. Yan J, Mamula MJ: B and T cell tolerance and autoimmunity in autoantibody transgenic mice. Int Immunol 14:963–971, 2002.

167. Mamula MJ, Fatehnejad S, Craft J: B-cells process and present lupus autoantigens that initiate autoimmune T-cell responses. J Immunol 152:1453–1461, 1994.

168. Xu H, Li H, Suri-Payer E, et al: Regulation of anti-DNA B cells in recombination-activating gene-deficient mice. J Exp Med 188:1247–1254, 1998.

169. Seo S, et al: The impact of T helper and T regulatory cells on the regulation of anti-double-stranded DNA B cells. Immunity 16:535–546, 2002.

170. Metcalf ES, Schrater AF, Klinman NR: Murine models of tolerance induction in developing and mature B cells. Immunol Rev 43:143, 1979.

171. Fulcher DA, et al: The fate of self-reactive B cells depends primarily on the degree of antigen receptor engagement and availability of T cell help. J Exp Med 183:2313–2328, 1996.

172. Cooke MP, et al: Immunoglobulin signal transduction guides the specificity of B cell-T cell interactions and is blocked in tolerant self-reactive B cells. J Exp Med 179:425–438, 1994.

173. Goodnow CC, Brink R, Adams E: Breakdown of self-tolerance in anergic B lymphocytes. Nature 352:532–536, 1991.

174. Giese T, Davidson WF: Evidence for early onset polyclonal activation of T cell subsets in mice homozygous for lpr. J Immunol 149:3097–3106, 1992.

175. Yi Y, McNerney M, Datta S: Regulatory defects in cbl and mitogen-activated protein kinase: Extracellular signal-related kinase pathways cause persistent hyperexpression of CD40 ligand in human lupus T cells. J Immunol 165:6627–6634, 2000.

176. Mohan C, Adams S, Stanik V, Datta SK: Nucleosome: A major immunogen for pathogenic autoantibody-inducing T cells of lupus. J Exp Med 177:1367–1381, 1993.

177. Rosen A, Casciola-Rosen L: Clearing the way to mechanisms of autoimmunity. Nat Med 7:664–665, 2001.

178. Leadbetter EA, et al: Chromatin-IgG complexes activate B cells by dual engagement of IgM and Toll-like receptors. Nature 416:603–607, 2002.

179. Katsiari C, Tsokos G: Re-establishment of tolerance: The prospect of developing specific treatment for human lupus. Lupus 13:485–488, 2004.

180. Shlomchik MJ, Madaio MP, Ni D, et al: The role of B cells in lpr/lpr-induced autoimmunity. J Exp Med 180:1295–1306, 1994.

181. Chan OT, Hannum LG, Haberman AM, et al: A novel mouse with B cells but lacking serum antibody reveals an antibody-independent role for B cells in murine lupus. J Exp Med 189:1639–1648, 1999.

182. Chan OT, Madaio MP, Shlomchik MJ: The central and multiple roles of B cells in lupus pathogenesis. Immunol Rev 169:107–121, 1999.

183. Harris DP, et al: Reciprocal regulation of polarized cytokine production by effector B and T cells. Nat Immunol 1:475–482, 2000.

184. Linton PJ, Harbertson J, Bradley LM: A critical role for B cells in the development of memory CD4 cells. J Immunol 165:5558–5565, 2000.

185. Duddy ME, Alter A, Bar-Or A: Distinct profiles of human B cell effector cytokines: A role in immune regulation? J Immunol 172:3422–3427, 2004.

186. Tumanov A, et al: Distinct role of surface lymphotoxin expressed by B cells in the organization of secondary lymphoid tissues. Immunity 17:239–250, 2002.

187. Chan O, Shlomchik MJ: A new role for B cells in systemic autoimmunity: B cells promote spontaneous T cell activation in MRL-lpr/lpr mice. J Immunol 160:51–59, 1998.

188. Chan O, Shlomchik M: Cutting edge: B cells promote CD8$^+$ T cell activation in MRL-Faslpr mice independently of MHC class I antigen presentation. J Immunol 164:1658–1662, 2000.

189. Sato T, et al: Aberrant B1 cell migration into the thymus results in activation of CD4 T cells through its potent antigen-presenting activity in the development of murine lupus. Eur J Immunol 34:3346–3358, 2004.

190. Ito T, et al: Defective B1 cell homing to the peritoneal cavity and preferential recruitment of B1 cells in the target organs in a murine model for systemic lupus erythematosus. J Immunol 172:3628–3634, 2004.

191. Cassese G, et al: Inflamed kidneys of NZB/W mice are a major site for the homeostasis of plasma cells. Eur J Immunol 31:2726–2732, 2001.

192. Sekine H, Watanabe H, Gilkeson GS: Enrichment of anti-glomerular antigen antibody-producing cells in the kidneys of MRL/MpJ-Faslpr mice. J Immunol 172:3913–3921, 2004.

193. Ehrenstein MR, Cook HT, Neuberger MS: Deficiency in serum immunoglobulin IgM predisposes to development of IgG autoantibodies. J Exp Med 191:1253–1258, 2000.

194. Berden JHM: Lupus nephritis. Kidney Int 52:538–558, 1997.

195. Foster MH, Cizman BC, Madaio MP: Nephritogenic autoantibodies in systemic lupus erythematosus: Immunochemical properties mechanisms of immune deposition and genetic origins. Lab Invest 69:494–507, 1993.

196. Foster MH, Kelley VR: Lupus nephritis: Update on pathogenesis and disease mechanisms. Semin Nephrol 19:173–181, 1999.

197. Vlahakos DV, et al: Anti-DNA antibodies form immune deposits at distinct glomerular and vascular sites. Kidney Int 41:1690–1700, 1992.

198. Ehrenstein MR, et al: Human IgG anti-DNA antibodies deposit in kidneys and induce proteinuria in SCID mice. Kidney Int 48:705–711, 1995.

199. Pankewycz OG, Migliorini P, Madaio MP: Polyreactive autoantibodies are nephritogenic in murine lupus nephritis. J Immunol 139:3287–3294, 1987.

200. Foster MH, et al: Molecular analysis of nephrotropic anti-laminin antibodies from an MRL/lpr autoimmune mouse. J Immunol 151:814–824, 1993.

201. Madaio MP, et al: Murine monoclonal anti-DNA antibodies bind directly to glomerular antigens and form immune deposits. J Immunol 138:2883–2889, 1987.

202. Mostoslavsky G, et al: Lupus anti-DNA autoantibodies cross-react with a glomerular structural protein: A case for tissue injury by molecular mimicry. Eur J Immunol 31:1221–1227, 2001.

203. Pratesi F, et al: Autoantibodies specific for alpha-enolase in systemic autoimmune disorders. J Rheumatol 27:109–115, 2000.

204. Koren E, et al: Murine and human antibodies to native DNA that cross-react with the A and D SnRNP polypeptides cause direct injury of cultured kidney cells. J Immunol 154:4857–4864, 1995.

205. Vlahakos DV, et al: Murine monoclonal anti-DNA antibodies penetrate cells bind to nuclei and induce glomerular proliferation and proteinuria in vivo. J Am Soc Nephrol 2:1345–1354, 1992.
206. Putterman C: New approaches to the renal pathogenicity of anti-DNA antibodies in systemic lupus erythematosus. Autoimmun Rev 3:7–11, 2004.
207. Zavala F, et al: Granulocyte-colony stimulating factor treatment of lupus autoimmune disease im MRL-lpr/lpr mice. J Immunol 163:5125–5132, 1999.
208. Matsumoto K, et al: Fc receptor-independent development of autoimmune glomerulonephritis in lupus-prone MRL/lpr mice. Arthritis Rheum 48:486–494, 2003.
209. Takai T: Roles of Fc receptors in autoimmunity. Nat Rev Immunol 2:580–592, 2002.
210. Boule MW, et al: Toll-like receptor 9-dependent and -independent dendritic cell activation by chromatin-immunoglobulin G complexes. J Exp Med 199:1631–1640, 2004.
211. Bolland S, Yim Y, Tus K, Wakeland E, Ravetch J: Genetic modifiers of systemic lupus erythematosus in FcgammaRIIB-/- mice. J Exp Med 195:1167–1174, 2002.
212. Manderson AP, Botto M, Walport MJ: The role of complement in the development of systemic lupus erythematosus. Annu Rev Immunol 22:431–456, 2004.
213. Chen Z, Koralov SB, Kelsoe G: Complement C4 inhibits systemic autoimmunity through a mechanism independent of complement receptors CR1 and CR2. J Exp Med 192:1339–1352, 2000.
214. Einav S, Pozdnyakova OO, Ma M, Carroll MC: Complement C4 is protective for lupus disease independent of C3. J Immunol 168:1036–1041, 2002.
215. Mitchell D, et al: C1q deficiency and autoimmunity: The effects of genetic background on disease expression. J Immunol 168:2538–2543, 2002.
216. Paul E, Pozdnyakova OO, Mitchell E, Carroll MC: Anti-DNA autoreactivity in C4-deficient mice. Eur J Immunol 32:2672–2679, 2002.
217. Mitchell DA, et al: Cutting edge: C1q protects against the development of glomerulonephritis independently of C3 activation. J Immunol 162:5676–5679, 1999.
218. Watanabe H, et al: Modulation of renal disease in MRL/lpr mice genetically deficient in the alternative complement pathway factor B. J Immunol 15:786–794, 2000.
219. Elliott MK, et al: Effects of complement factor D deficiency on the renal disease of MRL/lpr mice. Kidney Int 65:129–138, 2004.
220. Croix D, et al: Antibody response to a T-dependent antigen requires B cell expression of complement receptors. J Exp Med 183:1857–1864, 1996.
221. Bao L, et al: Administration of a soluble recombinant complement C3 inhibitor protects against renal disease in MRL/lpr mice. J Am Soc Nephrol 14:670–679, 2003.
222. Sekine H, et al: Complement component C3 is not required for full expression of immune complex glomerulonephritis in MRL/lpr mice. J Immunol 166:6444–6551, 2001.
223. Wang Y, et al: Amelioration of lupus-like autoimmune disease in NZB/WF1 mice after treatment with a blocking monoclonal antibody specific for complement component C5. Proc Natl Acad Sci U S A 93:8563–8568, 1996.
224. Miwa T, et al: Deletion of decay-accelerating factor CD55 exacerbates autoimmune disease development in MRL/lpr mice. Am J Pathol 161:1077–1086, 2002.
225. Tesch GH, et al: Monocyte chemoattractant protein-1 promotes macrophage-mediated tubular injury but not glomerular injury in nephrotoxic serum nephritis. J Clin Invest 103:73–80, 1999.
226. Duffield JS, et al: Activated macrophages direct apoptosis and suppress mitosis of mesangial cells. J Immunol 164:2110–2119, 2000.
227. Lenda DM, Kikawada E, Stanley ER, Kelley VR: Reduced macrophage recruitment proliferation and activation in colony-stimulating factor-1-deficient mice results in decreased tubular apoptosis during renal inflammation. J Immunol 170:3254–3262, 2003.
228. Yui MA, Brissette WH, Brennan DC, et al: Increased macrophage colony-stimulating factor in neonatal and adult autoimmune MRL-lpr mice. Am J Pathol 139:255–261, 1991.
229. Bloom RD, Florquin S, Singer GG, et al: Colony stimulating factor-1 in the induction of lupus nephritis. Kidney Int 43:1000–1009, 1993.
230. Naito T, Griffiths RC, Coffman TM, Kelley VR: Transplant approach establishes that kidneys are responsible for serum CSF-1 but require a stimulus in MRL-lpr mice. Kidney Int 49:67–74, 1996.
231. Wada T, Naito T, Griffiths RC, et al: Systemic autoimmune nephritogenic components induce CSF-1 and TNF-alpha in MRL kidneys. Kidney Int 52:934–941, 1997.
232. Naito T, et al: Macrophage growth factors introduced into the kidney initiate renal injury. Mol Med 2:297–312, 1996.
233. Matsuda M, Shikata K, Makino H, et al: Glomerular expression of macrophage colony-stimulating factor and granulocyte-macrophage colony-stimulating factor in patients with various forms of glomerulonephritis. Lab Invest 75:403–412, 1996.
234. Lenda D, Kikawada E, Stanley ES, Kelley VR: Reduced Mø recruitment proliferation and activation in CSF-1 deficient mice results in decreased tubular apoptosis during renal inflammation. J Immunol 2004.
235. Moore KJ, Naito T, Martin C, Kelley VR: Enhanced response of macrophages to CSF-1 in autoimmune mice: A gene transfer strategy. J Immunol 157:433–440, 1996.
236. Levine J, Hartwell D, Beller DI: Imbalanced cytokine production by macrophages from autoimmune-prone mice. Immunol Lett 30:183–192, 1991.
237. Hartwell DW, Fenton MJ, Levine JS, Beller DI: Aberrant cytokine regulation in macrophages from young autoimmune-prone mice: Evidence that the intrinsic defect in MRL macrophage IL-1 expression is transcriptionally controlled. Mol Immunol 32:743–751, 1995.
238. Liu J, Beller DI: Distinct pathways for NF-kappa B regulation are associated with aberrant macrophage IL-12 production in lupus- and diabetes-prone mouse strains. J Immunol 170:4489–4496, 2003.
239. Dang-Vu AP, Pisetsky DS, Weinberg JB: Functional alterations of macrophages in autoimmune MRL-lpr/lpr mice. J Immunol 138:1757–1761, 1987.
240. Licht R, Dieker JW, Jacobs CW, et al: Decreased phagocytosis of apoptotic cells in diseased SLE mice. J Autoimmun 22:139–145, 2004.
241. Baumann I, et al: Impaired uptake of apoptotic cells into tingible body macrophages in germinal centers of patients with systemic lupus erythematosus. Arthritis Rheum 46:191–201, 2002.
242. Davidson WF, Dumont FJ, Bedigian HG, et al: Phenotypic functional and molecular genetic comparisons of the abnormal lymphoid cells of C3H-lpr/lpr and C3H-gld/gld mice. J Immunol 136:4075–4084, 1986.
243. Dumont FJ, Habbersett RC, Nichols EA, et al: A monoclonal antibody 100C5 to the Lyt-2-T cell population expanding in MRL/Mp-lpr/lpr mice detects a surface antigen normally expressed on Lyt-2+ cells and B cells. Eur J Immunol 13:455–459, 1983.
244. Huang L, Soldevila G, Leeker M, et al: The liver eliminates T cells undergoing antigen-triggered apoptosis in vivo. Immunity 1:741–749, 1994.
245. Hughes DP, Hayday A, Craft JE, et al: T cells with gamma/delta T cell receptors TCR of intestinal type are preferentially expanded in TCR-alpha-deficient lpr mice. J Exp Med 182:233–241, 1995.

246. Crispe IN, Huang L: Neonatal moribund and undead T cells: The role of the liver in T cell development. Semin Immunol 6:39–41, 1994.

247. Yamagiwa S, et al: The primary site of CD4- 8- B220+ alphabeta T cells in lpr mice: The appendix in normal mice. J Immunol 160:2665–2674, 1998.

248. Watanabe D, Suda T, Hashimoto H, Nagata S: Constitutive activation of the Fas ligand gene in mouse lymphoproliferative disorders. EMBO J 14:12–18, 1995.

249. Diaz Gallo C, et al: Autoreactive kidney-infiltrating T-cell clones in murine lupus nephritis. Kidney Int 42:851–859, 1992.

250. Christianson GJ, et al: Beta2-microglobulin dependence of the lupus-like autoimmune syndrome of MRL-lpr mice. J Immunol 156:4932–4939, 1996.

251. Christianson GJ, et al: Beta 2-microglobulin-deficient mice are protected from hypergammaglobulinemia and have defective antibody responses because of increased IgG catabolism. J Immunol 159:4781–4792, 1997.

252. Wada T, Schwarting A, Chesnutt MS, et al: Nephritogenic cytokines and disease in MRL-Faslpr kidneys are dependent on multiple T-cell subsets. Kidney Int 59:565–578, 2001.

253. Wang JKM, Zhu B, Ju ST, et al: CD4+ T cells reactivated with superantigen are both more sensitive to FasL-mediated killing and express a higher level of FasL. Cell Immunol 179:153–164, 1997.

254. Duan JM, Fagard R, Madaio MP: Abnormal signal transduction through CD4 leads to altered tyrosine phosphorylation in T cells derived from MRL-lpr/lpr mice. Autoimmunity 23:231–243,1996.

255. Bretscher P, Cohn M: A theory of self-nonself discrimination. Science 169:1042–1049, 1970.

256. Janeway CA, Bottomly K: Signals and signs for lymphocyte responses. Cell 76:275–285, 1994.

257. Linsley PS, Ledbetter JA: The role of the CD28 receptor during T cell responses to antigen. Annu Rev Immunol 11:191–212, 1993.

258. Bluestone JA: New perspectives of CD28-B7-mediated T cell costimulation. Immunity 2:555–559, 1995.

259. Thompson CB: Distinct roles for the costimulatory ligands B7-1 and B7-2 in T helper cell differentiation. Cell 81:979–982, 1995.

260. Sayegh MH, Turka LA: The role of T-cell costimulatory activation pathways in transplant rejection. N Engl J Med 338:1813–1821, 1998.

261. Yamada A, Salama AD, Sayegh MH: The role of novel T cell costimulatory pathways in autoimmunity and transplantation. J Am Soc Nephrol 13:559–575, 2002.

262. Yamada A, et al: CD28 independent costimulation of T cells in alloimmune responses. J Immunol 167:140–146, 2001.

263. Linsley PS, et al: CTLA-4 is a second receptor for the B cell activation antigen B7. J Exp Med 174:561–569, 1991.

264. Walunas TL, et al: CTLA-4 can function as a negative regulator of T cell activation. Immunity 1:405–413, 1994.

265. Waterhouse P, et al: Lymphoproliferative disorders with early lethality in mice deficient in CTLA4. Science 270:985–988, 1995.

266. Tivol EA, et al: Loss of CTLA-4 leads to massive lymphoproliferation and fatal multiorgan tissue destruction revealing a critical negative regulatory role of CTLA-4. Immunity 3:541–547, 1995.

267. Bluestone JA: Is CTLA-4 a master switch for peripheral T cell tolerance? J Immunol 158:1989–1993, 1997.

268. Kinoshita K, et al: Costimulation by B7-1 and B7-2 is required for autoimmune disease in MRL-Faslpr mice. J Immunol 164:6046–6056, 2000.

269. Takiguchi M, et al: Blockade of CD28/CTLA4-B7 pathway prevented autoantibody-related diseases but not lung disease in MRL/lpr mice. Lab Invest 79:317–326, 1999.

270. Tada Y, et al: Role of the costimulatory molecule CD28 in the development of lupus in MRL/lpr mice. J Immunol 163:3153–3159, 1999.

271. Daikh DI, Wofsy D: Cutting edge: Reversal of murine lupus nephritis with CTLA4Ig and cyclophosphamide. J Immunol 166:2913–2916, 2001.

272. Hutloff A, et al: ICOS is an inducible T-cell co-stimulator structurally and functionally related to CD28. Nature 397:263–266, 1999.

273. Yoshinaga SK, et al: T-cell co-stimulation through B7RP-1 and ICOS. Nature 402:827–832, 1999.

274. Brodie D, et al: LICOS a primordial costimulatory ligand? Curr Biol 10:333–336, 2000.

275. Ling V, et al: Cutting edge: Identification of GL50 a novel B7-like protein that functionally binds to ICOS receptor. J Immunol 164:1653–1657, 2000.

276. Mages HW, et al: Molecular cloning and characterization of murine ICOS and identification of B7h as ICOS ligand. Eur J Immunol 30:1040–1047, 2000.

277. Aicher A, et al: Characterization of human inducible costimulator ligand expression and function. J Immunol 164:4689–4696, 2000.

278. Coyle AJ, et al: The CD28-related molecule ICOS is required for effective T cell- dependent immune responses. Immunity 13:95–105, 2000.

279. McAdam AJ, et al: Mouse inducible costimulatory molecule ICOS expression is enhanced by CD28 costimulation and regulates differentiation of CD4+ T cells. J Immunol 165:5035–5040, 2000.

280. Coyle AJ, Gutierrez-Ramos JC: The expanding B7 superfamily: Increasing complexity in costimulatory signals regulating T cell function. Nat Immunol 2:203–209, 2001.

281. Khayyamian S, et al: ICOS-ligand expressed on human endothelial cells costimulates Th1 and Th2 cytokine secretion by memory CD4+ T cells. Proc Natl Acad Sci U S A 99:6198–6203, 2002.

282. Dong C, et al: ICOS co-stimulatory receptor is essential for T-cell activation and function. Nature 409:97–101, 2001.

283. Rottman JB, et al: The costimulatory molecule ICOS plays an important role in the immunopathogenesis of EAE. Nat Immunol 2:605–611, 2001.

284. Wahl P, Bilic G, Neuweiler J, et al: B7RP-1 a novel renal tubular epithelial antigen with costimulatory function. J Am Soc Nephrol 12:643A, 2001.

284a. Jang WH, Herber DM, Jiang Y, et al: Distinct in vivo roles of colony stimulating factor-1 isoforms in renal inflammation. Immunol 177:4055–4063, 2006.

285. Freeman GJ, et al: Engagement of the PD-1 immunoinhibitory receptor by a novel B7 family member leads to negative regulation of lymphocyte activation. J Exp Med 192:1027–1034, 2000.

286. Latchman Y, et al: PD-L2 is a second ligand for PD-I and inhibits T cell activation. Nat Immunol 2:261–268, 2001.

287. Nishimura H, Honjo T, Minato N: Facilitation of beta selection and modification of positive selection in the thymus of PD-1-deficient mice. J Exp Med 191:891–898, 2000.

288. Wuthrich RP, et al: Enhanced MHC class II expression in renal proximal tubules precedes loss of renal function in MRL/lpr mice with lupus nephritis. Am J Pathol 134:45–51, 1989.

289. Wuthrich RP, et al: MHC class II antigen presentation and tumor necrosis factor in renal tubular epithelial cells. Kidney Int 37:783–792, 1990.

290. Singer GG, et al: Stimulated renal tubular epithelial cells induce anergy in CD4+ T cells. Kidney Int 44:1030–1035, 1993.

291. Yokoyama H, Zheng X, Strom TB, et al: B7+-transfectant tubular epithelial cells induce T cell anergy ignorance or proliferation. Kidney Int 45:1105–1112, 1994.

292. Diaz-Gallo C, Kelley VR: Self-regulation of autoreactive kidney-infiltrating T cells in MRL-lpr nephritis. Kidney Int 44:692–699, 1993.

Chapter 30

Molecular and Genetic Aspects of Ischemic Acute Kidney Injury

Joseph V. Bonventre

Ischemic acute kidney injury (AKI) is a condition that results from a mismatch between oxygen and nutrient delivery to the nephrons and energy demand of the nephrons. At times there is a clearly defined transient drop in total or regional blood flow to the kidney that results from compromise of the systemic circulation; at other times, for example in the setting of sepsis, the reduction in perfusion may not be associated with systemic signs of hypotension or circulatory compromise. AKI is frequently associated with multiple-organ failure and sepsis. Despite advances in preventative strategies and support measures, this syndrome continues to be associated with significant morbidity and mortality. The pathophysiology of AKI is complex. Figure 30-1 summarizes a complex interplay of vascular and tubular processes that ultimately lead to organ dysfunction. AKI is a state characterized by enhanced vasoconstriction, which is manifest in response to enhanced renal nerve activity and increased tissue concentrations of vasoconstrictive agents such as angiotensin II and endothelin. At the same time there is decreased responsiveness of the resistance vessels to vasodilators such as acetylcholine, bradykinin, and nitric oxide, and lower production levels of some of the vasodilators. These effects on the resistance vessels are complemented by enhanced leukocyte-endothelial adhesion, particularly in the post-capillary venules, resulting in small-vessel occlusion and activation of the leukocytes with resultant inflammation providing a positive-feedback network. The inflammation will act to result in increased amounts of mediators, which increase the interactions between leukocytes and endothelial cells and activate the coagulation pathways. The resultant effects on O_2 and nutrient delivery to the epithelial cells results in damage to those cells.

The processes of injury and repair to the kidney epithelium is depicted schematically in Figure 30-2. Ischemia results in rapid loss of cytoskeletal integrity and cell polarity. There is shedding of the proximal tubule brush border, loss of polarity with mislocalization of adhesion molecules and other membrane proteins such as the Na^+/K^+-ATPase and β-integrins,[1] as well as apoptosis and necrosis.[2] With severe injury viable and nonviable cells are desquamated, leaving regions where the basement membrane remains as the only barrier between the filtrate and the peritubular interstitium. This allows for back-leak of the filtrate, especially under circumstances in which the pressure in the tubule is increased because of intratubular obstruction resulting from cellular debris in the lumen interacting with proteins such as fibronectin that enter the lumen.[3] This injury to the epithelium results in the generation by this tubular cells of inflammatory and vasoactive mediators, which can feed back on the vasculature to worsen the vasoconstriction and inflammation. Thus inflammation contributes in a critical way to the pathophysiology of AKI.[4]

In contrast to the heart or brain, the kidney can completely recover from an ischemic or toxic insult that results in cell death. Surviving cells that remain adherent undergo repair with the potential to recover normal renal function. When the kidney recovers from acute injury it relies on a sequence of events that include epithelial cell spreading and possibly migration to cover the exposed areas of the basement membrane, cell dedifferentiation and proliferation to restore cell number, followed by differentiation, which results in restoration of the functional integrity of the nephron.[5] The kidney also probably relies on processes to repair the damaged endothelium and replace blood vessels if the injury has been severe enough to result in vascular loss. This review will focus on some of the molecular and genetic aspects of AKI.

VASCULAR REACTIVITY

The vasculature plays a critical role in the pathophysiology of AKI. Clearly the vasculature is instrumental in initation of the injury in the case of ischemia but also probably in the case of most other causes of AKI. In addition, the intrinsic capabilities of the kidney epithelium to repair, as introduced above, depends on the delivery of O_2 and other nutrients to the epithelial cell. Whereas systemic or localized disturbance of renal blood flow is a major contributor to the etiology of AKI, intrinsic renal factors contribute to the pathogenesis of the disease. Two foci of persistent vasoconstriction following injury have been identified. Persistence of pre-glomerular vasoconstriction is proposed to be triggered by a high salt load arriving in the distal tubule as a result of inadequate Na^+ reabsorption in the injured, more proximal parts of the tubule. In addition, studies of regional renal blood flow reveal reductions in local blood flow to the outer medulla that persist for many hours after renal injury in both experimental models of injury in rodents and in human biopsy specimens.[6-12] Three variables may contribute to a reduction in perfusion in the outer medulla. The medullary blood flow is post capillary, and hence low pressure. Injured endothelial cells swell and, in combination with leukocyte adhesion to the injured endothelium, will impede low-pressure blood flow. In addition, coagulation cascades may become activated. The inflammatory aspects of this response will be discussed in the next section of this review. This section focuses on the vasoconstriction. Reduced blood flow to the outer medulla can have particularly detrimental effects on the tubular cells in that region of the kidney, because the outer medulla is normally hypoxic as a result of the countercurrent exchange properties of the vasa recta.[13]

Local production of vasoconstrictors is markedly upregulated following ischemic injury. Measurement of renal blood

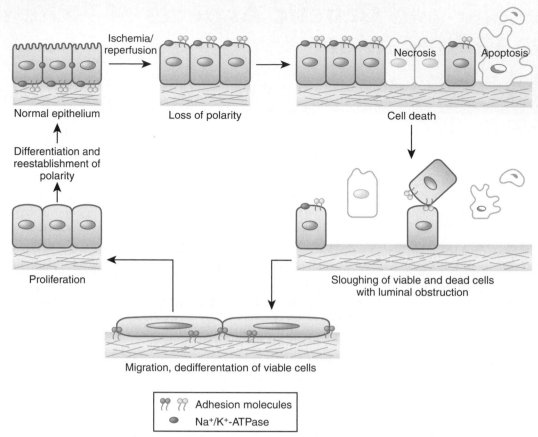

Figure 30-1 Injury and repair to the epithelial cell of the kidney with ischemia/reperfusion. As a very early response of the epithelium to injury, the normally highly polar epithelial cell loses its polarity. This can be demonstrated by alterations in the location of adhesion molecules and Na+/K+-ATPase. In addition, early with ischemia there is a loss of the brush border of the proximal epithelial cell. With increasing time of ischemia there is cell death by either necrosis or apoptosis. Some of the necrotic debris is then released into the lumen, where it can ultimately result in obstruction, because it interacts with lumenal proteins. In addition, because of the mislocation of adhesion molecules, viable epithelial cells lift off the basement membrane and are found in the urine. The kidney responds to the injury by initiating a repair process, if there are sufficient nutrients and sufficient O_2 delivery subsequent to the ischemia period. Viable epithelial cells migrate and cover denuded areas of the basement membrane. These cells are dedifferentiated and express proteins that are not normally expressed in an adult mature epithelial cell. The cells then undergo division and replace lost cells. Ultimately, the cells go on to differentiate and reestablish the normal polarity of the epithelium. The role of a subpopulation of stem/progenitor cells in this process of repair is controversial.

flow in rats 1 week after ischemic injury points to persistent dysregulation of vascular tone at rest and in response to vasodilators and constrictors. In essence, the renal vasculature is tonically more constricted, is hyper-responsive to vasoconstrictors, hyporesponsive to vasodilators, and inappropriately responsive to a fall in perfusion pressure by vasoconstriction (Fig. 30-3).[6,7]

Endotoxemia is characterized by systemic nonrenal vasodilation and renal vasoconstriction. Early in sepsis-associated AKI in animals the predominant response is vasoconstriction with relative preservation of tubular function.[14] Over time, however, endotoxemia induces a hemodynamic form of AKI in animals with enhanced production of peripheral vasodilatory influences including inflammatory cytokines such as tumor necrosis factor α (TNFα) and interleukin-1 (IL-1) as well as inducible nitric oxide synthase (iNOS) activation with enhanced production of nitric oxide (NO). To counter-regulate this vasodilatation there are increased systemic levels of catecholamines and activation of the renin-angiotensin system at least partially in

response to this systemic vasodilation, and these events can contribute to intrarenal vasoconstriction. Furthermore, the renal nerves are believed to participate in the intrarenal vasoconstriction, because denervation markedly protects the kidney against a decrease in glomerular filtration rate seen with endotoxemia.[14] In animal models of endotoxemia the reactivity of renal microvasculature to vasoconstrictor agents is normal or enhanced, in contrast to nonrenal beds, where response to vasoconstrictor agents is diminished.[15] Zager et al evaluated the effects of levosimendan, an ATP-sensitive K+ (K_{ATP}) channel agonist, on endotoxin-induced injury.[16] This agent has potent vasodilatory effects because K_{ATP} channel activation hyperpolarizes the plasma membrane of the vascular smooth muscle cell[17] and levosimendan attenuates Ca^{2+} entry through voltage-sensitive L-type channels that normally occurs in response to vasoconstrictor influences. The authors found that this agent had no effect on endotoxin-induced inflammation or NO production and did not protect isolated proximal tubules in vitro against hypoxia-reoxygenation injury but did

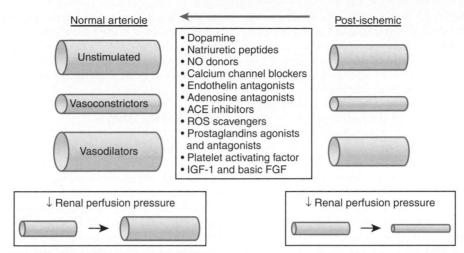

Figure 30-2 Effects of ischemia/reperfusion on arteriolar tone. In studies performed by John Conger and his group at the University of Colorado, it was found that the post-ischemic arteriole is more sensitive to vasoconstrictive agents and less sensitive to vasodilatory agents. In addition, whereas a normal arteriole will dilate in response to a decrease in perfusion pressure, the post-ischemic arteriole constricts. Given these properties of the microvasculature of the kidney after ischemia, several investigators have attempted to use various vasodilatory agents (some of which are listed in the box) as potential therapeutic agents to target the vessels and relieve this vasoconstrictive tendency.

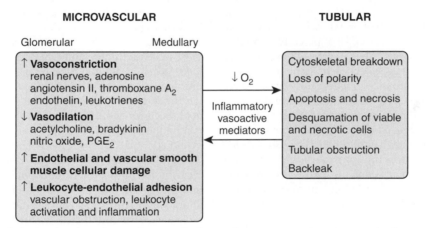

Figure 30-3 Summary of the pathophysiology of AKI, which can be recognized as having both microvascular and tubular components. Furthermore, the microvascular component can be further classified into pre-glomerular and outer medullary vessel components. With AKI there is enhanced vasoconstriction in response to several agents listed in this figure. In addition, there is decreased vasodilatation to agents that are present in the post-ischemic kidney. Furthermore, the combined occurrence of increased endothelial and vascular smooth muscle cellular damage and increased leukocyte-endothelial adhesion results in activation of the coagulation system and vascular obstruction with leukocyte activation and potentiation of inflammation. At the level of the tubule there is cytoskeletal breakdown and loss of polarity, followed by, as described in Figure 30-1, apoptosis and necrosis, intratubular obstruction, and backleak of glomerular filtrate through a denuded basement membrane. In addition, the tubule cells generate inflammatory vasoactive mediators that in turn can affect the vasculature to enhance vascular compromise. This then results in a positive-feedback mechanism whereby the vascular compromise results in decreased O_2 delivery to the tubules, which in turn generate more vasoactive inflammatory mediators that enhance the vasoconstriction and the endothelial-leukocyte interactions.

protect the kidney against lipopolysaccharide-induced AKI. This agent had no effect on AKI induced by occluding the blood supply to the kidney for 12.5 or 20 minutes. The authors conclude the effect of levosimendan was related to a reduction in renal vascular resistance.

Other potent vasoconstrictors have been identified in the ischemic kidney, including endothelin-1, angiotensin II, thromboxane A_2, prostaglandin H_2, leukotrienes C_4, D_4,

adenosine, and sympathetic nerve stimulation.[18,19] This may not be limited to the acute ischemic phase, in that a recent study has revealed that 5 to 8 weeks after acute ischemia in the rat there was increased responsiveness of microvessels and resistance vessels of the skeletal vascular beds to angiotensin II.[20] Several studies indicate that blockade of endothelin receptors before an ischemic insult protects the rat kidney from injury.[21–24] There are two vascular smooth muscle cell receptors for endothelin: ER-A and ER-B. The former seems to function primarily in vasoconstriction, and selective blockade in rats has proven beneficial to recovery. By contrast, angiotensin receptor blockade is widely implicated in the deterioration of renal function in susceptible individuals through paralysis of post-glomerular arterioles.[25,26]

In the rodent model of ischemia in which the renal artery is clamped, the proximal tubule in the outer medulla is most affected after ischemic injury.[27,28] Even when total perfusion to the kidney is normalized, the outer medulla fails to recover normal blood flow promptly. In the outer medulla, the S3 portion of proximal tubules and the medullary thick ascending limb of Henle dominate. Both nephron segments require substrates for high levels of adenosine triphosphate (ATP) production. Cell injury is most apparent in the S3 segment of the proximal tubule in most animal models. There is some controversy as to the relative extent of proximal versus distal tubule injury in humans with AKI.[1]

An important finding in animal models of ischemic renal injury is that previous ischemic injury protects from future injury. This "preconditioning" effect lasts for several weeks. These studies indicate that the kidney can activate endogenous protective mechanisms. These mechanisms seem to protect vessels as well as tubules from injury.[29–31] Exploiting these mechanisms will probably lead to new therapies. Although the deliberate induction of sublethal renal ischemia has little practical application to patients, studies of preconditioning in the myocardium have shown that several pharmacologic agents can mediate the same protection as ischemic preconditioning.[32–37] During coronary bypass surgery ischemic injury sufficient to induce atrial fibrillation (5 minutes) protected the myocardium during subsequent surgery. In addition, the use of diazoxide to pharmacologically precondition the myocardium for 5 minutes before surgery has also afforded marked benefit to the myocardium during surgery.[38,39] Cardiac studies have highlighted signaling pathways involving protein kinase A, protein kinase D, and mitogen-activated protein kinase (MAPK) pathways in preconditioning. We have found that NO, a pluripotential molecule derived from iNOS is a key mediator of protection in the kidney.[40] Intrinsic cells of the kidney continue to generate NO through increased activation of iNOS for several weeks after injury. NO is the most potent vasodilator yet described. In inflammatory diseases, iNOS-derived NO has been shown to take over the function of endothelial NOS (eNOS)–derived NO in regulating vascular tone.[41] One mechanism by which iNOS-derived NO protects the kidney from injury is by preventing inappropriate vasoconstriction directly as a vasodilator and indirectly by preventing upregulation of vasoconstrictors.[42] In support of this, Yamashita and colleagues indicate that in the preconditioned kidney, production of the vasoconstrictor endothelin-1 is markedly attenuated during ischemia.[43] Because ischemic preconditioning is probably not explained entirely by changes in vascular reactivity, a later section of this review is devoted specifically to this topic.

Successful reduction of post-injury vasoconstriction in animal models with improved functional response has not translated into practical therapies for humans thus far.[44] This may be because animal studies are performed in a background of normal vasculature, whereas most patients with AKI have at least some degree of underlying vascular disease that could alter the response to vasodilatory drugs. In addition, the agents are given much later in the disease course in humans than they are in animals. It is the author's opinion that, although these factors are important, in humans AKI inflammation plays a critical role, and therapy directed toward the vasoconstriction alone will not be effective once there is tubular injury.

ENDOTHELIUM

Damage to the endothelium can contribute to the pathobiology of ischemic AKI in many ways. A damaged endothelial layer would contribute to vasoconstriction by less production of vasodilatory substances such as NO. If vessels are lost with ischemia and angiogenesis is inadequate, then there will be problems with repair. Injured endothelium will also contribute to the inflammatory response through upregulation of adhesion molecules whose counter-receptors are on circulating leukocytes. The enhanced interaction resulting from the upregulation of these adhesion molecules will then result in local small-vessel obstruction and enhanced activation of the leukocytes, leading to potentiation of the inflammation. The role of endothelial cells in inflammation will be discussed more extensively in the next section of this review. The concept that endothelial cells play an important role in post-ischemic renal injury was suggested as early as 1972 by Leaf and colleagues when they described endothelial swelling and narrowing of the blood vessel lumen as important features of post-ischemic injury and suggested that "no-reflow" in the post-ischemic period could be an important contributor to the injury and could contribute to inhibition of the ability of the kidney to recover.[45] This "no-reflow" phenomenon had been previously proposed to be important for the pathophysiology of ischemic brain injury by Ames et al.[46] Although total kidney blood flow returns to near-normal levels after release of a clamp interrupting this flow, the distribution of blood flow does not return to normal. There is marked congestion of the outer medulla and reduction in blood flow to this region of the kidney after ischemia.[47]

Evidence for endothelial dysfunction in the cortex has also been presented in studies that demonstrated retrograde blood flow through peritubular capillaries upon reperfusion after ischemia.[48] With reperfusion, a partial transient compromise of the patency of the peritubular capillaries was also present. When human umbilical vein endothelial cells or human embryonic kidney cells stably expressing eNOS were administered either intravenously or into the renal artery after ischemia, these cells implanted into the kidney and resulted in partial functional protection against injury.[48] In addition, after prolonged ischemia (60 minutes) in the rat, peritubular capillaries undergo permanent damage.[49] The number of microvessels in the inner stripe of the outer medulla declines, with the reduction in number associated with increased tubulointerstitial fibrosis and altered concentrating ability.

INFLAMMATION

The Immune Response

The immune response has an innate component and an adaptive component, both of which are important contributors to the pathobiology of ischemic injury. The innate component is responsible for the early response to infection or injury and is independent of foreign antigens. Toll-like receptors (TLRs) detect exogenous microbial products, leading to activation of innate immunity[50] and development of antigen-dependent adaptive immunity.[51] It has been recognized that TLRs also recognize host material released during injury.[52] Although TLRs are present on antigen-presenting cells such as monocytes/macrophages and dendritic cells as well as neutrophils, in the kidney the majority of the TLR messenger RNA (mRNA) is present on proximal and distal tubular epithelial cells as well as Bowman's capsule. Proximal epithelial cells stained more intensely for TLR4 mRNA than distal epithelial cells. Ischemia/reperfusion markedly enhance levels of TLR2 and TLR4 mRNA in the distal tubular epithelium, the thin limb of Henle's loop, and collecting ducts, perhaps associated with the increases in TNFα[53] and interferon-γ in the kidney after ischemia/reperfusion.[54] There was little change in the proximal tubule or glomerular capsule TLR2 or 4 mRNA levels. Whereas protein expression of TLR4 was confirmed to be upregulated by western blot analysis, the cellular localization of protein expression upregulation was unclear. The role of TLRs was further evaluated using an ischemia/reperfusion model in $Tlr2^{-/-}$ and $Tlr^{+/+}$ mice.[55] Significantly fewer granulocytes were present in the interstitium of the kidney 1 day after ischemia/reperfusion in the $Tlr2^{-/-}$ mice, and fewer macrophages were present 1 to 5 days after ischemia/reperfusion. Kidney homogenate cytokines KC, MCP-1 IL-1b, and IL-6 were also significantly lower in the $Tlr2^{-/-}$ animals as compared with the $Tlr2^{+/+}$ mice. Hence the absence of Tlr2 clearly had an anti-inflammatory effect on the response to ischemia/reperfusion. This anti-inflammatory effect was associated with a functional protection, as measured by serum creatinine at 1 day after ischemia/reperfusion and blood urea nitrogen and tubular injury score 1 and 5 days after ischemia/reperfusion.

Leukocyte-Endothelial Interactions

With ischemia/reperfusion endothelial cells upregulate integrins, selectins, and members of the immunoglobulin superfamily, including intercellular adhesion molecule 1 (ICAM-1) and vascular cell adhesion molecule (Fig. 30-4). Several vasoactive compounds may also affect leukocyte-endothelial interactions. In fact, protective effects of agents that have been used primarily to block vasoconstriction in animal models of ischemia such as endothelin antagonists may also have an effect on neutrophil adhesion or other aspects of leukocyte-endothelial

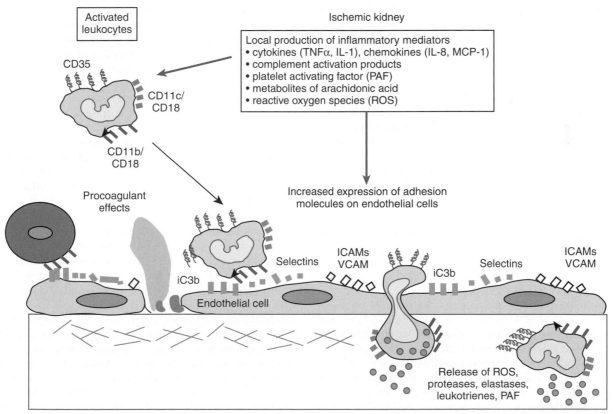

Figure 30-4 The role of inflammation in the pathophysiology of ischemia/reperfusion. Some of the aspects of inflammation that are prevalent in the post-ischemic kidney include the generation of inflammatory mediators by cells in the kidney, which results in increased expression of adhesion molecules on endothelial cells that are themselves injured in response to the ischemia. Systemic and local factors are also released, leading to activation of leukocytes. Furthermore, there is activation of the coagulation pathway, with activation of platelets and formation of microthrombi, further compromising the small vessels. Activated leukocytes interact through their upregulated membrane proteins with counter-receptors on the vascular endothelium to result in further activation of the leukocytes, and further potentiation of small-vessel obstruction. As a result of this activation of the leukocytes greater amounts of inflammatory mediators are released, and these inflammatory mediators then serve in a positive-feedback process to further activate the pro-adhesive characteristics and add to vasoconstriction of the vessels. The leukocytes involved include neutrophils, monocytes/microphages, and T cells.

interactions with implications for inflammation.[56] Vasodilators, such as NO, also can have effects to decrease inflammation. NO inhibits adhesion of neutrophils to endothelial cells, stimulated by TNFα, which would also be protective.[57] As discussed previously, it has been known for quite some time now that there is less flow to the medullary than the cortical region in the post-ischemic kidney.[11] In addition, as endothelial cells are injured with resulting cell swelling and increased expression of cell adhesion molecules, so also are leukocytes activated. Enhanced leukocyte-endothelial interactions can result in cell-cell adhesion, which can physically impede blood flow.[44] Furthermore, these interactions will additionally activate both leukocytes and endothelial cells and contribute to the generation of local factors that promote vasoconstriction especially in the presence of other vasoactive mediators, resulting in compromised local blood flow and impaired tubule cell metabolism.[58] Because of the anatomy of the vascular-tubular relationships in the outer medulla prone to congestion, these leukocyte-endothelial interactions probably affect the outer medulla to a greater extent than the cortex.

In an early study to evaluate the significance of endothelial-leukocyte interactions and inflammation to the pathobiology of ischemic injury, we administered antibodies to ICAM-1 and found that when they were administered before or 2 hours after renal ischemia/reperfusion they protected the kidney from injury.[59] We further confirmed these results in finding that kidneys of ICAM-1 knockout mice also are protected.[53] We proposed that this upregulation of ICAM-1 was related to the upregulation of the pro-inflammatory cytokines TNFα and IL-1, which we measured to be increased by ischemia/reperfusion. This protection was associated with decreased tissue myeloperoxidase (MPO) reflective of decreased trapped leukocytes. Dragun et al[60] found that pretreatment of donor kidneys with antisense deoxyoligonucleotides directed to ICAM-1 before transplantation into rats resulted in better long-term survival of the recipients, lower serum creatinine concentrations, and reduced interstitial fibrosis and other changes seen with chronic graft rejection as a consequence of delayed graft function. Administration of antisense deoxyoligonucleotides to recipient rats resulted in prolonged survival of kidney allografts and synergized with cyclosporin in further prolongation of graft survival.[61] This same group then perfused kidneys of cynomolgus monkeys ex situ with unformulated "naked" ICAM antisense deoxyoligonucleotides and exposed to 30 minutes of cold and 30 minutes of warm ischemic time. ICAM-1 protein expression was reduced and graft function was improved, as measured by glomerular filtration rate and blood creatinine 24 hours after grafting.[62] Troncoso et al[63] recently reported that the administration of ICAM-1 antisense oligonucleotides resulted in less functional and morphologic chronic graft damage secondary to ischemia/reperfusion in the rat. A randomized trial was conducted to evaluate the use of a mouse monoclonal antibody against ICAM-1 to prevent acute rejection and delayed graft function in cadaveric renal transplantation in humans.[64] No difference was found in the incidence of delayed graft function between the two groups. There are concerns about the study, however, because it was underpowered and the antibody did not inhibit leukocyte adhesion to human endothelial cells whereas its Fab fragment did. Furthermore a phase I multicenter study of a monoclonal antibody specific to LFA-1 (LFA-1 is a leukocyte ligand for ICAM-1) as induction therapy showed equivalent efficacy to ATG and a tendency to reduction in the incidence of delayed graft function.[65]

Leukocyte Subgroups

There are many additional mechanisms by which leukocytes can potentiate renal injury. Leukocytes are activated by inflammatory mediators, including cytokines, chemokines, eicosanoids, and reactive oxygen species (ROS), which upregulate adhesion molecules that engage counter-receptors on the activated endothelium. Leukocytes are recruited and activated by chemokines, which are upregulated by the proinflammatory cytokines IL-1 and TNFα. TNFα, IL-1, and interferon γ produce a number of injurious changes in proximal tubular epithelial cells (see later). These cytokines also disrupt cell matrix adhesion dependent on β_1-integrin, inducing cell shedding into the lumen.

Leukocyte subgroups contribute in different ways to ischemia/reperfusion injury. MPO activity is elevated soon after ischemic insult and may originate from macrophages and/or neutrophils.[47] We showed that neutrophils are seen in the interstitium early after ischemic injury in the mouse,[53] as have others subsequently.[66] If neutrophil accumulation is prevented, tissue injury is ameliorated.[53] It is possible that neutrophil depletion models, however, may not adequately differentiate involvement of neutrophils from that of T lymphocytes and macrophages. In a recent study Mizuno and Nakamura found that administration of hepatocyte growth factor prevents neutrophil accumulation in the mouse exposed to ischemia/reperfusion.[67] This reduction in tissue neutrophil accumulation is associated with reduced vascular ICAM-1 expression, reduced tubular cell apoptosis, and reduced blood urea nitrogen levels 3 and 18 hours after ischemia.

Later phases of AKI are characterized by infiltration of macrophages and T lymphocytes, which predominate over neutrophils. Knockout mice lacking CD4 and CD8, cell adhesion receptors on T lymphocytes, are protected from ischemia/reperfusion injury,[68] suggesting a causal role for T lymphocytes in mediating injury. Mice deficient in T cells (nu/nu mice) are both structurally and functionally protected against ischemic injury, and mice deficient in CD4+ cells, but not mice deficient in CD8+ cells, were protected against ischemic injury.[69] Addition of T cells to the nu/nu mice reconstituted susceptibility to ischemia, as did addition of CD4+ T cells to CD4-deficient mice. In addition, blockade of T-cell CD28-B7 co-stimulation protects against ischemic injury in rats and significantly inhibits T-cell and macrophage infiltration and activation in situ.[70] The role of the T cell, however, has been recently questioned. Mice deficient in recombination-activating gene 1 (Rag1) lack T and B cells and do not produce immunoglobulins or T-cell receptor (TCR) proteins. In the absence of these cells and their receptors, some investigators have found that Rag1-deficient mice are not protected from AKI induced by ischemia. Tubular necrosis and neutrophil infiltration are present to a degree comparable to that seen in wild-type mice.[71,72] One group has found that mice deficient in the T-cell receptor had structural and functional protection against ischemic injury, associated with decreased levels of TNFα and IL-6 but unchanged macrophage or neutrophil infiltration patterns.[73] Another group, however, has found that injury in the TCRα mice is similar to that in in wild-type animals.[74]

Complement

Complement activation is a characteristic of ischemia/reperfusion injury in several organs, but the kidney is unique in that activation after ischemia/reperfusion occurs predominantly if not exclusively by the alternative pathway.[75] Complement may also potentiate leukocyte-endothelial interactions. In several different tissues exposed to ischemia/reperfusion, complement-dependent upregulation of endothelial cell adhesion molecules, with resulting neutrophil accumulation in the vasculature, has been implicated as a mechanism for complement-mediated injury.[76] Others, however, suggest that the primary effect of complement in kidney ischemia/reperfusion is on the epithelial cell as a result of a direct effect of the membrane attack complex of complement.[77] Farrar et al explored the role of local intrarenal production of the third complement component C3 as distinguished from circulating C3 by using a mouse isograft model.[78] They found a close relationship between cold ischemia-induced injury and intrarenal C3 expression. Ischemic C3[+] donor kidneys transplanted into C3[−] recipients developed widespread tissue injury and severe functional impairment. By contrast, ischemic C3[−] isografts transplanted into C3[+] recipients developed mild structural and functional deficiencies. In humans there is deposition of C3d along a significant number of tubules in biopsy specimens from patients with AKI.[75]

Reactive Oxygen Species

ROS that are generated during reperfusion and as a contributor to the inflammatory response then play a major role in cell injury with ischemia. The superoxide radical as well as H_2O_2 and hydroxyl radical are increased in renal tissue after ischemia/reperfusion. In addition, NO reacts with superoxides to generate the highly reactive peroxynitrite molecule. One of the sites of this interaction between ROS and NO has been recently reported to be at the inner mitochondrial membrane in the kidney.[79] Both ROS and NO are generated within mitochondria, and the resultant formation of peroxynitrite is proposed to lead to cytochrome c release and apoptosis in ischemia/reperfusion.

ROS are generated by activated infiltrating leukocytes and by epithelial cells. ROS are directly toxic to tubular epithelial cells, with ROS-generating systems mimicking the effects of ischemic injury.[80] In some cases, scavengers (superoxide dismutase, glutathione, edaravone, vitamin E) and inhibitors of ROS (deferoxamine) have been found to protect against renal injury.[81–86] The presence of ROS can result in the peroxidation of lipids in cell membranes, protein denaturation, and DNA strand breaks. Lipid peroxidation by ROS enhances membrane permeability and impairs function of membrane enzymes and ion pumps. ROS disrupt the cellular cytoskeleton and cellular integrity, and break down DNA.[82,87,88]

ROS-induced strand breaks in DNA lead to activation of DNA repair mechanisms, including the nuclear enzyme poly(ADP-ribose) polymerase (PARP) and subsequent ATP depletion. PARP is a zinc-finger DNA-binding protein that detects DNA strand breaks or nicks and transfers ADP-ribose from nicotinamide adenine diphosphate (NAD) to nuclear proteins. Subsequent to ischemia/reperfusion, PARP is activated, NAD is depleted, and generation of cellular ATP is inhibited, worsening the injury. This amplification of injury may be the major mechanism by which ROS are directly toxic to cells. Inhibiting PARP protects renal[89] cells against ROS-induced injury in particular, resulting from ischemia/reperfusion. Mice genetically deficient in PARP are protected against ischemia/reperfusion injury even though the levels of ROS and the DNA damage were similar in Parp-knockout and wild-type mice.[90] There was decreased inflammation in the Parp-knockout mice as demonstrated by diminished neutrophil infiltration and decreased expression of ICAM-1 as well as TNFα and IL-1.

Lipid peroxidation and production of ROS are regulated by various extracellular and intracellular antioxidant enzymes. A contributing factor to the increase of ROS levels after ischemia/reperfusion is the reduction of antioxidant enzyme activity. It has been reported that catalase activity is decreased after ischemia/reperfusion.[82] Superoxide dismutase (SOD) is an important free radical mediating cellular damage. It is scavenged by CuZnSOD located in cytoplasm and manganese superoxide dismutase (MnSOD) in mitochondria. MnSOD is the major antioxidant enzyme located in mitochondria and is essential for life.[91,92] Chien and colleagues reported that intravenous treatment with SOD in rats resulted in reduced apoptotic cell death and ROS production after kidney ischemia/reperfusion.[92a] Mice expressing only 50% of the normal complement of MnSOD demonstrate increased susceptibility to oxidative stress and severe mitochondrial dysfunction resulting from elevation of ROS.[93] MnSOD is susceptible to nitrotyrosylation, which results in enzyme inactivation.[94,95] Overexpression of MnSOD enzyme protects the heart after ischemia/reperfusion injury.[96] We found that MnTMPyP, a SOD mimetic, reduced post-ischemic lipid peroxidation and the tissue levels of H_2O_2 in the kidney and protected the kidney against functional injury as measured by a reduced level of serum creatinine after ischemia.[97] Transgenic mice overexpressing the antioxidants, intracellular and extracellular glutathione peroxidases, are protected against ischemic injury.[98] These animals have less induction of the chemokines, interleukin-8 (IL-8) and monocyte chemotactic protein-1 (MCP-1), less neutrophil infiltration, and less functional injury compared to the wild-type controls, suggesting that the effects of ROS are mediated by chemokines. Exposure of leukocytes to circulating cytokines reduces their deformability and enhances their tendency to be sequestered.[99] Sequestered leukocytes can then potentiate injury by further generating more ROS and eicosanoids, enhancing inflammation and vascular tone.

Tubule Contribution to Inflammatory Injury

Both the S3 segment of the proximal tubule and the medullary thick ascending limb are located in the outer stripe of the outer medulla. This region of the kidney is marginally oxygenated under normal conditions, and after an ischemic insult oxygenation is further compromised because the return in blood flow is delayed. Both segments of the nephron contribute to the inflammatory response in acute renal failure.[100] As previously described, the tubule cell express TLRs. The tubule epithelial cells are known to generate pro-inflammatory and chemotactic cytokines such as TNFα, MCP-1, IL-8, interleukin-6 (IL-6), interleukin-1β (IL-1β), and transforming growth factor-β, MCP-1, IL-8, RANTES, and ENA-78.[4]

Proximal tubular epithelia may respond to T-lymphocyte activity through activation of receptors for T-cell ligands that are expressed on the proximal tubule cell.[101] CD4[+] cells express CD40 ligand. When CD40 is ligated in response to interaction with CD154, CD40 ligation stimulates MCP-1 and IL-8 production, TRAF6 recruitment, and MAPK activation.[101] CD40 also induces RANTES production by human renal tubular epithelia, an effect that is amplified by production of IL-4 and IL-13 by Th2 cells, a subpopulation of T cells.[102] CD40 ligation, however, also generates an anti-inflammatory response.[103] There is an increase in heme oxygenase-1 promoter activity as a result of CD40 ligation. Heme oxygenase-1 in most cases has been demonstrated to protect against ischemia/reperfusion injury.[104] B7-1 and B7-2 can be induced on proximal tubule epithelial cells in vivo and in vitro. After B7-1 and B7-2 induction, proximal tubule epithelial cells co-stimulate CD28 on T lymphocytes, resulting in cytokine production.[105]

The proximal tubule epithelial cells also are involved in complement activation with ischemia/reperfusion. Loss of polarity of the cell results in loss of the normal distribution of the only complement inhibitor expressed on the surface of renal tubular cells, complement receptor 1-related protein (Crry). Normally Crry is expressed on the basolateral aspects of the cell, but after ischemia this polar distribution is lost and Crry is seen within the tubular lumen. This loss of basolateral localization occurs primarily in the proximal tubule and precedes the deposition of C3 along the circumference of the tubule.[106] Furthermore *Crry[−/−]* mice are more susceptible to ischemia/reperfusion injury than are wild-type control mice.

PROTECTION AGAINST INJURY BY ISCHEMIC PRECONDITIONING

An area of increasing interest is the possibility of rendering an organ resistant to subsequent injury by a prior insult or preconditioning maneuver. Ischemic preconditioning of the kidney confers protection against a subsequent ischemic attack (Fig.30-5).[30] This protective effect decreases with an increasing time interval between the preconditioning insult and the subsequent insult, but protection can be measured as long as 12 weeks after the initial insult (Fig. 30-6).[40] Prior ischemia has a marked effect to decrease tissue inflammation that occurs after the subsequent ischemia/reperfusion. This is reflected by the marked reduction in MPO accumulation in the kidney after the second ischemia/reperfusion (Fig. 30-7). Identification of the mechanisms responsible for renal ischemic preconditioning will probably facilitate our understanding of the pathophysiology of ischemic injury and guide the development of novel therapeutics aimed at mimicking the protective mechanism(s). Several candidates that could potentially serve as mediators of preconditioning have been identified. We have implicated activation of NOS[40] and phosphatidylinositol 3-kinase (PI 3-kinase)/Akt/PKB pathways, reduction in the relative activation of Jun N-terminal kinase (JNK) as compared with extracellular signal-regulated kinases (ERK) 1/2,[12,47] induction of HSPs, heme oxygenase, and endoplasmic reticulum (ER) stress proteins.[29] A recent review discusses many of these candidate mediators of preconditioning in more detail.[30]

Of these potential mediators, the NOS pathway is particularly important to consider. We demonstrated that iNOS is responsible for a component of the long-term protection

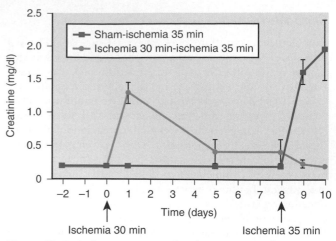

Figure 30-5 A demonstration of ischemic preconditioning in the kidney. A 30-minute period of bilateral renal ischemia at *t* = 0 results in an increase in serum creatinine concentration followed by recovery of renal function. When a second bout of ischemia is introduced at 8 days after the first ischemic period, even when the second ischemic period is longer than the first (35 minutes), there is no increase in serum creatinine. By contrast the control animal that received sham ischemia surgery on day 0 and was subsequently exposed to bilateral ischemia on day 8 had a very significant increase in serum creatinine concentration. (Redrawn from Park KM, Kramers C, Vayssier-Taussat M, et al: Prevention of kidney ischemia/reperfusion-induced functional injury, MAPK and MAPK kinase activation, and inflammation by remote transient ureteral obstruction. J Biol Chem 277:2040–2049, 2002.

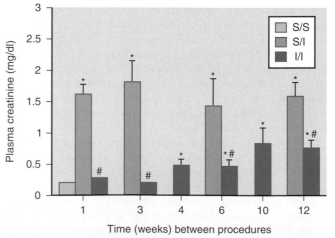

Figure 30-6 Protection afforded by preconditioning is present for an extended period of time. This histogram shows that mice treated with ischemia at time 0 had significant protection against bilateral ischemia (I) even as long as 12 weeks after the first procedure. Renal function was measured by monitoring plasma creatinine levels, and it can be seen that the increase in creatinine concentration in the I/I group is not as great as that seen with animals that have undergone sham surgery (S) at time 0 and subsequent exposure to bilateral renal ischemia. Creatinine measurements were made 24 hours after the second procedure. (Redrawn from Park KM, Byun JY, Kramers C, et al: Inducible nitric oxide synthase is an important contributor to prolonged protective effects of ischemic preconditioning in the mouse kidney. J Biol Chem 278: 27256–27266, 2003.)

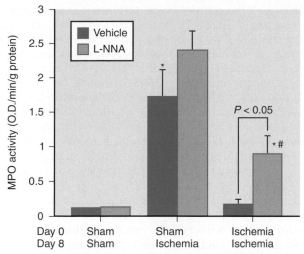

Figure 30-7 Effect of L-NNA on mouse kidney myeloperoxidase levels with preconditioning. Tissue myeloperoxidase (MLO) is a measure of tissue leukocytes and hence a marker for inflammation. A previous period of ischemia followed by a second period of ischemia results in a marked reduction in MLO 24 hours after the second ischemic period when compared with animals that have been rendered ischemic on day 8 after a sham procedure on day 0. When one interferes with NO synthesis using L-NNA, a second period of ischemia results in more MPO in the kidney than if this compound is not present. This provides evidence that NO synthesis is necessary to achieve the marked reduction in MPO after the second period of ischemia. O.D., optical density. (Redrawn from Park KM, Byun JY, Kramers C, et al: Inducible nitric oxide synthase is an important contributor to prolonged protective effects of ischemic preconditioning in the mouse kidney. J Biol Chem 278: 27256–27266, 2003.)

afforded the kidney by ischemic preconditioning.[40] Thirty minutes of prior ischemia results in a prolonged increase in the expression of iNOS and eNOS as well as HSP-25. In addition, there is increased interstitial expression of α-smooth muscle actin, an indicator of long-term renal interstitial changes. Gene deletion of iNOS, but not eNOS, increased kidney susceptibility to ischemia, as did treatment with pharmacologic inhibitors of NO synthesis, including N-nitro-L-arginine (L-NNA) and L-N_6-(1-iminoethyl)lysine (L-NIL), the latter a specific inhibitor of iNOS. L-NNA partially blocked the protective effect of prior ischemia on leukocyte infiltration after the second period of ischemia (Fig. 30-7). When the initial period of ischemia was reduced (15 minutes), there was less protection of the kidney from subsequent ischemia on day 8. Under these conditions there was no sustained increase in iNOS or eNOS expression, and protection was not abolished by L-NIL treatment, suggesting that the residual protection was not related to iNOS. In addition, renal function was not impaired and expression of interstitial α-smooth muscle actin did not change. The data indicate that iNOS plays an important role in kidney protection afforded by prolonged ischemic preconditioning and that persistent long-term changes in the renal interstitium may be critical in affording this protection by sustaining iNOS synthesis. In addition, this study is the first to demonstrate in any organ system that partial protection persists as long as 12 weeks after

an initial ischemic event. The iNOS-independent protection associated with preconditioning may be related, at least in part, to an upregulation of HSP-25.

We also proposed that MAPKs are also likely to be involved in affording protection following ischemic preconditioning.[47] MAPKs are ubiquitously expressed serine/threonine kinases that, in mammalian cells, play central roles in determining if the response to multiple signaling inputs will be proliferation, differentiation, or apoptosis. They also play a major role in inflammation.[107] In mammalian cells there are three common MAPK pathways. The best studied of these include the ERK cascade, involved in cell proliferation and differentiation in a variety of cell types. The ERK pathway is activated by growth factors and many other agonists, including vasoactive peptides. JNK, also known as stress-activated protein kinase (SAPK), and p38 are components of the two other MAPK cascades. Each pathway, when activated, involves activation of several closely related MAPK enzymes, for example ERK1 and ERK2 or JNK1, JNK2, and JNK3. JNK and p38 are activated by inflammatory cytokines (TNF and IL-1) and cellular stress, including genotoxic stress and osmolar stress. They are only minimally activated by growth factors. JNK has been implicated in proximal tubular cell injury and is increased after ATP depletion in vitro and ischemia/reperfusion injury in vivo.[108] Interestingly, ERK is activated predominantly in distal cells (medullary thick ascending limb),[109] perhaps explaining in part the differential susceptibility to injury of the proximal and distal nephron segments. ERK has been proposed to be protective in the distal tubule, and its absence in the proximal tubule has been implicated in the increased susceptibility of this segment of the nephron to ischemic injury.[110] The cyclic adenosine monophosphate–responsive element binding protein (CREB) has been proposed to act downstream of ERK and mediate survival in response to oxidant stress.[111]

It has been proposed in neurons[112] and proximal tubule cells[110] that the relative extent of JNK, p38, and ERK activation may determine cell fate, with JNK activation associated with cell death and ERK activity protective. JNK has been implicated in the mitochondrial death pathway.[112] When the kidney is preconditioned by ischemia, we have reported that activation of JNK and p38 is markedly reduced, as is activation of their upstream MAPK kinases (MKK7, MKK4, and MKK3/6). By contrast, activation of ERK1/2 and its upstream MAPKK activator, MKK3/4, is unaltered by preconditioning. Thus, the relative ratio of ERK1/2 activation to JNK or p38 activation is enhanced in the preconditioned post-ischemic kidney.

We explored the relationship between ERK1/2 activation and susceptibility of kidney epithelial cells to oxidative injury extensively.[29] We established a preconditioning model in vitro using ER stress. Ischemia/reperfusion induces ER stress.[113] The lumen of the ER is a location within the cell in which the microenvironment is conducive to proper folding of proteins that will ultimately be secreted or located at the cell surface. Ischemia/reperfusion results in activation of an evolutionarily conserved "unfolded protein response". Abnormal Ca^{2+} homeostasis in the ER contributes to this response, which involves three Ca^{2+}-dependent chaperones (GRP78, GRP94, and calreticulin), which exist in high concentration in the ER. A mild insult to the cell activates the unfolded protein response to deal with the burden of unfolded or improperly folded proteins in the ER. Transcriptional programs are turned on to enhance protein folding and promote degradation of improperly folded proteins. In addition, overall transcription in the cell is reduced so as to reduce the influx of new proteins in the ER. Increased amounts of RNA transcripts for GRP78 and other ER stress proteins are characteristic of rat models of brain, kidney, and heart ischemia/ reperfusion.[114-117]. We proposed that the epithelial cell might take advantage of this response as a way to protect itself and considered that this response may contribute to the protection afforded by preconditioning.

We investigated the role of the ER stress response on intracellular Ca^{2+} regulation, MAPK activation, and cytoprotection in LLC-PK1 renal epithelial cells in an attempt to identify the mechanisms of protection afforded by ER stress. Cells preconditioned with DTTox, tunicamycin, thapsigargin, or A23187 express ER stress proteins and are resistant to subsequent H_2O_2-induced cell injury. In addition, ER stress preconditioning prevents the increase in intracellular free Ca^{2+} concentration ($[Ca^{2+}]_i$) that normally follows H_2O_2 exposure. Overexpression of calreticulin protects LLC-PK1 cells against H_2O_2-induced cell injury and an increase in $[Ca^{2+}]_i$. This fact that increasing ER Ca^{2+} buffering protects against oxidative injury supports the proposal that the protective effect of ER stress is due, in part, to better Ca^{2+} buffering, decreased Ca^{2+} release, or indirect mechanisms involving cooperation between Ca^{2+} uptake by ER and/or extrusion across the plasma membrane. Each of these mechanisms could prevent a change in $[Ca^{2+}]_i$. Stable transfection of cells with antisense RNA targeted against GRP78 (pkASgrp78 cells) prevents GRP78 induction, disables the ER stress response, sensitizes cells to H_2O_2-induced injury, and prevents the development of tolerance to H_2O_2 that normally occurs with preconditioning.

ERK and JNK are transiently (30–60 minutes) phosphorylated in response to H_2O_2. ER stress–preconditioned cells have more phospho-ERK, more phospho-MEK1/2 (the upstream activator of ERK), and less JNK phosphorylation than control cells in response to H_2O_2 exposure (Fig. 30-8). Pre-incubation with a specific inhibitor of JNK activation or adenoviral infection with a construct that encodes constitutively active MEK1 also protects cells against H_2O_2 toxicity. In contrast, the pkASgrp78 cells have less ERK and more JNK phosphorylation with H_2O_2 exposure (Fig. 30-9). The ability of ER stress to suppress JNK activation in response to subsequent oxidative stress might be related to the prevention of an increase in $[Ca^{2+}]_i$ by GRP78 and other ER stress proteins. There is precedent for an interaction among proteins that regulated oxidative stress, $[Ca^{2+}]_i$ and JNK activation. Under normal conditions the redox regulatory protein thioredoxin (Trx) has been shown to bind and inhibit the activity of apoptosis signal-regulated kinase 1 (ASK-1), a MAPKK involved in both JNK and p38 kinase activation.[118] Furthermore, in HaCaT keratinocytes, increased $[Ca^{2+}]_i$ leads to oxidation of Trx, dissociation of the Trx-ASK1 complex, and activation of JNK.[119] By preventing a rise in $[Ca^{2+}]_i$, the ER stress response, including upregulation of GRP78 expression, could prevent this dissociation of the Trx-ASK1 complex and diminish activation of the JNK pathway. Although such a mechanism is speculative at this time, it represents one plausible mechanism linking oxidative stress and deregulation of $[Ca^{2+}]_i$ to JNK activation and cell death. An increase in $[Ca^{2+}]_i$, however, is not the only contributor to the increased phosphorylation of JNK. This is demonstrated by our experiment with calreticulin-overexpressing cells. The cells are protected against H_2O_2-induced cell injury associated with prevention of an increase

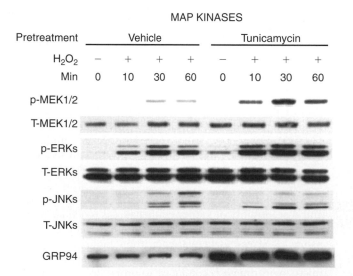
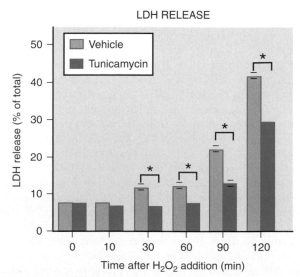

Figure 30-8 ER stress due to tunicamycin modulates MAPK signaling responses to oxidative stress. Non-pretreated LLC-PK1 cells or cells preconditioned with tunicamycin (1.5 mg/mL, 16 hours) to induce ER stress were then exposed to 250 µM H_2O_2. Cell injury at various times was determined by lactate dehydrogenase (LDH) release. MEK1/2, ERK, and JNK activation were determined with phosphospecific antibodies in western blots of cell lysates. Total (T) MEK1/2, ERK, and JNK were also measured with specific antibodies. Expression of GRP94 confirmed the induction of ER stress by tunicamycin. MAPK, mitogen-activated protein kinase; ERK, extracellular signal–regulated protein kinase; JNK, c-Jun N-terminal protein kinase; MEK, mitogen-activated protein kinase/extracellular signal-regulated kinase kinase; GRP78, glucose-regulated protein 78. (Redrawn from Hung CC, Takaharu I, Stevens JL, Bonventre JV: Protection of renal epithelial cells against oxidative injury by endoplasmic reticulum stress preconditioning is mediated by ERK1/2 activation. J Biol Chem 278: 29317–29326, 2003.)

in $[Ca^{2+}]_i$. Despite the absence of a change in $[Ca^{2+}]_i$, JNK phosphorylation is increased in the cells to an extent equivalent to the increase seen in control cells.

Expression of constitutively active MEK (MEK-DD) using an adenovirus also confers protection on native as well as pkASgrp78 cells (Fig. 30-10). These results indicate that GRP78 plays an important role in the ER stress response and cytoprotection. ER stress preconditioning attenuates H_2O_2-induced cell injury in LLC-PK1 cells by preventing an increase in $[Ca^{2+}]_i$, potentiating ERK activation and decreasing JNK activation. Thus, the ER stress response modulates the balance between ERK and JNK signaling pathways to prevent cell death after oxidative injury. Furthermore, ERK activation is also an important downstream effector mechanism for cellular protection by ER stress.[29]

Although the epithelial cell itself may be protected against subsequent injury by preconditioning, we demonstrated that the protection against ischemia was not related to the generation of new cells that were "younger" and hence less susceptible to O_2 deprivation. We showed that transient urinary tract obstruction, which did not result in cell death and replacement of tubular cells, also resulted in marked protection against ischemic injury 8 days after the transient obstruction (Fig. 30-11).[12,47] In both the case of ischemia-related preconditioning and of obstruction-related preconditioning there was a marked decrease in outer medullary vascular congestion and leukocyte accumulation in the outer medulla after ischemia. We proposed in 2001[47] that the marked reduction in post-ischemic outer medullary congestion in the kidney previously exposed to ischemia argues for an important effect of

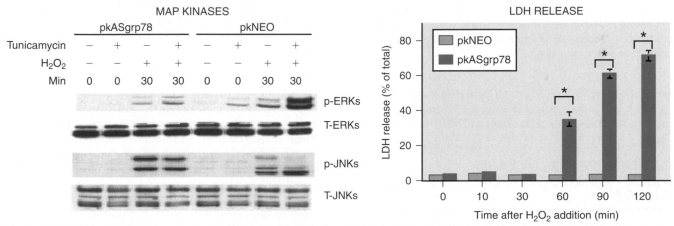

Figure 30-9 Cells expressing antisense-GRP78 were not protected against H_2O_2. Toxicity to H_2O_2 (250 mM) was much greater in LLC-PK1 cells if they expressed antisense-GRP78. Toxicity was measured by lactate dehydrogenase (LDH) release at different time points. H_2O_2-induced p-ERK is reduced in tunicamycin-pretreated cells if they express antisense-GRP78. Likewise p-JNKs are activated more in the tunicamycin-treated cells expressing antisense-GRP78. (Redrawn from Hung CC, Takaharu I, Stevens JL, Bonventre JV: Protection of renal epithelial cells against oxidative injury by endoplasmic reticulum stress preconditioning is mediated by ERK1/2 activation. J Biol Chem 278: 29317–29326, 2003.)

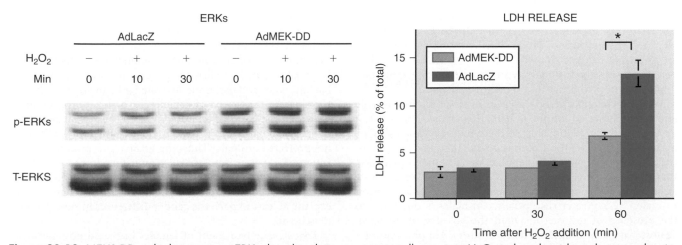

Figure 30-10 MEK1-DD, which increases ERK phosphorylation, protects cells against H_2O_2-induced oxidant damage despite inhibition of GRP78. Constitutively active MEK1-DD, the upstream activator of ERK, when administered via adenovirus (Ad), protected antisense-GRP–expressing LLC-PK1 cells against oxidant-induced injury, as measured by lactate dehydrogenase (LDH) release. (Redrawn from Hung CC, Takaharu I, Stevens JL, Bonventre JV: Protection of renal epithelial cells against oxidative injury by endoplasmic reticulum stress preconditioning is mediated by ERK1/2 activation. J Biol Chem 278: 29317–29326, 2003.)

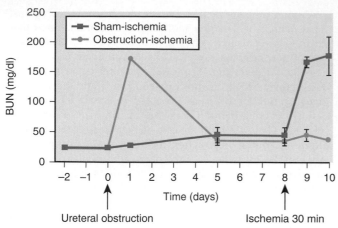

Figure 30-11 Prior ureteral obstruction results in protection of mouse kidneys rendered ischemic 8 days later. Both ureters were clamped for 24 hours and then released. Another group received sham surgery. In the previously obstructed animals ischemia induced 8 days later resulted in very little increase in blood urea nitrogen as compared with the animals previously undergoing sham surgery.

preconditioning to prevent small-vessel leukocyte- and perhaps platelet-endothelial interactions and therefore may be explained to a large extent by decreased inflammation.

GENDER DIFFERENCES IN SUSCEPTIBILITY TO ISCHEMIC KIDNEY INJURY

Gender differences characterize the susceptibility or expression of many diseases. In general, these differences have been attributed to estrogen-mediated protection against pathologic conditions.[121-124] Male hormones, however, may also play important roles in gender differences in disease susceptibility.[125-127] Steroid hormones, including sexual hormones, regulate inflammation and hence could be expected to contribute to the pathophysiology of ischemia/reperfusion-induced tissue injury.[12,47,58,128] An important endogenous modulator of ischemia/reperfusion-induced tissue injury is NO,[40,129] the product of NOSs. Furthermore, sex hormones are known to regulate NO synthesis,[130,131] which, as described before, possesses anti-inflammatory, vasodilatory activity, and is anti-apoptotic through Akt signaling pathways.[40,129,132-134]

We have characterized differences in susceptibility of male and female mice to kidney ischemia/reperfusion injury and have studied the relationship of these differences to estrogen or testosterone.[135] Our findings reveal that the kidneys of males are much more susceptible to ischemia/reperfusion than those of females (Fig. 30-12). There is increased post-ischemic proximal tubule injury, apoptosis, and inflammation in males. This greater susceptibility in males is due more to the presence of testosterone than the absence of estrogen. Testosterone acts to inhibit NOS activation, Akt phosphorylation, and the post-ischemic increase in the ratio of ERK to JNK activation, leading to greater inflammatory responses. The differences in susceptibility to ischemia between male and female kidneys were eliminated by treatment of females with testosterone or dihydrotestosterone (Fig. 30-13), which

cannot be aromatized to estrogen, or orchiectomy of males (Fig. 30-14). The effects of testosterone and dihydrotestosterone were not inhibited by androgen receptor antagonists.

We found that ICAM-1 expression, post-ischemic MPO activity (a measure of leukocyte accumulation in the kidney), and RAW 264.7 cell trapping after ischemia/reperfusion were greater in males than in females. Ovariectomy did not increase ICAM-1 expression or MPO activity in females, consistent with the absence of an effect of ovariectomy on renal functional impairment. By contrast, testosterone treatment of females resulted in increased ICAM-1 expression and MPO activity with ischemia, whereas orchiectomy of males resulted in reduced post-ischemic ICAM-1 expression and MPO activity. Thus, our results suggest that functionally significant post-ischemic kidney inflammatory responses probably depend more on testosterone than estrogen.[135] Testosterone has been shown to accentuate vascular responses to vasopressor agents,[136] increase the thromboxane-to-prostaglandin ratio,[137] increase platelet aggregation,[138] and increase monocyte adhesion to endothelial cells,[139] properties that can contribute to vasoconstriction, small-vessel occlusion, and AKI.[58]

Expression of eNOS and iNOS in the medulla has been reported to be greater in female rats than in males.[131] We found that both Ca^{2+}-dependent (cNOS) and Ca^{2+}-independent NOS (ciNOS) activities were greater in females than in males.[135] Testosterone treatment of females resulted in a mitigated increase of post-ischemic cNOS and ciNOS activity, whereas orchiectomy in males enhanced cNOS and ciNOS activation. This effect of testosterone in vivo was mimicked in vitro in RAW 264.7 cells, where we found that testosterone reduced NO synthesis when cells are activated by lipopolysaccharide, whereas estrogen enhanced NO synthesis. We proposed that testosterone-induced inhibition of NO production is an important contributor to the gender differences in functional consequences of ischemia, although, as reflected by the effects of L-NNA in females and L-arginine in males, NO is not the only contributor to gender differences in susceptibility to ischemic injury of the kidney.[135]

NO has been reported to protect against apoptotic cell death through the PI 3-kinase/Akt pathway.[140] Camper-Kirby et al reported that young women possess higher levels of activated Akt than comparably aged men or postmenopausal women, and sexually mature female mice have higher levels of activated Akt than male mice.[122] In our studies, pre- and post-ischemic levels of activated Akt in kidney were much greater in females than in males. Castration increased the levels of baseline and post-ischemic activated Akt in males, whereas testosterone treatment of females or orchiectomy of males decreased the levels of activated Akt.[135] The Akt activation in the protected animals is greater and sustained longer than in nonprotected animals. Thus, the greater and prolonged activation of Akt after ischemia may contribute to gender-related kidney resistance to ischemia, and the sustained activation of Akt may be downregulated by testosterone. These would explain, at least in part, the gender differences in susceptibility to ischemia.

Testosterone treatment of females increased post-ischemic JNK phosphorylation and decreased ERK phosphorylation. Orchiectomy increased the ratio of ERK to JNK phosphorylation. Thus, testosterone-induced potentiation of post-ischemic injury is associated with the downregulation of NOS enzymes, resulting in less NO and hence less Akt phosphorylation,

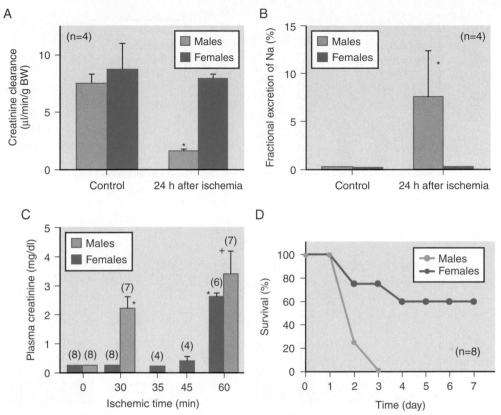

Figure 30-12 Effect of gender on ischemia-induced kidney injury. BALB/c male and female mice were exposed to 30 minutes (**A** and **B**), 60 minutes (**D**), or varying times of ischemia (**C**). Creatinine clearance (**A**), fractional excretion of Na⁺ (**B**), plasma creatinine (**C**) 24 hours after reperfusion, and survival (**D**) over time were then evaluated. Using these multiple metrics, female mice were protected against ischemic injury. *$P < 0.05$ versus control; †$P < 0.05$ versus female group after 60 minutes of ischemia, respectively. (From Park KM, Kim JI, Ahn Y, et al: Testosterone is responsible for enhanced susceptibility of males to ischemic renal injury. J Biol Chem 279:52282–52292, 2004.)

which results in reduced cellular stress and reduced activation of the JNK kinases.

It is possible that the forkhead family of transcription factors, which we have found to be upregulated with ischemia in males,[141] are involved in this effect of Akt. Forkhead proteins are transcription factors involved in the regulation of cellular survival and cell cycle control.[142–144] The three forkhead (or Fox) proteins FKHRL1 (FOXO3a), FKHR (FOXO1a), and AFX (FOXO4), belonging to the "O" subfamily of the Fox proteins, contain the "forkhead" DNA-binding domain and the conserved Akt phosphorylation sites. These three members are phosphorylated at several serines and one threonine by Akt.[144,145] We found that one of the forkhead proteins, FKHR, is phosphorylated after ischemia/ reperfusion in the rat kidney. The time course of phosphorylation is similar to the time course of activation of the forkhead protein kinase Akt/PKB kinase, with maximal phosphorylation at 24 to 48 hours after reperfusion when the process of regeneration peaks. In studies in vitro we found that phosphorylation of Akt, FKHR, and FKHRL1 were PI 3-kinase dependent, in that phosphorylation was reduced by the PI 3-kinase inhibitors, wortmannin, or LY294002. Inhibition of MAPK/ERK kinase (MEK1/2), the upstream activator of ERK1/2, had no effect on forkhead protein phosphorylation after chemical anoxia/dextrose addition. We concluded that PI 3-kinase and Akt are activated after renal ischemia/reperfusion and that Akt phosphorylation

leads to phosphorylation of FKHR and FKHRL1, which may affect epithelial cell fate in acute kidney injury.[141]

Recently we reported that the orchiectomized male mouse has significantly less lipid peroxidation and production of H_2O_2 in the kidney 4 and 24 hours after 30 minutes of bilateral renal ischemia when compared with intact or dihydrotestosterone-treated orchiectomized males.[97] The post-ischemic kidney expression and activity of MnSOD in orchiectomized mice were much greater than in intact or dihydrotestosterone-administered orchiectomized mice. Four hours after 30 minutes of bilateral ischemia superoxide formation was significantly lower in orchiectomized mice than in intact mice. We used Madin-Darby canine kidney cells, a kidney epithelial cell line, to evaluate whether we could see an effect of testosterone in vitro on kidney epithelial cells. One millimolar H_2O_2 decreased MnSOD activity, an effect that was potentiated by pretreatment with dihydrotestosterone. In addition, orchiectomy prevented the post-ischemic decrease of catalase activity. Treatment of male mice with Mn(III) tetrakis (1-methyl-4-pyridyl) porphyrin, a SOD mimetic, reduced the post-ischemic increase of plasma creatinine, lipid peroxidation, and tissue H_2O_2. These results suggest that orchiectomy accelerates the post-ischemic activation of MnSOD and reduces ROS and lipid peroxidation, resulting in reduced levels of toxic and pro-inflammatory ROS and reduced kidney susceptibility to ischemia/reperfusion injury.

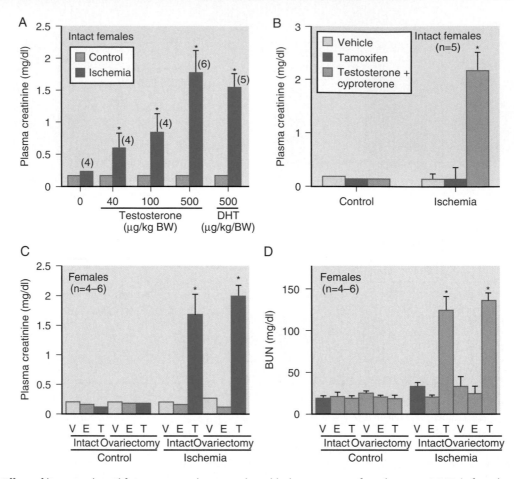

Figure 30-13 Effect of hormonal modification on ischemia-induced kidney injury in female mice. BALB/c female mice were used. Some were ovariectomized on day 0 and some were treated with testosterone (T, 500 μg/kg unless specifically stated otherwise) or dihydrotestosterone (DHT, 500 μg/kg) daily for 14 days subcutaneously. Nonovariectomized animals are indicated as "Intact". Others were treated with an estrogen receptor antagonist for 14 days. Some animals were treated with T and cyproterone (5 mg/kg), an antagonist of the androgen receptor, for 14 days. On day 15 animals were subjected to 30 minutes of bilateral renal ischemia. Plasma creatinine (**A–C**) and blood urea nitrogen (BUN) (**D**) concentrations were determined 24 hours after reperfusion. *$P < 0.05$ as compared with intact females treated with vehicle (V). E, treated with 17β-estradiol; T, treated with testosterone. (From Park KM, Kim JI, Ahn Y, et al: Testosterone is responsible for enhanced susceptibility of males to ischemic renal injury. J Biol Chem 279:52282–52292, 2004.)

We evaluated whether lower susceptibility to ischemia/reperfusion injury seen in orchiectomized mice was associated with changes in Hsp expression.[146] Hsp expression was measured in the kidney isolated from intact, orchiectomized, and dihydroxytestosterone-treated orchiectomized mice before and 4 hours after ischemia/reperfusion. Orchiectomy increased the expression of Hsp-27 in tubular epithelial cells in kidneys before and 4 hours after reperfusion but had no effect on Hsp-72, glucose-regulated protein (GRP-78) or GRP-94. Dihydrotestosterone treatment of orchiectomized animals resulted in prevention of this increase in Hsp-27 production. Thus, the greater resistance to ischemia/reperfusion seen in orchiectomized mice is associated with an increased expression of Hsp-27, which stabilizes the actin cytoskeleton in the proximal tubular epithelial cell.[147] This may contribute to reductions in post-ischemic histologic damage and functional impairment.

REPAIR OF THE KIDNEY AFTER ACUTE INJURY

When the kidney recovers from acute injury it manifests a sequence of events that include epithelial cell spreading and possibly migration to cover the exposed areas of the basement membrane, cell dedifferentiation and proliferation to restore cell number, followed by differentiation, which results in restoration of the functional integrity of the nephron.[2] Repair of the kidney parallels kidney organogenesis in the high rate of DNA synthesis and apoptosis and in patterns of gene expression. Vimentin, a filament protein that is expressed in mesenchymal cells but not in the uninjured mature nephron, is detectable in proximal tubules for more than 5 days after ischemia/ reperfusion injury.[148] The neural cell adhesion molecule, which is expressed in metanephric mesenchyme but not in normal mature kidneys, is abundantly expressed in

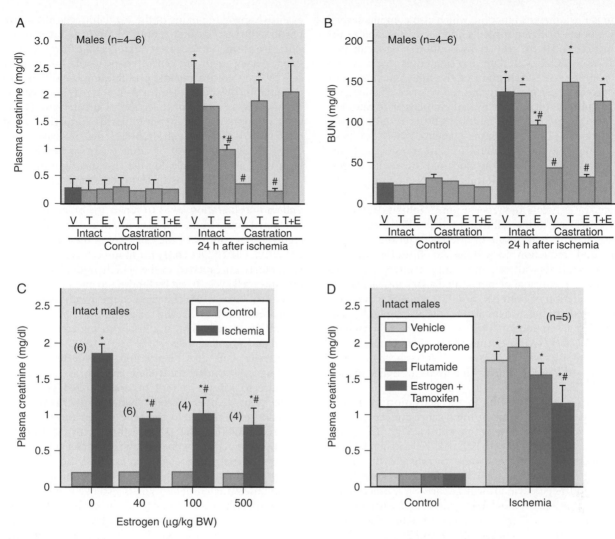

Figure 30-14 Effect of hormonal modification on ischemia-induced kidney injury in male mice. Some male BALB/c mice were castrated on day 0. Noncastrated male animals are indicated as "Intact". Some were treated with testosterone (T, 500 μg/kg) or 17β-estradiol (E, 40 μg/kg), and/or tamoxifen (5 μg/kg). Some animals were treated with flutamide or cyproterone (5 mg/kg), both antagonists of the androgen receptor, or with vehicle (V). All treatments were daily for 14 days administered subcutaneously. On day 15 animals were subjected to 30 minutes of bilateral renal ischemia. Plasma creatinine (**A, C, D**) and blood urea nitrogen (BUN) (**B**) concentrations were determined 24 hours after reperfusion. *,#$P < 0.05$ compared with control and intact males treated with vehicle, respectively. (From Park KM, Kim JI, Ahn Y, et al: Testosterone is responsible for enhanced susceptibility of males to ischemic renal injury. J Biol Chem 279:52282–52292, 2004.)

proximal tubules 5 days after reperfusion of post-ischemic rat kidneys.[149] Thus, a molecule not expressed by normal mature renal tubule epithelial cells is expressed in proximal tubular cells during recovery from ischemia, recapitulating its expression in early renal development.

The loss of the differentiated phenotype of the epithelial cell of the proximal tubule S3 segment is reflected in several ways. The brush border breaks down,[150] with loss of microvilli, blebbing of the apical membrane, fragmentation, and release into the lumen, as well as endocytosis and a rapid change in cell polarity.[151] Abnormalities are present in the apical cortical cytoskeleton as reflected by changes in actin localization from apical to lateral cell membrane.[152,153]. With ATP depletion cellular free-Ca^{2+} concentration increases, resulting in activation of proteases and phospholipases, which in turn contribute to the disruption of the cytoskeleton and further impair

mitochondrial energy metabolism, interfering with production of ATP.[87] The apical brush border protein, villin, an actin bundling and severing protein, appears at the basolateral pole of proximal tubule cells within 1 hour after reperfusion.[153] Ezrin is dephosphorylated with ischemia, resulting in loss of its ability to tether the actin cytoskeleton to the membrane.[154] There is dephosphorylation and activation of actin-depolymerizing factor, which translocates to the apical region of the cell and enhances microvillar F-actin filament severing and depolymerization.[155]

ATP depletion of the S3 segment of the proximal tubule[153,156] also results in disruption of cell-cell junctional complexes. The tight junction serves as a boundary between the apical and basolateral plasma membrane and also as a scaffold for trafficking and signaling molecules.[157] The tight junction probably does not act alone. Immediately basal to the tight junction is the adherens junction, which also contains several transmembrane-bridging proteins and serves to stabilize the tight junction.[158] Altered cellular distribution of tight-junction proteins ZO-1, ZO-2, occluding, and cingulin is observed with ATP depletion.[159–161] Disruption of the tight junction alters both paracellular permeability and cell polarity. The increase in permeability results in backleak of glomerular filtrate. The change in cell polarity has multiple effects resulting from incorrect targeting of membrane proteins. Na^+/K^+-ATPase, usually confined to the basolateral domain, translocates to the apical membrane resulting in impaired transcellular Na^+ transport and an increase in intraluminal Na^+ delivery to the distal tubule. The group IV cytosolic phospholipase A_2, which is activated by ischemia and reperfusion,[162] inhibits trafficking of Na^+/K^+-ATPase to the cell membrane.[163] Enhanced phospholipase activity may result in afferent arteriole vasoconstriction and reduction in glomerular filtration rate. In transplant recipients with ischemic injury resulting in delayed graft function, Kwon et al demonstrated a striking increase in fractional excretion of both Na^+ and Li^+, which are normally co-transported in the proximal and distal tubules.[164] The observed changes in fractional Na^+ and Li^+ excretion coincide with loss of Na^+/K^+-ATPase from the basolateral membrane of proximal tubules with ischemia.[152,164] It has been proposed that Na^+/K^+-ATPase is directly involved in tight-junction assembly.[165,166]

Ischemia/reperfusion results in the activation of a large number of genes.[167,168] Some of these genes are expressed at increased levels in the developing kidney.[148,169] The genes whose expression is altered with ischemia/reperfusion fall into several functional categories. Some encode growth factors (e.g., insulin-like growth factor-1,[170,171] fibroblast growth factors,[172–175] and hepatocyte growth factor[176,177]), others transcription factors (e.g., paired box gene 2 and early growth response factor 1).[178,179] Some encoded proteins (e.g., B-cell leukemia/lymphoma protein 2, or BCL2, and BCL2-associated X protein) that have been implicated in regulation of apoptosis, a property characteristic of many renal proximal epithelial cells both during development[180,181] and after injury.[182] Other growth factors, such as epidermal growth factor,[179,183] and nuclear DNA-binding proteins such as Kid-1[184] are downregulated in both kidney development and repair after injury. When and how these genes regulate the differentiation state of the cell are ill-defined. A more complete analysis of this genomic approach to understanding the pathophysiology of AKI is currently somewhat premature, because attempts to derive insight from microarray analyses have been disappointing.[168]

Under normal circumstances human proximal tubule cells divide at a low rate, as evaluated by proliferative cell nuclear antigen and Ki-67 immunoreactivity.[185] This cell production balances the loss of tubular epithelial cells into the urine.[186] This turnover rate must be under tight control, because a small imbalance between cell loss and cell division would soon lead to nephron loss or marked increases in nephron and kidney size over time. This low rate of cell turnover changes markedly after an ischemic insult where there is cell death by necrosis and apoptosis and a response to replace these cells. As we have shown in proliferative cell nuclear antigen and 5-bromo 2'-deoxyuridine (BrdU) labeling studies,[149] and in unpublished studies by counting mitotic spindles identified by labeling them with antibodies to tubulin, this response is rapid and

extensive, involving many of the surviving cells of the straight portion of the proximal tubule.[148] We have interpreted this extensive proliferative capacity to reflect the intrinsic ability of the surviving epithelial cell to adapt to the loss of adjacent cells by dedifferentiating and proliferating. We will discuss the potential involvement of intrarenal and extrarenal stem cells in this process in the next section of this review. The mitogenic response may be driven in part by autocrine and paracrine growth factors at the tubular sites of severe injury.[187] This mitogenic potential of adult proximal tubule cells has been used as a rationale for the therapeutic use of growth factors to accelerate recovery from acute renal failure.[188]

Although it is important that the surviving epithelial cells undergo proliferation so as to repair the organ and restore a functional epithelium, it is also important that there be fine regulation of control of the cell cycle in the repair process.[189] p21WAF1/CIP1/SDI1 (p21) promotes cell cycle arrest and yet is markedly upregulated in the acutely injured kidney.[190] p21 promotes cell cycle arrest by binding to and inhibiting cyclin-dependent kinases, which, when coupled with specific cyclins, facilitates the cell cycle. The upregulation of p21 may prevent replication of cells that, if allowed to undergo cell division, would undergo apoptosis.

Epithelial cell dedifferentiation is a feature of rapidly dividing cells under controlled growth, as in the case of response to injury or that of uncontrolled growth, as in cancer. This dedifferentiated phenotype in many ways is a reflection of a change in the gene expression pattern of the cell, recapitulating the pattern that occurs during kidney development before the mesenchymal-epithelial transition has occurred. Renal mesenchymal cells are dedifferentiated and highly proliferative throughout the developmental period.[191] The dedifferentiated phenotype is also likely to be important for the spreading migratory behavior of the viable epithelial cells as they cover the basement membrane during the repair process. The factors responsible for and the significance of reversion to a less differentiated cell phenotype as well as its relationship to the proliferative and migratory response after renal epithelial cell injury are poorly understood.

The dedifferentiation of renal tubular cells with associated recapitulation of gene expression patterns typical of the developing nephron has major implications for the regulation of renal repair; however, the relationships between proliferation and alterations in the state of cellular differentiation have not been defined. For example, it is not clear to what stage of development the tubule cells revert and how the temporal patterns that evolve may relate to injury, proliferation, and final redifferentiation of the cell. It is not clear to what extent the inductive interactions that occur during kidney development are critical for the repair of the proximal nephron.[191]

Dedifferentiation of the epithelial cell may play an important role in spreading and migration of cells over the denuded basement membrane early in the recovery process. In a model in vitro of this process, Toback and colleagues scratched cells off the tissue culture plate and monitored the migration of the cells into the denuded area, as well as the gene expression pattern of the cells.[192] After "wounding" of the monolayer there was upregulation of the immediate-early genes encoding early growth response factor 1, the transcription factors c-fos and NAK-1, and the cytokine GRO at 1 hour, followed by peak levels of mRNA encoding connective tissue growth factor (CTGF) and c-myc at 4 hours. mRNA levels of urokinase-type plasminogen activator (u-PA) and its inhibitor (PAI-1) and HSP-70 were markedly raised 4 to 8 hours after wounding. By contrast, mRNA levels for osteopontin, epidermal growth factor, and hepatocyte growth factor (c-met) receptors, were reduced. NAK-1, PAI-1, and HSP-70 were induced or stimulated only in cells at the wound edge. Adenosine diphosphate, a potent stimulator of cell migration, stimulated expression of u-PA and PAI-1 after wounding. The RET-glial cell–derived neurotrophic factor (GDNF) pathway stimulates migration of renal epithelial cells[193] and may play a role in regulation of migration, but this has not been studied after ischemic injury. GDNF expression is upregulated in renal epithelial cells of the dysplastic human kidney associated with obstruction and high levels of proliferation.[194] Another protein, CD44, which is upregulated in the S3 cell with ischemia/reperfusion,[195] and its ligands, osteopontin and hyaluronic acid, are expressed at wound margins associated with cellular proliferation and migration of injured mucosal and vascular endothelial tissues. CD44 peptide is localized to the basal and lateral cell membranes. CD44 expression is markedly upregulated in the kidney with ischemia/reperfusion, and this upregulation persists for at least 7 days.[196,197] It is upregulated on the apical membrane of regenerating, not fully differentiated tubule cells and some interstitial cells. CD44 is also prominently expressed on infiltrating neutrophils. In addition to its role in inflammation, CD44 may be involved in migration through interactions between expressing epithelial cells and matrix proteins.

Matrix molecules probably play an important role in the migration that occurs during the repair process. Within 3 hours of reperfusion after ischemia, cellular fibronectin is deposited.[3] This may stimulate dedifferentiation, as suggested by studies carried out in the skin, gastrointestinal tract, and cornea. At 1 day after ischemic injury, hyaluronic acid is upregulated in the interstitium surrounding regenerating tubules. Osteopontin is upregulated in the proximal tubules after acute ischemic injury.[195,198] Immunoreactive osteopontin peptide continues to be localized in those tubules still undergoing repair for as long as 7 days after the injury. At later times after ischemic injury, laminin isoforms are expressed. It has been proposed that laminin deposition may regulate redifferentiation and repolarization of the epithelium.[199]

Are Stem Cells Involved in Recovery from Acute Kidney Injury?

There are several possibilities for the origin of regenerating epithelial cells after injury. First, as we have discussed above, epithelial cells may dedifferentiate, proliferate, then redifferentiate into mature tubular cells, as a survival response to injury; second, bone marrow (BM) stem cells may home to the injured epithelium, where local cues trigger differentiation; third, a population of intrarenal progenitor cells may replenish the epithelial cell population after injury. Several reports have suggested that BM-derived cells participate in the repair response by directly replacing cells that have been lost.[200–202] One study identified these cells as hematopoietic stem cells,[201] another as mesenchymal stromal stem cells (MSCs).[203] In addition to a potential role of cells from the BM to directly replace lost epithelial cells, BM-derived cells can potentially participate in the repair process by infiltrating the interstitium of the kidney and generating paracrine factors, such as growth factors, which may facilitate repair of the

epithelium and endothelium and also may participate directly in the replacement of dead endothelial cells (Fig. 30-15). We studied kidney repair in chimeric mice expressing green fluorescent protein (GFP) or bacterial β-galactosidase (β-gal), or harboring the male Y chromosome, exclusively in BM-derived cells.[204,212] We generated chimeric mice by treating wild-type recipient mice with lethal doses of irradiation and then transferring whole BM from male mice, or mice transgenic for β-gal or enhanced GFP (eGFP). Ten million cells were injected into the lateral tail vein of recipients 2 hours after irradiation. The mice were then allowed to recover for 6 weeks, after which they were subjected to either 30 minutes (males) or 45 minutes (females) of bilateral ischemia. In GFP chimeras, some interstitial cells but no tubular cells expressed GFP after ischemic injury. More than 99% of GFP+ interstitial cells were leukocytes. In female mice with male BM, occasional tubular cells (0.06%) appeared positive for the Y chromosome, but deconvolution microscopy revealed these to be artifactual. In β-gal chimeras, some tubular cells also appeared to express β-gal by X-gal staining, but subsequent to suppression of endogenous (mammalian) β-gal, no tubular cells could be found that stained with X-gal after ischemic injury. In contrast to the absence of BM-derived tubular cells, many tubular cells expressed proliferative cell nuclear antigen, reflective of a high proliferative rate of endogenous surviving tubular cells. The report of Lin et al[205] supported our conclusion that prior studies with β-gal were unreliable because of significant overestimation of the role of BM-derived cells to directly replace epithelial cells. There may be increased endogenous staining for β-gal activity with X-gal as we proposed, or there may be release of β-gal by infiltrating inflammatory cells which is then taken up by the tubular cells.[206] Although there was no evidence for eGFP+ tubular cells using the eGFP reporter, these experiments provided evidence for direct BM

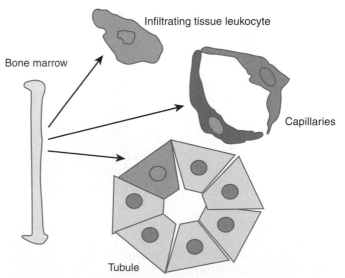

Figure 30-15 Possible fates of bone marrow cells involved in kidney repair. The cells might directly replace lost tubular epithelial cells. They might replace lost endothelial cells or otherwise participate in the angiogenesis that follows an ischemic period. Alternatively, the cells can infiltrate the tissues and participate in the repair process via a paracrine effect.

stem cell involvement in making a small contribution to repopulation of the injured vascular endothelium, which could indirectly affect tubule regeneration.[212] These results were supported by examination of sex-mismatched chimeras. To determine the proportion of endothelial cells expressing eGFP, serial high power fields in the cortex were scored for green fluorescent cells that also expressed either vWF or CD31, two endothelial cell markers. 0.3 ± 0.3% of endothelial cells in contralateral kidneys and 1.6 ± 0.4% in 7-day post-ischemic kidneys co-expressed vWF and eGFP. Similar percentages of CD31[+] and eGFP[+] cells were found (Fig. 30-16). Together these data suggest that endothelial cell replacement by BM stem cells or fusion with BM-derived cells occurs at a low level in response to the vascular injury resulting from ischemia.

These results do not rule out, however, a role for BM-derived cells that are seen in the interstitium, in the production of paracrine factors that may facilitate repair of the epithelium. It has become clear that the injection of cell populations before or just after renal injury may prevent renal damage by stem cell–independent mechanisms. We evaluated whether BM-derived MSCs could exert a benefit to protect the kidney against ischemic injury, as measured functionally by evaluating the effect of BM cells on post-ischemic serum creatinine increases. Intravenous injection of BM MSCs reduced post-ischemic functional renal impairment without evidence of differentiation of these cells into tubular cells of the kidney. Thus, our data indicate that intrinsic tubular cell proliferation accounts for replenishment of the tubular epithelium subsequent to ischemia. Another group has also found that MSCs protect against ischemic renal injury by a differentiation-independent mechanism.[207] Injection of certain cell types just after renal injury may be reno-protective by an immuno-modulatory mechanism, because injected cells may be rapidly

ingested by immune cells in the spleen, liver, and lungs. MSCs, when cultured in vitro under certain conditions, may home to the kidney or another side and secrete factors that may act as pro-survival factors for the epithelium and/or the endothelium, may be pro-proliferative increasing the rate of regeneration, may suppress inflammation, or may recruit the influx and differentiation of endogenous kidney progenitor cells. These cells may either act from a kidney site or a distant site.

These data on BM-derived cells do not rule out the possibility that there are intrinsic kidney stem cells that participate in the repair process. Oliver et al have used a BrdU labeling approach to identify putative adult renal stem cells after kidney injury. They labeled 3-day-old rat pups with BrdU followed by a long chase of at least 2 months. A population of papillary label-retaining cells were identified in the renal papilla.[208] These cells were primarily interstitial, although a small fraction were intratubular and co-expressed renal epithelial markers. After transient renal ischemia, BrdU label was lost in the absence of apoptosis, suggesting that these stem cells proliferated in response to injury. The authors suggest that the renal papilla is a niche for progenitor cells. The use of BrdU is fraught with some concerns, however, given that it is released by dying cells and can be taken up by adjacent, dividing cells.[209]

Recently Challen et al reported that the "side population" of putative renal progenitor cells composed 0.1% to 0.2% of the total viable kidney cell population.[210] Hematopoietic stem cells are characterized by low fluorescence uptake after incubation of cells with Hoechst 33342 and Rhodamine 123. Hoechst low-fluorescence cells are designated the "side population" by virtue of their location on fluorescent-activated cell sorting dot plots. It has been proposed that this "side population" would also define a stem cell population in solid organs as well.[211] When Challen et al carried out mRNA expression profiling on the side population they implicated a role for Notch signaling in these cells, and in situ hybridization supported the existence of a tubular "niche" but also revealed heterogeneity, including the presence of renal macrophages in the side population. Adult kidney side population cells demonstrated multilineage differentiation in vitro, whereas microinjection of the side population cells into mouse metanephrons showed a 3.5- to 13-fold greater potential to contribute to developing kidney than non–side population cells. Introduction of these cells into an adriamycin-nephropathy model reduced albuminuria-to-creatinine ratios but did not integrate into the tubules, suggesting that the functional benefit was due to a humoral effect in renal repair.[210]

It is difficult to envision that the putative renal stem cells identified by Oliver et al[208] or the side population identified by Challen et al[210] are the only source of new epithelial cells in regenerating kidney, given the rapid epithelial proliferation seen in post-ischemic kidney 24 to 48 hours after injury. Additional studies are necessary to validate the presence of progenitor or stem cells within the kidney itself and to determine the contribution of these cells relative to the contribution of resident tubular differentiated cells that undergo dedifferentiation and proliferation in response to injury.

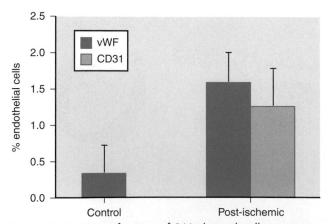

Figure 30-16 Quantification of BM–derived cells expressing markers of endothelial cells (vWF and CD31). Data are presented as percentage of vWF-positive or CD31-positive cells that express eGFP 7 days after ischemia. Donor BM eGFP-positive cells were transplanted into a recipient animal after exposure of the recipient to a lethal dose of radiation. eGFP-chimeric animals were then exposed to ischemia 6 weeks later. (Redrawn from Duffield JS, Park KM, Hsiao LL, et al: Restoration of tubular epithelial cells during repair of the postischemic kidney occurs independently of bone marrow–derived stem cells. J Clin Invest 115:1743–1755, 2005.)

ORGAN CROSSTALK

Often when we consider the cellular and molecular aspects of AKI we focus exclusively on the kidney, ignoring the effects of other organs. Many of our patients with AKI have multiple-organ failure, and many are on positive pressure mechanical ventilation. We have reported that ventilation of the lung has distal effects on the kidney even if the kidney has not been manipulated in the rat.[213] Positive pressure ventilation resulted in increased microvascular leak in the lung that is dependent on NOS expression. Rats were ventilated with room air at 85 breaths/min for 2 hours with a tidal volume of either 7 or 20 mL/kg. There was significant microvascular leak in both lung and kidney with large tidal-volume (20 mL/kg) ventilation. Kidney microvascular leak was assessed by measuring 24-hour urine protein and albuminuria (Fig. 30-17) and Evans blue dye. Injection of 0.9% NaCl prevented any hypotension and the decreased cardiac output related to large tidal volume, but it did not attenuate microvascular leak of lung and kidney. Serum vascular endothelial growth factor was significantly elevated in the higher tidal-volume groups. Endothelial NOS expression significantly increased in the lung and kidney tissue with large tidal-volume ventilation but not inducible NOS. The NOS inhibitor, N-nitro-L-arginine methyl ester (L-NAME), attenuated the microvascular leak of lung and kidney and the proteinuria associated with ventilation. Endothelial NOS may mediate the systemic microvascular leak of this model of ventilation-induced lung injury. This finding may have important implications for the pathophysiology of ischemic acute tubular injury, in that enhanced microvascular permeability in the renal parenchyma of the outer medulla could be expected to contribute to outer medullary congestion and impaired blood flow through the microcapillary bed supplying the tubule structures in that region of the kidney.

Another important organ-organ crosstalk that has been appreciated to be potentially important for morbidity and mortality in patients is the kidney-heart interaction. In recent years it has become increasingly recognized that even minor changes in kidney function can be powerful cardiovascular risk factors.[214] In animal models ischemia to the kidney has important effects on the heart. Ischemia/reperfusion results in increased levels of immunoreactive TNF-α, IL-1, and ICAM-1 mRNA and MPO levels in the heart.[215] This increase in MPO was also seen in the lungs. There were increases in left ventricular end-diastolic diameter and decreased fractional shortening by echocardiography. Ischemia/reperfusion also resulted in increased apoptosis of cardiac cells, even when the ischemic period was insufficient to cause uremia, ruling out uremia as the cause of the distant effects.

GENETICS OF ACUTE KIDNEY INJURY

Genetics may be a useful tool to study the propensity of patients for the development of AKI. Because, as discussed above, inflammation plays a critical role in the pathophysiology of AKI, it is reasonable to consider whether there are genetic variations that would account for differences in the inflammatory response and hence the development of vascular activation, tubular injury, and organ dysfunction. Polymorphisms in the TNF-α gene have been studied extensively in sepsis and have been associated with adverse clinical outcomes.[216,217] In other studies the association with development of sepsis is less clear.[218] In one study of patients with AKI requiring dialysis, carriers of the A allele in the TNF-α promoter (position −308) had greater TNF-α production by endotoxin-treated leukocytes, a higher APACHE II score, and increased mortality.[219] In this study by Jaber et al, patients who carried the G allele at position −1082 of the IL-10 promoter had higher IL-10 production and a lower risk of death after adjustment for APACHE II score, multiple-organ failure

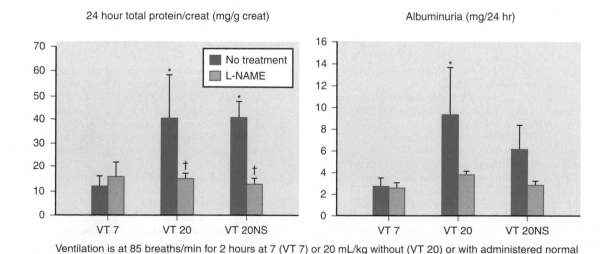

24 hour total protein/creat (mg/g creat)

Albuminuria (mg/24 hr)

Ventilation is at 85 breaths/min for 2 hours at 7 (VT 7) or 20 mL/kg without (VT 20) or with administered normal saline (VT 20NS)

Figure 30-17 Effects of mechanical ventilation with high tidal volumes on urine protein excretion. Ventilation was with 85 breaths per minute for 2 hours at 7 (V_T 7) or 20 mL/kg without (V_T 20) or with administered normal saline (V_T 20NS). Large-V_T (20 mL/kg) ventilation caused significant proteinuria as compared with lower V_T (7 mL/kg), which was attenuated by L-NAME administration in the rats ventilated with a large V_T. The increased total proteinuria was associated with an increase in urinary albuminuria in the V_T 20 group as compared with the V_T 7 group. *$P < 0.05$ versus V_T 7; †$P < 0.05$ versus no treatment at the same V_T. (Redrawn from Choi WI, Quinn DA, Park KM, et al: Systemic microvascular leak in an in vivo rat model of ventilator-induced lung injury. Am J Respir Crit Care Med 167:1627–1632, 2003.)

score, and sepsis.[219] This is a nascent area of investigation. There are many candidate polymorphisms to explore in several genes encoding molecules that are important for the inflammatory response, including members of the IL-1 family, chemokines such as IL-8 and MCP-1, TLRs, HSPs, and oxidant stress-related proteins. The rationale behind examining these genes for polymorphisms in patients with AKI is presented in a recent review.[220]

CONCLUSION

Ischemic renal injury is a dynamic process that often exists in the context of multiple-organ failure and involves hemodynamic alterations, inflammation, and direct injury to the tubular epithelium followed by a repair process that restores epithelial differentiation and function. Inflammation is a significant component of this disease, playing a considerable role in its pathophysiology. Although significant progress has been made in defining the major components of this process, the complex molecular and cellular interactions among endothelial cells, inflammatory cells and the injured epithelium are poorly understood, although we are gaining ground in this quest. A better understanding of the molecular, cellular, and genetic aspects underlying the response to influences that adversely affect the kidney will result in more targeted therapies to prevent the injury and hasten the repair. Progress is being made on multiple fronts, but we continue to be humbled by this disease whose mortality rate has changed little over four decades.

Acknowledgments

This work was supported by the National Institutes of Health (grants DK 39773, DK 38452, NS 10828, DK54741, DK 46267).

References

1. Zuk A, Bonventre JV, Brown D, Matlin KS: Polarity, integrin and extracellular matrix dynamics in the post-ischemic rat kidney. Am J Physiol Cell Physiol 275:C711–C731, 1998.
2. Thadhani R, Pascual M, Bonventre JV: Acute renal failure. N Engl J Med 334:1448–1460, 1996.
3. Zuk A, Bonventre JV, Matlin KS: Expression of fibronectin splice variants in the postischemic rat kidney. Am J Physiol Renal Physiol 280:F1037–F1053, 2001.
4. Bonventre JV, Zuk A: Ischemic acute renal failure: an inflammatory disease? Kidney Int 66:480–485, 2004.
5. Bonventre JV: Dedifferentiation and proliferation of surviving epithelial cells in acute renal failure. J Am Soc Nephrol 14 (Suppl 1):S55–S61, 2003.
6. Conger JD: Vascular abnormalities in the maintenance of acute renal failure. Circ Shock 11:235–244, 1983.
7. Conger JD, Schrier RW: Renal hemodynamics in acute renal failure. Annu Rev Physiol 42:603–614, 1980.
8. Conger J, Robinette J, Villar A, et al: Increased nitric oxide synthase activity despite lack of response to endothelium-dependent vasodilators in postischemic acute renal failure in rats. J Clin Invest 96:631–638, 1995.
9. Vetterlein F, Hoffmann F, Pedina J, et al: Disturbances in renal microcirculation induced by myoglobin and hemorrhagic hypotension in anesthetized rat. J Clin Invest 268:F839–F846, 1995.
10. Vetterlein F, Bludau J, Petho-Schramm A, Schmidt G: Reconstruction of blood flow distribution in the rat kidney during postischemic renal failure. Nephron 66:208–214, 1994.
11. Vetterlein F, Petho A, Schmidt G: Distribution of capillary blood flow in rat kidney during postischemic renal failure. Am J Physiol 251:H510–H519, 1986.
12. Park KM, Kramers C, Vayssier-Taussat M, et al: Prevention of kidney ischemia/reperfusion-induced functional injury, MAPK and MAPK kinase activation, and inflammation by remote transient ureteral obstruction. J Biol Chem 277:2040–2049, 2002.
13. Brezis M, Rosen S, Silva P, Epstein FH: Renal ischemia: a new perspective. Kidney Int 26:375–383, 1984.
14. Schrier RW, Wang W: Acute renal failure and sepsis. N Engl J Med 351:159–169, 2004.
15. Boffa JJ, Arendshorst WJ: Maintenance of renal vascular reactivity contributes to acute renal failure during endotoxemic shock. J Am Soc Nephrol 16:117–124, 2005.
16. Zager RA, Johnson AC, Lund S, et al: Levosimendan protects against experimental endotoxemic acute renal failure. Am J Physiol Renal Physiol 290:F1453–F1462, 2006.
17. Chen SJ, Wu CC, Yang SN, et al: Hyperpolarization contributes to vascular hyporeactivity in rats with lipopolysaccharide-induced endotoxic shock. Life Sci 68:659–668, 2000.
18. Conger J: Hemodynamic factors in acute renal failure. Adv Renal Replace Ther 4 (2 Suppl 1):25–37, 1997.
19. Brooks DP: Role of endothelin in renal function and dysfunction. Clin Exp Pharmacol Renal Physiol 23:345–348, 1996.
20. Basile DP, Donohoe DL, Phillips SA, Frisbee JC: Enhanced skeletal muscle arteriolar reactivity to ANG II after recovery from ischemic acute renal failure. Am J Physiol Regul Integr Comp Physiol 289:R1770–R1776, 2005.
21. Nishida M, Ieshima M, Konishi F, et al: Role of endothelin B receptor in the pathogenesis of ischemic acute renal failure. J Cardiovasc Pharmacol 40:586–593, 2002.
22. Huang C, Hestin D, Dent PC, et al: The effect of endothelin antagonists on renal ischaemia-reperfusion injury and the development of acute renal failure in the rat. Nephrol Dial Transplant 17:1578–1585, 2002.
23. Inman SR, Plott WK, Pomilee RA, et al: Endothelin-receptor blockade mitigates the adverse effect of preretrieval warm ischemia on posttransplantation renal function in rats. Transplantation 75:1655–1659, 2003.
24. Kato A, Hishida A: Amelioration of post-ischaemic renal injury by contralateral uninephrectomy: a role of endothelin-1. Nephrol Dial Transplant 16:1570–1576, 2001.
25. Camaiti A, Del Rosso A, Federighi G: [Acute renal failure caused by treatment with diuretics and ACE inhibitors in the absence of renal artery stenosis]. Minerva Med 83:371–375, 1992.
26. Toto RD: Renal insufficiency due to angiotensin-converting enzyme inhibitors. Miner Electrolyte Metab 20:193–200, 1994.
27. Jo SK, Hu X, Kobayashi H, et al: Detection of inflammation following renal ischemia by magnetic resonance imaging. Kidney Int 64:43–51, 2003.
28. Trillaud H, Degreze P, Combe C, et al: USPIO-enhanced MR imaging of glycerol-induced acute renal failure in the rabbit. Magn Reson Imaging 13:233–240, 1995.
29. Hung CC, Ichimura T, Stevens JL, Bonventre JV: Protection of renal epithelial cells against oxidative injury by endoplasmic reticulum stress preconditioning is mediated by ERK1/2 activation. J Biol Chem 278:29317–29326, 2003.
30. Bonventre JV: Kidney ischemic preconditioning. Curr Opin Nephrol Hypertens 11:43–48, 2002.
31. Ogawa T, Mimura Y, Hiki N, et al: Ischaemic preconditioning ameliorates functional disturbance and impaired renal

perfusion in rat ischaemia-reperfused kidneys. Clin Exp Pharmacol Physiol 27:997–1001, 2000.

32. Yellon DM, Downey JM: Preconditioning the myocardium: from cellular physiology to clinical cardiology. Physiol Rev 83:1113–1151, 2003.

33. Vaage J, Valen G: Preconditioning and cardiac surgery. Ann Thorac Surg 75:S709–S714, 2003.

34. Asano G, Takashi E, Ishiwata T, et al: Pathogenesis and protection of ischemia and reperfusion injury in myocardium. J Nippon Med Sch 70:384–392, 2003.

35. Nicolini F, Beghi C, Muscari C, et al: Myocardial protection in adult cardiac surgery: current options and future challenges. Eur J Cardiothorac Surg 24:986–993, 2003.

36. Mozzicato S, Joshi BV, Jacobson KA, Liang BT: Role of direct RhoA-phospholipase D1 interaction in mediating adenosine-induced protection from cardiac ischemia. FASEB J 18:406–408, 2004.

37. Loubani M, Hassouna A, Galinanes M: Delayed preconditioning of the human myocardium: Signal transduction and clinical implications. Cardiovasc Res 61:600–609, 2004.

38. Ghosh S, Galinanes M: Protection of the human heart with ischemic preconditioning during cardiac surgery: Role of cardiopulmonary bypass. J Thorac Cardiovasc Surg 126:133–142, 2003.

39. Wang X, Wei M, Kuukasjarvi P, et al: Novel pharmacological preconditioning with diazoxide attenuates myocardial stunning in coronary artery bypass grafting. Eur J Cardiothoracic Surg 24:967–973, 2003.

40. Park KM, Byun JY, Kramers C, et al: Inducible nitric-oxide synthase is an important contributor to prolonged protective effects of ischemic preconditioning in the mouse kidney. J Biol Chem 278:27256–27266, 2003.

41. Fagan KA, Tyler RC, Sato K, et al: Relative contributions of endothelial, inducible, and neuronal NOS to tone in the murine pulmonary circulation. Am J Physiol 277:L472–L478, 1999.

42. Richard V, Hogie M, Clozel M, et al: In vivo evidence of an endothelin-induced vasopressor tone after inhibition of nitric oxide synthesis in rats. Circulation 91:771–775, 1995.

43. Yamashita J, Ogata M, Itoh M, et al: Role of nitric oxide in the renal protective effects of ischemic preconditioning. J Cardiovasc Pharmacol 42:419–427, 2003.

44. Bonventre JV, Weinberg JM: Recent advances in the pathophysiology of ischemic acute renal failure. J Am Soc Nephrol 14:2199–210, 2003.

45. Flores J, DiBona DR, Beck CH, Leaf A: The role of cell swelling in ischemic renal damage and the protective effect of hypertonic solutions. J Clin Invest 51:118–126, 1972.

46. Ames A, Wright RL, Kowada M, et al: Cerebral ischemia. II. The no-reflow phenomenon. Am J Pathol 52:437–453, 1968.

47. Park KM, Chen A, Bonventre JV: Prevention of kidney ischemia/reperfusion-induced functional injury and JNK, p38, and MAPK kinase activation by remote ischemic pretreatment. J Biol Chem 276:11870–11876, 2001

48. Brodsky SV, Yamamoto T, Tada T, et al: Endothelial dysfunction in ischemic acute renal failure: rescue by transplanted endothelial cells. Am J Physiol Renal Physiol 282:F1140–F1149, 2002.

49. Basile DP, Donohoe D, Roethe K, Osborn JL: Renal ischemic injury results in permanent damage to peritubular capillaries and influences long-term function. Am J Physiol Renal Physiol 281:F887–F899, 2001.

50. Aderem A, Ulevitch RJ: Toll-like receptors in the induction of the innate immune response. Nature 406:782–787, 2000.

51. Kaisho T, Akira S: Toll-like receptor function and signaling. J Allergy Clin Immunol 117:979–987; quiz 988, 2006.

52. Johnson GB, Brunn GJ, Platt JL: Activation of mammalian Toll-like receptors by endogenous agonists. Crit Rev Immunol 23:15–44, 2003.

53. Kelly KJ, Williams WW, Colvin RB, et al: Intercellular adhesion molecule-1 deficient mice are protected against renal ischemia. J Clin Invest 97:1056–1063, 1996.

54. Wolfs TG, Buurman WA, van Schadewijk A, et al: In vivo expression of Toll-like receptor 2 and 4 by renal epithelial cells: IFN-γ and TNF-α mediated up-regulation during inflammation. J Immunol 168:1286–1293, 2002.

55. Leemans JC, Stokman G, Claessen N, et al: Renal-associated TLR2 mediates ischemia/reperfusion injury in the kidney. J Clin Invest 115:2894–2903, 2005.

56. Sanz MJ, Johnston B, Issekutz A, Kubes P: Endothelin causes P-selectin-dependent leukocyte rolling and adhesion within rat mesenteric microvessels. Am J Physiol 277:H1823–H1830, 1999.

57. Linas S, Whittenburg D, Repine JE: Nitric oxide prevents neutrophil-mediated acute renal failure. Am J Physiol 272:F48–F54, 1997.

58. Sheridan AM, Bonventre JV: Cell biology and molecular mechanisms of injury in ischemic acute renal failure. Curr Opin Nephrol Hypertens 9:427–434, 2000.

59. Kelly KJ, Williams WW, Colvin RB, Bonventre JV: Antibody to intercellular adhesion molecule-1 protects the kidney against ischemic injury. Proc Natl Acad Sci U S A 91:812–816, 1994.

60. Dragun D, Lukitsch I, Tullius SG, et al: Inhibition of intercellular adhesion molecule-1 with antisense deoxynucleotides prolongs renal isograft survival in the rat. Kidney Int 54:2113–2122, 1998.

61. Stepkowski SM, Wang ME, Condon TP, et al: Protection against allograft rejection with intercellular adhesion molecule-1 antisense oligodeoxynucleotides. Transplantation 66:699–707, 1998.

62. Chen W, Bennett CF, Wang ME, et al: Perfusion of kidneys with unformulated "naked" intercellular adhesion molecule-1 antisense oligodeoxynucleotides prevents ischemic/reperfusion injury. Transplantation 68:880–887, 1999.

63. Troncoso P, Ortiz AM, Dominguez J, Kahan BD: Use of FTY 720 and ICAM-1 antisense oligonucleotides for attenuating chronic renal damage secondary to ischemia-reperfusion injury. Transplant Proc 37:4284–428, 2005.

64. Salmela K, Wramner L, Ekberg H, et al: A randomized multicenter trial of the anti-ICAM-1 monoclonal antibody (enlimomab) for the prevention of acute rejection and delayed onset of graft function in cadaveric renal transplantation: a report of the European Anti-ICAM-1 Renal Transplant Study Group. Transplantation 67:729–736, 1999.

65. Hourmant M, Bedrossian J, Durand D, et al: A randomized multicenter trial comparing leukocyte function-associated antigen-1 monoclonal antibody with rabbit antithymocyte globulin as induction treatment in first kidney transplantations. Transplantation 62:1565–1570, 1996.

66. Awad AS, Ye H, Huang L, et al: Selective sphingosine 1-phosphate 1 receptor activation reduces ischemia-reperfusion injury in mouse kidney. Am J Physiol Renal Physiol 290:F1516–F1524, 2006.

67. Mizuno S, Nakamura T: Prevention of neutrophil extravasation by hepatocyte growth factor leads to attenuations of tubular apoptosis and renal dysfunction in mouse ischemic kidneys. Am J Pathol 166:1895–1905, 2005.

68. Rabb H, Daniels F, O'Donnell M, et al: Pathophysiological role of T lymphocytes in renal ischemia-reperfusion injury in mice. Am J Physiol Renal Physiol 279:F525–F531, 2000.

69. Burne MJ, Daniels F, El Ghandour A, et al: Identification of the CD4(+) T cell as a major pathogenic factor in ischemic acute renal failure. J Clin Invest 108:1283-90, 2001.

70. De Greef KE, Ysebaert DK, Dauwe S, et al: Anti-B7-1 blocks mononuclear cell adherence in vasa recta after ischemia. Kidney Int 60:1415–1427, 2001.

71. Park P, Haas M, Cunningham PN, et al: Injury in renal ischemia-reperfusion is independent from immunoglobulins and T lymphocytes. Am J Physiol Renal Physiol 282:F352–F357, 2002.

72. Burne-Taney MJ, Yokota-Ikeda N, Rabb H: Effects of combined T- and B-cell deficiency on murine ischemia reperfusion injury. Am J Transplant 5:1186–1193, 2005.

73. Savransky V, Molls RR, Burne-Taney M, et al: Role of the T-cell receptor in kidney ischemia-reperfusion injury. Kidney Int 69:233–238, 2006.

74. Faubel S, Ljubanovic D, Poole B, et al: Peripheral CD4 T-cell depletion is not sufficient to prevent ischemic acute renal failure. Transplantation 80:643-9, 2005.

75. Thurman JM, Lucia MS, Ljubanovic D, Holers VM: Acute tubular necrosis is characterized by activation of the alternative pathway of complement. Kidney Int 67:524–530, 2005.

76. Homeister JW, Lucchesi BR: Complement activation and inhibition in myocardial ischemia and reperfusion injury. Annu Rev Pharmacol Toxicol 34:17–40, 1994.

77. Zhou W, Farrar CA, Abe K, et al: Predominant role for C5b-9 in renal ischemia/reperfusion injury. J Clin Invest 105:1363–1371, 2000.

78. Farrar CA, Zhou W, Lin T, Sacks SH: Local extravascular pool of C3 is a determinant of postischemic acute renal failure. FASEB J 20:217–226, 2006.

79. Vinas JL, Sola A, Hotter G: Mitochondrial NOS upregulation during renal I/R causes apoptosis in a peroxynitrite-dependent manner. Kidney Int 69:1403–1409, 2006.

80. Malis CD, Weber PC, Leaf A, Bonventre JV: Incorporation of marine lipids into mitochondrial membranes increases susceptibility to damage by calcium and reactive oxygen species: evidence for enhanced activation of phospholipase A_2 in mitochondria enriched with n-3 fatty acids. Proc Natl Acad Sci U S A 87:8845–8849, 1990.

81. Tahara M, Nakayama M, Jin MB, et al: A radical scavenger, edaravone, protects canine kidneys from ischemia-reperfusion injury after 72 hours of cold preservation and autotransplantation. Transplantation 80:213–221, 2005.

82. Dobashi K, Ghosh B, Orak JK, et al: Kidney ischemia-reperfusion: modulation of antioxidant defenses. Mol Cell Biochem 205:1–11, 2000.

83. Eltzschig HK, Collard CD: Vascular ischaemia and reperfusion injury. Br Med Bull 70:71–86, 2004.

84. Land W, Schneeberger H, Schleibner S, et al: The beneficial effect of human recombinant superoxide dismutase on acute and chronic rejection events in recipients of cadaveric renal transplants. Transplantation 57:211–217, 1994.

85. Gurel A, Armutcu F, Sahin S, et al: Protective role of α-tocopherol and caffeic acid phenethyl ester on ischemia-reperfusion injury via nitric oxide and myeloperoxidase in rat kidneys. Clin Chim Acta 339:33–41, 2004.

86. Inal M, Altinisik M, Bilgin MD: The effect of quercetin on renal ischemia and reperfusion injury in the rat. Cell Biochem Funct 20:291–296, 2002.

87. Bonventre JV: Mechanisms of ischemic acute renal failure. Kidney Int 43:1160–1178, 1993.

88. Toyokuni S: Reactive oxygen species-induced molecular damage and its application in pathology. Pathol Int 49:91–102, 1999.

89. Chatterjee PK, Zacharowski K, Cuzzocrea S, et al: Inhibitors of poly(ADP-ribose) synthetase reduce renal ischemia-reperfusion injury in the anesthetized rat in vivo. FASEB J 14:641–651, 2000.

90. Zheng J, Devalaraja-Narashimha K, Singaravelu K, Padanilam BJ: Poly(ADP-ribose) polymerase-1 gene ablation protects mice from ischemic renal injury. Am J Physiol Renal Physiol 288:F387-98, 2005.

91. Li Y, Huang TT, Carlson EJ, et al: Dilated cardiomyopathy and neonatal lethality in mutant mice lacking manganese superoxide dismutase. Nat Genet 11:376–381, 1995.

92. Lebovitz RM, Zhang H, Vogel H, et al: Neurodegeneration, myocardial injury, and perinatal death in mitochondrial superoxide dismutase–deficient mice. Proc Natl Acad Sci U S A 93:9782–9787, 1996.

92a. Chien CT, Lee PH, Chen CF, et al: De novo demonstration and colocalization of free-radical production and apoptosis formation in rat kidney exposed to ischemia/reperfusion. J Am Soc Nephrol 12:973–982, 2001.

93. Macmillan-Crow LA, Cruthirds DL: Invited review: manganese superoxide dismutase in disease. Free Radic Res 34:325–336, 2001.

94. MacMillan-Crow LA, Cruthirds DL, Ahki KM, et al: Mitochondrial tyrosine nitration precedes chronic allograft nephropathy. Free Radic Biol Med 31:1603–1608, 2001.

95. MacMillan-Crow LA, Crow JP, Kerby JD, et al: Nitration and inactivation of manganese superoxide dismutase in chronic rejection of human renal allografts. Proc Natl Acad Sci U S A 93:11853–11858, 1996.

96. Chen Z, Siu B, Ho YS, et al: Overexpression of MnSOD protects against myocardial ischemia/reperfusion injury in transgenic mice. J Mol Cell Cardiol 30:2281–2289, 1998.

97. Kim J, Kil IS, Seok YM, et al: Orchiectomy attenuates post-ischemic oxidative stress and ischemia/reperfusion injury in mice. A role for manganese superoxide dismutase. J Biol Chem 281:20349–20356, 2006.

98. Ishibashi N, Weisbrot-Lefkowitz M, Reuhl K, et al: Modulation of chemokine expression during ischemia/reperfusion in transgenic mice overproducing human glutathione peroxidases. J Immunol 163:5666–5677, 1999.

99. Suwa T, Hogg JC, Klut ME, et al: Interleukin-6 changes deformability of neutrophils and induces their sequestration in the lung. Am J Respir Crit Care Med 163:970–976, 2001.

100. Bonventre JV, Brezis M, Siegel N, et al: Acute renal failure. I. Relative importance of proximal vs. distal tubular injury. Am J Physiol 275:F623–F631, 1998.

101. Li H, Nord EP: CD40 ligation stimulates MCP-1 and IL-8 production, TRAF6 recruitment, and MAPK activation in proximal tubule cells. Am J Physiol Renal Physiol 282:F1020–F1033, 2002.

102. Deckers JG, De Haij S, van der Woude FJ, et al: IL-4 and IL-13 augment cytokine- and CD40-induced RANTES production by human renal tubular epithelial cells in vitro. J Am Soc Nephrol 9:1187–1193, 1998.

103. Laxmanan S, Datta D, Geehan C, et al: CD40: a mediator of pro- and anti-inflammatory signals in renal tubular epithelial cells. J Am Soc Nephrol 16:2714–2723, 2005.

104. Nath KA: Heme oxygenase-1: a provenance for cytoprotective pathways in the kidney and other tissues. Kidney Int 70:432–443, 2006.

105. Niemann-Masanek U, Mueller A, Yard BA, et al: B7-1 (CD80) and B7-2 (CD 86) expression in human tubular epithelial cells in vivo and in vitro. Nephron 92:542–556, 2002.

106. Thurman JM, Royer PA, Ljubanovic D, et al: Treatment with an inhibitory monoclonal antibody to mouse factor B protects mice from induction of apoptosis and renal ischemia/reperfusion injury. J Am Soc Nephrol 17:707–715, 2006.

107. Karin M: Inflammation-activated protein kinases as targets for drug development. Proc Am Thorac Soc 2:386–390; discussion 394–395, 2005.

108. Pombo CM, Bonventre JV, Avruch J, et al: The stress activated protein kinases are major c-jun amino-terminal kinases activated by ischemia and reperfusion. J Biol Chem 269:26545–26551, 1994.

109. Safirstein RL, Bonventre JV. A molecular response to ischemic and nephrotoxic acute renal failure. In Schlöndorff D, Bonventre JV (eds): Molecular Nephrology. New York, Marcel Dekker, 1995, pp 839–854).

110. di Mari JF, Davis R, Safirstein RL: MAPK activation determines renal epithelial cell survival during oxidative injury. Am J Physiol 277:F195–203, 1999.

111. Arany I, Megyesi JK, Reusch JE, Safirstein RL: CREB mediates ERK-induced survival of mouse renal tubular cells after oxidant stress. Kidney Int 68:1573–1582, 2005.

112. Tournier C, Hess P, Yang DD, et al: Requirement of JNK for stress-induced activation of the cytochrome *c*-mediated death pathway. Science 288:870–874, 2000.

113. Xu C, Bailly-Maitre B, Reed JC: Endoplasmic reticulum stress: cell life and death decisions. J Clin Invest 115:2656–2664, 2005.

114. Bush KT, Keller SH, Nigam SK: Genesis and reversal of the ischemic phenotype in epithelial cells. J Clin Invest 106:621–626, 2000.

115. Benjamin IJ, McMillan DR: Stress (heat shock) proteins: molecular chaperones in cardiovascular biology and disease. Circ Res 83:117–132, 1998.

116. Paschen W: Dependence of vital cell function on endoplasmic reticulum calcium levels: implications for the mechanisms underlying neuronal cell injury in different pathological states. Cell Calcium 29:1-11, 2001.

117. Kuznetsov G, Bush KT, Zhang PL, Nigam SK: Perturbations in maturation of secretory proteins and their association with endoplasmic reticulum chaperones in a cell culture model for epithelial ischemia.Proc Natl Acad Sci U S A 93:8584–8589, 1996.

118. Martindale JL, Holbrook NJ: Cellular response to oxidative stress: signaling for suicide and survival. J Cell Physiol 192:1–15, 2002.

119. Gitler C, Zarmi B, Kalef E, et al: Calcium-dependent oxidation of thioredoxin during cellular growth initiation. Biochem Biophys Res Commun 290:624–628, 2002.

120. Park HS, Cho SG, Kim CK, et al: Heat shock protein hsp72 is a negative regulator of apoptosis signal-regulating kinase 1. Mol Cell Biol 22:7721–7730., 2002.

121. Fukuda K, Yao H, Ibayashi S, et al: Ovariectomy exacerbates and estrogen replacement attenuates photothrombotic focal ischemic brain injury in rats. Stroke 31:155–160, 2000.

122. Camper-Kirby D, Welch S, Walker A, et al: Myocardial Akt activation and gender: increased nuclear activity in females versus males. Circ Res 88:1020–1027, 2001.

123. Squadrito F, Altavilla D, Squadrito G, et al: 17β-oestradiol reduces cardiac leukocyte accumulation in myocardial ischaemia reperfusion injury in rat. Eur J Pharmacol 335:185–92, 1997.

124. Sugden PH, Clerk A: Akt like a woman: gender differences in susceptibility to cardiovascular disease. Circ Res 88:975–977, 2001.

125. Ling S, Dai A, Williams MR, et al: Testosterone (T) enhances apoptosis-related damage in human vascular endothelial cells. Endocrinology 143:1119–1125, 2002.

126. Muller V, Losonczy G, Heemann U, et al: Sexual dimorphism in renal ischemia-reperfusion injury in rats: possible role of endothelin. Kidney Int 62:1364–1371, 2002.

127. Yang SH, Perez E, Cutright J, et al: Testosterone increases neurotoxicity of glutamate in vitro and ischemia-reperfusion injury in an animal model. J Appl Physiol 92:195–201, 2002.

128. Kelly KJ, Williams WJ, Colvin RB, et al: Intercellular adhesion molecule-1-deficient mice are protected against ischemic renal injury. J Clin Invest 97:1056–1063, 1996.

129. Simoncini T, Hafezi MA, Brazil DP, et al: Interaction of oestrogen receptor with the regulatory subunit of phosphatidylinositol-3-OH kinase. Nature 407:538–541, 2000.

130. Friedl R, Brunner M, Moeslinger T, Spieckermann PG: Testosterone inhibits expression of inducible nitric oxide synthase in murine macrophages. Life Sci 68:417–429, 2000.

131. Neugarten J, Ding Q, Friedman A, et al: Sex hormones and renal nitric oxide synthases. J Am Soc Nephrol 8:1240–1246, 1997.

132. Schramm L, La M, Heidbreder E, et al: L-arginine deficiency and supplementation in experimental acute renal failure and in human kidney transplantation. Kidney Int 61:1423–1432, 2002.

133. Alexander BT, Cockrell K, Cline FD, Granger JP: Inducible nitric oxide synthase inhibition attenuates renal hemodynamics during pregnancy. Hypertension 39:586–590, 2002.

134. Hickey MJ: Role of inducible nitric oxide synthase in the regulation of leucocyte recruitment. Clin Sci (Lond) 100:1–12, 2001.

135. Park KM, Kim JI, Ahn Y, et al: Testosterone is responsible for enhanced susceptibility of males to ischemic renal injury. J Biol Chem 279:52282–52292, 2004.

136. Baker P, Ramey ER, Ramwell PW: Androgen-mediated sex differences of cardiovascular responses in rats. Am J Physiol 235:H242–H246, 1978.

137. Wakasugi M, Noguchi T, Kazama YI, et al: The effects of sex hormones on the synthesis of prostacyclin (PGI2) by vascular tissues. Prostaglandins 37:401–410, 1989.

138. Milewich L, Chen GT, Lyons C, et al: Metabolism of androstenedione by guinea-pig peritoneal macrophages: synthesis of testosterone and 5 alpha-reduced metabolites. J Steroid Biochem 17:61–65, 1982.

139. McCrohon JA, Jessup W, Handelsman DJ, Celermajer DS: Androgen exposure increases human monocyte adhesion to vascular endothelium and endothelial cell expression of vascular cell adhesion molecule-1. Circulation 99:2317–2322, 1999.

140. Ha K, Kim K, Kwon Y, et al: Nitric oxide prevents 6-hydroxydopamine-induced apoptosis in PC12 cells through cGMP-dependent PI3 kinase/Akt activation. FASEB J 17:1036–1047, 2003.

141. Andreucci M, Michael A, Kramers C, et al: Renal ischemia/reperfusion and ATP depletion/repletion in LLC-PK1 cells result in phosphorylation of FKHR and FKHRL1. Kidney Int 64:1189–1198, 2003.

142. Coffer PJ, Burgering BM: Forkhead-box transcription factors and their role in the immune system. Nat Rev Immunol 4:889–899, 2004.

143. Wijchers PJ, Burbach JP, Smidt MP: In control of biology: of mice, men and Foxes. Biochem J 397:233–246, 2006.

144. Brunet A, Bonni A, Zigmond MJ, et al: Akt promotes cell survival by phosphorylating and inhibiting a Forkhead transcription factor. Cell 96:857–868, 1999.

145. Accili D, Arden KC: FoxOs at the crossroads of cellular metabolism, differentiation, and transformation. Cell 117:421–46, 2004.

146. Park KM, Cho HJ, Bonventre JV: Orchiectomy reduces susceptibility to renal ischemic injury: a role for heat shock proteins. Biochem Biophys Res Commun 328:312–317, 2005.

147. Aufricht C, Ardito T, Thulin G, et al: Heat-shock protein 25 induction and redistribution during actin reorganization after renal ischemia. Am J Physiol 274:F215–F22, 1998.

148. Witzgall R, Brown D, Schwarz C, Bonventre JV: Localization of proliferating cell nuclear antigen, vimentin, c-Fos, and clusterin in the post-ischemic kidney. Evidence for a heterogeneous genetic response among nephron segments, and a large pool of mitotically active and dedifferentiated cells. J Clin Invest 93:2175–2188, 1994.

149. Abbate M, Brown D, Bonventre JV: Expression of NCAM recapitulates tubulogenic development in kidneys recovering from acute ischemia. Am J Physiol 277:F454–F463, 1999.

150. Solez K, Morel-Maroger L, Sraer JD: The morphology of "acute tubular necrosis" in man: analysis of 57 renal biopsies and a comparison with the glycerol model. Medicine (Baltimore) 58:362–376, 1979.

151. Molitoris BA, Hoilien CA, Dahl R, et al: Characterization of ischemia-induced loss of epithelial polarity. J Membr Biol 106:233–242, 1988.

152. Molitoris BA, Dahl R, Geerdes A: Cytoskeleton disruption and apical redistribution of proximal tubule Na$^+$/K$^+$-ATPase during ischemia. Am J Physiol 263:F488–F495, 1992.

153. Brown D, Lee R, Bonventre JV: Redistribution of villin to proximal tubule basolateral membranes after ischemia and reperfusion. Am J Physiol 273:F1003–F1012, 1997.

154. Chen J, Cohn JA, Mandel LJ: Dephosphorylation of ezrin as an early event in renal microvillar breakdown and anoxic injury. Proc Natl Acad Sci U S A 92:7495–7499, 1995.

155. Ashworth SL, Sandoval RM, Hosford M, et al: Ischemic injury induces ADF relocalization to the apical domain of rat proximal tubule cells. Am J Physiol Renal Physiol 280:F886–F894, 2001.

156. Abbate M, Bonventre JV, Brown D: The microtubule network of renal epithelial cells is disrupted by ischemia and reperfusion. Am J Physiol 267:F971–F978, 1994.

157. Lee DB, Huang E, Ward HJ: Tight junction biology and kidney dysfunction. Am J Physiol Renal Physiol 290:F20–F34, 2006.

158. Gumbiner B, Stevenson B, Grimaldi A: The role of the cell adhesion molecule uvomorulin in the formation and maintenance of the epithelial junctional complex. J Cell Biol 107:1575–1587, 1988.

159. Gumbiner B, Garfinkel A, Monke S, et al: ATP depletion: a novel method to study junctional properties in epithelial tissues. I. Rearrangement of the actin cytoskeleton. J Cell Sci 107 (Pt 12):3301–3313, 1994.

160. Gopalakrishnan S, Raman N, Atkinson SJ, Marrs JA: Rho GTPase signaling regulates tight junction assembly and protects tight junctions during ATP depletion. Am J Physiol 275:C798–C809, 1998.

161. Tsukamoto T, Nigam SK: Tight junction proteins form large complexes and associate with the cytoskeleton in an ATP depletion model for reversible junction assembly. J Biol Chem 272:16133–16139, 1997.

162. Nakamura H, Nemenoff RA, Gronich JH, Bonventre JV: Subcellular characteristics of phospholipase A$_2$ activity in the rat kidney. Enhanced cytosolic, mitochondrial, and microsomal phospholipase A$_2$ enzymatic activity after renal ischemia and reperfusion. J Clin Invest 87:1810–1818, 1991.

163. Choukroun GJ, Marshansky V, Gustafson CE, et al: Cytosolic phospholipase A$_2$ regulates Golgi structure and modulates intracellular trafficking of membrane proteins. J Clin Invest 106:983–993, 2000.

164. Kwon O, Corrigan G, Myers BD, et al: Sodium reabsorption and distribution of Na$^+$/K$^+$-ATPase during postischemic injury to the renal allograft. Kidney Int 55:963–975, 1999.

165. Rajasekaran AK, Rajasekaran SA: Role of Na$^+$/K$^+$-ATPase in the assembly of tight junctions. Am J Physiol Renal Physiol 285:F388–F396, 2003.

166. Rajasekaran SA, Hu J, Gopal J, et al: Na$^+$,K$^+$-ATPase inhibition alters tight junction structure and permeability in human retinal pigment epithelial cells. Am J Physiol Cell Physiol 284:C1497–1507, 2003.

167. Villanueva S, Cespedes C, Vio CP: Ischemic acute renal failure induces the expression of a wide range of nephrogenic proteins. Am J Physiol Regul Integr Comp Physiol 290:R861–R870, 2006.

168. Yuen PS, Jo SK, Holly MK, et al: Ischemic and nephrotoxic acute renal failure are distinguished by their broad transcriptomic responses. Physiol Genomics 25:375–386, 2006.

169. Ronco P, Antoine M, Baudouin B, et al: Polarized membrane expression of brush-border hydrolases in primary cultures of kidney proximal tubular cells depends on cell differentiation and is induced by dexamethasone. J Cell Physiol 145:222–237, 1990.

170. Andersson G, Jennische E: IGF-I immunoreactivity is expressed by regenerating renal tubular cells after ischaemic injury in the rat. Acta Physiol Scand 132:453–457, 1988.

171. Rogers SA, Ryan G, Hammerman MR: Insulin-like growth factors I and II are produced in the metanephros and are required for growth and development in vitro. J Cell Biol 113:1447–1453, 1991.

172. Dudley AT, Godin RE, Robertson EJ: Interaction between FGF and BMP signaling pathways regulates development of metanephric mesenchyme. Genes Dev 13:1601–1613, 1999.

173. Ichimura T, Finch PW, Zhang G, et al: Induction of FGF-7 after kidney damage: a possible paracrine mechanism for tubule repair. Am J Physiol 271:F967–F976, 1996.

174. Ichimura T, Maier JA, Maciag T, et al: FGF-1 in normal and regenerating kidney: expression in mononuclear, interstitial, and regenerating epithelial cells. Am J Physiol 269:F653–F662, 1995.

175. Qiao J, Uzzo R, Obara-Ishihara T, et al: FGF-7 modulates ureteric bud growth and nephron number in the developing kidney. Development 126:547–54, 1999.

176. Nagaike M, Hirao S, Tajima H, et al: Renotropic function of hepatocyte growth factor in renal regeneration after unilateral nephrectomy. J Biol Chem 266:22781–22784, 1991.

177. Davies JA, Fisher CE: Genes and proteins in renal development. Exp Nephrol 10:102–113, 2002.

178. Ouellette AJ, Malt RA, Sukhatme VP, Bonventre JV: Expression of two "immediate early" genes, *Egr-1* and c-*fos*, in response to renal ischemia and during compensatory renal hypertrophy in mice. J Clin Invest 85:766–771, 1990.

179. Rackley RR, Kessler PM, Campbell C, Williams BR: In situ expression of the early growth response gene-1 during murine nephrogenesis. J Urol 154:700–705, 1995.

180. Coles HS, Burne JF, Raff MC: Large-scale normal cell death in the developing rat kidney and its reduction by epidermal growth factor. Development 118:777–784, 1993.

181. Koseki C, Herzlinger D, Al-Awqati Q: Apoptosis in metanephric development. J Cell Biol 119:1327–1333, 1992.

182. Lieberthal W, Levine J: Mechanisms of apoptosis and its potential role in renal tubular epithelial injury. Am J Physiol 271:F477–F488, 1996.

183. Safirstein R, Zelent A, Price P: Reduced preproEGF mRNA and diminished EGF excretion during acute renal failure. Kidney Int 36:810–815, 1989.

184. Witzgall R, O'Leary E, Gessner R, et al: *Kid-1*, a putative renal transcription factor: regulation during ontogeny, and in response to ischemia and toxic injury. Mol Cell Biol 13:1933–1942, 1993.

185. Nadasdy T, Laszik Z, Blick KE, et al: Proliferative activity of intrinsic cell populations in the normal human kidney. J Am Soc Nephrol 4:2032–2039, 1994.

186. Prescott LF: The normal urinary excretion rates of renal tubular cells, leucocytes and red blood cells. Clin Sci 31:425–435, 1966.

187. Toback FG: Regeneration after acute tubular necrosis. Kidney Int 41:226–246, 1992.

188. Ichimura T, Bonventre, JV: Growth factors, signaling, and renal injury and repair. In Molitoris BA, Finn WF (eds): Acute Renal Failure. Philadelphia, WB Saunders Co., 2001, pp 101–118.

189. Megyesi J, Andrade L, Vieira JM, Jr, et al: Coordination of the cell cycle is an important determinant of the syndrome of acute renal failure. Am J Physiol Renal Physiol 283:F810–F816, 2002.

190. Megyesi J, Andrade L, Vieira JM, Jr, et al: Positive effect of the induction of p21WAF1/CIP1 on the course of ischemic acute renal failure. Kidney Int 60:2164–2172, 2001.

191. Bard JB: Growth and death in the developing mammalian kidney: signals, receptors and conversations. Bioessays 24:72–82, 2002.

192. Pawar S, Kartha S, Toback FG: Differential gene expression in migrating renal epithelial cells after wounding. J Cell Physiol 165:556–565, 1995.

193. Tang MJ, Worley D, Sanicola M, Dressler GR: The RET-glial cell-derived neurotrophic factor (GDNF) pathway stimulates migration and chemoattraction of epithelial cells. J Cell Biol 142:1337–1345, 1998.

194. El-Ghoneimi A, Berrebi D, Levacher B, et al: Glial cell line derived neurotrophic factor is expressed by epithelia of human renal dysplasia. J Urol 168:2624–2628, 2002.

195. Lewington AJ, Padanilam BJ, Martin DR, Hammerman MR: Expression of CD44 in kidney after acute ischemic injury in rats. Am J Physiol Regul Integr Comp Physiol 278:R247–R254, 2000.

196. Decleves AE, Caron N, Nonclercq D, et al: Dynamics of hyaluronan, CD44, and inflammatory cells in the rat kidney after ischemia/reperfusion injury. Int J Mol Med 18:83–94, 2006.

197. Rouschop KM, Roelofs JJ, Claessen N, et al: Protection against renal ischemia reperfusion injury by CD44 disruption. J Am Soc Nephrol 16:2034–2043, 2005.

198. Kleinman JG, Worcester EM, Beshensky AM, et al: Upregulation of osteopontin expression by ischemia in rat kidney. Ann NY Acad Sci 760:321–323, 1995.

199. Zuk A, Matlin KS: Induction of a laminin isoform and $\alpha_3\beta_1$-integrin in renal ischemic injury and repair in vivo. Am J Physiol Renal Physiol 283:F971–F984, 2002.

200. Poulsom R, Forbes SJ, Hodivala-Dilke K, et al: Bone marrow contributes to renal parenchymal turnover and regeneration. J Pathol 195:229–235, 2001.

201. Kale S, Karihaloo A, Clark PR, et al: Bone marrow stem cells contribute to repair of the ischemically injured renal tubule. J Clin Invest 112:42–49, 2003.

202. Lin F, Cordes K, Li L, et al: Hematopoietic stem cells contribute to the regeneration of renal tubules after renal ischemia-reperfusion injury in mice. J Am Soc Nephrol 14:1188–1199, 2003.

203. Morigi M, Imberti B, Zoja C, et al: Mesenchymal stem cells are renotropic, helping to repair the kidney and improve function in acute renal failure. J Am Soc Nephrol 15:1794–1804, 2004.

204. Duffield JS, Bonventre JV: Kidney tubular epithelium is restored without replacement with bone marrow-derived cells during repair after ischemic injury. Kidney Int 68:1956–1961, 2005.

205. Lin F, Moran A, Igarashi P: Intrarenal cells, not bone marrow-derived cells, are the major source for regeneration in postischemic kidney. J Clin Invest 115:1756–1764, 2005.

206. Krause D, Cantley LG: Bone marrow plasticity revisited: protection or differentiation in the kidney tubule? J Clin Invest 115:1705–1708, 2005.

207. Togel F, Hu Z, Weiss K, et al: Administered mesenchymal stem cells protect against ischemic acute renal failure through differentiation-independent mechanisms. Am J Physiol Renal Physiol 289:F31–F42, 2005.

208. Oliver JA, Maarouf O, Cheema FH, et al: The renal papilla is a niche for adult kidney stem cells. J Clin Invest 114:795–804, 2004.

209. Burns TC, Ortiz-Gonzalez XR, Gutierrez-Perez M, et al: Thymidine analogs are transferred from pre-labeled donor to host cells in the central nervous system after transplantation: a word of caution. Stem Cells 24:1121–1127, 2006.

210. Challen GA, Bertoncello I, Deane JA, et al: Kidney side population reveals multilineage potential and renal functional capacity but also cellular heterogeneity. J Am Soc Nephrol 17:1896–1912, 2006.

211. Challen GA, Little MH: A side order of stem cells: the SP phenotype. Stem Cells 24:3–12, 2006.

212. Duffield JS, Park KM, Hsiao LL, et al: Restoration of tubular epithelial cells during repair of the postischemic kidney occurs independently of bone marrow-derived stem cells. J Clin Invest 115:1743–1755, 2005.

213. Choi WI, Quinn DA, Park KM, et al: Systemic microvascular leak in an in vivo rat model of ventilator-induced lung injury. Am J Respir Crit Care Med 167:1627–1632, 2003.

214. Amann K, Wanner C, Ritz E: Cross-talk between the kidney and the cardiovascular system. J Am Soc Nephrol 17:2112–2119, 2006.

215. Kelly KJ: Distant effects of experimental renal ischemia/reperfusion injury. J Am Soc Nephrol 14:1549–1558, 2003.

216. Tang GJ, Huang SL, Yien HW, et al: Tumor necrosis factor gene polymorphism and septic shock in surgical infection. Crit Care Med 28:2733–2736, 2000.

217. Mira JP, Cariou A, Grall F, et al: Association of TNF2, a TNF-α promoter polymorphism, with septic shock susceptibility and mortality: a multicenter study. JAMA 282:561–568, 1999.

218. Gordon AC, Lagan AL, Aganna E, et al: TNF and TNFR polymorphisms in severe sepsis and septic shock: a prospective multicentre study. Genes Immun 5:631–640, 2004.

219. Jaber BL, Rao M, Guo D, et al: Cytokine gene promoter polymorphisms and mortality in acute renal failure. Cytokine 25:212–219, 2004.

220. Jaber BL, Pereira BJ, Bonventre JV, Balakrishnan VS: Polymorphism of host response genes: implications in the pathogenesis and treatment of acute renal failure. Kidney Int 67:14–33, 2005.

Index

Note: Page numbers followed by *f* and *t* indicate figures and tables, respectively.

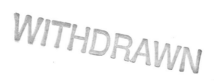